Paramedic Care: Principles & Practice

Fifth Edition

Volume 1
Introduction to Paramedicine

BRYAN E. BLEDSOE, DO, FACEP, FAAEM, EMT-P
Professor of Emergency Medicine
University of Nevada, Las Vegas School of Medicine
University of Nevada, Reno School of Medicine
Attending Emergency Physician
University Medical Center of Southern Nevada
Medical Director, MedicWest Ambulance
Las Vegas, Nevada

RICHARD A. CHERRY, MS, EMT-P
Training Consultant
Northern Onondaga Volunteer Ambulance
Liverpool, New York

LEGACY AUTHOR

ROBERT S. PORTER

PEARSON

Boston   Columbus   Indianapolis   New York City   San Francisco
Amsterdam   Cape Town   Dubai   London   Madrid   Milan   Munich   Paris   Montréal   Toronto
Delhi   Mexico City   São Paulo   Sydney   Hong Kong   Seoul   Singapore   Taipei   Tokyo

Publisher: Julie Levin Alexander
Publisher's Assistant: Sarah Henrich
Editor: Sladjana Repic Bruno
Editorial Assistant: Lisa Narine
Development Editors: Sandra Breuer and Deborah Wenger
Director, Publishing Operations: Paul DeLuca
Team Lead, Program Management: Melissa Bashe
Team Lead, Project Management: Cynthia Zonneveld
Manufacturing Buyer: Maura Zaldivar-Garcia
Art Director: Mary Siener
Cover and Interior Designer: Mary Siener
Managing Photography Editor: Michal Heron
Vice President of Sales & Marketing: David Gesell

Vice President, Director of Marketing: Margaret Waples
Senior Field Marketing Manager: Brian Hoehl
Marketing Assistant: Amy Pfund
Senior Producer: Amy Peltier
Media Producer and Project Manager: Lisa Rinaldi
Full-Service Project Manager: Amy Kopperude/
  iEnergizer Aptara®, Ltd.
Composition: iEnergizer Aptara®, Ltd.
Printer/Binder: LSC Communications
Cover Printer: Phoenix Color
Cover Image: ollo/Getty Images, Rudi Von Briel/Getty Images
Chapter Opener Photo: Madison Avenue rain © Rudi Von
  Brie/Stockbyte/Getty Images

Notice

The author and the publisher of this book have taken care to make certain that the information given is correct and compatible with the standards generally accepted at the time of publication. Nevertheless, as new information becomes available, changes in treatment and in the use of equipment and procedures become necessary. The reader is advised to carefully consult the instruction and information material included in each piece of equipment or device before administration. Students are warned that the use of any techniques must be authorized by their medical advisor, where appropriate, in accordance with local laws and regulations. The publisher disclaims any liability, loss, injury, or damage incurred as a consequence, directly or indirectly, of the use and application of any of the contents of this book.

Cataloging-in-Publication data is on file with the Library of Congress.

Brady
is an imprint of

www.bradybooks.com

ISBN 10:   0-13-457203-3
ISBN 13: 978-0-13-457203-1

25 2022

This text is respectfully dedicated to all EMS personnel who have made the ultimate sacrifice. Their memory and good deeds will forever be in our thoughts and prayers.

BEB, RAC

Contents

14 Intravenous Access
and Medication
Administration 440

15 Airway Management and Ventilation   **512**

Preface to Volume 1

Modern EMS is based on sound principles and practice. Today's paramedic must be knowledgeable in all aspects of EMS. This begins with a fundamental understanding of EMS operations, basic medical science, and basic procedures. We have followed the *National EMS Education Standards* and the accompanying *Paramedic Instructional Guidelines* to provide the appropriate introductory material in *Volume 1, Introduction to Paramedicine.*

This volume provides paramedic students with the principles of advanced prehospital care and EMS operations. The first four chapters detail EMS systems and paramedic roles and responsibilities with added emphasis on personal wellness and injury and illness prevention. The next chapters deal with EMS research and the importance of evidence-based medicine, the EMS role in public health, the medical/legal aspects of emergency care, and ethics in paramedicine. The next two chapters deal with EMS system communications and documentation of patient care. The final chapters of this volume cover life span development, pathophysiology, emergency pharmacology, intravenous access and medication administration, and airway management and ventilation.

Overview of the Chapters . . . and What's New in the 5th Edition?

CHAPTER 1   Introduction to Paramedicine introduces the paramedic student to the world of paramedicine. It summarizes the importance of professionalism and the expanding roles of the paramedic.

New in the 5th Edition: An introduction to **Mobile Integrated Health Care** and **Community Paramedicine**, both concepts relating to paramedicine expanding beyond emergency response and transport to community health initiatives.

CHAPTER 2   EMS Systems reviews the history of EMS and provides an overview of EMS today. It details the aspects of EMS system design and operation. It emphasizes the importance of medical direction in all aspects of prehospital care.

New in the 5th Edition: A new section **Healthcare System Integration**, emphasizing, per newest AHA guidelines, the role of EMS in all types of cardiac emergencies, especially in the identification of acute coronary syndrome and ST-segment myocardial infarction (STEMI).

CHAPTER 3   Roles and Responsibilities of the Paramedic is a detailed discussion of the expectations and responsibilities of the modern paramedic. It emphasizes the various aspects of professionalism as they pertain to the paramedic.

New in the 5th Edition: A note acknowledging that aspects of the **Affordable Care Act of 2010** have changed health care in numerous ways.

CHAPTER 4   Workforce Safety and Wellness presents material crucial to the survival of the paramedic in EMS. It addresses such important issues as prevention of work-related injuries, personal protection from disease, and safety concerns. It discusses physical fitness and nutrition. It discusses ways of dealing with death and dying, details the role of stress in EMS, and presents important coping strategies.

New in the 5th Edition: Notes on diseases introduced by international travel. A new section **Ebola virus disease**, how it is carried, and how to protect against an exposure. A new section on **post-traumatic stress disorder**.

CHAPTER 5   EMS Research discusses the importance of research and evidence-based practices in EMS. It emphasizes ethical considerations in human research. Additionally, it explains how to read, evaluate, and participate in research.

New in the 5th Edition: Updated **American Heart Association Levels of Evidence.**

CHAPTER 6   Public Health discusses the increasingly important role of EMS in public health, public education, and prevention of illness and injury—stopping injuries and illnesses before they happen.

CHAPTER 7 Medical/Legal Aspects of Prehospital Care is a detailed treatise on law and emergency care. In addition to an overview of the law and the legal system, this chapter discusses how the legal system can impact the paramedic. It also provides important tips on how the paramedic can avoid liability in a malpractice action.

> **New in the 5th Edition:** Emphasis that **EMS laws and regulations differ** between states and even between cities and counties. Emphasis on the importance of individual **liability insurance.** Emphasis on **invasion of privacy issues concerning cell phone cameras and social media.** A new section on **physician orders for life-sustaining treatment (POLST).**

CHAPTER 8 Ethics in Paramedicine presents the fundamentals of medical ethics. As EMS becomes more sophisticated, the paramedic will be faced with an ever-increasing number of ethical dilemmas. This chapter provides the paramedic student with an overview of medical ethics so as to be able to make sound decisions when confronted with ethical problems.

CHAPTER 9 EMS System Communications discusses communication as the key component linking all phases of an EMS run, discusses the current state of EMS communications, and presents anticipated advances in EMS communications and communications technology.

CHAPTER 10 Documentation explains how to write a prehospital care report (PCR), including examples of narrative report-writing styles, and discusses the elements and uses of electronic patient care records.

CHAPTER 11 Pathophysiology provides a detailed description of basic pathophysiology. The first part of the chapter introduces the concept of disease, including predisposing factors to disease and classifications of disease. The next parts of the chapter discuss disease at the chemical level, the cellular level, the tissue level, and the organ level. Finally, the chapter details the body's defenses against disease and injury.

CHAPTER 12 Human Life Span Development provides an overview of physiologic and psychosocial developmental and age-related changes from infancy to late adulthood.

CHAPTER 13 Emergency Pharmacology is a comprehensive chapter covering the various medications used in medical practice, especially paramedic practice. It presents an overview of pharmacology, followed by a discussion of drug classifications.

> **New in the 5th Edition:** Tables listing **antiarrhythmic and hormone-related drugs updated per latest American Heart Association guidelines.**

CHAPTER 14 Intravenous Access and Medication Administration is presented in three parts, the first part detailing principles and routes of medication administration; the second part concerning intravenous access, blood sampling, and intraosseous infusion; and the final part giving an overview of medical mathematics and dose calculation.

> **New in the 5th Edition:** An updated section on **Venous Access Devices,** including tunneled catheters, medication ports, and peripherally inserted central catheters (PICCs). A new section on **Ultrasound-Guided Intravenous Access.**

CHAPTER 15 Airway Management and Ventilation presents the crucial prehospital skill of airway management. The first part of the chapter deals with respiratory anatomy, physiology, and assessment. The chapter then goes on to address both basic manual and advanced airway management techniques. In addition, this chapter details patient positioning, oxygenation, ventilation techniques, suction, rapid sequence intubation, surgical airways, the difficult airway, and other airway and ventilation issues and techniques.

> **New in the 5th Edition:** A segment on **apneic oxygenation,** a new strategy used to minimize the likelihood of hypoxia during endotracheal intubation.

Bryan Bledsoe
Richard Cherry

Acknowledgments

Chapter Contributors

We wish to acknowledge the remarkable talents of the following people who contributed to this five volume series. Individually, they worked with extraordinary commitment. Together, they form a team of highly dedicated professionals who have upheld the highest standards of EMS instruction.

Paul Ganss, MS, NRP (Volume 1, Chapter 2)

Michael F. O'Keefe (Volume 1, Chapter 5)

Wes Ogilvie, MPA, JD, LP (Volume 1, Chapter 7)

Kevin McGinnis, MPS, EMT-P (Volume 1, Chapter 9)

Jeff Brosious, EMT-P (Volume 1, Chapter 10)

W.E. Gandy, JD, NREMT-P (Volume 1, Chapter 15)

Darren Braude, MD, MPH, FACEP (Volume 1, Chapter 15)

Joseph R. Lauro, MD, EMT-P (Volume 2, Chapter 6)

Brad Buck, NRP, CCEMT-P (Volume 3, Chapter 10)

Bryan Bledsoe, DO, FACEP, FAAEM, EMT-P (Volume 4, Chapter 10)

Andrew Schmidt, DO, MPH (Volume 4, Chapter 10)

Justin Sempsrott, MD (Volume 4, Chapter 10)

David Nelson, MD, FAAP, FAAEM (Volume 5, Chapter 4)

Mike Abernethy, MD, FAAEM (Volume 5, Chapter 10)

Ryan J. Wubben, MD, FAAEM (Volume 5, Chapter 10)

Louis Molino, NREMT-I (Volume 5, Chapter 11)

Dale M. Carrison, DO, FACEP, FACOEP (Volume 5, Chapter 14)

Dan Limmer, AS, NRP (Volume 5, Chapter 14)

Deborah J. McCoy-Freeman, BS, RN, NREMTP (Volume 5, Chapter 15)

BEB, RAC

Instructor Reviewers

The reviewers of this edition of *Paramedic Care: Principles & Practice* have provided many excellent suggestions and ideas for improving the text. The quality of the reviews has been outstanding, and the reviews have been a major aid in the preparation and revision of the manuscript. The assistance provided by these EMS experts is deeply appreciated.

Fifth Edition

Michael Smith, MS, Educator, Kilgore College, Longview, TX

Edward Lee, A.A.S., BS, Ed.S., NRP, CCEMT-P, EMT Paramedic Program Coordinator, Trident Technical College, Summerville, SC

Ryan Batenhorst, BA, NRP, EMS-I, Program Director, Paramedic Program, Southeast Community College, Milford, NE

Brett Peine, BS, NRP, Director, Southern State University, Joplin, MO

Fourth Edition

Ronald R. Audette, NREMT-P
Vice President
Educational Resource Group LLC
East Providence, RI

Troy Breitag, BS, NREMT-P, Fire Lt.
Department Supervisor – Med/Fire Rescue
Lake Area Technical Institute
Watertown, SD

Joshua Chan, BA, NREMT-P
EMS Educator
Cuyuna Regional Medical Center
Crosby, MN

Thomas E. Ezell, III, NREMT-P, CCEMT-P, CHpT
Fire/Rescue Captain (Ret.)
James City County Fire Department
Williamsburg, VA

Sean P. Haaverson, AA, NR/CCEMT-P
EMS Faculty
Central New Mexico Community College
Albuquerque, NM

L. Kelly Kirk, III, AAS, BS, EMT-P
Director of Distance Education
Randolph Community College
Asheboro, NC

Paul Salway, CCEMT-P, NREMT-P
Firefighter/EMT-P
South Portland Fire Department
South Portland, ME

R. Thomy Windham, BS
Director
Pee Dee Regional Community Training
Center
Florence, SC

We also wish to express appreciation to the following EMS professionals who reviewed the third edition of Paramedic Care: Principles & Practice. *Their suggestions and perspectives helped to make this program a successful teaching tool.*

Mike Dymes, NREMT-P
EMS Program Director
Durham Technical Community College
Durham, NC

Wes Hamilton, RN, BSN, CCRN, CFRN, CTRN, NREMT-P, FP-C
Clinical Educator
Clinical Care Services Division
Air-Evac Lifeteam
West Plains, MO

Sean Kivlehan, EMT-P
St. Vincent's Hospital, Manhattan
New York, NY

Darren P. Lacroix, AAS, EMT-P
Del Mar College
Emergency Medical Service Professions
Corpus Christi, TX

Mike McEvoy, PhD, REMT-P, RN, CCRN
EMS Coordinator
Saratoga County, NY

Greg Mullen, MS, NREMT-P
National EMS Academy
Lafayette, LA

Deborah L. Petty, BS, EMT-P I/C
Training Officer
St. Charles County Ambulance District
St. Peter's, MO

B. Jeanine Riner, MHSA, BS, RRT, NREMT-P
GA Office of EMS and Trauma
Atlanta, GA

Michael D. Smith, LP
Kilgore College
Longview, TX

Allen Walls
Department of Fire & EMS
Colerain Township, OH

Brian J. Wilson, BA, NREMT-P
Education Director
Texas Tech School of Medicine
El Paso, TX

Photo Acknowledgments

All photographs not credited adjacent to the photograph or in the photo credit section below were photographed on assignment for Brady/Pearson Education.

Organizations

We wish to thank the following organizations for their valuable assistance in creating the photo program for this edition:

Canandaigua Emergency Squad
Canandaigua, NY

Flower Mound Fire Department
Flower Mound, TX

Children's Hospital St. Louis/BJC Health Care
St. Louis, MO

Christian Hospital/BJC Health Care
St. Charles, MO

MedicWest Ambulance
Las Vegas, NV

Tyco Health Care/Nellcor Puritan Bennet
Pleasanton, CA

Wolfe Tory Medical
Salt Lake City, UT

Models

Thanks to the following people from the Flower Mound Fire Department, Flower Mound, Texas, who provided locations and/or portrayed patients and EMS providers in our photographs.

FAO/Paramedic Wade Woody
FF/Paramedic Tim Mackling
FF/Paramedic Matthew Daniel
FF/Paramedic Jon Rea
FF/Paramedic Waylon Palmer
FF/EMT Jesse Palmer
Captain/EMT Billy McWhorter

About the Authors

BRYAN E. BLEDSOE, DO, FACEP, FAAEM, EMT-P

Dr. Bryan Bledsoe is an emergency physician, researcher, and EMS author. Presently he is Professor of Emergency Medicine at the University of Nevada School of Medicine and an Attending Emergency Physician at the University Medical Center of Southern Nevada in Las Vegas. He is board-certified in emergency medicine and emergency medical services. Prior to attending medical school, Dr. Bledsoe worked as an EMT, a paramedic, and a paramedic instructor. He completed EMT training in 1974 and paramedic training in 1976 and worked for six years as a field paramedic in Fort Worth, Texas. In 1979, he joined the faculty of the University of North Texas Health Sciences Center and served as coordinator of EMT and paramedic education programs at the university.

Dr. Bledsoe is active in emergency medicine and EMS research. He is a popular speaker at state, national, and international seminars and writes regularly for numerous EMS journals. He is active in educational endeavors with the United States Special Operations Command (USSOCOM) and the University of Nevada at Las Vegas. Dr. Bledsoe is the author of numerous EMS textbooks and has in excess of 1 million books in print. Dr. Bledsoe was named a "Hero of Emergency Medicine" in 2008 by the American College of Emergency Physicians as a part of their 40th anniversary celebration and was named a "Hero of Health and Fitness" by *Men's Health* magazine as part of their 20th anniversary edition in November of 2008. He is frequently interviewed in the national media. Dr. Bledsoe is married and divides his time between his residences in Midlothian, TX, and Las Vegas, NV.

RICHARD A. CHERRY, MS, EMT-P

Richard Cherry is a Training Consultant for Northern Onondaga Volunteer Ambulance (NOVA) in Liverpool, New York, a suburb of Syracuse. He is also a program reviewer for The Continuing Education Coordinating Board for Emergency Medical Services (CECBEMS). He formerly held positions in the Department of Emergency Medicine at Upstate Medical University as Director of Paramedic Training, Assistant Emergency Medicine Residency Director, Clinical Assistant Professor of Emergency Medicine, and Technical Director for Medical Simulation. His experience includes years of classroom teaching and emergency fieldwork. A native of Buffalo, Mr. Cherry earned his bachelor's degree at nearby St. Bonaventure University in 1972. He taught high school for the next ten years while he earned his master's degree in education from Oswego State University in 1977. He holds a permanent teaching license in New York State.

Mr. Cherry entered the emergency medical services field in 1974 with the DeWitt Volunteer Fire Department, where he served his community as a firefighter and EMS provider for more than 15 years. He took his first EMT course in 1977 and became an ALS provider two years later. He earned his paramedic certificate in 1985 as a member of the area's first paramedic class. He then worked both as a paid and volunteer paramedic for the next 15 years.

Mr. Cherry has authored several books for Brady. Most notable are *Paramedic Care: Principles & Practice, Essentials of Paramedic Care, Intermediate Emergency Care: Principles & Practice,* and *EMT Teaching: A Common Sense Approach.* He has made presentations at many state, national, and international EMS conferences on a variety of EMS clinical and teaching topics. He and his wife, Sue, reside in Sun City West, Arizona. In addition to riding horses, hiking, and playing softball, they volunteer their time at Banner Del Webb Medical Center. Mr. Cherry also plays lead guitar in a Christian band.

A GUIDE TO KEY FEATURES

Emphasizing Principles

LEARNING OBJECTIVES

Terminal Performance Objectives and a separate set of Enabling Objectives are provided for each chapter.

KEY TERMS

Page numbers identify where each key term first appears, boldfaced, in the chapter.

Chapter 1

Introduction to Paramedicine

Bryan Bledsoe, DO, FACEP, FAAEM

STANDARD
Preparatory (EMS Systems)

COMPETENCY
Integrates comprehensive knowledge of EMS systems, the safety and well-being of the paramedic, and medical–legal and ethical issues, which is intended to improve the health of EMS personnel, patients, and the community.

∨ Learning Objectives

Terminal Performance Objective: After reading this chapter your should be able to discuss the characteristics of the profession of paramedicine.

Enabling Objectives: To accomplish the terminal performance objective, you should be able to:

1. Define key terms introduced in this chapter.
2. Compare and contrast the four nationally recognized levels of EMS providers in the United States.
3. Describe the requirements that must be met for EMS professionals to function at the paramedic level.
4. Discuss the traditional and emerging roles of the paramedic in health care, public health, and public safety.
5. List and describe the various health care settings paramedics may practice in with an expanded scope of practice.

KEY TERMS

Advanced Emergency Medical Technician (AEMT), p. 3

community paramedicine, p. 4

critical care transport, p. 7

Emergency Medical Responder (EMR), p. 3

Emergency Medical Services (EMS) system, p. 2

Emergency Medical Technician (EMT), p. 3

mobile integrated health care, p. 4

National Emergency Medical Services Education Standards: Paramedic Instructional Guidelines, p. 5

Paramedic, p. 3

paramedicine, p. 4

1

more rapid are the pulse and respiratory rates.

3.0 and 3.5 kg. Because of the excretion of extracellular

As newborns make the transition from fetal to pulmonary circulation in the first few days of life, several important

Table 11-1 Normal Vital Signs

	Pulse (Beats per Minute)	Respiration (Breaths per Minute)	Blood Pressure (Average mmHg)	Temperature	
Infancy:					
At birth:	100–180	30–60	60–90 systolic	98–100°F	36.7–37.8°C
At 1 year:	100–160	30–60	87–105 systolic	98–100°F	36.7–37.8°C
Toddler (12 to 36 months)	80–110	24–40	95–105 systolic	96.8–99.6°F	36.0–37.5°C
Preschool age (3 to 5 years)	70–110	22–34	95–110 systolic	96.8–99.6°F	36.0–37.5°C
School-age (6 to 12 years)	65–110	18–30	97–112 systolic	98.6°F	37°C
Adolescence (13 to 18 years)	60–90	12–26	112–128 systolic	98.6°F	37°C
Early adulthood (19 to 40 years)	60–100	12–20	120/80	98.6°F	37°C
Middle adulthood (41 to 60 years)	60–100	12–20	120/80	98.6°F	37°C
Late adulthood (61 years and older)	*	*	*	98.6°F	37°C

*Depends on the individual's physical health status.

TABLES

A wealth of tables offers the opportunity to highlight, summarize, and compare information.

components of the rule of threes. Whenever BVM ventilation is difficult, however, the rule of threes should be employed.

CONTENT REVIEW
➤ The Rule of Threes for Optimal BVM Ventilation
  • Three providers
  • Three inches
  • Three fingers
  • Three airways
  • Three PSI
  • Three PEEP

• *Three providers.* One provider on the mask, one on the bag, and one for cricoid pressure.

• *Three inches.* A reminder to place the patient in the sniffing position (elevate the head three inches) if not contraindicated.

• *Three fingers.* Three fingers on the cricoid cartilage to perform cricoid pressure.

• *Three airways.* In a worst-case scenario, the airway can be maintained, if necessary, with an oropharyngeal airway and two nasopharyngeal airways (one in each nostril).

CONTENT REVIEW

Content review boxes set off from the text are interspersed throughout the chapter. They summarize key points and serve as a helpful study guide—in an easy format for quick review.

PHOTOS AND ILLUSTRATIONS

Carefully selected photos and a unique art program reinforce content coverage and add to text explanations.

index, and middle finger of one hand. If a lesser-trained provider is performing the maneuver, you should confirm that they are in the correct position (Figure 15-47).

Use caution not to apply so much pressure as to deform and possibly obstruct the trachea; this is a particular danger in infants. The necessary pressure has been estimated as the amount of force that will compress a capped 50-mL syringe from 50 mL to the 30 mL marking. In the event that the patient actively vomits, it is imperative to release the pressure to avoid esophageal rupture. Similarly, if cricoid pressure is being performed during intubation, reduce or release the pressure if the intubator is having difficulty visualizing the vocal cords.

Optimal BVM Ventilation Using the Rule of Threes

The *rule of threes* was developed to help providers recall the components of optimal BVM ventilation. Many patients can be easily oxygenated and ventilated without using all

FIGURE 15-47 Cricoid pressure.

Thyroid cartilage (Adam's apple)
Cricothyroid membrane
Trachea
Esophagus
Cricoid cartilage occluding esophagus

• *Three PSI.* A gentle reminder to use the lowest pressure necessary to see the chest rise.

• *Three seconds.* A reminder to ventilate slowly and allow time for adequate exhalation.

• *Three PEEP.* Or up to 15 cm/H_2O positive-end expiratory pressure (PEEP) as needed to improve oxygen saturations.

Bag-Valve Ventilation of the Pediatric Patient

The differences in the pediatric patient's anatomy require some variation in ventilation technique. First, the child's relatively flat nasal bridge makes achieving a mask seal more difficult. Pressing the mask against the child's face to improve the seal can actually obstruct the airway, which is more compressible than an adult's. You can best achieve the mask seal with the two-person BVM technique, using a jaw-thrust to maintain an open airway.

For BVM ventilation, the bag size depends on the child's age. Full-term neonates and infants will require a pediatric BVM with a capacity of at least 450 mL. For children up to 8 years of age, the pediatric BVM is preferred, although for patients in the upper portion of that age range you can use an adult BVM with a capacity of 1,500 mL if you do not maximally inflate it. Children older than 8 years require an adult BVM to achieve adequate tidal volumes. Additionally, be

Summary

The scene size-up is the initial step in the patient care process. Sizing up the scene and situation begins at your initial dispatch and does not end until you are clear of the call. As the call unfolds, you should be making constant observations and adjustments to your plan of action. Remember that your safety and the safety of your partner are paramount—it is hard to effectively treat both yourself and others.

Scene size-up should be practiced so much that it becomes second nature to you. It is like noticing veins on people in public after you begin starting IVs. (You have all done it—looked across the room at the back of someone's hand and noticed what nice veins they had.) Sizing up a scene is no different. After a while, you begin to notice mechanisms of injury and other important details almost subconsciously. But be careful and do not get complacent! Always make it a point to pause for just a few seconds and consciously look around the scene before proceeding into any situation.

Scene size-up is not a step-by-step process, but a series of decisions you make when confronted with a variety of circumstances that are often beyond your control. It is a way to make order out of chaos, keep yourself and your crew safe, and ensure that all necessary resources are focused on patient care and outcomes. With time and experience, you will learn to perform a scene size-up quickly and focus on important issues. Your careful size-up lays the foundation for an organized and timely approach toward patient care and scene management. And always remember that scene size-up is not a one-time occurrence. It is an ongoing process.

SUMMARY

This end-of-chapter feature provides a concise review of chapter information.

airway management in every patient, you should learn and use advanced skills such as intubation, RSI, and cricothyrotomy. You must maintain proficiency in all airway skills, especially the more advanced techniques, through ongoing continuing education, physician medical direction, and testing with each EMS service. If you cannot do this, it is in the patient's best interest to focus on less sophisticated airway skills. If you anticipate that every airway will be complicated, apply basic airway skills before using advanced procedures, and perform frequent reassessments, you will give the patient his best chance for meaningful survival.

You Make the Call

You and your paramedic partner, Preston Connelly, are assigned to District 4, a quiet suburban neighborhood, on a warm Saturday in June. At 2:00 P.M., you are dispatched to care for a choking child at the Happy Hotdog Restaurant on Main Street. On your way to the location, the dispatcher advises you that they are currently giving prearrival choking instructions to the bystanders at the scene. On arrival, you find a frantic mother who tells you that her 6-year-old son was eating a hot dog and drinking a soda when he started coughing and gasping for air. She keeps yelling for you to do something. Bystanders surround the child and are attempting to perform the Heimlich maneuver without success. On your primary assessment, you find a 6-year-old boy lying on the floor, unconscious and apneic, with a pulse rate of 130. There is cyanosis surrounding his lips and fingernail beds, with a moderate amount of secretions coming from his mouth. There are no signs of trauma. You and Preston immediately start management of this child.

1. What is your primary assessment and management of this child?

2. What are your first actions?

3. What are your options for managing the airway after the obstruction is relieved?

4. What are the major anatomic differences between pediatric and adult patients in terms of airway management?

See Suggested Responses at the back of this book.

YOU MAKE THE CALL

A scenario at the end of each chapter promotes critical thinking by requiring students to apply principles to actual practice.

REVIEW QUESTIONS

These questions ask students to review and recall key information they have just learned.

Review Questions

1. When you couple the physical assessment findings with the patient's medical history, you are able to derive a list of _____
   a. clinical diagnostics.
   b. field prognoses.
   c. chief complaints
   d. differential field diagnoses.

2. The pain, discomfort, or dysfunction that caused your patient to request help is known as the _____
   a. primary problem.
   b. nature of the illness.
   c. differential diagnosis.
   d. chief complaint.

3. You are assessing a patient who complains of cardiac-type chest pain that is felt in the jaw and down the left arm. This pattern of pain is known as _____
   a. sympathetic pain.
   b. tenderness.
   c. referred pain.
   d. associated pain.

4. Your patient has smoked 2 packs of cigarettes each day for the past 35 years. He is a _____ pack/year smoker.
   a. 35   c. 730
   b. 70   d. 25,550

5. The CAGE questionnaire is used as an evaluation tool to assess a patient with what type of history?
   a. Alcoholism   c. Allergies
   b. Lung disease   d. Pregnancy

6. What interviewing mnemonic should be used for each presenting problem a patient has?
   a. SAMPLE
   b. DCAP–BTLS
   c. OPQRST–ASPN
   d. AEIOU–TIPS

7. The mnemonic GPAL is used to evaluate a patient's _____
   a. alcoholism.
   b. allergies.
   c. pregnancy history.
   d. endocrine dysfunction.

Match the following elements of the present illness of the patient with a chief complaint of chest pain with their respective examples:

1. O   a. Pain is 6 on a scale of 1–10
2. P   b. Patient also complains of shortness of breath and nausea
3. Q   c. Pain had a sudden onset
4. R   d. Pain began 2 hours ago
5. S   e. Pain worsens while lying down
6. T   f. Patient denies dizziness
7. AS   g. Pain goes through to the back
8. PN   h. Pain is heavy and vise-like

See Answers to Review Questions at the back of this book.

6. Which radio frequencies may be used by cities and municipalities for their ability to better transmit through concrete and steel?
   a. UHF   c. 800-mHz
   b. VHF   d. none of the above

7. Which frequency band is typically used by county and suburban agencies due to its ability to transmit over various terrains and longer distances?
   a. UHF   c. 800-mHz
   b. VHF   d. none of the above

8. What is the name of the basic communications system that uses the same frequency to both transmit and receive?
   a. Multiplex   c. Simplex
   b. Duplex   d. Complex

9. A communications system that uses a different transmit and receive frequency allowing for simultaneous communications between two parties is called _____
   a. multiplex.
   b. duplex.
   c. simplex.
   d. complex.

10. _____ communications systems are capable of transmitting both voice and electronic patient data simultaneously.
   a. Multiplex   c. Simplex
   b. Duplex   d. Complex

See answers to Review Questions at the back of this book.

REFERENCES

This listing is a compilation of source material providing the basis of updated data and research used in the preparation of each chapter.

References

1. Department of Homeland Security. SAFECOM. (Available at http://www.dhs.gov/safecom/)
2. National EMS Information System (NEMSIS). The NEMSIS Technical Assistance Center (TAC). (Available at http://www.nemsis.org/./.)
3. American College of Emergency Physicians (ACEP). "Automatic Crash Notification and Intelligent Transportation Systems." *Ann Emerg Med* 55 (2010): 397.
4. National Emergency Number Association (NENA). National Emergency Number Association. (Available at: http://www.nena.org)
5. Association of Public-Safety Communications Officials (APCO). [Available at http://www.apco911.org/]
6. Department of Transportation, Research and Innovative Technology Administration. Next Generation 911. (Available at: http://www.its.dot.gov/ng911/.)
7. Centers for Disease Control and Prevention. Recommendations from the Expert Panel: Advanced Automatic Collision Notification and Triage of the Injured Patient. (See NHTSA summary at http://www.nhtsa.gov/Research/Biomechanics+&+Trauma/Advanced+Automatic+Collision+Notification+-+AACN)

8. Wilson, S., M. Cooke, R. Morrell et al. "A Systematic Review of the Evidence Supporting the Use of Priority Dispatch of Emergency Ambulances." *Prehosp Emerg Care* 6 (2002): 42–29.
9. Billittier, A. J., 4th, E. B. Lerner, W. Tucker, and J. Lee. "The Lay Public's Expectations of Prearrival Instructions When Dialing 911." *Prehosp Emerg Care* 4 (2000): 234–237.
10. Munk, M. D., S. D. White, M. L. Perry, et al. "Physician Medical Direction and Clinical Performance at an Established Emergency Medical Services System." *Prehosp Emerg Care* 13 (2009): 185–192.
11. Cheung, D. S., J. J. Kelly, C. Beach, et al. "Improving Handoffs in the Emergency Department." *Ann Emerg Med* 55 (2010): 171–180.
12. Chan, T. C., J. Killeen, W. Griswold, and L. Lenert. "Information Technology and Emergency Medical Care during Disasters." *Acad Emerg Med* 11 (2004): 1229–1236.
13. DREAMS Ambulance Project. (See article at https://www.ems1.com/ems-products/technology/articles/1183110-DREAMS-revolutionize-communication-between-ER-and-ambulance/.)
14. Haskins, P. A., D. G. Ellis, and J. Mayrose. "Predicted Utilization of Emergency Medical Services Telemedicine in Decreasing Ambulance Transports." *Prehosp Emerg Care* 6 (2002): 445–448.

FURTHER READING

This list features recommendations for books and journal articles that go beyond chapter coverage.

Further Reading

Bass, R., J. Potter, K. McGinnis, and T. Miyahara. "Surveying Emerging Trends in Emergency-related Information Delivery for the EMS Profession." *Topics in Emergency Medicine* 26 (April–June 2004): 2, 93–102.

Fitch, J. "Benchmarking Your Comm Center." *JEMS* 2006: 98–112.

McGinnis, K. K. "The Future of Emergency Medical Services Communications Systems: Time for a Change." *N C Med J* 68 (2007): 283–285.

McGinnis, K. K. *Future EMS Technologies: Predicting Communications Implications.* National Public Safety Telecommunications Council,

National Association of State EMS Officials, National Association of EMS Physicians, June, 2010.

McGinnis, K. K. "The Future Is Now: Emergency Medical Services (EMS) Communications Advances Can Be as Important as Medical Treatment Advances When It Comes to Saving Lives." *Interoperability Today* (SafeCom, U.S. Department of Homeland Security), Volume 3, 2005.

McGinnis, K. K. *Rural and Frontier Emergency Medical Services Agenda for the Future.* National Rural Health Association Press: October 2004.

cleaning, p. 70
Code Green Campaign, p. 78
disinfection, p. 70
exposure, p. 70

isotonic exercise, p. 61
pathogens, p. 65
personal protective equipment (PPE), p. 66

sterilization, p. 70
stress, p. 74
stressor, p. 74
Tema Conter Memorial Trust, p. 78

CASE STUDY

This feature at the start of each chapter draws students into the reading and creates a link between text content and real-life situations.

Case Study

Howard is a 15-year veteran of a high-volume, inner-city EMS service. When he first started his career, Howard thought he knew what he was getting into, but the years have taught him differently.

Right now, Howard is in the spotlight for saving the life of a police officer who was shot in a hostage situation. "That call forced me to reflect on a few important things," he says. "Two years ago, I had a minor heart problem, and it was a good wake-up call. Since then I've been lifting weights and running, so I was able to get to the officer with enough strength to carry him to safety.

"Another thing is that I always use personal protective equipment. I never go to work without steel-toed boots and I never leave the ambulance without a pair of disposable gloves. Can you believe there are still paramedics who knock the concept of infection control? If any one of my partners sticks a needle into the squad bench in my ambulance, they know I'll speak up."

Howard, a mild-mannered, nondescript man, doesn't realize that his young colleagues regard him as a role model. They've seen him handle himself at chaotic scenes as well as when a situation demands sensitivity, patience, and gentleness. "Howard is the man I'd want to tell bad news to my mother," one of his partners says. "He can handle people involved in just about any circumstance—death situations, panicked parents, lonely elderly people, and even hostile drunks. I've never seen anyone treat others with such dignity and respect. He's the best partner anyone could want, especially when we have to manage patients who are thrashing around. But that was not always so, was it, Howard?"

"No, it wasn't," Howard replies. "There was a time when no one wanted to work with me. I was a rebel, and I figured there was only one way to do things: my way. But an incident that occurred a few years ago changed all that. It's a long story. But the upshot is that when I recovered from the stress, my outlook had been altered. I realized that though I couldn't save the world, I could save myself. That's when I learned how to deal with the effects of a stressful job. I started eating right, lost a lot of weight, and adopted a new attitude. Anyway, if I can maintain my own well-being, I can do a lot more to help others. Right? Isn't that what we're about?"

Introduction

The safety and well-being of the workforce is a fundamental aspect of top-notch performance in EMS.[1] As a paramedic, it includes your physical well-being as well as your mental and emotional well-being. If your body is fed well and kept fit, if you use the principles of safe lifting, observe safe driving practices, and avoid potentially addictive and insidious infections. If you let your spirit appreciate the fear and sadness on other faces, you will find ways to combat your prejudices and treat people with dignity and respect. By doing all these things, you will also be able to promote the benefits of well-being to your EMS colleagues.

Death, dying, stress, injury, infection, fear—all these threaten your wellness and conspire to interfere with your good intentions. However, you can do something about

PROCEDURE SCANS

Visual skill summaries provide step-by-step support in skill instruction.

Procedure 7-4 Reassessment

7-4a Reevaluate the ABCs.

7-4b Take all vital signs again.

7-4c Perform your focused assessment again.

7-4d Evaluate your interventions' effects.

laryngospasm may be occurring. Airway and breathing management requires constant reevaluation.

oxygenation. Lip cyanosis indicates central hypoxia (overall oxygen status), whereas peripheral cyanosis indicates decreased oxygen to the tissues. Pallor and coolness sug-

---

Special Features

the present illness. Common sense and clinical experience will determine how much of the following history to use.

Preliminary Data

For documentation, always record the date and time of the physical exam. Determine your patient's age, sex, race, birthplace, and occupation. This provides a starting point for the interview and establishes you as the interviewer. Who is the source of the information you receive about your patient? Is it the competent patient himself, his spouse, a friend, or a bystander? Are you receiving a report from a first responder, the police, or another health care worker? Do you have the medical record from a transferring facility?

After you have gathered the information, you should establish its reliability, which will vary according to the source's knowledge, memory, trust, and motivation. Again, reconfirm the information with the patient, if possible. This is a judgment call based on your experience. For example, if the patient information you received from a particular EMT first responder has been accurate in the past, you probably will trust it again. On the other hand, if the nurse at a physician's office has repeatedly provided you with erroneous information, you probably will doubt its accuracy.

scious patient, the chief complaint becomes what someone else identifies or what you observe as the primary problem. In some trauma situations, for instance, the chief complaint might be the mechanism of injury, such as "a penetrating wound to the chest" or "a fall from 25 feet."

Patho Pearls

The renowned Canadian physician Sir William Osler said, "Listen to the patient, and he will tell you what is wrong." This advice is as true today as it was 100 years ago. A great deal of information can be determined from a skillful history taking. As you listen to a patient's medical history, try to understand the underlying pathophysiologic processes that might cause the symptoms the patient describes. This will help you to fully comprehend the disease process or processes affecting the patient.

For example, consider the following case. Mrs. J. Franklin is a 72-year-old pensioner, twice widowed, who lives in an older section of town. She summons EMS with what initially seem like vague complaints. She reports to the dispatcher, when queried, that she is "just sick." You arrive and begin an assessment, starting with a pertinent history. The patient reports that her symptoms began about two weeks ago after several family members came to her house with dinner, which included a baked ham. Since that time, she has developed some fatigue, progressive dyspnea, and occasional chest pain. She now reports that she often wakes up at 3:00 A.M. with breathing trouble that resolves when she walks around the room or

PATHO PEARLS

Offer a snapshot of pathological considerations students will encounter in the field.

FIGURE 2-11 Patients may be transported by ground or air. Medical helicopter transport was introduced in the 1950s during the Korean War. *(© Ed Effron)*

Vietnam, and success of military evacuation procedures led to their use in civilian ambulance systems. In 1970, the Military Assistance to Safety and Traffic (MAST) program was established. This demonstration project set up 35 helicopter transportation programs nationwide to test the feasibility of using military helicopters and paramedics in

Legal Considerations

Emergency Department Closures. Numerous factors have resulted in emergency department closures and ambulance diversions. This can have a significant impact on the EMS system. All systems must address this situation so that patient care does not suffer.

In 1974, in response to a request from the DOT, the General Services Administration (GSA) developed the "KKK-A-1822 Federal Specifications for Ambulances." This was the first attempt at standardizing ambulance design to permit intensive life support for patients en route to a definitive care facility. The act defined the following basic types of ambulance:

- *Type I (Figure 2-13).* This is a conventional cab and chassis on which a module ambulance body is mounted, with no passageway between the driver's and patient's compartments.
- *Type II (Figure 2-14).* A standard van, body, and cab form an integral unit. Most have a raised roof.

LEGAL CONSIDERATIONS

Offer a snapshot of pathological considerations students will encounter in the field.

An important part of patient assessment is gathering information that is accurate, complete, and relevant to the present emergency. To begin, you must identify the patient's chief complaint. Although dispatch probably will have given you an idea of what the emergency is about, it is

Cultural Considerations

Eye contact is a major form of nonverbal communication. Short eye contact is often seen as friendly, whereas prolonged eye contact may be interpreted as threatening. Thus, timing is an important factor in how a person interprets eye contact.

One's culture also influences how eye contact is interpreted. Eye contact can mean respect in one culture and disrespect in another. Often, Asians will avoid eye contact even when they have nothing to hide. Eye contact between people of different sexes is problematic in Muslim cultures, in which a prolonged look in the face of a member of the opposite sex might be misinterpreted. Because of this, people in Middle Eastern countries might look a person of the same sex in the eye and not look into the eyes of a person of the opposite sex.

If you work in a culturally diverse community, you should learn the customs of eye contact and other forms of nonverbal communication of those you might encounter during the course of your work.

unexpected but important facts. For example, instead of asking your patient with abdominal pain, "Did you have breakfast today?" which can be answered with either a "yes" or a "no," ask: "What have you eaten today?"

- *Use direct questions when necessary.* Direct questions, or **closed questions**, ask for specific information. ("Did you take your pills today?" or "Does the abdominal pain come and go like a cramp, or is it constant?") These questions are good for three reasons: They fill in information generated by open-ended questions. They help to answer crucial questions when time is limited. And they can help to control overly talkative patients, who might want to tell you about their gallbladder surgery in 1969 when their chief complaint is a sprained ankle.
- *Ask only one question at a time, and allow the patient to complete his answers.* If you ask more than one question, the patient may not know which one to answer and may leave out portions of information or become confused. Equally important is having one person do the interview. Don't force your patient to discern questions from multiple interviewers.
- *Listen to the patient's complete response before asking the next question.* By doing so, you might find that

CULTURAL CONSIDERATIONS

Provide an awareness of beliefs that might affect patient care.

ASSESSMENT PEARLS

Offer tips, guidance, and information to aid in patient assessment.

PEDIATRIC PEARLS

Offer tips, guidance, and information on how to deal with pediatric patients encountered in the field.

CUSTOMER SERVICE MINUTE

Shows how extending extra kindness and compassion can make an important difference to patients and families coping with an emergency.

IN THE FIELD

Provides extra tips that can help ensure success in real-life emergency situations.

Image by Christof VanDerWalt

MyBRADYLab®

Our goal is to help every student succeed.
We're working with educators and institutions to improve results for students everywhere.

MyLab & Mastering is the world's leading collection of online homework, tutorial, and assessment products designed with a single purpose in mind: to improve the results of higher education students, one student at a time. Used by more than 11 million students each year, Pearson's MyLab & Mastering programs deliver consistent, measurable gains in student learning outcomes, retention, and subsequent course success.

Highlights of this Fully Integrated Learning Program

- **Gradebook:** A robust gradebook allows you to see multiple views of your classes' progress. Completely customizable and exportable, the gradebook can be adapted to meet your specific needs.

- **Multimedia Library:** allows students and instructors to quickly search through resources and find supporting media.

- **Pearson eText:** Rich media options let students watch lecture and example videos as they read or do their homework. Instructors can share their comments or highlights, and students can add their own, creating a tight community of learners in your class.

- **Decision-Making Cases:** take Paramedic students through real-life scenarios that they typically face in the field. These cases give students the opportunity to gather patient data and make decisions that would affect their patient's health.

**For more information,
please contact your BRADY sales representative at 1-800-638-0220,
or visit us at www.bradybooks.com**

Chapter 1
Introduction to Paramedicine

Bryan Bledsoe, DO, FACEP, FAAEM

STANDARD
Preparatory (EMS Systems)

COMPETENCY
Integrates comprehensive knowledge of EMS systems, the safety and well-being of the paramedic, and medical–legal and ethical issues, which is intended to improve the health of EMS personnel, patients, and the community.

 Learning Objectives

Terminal Performance Objective: After reading this chapter your should be able to discuss the characteristics of the profession of paramedicine.

Enabling Objectives: To accomplish the terminal performance objective, you should be able to:

1. Define key terms introduced in this chapter.

2. Compare and contrast the four nationally recognized levels of EMS providers in the United States.

3. Describe the requirements that must be met for EMS professionals to function at the paramedic level.

4. Discuss the traditional and emerging roles of the paramedic in health care, public health, and public safety.

5. List and describe the various health care settings paramedics may practice in with an expanded scope of practice.

KEY TERMS

Advanced Emergency Medical Technician (AEMT), p. 3

community paramedicine, p. 4

critical care transport, p. 7

Emergency Medical Responder (EMR), p. 3

Emergency Medical Services (EMS) system, p. 2

Emergency Medical Technician (EMT), p. 3

mobile integrated health care, p. 4

National Emergency Medical Services Education Standards: Paramedic Instructional Guidelines, p. 5

Paramedic, p. 3

paramedicine, p. 4

Case Study

Marcus Ward is a 65-year-old attorney who is celebrating his recent retirement with a week-long trip to Las Vegas. He has taken in the shows, eaten the fine food, and is spending his last night in town in one of the casinos on the famous Las Vegas strip. He sits down at a blackjack table and lights a cigarette. As the dealer is shuffling the cards, Marcus starts to feel warm. He turns to his friend Ray and says, "Does it feel warm in here to you?" Then, without another word, Marcus grasps at the collar of his shirt and collapses to the floor. Initially, Ray thinks his friend has slipped on the stool. Quickly, though, he realizes the situation is much worse. He starts screaming for help. The dealer presses a security button and several security officers immediately come to the table. After a quick exam, the security staff moves Marcus to a beverage area off the casino floor and calls 911. There they start CPR and immediately apply an automated external defibrillator (AED) to Marcus. The AED detects ventricular fibrillation and delivers a shock. Immediately, Marcus starts moving and soon opens his eyes. The security staff closely monitors Marcus, and soon a paramedic fire crew arrives. Shortly thereafter, paramedics from the ambulance service arrive.

The paramedics assess Marcus and obtain a 12-lead ECG. The ECG is consistent with an acute anterior ST-segment elevation myocardial infarction (STEMI). The ECG monitor electronically transmits Marcus's ECG to the hospital emergency department and the on-call STEMI team. The cardiologist reviews the ECG and calls for a "Code STEMI," after which the team is activated. Paramedics insert an IV and administer nitroglycerin and 325 mg of aspirin. Marcus is quickly moved to the ambulance and transported to the designated hospital.

Once Marcus arrives at the emergency department, he is quickly evaluated by the interventional cardiologist and an emergency physician. Finding no contraindications, the cardiologist has Marcus immediately moved to the cardiac catheterization suite. After he arrives in the lab, the team goes to work. Marcus is moved to the table. A nurse shaves his groin and applies an antiseptic soap. An anesthesiologist sedates Marcus and monitors his vital signs. The cardiologist quickly inserts a catheter into Marcus's femoral artery and threads it up the aorta to the heart. He injects a dye, and immediately Marcus's coronary arteries can be seen on the monitor. As expected, part of the left anterior descending coronary artery is blocked. The cardiologist then inserts a balloon catheter into the diseased artery and restores blood flow to the affected part of the heart. Some ventricular irritability and premature ventricular contractions follow, but these soon abate and the cardiologist then inserts a drug-eluting stent to keep the artery open. Additional dye is injected, blood flow through the stent looks good, and no other lesions require treatment. Marcus is moved to the coronary care unit, where he ultimately recovers and flies back to Irvine, California, four days later.

Marcus survived because the EMS and emergency health care system worked together cohesively. When he collapsed at the blackjack table, he was defibrillated within 3 minutes of his collapse. His STEMI was promptly identified and treated by prehospital personnel, who also notified and activated the STEMI team at the hospital. The time interval from Marcus's arrival at the hospital until blood flow was restored to his diseased artery (door-to-balloon time) was 31 minutes.

Back in Irvine, Marcus has vowed to improve his life and appears to be making important changes. He has quit smoking and has begun an exercise regimen. He now sees a local cardiologist on a regular basis. He and his wife have made major changes in their diet. His prognosis is good, and he should enjoy many more years of his retirement. A month after his cardiac arrest, Marcus purchased an AED and donated it to the fitness center where he now exercises. Moreover, he has developed a new understanding and appreciation for the EMS system.

Introduction

Congratulations on your decision to become a Paramedic. Before you begin this long but rewarding endeavor, it is important to understand what the job of a paramedic in the twenty-first century entails. As a member of the allied health professions (ancillary health care professions, apart from physicians and nurses), the paramedic is highly regarded by society (Figure 1-1).

The **Emergency Medical Services (EMS) system** has made significant advances over the past 30 years. Understandably, the roles and responsibilities of the paramedic have advanced accordingly. Not that long ago, the ambulance was simply a vehicle that provided rapid, horizontal transportation to the hospital. Today, equipped with the latest in equipment and technology, the modern ambulance is truly a mobile emergency room that brings sophisticated emergency medical care to the patient. The

FIGURE 1-1 The paramedic of the twenty-first century is a highly trained health care professional.

paramedic of the twenty-first century is a highly trained health care professional who provides comprehensive, compassionate, and efficient prehospital emergency medical care.

Description of the Profession

The paramedic is the highest level of prehospital care provider and the leader of the prehospital care team.[1] There are four nationally recognized levels of EMS providers in the United States:

- *Emergency Medical Responder (EMR).* The primary focus of the **Emergency Medical Responder (EMR)** is to initiate immediate lifesaving care to critical patients who access the emergency medical system. This individual possesses the basic knowledge and skills necessary to provide lifesaving interventions while awaiting additional EMS response and to assist higher level personnel at the scene and during transport. EMRs must successfully complete an accredited EMR educational program.

- *Emergency Medical Technician (EMT).* The primary focus of the **Emergency Medical Technician (EMT)** is to provide basic emergency medical care and transportation for critical and emergent patients who access the emergency medical system. The EMT possesses the basic knowledge and skills necessary to provide patient care and transportation. EMTs perform interventions with basic equipment and are an essential link in the prehospital emergency care continuum. EMTs must successfully complete an EMT educational program.

- *Advanced EMT (AEMT).* The primary focus of the **Advanced Emergency Medical Technician (AEMT)** is to provide basic and limited advanced emergency medical care and transportation for critical and emergent patients who access the EMS system. The AEMT possesses the basic knowledge and skills necessary to provide patient care and transportation. In addition, AEMTs perform interventions with both basic and advanced equipment. The AEMT must successfully complete an accredited EMT educational program.

- *Paramedic.* The **Paramedic** is an allied health professional whose primary focus is to provide advanced emergency medical care for critical and emergent patients who access the EMS system. The paramedic possesses the complex knowledge and skills necessary to provide patient care and transportation. Paramedics function as part of a comprehensive EMS response under medical oversight. Paramedics perform interventions with both basic and advanced equipment typically found on an ambulance. The paramedic is an essential link in the emergency care system. Because of the amount of complex decision making, paramedics must successfully complete a comprehensive accredited paramedic education program at the certificate or associate's degree level.[2]

The Modern Paramedic

The roles and responsibilities of the paramedic are diverse and encompass the disciplines of health care,

> **CONTENT REVIEW**
>
> ➤ Levels of EMS Providers
>   - Emergency Medical Responder (EMR)
>   - Emergency Medical Technician (EMT)
>   - Advanced Emergency Medical Technician (AEMT)
>   - Paramedic
> ➤ The paramedic is the highest level of prehospital care provider and the leader of the prehospital care team.

> **CONTENT REVIEW**
>
> ➤ Emerging Roles of the Paramedic
>   - Public education
>   - Health promotion
>   - Illness and injury prevention

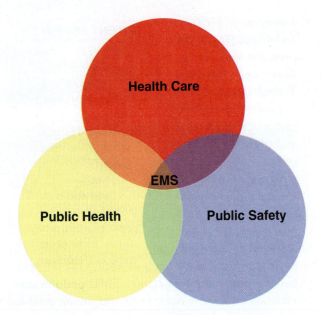

FIGURE 1-2 Modern EMS is a combination of public health, public safety, and health care.

FIGURE 1-3 The paramedic must always be an advocate for the patient.

public health, and public safety. Any of these might come into play on a given day. As EMS research evolves, it is becoming clear that illness and injury prevention are just as important as acute health care and public safety responsibilities (Figure 1-2). The totality of these roles and responsibilities of paramedic practice is known as **paramedicine**.

The primary task of the paramedic is to provide emergency medical care in an out-of-hospital setting. As a paramedic, you will use your advanced training and equipment to extend the care of the emergency physician to the patient in the field. However, you must also be able to make accurate independent judgments. The ability to do this in a timely manner is essential, as it can mean the difference between life and death for the patient.

To function as a paramedic—to practice the art and science of out-of-hospital medicine in conjunction with physician medical oversight—you must have fulfilled the prescribed requirements of the appropriate licensing or credentialing body. Licensing or credentialing is typically provided by a state or provincial agency. All paramedics must be licensed, registered, or otherwise credentialed by the appropriate agency in the area where they work.

Paramedics may function only under the direction of the EMS system's medical director. Because of this, in addition to being appropriately licensed or credentialed, the system's medical director must also approve and credential the paramedic before being permitted to practice advanced prehospital care. Paramedics must possess knowledge, skills, and attitudes consistent with the expectations of the public and the profession.

As a paramedic, you must recognize that you are an essential component in the continuum of care. Furthermore, paramedics often serve as a link between various

health resources in the community. In the future, there will be a continuing demand to control or cut health care costs. As a consequence, paramedics may find themselves in the role of gatekeepers to the health care system. For example, you may be charged with the responsibility of ensuring that your patient gets to the appropriate health care facility in a timely manner, even though the appropriate health care facility may not be a hospital emergency department.

Paramedics must always strive toward maintaining high-quality health care at a reasonable cost. Nevertheless, you must always be an advocate for your patient and ensure that the patient receives the best possible care—without regard to the patient's ability to pay or insurance status (Figure 1-3).

Paramedics of the twenty-first century will continue to fill the well-defined and traditional role of 911 response, but they will also find themselves taking on a wide variety of additional responsibilities. The emerging roles and responsibilities of the paramedic include public education, health promotion, and participation in injury and illness prevention programs. One rapidly expanding role of paramedics is **mobile integrated health care**. Mobile integrated health care, also called **community paramedicine**, is a new and evolving aspect of community-based health care in which paramedics function outside their customary emergency response and transport roles in ways that facilitate more appropriate use of emergency care resources (Figure 1-4). Paramedics also serve to enhance access to primary care for medically underserved populations and help to ensure that all members of the community have access to some level of health care.[3] As the scope of paramedic service continues to expand, the paramedic will function as a facilitator of access to care, as well as an individual treatment provider.

Paramedics are responsible and accountable to the system medical director, their agency, the public, and their peers. Although this may seem like a difficult standard to meet, if you always act in the best interest of the patient, you will seldom run into problems.

FIGURE 1-4 The modern EMS system has begun a new nontraditional role in nonemergent care through such programs as community paramedicine and mobile integrated health care.

(Photo courtesy © Dallas Fire-Rescue Department)

Paramedic Characteristics

There are many different types of EMS system designs and operations. As a paramedic, you may work for a fire department, private ambulance service, third city service, hospital, police department, or other operation. Regardless of the type of service provider you work for, you must be flexible to meet the demands of the ever-changing emergency scene.

As a paramedic, you must be a confident leader who can accept the challenge and responsibility of the position. You must have excellent judgment and be able to prioritize decisions to act quickly in the best interest of the patient. You must be able to develop rapport with a wide variety of patients so that, for example, you can safely interview hostile patients and communicate with members of diverse cultural groups and the various ages within those groups. Overall, you must be able to function independently at an optimum level in a nonstructured, constantly changing environment. The job is never easy and always challenging.

The Paramedic: A True Health Professional

Despite its relative youth as a profession, the field of emergency medical services is now recognized as an important part of the health care system. With this, paramedics are now highly respected members of the health care team. As a paramedic, you must never take this status for granted. Instead, you must always strive to earn your acceptance as a health care professional.

You should consider the completion of your initial paramedic course to be the start of your professional education, not the end. You should participate in various continuing education programs when they become available. Frequently review and practice skills that are infrequently

Legal Considerations

Which Hat Are You Wearing? The modern paramedic, whether career or volunteer, must wear several hats. Many paramedics are also cross trained as firefighters or police officers. The role of each of these professions is different, but there is often significant overlapping of duties. Paramedics may participate in rescue operations, directing traffic, firefighting, and other tasks on an emergency scene. However, it is essential that, when functioning in the role of paramedic, you remember that your primary responsibility is the patient and patient care. You must also be an advocate for the patient.

If you are cross trained, this can cause a certain degree of confusion and conflict. For example, if you are a cross-trained police officer/paramedic who is treating an intoxicated driver, you may have conflicting responsibilities. However, as already noted, when you are functioning as a paramedic your priority should be the patient. Legal issues and other tasks normally addressed by police officers must be handled by other police officers on scene or dealt with after the patient has been treated and transported. Similarly, paramedics who are cross trained may learn information about a patient that is protected from disclosure by the Health Insurance Portability and Accountability Act (HIPAA) and other medical privacy laws and regulations. In a case like this, you may not be able to disclose certain information to your law enforcement colleagues despite the fact that you are also a police officer.

Laws regarding responsibilities of cross-trained individuals vary from state to state. You must be familiar with the laws of the state where you are employed. Remember: When you function as a paramedic, you must put care of the patient above all other tasks—and always remember which hat you are wearing.

used to ensure competency when the skill is needed. As a rule, the less a skill or procedure is used, the more frequent should be the review of that skill or procedure. Most quality continuing education programs acknowledge this by scheduling periodic review and practice of infrequently used skills or procedures. Professional development should be a never-ending, career-long pursuit. Additionally, you should participate in routine peer-evaluation and assume an active role in professional and community organizations (Figure 1-5).

A major step toward the development of EMS as a true health care profession has been to raise the standards of education for out-of-hospital personnel. A significant advance was the 2009 publication by the U.S. Department of Transportation of the ***National Emergency Medical Services Education Standards: Paramedic Instructional Guidelines***.[4] These instructional guidelines have taken paramedic education to a much higher level and were based on a national EMS practice analysis completed by the National Registry of Emergency Medical Technicians in 2004.[5] An anatomy

(a)

(b)

FIGURE 1-5 (a and b) Public education is an important part of the paramedic's job.

and physiology course is now a prerequisite to the paramedic course. The paramedic course itself requires a far more extensive foundation of medical knowledge to underlie the required skills. In particular, the curriculum provides for an improved understanding of the pathophysiology of the various illness and injury processes paramedics encounter in their work. The materials presented in the 2009 DOT EMS Instructional Guidelines are the foundation for this textbook.

As a paramedic, you must actively participate in the design, development, evaluation, and publication of research on topics relevant to your profession. For years, paramedic practice was based on anecdotal data and tradition. Only during the past two decades did we truly begin applying the scientific method to various aspects of prehospital practice. Surprisingly, we found that there were little or no scientific data to support many of our prehospital practices. As a result of research, many traditional EMS treatments have been abandoned or refined. There are still many unanswered questions about paramedic practice, and these can be answered only by sound scientific research.

An essential aspect of a health professional is acceptance and adherence to a code of professional ethics and etiquette. Ethics are standards of right or honorable

behavior, whereas etiquette refers to good manners. Both can apply to all human relationships. However, you will find that questions of ethics most often arise in relationships with patients and the public, whereas etiquette more often relates to behavior between health professionals.

The public must feel confident that, for the paramedic, the patient's and public's interests are always placed above personal, corporate, or financial interests. You must never forget that the emergency patient is your primary concern. Emergency patients are vulnerable and in need. Always keep this in mind and serve as their advocate until you turn patient care over to another health care professional.

Expanded Scope of Practice

Paramedics have a very bright future. New technologies and therapies can literally bring the emergency department to the patient. Paramedics must be willing to step up to these expanding roles, or persons from other health care disciplines will fill them.[6] There are many aspects of out-of-hospital care that can provide you with the opportunity to work in an environment other than the typical 911 response vehicle. These include:

- Critical care transport
- Helicopter air ambulance
- Tactical EMS
- Primary care
- Industrial medicine
- Sports medicine
- Corrections
- Hospital emergency departments

Paramedics are now stepping into nontraditional roles such as these because of their unique education and ability to think and work independently.

Critical Care Transport (CCT)

As a result of the specialization of health care facilities that began to occur in the 1990s, an increasing number of

FIGURE 1-6 The modern critical care transport vehicle provides virtually all the capabilities of the hospital intensive care unit.

FIGURE 1-8 The helicopter has become an important part of the modern EMS system.

(© REACH Air medical Services, LLC)

patients are being moved from one health care facility to another for specialized care. Many of these patients are critically ill and require equipment and care more sophisticated than that available on standard ambulances. Because of this, many EMS systems have developed specialized **critical care transport** vehicles to move these patients between facilities.

These vehicles include specialized ground ambulances, fixed-wing aircraft, and helicopters. Many services have elected to use large vehicles mounted on truck chassis to provide the added space needed for critical care transport (Figure 1-6). To staff these vehicles, paramedics have been educated in various aspects of critical care medicine. These include advanced airway management, ventilator management, fluid and electrolyte therapy, advanced pharmacology, specialized monitoring, operation of intra-aortic balloon pumps, and other techniques usually found in an intensive care setting. This provides a safe and efficient way to move critical patients between facilities without compromising hospital staffing (Figure 1-7).

Helicopter Air Ambulance (HAA)

Helicopters have been a part of the EMS system for more than 30 years and play an important role—especially in

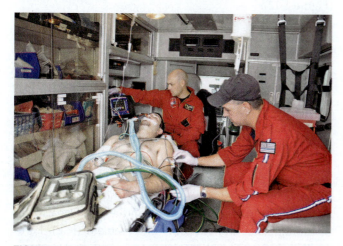

FIGURE 1-7 Critical care transport provides for the safe transfer of critically ill or injured patients between health care facilities.

(© Edward T. Dickinson, MD)

rural areas. Most helicopter air ambulance (HAA) programs staff the helicopter with two medical crew members and often include paramedics. The flight paramedic typically will respond to both scene calls and interfacility transfers. The skills of the flight paramedic are very similar to those of a critical care paramedic, but must include additional education in flight physiology, aircraft operations, flight safety, and similar areas. (Figure 1-8).

Tactical EMS

Over the past decade or so there has been a trend to use EMS personnel in tactical situations. Tactical EMS is designed to enhance the safety of special operations personnel and the public. In some situations, tactical paramedics are cross trained as police officers and carry weapons. The role of the tactical paramedic is to provide life-saving care, sometimes in dangerous environments, until the patient can be safely evacuated to the general EMS system. Many of the practices and techniques of tactical EMS were drawn from experience with the military—particularly with special operations (Figure 1-9).

Mobile Integrated Health Care

Today, many patients can receive primary care outside the hospital at far less cost—for example, in physicians' offices and minor-care or outpatient clinics.[7] Additionally, many patients can be cared for at home. In certain cases, paramedics, in close contact with medical direction, can provide care at the scene without transport to the hospital (e.g., to treat simple lacerations or to change dressings or gastrostomy tubes). Several EMS systems have designated specialized crews to periodically assess and monitor high-risk patients in their community (Figure 1-10).

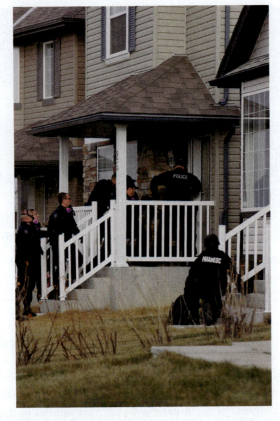

FIGURE 1-9 The tactical paramedic must often provide life-saving care in austere and dangerous situations.

(© Kevin Link/Science Source)

Industrial Medicine

Paramedics have long been the principal health care providers on oil rigs, movie sets, and similar industrial operations. Paramedics are specially trained for the industry in question and often assume additional responsibilities, including safety inspection, accident prevention, medical screening of employees, and vaccinations and immunizations. Many industries use paramedics to assist with sick

FIGURE 1-10 Paramedics play an important role in ensuring the health of the community they serve—especially high-risk patients.

FIGURE 1-11 The industrial paramedic provides several important services in addition to emergency care.

calls and minor medical care. Having paramedics on site allows for increased employee safety and decreased time lost from work (Figure 1-11).

Sports Medicine

Another area in the expanded scope of paramedic practice is sports medicine. Many teams, including those in professional sports, have found that paramedics complement their athletic trainers. In this role, paramedics assume considerably more responsibility for injury prevention. They are also trained to deal with injuries specific to the sport in question. For example, paramedics working with a football team will assist in pregame preparation of players. During the game, they provide any needed emergency medical care. They can also advise the staff whether an injured or ill player may return to the game. Paramedics working with hockey teams, for example, often learn to perform simple laceration repairs and provide care for orthopedic injuries to safely return the players to action as soon as possible (Figure 1-12).

Corrections Medicine

Many states and the federal government have begun to use paramedics as emergency and medical care providers in jails and prisons. In these institutions, paramedics will often do the initial prisoner medical intake assessment and oversee the medical needs of the prison population. They are also responsible for responding to emergencies within the prison. Because of this, they must also have training in correctional operations and similar issues. Paramedics also play a major role in the U.S. Department of Immigration and Customs Enforcement (ICE). Paramedics often work with Border Patrol agents and Customs agents as they endeavor to maintain homeland security (Figure 1-13).

FIGURE 1-12 Injuries and medical emergencies are common at sporting events, and many teams and facilities have paramedics readily available.

(© Ray Kemp/Science Source)

Hospital Emergency Departments

Faced with a nursing shortage, many hospitals have found paramedics to be very suitable providers for emergency departments and minor care centers. The role of the paramedic in these settings varies significantly from state to state, based on local laws. In some situations, the paramedic will function in a role comparable to nursing. In others, they will work in a more technical role, assisting the

FIGURE 1-13 Paramedics often accompany U.S. Border Patrol agents and provide care to both officers and detainees.

(Photo used by permission. Courtesy of the Office of Border Patrol, Field Communications Branch)

medical and nursing staff with skills and responsibilities within the scope of paramedicine. Many paramedics enjoy the diversity and work experience of a busy emergency department (Figure 1-14).

FIGURE 1-14 Hospitals are increasingly turning to paramedics to help staff at busy emergency departments and trauma centers.

Summary

Even though it is still a young profession, EMS is now recognized as a staple in the health care system. Paramedics have been identified as underutilized medical experts and are being offered opportunities that were unheard of just a few years ago.

As the scope of practice for paramedicine continues to expand, so will the demand for skilled practitioners. It is truly an exciting time for EMS and paramedicine. The paramedic of the twenty-first century can have a more significant impact on health care than ever before. The paramedic is often the first member of the health care system with whom the patient interacts, and the results of those interactions can affect the patient's opinion of the health care system in general.

EMS is a profession in which you can make a difference. Every call and every patient interaction has the potential to make the difference between life and death for the patient. Few professions carry such awesome responsibility.

You Make the Call

Finally, after two straight years of urban EMS work without a vacation, you and two of your best paramedic friends, Eileen and Dee Dee, are taking the trip you've been planning for some time. The small airplane grinds to a bumpy halt as you land on a tiny speck of land in the midst of a bright turquoise sea. The ride from the mainland was rough, and Eileen has thrown up. To make matters worse, two of your bags didn't make it aboard the plane. You question the ticket agent who says, "Maybe a plane come Monday. No plane Sunday." Your dream vacation is quickly turning into a nightmare.

After standing in the sun for 45 minutes waiting for a taxi, a 1995 Kia shows up. The driver tells you that your hotel is about 45 minutes away. He throws your bags into the trunk, ties the trunk shut with a piece of rope, and takes off like a dragster from the starting line. You and your friends hang on for dear life as the cab speeds through the winding streets. You try to remember whether people on this island drive on the left side or the right. You certainly can't tell based on your driver's actions. The driver seems to know everybody and honks accordingly. Loud island music crackles through the small speakers in the cab. Dee Dee, the friend who managed not to vomit on the plane, leans over to you and tells you that she thinks she needs to vomit now.

Suddenly, you see a plume of smoke billowing up on the road ahead. As the cab slows, you spot what appears to be an accident. On closer inspection, you see that another cab has plowed into a station wagon at an intersection. Several people are lying on the ground, and there is the general appearance of pandemonium. Dee Dee throws up.

The three of you, experienced paramedics, get out of the cab to take a look. The scene appears safe to approach. Unfortunately, the accident looks severe, with several persons suffering serious injuries. Bystanders begin to reach inside the station wagon and drag the occupants out to a nearby shade tree. You try to offer some advice on providing cervical spine precautions, but they aren't paying any attention to you. You cringe as you see a patient's head fall back and strike the ground.

Before long, all six victims are spread out under a large magnolia tree. A woman is crying loudly and reciting a prayer. A dog walks among the victims. One of the bystanders says that the police should be there "pretty soon." You ask if anyone has called the fire department. The bystander responds with a confused look on his face. "Why do we call the fire department?" he asks. "I do not see a fire."

One victim is obviously dead of a massive head injury. The others are alive but with various injuries. You and your friends try to provide what care you can with absolutely no medical equipment available. Before long, you hear the shrill siren of an approaching police car. The police officers get out of their vehicle and take a significant amount of time putting their hats on. One officer goes to the vehicles. The other goes to the magnolia tree, where he proceeds to get into a heated argument with one of the bystanders. Nobody is paying much attention to the victims except you and your friends.

Before long, there is some excitement as another vehicle pulls up. It seems to be some sort of ambulance. It is an old delivery van painted white with a large orange cross on the side. There are two attendants dressed in white smocks. They carry a canvas litter and, again with no spinal precautions and in no particular order, they begin to load up the victims. You and your friends try to relay the results of your assessment and care. The attendants continue with their tasks, both disinterested and unimpressed with your work. From what you can tell, absolutely no medical care is being provided.

When the last victim is loaded with the other five in the van, both attendants take their seats in the front of the van and leave for the hospital. The shrill sound of the siren slowly fades into the distance, and you and your friends go on to the hotel. You look at the local paper each day, hoping to find out something about the crash victims, but you never find a story about the accident.

Although you are still upset about the accident and the unsophisticated level of medical care you witnessed—and after your bags finally arrive—you, Dee Dee, and Eileen have a nice vacation with no further adverse events.

1. Discuss the vast differences between EMS and paramedic care in the United States, Canada, and other economically developed nations compared with those that exist in some less developed countries of the world. How should awareness of such differences affect your attitude about your work?

See Suggested Responses at the back of this book.

Review Questions

1. Paramedics may function only under the direction and license of the EMS system's _____
   a. town council.
   c. medical director.
   b. company owner.
   d. board of directors.

2. The emerging roles and responsibilities of the paramedic include _____
   a. public education.
   b. health promotion.
   c. participation in injury and illness prevention programs.
   d. all of the above.

3. The rules, standards, and expected actions governing the activities of a group or profession are called _____
   a. ethics.
   c. manners.
   b. morals.
   d. etiquette.

4. Which of the following is an aspect of professionalism?
   a. Being well groomed
   b. Maintaining patient confidentiality
   c. Attending continuing education sessions
   d. All of the above

5. All of the following are considered new, nontraditional roles for the paramedic *except* _____
   a. primary care.
   b. sports medicine.
   c. family practitioner.
   d. industrial medicine.

See answers to Review Questions at the back of this book.

References

1. U.S. Department of Transportation/National Highway Traffic Safety Administration. National EMS Scope of Practice Model. Washington, DC: 2006.

2. Patterson, P. D., J. C. Probst, K. H. Leith, S. J. Corwin, and M. P. Powell. "Recruitment and Retention of Emergency Medical Technicians: A Qualitative Review." *J Allied Health* 34 (2005): 153–162.

3. Bigham, B., S. Kennedy, I. Drennan, L. Morrison, "Expanding Paramedic Scope of Practice in the Community: A Systematic Review of the Literature." *Prehosp Emerg Care* (2013);17: 161–372.

4. U.S. Department of Transportation/National Highway Traffic Safety Administration. National Emergency Medical Services Educational Standards: Paramedic Instruction Guidelines. Washington, DC: 2009.

5. National Registry of Emergency Medical Technicians. 2004 National EMS Practice Analysis. Columbus, OH: 2004.

6. Cooper, S., B. Barrett, S. Black, et al. "The Emerging Role of the Emergency Care Practitioner." *Emerg Med J* 21 (2004): 614–618.

7. Ball, L. "Setting the Scene for the Paramedic in Primary Care: A Review of the Literature." *Emerg Med J* 22 (2005): 896–900.

Further Reading

Bledsoe, B. E. "EMS Needs a Few More Cowboys." *Journal of Emergency Medical Services* (JEMS) 28(12) (2003): 112–113.

Bledsoe, B. E. "Where Are the Wise Men?" Emergency Medical Services (EMS) 31(10) (2002): 172.

Grayson, S. *En Route: A Paramedic's Stories of Life, Death, and Everything in Between.* New York, NY: Kaplan Publishing, 2009.

Page, J. O. *Simple Advice.* Carlsbad, CA: JEMS Publishing, 2002.

Page, J. O. *The Magic of 3 A.M.: Essays on the Art and Science of Emergency Medical Services.* Carlsbad, CA: JEMS Publishing, 2002.

Page, J. O. *The Paramedics.* Morristown, N.J.: Backdraft Publications, 1979.

Perry, M. *Population 485: Meeting Your Neighbors One Siren at a Time.* New York: Harper-Collins, 2002.

Chapter 2
EMS Systems

Bryan Bledsoe, DO, FACEP, FAAEM

Paul Ganss, MS, NRP

STANDARD
Preparatory (EMS Systems)

COMPETENCY
Integrates comprehensive knowledge of EMS systems, the safety and well-being of the paramedic, and medical-legal and ethical issues, which is intended to improve the health of EMS personnel, patients, and the community.

 Learning Objectives

Terminal Performance Objective: After reading this chapter you should be able to discuss the characteristics, components, and functions of emergency medicine services (EMS) systems.

Enabling Objectives: To accomplish the terminal performance objective, you should be able to:

1. Define key terms introduced in this chapter.

2. List the out-of-hospital and in-hospital components of EMS systems.

3. Link key events in the history of EMS to the development of the modern EMS system.

4. Discuss the importance of the 1966 publication *Accidental Death and Disability: The Neglected Disease of Modern Society* as it relates to the development of EMS in the United States.

5. Describe each of the ten components of EMS systems according to the Statewide EMS Technical Assessment Program.

6. Identify and discuss the vision and documents that are guiding EMS into the future.

7. Discuss the contemporary problems facing EMS as described in the Institute of Medicine document, *Emergency Medical Services: At the Crossroads*.

8. Provide examples of various configurations of EMS systems in the United States and how they integrate into the chain of survival.

9. List and describe the purposes of the national documents guiding EMS education and practice.

10. Discuss typical components that should be established for local and state-level EMS systems.

11. Describe the similarities, differences, and general purposes of the professional organizations and professional journals related to the practice of EMS.

12. Describe the intent of the General Services Administration KKK-A-1822 Federal Specifications for Ambulances.

13. Describe the purpose of categorizing receiving hospital facilities by their capabilities.

14. Explain the purpose and components of an effective continuous quality improvement program.

15. Describe how you can contribute to greater patient safety in emergency medical services.

16. Explain the role of research in EMS.

17. Discuss how evidence-based medicine is enhancing EMS.

KEY TERMS

accreditation, p. 28

bystander, p. 14

certification, p. 29

chain of survival, p. 23

clinical protocols, p. 25

Department of Homeland Security, p. 21

Emergency Medical Dispatcher (EMD), p. 27

ethics, p. 35

evidence-based medicine (EBM), p. 37

helicopter air ambulances (HAA), p. 20

interoperability, p. 27

intervener physician, p. 25

licensure, p. 29

medical director, p. 25

medical oversight, p. 25

National Highway Traffic Safety Administration (NHTSA), p. 20

National Incident Management System (NIMS), p. 21

National Transportation Safety Board (NTSB), p. 22

off-line medical oversight, p. 25

on-line medical direction, p. 25

Ontario Prehospital Advanced Life Support (OPALS) study, p. 20

peer review, p. 25

prearrival instruction, p. 28

profession, p. 29

professionalism, p. 34

prospective medical oversight, p. 25

quality improvement (QI), p. 20

reciprocity, p. 29

registration, p. 29

research, p. 36

retrospective medical oversight, p. 25

rules of evidence, p. 34

scope of practice, p. 24

standing orders, p. 26

teachable moment, p. 26

tiered response, p. 14

trauma, p. 33

trauma center, p. 20

Case Study

It is a beautiful Fourth of July. You and your family are traveling down the interstate on your way to a concert and fireworks show. Just an hour from your destination, a tire blows out on the BMW ahead of you, and you see it skid into the median and crash into some pine trees. You pull onto the shoulder. As an experienced paramedic, you ensure scene safety before approaching the mangled car. You see no movement inside the passenger compartment.

Your daughter grabs her cell phone and calls 911. The dispatcher asks for the location of the crash and transfers your call to the 911 call center for that area. The emergency medical dispatcher gathers the appropriate information and dispatches the local volunteer fire service and a paramedic ambulance. While you attempt to gain access to the patients, your daughter continues to

provide the dispatcher with information that he, in turn, relays to the responding units.

The local volunteer fire and rescue team arrives on scene in about 7 minutes. You provide a verbal report to the arriving rescuers. They do their own scene safety check, approach the car, and determine that there are four patients. Two are priority-1 patients (one of these is a 2-year-old child), and two are priority-3 patients. Based on the primary assessment, Rescuer Lt. C. J. Greenlee requests a medical helicopter and a second paramedic unit. Approximately 2 minutes later, a fire truck crew arrives. They reroute traffic and establish a landing zone for the helicopter.

When all EMS personnel summoned are on scene, they decide that the 2-year-old patient will be flown to Children's Hospital, a pediatric specialty center. The other immediate patient will be transported by ground to the closest Level I trauma center. The patients with minor injuries will be taken to the local hospital by ground transport. Working as a team, the fire and ambulance personnel extricate the patients and package them for transport.

Approximately 22 minutes after the arrival of the first paramedic unit, all patients have been extricated and are en route to a receiving facility capable of providing the level of care they need. Within 15 minutes of arrival at the pediatric trauma center and just 31 minutes after the crash, the 2-year-old is moved to surgery for the repair of a ruptured liver and spleen. The other patients are being treated at their destinations as well.

Introduction

As discussed in the preceding chapter, the emergency medical services (EMS) system is a comprehensive network of personnel, equipment, and resources established to deliver aid and emergency medical care to the community. To meet the needs of the community it serves, an EMS system must function as a unified whole. In general, an EMS system is composed of both out-of-hospital and in-hospital components. The out-of-hospital component includes:

- Members of the community who are trained in first aid and CPR
- A communications system that allows public access to emergency services dispatch and allows EMS providers to communicate with one another
- EMS providers, including paramedics
- Fire/rescue and hazardous-materials services
- Law enforcement officers
- Public utilities, such as power and gas companies
- Resource centers, such as regional poison control centers

The in-hospital component includes:

- Emergency nurses
- Advanced-practice providers (physicians' assistants and advanced-practice nurses)
- Emergency physicians and specialty physicians
- Ancillary services, such as radiology and respiratory therapy
- Specialty physicians, such as trauma surgeons and cardiologists
- Social workers
- Mental health providers
- Rehabilitation services

Every EMS system must rely on the strength of its components. A weakness in one component will diminish the overall quality of patient care. For example, a typical EMS operation begins with citizen activation. That is, a

bystander—a family member, friend, or a stranger to the patient—initiates contact with an emergency dispatch center. EMS dispatch is then responsible for collecting essential information and sending out the closest appropriately staffed and equipped unit. In many EMS systems, the dispatcher also provides prearrival instructions (discussed later in the chapter) to the patient or caller so that care may begin immediately.

Usually, the first EMS provider to respond to the scene of an emergency is a police officer, firefighter, lifeguard, teacher, or other community member who has received basic medical training in an approved Emergency Medical Responder program. That person's role is to stabilize the patient until more advanced EMS personnel arrive.

The next EMS provider likely to arrive on scene depends on the type of EMS system involved. In most areas, the dispatcher will send an EMT-level or paramedic-level ambulance. In other areas of the country, EMS uses a **tiered response**, sending multiple levels of emergency care personnel to the same incident.[1] In still other areas of the country, paramedic personnel may respond to every incident regardless of the level of care needed to treat a patient (Figure 2-1).

Once emergency care has been initiated, EMS providers must quickly decide on the medical facility to which the patient should be transported. This decision is based on the type of care needed, transport time, and local protocols. In a comprehensive EMS system in which specialty centers have been designated (such as pediatric, trauma, and burn centers), it may be necessary to transport the patient to a facility other than the closest hospital.

On arrival at the receiving medical facility, where an emergency nurse or physician assumes responsibility for the patient, the patient is assigned a priority of care. If needed, a surgeon or other specialist will be summoned.

History of EMS

The Emergency Medical Services (EMS) system, as we know it today, developed from the traditional and scientific beliefs of many cultures. To understand EMS today, it

Tiered Response

Basic life support (BLS)

Advanced life support (ALS)

Fire/rescue

Alternative Response

Basic and advanced
life support

FIGURE 2-1 Some systems elect to use a tiered response whereby EMT providers provide initial on-scene care while paramedic care arrives later. Other systems send an paramedic provider to each call.

is first important to know its history. Certainly, the most significant advances in EMS have occurred during the past 50 years (see Table 2-1).

Early Development

Ancient Times

There is evidence that emergency medicine has a very long history. In fact, it may be traced back to biblical times, when it was recorded that a "good Samaritan" provided care to a wounded traveler by the side of a road.

Approximately 4,000 to 5,000 years ago, scribes in Sumer, a civilization in Mesopotamia (in southwest Asia), inscribed clay tablets with some of the earliest medical records. Similar to protocols that EMS uses today, the ancient tablets provided healers with step-by-step instructions for patient care based on the patient's description of symptoms. The tablets also included instructions on how to create the medications needed to cure the patient and explained how and when to administer them. The most striking difference between these first "protocols" and EMS today is the absence of a physical exam.

In 1862, the Egyptologist Edwin Smith purchased a papyrus scroll dating back to about 1500 B.C.E. It contained 48 medical case histories with data arranged in head-to-toe order and in order of severity, an arrangement very similar to today's patient assessment. Each case also had a particular format, including a title, specific instructions to the healer, and a projection of possible outcomes.

One section, called the "Book of Wounds," explains the treatment of injuries such as fractures and dislocations. It includes descriptions of the materials needed for making bandages and splints, as well as information about sutures and solutions that may be used to clean wounds.

At about the same time, in another civilization in the Mesopotamian region, King Hammurabi of Babylon commissioned a large painting of 282 case laws known today as the "Code of Hammurabi." That code governed criminal and civil matters, and it established strict penalties for violations, a concept called *lex talionis* or "law of the claw" (very similar to the idea of "an eye for an eye").

One section of the code was devoted to the regulation of medical fees and penalties, which were based on the social class of the patient. For example, if a surgeon operated successfully on a commoner, he would be paid only half of what his fee would be if he had operated on a rich man. Social class was also the basis for penalties. If a surgeon caused the death of a rich man, the surgeon's hand would be cut off, but if a slave died under his care, he only had to replace the slave.

EMS came from humble beginnings. Initially, out-of-hospital care involved nothing more than transport. Around 900 C.E., the Anglo-Saxons used a hammock suspended across a horse-drawn wagon. By 1100, the Normans had devised a litter that was carried between two horses to transport patients. The first recorded use of an ambulance was in the Siege of Malaga in 1487. Queen Isabella of Spain designated certain wagons for

Table 2-1 An EMS Timeline

1797	Napoleon's chief physician implements a prehospital system designed to triage and transport the injured from the field to aid stations.
1860s	Civilian ambulance services begin in Cincinnati and New York City.
1891	Dr. Friedrich Maass performs the first equivocally documented chest compression in humans.
1915	First-known air medical transport occurs during the retreat of the Serbian army from Albania.
1920	First volunteer rescue squads organize in Roanoke, Virginia, and along the New Jersey coast.
1947	Claude Beck develops first defibrillator and first human saved with defibrillation.
1958	Dr. Peter Safar demonstrates the efficacy of mouth-to-mouth ventilation.
1960	Cardiopulmonary resuscitation (CPR) is shown to be efficacious.
1965	J. Frank Pantridge converts an ambulance into a mobile coronary care unit with a portable defibrillator and recorded ten prehospital resuscitations with a 50 percent long-term survival rate.
1966	The National Academy of Sciences, National Research Council publishes *Accidental Death and Disability: The Neglected Disease of Modern Society.*
1966	Highway Safety Act of 1966 establishes the Emergency Medical Services Program in the Department of Transportation.
1967	Star of Life is patented by the American Medical Association.
1968	AT&T designates 911 as its new national emergency number.
1970	National Registry of EMTs is founded.
1970	Television show *Emergency!* debuts on NBC.
1972	Department of Health, Education, and Welfare allocates $16 million to EMS demonstration programs in five states.
1973	The Emergency Medical Services Systems (EMSS) Act provides additional federal guidelines and funding for the development of regional EMS systems; the law establishes 15 components of EMS systems.
1975	National Association of EMTs is organized.
1979	First automated external defibrillators (AEDs) become available.
1981	The Omnibus Budget Reconciliation Act consolidates EMS funding into state preventive health and health services block grants, and eliminates funding under the EMSS Act.
1981	Prehospital trauma life support (PHTLS) is developed.
1981	International trauma life support (ITLS), formerly basic trauma life support (BTLS), is developed.
1984	The EMS for Children program, under the Public Health Act, provides funds for enhancing the EMS system to better serve pediatric patients.
1985	National Research Council publishes *Injury in America: A Continuing Public Health Problem*, describing deficiencies in the progress of addressing the problem of accidental death and disability.
1988	The National Highway Traffic Safety Administration initiates the Statewide EMS Technical Assessment program based on ten key components of EMS systems.
1990	The Trauma Care Systems and Development Act encourages development of inclusive trauma systems and provides funding to states for trauma system planning, implementation, and evaluation.
1993	The Institute of Medicine publishes *Emergency Medical Services for Children*, which points out deficiencies in our health care system's ability to address the emergency medical needs of pediatric patients.
1995	Congress does not reauthorize funding under the Trauma Care Systems and Development Act.
1999	President Clinton signs bill designating 911 as national emergency number.
2003	Health Insurance Portability and Accountability Act (HIPAA) becomes effective, strictly regulating the flow of confidential information.
2006	The National Highway Traffic Safety Administration publishes *Emergency Medical Services: Agenda for the Future* to guide the development of EMS in the United States in the twenty-first century.

the transport of injured soldiers. Her grandson, King Charles V, reportedly again used field ambulances in 1553 in the Siege of Metz.

The Napoleonic Wars

In the wars between Napoleon's French Empire and other European countries from 1803 to 1815, ambulances were often used to evacuate the wounded. Military surgeon Dominique-Jean Larrey, one of Napoleon's chief surgeons, devised this idea. Larrey became distressed to see that many of the wounded were neglected for a long period of time and that most died before reaching a hospital. He subsequently developed a light carriage that allowed the movement of injured soldiers from the battlefield. These carriages came to be called *ambulances volantes*, or "Larrey's Flying Ambulances," because they were positioned with the French "flying artillery" on the battlefield. Even though the *ambulance volante* was little more than a covered horse-drawn cart, Larrey is credited with the development of the first prehospital system that used both triage and transport. Larrey was also credited with being the first to place a medical attendant in an ambulance.[2]

Although the first use of aircraft for medical evacuation is lost to history, there are records of hot air balloons being used to evacuate wounded from the Prussian Siege of Paris in 1870. During the retreat of the Serbian Army from Albania in 1915, unmodified French fighter aircraft were used to ferry the injured.

The United States in the Nineteenth Century

The development of ambulances in the United States occurred in the first part of the nineteenth century. In 1861, during the Civil War, surgeon Jonathan Letterman reorganized battlefield medical care and initiated the use of ambulances for the evacuation of battlefield casualties. In 1864, President Abraham Lincoln signed into law an act that firmly established a uniform army ambulance plan. This act separated ambulance transport from all other transport services in the Army and placed it under the medical command.

Between 1861 and 1865, a nurse named Clara Barton coordinated care for the sick and injured at Civil War battlefield sites along the East Coast. Defying army leaders, she persisted in going to the front, where wounded men suffered and often died from lack of the simplest medical attention. She continued the concept of the *ambulance volante* by organizing the triage and transport of injured soldiers to improvised hospitals in nearby houses, barns, and churches away from the battlefield.[3]

Following the success of ambulances in the Civil War, several communities and hospitals began to develop civilian ambulance services. The first civilian ambulance was established in 1860 (before the Civil War) in Cincinnati,

Ohio, by Commercial Hospital. In 1869, Bellevue Hospital, on the island of Manhattan in New York City, began to operate an ambulance service. The ambulances of both services were specially designed horse-drawn carts that were staffed with physician interns from the various hospital wards. By 1899, Michael Reese Hospital in Chicago began to operate a motorized ambulance.[4]

The Twentieth Century

From World War I to World War II

During World War I, a high mortality rate of soldiers was associated with an average evacuation time of 18 hours. As a result, in World War II a system of transportation to increasing echelons (levels) of care was created. Battlefield ambulance corps transported wounded soldiers from the front lines to the echelons of care. However, many of the echelons were so far from the battlefield and from each other that there were huge delays in patient care. In many cases, it was often days from the injury itself to definitive surgery.

There were some developments in American civilian ambulance services after World War I. Some hospitals experimented with placing physician interns on ambulances. In 1926, the Phoenix Fire Department began providing "inhalator" service and officially entered into the realm of medical care. In 1928, the first bona fide rescue squad, called the Roanoke Life Saving Crew, was started in Roanoke, Virginia. However, in 1929, the United States entered the severe economic crisis known as the Great Depression, which lasted until the start of American involvement in World War II in 1941. Little changed in the civilian ambulance service during this period.

Effects of World War II

Following the bombing of Pearl Harbor on December 7, 1941, the United States entered World War II. Because of the demands of war, many hospital-based ambulance services shut down. Many city governments turned ambulance services over to local police and fire departments. Unfortunately, there were no requirements for minimal training or care. In fact, ambulance work was often seen as a punishment, and many departments were quick to eliminate ambulance service as soon as they could.

Post-World War II

The end of World War II brought prosperity to the United States. Several medical advances occurred subsequently, improving the lives of the public. Not long after World War II, however, the United States found itself at war again—this time on the Korean peninsula.

The 1950s

Korea is a mountainous country that lacked an organized system of highways and roads. Because of this, the U.S. Army began using helicopters to move the injured from the front lines to mobile army surgical hospitals (MASHs) located fairly close to the front lines. Thus, injured soldiers were being promptly evacuated to a surgical center and were receiving emergency care and surgery shortly after their injury. This practice resulted in significant improvements in battlefield mortality.[5]

Similarly, in the late 1950s the United States entered the Vietnam War. This time, the battles took place in the jungles of Southeast Asia. As in Korea, there were few roads, and jungles slowed movement of the injured. Again, helicopters were called on to evacuate the wounded to forward-placed surgical hospitals. In Vietnam, in many cases, evacuation occurred within 10 to 20 minutes of injury (Figure 2-2). Once stabilized and able to be moved (generally within 24 to 48 hours), the patients would be flown by jet to Clark Air Force Base in the Philippines, where they would receive any necessary further treatment. The decrease in the amount of time to definitive care plus advances in medical procedures significantly reduced mortality rates. This strategy also set the stage for trauma system development in the United States.[6]

Several significant medical developments occurred in the 1950s. In 1956, physicians Peter Safar and James Elam pioneered the use of mouth-to-mouth resuscitation. In 1959, the first portable defibrillator was used at Johns Hopkins Hospital in Baltimore.[7] In 1960, cardiopulmonary resuscitation (CPR) was refined and deemed to be effective for human resuscitation.[8]

The 1960s

Throughout history, significant advances in trauma care occurred during wartime. However, until the late 1960s,

FIGURE 2-2 Medical evacuation helicopters, colloquially called "Dustoff," saved many lives during the Vietnam War.

(Dust off © Joe Kline Aviation Art)

few areas of the United States provided adequate civilian prehospital emergency care similar to what was provided to soldiers and sailors during war. The prevailing thought was that medical care began in the hospital emergency department. Rescue techniques were crude, ambulance attendants poorly educated, and equipment minimal. Police, fire, and EMS personnel often had no radio communication. Proper medical direction was not available, and the only interaction between physicians and EMS personnel was at the receiving facility.

Eventually, as costs and demand for additional services forced many rural mortician-operated ambulances to withdraw, local police and fire departments found that they had to provide the ambulance service. In many areas, volunteer ambulance services made up of local, independent EMS provider agencies proliferated. In urban settings, the increased demand on hospital-based EMS systems resulted in the development of municipal services, which were operated on city, county, or regional levels. However, because they could not communicate with one another, it was impossible to coordinate a response to any but the simplest local calls.

In 1966, the publication of *Accidental Death and Disability: The Neglected Disease of Modern Society* by the National Academy of Sciences, National Research Council, focused attention on the problem. The "White Paper," as the report was called, spelled out the deficiencies in prehospital emergency care.[9] It suggested guidelines for the development of EMS systems, the training of prehospital emergency medical providers, and the upgrading of ambulances and their equipment. The problems identified in the study included:

- Lack of uniform laws and standards for prehospital care
- Poorly equipped ambulances
- Poor-quality ambulances
- Lack of communications between the ambulance and the hospital
- Inadequate training of ambulance personnel
- Inadequate physician and nursing staffing of hospital emergency departments

CONTENT REVIEW

➤ 1973 EMSS Act: Fifteen Components of EMS Systems
- Manpower
- Training
- Communications
- Transportation
- Emergency facilities
- Critical care units
- Public safety agencies
- Consumer participation
- Access to care
- Patient transfer
- Standardized record keeping
- Public information and education
- System review and evaluation
- Disaster management plans
- Mutual aid

Civilian EMS, as we know it today, started to evolve significantly in the 1960s. In 1960, the Los Angeles Fire Department placed medical personnel with every engine, ladder, and rescue company. It was one of the first large fire departments to embrace the concept of emergency medical care.

In 1966, the Highway Safety Act promulgated initial EMS guidelines for the United States. The same year, Dr. J. Frank Pantridge developed a mobile coronary response unit in Belfast, Northern Ireland. Using a portable defibrillator, he treated ten cardiac arrest patients, five of whom enjoyed long-term survival.[10] In 1969, the first paramedic program began in Miami, Florida, by Dr. Eugene Nagel.[11]

The 1970s

The 1970s were the decade when EMS truly came into its own. The National Registry of Emergency Medical Technicians was established in 1970. Interestingly, EMS got one of its biggest boosts from Hollywood. On January 15, 1972, the television show *Emergency!* made its debut on NBC. The show, produced by Hollywood legend Jack Webb, featured two Los Angeles County Fire Department paramedics and the new paramedic program in southern California (Figure 2-3). The show brought public attention to the concept of prehospital care and provided considerable encouragement for development of the modern EMS system.[12]

Then, in 1973, Congress passed the Emergency Medical Services Systems Act, which provided funding for a series of projects related to the delivery of trauma care.

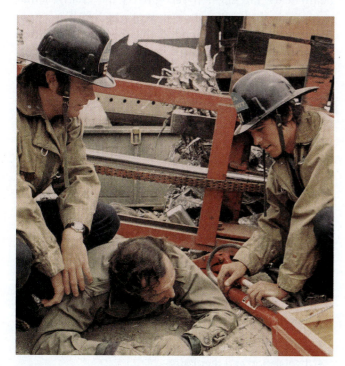

FIGURE 2-3 The television show *Emergency!* played a major role in bringing the world of EMS into the public spotlight.

(Larry Barbier/NBCU Photo Bank via AP Images)

This enabled the development of regional EMS systems that took place from 1974 through 1981. A total of $300 million was allocated to study the feasibility of EMS planning, operations, expansion, and research.[13]

To be eligible for this funding, an EMS system had to include the following 15 components: manpower, training, communications, transportation, emergency facilities, critical care units, public safety agencies, consumer participation, access to care, patient transfer, standardized record keeping, public information and education, system review and evaluation, disaster management plans, and mutual aid. As farsighted as these criteria were, the designers of the legislation unfortunately omitted two key components: system financing and medical direction.

When federal funding was significantly reduced in the early 1980s, many EMS systems faced economic disaster. Subsequently, the Emergency Medical Services Systems Act was amended in 1976 and again in 1979, and a total of $215 million was appropriated over a seven-year period toward the establishment of regional EMS systems. However, many systems were still operating without medical direction.

The 1980s

In 1981, the passage of the Consolidated Omnibus Budget Reconciliation Act (COBRA) essentially wiped out federal funding for EMS. The small amount of funding that remained was placed into state preventive-health and health-services block grants. The National Highway Traffic Safety Administration (NHTSA) attempted to sustain the efforts of the Department of Health and Human Services, but with its other EMS responsibilities and no additional funding, the momentum for continued development was lost.

In 1988, the Statewide EMS Technical Assessment Program was established by the NHTSA. It defines elements necessary to all EMS systems. Briefly, they are:

- ***Regulation and policy.*** Each state must have laws, regulations, policies, and procedures that govern its EMS system. It also is required to provide leadership to local jurisdictions.

- ***Resources management.*** Each state must have central control of EMS resources so all patients have equal access to acceptable emergency care.

- ***Human resources and training.*** Qualified instructors should teach a standardized EMS curriculum, and all personnel who transport patients in the prehospital setting should be adequately trained.

- *Transportation.* Patients must be safely and reliably transported by ground or air ambulance.

- *Facilities.* Every seriously ill or injured patient must be delivered in a timely manner to an appropriate medical facility.

- *Communications.* A system for public access to the EMS system must be in place. Communication among dispatchers, the ambulance crew, and hospital personnel must also be possible.

- *Trauma systems.* Each state should develop a system of specialized care for trauma patients, including one or more **trauma centers** and rehabilitation programs. It also must develop systems for assigning and transporting patients to those facilities.

- *Public information and education.* EMS personnel should participate in programs designed to educate the public. The programs are to focus on the prevention of injuries and how to properly access the EMS system.

- *Medical direction.* Each EMS system must have a physician as its medical director. This physician delegates medical practice to nonphysician caregivers and oversees all aspects of patient care.

- *Evaluation.* Each state must have a **quality improvement (QI)** system in place for continuing evaluation and upgrading of its EMS system.

Helicopter air ambulances (HAA) began to develop in the early 1980s. A hospital or consortium of hospitals operated most helicopter programs. These services initially used all-nurse crews. However, as the operations matured, a paramedic was often used in place of one of the nurses on the flight. HAA is primarily used for both scene-to-hospital and interhospital transfer of critically ill or injured patients.

The 1990s

Further improvements were made to EMS during the 1990s. In 1990, Congress passed the Trauma Care Systems and Development Act. This Act provided funding to states for trauma system planning, development, implementation, and evaluation.

In 1993, the Institute of Medicine published *Emergency Medical Services for Children*. This document pointed out the deficiencies in pediatric emergency care in the United States. A small amount of federal funding subsequently financed the Emergency Medical Services for Children (EMSC) program.

In 1995, Congress did not reauthorize the Trauma Care Systems and Development Act, and the funding for trauma systems fell back on the states. This resulted in significant variability in trauma system care across the United States.

By the late 1990s, EMS systems and EMS practice had started to mature. It was at this point that self-assessment of EMS began to occur. Researchers and systems began to link patient outcomes (morbidity and mortality—illness and death) with various EMS practices. Surprisingly, some practices that had seemed intuitive did not hold up to the test of science. One of the largest studies of prehospital practices and outcomes was the **Ontario Prehospital Advanced Life Support (OPALS) study** that was conducted in various regions of the province of Ontario, Canada. The study has provided significant information about early defibrillation, response times, advanced life support procedures, and much more.[14]

EMS Agenda for the Future

The **National Highway Traffic Safety Administration (NHTSA)** published the *EMS Agenda for the Future* in 1996.[15] This document examined what had been learned during the prior three decades of EMS and endeavored to create a vision for the future of EMS in the United States. It was published at an important time, when those agencies, organizations, and individuals that affect EMS were evaluating their respective roles in the context of a rapidly evolving health care system—a process of evaluation that is ongoing.

NHTSA is a division of the U.S. Department of Transportation (DOT) and the Health Resources and Services Administration (HRSA), Maternal and Child Health Bureau. *The EMS Agenda for the Future* focused on aspects of EMS related to emergency care outside traditional health care facilities. It recognized the changes that occurred in the health care system of which EMS is a part. The document recommended that EMS of the future would be a community-based health management system that would be fully integrated into the overall health care system. EMS of the future would have the ability to identify and modify illness and injury risks, provide acute illness and injury care and follow-up, and contribute to the treatment of chronic conditions and to community health monitoring. EMS would be integrated with other health care providers and public health and public safety agencies in the effort to improve community health, which would result in more appropriate use of acute health care resources. Overall, EMS would remain the public's emergency medical safety net.

To realize this vision, *The EMS Agenda for the Future* proposed continued development of 14 core EMS attributes. They were:

- Integration of health services
- EMS research
- Legislation and regulation
- System finance
- Human resources

- Medical direction
- Education systems
- Public education
- Prevention
- Public access
- Communication systems
- Clinical care
- Information systems
- Evaluation

Although many of the recommendations proposed by the *EMS Agenda for the Future* have been realized, many have not. Despite this, this document continues to serve as a guide for EMS providers, health care organizations and institutions, governmental agencies, and policy makers who must be committed to improving the health of their communities and to ensuring that EMS efficiently contributes to that goal. They must invest the resources necessary to provide the nation's population with emergency health care that is reliably accessible, effective, subject to continuous evaluation, and integrated with the remainder of the health care system.

The Twenty-First Century

The United States has changed significantly following the terrorist attacks of September 11, 2001 (Figure 2-4). Among other things that occurred as a result of 9/11, review of the public safety system found numerous flaws. President George W. Bush established the **Department of Homeland Security** to coordinate the various agencies responsible for protecting the country. With this came the **National Incident Management System (NIMS)** and other strategies to prepare the country for terrorist attacks and other threats.[16]

FIGURE 2-4 The attacks on New York City and Washington on September 11, 2001, forever changed the face of EMS.

(© Reuters)

In 2005, two devastating hurricanes (Katrina and Rita) hit several Gulf Coast states, causing massive damage and loss of life. The emergency response, in some cases, was less than ideal. Additional changes were made to improve the Federal Emergency Management Agency (FEMA) and other governmental agencies following these disasters. A significant economic downturn in 2008 forced many cities to cut back on EMS and fire operations. As in most times of economic distress, EMS and hospital emergency departments were faced with less funding and more patients.

In the 2010s, EMS began to fill nontraditional roles, including some primary care roles, through community paramedicine and mobile integrated health care programs. The driving forces for these endeavors vary. In some communities, primary care is limited, so EMS providers have stepped up and assumed part of the role. In other communities, building codes and fire prevention strategies have significantly reduced the incidence of fires. Because of this, some fire departments have looked to expand their services beyond traditional firefighting roles. Community paramedicine has seemed to be a natural fit.

EMS at the Crossroads

In 2006, the National Academies Institute of Medicine published another evaluation of the status of emergency services in the United States. This document, titled *Emergency Medical Services: At the Crossroads,* was critical of many EMS practices. The study found that there were significant problems at the federal level. Despite the advances made in EMS, sizable challenges remained. At the federal policy level, government leadership in emergency care was found to be fragmented and inconsistent. As it is currently organized, responsibility for prehospital and hospital-based emergency and trauma care is scattered across multiple agencies and departments. Similar divisions are evident at the state and local levels. In addition, the current delivery system suffers in a number of key areas:

- *Insufficient coordination.* EMS care is highly fragmented, and often uncoordinated among providers. Multiple EMS agencies serving within a single population center do not operate cohesively. Agencies in adjacent jurisdictions often are unable to communicate with one another. In many cases, EMS and other public safety agencies cannot talk to one another because they operate with incompatible communications equipment or on different frequencies.

- *Coordination of transport within regions is limited.* The management of the regional flow of patients is poor, and patients may not be transported to facilities that are optimal and ready to receive them. Communications and hand-offs between EMS and hospital personnel are frequently ineffective and often omit important clinical information.

- *Disparities in response times.* The speed with which ambulances respond to emergency calls is highly variable. In some cases, this variability is related to geography. In dense population centers, for example, the distances ambulances must travel are small, but traffic and other problems can cause delays. In contrast, rural areas involve longer travel times, sometimes over difficult terrain. This is further worsened by problems in the organization and management of EMS services, the communications and coordination between 911 dispatch and EMS responders, and the priority placed on response time given the resources available.

- *Uncertain quality of care.* Very little is known about the quality of care delivered by EMS services in the United States because there are no standardized measures of EMS quality, no nationwide standards for the training and certification of EMS personnel, no accreditation of institutions that educate EMS personnel, and virtually no accountability for the performance of EMS systems. Even though most Americans assume that their communities are served by competent EMS services, the public has no idea whether this is true, and no way to know.

- *Lack of readiness for disasters.* Although EMS personnel are among the first to respond in the event of a disaster, they are the least prepared component of community response teams. Most EMS personnel have received little or no disaster response training for terrorist attacks, natural disasters, or other public health emergencies. Despite the massive amounts of federal funding directed to homeland security, only a tiny proportion of those funds have been directed to medical response. Furthermore, EMS representation in disaster planning at the federal level has been highly limited.

- *Divided professional identity.* EMS is a unique profession, one that straddles both medical care and public safety. Among public safety agencies, however, EMS is often regarded as a secondary service, with police and fire taking more prominent roles; within medicine, EMS personnel often lack the respect afforded to other professionals, such as physicians and nurses. Despite significant investments in education and training, salaries for EMS personnel are often well below those for comparable positions, such as police officers, firefighters, and nurses. In addition, there is a cultural divide among EMS, public safety, and medical care workers that contributes to the fragmentation of these services.

CONTENT REVIEW

➤ Types of EMS Services
  - Fire-based
  - Third service
  - Private
  - Hospital-based
  - Volunteer
➤ Regardless of the delivery type, all emergency operations must be closely integrated and work together.

- *Limited evidence base.* The evidence base for many practices routinely used in EMS is limited. Strategies for EMS have often been adapted from settings that differ substantially from the prehospital environment and, consequently, their value in the field is questionable, and some may even be harmful. For example, field intubation of children, still widely practiced, has been found to do more harm than good in many situations.[17] Although some recent research has added to the EMS evidence base, a host of critical clinical questions remain unanswered because of limited federal research support, as well as inherent difficulties associated with prehospital research due to its sporadic nature and the difficulty of obtaining informed consent for the research.[18]

National Report Card on the State of Emergency Medicine

The American College of Emergency Physicians (ACEP) in 2006 published a study similar to EMS at the Crossroads. The paper, *The National Report Card on the State of Emergency Medicine: Evaluating the Environment of Emergency Care Systems State by State*, pointed out the significant problems that existed in all aspects of emergency care.[19] This paper primarily addressed problems in hospital emergency departments but also addressed EMS issues. Overall, the report detailed that emergency services in the United States are so overstressed that the quality of care has been compromised. Multiple causes were indentified and included such things as inadequate funding, patient overcrowding, lack of alternate care facilities, problems with medical liability, the effect of illegal immigration, and many other factors. Each state was given a letter grade that reflected the reported standard of emergency care in that state.

Helicopter Air Ambulance Recommended Improvements

In 2001, federal reimbursement for medical helicopters improved, and the national medical helicopter fleet expanded from 300 aircraft to almost 900 in a matter of years. With the increase in helicopters came an increase in accidents and overutilization. In 2008, there were a record number of helicopter air ambulance crashes with related fatalities. As a result, the **National Transportation Safety Board (NTSB)** held hearings in 2009 and later recommended sweeping improvements for the helicopter air ambulance industry.

Today's EMS Systems

The EMS system of today remains a mixture of various types of operations. The modern EMS system is now fairly well integrated with the health care system and, to a lesser degree, with the public safety system. Despite some federal oversight, the provision of EMS is still primarily a local government responsibility. Because of the differences among localities, there are significantly different approaches to the provision of EMS across the United States. Government entities have elected to operate various service types of EMS. These include:

- Fire-based
- Third service
- Private (profit or nonprofit)
- Hospital-based
- Volunteer
- Hybrid (combination of any of these)

Regardless of the delivery type, the lessons of 9/11 have shown that all emergency operations must be closely integrated and able to work together. The rapid development of EMS technology is making this possible and has simplified many aspects of EMS.

Chain of Survival

Traditionally, emergency health care was considered to begin at the time of the emergency. More recently, however, it has been shown that emergency health care may actually begin long before an emergency occurs. In this regard, EMS and emergency medicine practitioners are embracing preventive health care measures that may help to reduce emergency illnesses and accidents. It also now includes such innovative measures as EMS personnel periodically visiting high-risk and homebound citizens and assessing their health status and needs.

Aside from such preventive activities, the EMS system is part of a continuum of care that begins once an emergency occurs and ends when the patient completes care and returns to his normal activities of daily living. This continuum is often referred to as the **chain of survival**. As defined by the American Heart Association (AHA), the chain of survival consists of the five most important factors affecting survival of a cardiac arrest patient: (1) immediate recognition and activation of EMS; (2) early CPR; (3) rapid defibrillation; (4) effective advanced life support; and (5) integrated post-cardiac arrest care. A similar continuum of events, essential to the optimal care of any emergency patient, might include, but would not be limited to, the following:

- Bystander care
- Dispatch
- Response
- Prehospital care

- Transportation
- Emergency department care
- Definitive care
- Rehabilitation

To achieve this continuum, several components of the EMS system must be in place.

Essential Components for Continuum of Care

Health Care System Integration

It is now recognized that EMS is a major component of the modern health care system. Interestingly, the original purpose of EMS was to address cardiac emergencies—particularly cardiac arrest. Now, almost forty years later, there is renewed emphasis of the roles and responsibilities of the EMS system in all types of cardiac emergencies. These responsibilities begin with the public service access points (PSAPs) that are typically the 911 call centers. PSAPs are now the primary interface between the EMS system and the communities it serves. Now, dispatchers can give basic first aid and emergency care instructions, including CPR instructions, to the caller until the EMS providers arrive (Figure 2-5).

The role of the EMS system is now extremely important in the identification of acute coronary syndrome and

FIGURE 2-5 Emergency Medical Dispatchers can give prearrival instructions to a caller, including how to perform CPR.

(From Advanced MPDS v13.0 © 1979-2015 International Academies of Emergency Dispatch and ProQA Paramount v5.1 © 2007–2015 Priority Dispatch Corp. All Rights Reserved. Used by permission.)

ST-segment elevation myocardial infarction (STEMI). The standard of care has quickly shifted—now, in many cases, paramedics make the decision to activate a cardiac catheterization team based on their interpretation of a prehospital ECG. This has significantly decreased the time from onset of symptoms to primary percutaneous coronary intervention (PPCI). Evidence is beginning to show that many cardiac arrest patients may benefit from PPCI, and certain health care facilities are now devoting resources to the specific care of cardiac arrest that may include PPCI.

Finally, EMS is stepping up and assuming an important role as the initial component and gatekeeper of the modern health care system.

Levels of Licensure/Certification

As noted in the preceding chapter, the *National EMS Scope of Practice Model* defines and describes four levels of EMS licensure:

- Emergency Medical Responder (EMR)
- Emergency Medical Technician (EMT)
- Advanced EMT (AEMT)
- Paramedic

Each level represents a unique role, set of skills, and knowledge base.[20] In 2009,*National EMS Education Instructional Guidelines* were developed and published for each of these four levels.[21] These instructional guidelines replace the various curricula that had been previously published to guide EMS education. The use of instructional guidelines, as opposed to a rote curriculum, allows EMS educators to adapt their educational strategies to the specific student population they serve. When used in conjunction with the *National EMS Core Content*, national EMS certification, and National EMS Education program accreditation, the *National EMS Scope of Practice Model* and the *National EMS Education Standards* create a strong and interdependent system that provides the foundation to ensure the competency of out-of-hospital emergency medical personnel throughout the United States.

Quality of Education

One of the fundamental principles of quality EMS is a solid education program for providers. EMS education has evolved significantly in the past two decades. Now, there are more educators with advanced degrees and EMS is being recognized in the academic community. Despite the advances, however, there remains considerable variation in EMS educational programs across the country.

In response to *The EMS Agenda for the Future*, several documents have been prepared to guide EMS education. The first of these was the *National EMS Core Content*, published by NHTSA in 2005.[22] This document defined the

body of knowledge, skills, and abilities desired in EMS personnel. It was followed shortly thereafter by *The National EMS Scope of Practice,* also published in 2005, which helped to define the future roles of EMS providers. This consensus document supported a system of EMS personnel licensure that was common in other allied health professions and was designed to serve as a guide for states and territories in developing their **scope of practice** legislation, rules, and regulations. States following the *National EMS Scope of Practice* model as closely as possible would increase the consistency of the nomenclature and competencies of EMS personnel nationwide, facilitate reciprocity, improve professional mobility, and enhance the name recognition and public understanding of EMS. Some states have adopted the *National EMS Scope of Practice* model in its entirety, whereas others have adopted only parts of it.

Oversight by Local- and State-Level Agencies

The efficient delivery of emergency medical care requires a systematic approach and team effort to make the best use of existing resources. That means each community must develop an EMS system that best meets its needs. Although EMS systems across the country and the world will vary, certain elements are essential to ensure the best possible patient care.

At the municipal and regional levels, the first step in developing a comprehensive EMS system is to establish an administrative oversight agency. This agency is responsible for managing the local system's resources, developing operational protocols, and establishing standards and guidelines. Within the agency, a planning board is often formed. The planning board should be composed of community representatives, including emergency physicians, the emergency nurse association, the firefighter association, state and local police, and consumers. The planning board develops a budget and selects a qualified administrative staff capable of managing an EMS agency.

Once established, the agency designates who may function within the system and develops policies consistent with existing state requirements. It also creates a quality assurance or quality improvement program to evaluate the system's effectiveness and to ensure that the best interests of the patient are always a top priority. State EMS agencies are typically responsible for allocating funds to local systems, enacting legislation concerning the out-of-hospital practice of medicine, licensing and certification of field providers, enforcing all state EMS regulations, and appointing regional advisory councils.

In essence, EMS is made up of a series of systems within a system. The integration of these systems and the cooperation of all participants help to result in the best quality of emergency care.

Medical Oversight

An EMS system must retain a **medical director**—a physician who is legally responsible for all clinical and patient-care aspects of the system. The medical director serves as the de facto conscience of the EMS system and must first be an advocate for quality patient care. Prehospital medical care provided by nonphysicians is considered a delegated practice of the system medical director; that is, prehospital care providers are the medical director's designated agents, regardless of who their employers may be.

The medical director's roles in an EMS system are to:

- Educate and train personnel
- Participate in personnel and equipment selection
- Develop clinical protocols in cooperation with expert EMS personnel
- Participate in quality improvement and problem resolution
- Provide direct input into patient care
- Interface between the EMS system and other health care agencies
- Advocate within the medical community
- Serve as the "medical conscience" of the EMS system, including advocating for quality patient care

In addition to the responsibilities just listed, the medical director is the ultimate authority for all medical issues within the system. Traditionally, **medical oversight** has been divided into an on-line (direct) component and an off-line (indirect) component. The trend has been to decrease on-line activities and to bolster the off-line component.[23]

On-Line Medical Direction

On-line medical direction occurs when a qualified physician gives direct orders to a prehospital care provider by either radio or telephone (Figure 2-6). Medical direction may be delegated to a mobile intensive care nurse (MICN),

FIGURE 2-6 The medical director can provide on-line guidance to EMS personnel in the field.

(© Dr. Bryan E. Bledsoe)

advanced practice practitioner, or paramedic. In all circumstances, ultimate on-line responsibility remains with the medical director.

On-line medical direction offers several benefits to the patient. It gives the EMS provider direct and immediate access to medical consultation for specific patient care. It also allows for the transmission of essential data, such as 12-lead ECGs. The transmission of physiologic data provides the on-line physician with diagnostic information that can be used to make critical decisions while the patient is still on scene or en route. Most EMS systems have the equipment to record on-line consultations. Those recordings can then be used for **peer review** and other continuous quality improvement activities.

When at the scene of an emergency, the health care provider with the most knowledge and experience in the delivery of prehospital emergency care should be in charge. When a nonaffiliated physician or **intervener physician** is on scene and on-line medical direction may not exist, the paramedic should relinquish responsibility to the physician. However, the intervener physician must first identify himself, demonstrate a willingness to accept responsibility, and document the intervention as required by the local EMS system. If the treatment differs from established protocols, the intervener physician must accompany the patient in the ambulance to the hospital.

If an intervener physician is on scene and on-line medical direction does exist, the on-line physician is ultimately responsible. In case of a disagreement, the paramedic must take orders from the on-line physician.

Off-Line Medical Oversight

Off-line medical oversight refers to medical policies, procedures, and practices that a system medical director has established in advance of a call. It includes **prospective medical oversight** such as guidelines on the selection of personnel and supplies, training and education, and protocol development. An important part of medical oversight is participation in the selection of medical equipment. Off-line medical oversight also includes **retrospective medical oversight**, such as auditing, peer review, conflict resolution, and other quality assurance processes.

Clinical protocols are the policies and procedures of all medical components of an EMS system and are the responsibility of the medical director. Many EMS systems use committees, often made up of physicians within the community, to develop medical treatment protocols. EMS protocols provide a standardized approach to common patient problems and a consistent level of medical care, as well as a standard for accountability. When treatment is undertaken based on such protocols, the on-line physician, if needed, can assist prehospital personnel in interpreting the patient's complaint, understanding the findings of their evaluations, and providing the appropriate treatment.[24] Protocols are designed around the four "Ts" of emergency care:

- *Triage.* Guidelines that address patient flow through an EMS system, including how system resources are allocated to meet the needs of patients.
- *Treatment.* Guidelines that identify procedures to be performed on direct order from medical direction and procedures that are preauthorized protocols called **standing orders**.
- *Transport.* Guidelines that address the mode of travel (air vs. ground) based on the nature of the patient's injury or illness, the condition of the patient, the level of care required, and estimated transport time.
- *Transfer.* Guidelines that address receiving facilities to ensure that the patient is admitted to the one most appropriate for definitive care.

Protocols also are established for special circumstances, such as the proper handling of "Do Not Resuscitate" orders, patients who refuse treatment, sexual abuse, abuse of children or elderly people, termination of CPR, and intervener physicians. Although protocols standardize field procedures, they should allow the paramedic the flexibility necessary to improvise and adapt to special circumstances.

Public Information and Education

The public is an essential, yet often overlooked, component of an EMS system. EMS should have a plan to educate the public on recognizing an emergency, accessing the system, and initiating basic life support procedures. Because of this, public education has become an increasingly important role for EMS. As already noted, patient education can occur before the emergency occurs (prevention) through activities such as bicycle safety programs, infant car seat programs, and similar strategies (Figure 2-7). In addition, it has been found that patients are more likely to listen to advice and consider lifestyle changes following an emergency. This is often referred to as a **teachable moment**. A teachable moment is an unplanned opportunity to present information when the circumstances are such that a person is likely to understand and accept the information. EMS public education can take several forms, including role modeling, community involvement, leadership, and prevention.

One of the most fundamental components of EMS public education is to help members of the public to recognize an emergency when it occurs and to learn how to access the EMS system. Prompt recognition of an emergency can save lives. For example, the American Heart Association (AHA) estimates that more than 300,000 cardiac arrests per year occur before the patient reaches the

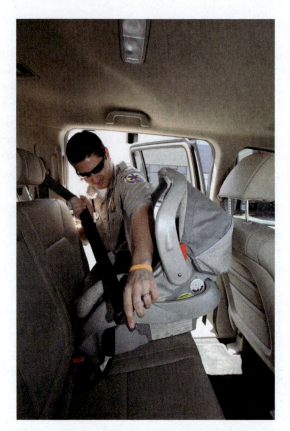

FIGURE 2-7 Providing disease and injury prevention education to the public has become an important role of EMS in the twenty-first century.
(© Dr. Bryan E. Bledsoe)

hospital. Such arrests are called "sudden death" because most happen within 2 hours of the onset of cardiac symptoms. Many patients delay calling for help when symptoms occur. If the patient and bystanders are taught to recognize the emergency and call for help in time, many cases of sudden death could be prevented.

The second aspect of public education is system access. Citizens must know how to activate EMS in an emergency to prevent life-threatening delays. Whether access is by way of 911 or a local seven-digit phone number, the number should be well publicized, and citizens should be taught how to give the necessary information to the emergency medical dispatcher.

Finally, after recognizing an emergency and activating EMS, citizens must know how to provide basic life support assistance, such as cardiopulmonary resuscitation (CPR) and bleeding control after major trauma. Abundant research indicates that a relationship exists between rapid emergency care and mortality (death) rates of patients—especially with cardiac arrest. Communities have proven that when many citizens are trained in basic life support and early defibrillation—and there is a rapid paramedic response—a larger number of patients can be successfully resuscitated. The AHA estimates that thousands of lives could be saved each year with implementation of bystander CPR programs and rapid paramedic response. Because of the widespread availability of automated external defibrillators (AEDs) in private homes and public places, early defibrillation has become more commonplace and more successful. Cardiac arrest survival takes a fully engaged public and an effective EMS system.

Effective Communications

The communications network is the heart of a regional EMS system (Figure 2-8). Coordinating the components into an organized response to urgent medical situations requires a comprehensive, flexible communications plan. Such a plan should include the following:

FIGURE 2-8 The EMS communications center is truly the heart of the modern EMS system.

- *Citizen access.* A well-publicized universal number, such as 911, provides direct citizen access to emergency services. Multiple community numbers only add life-threatening minutes to emergency response times. Enhanced 911, or E-911, gives automatic location of the caller, instant routing of the call to the appropriate emergency service (fire, police, or EMS), and instant callback capability. The proliferation of cell telephone and Internet-based phone lines (voice over Internet protocol, or VOIP) has made caller location more difficult, although strategies have been developed to address these issues.

- *Single control center.* One control center that can communicate with and direct all emergency vehicles within a large geographical area is best. Ideally, all public service agencies should be dispatched from the same communications center to ensure the best use of resources in an emergency response.

- *Operational communications capabilities.* With these, EMS dispatch can manage all aspects of system response and assess the system's readiness for the next response. Emergency units can communicate with one another and with other agencies during mutual aid and disaster operations. Hospitals also can communicate with other hospitals in the region to assess specialty capabilities.

- *Medical communications capabilities.* EMS providers can communicate with the receiving facility and, in many areas, transmit ECG and other patient information to the hospital or a physician's office. Newer technologies can send patient information to designated sites at the same time the information is obtained. The growth in communications technology has been one of the biggest advances in EMS in recent years.

- *Communications hardware.* The North American communications infrastructure has changed drastically. The utility of the Internet has changed the way we send and receive information. The massive development of the cell telephone network has affected this as well. EMS communications uses all these technologies as well as more typical radio communications systems. Most ambulances now have notebook computers and global positioning system (GPS) and vehicle tracking system capabilities. As a result of the terrorist attacks of 2001, there has been considerable federal emphasis on updating and improving the national emergency and public safety communications system. An important related directive has been to ensure **interoperability**—a feature that allows personnel from different jurisdictions and systems to communicate with one another effectively.

- *Communications software.* This includes the radio frequencies needed for in-system communication and, in many systems, the satellite and high-tech computer programs that track ambulances. Radio procedures, policies consistent with FCC standards and local protocols, and backup communication plans for disaster operations are essential to the modern EMS operation.

An EMS system must have an effective and efficient communications network in place. Because no single design will meet the needs of all communities, each system should design a network that is simple, flexible, and practical.

Emergency Medical Dispatcher

The activities of the **Emergency Medical Dispatcher (EMD)** are crucial to the efficient operation of EMS (Figure 2-9). EMDs not only send ambulances to the scene, but they also make sure that system resources are in constant readiness

FIGURE 2-9 The modern EMS dispatcher plays a major role in EMS system operations and can affect the quality of emergency care provided.

to respond. EMDs must be both medically and technically trained. Their training should cover basic telecommunication skills, medical interrogation (questioning), giving prearrival instructions, and dispatch prioritization. The course should be standardized, and it should include certification by a government agency.

EMS Dispatch

Emergency medical dispatching is the nerve center of an EMS system. It is the means of assigning and directing appropriate medical care to patients and should be under the full control of the medical director and the EMS agency. An emergency medical dispatch plan should include interrogation protocols, response configurations, system status management, and prearrival caller instructions.

Another management method is called "priority dispatching," which was first used by the Salt Lake City Fire Department. Using a set of medically approved protocols, EMDs are trained to medically interrogate a distressed caller, prioritize symptoms, select an appropriate response, and give life-saving prearrival instructions.[25]

In 1974, the Phoenix Fire Department introduced a **prearrival instruction** program developed by medically trained dispatchers. In that program, callers initiate lifesaving first aid with the dispatcher's help while they wait for emergency units to arrive on scene. In 1985, the Seattle EMS system initiated a successful program of instructing callers in CPR. Critics point out that prearrival instruction programs may result in increased liability. Even so, the increased liability of *not* providing such a service may far outweigh the risk of providing it.

An effective EMS dispatch system places the first responding units on scene within minutes of the onset of the emergency. The American Heart Association reports that brain resuscitation will not be successful if response time exceeds 4 minutes unless there was proper basic life support (BLS) intervention (CPR). Many studies have

shown that defibrillation is most effective when delivered in 4 minutes or less after patient collapse. If EMS responders arrive more than 4 minutes after patient collapse, patient outcomes are better if the patient receives at least 90 seconds of CPR prior to defibrillation. For many years, the desired EMS response time was established at 8 minutes, but recent studies have shown that a response time of 8 minutes has not been associated with improved outcomes. A response time of 4 minutes or less has been highly associated with improved outcomes in cardiac arrest. However, few EMS systems can routinely deliver response times of 4 minutes or less. Further research is needed to determine the best desired response times for a specific EMS system[26,27] and how to achieve them.

Initial and Continuing Education Programs

The two kinds of EMS education programs for EMS personnel are initial education and continuing education. *Initial education* programs are the original courses for prehospital providers. They involve the completion of a standardized course that meets or exceeds recommended standards. (As noted earlier, instead of various curricula for the various levels of EMS, the *National EMS Instructional Guidelines* now allow instructors more latitude in instructional strategies.) *Continuing education* programs include refresher courses for recertification and periodic in-service training sessions. All education programs should have medical oversight and a medical director who is involved in the process. The EMS agency is responsible for ensuring funding for its education programs.

Initial Education

A paramedic's initial education is accomplished by successfully completing a course following the most recent *National EMS Education Instructional Guidelines* published by the U.S. DOT. The guidelines establish the minimum content for the course and set a standard for paramedic programs across the country. The Instructional Guidelines offer guidance of three specific learning domains:

- *Cognitive,* which consists of facts, or information knowledge
- *Affective,* which requires students to assign emotions, values, and attitudes to that information
- *Psychomotor,* which consists of hands-on skills students learn while in laboratory and clinical settings

There is a national effort to have all paramedic education programs accredited. The **accreditation** process ensures that all paramedic education programs meet minimal guidelines in regard to faculty, facilities, equipment, medical oversight, clinical affiliations, and financial stability.[28] The primary accrediting organization in EMS is the

Committee on Accreditation of Educational Programs for the Emergency Medical Services Professions (CoAEMSP), an entity of the Commission on Accreditation of Allied Health Programs (CAAHEP). Some states have their own program accreditation processes.

Continuing Education

Once a paramedic has completed the initial education program, he must remain current on changes in EMS care. To achieve this, a continuing education program is essential. Various methods are available for a paramedic to attain the necessary continuing education. These include traditional lectures and prepackaged programs but also include innovative strategies such as web-based programs, podcasts, videos, and similar alternative delivery models. Most continuing education programs must be accredited or approved by an oversight body. The *Continuing Education Coordinating Board for Emergency Medical Services (CECBEMS)* is a national continuing education certifying body, although some states provide their own continuing education certifying process.

Continuing education is mandatory and is just as important as the initial paramedic education program. EMS is a relatively young **profession** and information and technology changes rapidly. More important, continuing education allows you to stay abreast of the changes in emergency care procedures to ensure that you are providing the best patient care possible. The best paramedics are those who seek and complete quality continuing education.

Licensure, Certification, Registration, and Reciprocity

Once initial education is completed, the paramedic will become either certified or licensed, depending on the laws governing EMS in the particular state.

Licensure is a process of occupational regulation. Through licensure, a governmental agency (usually a state agency) grants permission to engage in a given trade or profession to an applicant who has attained the degree of competency required to ensure the public's protection. Some states choose to license paramedics instead of certifying them. (There is an unfounded general belief that a licensed professional has greater status than one who is certified or registered. However, a certification granted by a state, conferring a right to engage in a trade or profession, is, in fact, a license.)

Regardless of what it is called, the paramedic must realize that the authority granted to him by the state is a privilege and his personal responsibility. He must take a proactive role in maintaining his good standing through continuing education, conduct his practice in a manner to uphold the public trust he has been given, and protect this privilege. The paramedic should never assume that anyone else would take over this responsibility for him.

Certification is the process by which an agency or association grants recognition to an individual who has met its qualifications. Many states certify paramedics. After attaining state certification, paramedics are permitted to work within an established EMS system under the direct supervision of a physician medical director.

Registration is accomplished by entering one's name and essential information within a particular record. Paramedics are registered so the state can verify the provider's initial certification and monitor recertification. Almost every state has an EMS office that tracks the registration of emergency care providers. Whereas some states track only paramedic providers, others maintain registers on the certifications of Emergency Medical Responders, EMTs, Advanced EMTs, and Paramedics.

Reciprocity is the process by which an agency grants automatic certification or licensure to an individual who has comparable certification or licensure from another agency. For example, some states grant reciprocity to paramedics who are certified in another state. In some states, certification or licensure is not automatic. In these cases, the state may grant certification or licensure through *equivalence* or *legal recognition*, under which the state determines that the out-of-state paramedic's initial education meets the requirements of the state, and the paramedic is then allowed to participate in a licensure examination or other activity to gain licensure or certification.

National Registry of EMTs

The National Registry of Emergency Medical Technicians (NREMT) is a nonprofit entity based in Columbus, Ohio. It prepares and administers standardized tests for the various EMS provider levels. The National Registry establishes the qualifications for registration and biennial reregistration and serves as a vehicle for establishing a national minimum standard of competency. Through these services, the National Registry serves as a major tool for reciprocity by providing a process for paramedics to become certified when moving from one state to another. The National Registry also supports the development and evaluation of EMS education programs with the goal of developing nationwide professional standards for EMS providers.

Currently, in the majority of states, National Registry examinations are being used at some level by EMS regulators. Several states offer locally developed examinations because their levels of certification or licensure differ from those recognized by the National Registry. The states that use the National Registry examinations benefit from savings that result from spreading exam development costs over a large user base as well as from the assurance that the examinations are widely recognized as providing a national standard.

Staying Abreast

In EMS, it is important to stay abreast of new developments and information. Professional organizations, professional publications, and the Internet provide opportunities to keep yourself professionally up to date.

Professional Organizations

The public image of EMS is often shaped by the professional organizations that represent that profession. Membership in professional organizations is a great way to stay abreast of changes in the profession and to interact with members from other parts of the country. It also provides an excellent opportunity to share ideas. National EMS organizations include the following:

- National Association of Emergency Medical Technicians (NAEMT)
- National Association of Search and Rescue (NASAR)
- National Association of EMS Educators (NAEMSE)
- National Association of EMS Physicians (NAEMSP)
- International Flight Paramedics Association (IFPA)
- National EMS Management Association (NEMSMA)
- National Council of State EMS Training Coordinators (NCSEMSTC)

In addition to these, most states have EMS organizations that provide information and assistance at a state or local level.

These are just some examples of organizations through which paramedics, emergency physicians, and nurses can enrich themselves and pursue their particular interests. Such organizations assist in the development of educational programs, operational policies and procedures, and the implementation of EMS. They establish guidelines with input from the public and the profession, which ensure that the public interest is served in the delivery of emergency medical services. They also provide a means to promote and enhance the status of EMS within the health care community, and their efforts help to create a unified voice for EMS providers.

Professional Journals and Magazines

A variety of journals are available to keep the paramedic aware of the latest developments in this ever-changing industry. These journals provide an abundant source of continuing-education material, as well as an excellent opportunity for EMS professionals to write and publish articles. The following is just a partial list of journals that routinely publish articles relating to the medical care of patients in EMS:

- *Academic Emergency Medicine*
- *American Journal of Emergency Medicine*
- *Annals of Emergency Medicine*
- *Emergency Medical Services*
- *Journal of Emergency Medical Services (JEMS)*
- *Journal of Pediatric Emergency Medicine*
- *Journal of Trauma: Injury, Infection and Critical Care*
- *Prehospital Emergency Care*

The Internet

The Internet has changed the world and certainly has changed EMS. There are now numerous websites designed for EMS providers. Many trade magazines and similar entities offer websites with constantly updated content and news. There are numerous websites that provide quality, accredited continuing education programs. There has been a similar trend in placing much of the didactic portion of initial EMS education on the Internet. This allows students to receive initial and continuing education in their local communities. Interestingly, several EMS-oriented social communities have been developed. These have allowed international EMS discussions and networking and have a considerable following among EMS providers (Figure 2-10).

Effective Patient Transportation

Patients who are transported under the direction of an EMS system should be taken to the nearest appropriate medical facility whenever possible. Medical oversight should designate that facility, based on the needs of the patient and the availability of services. In some cases, the patient's need for special services (such as care for burns) means designating a facility that is not nearby. At other times, the closest facility will be designated for stabilization of the patient while transfer is arranged. The ultimate authority for this decision remains with on-line medical direction.

Air Transport

Patients may be transported by ground or air (Figure 2-11). As noted earlier, use of helicopters for medical transport was introduced during the Korean War and expanded in

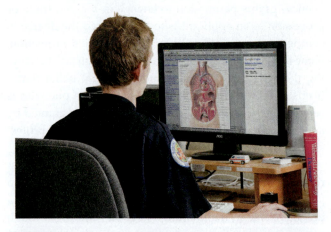

FIGURE 2-10 The Internet has allowed paramedics, regardless of their location, to obtain quality continuing education.

FIGURE 2-11 Patients may be transported by ground or air. Medical helicopter transport was introduced in the 1950s during the Korean War.
(© Ed Effron)

Vietnam, and success of military evacuation procedures led to their use in civilian ambulance systems. In 1970, the Military Assistance to Safety and Traffic (MAST) program was established. This demonstration project set up 35 helicopter transportation programs nationwide to test the feasibility of using military helicopters and paramedics in civilian medical emergencies.[29]

Today, trauma care systems use law enforcement, municipal, hospital-based, private, and military helicopter transport services to transfer patients. Fixed-wing aircraft also are used when patients must be transported long distances, usually more than 200 miles (Figure 2-12).

Ambulance Standards

All transport vehicles must be licensed and meet local and state EMS requirements. Equipment lists should be consistent with systemwide standards. There are various national and regional standards regarding what equipment and technologies should be available on both emergency and nonemergency ambulances. Regional standardization of equipment and supplies is most effective in facilitating interagency efforts during disaster operations.

FIGURE 2-12 Fixed-wing aircraft, as well as helicopters, have become an important part of patient transport in the modern EMS system.
(© REACH Air Medical Services)

In 1974, in response to a request from the DOT, the General Services Administration (GSA) developed the "KKK-A-1822 Federal Specifications for Ambulances." This was the first attempt at standardizing ambulance design to permit intensive life support for patients en route to a definitive care facility. The act defined the following basic types of ambulance:

- *Type I (Figure 2-13).* This is a conventional cab and chassis on which a module ambulance body is mounted, with no passageway between the driver's and patient's compartments.
- *Type II (Figure 2-14).* A standard van, body, and cab form an integral unit. Most have a raised roof.

FIGURE 2-13 Type I ambulance.

FIGURE 2-14 Type II ambulance.

FIGURE 2-15 Type III ambulance.

- *Type III (Figure 2-15).* This is a specialty van with forward cab and integral body. It has a passageway from the driver's compartment to the patient's compartment.

Only these certified ambulances may display the registered "Star of Life" symbol as defined by the National Highway Traffic Safety Administration (NHTSA). The word *ambulance* should appear in mirror image on the front of the vehicle so that other drivers can identify the ambulance in their rear-view mirrors.

Many services now place a variety of specialized equipment on board ambulances, including specialty rescue, hazardous materials (hazmat), and additional advanced life support equipment. This has often meant exceeding the gross vehicle weight and has resulted in introduction of a medium-duty truck chassis built for rugged durability and large storage and work areas (Figure 2-16). Another newer type of ambulance, developed for fuel economy and enhanced safety, is the diesel ambulance (Figure 2-17). Ambulance standards will continue to evolve. Concerns about the future of the environment have

FIGURE 2-16 Some EMS systems have elected to use medium-duty ambulances that are built on a commercial truck chassis.

(© Pat Songer)

FIGURE 2-17 The diesel, unibody ambulance is becoming increasingly popular because of cost, fuel economy, and safety.

(© Acadian Ambulance Services)

led to a trend to consider vehicle emissions (exhaust and carbon footprint) in ambulance design.

In 1980, the revision "KKK-A-1822A" aimed at improving ambulance electrical systems by designing a low-amp lighting system to replace antiquated light bars and beacons. This standard helped to reduce electrical system overloads. In 1985, another revision, "KKK-A-1822B," specified changes based on the National Institute for Occupational Safety and Health (NIOSH) standards. These include reduced internal siren noise, high engine temperatures, and exhaust emissions; safer cot-retention systems; wider axles; handheld spotlights; battery conditioners for longer life; and venting systems for oxygen compartments. In 2002, revision "KKK-A-1822E" provided guidelines to improve occupant protection in the patient compartment, including additional occupant restraints, more rounded interior corners, and more secure locations of the sharps container for needles and other potentially dangerous items. Revision "KKK-A-1822F" was published in 2007 and primarily addressed electrical systems, signage, and safety.[30]

All ambulances purchased with federal funds during the 1970s were required to comply with the KKK criteria. Since then, however, some states have adopted their own criteria.

Appropriate Receiving Facilities

Not all hospitals are equal in emergency and support service capabilities. So how do you get the right patient to the right facility in an appropriate amount of time? EMS systems organize hospitals into categories that identify the readiness and capability of each hospital and its staff to receive and effectively treat emergency patients. EMS coordinators can use these categories to quickly recognize the most appropriate medical facility for definitive treatment or life-saving stabilization.

FIGURE 2-18 The development of specialized trauma centers has resulted in significant improvements in trauma morbidity and mortality.

(© Dr. Bryan E. Bledsoe)

Categorization was initially designed to identify **trauma** care capabilites for hospitals. The hospitals that made a commitment to providing accredited trauma care were designated as trauma centers. As the system has evolved, other categorizations have been developed, including various categories of chest pain centers, stroke centers, and other specialized care capabilities.[31]

Once categorization has been established, regionalizing available services helps give all patients reasonable access to the appropriate facility. Burn, trauma, pediatric, psychiatric, perinatal, cardiac, spinal, and poison centers are examples of specialty service facilities that offer high-level care for specific groups of patients (Figure 2-18). Large EMS systems should designate a resource hospital that will coordinate specialty resources and ensure appropriate patient distribution.

Ideally, all receiving facilities should have the following capabilities: an emergency department with an emergency physician on duty at all times, surgical facilities, a lab and blood bank, medical imaging capabilities available around the clock, and critical and intensive care units. They should have a documented commitment to participate in the EMS system, a willingness to receive all emergency patients in transport regardless of their ability to pay, and medical audit procedures to ensure quality care and medical accountability. Finally, receiving facilities should exhibit a desire to participate in multiple-casualty preparedness plans.

Mutual Aid and Mass-Casualty Preparation

The resources of any one EMS system can be overwhelmed. A mutual-aid agreement ensures that help is available when needed. Such agreements may be between neighboring departments, municipalities, systems, or states. Cooperation among EMS agencies must transcend geographical, political, and historical boundaries.

Each EMS system should put a disaster plan in place for catastrophes that can overwhelm available resources. There should be a coordinated central management agency that identifies commanders within the framework of the incident command system and an existing mutual-aid agreement. The plan should integrate all EMS system components and have a flexible communications system. Frequent drills should test the plan's effectiveness and practicality. The communications and control systems should be capable of coordinating a systemwide response to a major medical incident without a major change in personnel, equipment, or operating protocol.

Quality Assurance and Improvement

An EMS system must be designed with the needs of the patient as its chief concern. The only acceptable level of quality is excellence, and systems should take the approach that they will never fully attain total excellence. For quality assurance and improvement programs to be effective, they must be dynamic and comprehensive. The EMS system must constantly monitor the community's expectations and standards of practice, and be willing to initiate, change, or eliminate its practices accordingly.

In 1997, the National Highway Traffic Safety Administration (NHTSA) released a manual called *A Leadership Guide to Quality Improvement for Emergency Medical Services Systems*. Its guidelines are based on the following components:

- Leadership
- Information and analysis
- Strategic quality planning

> **Legal Considerations**
>
> **9/11/01 and Beyond.** Since the attacks on the United States on September 11, 2001, disaster response and EMS have taken on significantly more and different responsibilities. All EMS personnel must be prepared for disasters, regardless of the cause. Biological and chemical agents pose significant risks to EMS personnel. Preparation and education are the keys to survival if such events are encountered.

> **CONTENT REVIEW**
>
> ➤ Guidelines for Quality Improvement
>   - Leadership
>   - Information and analysis
>   - Strategic quality planning
>   - Human resources development and management
>   - EMS process management
>   - EMS system results
>   - Satisfaction of patients and other stakeholders
> ➤ Customer satisfaction can be created or destroyed with a simple word or deed.

- Human resources development and management
- EMS process management
- EMS system results
- Satisfaction of patients and other stakeholders

Many EMS systems have developed ongoing quality assurance programs, while others have gone a step further with quality improvement programs. A quality assurance (QA) program is designed primarily to maintain continuous monitoring and measurement of the clinical care delivered to patients. It is in essence a problem-identifying mechanism. QA programs tend to look at the results, or the outputs, of the EMS system, much as a manufacturer looks at the finished product coming off the assembly line. QA programs document the effectiveness of the care provided after the fact. They help to identify problems and selected areas that need improvement. The limitation with QA is that it tends to address the actions of individuals within the system, and looks at established performance measurements. These performance measurements are often based on criteria that are set in an arbitrary manner. These criteria—for example, that an IV success rate will be greater than 80 percent—tend to become a ceiling. As long as the paramedics in the system are establishing 8 of 10 IV starts successfully, no one looks any further. If the success rate drops below 80 percent, however, the QA process may look at the individuals and miss that a change to new IV catheters has caused the decline. Furthermore, the QA system will probably not look at future improvements that could increase the success rate to 85 percent, 90 percent, or higher. A common complaint about QA programs is that they tend to identify only the problems and therefore focus only on punitive corrective action. Thus, prehospital personnel often view QA programs negatively.

As a result, many EMS systems have taken the quality process a step further with continuous quality improvement (CQI). In a CQI program, there is an ongoing effort to refine and improve the system to provide the highest level of service possible. CQI can be thought of as a problem-solving methodology. CQI programs are based on facts, data, and specifications, or management by fact. By its very nature, the statistical approach of CQI looks at the group as a whole, looking at the processes in an EMS system instead of the individual provider. In short, CQI is development of the "best possible" system, whereas the QA approach accepts a system that is "good enough."[32]

A CQI program emphasizes the improvement of the overall process that will, in turn, lead to improved patient care. The dynamic process of CQI includes a four-step cycle known as "plan, do, check, and act." In this process, data are analyzed and a *plan* of action developed. In the *do* phase, the plan is implemented; additional data are collected in the *check* phase to assess the viability of the changes. Finally, action is taken in the *act* phase to address

Legal Considerations

QI: A Risk Management Strategy. A good EMS quality improvement (QI) program is also an excellent risk management strategy. Problems in the system or with individual EMS providers can often be identified early through the QI program and remedied before patient care is harmed. Experience has shown that EMS services with an ongoing QI program have a decreased incidence of being sued. EMS cases can be divided into four areas of risk: high frequency/low risk; high frequency/high risk; low frequency/low risk; and low frequency/high risk. A good QI program should continuously monitor all high-risk cases and procedures, especially those that fall into the low-frequency category.

High-risk cases in EMS include cardiac arrest patients, patients who must be restrained, patients who refuse EMS care, those who later file a complaint about care, and others. High-risk procedures include endotracheal intubation, medication administration, and others. A good QI program will continuously monitor high-risk cases and procedures such as these at both the system and provider levels. If a provider is determined not to be managing these cases appropriately, that provider can be referred for additional education. Similarly, if it is learned that the system is not managing these cases appropriately, then changes must be made in the system to ensure that the problems are corrected.

Never look at an EMS QI program as punishment; look at it instead as an educational opportunity. If properly used, it will make you a better paramedic and your system a better EMS system.

the findings of the previous step, and the process repeats itself. This process helps to ensure that the improvement in the system is ongoing and does not stall.

In general, EMS quality can be divided into two categories: "good enough" quality and "best possible" quality.

"Take-It-for-Granted" Quality

People take it for granted that EMS will respond quickly to a 911 call. Because patients do not usually have medical training, they must assume that we are always acting in their best interests and at the highest level of **professionalism**. Thus, they also take it for granted that the care they receive from us is safe, appropriate, and the best that is available.

Quality improvement in this area is accomplished through continuous evaluation. Such clinical evaluation and improvement should be subject to rigorous examination prior to implementation and periodically thereafter. When considering a new medication, process, or procedure, for example, we must follow set rules before permitting its use in EMS. These rules, often called **rules of evidence**, were developed by Joseph P. Ornato, MD, PhD,. They include the following guidelines:

- *There must be a theoretical basis for the change.* That is, the change must make sense based on relevant anatomy, physiology, biochemistry, and other basic medical sciences.

- *There must be ample scientific human research to support the idea.* Any device or medication used in patient care must have adequate scientific human research to justify its use.

- *It must be clinically important.* The device, medication, or procedure must make a significant clinical difference to the patient. For example, a device such as an automated external defibrillator (AED) may mean the difference between living and dying for some patients, whereas color-coordinated stretcher linen has little clinical significance.

- *It must be practical, affordable, and teachable.* Some medical devices remain too expensive and too impractical for use in routine prehospital emergency care.

If a clinical innovation or improvement meets all these guidelines, then the change should be made. Only devices, medications, and procedures that pass these rigorous tests should be implemented.

Another way to accomplish "take-it-for-granted" quality improvement is through the ongoing education of personnel. Paramedics can improve their skills by reading, taking classes, soliciting feedback on clinical performance from receiving hospitals, and following up on patients. Peer review—the process of EMS personnel reviewing each other's patient reports, emergency care, and interactions with patients and families—is another way for paramedics to improve their knowledge and skills.

Ethics are the rules or standards that govern the conduct of members of a particular group or profession. Prehospital providers at all levels have an ethical responsibility to their patients and to the public. (See the chapter "Ethics in Paramedicine" for a detailed discussion of professional ethics.) The public expects excellence from the EMS system, and we should accept no less than excellence from ourselves.

Service Quality and Customer Satisfaction

In the business world, service quality is equated with "customer satisfaction." This is the kind of quality that individual customers get excited about, feel good about, and tell stories about. These are the little extras that exceed a customer's expectations and elicit thank-you letters. Prime examples of customer satisfaction include patient statements such as: "You fed my cat before we left." "You remembered my name and introduced me to the nurse." "You held my hand." "You seemed like a friend when I needed one."

Customer satisfaction can be created or destroyed with a simple word or deed. A significant part of the way we communicate with one another is through body language and tone of voice. Paramedics who genuinely care about

FIGURE 2-19 Our patients are our customers. We must strive to provide them with service that is compassionate and kind.

their patients communicate it in many subtle ways. From the patient's perspective, this is much more important than IVs, backboards, and ECGs. It is essential to remember the ultimate reason for our existence: to serve the patient by providing the highest quality service and care available (Figure 2-19).

Patient Safety

The primary tenet of medicine is *primum non nocere* (first, do no harm). The safety of the patient must be considered in any medical endeavor. This holds true for EMS as well. As the health care system becomes more complicated, the chances for errors and accidents increase. In 2000, the Institute of Medicine of the National Academies of Sciences published *To Err Is Human: Building a Safer Health System.* In this document, the institute estimated that between 44,000 and 98,000 Americans die annually because of medical errors. EMS is a part of the health care system—and medical errors occur.[33] Three areas have been identified as causes for medical errors:

- *Skills-based failures.* Skills-based failures occur because a health care worker failed to perform a skill or procedure properly. These often occur in a skill that is almost automatic to a provider and can occur when the provider's "routine" is interrupted.

- *Rules-based failures.* All health care systems, including EMS, have rules in place to ensure safety and prevent medical errors. Rules-based failures occur when a provider fails to follow the relevant rule, misapplies a good rule, or applies a bad rule.

- *Knowledge-based failures.* Knowledge-based failures are the most complex of the three causes of medical errors. They result primarily from insufficient information or misinterpreting the situation. They tend to occur when the provider is stressed or pressured. They can also occur when a provider thinks his judgment is "error proof"—a narcissistic trait.[34]

Although medical errors can occur at any time, some high-risk areas of EMS practice have been identified. These include:

- *Hand-off.* The transfer of patient care and the patient from an EMS crew to hospital staff is called the hand-off. During this time, essential information about the patient must be communicated. The failure to provide information by the EMS crew and the failure to receive (or ask for) information by the hospital staff can lead to misunderstanding and possible errors.[35]

- *Communications issues.* As with hand-off, the failure to communicate with family members, other responders, and hospital personnel can lead to misunderstandings and medical errors.

- *Medication issues.* Medications can heal, but they can also kill. Because of the large number of medications used in EMS, there is always the potential for error. Common errors include administering the wrong medication, administering the wrong dose of the right medication, or failing to administer a medication. Every paramedic must understand his responsibilities when given the authority to administer medications and treatment.

- *Airway issues.* Prehospital airway management has come under increased scrutiny following several studies that showed that patient outcomes are often not improved with endotracheal intubation.[36] The failure to recognize improper placement of an endotracheal tube (e.g., esophageal intubation) has been an ongoing issue in EMS and a source of malpractice litigation. Airway management is a skill that must be mastered, performed flawlessly, and documented carefully. Airway errors are often fatal and can be prevented.

- *Dropping patients.* Physically dropping a patient is not uncommon and not limited to emergency responses. There are several occasions in emergency care when patients are dropped—the most common being loading and unloading the patient into and out of the ambulance.

- *Ambulance crashes.* There has been an alarming increase in ambulance crashes in the past decade and the causes appear multifactorial. We are learning that most modern American ambulances are not particularly crashworthy, and strategies are being developed to address this. Most ambulance crashes can be avoided by following established guidelines and procedures.

- *Death pronouncements.* It is not uncommon for paramedics to encounter a patient who is clearly dead or who has what appears to be obviously mortal injuries. However, EMS personnel often arrive minutes after the onset of the problem and initial findings may not accurately indicate what will eventually happen to the patient. There have been many reports where paramedics have declared a patient dead and the patient was later found to be alive. Such an error is fodder for the media. EMS systems should have a protocol and practices to ensure that death pronouncement is accurate.

Medical error prevention is an important part of EMS. Several practices will help with this. One is to address possible EMS environmental issues that can lead to errors. To minimize these, an EMS system must have clear protocols, and they must be fully understood by all providers. When procedures are performed, there must be adequate lighting to ensure that the procedure can be carried out safely. There should be minimal interruptions (to the degree possible). Standardization and organization of drugs and their packaging can help to minimize medication errors—a major problem in EMS and health care.

Besides environmental strategies, the individual provider must also address medical error prevention. Medical errors can be minimized if providers always reflect on what they are planning to do. They should also constantly question assumptions. Often initial assumptions as to patient condition and necessary treatment change as more is learned about the patient and his condition. Tools to help in decision making and prompts (checklists, electronic reminders) can help reduce medical errors (a strategy gleaned from the aviation industry). Simply asking for help when a question arises can also effectively reduce medical errors. Although there has been a decrease in the routine use of on-line medical oversight, virtually all EMS systems have a medical director available to answer questions. A practice called "time outs" is now routinely used in the operating room to help minimize errors—particularly when high-risk procedures are involved. Before beginning the actual procedure, all involved take a "time out" and ensure that everything is in order—the right patient, the correct supplies, the correct personnel, and so on. This methodology can be applied to certain aspects of EMS, particularly high-risk procedures.

Medical errors are common and pose a clear and present danger for our patients. Just as airline pilots use strategies to maximize safety, EMS providers should also actively employ strategies and procedures that will help to minimize medical errors. One of the best strategies is simply: when in doubt, ask for help!

Research

A formal, ongoing **research** program is an essential component of the EMS system for moral, educational, medical,

FIGURE 2-20 The future of EMS will be driven by research and paramedics should try to participate in research projects when possible.

(© Dr. Bryan E. Bledsoe)

financial, and practical reasons. The future enhancement of EMS depends strongly on the availability of quality research.[37] Future changes in EMS procedures, techniques, and equipment must be evaluated to prove that they make a positive difference prior to implementation. The current trend of introducing "new and improved" ideas or new "high-tech" equipment to existing procedures must be evaluated scientifically. Unfortunately, many EMS protocols and procedures in use today have evolved without clinical evidence of usefulness, safety, or benefit to the patient.

One particular area that will rely heavily on research is funding. As managed care increases its influence on the delivery of emergency care, EMS systems will be forced to scientifically validate their effectiveness and necessity. The restrictions on reimbursement by managed care organizations, accountable care organizations (ACOs), and governmental agencies will drive the need for quality EMS research. Outcome studies will also be required to justify funding and ensure the future of EMS (Figure 2-20).

Future EMS research must address the following issues: Which prehospital interventions actually reduce morbidity and mortality? Are the benefits of certain field procedures worth the potential risks? What is the cost–benefit ratio of sophisticated prehospital equipment and procedures? Is field stabilization possible, or should paramedics begin immediate transport in every case?

Paramedics can play a valuable role in data collection, evaluation, and interpretation of research. The components of a research project include the following:

- Identify a problem, explain the reason for the proposed study, and state the hypothesis or a precise question.
- Identify the body of published knowledge on the subject.
- Select the best design for the study, clearly outline all logistics, examine all patient consent issues, and get

them approved through the appropriate investigational review process.

- Begin the study, and collect raw data.
- Analyze and correlate your data in a statistical application.
- Assess and evaluate the results against the original hypothesis or question.
- Write a concise, comprehensive description of the study for publication in a medical journal.

Current EMS practice must be justified by hard clinical data derived from an objective, valid program of ongoing research. EMS providers at all levels share the responsibility for identifying research opportunities, conducting peer review programs, and publishing the results of their projects. As leaders in the prehospital care environment, paramedics should set an example in the development of and participation in research projects.[37]

For a more detailed discussion of research in EMS, see the chapter "EMS Research."

Evidence-Based Medicine

A movement has been building in the house of medicine called **evidence-based medicine (EBM)**. This movement has been widely embraced by those in emergency medicine. It is only logical that the principles of EBM be applied to EMS. After all, EMS is an extension of the practice of emergency medicine. There is really nothing all that new about EBM. Its roots can be traced back to the mid-nineteenth century and beyond. The current resurgence of EBM began in Great Britain and has spread throughout the medical world.

EBM is the conscientious, explicit, and judicious use of the current best scientific evidence in making decisions about the care of individual patients. It requires combining clinical expertise with the best available clinical evidence from systematic research. Thus, to practice effective EBM, EMS personnel must first be proficient in prehospital care and exercise sound clinical judgment. These traits can be developed only by following a comprehensive initial education program, followed by clinical experience and practice.

To move to the next level, prehospital personnel must be familiar with the current and past research pertinent to prehospital care and be able to integrate that knowledge into the care of individual patients. An essential skill is knowing how to read and interpret the scientific literature and to determine whether the information is sound. (Again, refer to the chapter "EMS Research," which discusses how to read and evaluate research.)

External clinical evidence can invalidate previously accepted treatments and procedures and replace them with new ones that are more powerful, more effective, and safer. Good paramedics can become excellent paramedics by using both their clinical expertise and the best available external evidence. In today's medical setting, neither clinical experience nor external evidence alone is enough; there must always be a balance between the two.

Some might say that EBM is simply "cookbook" medicine. This is simply not true. As previously noted, EBM requires paramedics to be, first, clinically proficient. Anybody can follow simple "cookbook" directions and provide some level of patient care. To achieve excellent patient care, however, external evidence can inform, but never replace, the individual paramedic's clinical expertise. Clinical expertise is required to form the best determination of the optimum treatment for each individual patient.

There has been a trend in EMS over the past decade or so to study the various practices and procedures of out-of-hospital care. When studied, some treatments, such as pneumatic anti-shock garments (PASG), did not stand up to the test. Likewise, some treatments, such as early defibrillation, were found to have significant positive impact on survival following out-of-hospital cardiac arrest. Looking at this from a different perspective, by using the best research data available, we were able to abandon a practice (PASG) that helped few, if any, patients. Later, we were able to embrace a practice (early defibrillation) that has saved countless lives through diverse programs that include bystander defibrillation.

Practicing EBM helps to ensure that we are providing our patients the best possible care at the lowest possible price.

System Financing

At present in the United States, there are a wide variety of EMS system designs. EMS can be hospital-based, fire or police department–based, a municipal service, a private commercial business, a volunteer service, or some combination. Major differences exist in methods of EMS system finance, too. They range from fully tax-subsidized municipal systems to all-volunteer squads supported solely by contributions.

EMS funding can come from many sources. However, the most common is fee-for-service revenue, which may be generated from Medicare, Medicaid, private insurance companies, specialty service contracts, or private paying patients. Most of these sources of revenue are referred to as "third-party payers," because payment comes from someone other than the patient. To date, almost all third-party payers require the patient to be transported or the EMS service will not be compensated for a response. Reimbursement may also be based on the level of care the patient receives during transport. For the most part, third-party reimbursement rarely covers the expenses of operating an EMS system. Because of this, many EMS systems are subsidized by local taxing entities (e.g., city or county government) to remain operational. For the most part, funding has been, and remains, one of the biggest problems faced by EMS systems.

Summary

The evolution of EMS has occurred over thousands of years. Many of its innovations are the result of lessons learned from military conflicts. EMS today is also largely the result of federal legislation and investment from private foundations.

A comprehensive EMS system has many components. EMS provides a continuum of care that extends from the EMT who conducts public education classes to the mechanic who keeps the ambulance fleet running; from the emergency medical dispatcher who calms a distressed caller to the emergency department physician, surgeon, and physical therapist who see the patient through to definitive care and rehabilitation. No one component, no one person, is more important than another. EMS is a total team effort.

EMS systems are designed with the patient as the highest priority. Each system has an administrative agency, which structures the system around the community's needs and grants the medical director ultimate authority in all issues of patient care.

Most EMS systems may be activated by way of a single, universal number (911). They rely on a centralized communications center, which handles all medical emergencies in the area and coordinates all levels of communication—operational and medical—within a region. The goal of an emergency response is BLS care in less than 4 minutes and advanced life support (ALS) care in less than 8 minutes after the onset of an event. Coordination of ground and air transport follows established protocols at the communications center.

Mutual-aid agreements ensure a continuum of care during multiple-casualty incidents. Disaster plans are formalized, rehearsed regularly, continuously evaluated, and revised when necessary. Hospitals are categorized according to their readiness to provide essential and specialty services within a region. EMS providers are trained according to the U.S. DOT Instructional Guidelines. Continuing education programs encourage providers to achieve excellence.

A continuous quality improvement program documents the EMS system's performance. Ongoing research validates the actions of prehospital providers through scientific evaluation. Finally, EMS systems flourish because of strong, stable financial plans that ensure consistent development on a regional, state, and national basis.

You Make the Call

While you and your family are watching a fireworks display, one of the rockets tips over, shoots into the air, and explodes just above the crowd. There is a mad rush of people, and moments later everyone has scattered, leaving 11 injured people lying on the ground. You and your family are unhurt and move to a safe distance from the scene.

Luckily, the local fire and ambulance service has units on stand-by at the show. The crews immediately call dispatch and request additional ground and air transport units. The 911 dispatcher puts the region's mass casualty plan into effect and dispatches the appropriate law enforcement and fire personnel.

Meanwhile, the EMS crews on scene are triaging the patients. Five minutes after the incident, a breakdown of patients is reported to the incident commander. There are seven injured adults: one immediate, three delayed, and three minor. There are four injured children: one delayed and three minor.

It isn't long before the top-priority patient is transported by helicopter to a regional burn center, which is 80 miles from the scene. As the ambulances arrive on scene, the remaining patients are loaded and transported to appropriate receiving facilities. During transport, EMS providers follow local protocols for patient care. One EMS provider radios medical direction for guidance in the care of the youngest injured child. All units radio the receiving facility to provide updated patient information and an estimated time of arrival.

1. Which of the "ten system elements" identified by NHTSA are mentioned in this scenario?

2. For what possible reason was the top-priority patient sent so far from the scene?

3. How important was the role played by the emergency medical dispatcher in this scenario? Explain.

4. How might the EMS system benefit from an evaluation of this incident?

See Suggested Responses at the back of this book.

Review Questions

1. EMS trauma care generally evolves following
   _____
   a. studies and scientific reviews.
   b. military conflicts.
   c. medical consortiums.
   d. quality improvement reviews.

2. Which document published in 1966 outlined the deficiencies in prehospital emergency care?
   a. National Standard Curriculum
   b. *Accidental Death and Disability: The Neglected Disease of Modern Society*
   c. *EMS Agenda for the Future*
   d. Consolidated Omnibus Budget Reconciliation Act

3. _____ is a project published in 1996 and supported by the National Highway Traffic Safety Administration.
   a. Emergency Medical Services for Children (EMS-C)
   b. *EMS Agenda for the Future*
   c. White Paper
   d. OPALS

4. The _____ was established following the terrorist attacks of September 11, 2001.
   a. National Highway Transportation and Safety Act
   b. Department of Homeland Security
   c. National Incident Improvement and Mitigation
   d. Federal Emergency Management Agency

5. An essential, yet often overlooked, component of an EMS system is _____
   a. the QI process.
   b. the public.
   c. the medical director.
   d. the training officer.

6. All of the following are components of the communications network of a regional EMS system except _____
   a. citizen access.
   b. dual control center.
   c. operational communications capabilities.
   d. medical direction.

7. Crucial to the efficient operations of EMS, _____ are responsible for sending ambulances to the scene and ensuring that system resources are in constant readiness.
   a. Emergency Medical Radio Technicians
   b. Emergency Telecommunications Operators
   c. Emergency Medical Dispatchers
   d. Paramedical Telecommunications

8. There are two types of education in EMS: _____ education.
   a. prehospital and hospital
   b. initial and continuing
   c. clinical and field
   d. initial and hospital

9. The act of receiving a comparable certification or licensure from another state or agency is known as _____
   a. registration.
   b. reciprocity.
   c. regulation.
   d. reciprocation.

10. Professional organizations that help shape the public perception of EMS include all of the following *except* _____
    a. NASAR.   c. NAEMSP.
    b. NAEMSE.   d. NFPA.

See answers to Review Questions at the back of this book.

References

1. Stout, J., P. E. Pepe, and V. N. Mosesso, Jr. "All Advanced-Life Support vs. Tiered Response Ambulance Systems." *Prehosp Emerg Care* 4 (2000): 1–6.

2. Skandalakis, P. N., P. Lainas, O. Zoras, et al. "'To Afford the Wounded Speedy Assistance': Dominique Jean Larrey and Napoleon." *World J Surg* 30 (2006): 1392–1399.

3. Evans, G. D. "Clara Barton: Teacher, Nurse, Civil War Heroine, Founder of the American Red Cross." *Int Hist Nurs J* 7 (2003): 75–82.

4. Barkley, K. T. *The Ambulance*. Kiamesha Lake, NY: Load N Go Press, 1978.

5. Apel, O. F., Jr. and P. Apel. *MASH: An Army Surgeon in Korea*. Lexington: University of Kentucky Press, 1998.

6. Allison, C. E. and D. D. Trunkey. "Battlefield Trauma, Traumatic Shock and Consequences: War-Related Advances in Critical Care." *Crit Care Clin* 25 (2009): 31–45, vii.

7. Elam, J. O., E. S. Brown, and J. D. Elder, Jr. "Artificial Respiration by Mouth-to-Mask Method: A Study of the Respiratory Gas Exchange of Paralyzed Patients Ventilated by Operator's Expired Air." *NEJM* 250 (1954): 749–754.

8. Safer, P., T. C. Brown, W. J. Holtey, and J. Wilder. "Ventilation and Circulation with Closed-Chest Cardiac Massage in Man." *JAMA* 176 (1961): 574–576.

9. National Academy of Sciences, National Research Council. *Accidental Death and Disability: The Neglected Disease of Modern Society*. Washington, DC: U.S. Department of Health, Education, and Welfare, 1966.

10. Pantridge, J. F. and J. F. Geddes. "A Mobile Intensive Care Unit in the Management of Myocardial Infarction." *Lancet* 290 (1967): 271–273.

11. Hirschman, J. C., S. R. Nussenfeld, and E. L. Nagel. "Mobile Physician Command: A New Dimension in Civilian Telemetry-Rescue Systems." *JAMA* 230 (1974): 255–258.

12. Page, J. O. *The Paramedics*. Morristown, NJ: Backdraft Publications, 1979.

13. Harvey, J. C. "The Emergency Medical Services Act of 1973." *JAMA* 230 (1974): 1139–1140.

14. Stiell, I. G., D. W. Spaite, G. A. Wells, et al. "The OPALS Study: Rationale and Methodology for Cardiac Arrest Patients." *Ann Emerg Med* 32 (1998): 180–190.

15. National Highway Traffic Safety Administration. *The EMS Agenda for the Future*. Washington, DC: National Highway Traffic Safety Administration, 1996 [available at http://www.nhtsa.dot.gov/people/injury/ems/agenda/emsman.html].

16. Department of Homeland Security, Federal Emergency Management Agency (FEMA). *About the National Incident Management System (NIMS)* [available at http://www.fema.gov/emergency/nims/AboutNIMS.shtm].

17. Gausche, M., R. J. Lewis, S. J. Stratton, et al. "Effect of Out-of-Hospital Pediatric Endotracheal Intubation on Survival and Neurological Outcome: A Controlled Clinical Trial." *JAMA* 283 (2000): 783–790.

18. Institute of Medicine of the National Academies. *Emergency Medical Services at the Crossroads*. Washington, DC: National Academies Press, 2006.

19. American College of Emergency Physicians. *The National Report Card on the State of Emergency Medicine*. Irving, TX: American College of Emergency Physicians, 2006.

20. U.S. Department of Transportation/National Highway Traffic Safety Administration. *National EMS Scope of Practice Model*. Washington, DC, 2006.

21. U.S. Department of Transportation/National Highway Traffic Safety Administration. *National Emergency Medical Services Educational Standards: Paramedic Instruction Guidelines*. Washington, DC, 2009.

22. U.S. Department of Transportation/National Highway Traffic Safety Administration. *National EMS Core Content*. Washington, DC, 2005.

23. Munk, M. D., S. D. White, M. L. Perry, et al. "Physician Medical Direction and Clinical Performance at an Established Emergency Medical Services System." *Prehosp Emerg Care* 13 (2009): 185–192.

24. Jensen, J. L., D. A. Petrie, A. H. Travers, and PEP Project Team. "The Canadian Prehospital Evidence-Based Protocols Project: Knowledge Translation in Emergency Medical Services Care." *Acad Emerg Med* 16 (2009): 668–673.

25. Wilson, S., M. Cook, R. Morrell, et al. "Systematic Review of the Evidence Supporting the Use of Priority Dispatch of Emergency Ambulances." *Prehosp Emerg Care* 6 (2002): 42–49.

26. Pons, P. T., J. S. Haukoos, W. Bloodworth, et al. "Paramedic Response Time: Does It Affect Patient Survival?" *Acad Emerg Med* 12 (2005): 594–600.

27. Blackwell, T. H., J. A. Kline, J. J. Willis, and J. M. Hicks. "Lack of Association between Prehospital Response Times and Patient Outcomes." *Prehosp Emerg Care* 13 (2009): 144–150.

28. Dickinson, P., D. Hostler, T. E. Platt, and H. E. Wang. "Program Accreditation Effect on Paramedic Credentialing Examination Success Rate." *Prehosp Emerg Care* 10 (2006): 224–228.

29. Schneider, C., M. Gomez, and R. Lee. "Evaluation of Ground Ambulance, Rotor-Wing and Fixed-Wing Aircraft Services." *Crit Care Clin* 8 (1992): 533–564.

30. United States General Services Administration. *Federal Specification for the Star-of-Life Ambulance: KKK-A-1822F*. Washington, DC: General Services Administration, 2007.

31. Demetriades, D., M. Martin, A. Salim, et al. "Relationship between American College of Surgeons Trauma Center Designation and Mortality in Patients with Severe Trauma (Injury Severity Score >15)." *J Am Coll Surg* 202 (2006): 212–215.

32. Goldstone, J. "The Role of Quality Assurance versus Continuous Quality Improvement." *J Vasc Surg* 28 (1998): 378–80.

33. National Academies of Science, Institute of Medicine. *To Err Is Human: Building a Safer Health System*. Washington, DC: National Academies Press, 2000.

34. Banja, J. *Medical Errors and Medical Narcissism*. Sudbury, MA: Jones and Bartlett, 2005.

35. Yong, G., A. W. Dent, and T. J. Welland. "Handover from Paramedics: Observations and Emergency Department Clinical Perceptions." *Emerg Med Australas* 20 (2008): 149–155.

36. Davis, D. P., J. Peay, M. J. Sise, et al. "The Impact of Prehospital Endotracheal Intubation on Outcome in Moderate to Severe Traumatic Brain Injury." *J Trauma* 58 (2005): 933–939.

37. Sayre, M. R., L. J. White, L. H. Brown, et al. National EMS Research Agenda. *Prehosp Emerg Care* 6 (2002): S1–S43.

Further Reading

Bledsoe, B. E. "The Golden Hour: Fact or Fiction?" *Emergency Medical Services (EMS)* 31 (2002): 105.

Bledsoe, B. E. "Searching for the Evidence behind EMS." *Emergency Medical Services (EMS)* 32 (2003): 63–67.

National Academies of Emergency Dispatch. *Emergency Telecommunicator Course Manual*. Sudbury, MA: Jones and Bartlett Publishers, 2001.

Walz, B. *Introduction to EMS Systems*. Albany, NY: Delmar/Thompson Learning, 2002.

Chapter 3
Roles and Responsibilities of the Paramedic

Bryan Bledsoe, DO, FACEP, FAAEM

STANDARD
Preparatory (EMS Systems)

COMPETENCY
Integrates comprehensive knowledge of EMS systems, the safety and well-being of the paramedic, and medical–legal and ethical issues, which is intended to improve the health of EMS personnel, patients, and the community.

 ## Learning Objectives

Terminal Performance Objective: After reading this chapter, you should be able to explain the roles and responsibilities of paramedics.

Enabling Objectives: To accomplish the terminal performance objective, you should be able to:

1. Define key terms introduced in this chapter.

2. Discuss each of the primary responsibilities of paramedics.

3. Give examples of additional responsibilities of paramedics.

4. Define and discuss how to integrate expected characteristics of professionalism into the practice of paramedicine.

5. Give examples of behaviors that demonstrate the expected professional attitudes and attributes of paramedics.

KEY TERMS

allied health professions, p. 51

mechanism of injury (MOI), p. 45

nature of the illness (NOI), p. 45

paramedicine, p. 43

pathophysiology, p. 43

primary care, p. 48

Case Study

The central dispatch center for your city receives a call for a medical emergency. The patient's name, address, and street number appear on the computer monitor, so the dispatcher clicks a mouse and a map of the city appears on screen. In this EMS system, satellites are used continuously to track and monitor the location and availability of emergency vehicles using Automatic Vehicle Location (AVL). The dispatcher selects Medic 49, the unit closest to the scene, and, by way of the computer-aided dispatch (CAD) system, gives the unit specific directions and patient information.

While the ambulance is responding, the dispatcher talks to the caller and provides him with emotional support and prearrival instructions for immediate patient care.

On arrival, the ambulance personnel find a 66-year-old female patient lying in bed, unable to speak clearly or move the right side of her body. The primary assessment reveals her to be disoriented. It also finds that she has an open airway, a normal rate of breathing, and strong radial and carotid pulses.

Paramedic Bobby Moore decides to work with his partner to rapidly prepare the patient for transport. Then he performs a rapid stroke assessment scoring system, after which he determines that the patient has had a stroke. The patient is immediately moved to the stretcher and placed into the ambulance. Paramedics determine that the onset of the stroke was probably within the past 45 minutes and the patient is well within the stroke interventional window of 4½ hours.

In the ambulance, the paramedics complete a more detailed assessment and determine that the patient requires transport to a hospital with interventional neurology and fibrinolytic capabilities. During transport, they radio the hospital and report the patient's condition and estimated time of arrival. The hospital activates its "Code Stroke" team to await the patient's arrival. Vital signs and pulse oximetry are continuously monitored and an ECG is performed.

After approximately 18 minutes en route, the patient is delivered to the emergency department, where the stroke team—the emergency physician, a neurologist, and a radiologist—is waiting for her. Forty-five minutes later, after an emergency CT scan of the brain, the patient is receiving interventional therapy to help minimize the size of the infarct in her brain. One week later, the patient is discharged to her home with a schedule of appointments for rehabilitation. A home health nurse is also scheduled to perform follow-up assessments twice each week.

Introduction

In the past several years, the United States has seen dramatic changes in the health care delivery system. The Patient Protection and Affordable Care Act was signed into law on March 23, 2010. This law was the most significant health care regulatory change since the establishment of Medicare and Medicaid in 1965, and is bringing important changes to the U.S. health care system. EMS has not been immune to these changes. Driving forces such as technology, cost, and trends in patient population are forcing change. One such change involves the paramedic, whose roles and responsibilities are dramatically different from what they were 10 or 15 years ago.

Today, **paramedicine** is an enormous responsibility for which you must be mentally, physically, and emotionally prepared. You will be required to have a strong knowledge of **pathophysiology** and of the most current medical technology. You will have to be capable of maintaining a professional attitude while making medical and ethical decisions about severely injured and critically ill patients. You will be required to provide not only competent emergency care, but also emotional support to your patients and their families.

As a paramedic, the most highly trained prehospital emergency care provider in the EMS system, you will often serve people who are unaware of your knowledge and skills. However, if self-satisfaction and pride in a job well done are rewards enough—and if you have a genuine desire to help people in need—then being a paramedic will be a very fulfilling career.

Primary Responsibilities

A paramedic's responsibilities are diverse. They include emergency medical care for the patient (Figure 3-1) and a variety of other responsibilities that are attended to before, during, and after a call.[1,2]

Preparation

Before responding to a call, you must be mentally, physically, and emotionally

CONTENT REVIEW

➤ Primary Responsibilities
- Preparation
- Response
- Scene size-up
- Patient assessment
- Treatment and management
- Disposition and transfer
- Documentation
- Clean-up, maintenance, and review

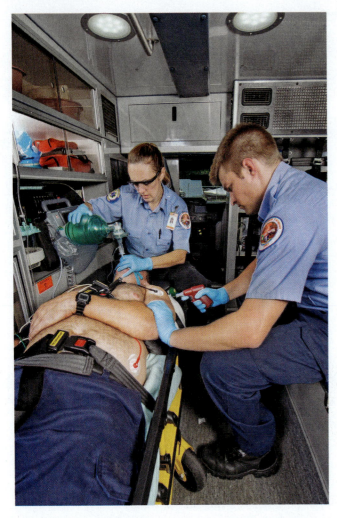

FIGURE 3-1 A paramedic provides emergency care to ill and injured patients—at the scene and in the ambulance.

able to meet the demands of the patient, the family, and other health care providers. Your ongoing training should include aerobics for cardiovascular fitness, exercises for muscle strength and endurance, stretching for increased flexibility, and an understanding of the biomechanics of lifting for prevention of lower-back injuries. Other keys to a successful career are recognizing the effects of stress and practicing ways to alleviate it.

You must be prepared. This means making sure that inspection and routine maintenance have been completed on your emergency vehicle and on all equipment. It means restocking medications and intravenous solutions and checking their expiration dates. In addition, you must be very familiar with the following:

- All local EMS protocols, policies, and procedures
- Communications system hardware (radios) and software (frequency utilization and communication protocols)
- Local geography, including populations during peak utilization times, and alternative routes during rush hours

- Support agencies, including services available from neighboring EMS systems, and the methods by which efforts and resources are coordinated

Response

During an emergency response, remember that personal safety is your number one priority. If your ambulance crashes en route to an incident because of speeding or running red traffic lights, you will be of no benefit to the patient. Responding safely to an emergency will reduce the risk to you, your partners, and other agencies responding to the same incident. Always follow basic safety precautions en route to an incident. Wear a seat belt, obey posted speed limits, and monitor the road for potential hazards.

Just as important as getting to the scene safely is getting to the scene in a timely manner. Make certain you know the correct location of the incident and that the appropriate equipment is en route. Also while you are en route, request any additional personnel or services that you think may be needed—for example, with alcohol- or drug-related issues. Waiting to ask for such assistance until you get to a chaotic scene can only delay the appropriate response. Learn to anticipate potential high-risk situations based on dispatch information and experience. For example, if any of the following is reported, you may need to call for assistance:

- Multiple patients
- Motor vehicle collisions
- Hazardous materials
- Rescue situations
- Violent individuals (patients or bystanders)
- Use of a weapon
- Knowledge of previous violence

Scene Size-Up

Your primary concern during scene size-up is the safety of your crew, the patient, and bystanders. Identify all potential hazards such as fire, smoke, traffic, bystanders, angry or distraught family members, unstable structures or vehicles, and hazardous materials (Figure 3-2). Never enter an unsafe scene until the hazards have been dealt with. Remember that any scene has the potential to deteriorate, so learn to anticipate problems and be prepared for anything.

When the scene is safe to enter, determine the number of patients. In medical emergencies, there usually is only one. However, in some cases—such as carbon monoxide poisoning or exposure to other toxic substances—it may be necessary to search the entire area for patients. Once the number of patients and the severity of their illnesses or injuries are determined, quickly request any additional or specialized services required to manage the incident.

FIGURE 3-2 Always assess the scene for potential hazards as you approach.
(© *Ed Effron*)

FIGURE 3-3 During the primary assessment of your patient, you will look for and immediately treat any life-threatening conditions.

The **mechanism of injury (MOI)** or the **nature of the illness (NOI)** also must be identified. For a trauma patient, some mechanisms of injury can be a cause for alarm. For example, a child struck by a fast-moving car is likely to have serious, multiple injuries. Knife and gunshot wounds suggest severe injury to internal organs and life-threatening internal bleeding. How far a patient is found from a collision or explosion, or how far a patient fell from a height, will also indicate how severe an injury may be. For a medical patient, clues identified at the scene can provide important insights into the nature of the illness. Identifying medications, such as insulin, or devices, such as an inhaler, may prevent misdiagnosis and speed the proper treatment of the patient.

Patient Assessment

One of the most critical skills you will learn is patient assessment. Although the order of the steps may vary for trauma and medical patients, the basic components are the same: primary assessment, patient history, secondary assessment, and ongoing assessment. (Volume 2 deals with patient assessment in detail.)

The primary assessment of a patient is usually performed in a scant minute or so. During this assessment, you must note your general impression of the patient's appearance. Then assess the patient's responsiveness—that is, determine whether the patient is alert, responding to verbal or painful stimuli, or not responding at all. Finally, you will assess the patient's airway, breathing, and circulation (Figure 3-3). If the patient is in cardiac arrest, circulation takes priority over airway and breathing. If you discover any life threats, you will treat them immediately.

As part of the primary assessment, you will decide whether to continue the assessment on scene or immediately transport the patient to a medical facility. The next step of assessment is gathering the facts of the patient's medical history from the patient and/or bystanders and performing a physical examination of the patient, with all information recorded and reported to the hospital. It is also the paramedic's responsibility to continuously monitor the patient and provide any additional emergency care needed until the patient is transferred to the care of the hospital's emergency department staff.

Recognition of Illness or Injury

Recognizing the nature of the illness or severity of injury, accomplished during the scene size-up and the primary assessment, is the first aspect of patient prioritization. Most commonly, patient priority is based on the urgency for transport. No matter what method of prioritization your EMS system uses, it is essential that you learn and practice it. Note that the method should be standardized so that all health care professionals within your system understand each other and can respond appropriately.

Patho Pearls

Research in EMS. As each year passes, we are learning more and more about EMS through research and scientific inquiry. Interestingly, some prehospital practices that seemed intuitive have not held up to scientific scrutiny. Because of this, EMS is adjusting so current practices reflect the current status of the science. Several things are becoming increasingly clear, especially in regard to the importance of early intervention: Paramedic-level measures appear to be most beneficial when provided early in the disease process. More lives are saved with the prehospital administration of aspirin than by all resuscitation measures combined. Other treatments, such as pain control and the use of continuous positive airway pressure (CPAP), benefit many more patients than once thought. As EMS evolves, there will be a decreased emphasis on raising the dead and a greater emphasis on intervening earlier in the disease spectrum.

Patient Management

Almost all EMS systems have a set of protocols or treatment guidelines that providers follow. As a paramedic, you must always follow your system's protocols. They ensure that various personnel, when presented with the same emergency, will respond in the same manner. Protocols related to patient care also specify when it is necessary for you to communicate with medical oversight. In response, medical direction will give you instructions on how to proceed with emergency care, permission to perform certain procedures, or alternatives to standard care.

Patient management includes the task of moving the patient from one location to another. To do so, you must make sure that the proper equipment is used and that there are adequate personnel available. Remember, back injury is the number one career injury in EMS. Ensure your own safety, and call dispatch for any additional assistance needed whenever you must lift or move a patient.

Appropriate Disposition

The paramedic must ensure, within the constraints of the EMS system and local protocols, that the patient gets to the appropriate facility by the appropriate mechanism of transport. With emergency department crowding on the increase, many EMS systems are looking at strategies to route patients to facilities that may be more appropriate for the patient's specific condition. In some situations, these facilities may not be traditional hospital emergency departments. Many factors affect ultimate patient disposition, including hospital capabilities, medical staffing, technology, transfer agreements, and reimbursement issues.

Transportation

A critical decision to be made is the mode of transportation for your patient. Time and distance are key factors to consider. For example, if an unstable patient needs to be taken to a facility that is far from the scene, an air medical service—helicopter or fixed-wing aircraft—rather than ground transport may be the best choice. However, there may be only a single receiving facility option if you practice in a rural setting. Know the resources available in your EMS system. Follow all local protocols on their use.

Receiving Facilities

Selecting the appropriate receiving facility for your patient is your responsibility. To do so, it is important for you to know which medical facilities in your area offer the following services:

- Fully staffed and equipped emergency department
- Trauma care capabilities

Legal Considerations

Gatekeeper to the Health Care System. The EMS system is often the initial point of contact for a person entering the health care system. Thus, to a certain extent, a paramedic frequently functions as a sort of gatekeeper to the health care system as a whole.

Part of a paramedic's responsibility is to ensure that a patient is taken to a facility that can appropriately care for the patient's condition. Today, hospitals have become more specialized—that is, some hospitals have chosen to provide certain services and not provide others. For example, one hospital may elect to specialize in cardiac care, another in stroke care, another in burn care, and so on. This is especially true in communities with multiple hospitals. Because of this, it is essential that paramedics understand the capabilities of the hospitals in the system where they work. Also, with overcrowding in modern emergency departments, diversion of ambulances by hospitals whose emergency departments are full has become commonplace.

For all these reasons, local EMS system protocols must be available to guide prehospital personnel in ensuring that each patient is delivered to a facility that can adequately care for the patient's condition.

- Operating suites available 24 hours a day and 7 days a week
- Critical care units, such as postanesthesia recovery rooms and surgical intensive care units
- Cardiac facilities with on-staff cardiologists (chest pain centers)
- Neurology department that provides a "stroke team"
- Acute hemodialysis capability
- Pediatric capabilities, including pediatric and neonatal intensive care units
- Obstetric capabilities, including facilities for high-risk delivery
- Radiological specialty capabilities, such as angiography, computerized tomography (CT), and magnetic resonance imaging (MRI)
- Burn specialization for infants, children, and adults
- Acute spinal cord and head injury management capability
- Rehabilitation staff and facilities
- Clinical laboratory services
- Toxicology, including hazmat decontamination facilities
- Hyperbaric oxygen therapy capability
- Microvascular surgical capabilities for replants
- Psychiatric facilities

Receiving facilities are categorized based on the level of care they can provide. For example, the American College of Surgeons categorizes trauma centers by levels:

Level I—The Level I facility is a regional resource trauma center and serves as a tertiary care facility for the trauma care system. Ultimately, all patients who require the resources of the Level I center should have access to it. This facility must have the capability of providing leadership and total care for every aspect of injury, from prevention through rehabilitation. In its central role, the Level I center must have adequate depth of resources and personnel.

A Level I trauma center requires a large number of personnel and an adequate facility for patient care, education, and research. Most Level I trauma centers are university-based teaching hospitals. Other hospitals willing to commit these resources, however, may meet the criteria for Level I recognition.

In addition to patient care responsibilities, Level I trauma centers have the major responsibility of providing leadership in education, research, and system planning. This responsibility extends to all hospitals caring for injured patients in their regions.

Medical education programs include residency program support and postgraduate training in trauma for physicians, nurses, and prehospital providers. Education can be accomplished through a variety of mechanisms, including classic continuing medical, trauma, and critical care fellowships, preceptorships, personnel exchanges, and other approaches appropriate to the local situation. Research and prevention programs, as defined in this document, are essential for a Level I trauma center.

Level II—The Level II trauma center is a hospital that also is expected to provide initial definitive trauma care, regardless of the severity of injury. Depending on geographic location, patient volume, personnel, and resources, the Level II trauma center may not be able to provide the same comprehensive care as a Level I trauma center. Therefore, patients with more complex injuries (for example, patients requiring advanced and extended surgical critical care) may have to be transferred to a Level I center. Level II trauma centers may be the most prevalent facilities in a community, however, managing the majority of trauma patients.

The Level II trauma center can be an academic institution or a public or private community hospital located in an urban, suburban, or rural area. In some areas where a Level I center does not exist, the Level II center should take on the responsibility for education and system leadership.

Level III—The Level III trauma center serves communities that do not have immediate access to a Level I or II institution. Level III trauma centers can provide prompt assessment, resuscitation, emergency operations, and stabilization, and also arrange for possible transfer to a facility that can provide definitive trauma care. General surgeons are required in a Level III facility. Planning for care of injured patients in these hospitals requires transfer agreements and standardized treatment protocols. Level III trauma centers are generally not appropriate in an urban or suburban area where Level I and/or Level II resources are available.

Level IV—Level IV trauma facilities provide advanced trauma life support before patient transfer in remote areas where no higher level of care is available. Such a facility may be a clinic rather than a hospital and may or may not have a physician available. Because of geographic isolation, however, the Level IV trauma facility is often the *de facto* primary care provider. If it is willing to make the commitment to provide optimal care, given its resources, the Level IV trauma facility should be an integral part of the inclusive trauma care system. As at Level III trauma centers, treatment protocols for resuscitation, transfer protocols, data reporting, and participation in system performance improvement are essential.

A Level IV trauma facility must have a good working relationship with the nearest Level I, II, or III trauma center. This relationship is vital to the development of a rural trauma system in which realistic standards must be based on available resources. Optimal care in rural areas can be provided by skillful use of existing professional and institutional resources supplemented by guidelines that result in enhanced education, resource allocation, and appropriate designation for all levels of providers. It is also essential for the Level IV facility to have the involvement of a committed health care provider who can provide leadership and sustain the affiliation with other centers.[3]

In addition to designated trauma centers, other facilities may offer unique services. They include burn, pediatric, psychiatric, perinatal, cardiac, spinal, and poison centers.

The best receiving facility is the one best able to care for your patient. Most patients request transportation to the nearest medical facility. However, patients enrolled in managed care programs, such as health maintenance organizations (HMOs) or designated provider groups, may request transport to a facility approved by their group, which may be a facility other than the nearest hospital. Other patients may ask you to transport them to a facility outside your run area. Even though the requested facility may be appropriate for the patient, there may be an equally appropriate hospital that is closer. Remember, you are responsible for patient care and therefore ultimately responsible for selecting the transport destination. When in doubt, contact on-line medical direction for advice and support.

Other Types of Disposition

In some areas, paramedics provide **primary care**. They have well-defined protocols that allow them to treat patients at the scene and transfer them to facilities other than a hospital. For example, consider a child who cuts his arm on a rusty nail. The father activates EMS by calling 911. When the paramedics arrive, they control the bleeding and perform a patient assessment. They find a simple 2-inch laceration on the child's forearm. Instead of transporting the patient to the hospital and using resources that are not needed for the treatment of this patient, the paramedics contact medical direction and request permission to transport the child to a local outpatient center for treatment. This decision saves the family from paying a costly emergency department fee, and it keeps the emergency department available for a more serious emergency.

Another type of disposition is called "treat and release." In this type of program, paramedics arrive on scene, assess the patient, and provide emergency care. If they determine that there is no need for further medical attention, they contact medical direction and request orders not to transport. In some systems, paramedics may then contact a specialized dispatch center, where an office appointment is made with a physician in the patient's area.[4]

While disposition systems such as these are not widely accepted, the increasing numbers of people in managed care programs (which generally attempt to achieve optimum care while finding ways to control costs) may change that. Innovative programs such as these are setting standards for the future of EMS.

Patient Transfer

The managed care environment has caused many people—both laypersons and health care providers—to occasionally question whether certain actions that are intended to reduce the cost of medical care are actually in the patient's best interest. For example, to avoid the cost of duplicating equipment and services in a number of facilities that serve the same geographic area, managed care systems have encouraged facilities to specialize and, often, to transfer patients to a facility that can provide the specific care needed.

Occasionally, there may be a question as to whether the transfer of a patient from one facility to another has been approved for cost reasons but may not actually be in the patient's best interest. When you are assigned to transport a patient, you share responsibility—with the receiving and accepting physician—for the treatment and care of the patient. When you are in doubt about the patient's stability for the duration of transport, or about the capabilities of the receiving facility, contact medical direction.

Before removing the patient from a hospital, request a verbal report from the primary care provider (usually a registered nurse or a physician). This report is often called the "hand-off." Also request a copy of essential parts of the patient's chart, including a summary of the patient's past and present medical history. However, if the results of diagnostic tests taken at the facility are not ready when you are prepared to leave, do not delay patient transport. The data can be faxed, e-mailed, or telephoned to the receiving facility.

Your first priority during transport is the patient. While en route, contact the receiving facility and provide them with an estimated time of arrival (ETA) and an update on the patient's condition. On arrival at your destination, seek out the contact person (usually a registered nurse or physician). Provide that person with an updated patient report, including any treatment or changes in status while en route. All documents provided by the sending facility should be turned over to the receiving care provider along with a copy of your run report. If required by your service, obtain appropriate billing/insurance information at this time.[5]

Documentation

Maintaining a complete and accurate written patient care report is essential to the flow of patient information, to research efforts, and to the quality improvement of your EMS system. The patient care report should be completed

---

Legal Considerations

What Is a Patient? Although this may seem like a rhetorical question, the answer is not as easy as one would think. For example, you arrive at the scene of a motor vehicle collision to find three people exchanging insurance information. All three deny injury and refuse assistance. Are they legally EMS patients? What if one of the drivers appears intoxicated? Is he a patient? What if one of the people is a 16-year-old female riding with an 18-year-old boyfriend? Is she a patient? The issue is certainly cloudy and most EMS systems have developed a statement in this regard. One example, developed by EMS medical directors in Texas, states:

A patient is any person who, on contact with an EMS system, presents with a complaint, circumstance, and/or condition that might require further assessment or treatment.

The standard of judgment is that of a reasonable and prudent medic.

The designated system Medical Director is responsible for promulgating specific criteria for designation of a patient within the above general guideline.

Certainly, the definition in your area may vary. However, EMS systems are encouraged to define this tricky issue, and EMS personnel should be aware of the definition used by their EMS system.

in its entirety as soon as emergency care has been completed—no later. Any brief notes that were taken during patient assessment—vital signs, for example—should be copied into the report.

The importance of accurate and complete documentation cannot be overemphasized. Proper record keeping helps to ensure continuity of patient care from the emergency scene to the hospital setting. To avoid potential legal problems and embarrassing court situations, record only your observations, not your opinions. For example, record "patient has an odor of alcohol on his breath," rather than "patient is drunk." The former cannot be disputed, and the latter cannot be proved.

Your final report should be complete, neat in appearance, and written legibly with no spelling errors. This ensures that other health care providers can readily understand your assessment and interventions as well as the patient's responses to your treatment. It is important to note that your patient care report will be a reflection of the emergency care you provided if a lawsuit is filed in the future.[6]

Returning to Service

Once you have completed patient care, turned the patient over to the hospital staff, and completed all documentation, immediately prepare to return to service (Figure 3-4). Clean and decontaminate the unit, properly discard disposable materials, restock supplies, and replace and stow away equipment. If necessary, refuel the unit on the way back to your station or post. Review the call with crew members, including any problems that may have occurred. Such a dialogue can lead to solutions that enhance the delivery of quality patient care. Finally, the paramedic team leader should check crew members for signs of critical incident stress and assist anyone who needs help.

FIGURE 3-4 A paramedic's responsibility does not end with providing patient care. Documentation, restocking, and cleaning of the ambulance and emergency equipment are equally important.

Additional Responsibilities

The role of the paramedic involves duties in addition to those associated with emergency response. They may include training civilians in CPR, running EMS demonstrations and seminars, teaching first aid classes, organizing prevention programs, and engaging in professional development activities. All involve taking an active role in promoting positive health practices in your community.

Administration

The paramedic has administrative duties that ensure that the EMS system operates as efficiently as possible. These include such things as station duties, record keeping and reporting, special projects, and developing interagency relationships. Station duties include such activities as stocking the ambulance, washing and cleaning the ambulance, and general housekeeping. EMS and fire stations are, in essence, a small community, and all members of that community must share housekeeping responsibilities. Record keeping is also extremely important to ensure that the system operates cohesively. Much of necessary EMS system record keeping and documentation is electronic; this allows easier data entry and faster sharing of information. Regardless of the type of record keeping used, it is an essential part of the job.

Community Involvement

Prehospital providers should take the lead in helping the public learn how to recognize an emergency, how to provide basic first aid measures, and how to properly access the EMS system. A successful effort can save lives. Providing educational programs, such as the American Heart Association's "prudent heart living" campaign, can also encourage positive health practices in the community. EMS injury prevention projects, such as seat belt awareness and the proper use of child safety seats, are essential to the reduction of long-term disability and accidental death.

To decide what injury prevention projects need to be developed in a community, EMS systems often conduct illness and injury risk surveys, both formally and informally. For example, consider an EMS service that reviews run reports for a six-month period. They might find that for a single county they responded to ten vehicle collisions at various railroad crossings. A public

CONTENT REVIEW

➤ Additional Responsibilities
- Community involvement
- Support for primary care
- Citizen involvement
- Personal and professional development

safety campaign directed at the safe crossing of railroad tracks may thus be appropriate. Once an EMS service has identified a problem and the target audience, EMS personnel should seek out community agencies—including the local political structure—to assist in the development, promotion, and delivery of the campaign.

Among the benefits of community involvement are the following: It enhances the visibility of EMS, promotes a positive image, and puts forth EMS personnel as positive role models. It also creates opportunities to improve the integration of EMS with other health care and public safety agencies through cooperative programs.

Support for Primary Care

Promoting wellness and preventing illness and injury will be important components of EMS in the future. Some systems have already begun to direct resources toward the development of prevention and wellness programs that decrease the need for emergency services. The theory is to reduce the cost of the services provided to the community by decreasing the burden on the system.[7]

One strategy is to establish protocols that specify the mode of transportation for nonemergency patients. Some systems already operate vans rather than ambulances to transport such patients to and from nursing facilities or from their residences to a doctor's office. Although it is an additional expense to the system, this service reduces emergency equipment costs and the demand for emergency personnel. The result is a decrease in the overall operating expense, which results in an increase in revenue.

Another strategy being used in many areas of the country is having EMS and hospitals team up to provide an alternative to the emergency department. They transport patients to freestanding outpatient centers or clinics, which ultimately reduces the cost of care to the patient and the system. The development of such alliances will undoubtedly continue. However, caution should be taken to ensure that the patient always receives the appropriate emergency care based on need, not cost.

Citizen Involvement in EMS

Citizen involvement in EMS helps to give "insiders" an outside, objective view of quality improvement and problem resolution. Whenever possible, members of the community should be used in the development, evaluation, and regulation of the EMS system. When considering the addition of a new service or the enhancement of

an existing one, community members should help to establish what is needed. After all, they are your "customers," and their needs are your priority.[8]

Personal and Professional Development

Only through continuing education and recertification can the public be assured that quality patient care is being delivered consistently. Therefore, after you are certified and/or licensed, you have an important responsibility to continue your personal and professional development. Remember, everyone is subject to the decay of knowledge and skills over time. Use this as a rule of thumb: As the volume of calls decreases, training should correspondingly increase. Refresher requirements and courses vary from state to state, but the goal is the same: to review previously learned materials and to receive new information.

Because EMS is a relatively young industry, new technology and data emerge rapidly. Make a conscious effort to keep up. A variety of journals, seminars, computer news groups, and learning experiences are available to help. So are professional EMS organizations, which exist at the local, state, and national levels.

There are other options for keeping up your interest and staying informed, too. By participating in activities designed to address work-related issues—such as case reviews and other quality improvement activities, mentoring programs, research projects, multiple-casualty incident drills, in-hospital rotations, equipment in-services, refresher courses, and self-study exercises—you can expect substantial career growth.

Alternative career paths may be open to you as well. For example, a career paramedic may decide to explore management by applying for a supervisory position or may take a critical care class to prepare for a job on a transport unit. Nontraditional careers for paramedics include working in the primary care setting, providing emergency care on offshore oil rigs, and taking on the occupational safety role in an industrial setting.

Professionalism

A paramedic is a member of the health care professions. Note that the word *profession* refers to the existence of a specialized body of knowledge or skills. Generally self-regulating, a profession will have recognized standards, including requirements for initial and ongoing education. When you have satisfied the initial education requirements for your training as a paramedic, you may then be either certified or licensed. The EMS profession has regulations that ensure that members maintain standards. For the paramedic, these regulations come in the form of periodic recertification with a specified amount of continuing education time.

In addition, the term *professionalism* refers to the conduct or qualities that characterize a practitioner in a particular field or occupation. Health care professionals promote quality patient care and generate pride in their profession. They set and strive for the highest standards. They earn the respect and confidence of team members and the public by performing their duties to the best of their ability. Attaining professionalism is not easy. It requires an understanding of what distinguishes the professional from the nonprofessional.[9]

Professional Ethics

Ethics are the rules or standards that govern the conduct of members of a particular group or profession. Physicians have long subscribed to a body of ethical standards developed primarily for the benefit of the patient. These standards cover the **allied health professions**, such as paramedic, respiratory therapist, and physical therapist. Ethics are not laws, but they are standards for honorable behavior. Conformity to ethical standards is expected. As members of an allied health profession, paramedics must recognize a responsibility not only to patients, but also to society, to other health professionals, and to themselves.[10]

In 1948, the World Medical Association adopted the "Oath of Geneva" (Figure 3-5). In 1978, the National Association of Emergency Medical Technicians adopted the "EMT Code of Ethics" (Figure 3-6). These documents detail the guiding principles for professional EMT service.

Professional Attitudes

A commitment to excellence is a daily activity. While on duty, health care professionals place their patients first; nonprofessionals place their egos first. True professionals establish excellence as their goal and never allow themselves to become complacent about their performance. They practice their skills to the point of mastery and then keep practicing them to stay sharp and improve. They also take refresher courses seriously, because they know they have forgotten a lot and because they are eager for new information. Nonprofessionals believe that their skills will never fade.

Professionals set high standards for themselves, their crew, their agency, and their system. Nonprofessionals aim for the minimum standard and can be counted on to take the path of least resistance. Professionals critically review their performance, always seeking ways to improve. Nonprofessionals look to protect themselves, hide their inadequacies, and place blame on others. Professionals check out all equipment prior to the emergency response. Nonprofessionals hope that everything will work, supplies will be in place, batteries will be charged, and oxygen levels will be adequate.

A professional paramedic is responsible for acting in a professional manner both on and off duty. Remember, the community you serve will judge other EMS providers, the service you work for, and the EMS profession as a whole by your actions.

Professionalism is an attitude, not a matter of pay. It cannot be bought, rented, or faked. Although it is a young industry, EMS has achieved recognition as a bona fide allied health profession. Gaining professional stature is the result of many hard-working, caring individuals who refused to compromise their standards. Always strive to maintain that level of performance and commitment.

OATH OF GENEVA

I solemnly pledge myself to consecrate my life to the service of humanity; I will give to my teachers the respect and gratitude which is their due; I will practice my profession with conscience and dignity; the health of my patient will be my first consideration; I will respect the secrets which are confided in me; I will maintain by all the means in my power the honor and noble traditions of the medical profession; my colleagues will be my brothers; I will not permit considerations of religion, nationality, race, party, politics, or social standing to intervene between my duty and my patient; I will maintain the utmost respect for human life from the time of conception; even under threat, I will not make use of my medical knowledge contrary to the laws of humanity. I make these promises solemnly, freely and upon my honor.

FIGURE 3-5 The Oath of Geneva.

EMT CODE OF ETHICS

Professional status as an Emergency Medical Technician-Paramedic is maintained and enriched by the willingness of the individual practitioner to accept and fulfill obligations to society, other medical professionals, and the profession of Emergency Medical Technician. As an Emergency Medical Technician at the basic level or an Emergency Medical Technician-Paramedic, I solemnly pledge myself to the following code of professional ethics:

A fundamental responsibility to the Emergency Medical Technician is to conserve life, to alleviate suffering, to promote health, to do no harm, and to encourage the quality and equal availability of emergency medical care.

The Emergency Medical Technician provides services based on human need, with respect for human dignity, unrestricted by consideration of nationality, race, creed, color, or status.

The Emergency Medical Technician does not use professional knowledge and skills in any enterprise detrimental to the public well being. The Emergency Medical Technician respects and holds in confidence all information of a confidential nature obtained in the course of professional work unless required by law to divulge such information.

The Emergency Medical Technician, as a citizen, understands and upholds the law and performs the duties of citizenship; as a professional, the Emergency Medical Technician has the never-ending responsibility to work with concerned citizens and other health care professionals in promoting a high standard of emergency medical care to all people.

The Emergency Medical Technician shall maintain professional competence and demonstrate concern for the competence of other members of the Emergency Medical Services health care team. An Emergency Medical Technician assumes responsibility in defining and upholding standards of professional practice and education.

The Emergency Medical Technician assumes responsibility for individual professional actions and judgement, both in dependent and independent emergency functions, and knows and upholds the laws which affect the practice of the Emergency Medical Technician.

The Emergency Medical Technician has the responsibility to be aware of and participate in matters of legislation affecting the Emergency Medical Technician and the Emergency Medical Services System.

The Emergency Medical Technician adheres to standards of personal ethics which reflect credit upon the profession.

Emergency Medical Technicians, or groups of Emergency Medical Technicians, who advertise professional services, do so in conformity with the dignity of the profession.

The Emergency Medical Technician has an obligation to protect the public by not delegating to a person less qualified, any service which requires the professional competence of an Emergency Medical Technician.

The Emergency Medical Technician will work harmoniously with and sustain confidence in Emergency Medical Technician associates, the nurse, the physician, and other members of the Emergency Medical Services health care team.

The Emergency Medical Technician refuses to participate in unethical procedures, and assumes the responsibility to expose incompetence or unethical conduct of others to the appropriate authority in a proper and professional manner.

National Association of Emergency Medical Technicians

FIGURE 3-6 The EMT Code of Ethics.

(Charles B. Gillespie, M.D. Adopted by the National Association of Emergency Medical Technicians (NAEMT), 1978. Reprinted with permission by NAEMT.)

Professional Attributes

There are several traits and attitudes that characterize a professional. True EMS professionals exemplify the traits detailed below (Table 3-1).

Leadership

Leadership is an important but often forgotten aspect of paramedic training. Paramedics are the prehospital team leaders (Figure 3-7). They must develop a leadership style that suits their personalities and gets the job done. Although there are many successful styles of leadership, certain characteristics are common to all great leaders. They include:

- Self-confidence
- Established credibility
- Inner strength
- Ability to remain in control
- Ability to communicate
- Willingness to make a decision
- Willingness to accept responsibility for the consequences of the team's actions

Table 3-1 Attributes of a Health Care Professional

Respects the patient

Provides quality patient care

Advocates for the patient (and the family)

Instills pride in the profession

Strives for high standards and has a commitment to excellence

Earns respect of others

Minimizes pain and suffering

Places patient safety above all but personal safety

Maintains a professional image and behavior

Is an excellent time manager

Works well with other team members

The successful team leader knows the members of the crew, including each one's capabilities and limitations. Ask crew members to do something beyond their capabilities and they will question your ability to lead, not their ability to perform.[11]

Integrity

Paramedics assume the leadership role for patient care in the prehospital setting. As a paramedic, you represent the EMS service and the health care system. The patient and other members of the health care team assume you are sincere and trustworthy. The single most important behavior that you will be judged by is honesty. The environment you work in will often put you in the patient's home or in charge of the patient's wallet and other personal possessions, such as jewelry and items left in a vehicle. You must be trustworthy. The easiest way for a paramedic to lose respect is to be dishonest.[12]

FIGURE 3-7 As leader of the EMS team, the paramedic must interact with patients, bystanders, and other rescue personnel in a professional and efficient manner.

A paramedic functions as an extension of the system's medical director, with authority delegated by the medical director. Because you may be practicing in an area that is remote from your medical director, you will be depended on to follow protocols and accurately document all patient care.

Empathy

Successfully interacting with a patient and family is a challenging skill to master. One of the most important components is empathy. To have empathy is to identify with and understand the circumstances, feelings, and motives of others. To be considered a professional, you will often have to place your own feelings aside to deal with others, even when you are having a bad day. Paramedics who act in a professional manner can show empathy by:

- Being supportive and reassuring
- Demonstrating an understanding of the patient's feelings and the feelings of the family
- Demonstrating respect for others
- Having a calm, compassionate, and helpful demeanor

Self-Motivation

The environment in which you work is often unsupervised, so it is up to you to be able to motivate yourself and establish a positive work ethic. The following are examples of a positive work ethic:

- Completing assigned duties without being asked or told to do so
- Completing all duties and assignments without the need for direct supervision
- Correctly completing all paperwork in a timely manner
- Demonstrating a commitment to continuous quality improvement
- Accepting constructive feedback in a positive manner
- Taking advantage of learning opportunities

Self-motivation is an internal drive for excellence. Remember, providing adequate patient care is not enough. You must strive for excellence in the care that you provide.

Appearance and Personal Hygiene

Society has high expectations for everyone in the allied health professions. From the moment you arrive at the scene of an emergency, you are being judged by the way you present yourself. Good appearance and personal hygiene are critical. If you do not look like a health care provider, then your patient may feel you must not be one. If you have a sloppy appearance, your patient may suspect that your medical care will be sloppy, too. Using slang, foul, abusive, or off-color language is not acceptable and will alienate you from your patients. Your appearance, as well as your behavior, is vital to establishing credibility and instilling confidence.

A paramedic should always wear a clean, pressed uniform and should always be well groomed. Hair should be kept off the collar. If facial hair is allowed, it should be kept neat and trimmed. A light-colored t-shirt may be worn under your uniform shirt, which should be buttoned up, with only the top collar button open. Jewelry—other than a wedding ring, a watch, or small plain earrings—is unprofessional. Long fingernails that have the potential to puncture protective gloves also should be avoided.

Self-Confidence

Having confidence in yourself and your abilities is very important. The patient and family will not trust you if they sense you do not trust yourself. A lack of self-confidence shows and is the basis of many lawsuits. The easiest way to gain self-confidence is to accurately assess your strengths and limitations, and then seek every opportunity to improve any weaknesses. Also, keep in mind that self-confidence does not equal cockiness. A self-confident paramedic who is presented with a complex situation will ask for assistance.

Communication

Communication is a skill often underestimated in EMS services. Providing emergency care in the out-of-hospital environment requires constant communication with the patient, family, and bystanders, as well as with other EMS providers and rescuers from other public agencies.

To be an effective communicator, the paramedic should remember to gather all patient information and present it in a clear and concise format. Speaking clearly, listening actively, and writing legibly are obviously very important skills. Remember, too, to speak in a way that is appropriate for your audience. For example, just as you would not refer to a laceration as a "booboo" when consulting with a physician, you should not use complicated medical terminology to explain a procedure to an injured child.

Being able to adjust your communication strategies to various situations is also an important skill. For example, learning a manual alphabet (sign language) or learning simple medical questions in foreign languages common in your area are just two ways to prepare yourself.

Time Management

Good time management skills are important to the paramedic. The experienced paramedic who plans ahead, prioritizes tasks, and organizes them to make maximum use of time will generally be more effective in the field. A paramedic with good time management skills is punctual for shifts and meetings and completes tasks such as paperwork and maintenance duties on or ahead of schedule.

Some simple time management techniques that you can use are making lists, prioritizing tasks, arriving at meetings or appointments early, and keeping a personal calendar. By implementing just one or two of these techniques, you may find your schedule to be more manageable and less stressful.

Teamwork and Diplomacy

The paramedic is a leader. Leadership implies the ability to work with other people—to foster teamwork. Teamwork requires diplomacy, or tact and skill, in dealing with people, even when you are under siege from the patient or family.

Diplomacy requires the paramedic to place the interest of the patient or team ahead of his own interests. It means listening to others, respecting their opinions, and being open-minded and flexible when it comes to change. A strong leader of any team realizes that he will be successful only if he has the support of all team members. A confident leader will do the following:

- Place the success of the team ahead of personal self-interests
- Never undermine the role or opinion of another team member
- Provide support for members of the team, both on and off duty
- Remain open to suggestions from team members and be willing to change for the benefit of the patient
- Openly communicate with everyone
- Above all, respect the patient, other care providers, and the community he serves

Respect

To respect others is to show—and feel—deferential regard, consideration, and appreciation for others. A paramedic respects all patients, and provides the best possible care to each and every one of them, no matter what their race, religion, sex, age, or economic condition. Showing that you care for a patient's or family member's feelings, being polite, and avoiding the use of demeaning or derogatory language toward even the most difficult patients are simple ways to demonstrate respect. By demonstrating respect, you will earn credit for yourself, your service, and the EMS profession.

Patient Advocacy

A paramedic is also an advocate for patients—defending them, protecting them, and acting in their best interests. For example, as a paramedic you should not allow your personal biases (religious, ethical, political, social, or legal) to interfere with proper emergency care of your patients. Except when your safety is threatened, you should always place the needs of your patient above your own self-interests. In addition, always keep a patient's health care information confidential. (Refer to the chapters "Medical/Legal Aspects of Emergency Care" and "Ethics in Emergency Medical Services" for details about patient confidentiality.)

Careful Delivery of Service

Professionalism requires the paramedic to deliver the highest quality of patient care with very close attention to detail. Examples of behaviors that demonstrate a careful delivery of service include:

- Mastering and refreshing skills
- Performing complete equipment checks
- Careful and safe ambulance operations
- Following policies, procedures, and protocols

Review of individual performance—and attitude—is also important in ensuring that all patients are receiving the proper care in the proper setting. Most EMS agencies have adopted or developed continuous quality improvement (CQI) programs to identify and correct substandard patient care.

Continuing Education

Maintaining certification is the responsibility of the paramedic. Most paramedics use continuing education programs to develop further knowledge or skills in a particular area of emergency health services. This type of education is most often acquired by attending lectures, seminars, conferences, and demonstrations. Each state, region, and local system may have its own policies, regulations, and procedures for recertification. Paramedics cannot work without satisfying those requirements.

There are many benefits to participating in as much continuing education as possible. The most obvious is the expansion of the paramedic's own personal knowledge and skills. Another important reason is to keep up with an emergency health care delivery system that is constantly being updated with more technologically advanced equipment and procedures.

Finally, the skills you learn in this course will need to be practiced. Continuing education programs provide the opportunity to review material and address weak points in patient care.

Summary

To become a paramedic, you must be willing to accept the responsibility of being a leader in the prehospital phase of emergency medical care. Your responsibilities include on-call emergency duties and off-duty preparation. When the emergency call comes in, you must already be prepared to respond. If not, you are likely to be too late.

Most of your time as a paramedic will be spent on preparing yourself to do the job properly—not providing emergency care. If you can accept this reality, and if you are willing to undertake the responsibility of preparing for this dynamic occupation, then you are ready to proceed with your education. Remember: The best paramedics are those who make a commitment to excellence.

You Make the Call

The First Response Ambulance Service receives a call for a patient experiencing chest pain and difficulty breathing. You, as a paramedic, and your EMT partner are immediately dispatched to the scene. While en route, the dispatcher tells you that the patient is a 55-year-old man who has had a sudden onset of chest pain while shoveling snow in his driveway and has audible labored breathing. The dispatcher also informs you that the patient has a history of heart disease and routinely takes multiple medications.

Approximately 7 minutes later, your ambulance arrives on scene. You observe that your patient, Mr. Yates, is sitting on his porch, clutching his chest. His wife and son are sitting beside him. As soon as you and your partner get out of the unit, the son runs to you and starts yelling, "Hurry!" and "Just get him to the hospital!"

While you are performing a primary assessment of the patient, the son continuously exclaims, "Just load my father and get him to the damn hospital!" In 2 minutes, the primary assessment is complete. Because of the cold weather, you decide to move the patient into the unit. Once inside the ambulance, you quickly complete the history and physical exam and begin to treat the patient. Meanwhile, the patient's wife and son are outside the ambulance yelling at your partner, "Leave immediately, or we'll sue you!" Your partner attempts to calm them, but is unsuccessful.

After assessing the patient and connecting him to the monitor, you open the door and ask the family if they are going to ride in the ambulance to the hospital. Mrs. Yates tells you that she will, and she attempts to enter the unit. She is stopped by your partner, who explains that if she is going to ride with the ambulance, she must ride up front in the passenger seat. She immediately and loudly protests. At this point, you ask your partner to sit with the patient. You exit the unit as your partner enters, and you close the unit door. You quickly but calmly explain to Mrs. Yates that First Response Ambulance Service has a policy that requires her to ride in a seat with a seat belt in place, and that the passenger seat is the only seat available. After you explain that during the transport you will keep her updated on her husband's condition, she reluctantly gets into the front seat.

While en route to the hospital, you establish an IV, administer nitroglycerin and aspirin, run numerous ECG strips, and maintain a close watch on the patient's vital signs. Every few minutes you stick your head up front to inform Mrs. Yates about her husband's condition. About 10 minutes from the hospital, you consult with the emergency department, providing an estimated time of arrival, the patient's medical history, and the patient's current status.

On arrival, your partner assists you in unloading the patient. After allowing her to talk with her husband, your partner escorts Mrs. Yates to the hospital waiting area. In the emergency department, you provide the hospital staff with a verbal report and assist them in moving the patient to a stretcher. Then you give a copy of the run report to the unit clerk who is responsible for placing it on the patient's chart. You then walk to the waiting area, where you find Mrs. Yates and her son. You take a minute to tell them that Mr. Yates is now in the care of Dr. Zimmer, and that he or one of the staff members will be out to speak with them as soon as an assessment is completed.

You and your partner meet outside the hospital and prepare the unit for the next call. The stretcher is made up, and the unit is cleaned and restocked. While driving back to the station, you discuss the difficulty you both had dealing with Mrs. Yates and her son.

1. What were your key responsibilities in the previously detailed scenario?

2. How should you have prepared yourself mentally and physically for this call?

3. Did you and your partner act professionally? Explain how you did or did not.

See Suggested Responses at the back of this book.

Review Questions

1. During an emergency response, remember that _____ _____ is your number one priority.
   a. patient care
   b. personal safety
   c. documentation
   d. medical direction

2. The force or forces that caused an injury define the _____
   a. nature of illness.
   b. chief complaint.
   c. mechanism of injury.
   d. primary illness.

3. _____ is the ability to identify with and understand the needs, motives, and emotions of others..
   a. Empathy
   b. Sympathy
   c. Ethics
   d. Equality

4. A _____ trauma center provides the highest level of trauma care.
   a. Level I
   b. Level II
   c. Level III
   d. Level IV

5. Maintaining a complete and accurate written patient care report is essential to _____
   a. research efforts.
   b. the flow of patient information.
   c. the quality improvement of EMS systems.
   d. all of the above.

6. Nontraditional careers for paramedics include _____
   a. working in the primary care setting.
   b. providing emergency care on offshore rigs.
   c. taking on the occupational safety role in an industrial setting.
   d. all of the above.

7. The term _____ refers to the conduct or qualities that characterize a practitioner in a particular field or occupation.
   a. licensure
   b. registration
   c. professionalism
   d. certification

8. _____ are the rules or standards that govern the conduct of members of a particular group or profession.
   a. Ethics   c. Etiquette
   b. Morals   d. Protocols

See answers to Review Questions at the back of this book.

References

1. U.S. Department of Transportation/National Highway Traffic Safety Administration. *National EMS Scope of Practice Model.* Washington, DC, 2006.

2. National Registry of Emergency Medical Technicians. 2004 National EMS Practice Analysis. Columbus, OH: National Registry of EMTs, 2005.

3. American College of Surgeons. *Verified Trauma Centers.* (Available at http://www.facs.org/trauma/verified.html.)

4. Feldman, M. J., J. L. Lukins, P. R. Verbeek, et al. "Use of Treat-and-Release Directives for Paramedics at a Mass Gathering." *Prehosp Emerg Care* 9 (2005): 213–217.

5. American College of Emergency Physicians. "Interfacility Transportation of the Critical Care Patient and Its Medical Direction." *Ann Emerg Med* 47 (2006): 305.

6. Harkins, S. "Documentation: Why Is It So Important?" *Emerg Med Serv* 31 (2002): 93–94.

7. Lerner, E. B., A. R. Fernandez, and M. N. Shah. "Do Emergency Medical Services Professionals Think They Should Participate in Disease Prevention?" *Prehosp Emerg Care* 13 (2009): 64–70.

8. Poliafico, F. "The Role of EMS in Public Access Defibrillation." *Emerg Med Serv* 32 (2003): 73.

9. Streger, M. R. "Professionalism." *Emerg Med Serv* 32 (2003): 35.

10. Klugman, C. M. "Why EMS Needs Its Own Ethics. What's Good for Other Areas of Healthcare May Not Be Good for You." *Emerg Med Serv* 36 (2007): 114–122.

11. Touchstone, M. "Professional Development. Part 1: Becoming an EMS Leader." *Emerg Med Serv* 38 (2009): 59–60.

12. Bledsoe, B. E. "EMS Needs a Few More Cowboys." *JEMS* 28 (2003): 112–113.

Further Reading

Bailey, E. D. and T. Sweeney. "Considerations in Establishing Emergency Medical Services Response Time Goals." *Prehosp Emerg Care* 7 (2003): 397–399.

Bledsoe, B. E. "Searching for the Evidence behind EMS." *Emerg Med Serv* 31 (2003): 63–67.

Heightman, A. J. "EMS Workforce. A Comprehensive Listing of Certified EMS Providers by State and How the Workforce Has Changed Since 1993." *JEMS* 5 (2000): 108–112.

Jaslow, D. J., J. Ufberg, and R. Marsh. "Primary Injury Prevention in an Urban EMS System." *J Emerg Med* 25 (2003): 167–170.

National Academy of Sciences, National Research Council. *Accidental Death and Disability: The Neglected Disease of Modern Society.* Washington, DC: U.S. Department of Health, Education, and Welfare, 1966.

Page, J. O. *The Magic of 3 AM.* San Diego, CA: JEMS Publishing, 2002.

Page, J. O. *The Paramedics.* Morristown, N.J.: Backdraft Publications, 1979. [No longer available for purchase except as a used book. Entire book can be viewed online at www.JEMS.com/Paramedics.]

Page, J. O. *Simple Advice.* San Diego, CA: JEMS Publishing, 2002.

Persse, D. E., C. B. Key, R. N. Bradley, et al. "Cardiac Arrest Survival as a Function of Ambulance Deployment Strategy in a Large Urban Emergency Medical Services System." *Resusc* 59 (2003): 97–104.

Chapter 4
Workforce Safety and Wellness

Bryan Bledsoe, DO, FACEP, FAAEM

STANDARD
Preparatory (Workforce Safety and Wellness)

COMPETENCY
Integrates comprehensive knowledge of EMS systems, the safety and well-being of the paramedic, and medical–legal and ethical issues, which is intended to improve the health of EMS personnel, patients, and the community.

Learning Objectives

Terminal Performance Objective: After reading this chapter, you should be able to select behaviors that promote EMS workforce safety and wellness.

Enabling Objectives: To accomplish the terminal performance objective, you should be able to:

1. Define key terms introduced in this chapter.

2. Explain the importance of preventing EMS workforce injuries and illnesses.

3. Describe the role and elements of basic physical fitness and nutrition in EMS workforce safety and wellness.

4. Explain the consequences of addictions and unhealthy habits as it pertains to the EMS provider.

5. Discuss techniques to ensure good back strength, and identify work habits that minimize the risk of back injuries.

6. Given a variety of scenarios, select proper Standard Precautions for infection control.

7. Discuss various patient, family, and EMS provider responses to death and dying.

8. Explain the pathophysiology of stress, including stressors, phases of the stress response, signs and symptoms, and consequences of prolonged exposure to stressors.

9. Describe effective stress management strategies the EMS provider can employ.

10. Discuss post-traumatic stress disorder (PTSD) as it relates to EMS providers and the role of mental health services.

11. Given a variety of scenarios, take steps to protect your personal safety, including effective interpersonal relationships and roadway safety precautions.

KEY TERMS

anchor time, p. 76

burnout, p. 76

circadian rhythms, p. 76

cleaning, p. 70

Code Green Campaign, p. 78

disinfection, p. 70

exposure, p. 70

incubation period, p. 65

infectious disease, p. 65

isometric exercise, p. 61

isotonic exercise, p. 61

pathogens, p. 65

personal protective equipment (PPE), p. 66

post-traumatic stress disorder, p. 77

Standard Precautions, p. 66

sterilization, p. 70

stress, p. 74

stressor, p. 74

Tema Conter Memorial Trust, p. 78

Case Study

Howard is a 15-year veteran of a high-volume, inner-city EMS service. When he first started his career, Howard thought he knew what he was getting into, but the years have taught him differently.

Right now, Howard is in the spotlight for saving the life of a police officer who was shot in a hostage situation. "That call forced me to reflect on a few important things," he says. "Two years ago, I had a minor heart problem, and it was a good wake-up call. Since then I've been lifting weights and running, so I was able to get to the officer with enough strength to carry him to safety.

"Another thing is that I always use personal protective equipment. I never go to work without steel-toed boots and I never leave the ambulance without a pair of disposable gloves. Can you believe there are still paramedics who knock the concept of infection control? If any one of my partners sticks a needle into the squad bench in my ambulance, they know I'll speak up."

Howard, a mild-mannered, nondescript man, doesn't realize that his young colleagues regard him as a role model. They've seen him handle himself at chaotic scenes as well as when a situation demands sensitivity, patience, and gentleness. "Howard is the man I'd want to tell bad news to my mother," one of his partners says. "He can handle people involved in just about any circumstance—death situations, panicked parents, lonely elderly people, and even hostile drunks. I've never seen anyone treat others with such dignity and respect. He's the best partner anyone could want, especially when we have to manage patients who are thrashing around. But that was not always so, was it, Howard?"

"No, it wasn't," Howard replies. "There was a time when no one wanted to work with me. I was a rebel, and I figured there was only one way to do things: my way. But an incident that occurred a few years ago changed all that. It's a long story. But the upshot is that when I recovered from the stress, my outlook had been altered. I realized that though I couldn't save the world, I could save myself. That's when I learned how to deal with the effects of a stressful job. I started eating right, lost a lot of weight, and adopted a new attitude. Anyway, if I can maintain my own well-being, I can do a lot more to help others. Right? Isn't that what we're about?"

Introduction

The safety and well-being of the workforce is a fundamental aspect of top-notch performance in EMS.[1] As a paramedic, it includes your physical well-being as well as your mental and emotional well-being. If your body is fed well and kept fit, if you use the principles of safe lifting, observe safe driving practices, and avoid potentially addictive and harmful substances, you stand a chance of having the physical strength and stamina to do the job.

If you seize the information about safe practices and apply them to your life, you will be better able to avoid harm from violent people, roadway hazards, ambulance accidents, and insidious infections. If you let your spirit appreciate the fear and sadness on other faces, you will find ways to combat your prejudices and treat people with dignity and respect. By doing all these things, you will also be able to promote the benefits of well-being to your EMS colleagues.

Death, dying, stress, injury, infection, fear—all these threaten your wellness and conspire to interfere with your good intentions. However, you can do something about them. Each person has choices about how to live. Every choice has outcomes and consequences. Many patients in nursing homes are living with their choices, paying for lifestyle decisions made decades ago when they were about your age. Is that what you want for yourself?

Most paramedic injuries are caused by lifting and being in and around motor vehicles. Those who train to be physically prepared for their jobs as paramedics stand a better chance of avoiding early forced retirement because of injured backs or knees. Those who train themselves to be mentally alert in the ambulance and at roadway scenes stand a better chance of staying alive and uninjured. Those who can inspire their colleagues to work toward a state of well-being are role models of the highest order.

This chapter introduces the many elements of well-being. If you listen now and enhance your knowledge later, you stand a good chance of enjoying a long and rewarding career of helping others—all because you helped yourself.

Prevention of Work-Related Injuries

Fortunately, in the twenty-first century there has been a renewed interest in EMS provider safety and injury prevention. Studies have shown that ambulance collisions are a major source of injury for paramedics. Strategies to minimize this have included improving the structural integrity and crashworthiness of emergency vehicles. In addition, restraint systems are now available to secure paramedics in the patient compartment while the vehicle is in motion. Because many ambulance accidents occur when emergency lights and sirens are in use, protocols and call screening schemes have been devised to limit the need for these types of responses to patients who actually have a time-critical condition.

The physical act of lifting and moving patients can injure paramedics—especially given the current obesity epidemic in North America. Fortunately, power-lift stretchers are now widely available. However, in many cases, paramedics must still lift patients onto the stretcher and lift the stretcher into the ambulance. Then, once at the hospital, they must lift the stretcher from the ambulance and move it to the ground. Finally, at the bedside, the crew must help move the patient to the hospital bed. Sometimes these lifts and moves are awkward and can result in injury to the provider. Specialized bariatric ambulances with large stretchers, a ramp, and a mechanical winch can help to move morbidly obese patients fairly safely. Properly and safely lifting and moving patients is an essential provider skill—regardless of level of training.

Historically, many EMS systems have placed personnel on long shifts, often 24 hours or more, to ensure 24-hour emergency coverage. However, as the volume of EMS calls continues to rise, many paramedics are finding themselves physically and mentally tired long before their shift is over. The lack of sleep has also been found to affect the provider's circadian rhythms, causing sleepiness, mental clouding, and lack of energy.[2] These factors can contribute to injury and increase the likelihood of provider injury and illness.[3]

In addition to sleep, nutrition and physical fitness play a role in long-term survival in EMS. Although the fire service has long embraced physical fitness, it has only recently been emphasized in EMS. Obese EMS providers caring for and lifting obese patients is a disaster waiting to happen. As EMS providers, it is time we embrace a healthy lifestyle. However, this decision is one that must be made by each individual.

Basic Physical Fitness

Unfortunately, physical fitness has not been a major emphasis in EMS. In a study of back injuries in EMS workers, researchers found that many EMS providers were significantly overweight. This and a lack of general physical fitness were associated with an increase in back injuries.[4] Another study found that physical fitness and satisfaction with current job assignment were modifiable risk factors associated with improvement of back health among EMS personnel.[5]

The benefits of achieving acceptable physical fitness are well known. They include a decreased resting heart rate and blood pressure, increased oxygen-carrying capacity, increased muscle mass and metabolism, and increased resistance to illness and injury. Exercise also slows the progression of osteoporosis, a condition that affects women more often than men. Quality of life is enhanced by physical fitness, too, because of the ability to do more, and there are positive correlations among fitness, personal appearance, and self-image. Other benefits of physical fitness are improved mental outlook and reduced anxiety levels. Finally, a physically fit body enhances a person's ability to maintain sound motor skills throughout life.

Core Elements

Core elements of physical fitness are muscular strength, cardiovascular endurance (aerobic capacity), and flexibility. As with a three-legged stool, if any one of the three is deficient, the whole becomes unstable. Each is equally important.

Be careful about plunging into a well-intended but

> **CONTENT REVIEW**
>
> ➤ Basics of Physical Fitness
>   - Cardiovascular endurance
>   - Strength and flexibility
>   - Nutrition and weight control
>   - Freedom from addictions
>   - Back safety
> ➤ Eat well, stay fit, and avoid addictive and harmful substances so you have the strength and stamina to do your job.

misguided effort to get into shape. For example, before starting an exercise or stretching regimen, it can be helpful to measure your current state of fitness. There are various methods of assessing the three core elements of fitness. Many EMS agencies have access to facilities where precise assessment methods—with trained personnel—are available. Take advantage of any information available to you.

Muscular strength is achieved with regular exercise that trains muscles to exert force and build endurance. Exercise may be isometric or isotonic. **Isometric exercise** is active exercise performed against stable resistance, where muscles are exercised in a motionless manner. **Isotonic exercise** is active exercise during which muscles are worked through their range of motion. Take time to get in-depth information about the best approach from a trainer or other knowledgeable person.

Weight lifting is an obvious way to achieve muscular strength, and it is excellent all-around training for the body. You can vary the amount of weight lifted, the number of times it is lifted, and the frequency of the demands on the muscle. Whatever type of strength-building exercise is best for you, consider rotating between training the muscles of your upper body and shoulders, muscles of the chest and back, and muscles of the lower body. Do abdominal exercises daily.

Cardiovascular endurance results from exercising at least three days a week vigorously enough to raise your pulse to its target heart rate (Table 4-1). Many people shy away from aerobic exercise, thinking the effort will be too great or the results will take too long. However, there is no need to become a marathon runner to gain aerobic capacity. Try a brisk walk or ride a stationary bike while watching TV. Make it a daily habit.

Even modest exercise programs, which can be done most days of the week, will improve cardiovascular endurance and muscular strength. Walking briskly from the outer reaches of the employee parking lot, using stairs whenever possible, and playing actively with your children can all "count" toward physical fitness.

Table 4-1 Finding Your Target Heart Rate

1. Measure your resting heart rate. (You will use this total later.)

2. Subtract your age from 220. This total is your estimated maximum heart rate.

3. Subtract your resting heart rate from your maximum heart rate, and multiply that figure by 0.7.

4. Add the figure you just calculated to your resting heart rate.

EXAMPLE: For a 44-year-old woman whose resting heart rate is 52, her maximum heart rate would be 176 (220 − 44). Her maximum heart rate minus resting heart rate is 124 (176 − 52). Multiply 124 by 0.7 for a value of 86.8. The resting heart rate plus the calculated figure is 138.8 (52 + 86.8). Rounded up, this person's target heart rate is 140 beats per minute.

Flexibility seems to be the forgotten element of fitness. Without an adequate range of motion, your joints and muscles cannot be used efficiently or safely. A body builder with tight hamstrings may be as much at risk for back injury as anyone else. To achieve (or regain) flexibility, stretch the main muscle groups regularly. Try to stretch daily. Never bounce when stretching; this causes micro tears in muscle and connective tissues. Hold a stretch for at least 60 seconds. A side benefit of good flexibility is prevention or reduction of back pain. Stretching is an excellent TV-time activity. If you are interested, consider studying yoga for improved flexibility.

Nutrition

It is a myth that people in EMS cannot maintain an adequate diet. Even so, the "hit-and-run" nature of emergency care requires planning and awareness of your options. The most difficult part of improving nutrition is altering established bad habits. A change in your behavior requires some commitment and self-discipline, understanding the change process, and patience with what will become long-term self-improvement. Set realistic goals, and understand that backsliding happens. Whatever your goals may be, such as reducing excess weight, gaining weight, or regularly eating more wholesome foods, it is helpful to be able to analyze your progress by using charts or daily intake tallies.

Patho Pearls

Obesity. Obesity has become a major problem in the United States and other industrialized countries. EMS personnel are not immune to this trend. In fact, EMS personnel are becoming, on the average, progressively more overweight. There are several factors inherent in EMS that can contribute to obesity. First, much of EMS work is sedentary. A great deal of time is spent seated in an ambulance or in a station. Second, physical activity on the job is usually limited to short periods of sometimes intense effort. Although these periods of work can be strenuous, they seldom last long enough to provide any significant degree of exercise. Third, the duties of the job often require EMS personnel to "eat on the run," which often means relying on fast food or processed food. These meals provide plenty of "empty calories" and contribute significantly to obesity.

Obesity can lead to numerous health problems, such as back pain, and can place paramedics at increased risk of sustaining a back injury. Obesity can also lead to cardiovascular disease, diabetes, and other long-term chronic problems. As an EMS professional, you must recognize that, to provide the best care for your patients—and to provide a good role model for your patients and the public—you must first care for yourself. This includes watching your weight, finding ways to eat a reasonable diet, and obtaining an adequate amount of exercise. More and more EMS employers are recognizing the obesity epidemic and are developing employee assistance and physical fitness programs designed to minimize the chances of obesity cutting an EMS career short.

FIGURE 4-1 Dietary guidelines from the U.S. Department of Agriculture are summarized in the ChooseMyPlate chart that uses a dinner-plate–shaped chart to represent appropriate food-group portions.

(U.S.Department of Agriculture, www.ChooseMyPlate.gov)

Good nutrition is fundamental to your well-being. The following are dietary guidelines published along with the ChooseMyPlate chart (Figure 4-1) by the U.S. Department of Agriculture.[6]

10 Tips to a Great Plate

1. *Balance calories.* Find out how many calories YOU need for a day. (Go to www.ChooseMyPlate.gov to find your calorie level.) Physical activity also helps balance calories.

2. *Enjoy your food but eat less.* Take the time to enjoy your food as you eat it. Pay attention to hunger and fullness clues.

3. *Avoid oversized portions.* Use a smaller plate. Portion out foods before you eat. When eating out, choose an appetizer-size portion, share a dish, or take some home for later.

4. *Eat certain foods more often.* Eat more fruits and vegetables, whole grains, and fat-free or low-fat dairy products.

5. *Make half your plate fruits and vegetables.* Choose red, orange, and dark green vegetables such as tomatoes, sweet potatoes, and broccoli. Add fruit to meals as part of main or side dishes or dessert.

6. *Switch to fat-free or low-fat (1%) milk.* These have the same nutrients as whole milk but fewer calories and less fat.

7. *Make half your grains whole grains.* Eat whole wheat bread instead of white bread. Eat brown rice instead of white rice. Eat oatmeal instead of a sugary cereal.

8. *Eat some foods less often.* Cut back on foods high in solid fats, added sugars, and salt. These include cakes, cookies, ice cream, candies, sweetened drinks, pizza, and fatty meats such as ribs, sausages, bacon, and hot dogs. Use these foods as occasional treats, not everyday foods.

9. *Compare sodium in foods.* Use the Nutrition Facts label to choose lower sodium versions of foods like soup, bread, and frozen meals. Select canned foods labeled "low sodium," "reduced sodium," or "no salt added."

10. *Drink water instead of sugary drinks.* Cut calories by drinking water or unsweetened beverages. Soda, energy drinks, and sports drinks are a major source of added sugar and calories.

The standardized Nutrition Facts label provides abundant information about nutritional content. Learn to read it. Be sure to check the serving size to avoid misinterpreting the food's overall nutritional value (Figure 4-2).

Eating on the run can be less detrimental if you plan ahead and carry a small cooler filled with whole-grain sandwiches, cut vegetables, fruit, and other wholesome foods. If you must obtain food during your shift, stop at a local market instead of the fast-food place next door. Buy fresh fruit, yogurt, and sensible deli selections. They are more nutritious and much cheaper than fast foods.

Finally, monitor your fluid intake. Your body needs plenty of fluids to flush food through your system and eliminate toxins. Pay attention to what you are drinking. Fill a "go-cup" with fresh ice water when you stop at the

---

CONTENT REVIEW

➤ Dietary Guidelines
  • Enjoy your food but avoid oversize portions.
  • Eat more fruits, vegetables, whole grains, and low-fat dairy items.
  • Eat less sodium and sugar.
➤ Avoid junk foods.

Serving size →
Number of servings per container →
Calories per serving →
Nutrients per serving as actual weight and as a % of daily diet

Nutrition Facts
Serving Size 8 fl oz (240 mL)
Servings Per Container 8

Amount Per Serving

Calories 110 Calories from Fat 0

	% Daily Value*
Total Fat 0g	**0%**
Sodium 0mg	**0%**
Potassium 450mg	**13%**
Total Carbohydrate 26g	**9%**
Sugars 22g	
Protein 2g	

Vitamin C 120% • Calcium 2%
Thiamin 10% • Niacin 4%
Vitamin B6 6% • Folate 15%

Not a significant source of saturated fat, cholesterol, dietary fiber, vitamin A and iron.

* Percent Daily Values are based on a 2,000 calorie diet.

FIGURE 4-2 Example of a standardized food label.

emergency department instead of spending your money on soft drinks. Water is more thirst quenching, cheaper, and much better for you.

Exercising and eating well can help you prevent both cancer and cardiovascular disease. For the typically youthful EMS provider, the likelihood of being hit by either of these diseases may seem remote, but it happens. You can do a lot to prevent these diseases. Minimizing stress through healthy stress management practices, for example, can work wonders. In addition, assess yourself and your family history.

Exercise will improve cardiovascular endurance, help lower blood pressure, and tip the balance of your body composition favorably—all good measures against cardiovascular disease. Know your cholesterol and triglyceride levels and keep them in check. For women who are menopausal, be informed of current research on the risks and benefits of hormone replacement therapy.

Diet can also do much to minimize the chances of getting certain cancers. Certain foods, such as broccoli and high-fiber foods, are thought to help reduce the incidence of cancer; others, such as charcoal-cooked foods, may increase it. The connection between sun exposure and skin cancer is well known. Therefore, take the precaution of using sunblocks, and wear sunglasses and a hat when you can. Watch out for the warning signs of cancer, such as blood in the stools (even in young people, especially men), a changing mole, unexplained weight loss, unexplained chronic fatigue, and lumps.

Be sure to include appropriate periodic risk-assessment screening and self-examination habits in your personal well-being program. That includes tests such as mammograms and prostate exams as you get older.

Habits and Addictions

Many people who work high-stress jobs overuse and abuse substances such as caffeine and nicotine. These bad habits are rampant in EMS. Each can contribute to long-term diseases such as cancer and cardiovascular disease. Choose a healthier life, and avoid overindulging in these and other harmful substances such as alcohol.

Smoking cessation programs are usually easily accessed in local areas or on the Internet. There are abundant approaches to this common addiction, including medications, behavior modification, nicotine replacement therapy ("patches"), aversion therapy, hypnotism, and going "cold turkey." Part of understanding your addiction is knowing whether it is a psychological dependency, sociocultural dependency, or a true physical addiction. Whatever it takes, the message is clear: Free yourself of addictions, particularly those that threaten your well-being. Substance-abuse programs, nicotine patches, 12-step groups, and the like all exist to help you help yourself. But the first step has to be yours.[7]

Legal Considerations

Substance Abuse in EMS. As in the rest of society, substance abuse in EMS is a growing problem. There is no evidence that substance abuse in EMS is any greater than in other professions. However, the subject has been inadequately studied, and we just don't know. Regardless, there has been an increase in media stories about paramedics stealing and abusing controlled substances such as morphine or fentanyl. Often, clandestine drug use such as this adversely affects patient care. The abuser will often remove the desired drug and replace the drug with water or saline. Another paramedic, unaware of the tampering, may administer the medication to a patient. In this case, the patient will not derive any benefit from the drug and could possibly develop a complication such as infection. In addition, if an impaired paramedic is allowed to continue to work, his decision making will ultimately be affected, which can adversely affect patient care.

Paramedics impaired by substance abuse must be immediately removed from patient care responsibilities while an objective investigation is completed. Substance abuse should be considered a medical condition—a disease—and should be treated as such. This attitude is not intended to excuse illegal behavior such as drug tampering, but rather to ensure the paramedic gets the help he needs. States should have a system in which impaired paramedics can self-report their addiction (or be referred) so they can obtain the necessary treatment and possibly salvage their careers. These programs, commonly referred to as *diversion programs*, usually require the impaired provider to enter and complete a substance abuse treatment program. Following completion of the program and other requirements, the paramedic may be allowed to return to work under a very strict surveillance program (called an aftercare contract) that includes periodic medical and addiction assessments, randomized observed drug screens, and, often, participation in 12-step or similar support programs.

Substance abuse is a real problem and must be dealt with swiftly, yet compassionately. However, our first consideration should always be the safety of the patient and of coworkers. Diversion programs must be available in each state to preserve the careers of those suffering substance abuse disorders.

Back Safety

EMS is a physically demanding endeavor. Of the host of movements required—scrambling down embankments, climbing ladders or trees, squeezing into narrow spaces, and so on—none will occur more frequently than lifting and carrying equipment and patients. To avoid back injury, you must keep your back fit for the work you do. You also must use proper lifting techniques each time you pick up a load, whether the load is heavy or light.

Back fitness begins with conditioning the muscles that support the spinal column. These are the "guy wires" that

FIGURE 4-3 Correct standing posture. Note the straight line from the ear through the shoulder, hip, and knee to the arch of the foot.

stabilize the spine, much the way cables help keep telephone poles upright. Note that the muscles of the abdomen are also crucial to overall spinal-column strength and safe lifting. Never perform old-fashioned sit-ups. They can seriously strain your lumbar spine. Instead, use abdominal crunches, which target only the stomach muscles. Consult an exercise coach or trainer for specifics.

Correct posture will minimize the risk of back injury (Figures 4-3 and 4-4). Good nutrition helps to maintain healthy connective tissue and intervertebral disks. Excess weight contributes to disk deterioration. So does smoking. Thus, proper weight management and smoking cessation are relevant to back health. Finally, adequate rest gives the spine non–weight-bearing time to nourish disks and repair itself.

Proper lifting techniques should ideally be taught by and practiced with a trainer who understands the variety of challenges faced by EMS providers.[8] Important principles of lifting are as follows (Figure 4-5):

- Move a load only if you can safely handle it.
- Ask for help when you need it—for *any* reason.
- Position the load as close to your body and center of gravity as possible.
- Keep your palms up whenever possible.

FIGURE 4-4 Correct sitting posture.

- Do not hurry. Take the time you need to establish good footing and balance. Keep a wide base of support, with one foot ahead of the other.
- Bend your knees, lower your buttocks, and keep your chin up. If your knees are bad, do not bend them more than 90 degrees.
- "Lock in" the spine with a slight extension curve, and tighten the abdominal muscles to support spinal positioning.

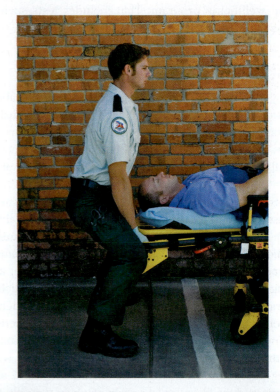

FIGURE 4-5 For back safety, always employ the important principles of lifting.

- Always avoid twisting and turning.
- Let the large leg muscles, not your back, do the work of lifting.
- Exhale during the lift. Do not hold your breath.
- Given a choice, push. Do not pull.
- Use help when moving patients up and down stairs and into and out of the ambulance.
- Look where you are walking or crawling. If you are walking, take only short steps. Move forward rather than backward whenever possible.
- When rescuers are working together as a team to lift a load, only one person should be in charge of verbal commands.

Heed your own body's signals. You are stronger on some days than on others. Know when you are physically depleted from exhaustion, lack of food, or minor illness. Use volunteers as helpers wisely, and be sure to ask whether their backs are strong enough for the job.

Never reach for an item and twist at the same time. Most back injuries occur because of the cumulative effect of such low-level everyday stresses. Everything you do on behalf of back safety adds up to choices that can mean the difference between a long and rewarding career in EMS, or one shortened by an injury. Be careful!

Personal Protection from Disease

In recent years, the emphasis on infection control has focused on the most devastating diseases, such as HIV/AIDS, hepatitis B, hepatitis C, tuberculosis, and influenza—and rightly so. There is enough risk in EMS without having to worry about dying of a disease you caught while caring for others. Fortunately, you can do a lot to minimize your risk of infection. A good first step is to develop a habit of doing the things promoted in this chapter. Eating well, getting adequate rest, and managing stress are among the building blocks of a good defense against infection. In addition, it is a good idea to periodically assess your risk for infection, such as noticing when you are run down or when your hands are dangerously chapped.

Infectious Diseases

Infectious diseases are caused by **pathogens** such as bacteria and viruses, which may be spread from person to person. For example, infection by way of bloodborne pathogens can occur when the blood of an infected person comes in contact with another person's broken skin (cuts, sores, chapped hands) or by way of parenteral contact (stick by a needle or other sharp object). Infection by airborne pathogens can occur when an infected person sneezes or coughs, causing body fluids in the form of tiny droplets to be inhaled or to come in contact with the mucous membranes of another person's eyes, nose, or mouth.

HIV/AIDS, hepatitis B, hepatitis C, and tuberculosis are diseases of great concern because they are life threatening. However, one may be exposed to many different infectious diseases. See Table 4-2 for some common ones, their modes of transmission, and their **incubation periods**.

New and emerging diseases also can pose threats to EMS personnel. International travel now allows individuals to move quickly between continents—sometimes bringing endemic diseases with them. In some instances, EMS personnel can inadvertently be exposed to rare and deadly diseases. Such was the case in 2004 when EMS providers in Dallas were exposed to the deadly Ebola virus in a patient who had recently flown from Liberia to Dallas and who then, feeling ill, had called EMS. Because of this and other such outbreaks—now more than ever—it is essential that EMS personnel receive training in disease prevention strategies and that they have the necessary equipment when suspect patients are encountered.

Even when someone is carrying pathogens for disease, signs of an illness may not be apparent. For this reason, *you must consider the blood and body fluids of every patient you treat as infectious.* Safeguards against infection are mandatory for all medical personnel.

Standard Safety Precautions

Each profession has its occupational hazards and risks. EMS is no different. EMS straddles the disciplines of health care and public safety and the associated risks of both. Anything you do as a paramedic should start with considerations about minimizing risk for you, your patient, your partners, other responders, and the community. Various strategies for this are discussed in detail in this chapter.

Infection Control Measures

Infection control practices are those procedures and practices used by health care personnel to minimize disease transmission and transmission of infectious agents. Infection control is a fundamental tenet of health care and must be practiced proficiently by all EMS personnel.

Table 4-2 Common Infectious Diseases

Disease	Mode of Transmission	Incubation Period
AIDS (acquired immune deficiency syndrome)	AIDS- or HIV-infected blood via intravenous drug use, semen and vaginal fluids, blood transfusions, or (rarely) needle sticks. Mothers also may pass HIV to their unborn children.	Several months or years
Hepatitis B, C	Blood, stool, or other body fluids, or contaminated objects.	Weeks or months
Tuberculosis	Respiratory secretions, airborne, or on contaminated objects.	2 to 6 weeks
Meningitis, bacterial	Oral and nasal secretions.	2 to 10 days
Pneumonia, bacterial and viral	Oral and nasal droplets and secretions.	Several days
Influenza	Airborne droplets, or direct contact with body fluids.	1 to 3 days
Staphylococcal skin infections	Contact with open wounds or sores or contaminated objects.	Several days
Chicken pox (varicella)	Airborne droplets, or contact with open sores.	11 to 21 days
German measles (rubella)	Airborne droplets. Mothers may pass it to unborn children.	10 to 12 days
Whooping cough (pertussis)	Respiratory secretions or airborne droplets.	6 to 20 days
SARS (severe acute respiratory syndrome)	Airborne droplets and personal contact.	4 to 6 days

Standard Precautions

Standard Precautions are strategies that include the major features of what were once called universal precautions (UP)—blood and body fluid precautions designed to reduce the risk of transmission of bloodborne pathogens—and body substance isolation (BSI)—precautions designed to reduce the risk of transmission of pathogens from moist body substances. Standard Precautions apply UP and BSI concepts to all patients receiving care regardless of their diagnosis or presumed infection status. Standard Precautions apply to:

- Blood
- All body fluids, secretions, and excretions except sweat, regardless of whether or not they contain visible blood
- Nonintact skin
- Mucous membranes

Standard Precautions are designed to reduce the risk of transmission of microorganisms from both recognized and unrecognized sources of infection in hospitals.

Standard Precautions dictate that all EMS personnel take the same (standard) precautions with every patient. To achieve this, appropriate **personal protective equipment (PPE)** should be available in every emergency vehicle. The minimum recommended PPE are the following:

- *Protective gloves.* Wear disposable protective gloves before initiating any emergency care. When an emergency involves more than one patient, change gloves between patients. When gloves have been contaminated, remove and dispose of them properly as soon as possible (Figure 4-6).

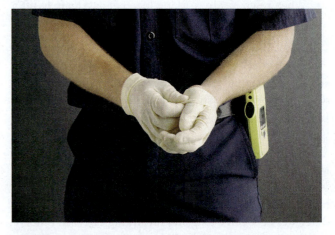

FIGURE 4-6A To remove gloves, first hook the gloved fingers of one hand under the cuff of the other glove. Then pull that glove off without letting your gloved fingers come in contact with bare skin.

FIGURE 4-6B Then slide the fingers of the ungloved hand under the remaining glove's cuff. Push that glove off, being careful not to touch the glove's exterior with your bare hand.

FIGURE 4-7 Proper gloves, mask, and eyewear prevent a patient's blood and body fluids from contacting a break in your skin or spraying into your eyes, nose, or mouth. (A) Combined mask and eye shield; (B) Mask and protective eyewear.

- *Masks and protective eyewear.* (Figure 4-7). These should be worn together whenever blood spatter is likely to occur, such as with arterial bleeding, childbirth, endotracheal intubation and other invasive procedures, oral suctioning, and cleanup of equipment that requires heavy scrubbing or brushing. Both you and your patient should wear masks whenever the potential for airborne transmission of disease exists.

- *HEPA and N-95 respirators.* (Figure 4-8). Because of the resurgence of tuberculosis (TB), you must protect yourself from infection through the use of a high-efficiency particulate air (HEPA) or N-95 respirator. Wear one whenever you care for a patient with confirmed or suspected TB. This is especially true during procedures that involve the airway, such as the administration of nebulized medications, endotracheal intubation, or suctioning.

- *Gowns.* Disposable gowns protect your clothing from splashes. If large splashes of blood are expected, such as with childbirth, wear an impervious gown.

- *Resuscitation equipment.* Use disposable resuscitation equipment as your primary means of artificial ventilation in emergency care. Such items should be used once, and then disposed of properly.[9]

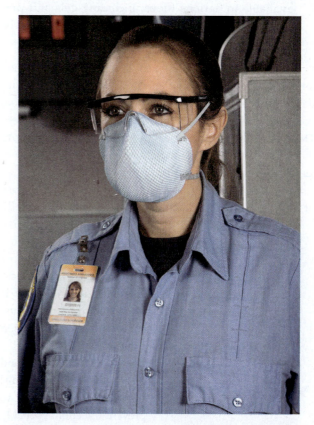

FIGURE 4-8A A high-efficiency particulate air (HEPA) respirator. .

FIGURE 4-8B An N-95 respirator.

- *Hand-washing supplies.* Non–water-based hand-washing solutions should be widely available for EMS personnel. These alcohol-based hand sanitizers are available in various forms, including gels and pre-wrapped hand towels. The prewrapped towels can be kept in a pocket for ready use.

The garments and equipment described previously are intended to protect against infection through contact with both potentially contaminated body substances, such as blood, vomit, and urine, and other agents such as airborne droplets. These garments and equipment will assist you in achieving, to the extent possible, the precautions recommended by the Centers for Disease Control and Prevention (CDC).

Infectious diseases also are minimized through the use of appropriate work practices and equipment especially engineered to minimize risk. For example, most invasive equipment is now used on a one-time, disposable basis. Of course, it is important to launder reusable clothing with infection control in mind.

General cleanliness and appropriate personal hygiene will do much to prevent infection. Probably the most important infection

FIGURE 4-9 To wash your hands properly, lather up well and be sure to scrub under your nails. When you rinse off your hands, point them downward so that soap and water run off away from your arms and body.

control practice is handwashing (Figure 4-9). As soon as possible after every patient contact and decontamination procedure, thoroughly wash your hands. To do so, first remove any rings or jewelry from your hands and arms. Then use soap and water. Lather your hands vigorously front and back for at least 15 seconds up to 2 or 3 inches above the wrist. Be sure to lather and rub between your fingers and in the creases and cracks of your knuckles. Scrub under and around the fingernails with a brush. Rinse your hands well under running water, holding your hands downward so that the water drains off your fingertips. Dry your hands on a clean towel.

Plain soap works perfectly well for handwashing. At those times when soap is not available, you might use an antimicrobial handwashing solution or an alcohol-based foam or towelette.

Ebola Virus Disease

The appearance of the Ebola virus in the United States in 2014 brought a new level of infectious disease threat to EMS providers. The Ebola virus is the causative agent of Ebola virus disease (EVD), formerly called Ebola hemorrhagic fever. People can contract EVD (through broken

CONTENT REVIEW

➤ Handwashing
- Lather with soap and water.
- Scrub for at least 15 seconds.
- Rinse under running water.
- Dry on a clean towel.

➤ Handwashing is perhaps the most important infection control practice.

skin or mucous membranes in, for example, the eyes, nose, or mouth) by direct contact with:

- Blood or body fluids (including but not limited to urine, saliva, sweat, feces, vomit, breast milk, and semen) of a person who is sick with or has died from EVD
- Objects (such s needles and syringes) that have been contaminated with body fluids from a person who is sick with EVD or the body of a person who has died from EVD
- Infected fruit bats or primates (apes and monkeys)
- Possibly, semen from a man who has recovered from EVD (for example, by having oral, vaginal, or anal sex).

Standard PPE alone is not sufficient to ensure protection from EVD. For protection from possible EVD the PPE must be such that no skin is exposed. Recommended PPE for EVD includes:

- *PAPR (powered air purifying respirator) or N95 respirator.* If a NIOSH-certified PAPR and a NIOSH-certified disposable N95 respirator are used in local protocols, ensure compliance, including fit testing, medical evaluation, and training of the health care worker.
  - *PAPR:* PAPR with a full face shield, helmet, or headpiece. Any reusable helmet or headpiece must be covered with a single-use (disposable) hood that extends to the shoulders, fully covers the neck, and is compatible with the selected PAPR. The facility should follow the manufacturer's instructions for decontamination of all reusable components and, based on those instructions, develop local protocols that include the designation of responsible personnel who ensure that the equipment is appropriately reprocessed and that batteries are fully charged before reuse.
    - A PAPR with a self-contained filter and blower unit integrated inside the helmet is preferred.
    - A PAPR with an external belt-mounted blower unit requires adjustment of the sequence for donning and doffing.
  - *N95 Respirator:* Single-use (disposable) N95 respirator in combination with single-use (disposable) surgical hood extending to shoulders and single-use (disposable) full face shield. If N95 respirators are used instead of PAPRs, careful observation is required to ensure that health care workers are not inadvertently touching their faces under the face shield during patient care.
- *Single-use (disposable) fluid-resistant or impermeable gown that extends to at least mid-calf or coverall without integrated hood.* Coveralls with or without integrated socks are acceptable. Consideration should be given to selecting gowns or coveralls with thumb hooks to secure sleeves over inner gloves. If gowns or coveralls

with thumb hooks are not available, personnel may consider taping the sleeve of the gown or coverall over the inner glove to prevent potential skin exposure from separation between sleeve and inner glove during activity. However, if taping is used, care must be taken to remove tape gently. Experience in some facilities suggests that taping may increase risk by making the doffing process more difficult and cumbersome.

- *Single-use (disposable) nitrile examination gloves with extended cuffs.* Two pairs of gloves should be worn. At a minimum, outer gloves should have extended cuffs.
- *Single-use (disposable), fluid-resistant or impermeable boot covers that extend to at least mid-calf or single-use (disposable) shoe covers.* Boot and shoe covers should allow for ease of movement and not present a slip hazard to the worker.
  - *Single-use (disposable) fluid-resistant or impermeable shoe covers* are acceptable only if they will be used in combination with a coverall with integrated socks.
- *Single-use (disposable), fluid-resistant or impermeable apron that covers the torso to the level of the mid-calf should be used if patients with EVD have vomiting or diarrhea.* An apron provides additional protection against exposure of the front of the body to body fluids or excrement. If a PAPR will be worn, consider selecting an apron that ties behind the neck to facilitate easier removal during the doffing procedure.

The CDC provides recommendations for PPE protection levels for EMS personnel based on a threat level determined by two major factors:

- The PPE wearer's possible exposure to Ebola
- Proximity to symptomatic patients (Table 4-3)

Table 4-3 Ebola PPE Protection

Patient's Ebola Exposure Level	Definition
Known or suspected exposure	Known disease, known contact with Ebola patient or travel within 21 days to an area with current Ebola cases
Possible exposure	Environmental or interpersonal exposure in an area with suspect or recent cases, except as outlined in previous box
No known exposure	No known exposure to EVD patients or travel to areas with a known outbreak of the disease

Signs/Symptoms	Definition
Asymptomatic	No symptoms relevant to an infectious disease.
Fever	Measured temperature ≥ 100.4°F.
Body fluids	Patient has fever with vomiting, diarrhea, blood in vomitus and/or feces, is incontinent of urine or stool, or is sweating, salivating, or otherwise producing blood and body fluids to which emergency responders could be exposed.

Vaccinations and Screening Tests

Immunizations against many illnesses are available. Get them. Even "nuisance" illnesses can be avoided if you get vaccinated. Immunizations that are available include those for rubella (German measles), measles, mumps, chicken pox, and other childhood diseases, as well as for tetanus/diphtheria, polio, influenza, hepatitis A, hepatitis B, and Lyme disease. Some, such as tetanus, may require booster shots periodically, so monitor your personal medical history well. Also arrange for routine tuberculosis (TB) screenings and record the results.

Influenza kills thousands of people each year. Some strains of influenza, such as H1N1 (swine flu) or H5N1 (bird flu), can quickly reach pandemic or epidemic states. Health care workers will be among the first to be exposed to novel viruses. Because of this, EMS personnel and other emergency responders are often the first to receive vaccines when a virus becomes a threat. It is important for EMS personnel to follow warnings and recommendations from the World Health Organization (WHO), the Centers for Disease Control and Prevention (CDC), and state and local public health officials.

Decontamination of Equipment

Any PPE designed for a single use should be properly disposed of after use. The same is true of contaminated medical devices designed for a single use. Such materials should be discarded in a red bag marked with a biohazard seal (Figure 4-10a). Needles and other sharp objects should be discarded in properly labeled, puncture-proof containers (Figure 4-10b). Once an item is placed in the appropriate container, the container should be disposed of according to local guidelines.

Nondisposable equipment that has been contaminated must be cleaned, disinfected, or sterilized:

- *Cleaning.* **Cleaning** refers to washing an object with soap and water. After caring for a patient, wash your work areas thoroughly with approved soaps. Throw away single-use cleaning supplies in a proper biohazard container.

- *Disinfection.* **Disinfection** means cleaning with a disinfecting agent, which should kill many microorganisms on the surface of an object. Disinfect equipment that had direct contact with the intact skin of a patient, such as backboards and splints. Use a commercial disinfectant or bleach diluted in water (one part bleach to 10 parts water), or follow local guidelines.

- *Sterilization.* **Sterilization** is the use of a chemical or a physical method such as pressurized steam to kill all microorganisms on an object. Items that were inserted into the patient's body (a laryngoscope blade, for example) should be sterilized by heat, steam, or radiation. There are also EPA-approved solutions for sterilization.

FIGURE 4-10A Dispose of biohazardous wastes in a bag that is properly marked.

FIGURE 4-10B Discard needles and other sharp objects in a properly labeled, puncture-proof container.

If your equipment needs more extensive cleaning, bag it and remove it to an area designated for this purpose. Disposable work gloves worn during cleaning and decontamination should be properly discarded. If your clothing has become contaminated, bag the items and wash them in accordance with local guidelines. After removing contaminated clothing, take a shower before dressing again.

Post-Exposure Procedures

By definition, an **exposure** is any occurrence of blood or body fluids coming in contact with nonintact skin or the eyes or other mucous membranes or by parenteral contact

INFECTIOUS DISEASE EXPOSURE PROCEDURE

Airborne Infection Such as TB (Tuberculosis)	Bloodborne Infection Such as HIV (AIDS virus) or HBV (Hepatitis B virus)
You transport a patient who is infected with a life-threatening airborne disease, such as TB, but you are not aware that the patient is infected.	You come into contact with blood or body fluids of a patient, and you wonder if that patient is infected with a life-threatening bloodborne disease such as HIV or HBV.
The medical facility diagnoses the disease in the patient you transported.	You seek immediate medical attention and document the incident for worker's compensation.
The medical facility must notify your designated officer within 48 hours.	You ask your designated officer to determine if you have been exposed to an infectious disease.
Your designated officer notifies you that you have been exposed.	Your designated officer (DO) must gather information and, if DO determines it is warranted, consult the medical facility to which the patient was transported.
Your employer arranges for you to be evaluated and followed up by a doctor or other appropriate health care professional.	The medical facility must gather information and report findings to your designated officer within 48 hours. Your DO notifies you of the findings.

FIGURE 4-11 A federal regulation called the Ryan White Comprehensive AIDS Resources Emergency (CARE) Act outlines procedures to follow after an occupational exposure to human immunodeficiency virus (HIV), hepatitis B, diphtheria, meningitis, plague, hemorrhagic fever, rabies, and tuberculosis.

(needle stick). In most areas, an EMS provider who has had an exposure should (Figure 4-11):

- Immediately wash the affected area with soap and water.
- Get a medical evaluation.
- Take the proper immunization boosters.
- Notify the agency's infection control liaison.
- Document the circumstances surrounding the exposure, including the actions taken to reduce chances of infection.

In general, the EMS provider should cooperate with the incident investigation and comply with all required reporting responsibilities and time frames.

Death and Dying

Most paramedics agree that of all out-of-hospital situations, those involving death or dying are among the most personally uncomfortable and challenging. There are many reasons for this. Of course, a death is normally a sad event. There is an air of unalterability, of finality. Each person experiences a death in an individual way because of that person's prior experiences of loss, coping skills, religious convictions, and other personal background. Paramedics encounter death much more frequently than most other people do. They often see it as it happens. This can lead to a cumulative sense of overload, which the smart paramedic recognizes and deals with in

Cultural Considerations

Responses to Death. The emotional response to the death of a friend or family member varies significantly among cultures as well as among individuals. Some people will accept the news quietly, whereas others will react with an emotional outburst. Use simple terms and avoid euphemisms. Realize that grieving is a cultural as well as a personal phenomenon, and that it is normal for people to respond to bad news in different ways.

a healthy manner through appropriate grief work and stress management.

Loss, Grief, and Mourning

For decades, discussing death and dying openly was difficult because of cultural taboos. This began to change when pioneer Elisabeth Kübler-Ross braved the backlash to meet with terminally ill hospital patients to discuss their feelings about death and dying.[10] Before then, it was assumed dying people did not want to talk about the experience. Kübler-Ross found that there are five predictable stages of grief:

- *Denial, or "Not me."* This is an inability or refusal to believe the reality of impending death. It is a defense mechanism, during which the patient puts off dealing with the inevitable end of life.

- *Anger, or "Why me?"* The patient's anger is really frustration related to his inability to control the situation. That anger could focus on anyone or anything.

- *Bargaining, or "Okay, but first let me . . ."* In the patient's mind, he tries to make a deal to "buy additional time" to put off or change the expected outcome.

- *Depression, or "Okay, but I haven't . . ."* The patient is sad and despairing, often mourning things not accomplished and dreams that will not come true. The patient withdraws or retreats into a private world, unwilling to communicate with others.

- *Acceptance, or "Okay, I'm not afraid."* The patient may come to realize his fate and achieve a reasonable level of comfort with the anticipated outcome. At this stage, the family may need more support than the patient does.

CONTENT REVIEW

➤ Stages of Grief
- Denial
- Anger
- Bargaining
- Depression
- Acceptance

A person experiencing any significant loss usually works through these stages, given enough time. Although there is a tendency to progress from one stage to the next in order, both dying patients and

their loved ones experience the stages in their own unique ways. They may jump around among the stages, they may go back and forth, or they may never finish them. It is important for you to remain flexible, so you can decide how best to help, if asked.

Because paramedics encounter death and dying often, there is a mistaken belief that they handle it better. However, paramedics are human, too. Let yourself deal with death and dying when they occur. Do not shirk the support of friends and family. Do not try to "tough it out." Use every opportunity to process a specific incident in a healthy manner by appropriately grieving losses that have an impact on you.

Grief is a feeling. Mourning is a process. A grieving person feels mostly sadness or distress. A person in mourning is immersed in the process of undergoing, perhaps displaying, and ultimately dissipating the feelings of grief. The sense of loss is predictably most intense immediately after the news is received. Although numerous models for the mourning process exist, a good rule of thumb is that after the loss of a close friend or relative, a period of one year of mourning is normal.

On initially hearing the news of a death, a person experiences a paralyzing, totally incapacitating surge of grief that is exactly comparable to the incapacitating pain of an acute blow to an eye or testicle—in that the whole world shrinks down to that acute pain. Typically, the feeling lasts for 5 to 15 minutes. When you deliver the news of a death, remember that a survivor cannot function during this grief spike. After delivering the news, wait until it is past and the survivor is ready and able to receive information and make decisions.

A period of intense feelings that continues for around four to six weeks follows the grief spike. Feelings may include loss, anger, resentment, sadness, and even guilt, depending on the relationship and the circumstances surrounding the death. Gradually, the intensity and immediacy of the loss fade into a phase dominated by a sense of loneliness, which lasts about six months. Finally, a period of recovery usually ensues. The survivor begins to view the loss more objectively and rediscovers an interest in living. Key to the process of mourning is the passage of significant dates and anniversaries, such as birthdays, holidays, and the monthly (then annual) date when the loss occurred.

People cope in various ways with difficult moments such as death. If you are dealing with a child, understand that children's perceptions are different from an adult's. (See Table 4-4 for a summary.) This is true of all the special populations you will encounter, such as the elderly and people with mental disabilities. The elderly, for example, may be particularly concerned about the effects of the loss on other family members, about further loss of their own independence, and about the costs of a funeral and burial.

Table 4-4 Needs and Expectations of Children Regarding Death

Age Range	Characteristics	Suggestions
Newborn to age 3	Senses that something has happened in the family, and notices that there is much activity in the household. Realizes that people are crying and sad. Watch for irritability and changes in eating, sleeping, or other behavioral patterns.	Be sensitive to the child's needs. Try to maintain consistency in routines. Maintain consistency with significant people in child's life.
Ages 3 to 6	Believes death is a temporary state, and may ask continually when the person will return. Believes in magical thinking, and may feel responsible for the death or that it is punishment for own behavior. May be fearful of catching the same illness and die, or may believe that everyone else he loves will die also. Watch for changes in behavior patterns with friends and at school, difficulty sleeping, and changes in eating habits.	Emphasize that the child was not responsible for the death. Reinforce that when people are sad, they cry, and that crying is normal and natural. Encourage the child to talk about and/or draw pictures of his feelings, or to cry.
Ages 6 to 9	May prefer to hide or disguise feelings to avoid looking babyish. Is afraid significant others will die. Seeks out detailed explanations for death, and differences between fatal illness and "just being sick." Has an understanding that death is real, but may believe that those who die are too slow, weak, or stupid. Fantasizes in an effort to make everything the way it was. Denial is the most helpful coping skill.	Talk about the normal feelings of anger, sadness, and guilt. Share your own feelings about death. Do not be afraid to cry in front of the child. This and other expressions of loss help to give the child permission to express his feelings.
Ages 9 to 12	Begins to understand the irreversibility of death. May seek details and specifics of the situation, and may need repeated, explicit explanations. Hard-won sense of independence becomes fragile, and may show concern about the practical matters of his lifestyle. May try to act "adult," but then regress to earlier stage of emotional response. When threatened, expresses anger toward the ill/deceased, himself, or other survivors.	Set aside time to talk about feelings. Encourage sharing of memories to facilitate grief response.
Ages 12 to 18	Demanding developmental processes are an awkward fit with the need to take on different family roles. Retreats to safety of childhood. Feels pressure to act as an adult, while still coping with skills of a child. Suppresses feelings in order to "fit in," leaving teen isolated and vulnerable.	Encourage talking, but respect need for privacy. See if a trusted, reliable friend or adult can provide appropriate support. Locate support group for teens.

There are a wide variety of responses to death among different peoples and cultures as well. Be flexible, and be ready for anything.

What to Say

As "Do Not Resuscitate" orders and other out-of-hospital death situations increase, EMS personnel are more often placed in the position of telling people that someone has died. It would be nice to have a script for those difficult moments, but the reality is that you have to assess the scene and the people in each situation to determine the safest and most compassionate way to deliver the sad news.

In terms of safety, you never know how people will respond, even if you know them. Most people accept the news quietly. However, some allow their grief to flood out of them in very physical ways, such as throwing things, kicking walls, screaming, or running in circles. Before speaking to any survivors, consciously position yourself between them and the door or other escape route. Remember, initially the grief spike has its grip on the survivors. There is little you can do but give them a safe, private place to get through it. Also, for safety, do not deliver the news to a large group. Ask the primary people (no more than four or five) to step aside with you to a private place. Let them tell the others in their own way.

Find out who is who among the survivors. Do not make assumptions. Then address the closest survivor, preferably in a way that shows compassion. That is, avoid standing above the survivor. Instead, sit or squat so that your eyes are at the same level. If the survivor is alone, call for a friend, neighbor, clergy member, or relative. If possible, wait to tell the survivor the news until that person has arrived.

Introduce yourself by name and function ("My name is Kate. I'm a paramedic with MedicWest EMS.") A careful choice of words is helpful. Although it may seem blunt, use the words "dead" and "died," rather than euphemisms that may be misinterpreted or misunderstood. Use gentle eye contact and, if appropriate, the comforting power of touching an arm or holding a hand. Basic elements of your message should include the following:

- A loved one has died.

- There is nothing more anyone could have done.

- You and your EMS service are available to assist the survivors if needed. (Sometimes, medical emergencies occur in survivors in the wake of such stressful news.)

- Give information about local procedures for out-of-hospital death, such as the inspection of the scene by the medical examiner or coroner, and so on.

Do not include statements about God's will or relief from pain or any subjective assumption. You do not know the people well enough to know the details about their relationship or their religious preferences.[11]

When It Is Someone You Know

Many paramedics serve in small communities where calls often involve people they know. Some elements of this are rewarding, and others are heart-wrenching. People may be greatly relieved to see a familiar, trusted face among the ambulance crew. There also is a lot of support for paramedics in small communities, because you are from the community itself and are there to help fellow community members during their most fearful moments. However, being involved when the life of someone you know is threatened—or lost—can have a powerful impact on your own emotions. If it is too much, you must find a way to manage the stress. Often, you must grieve as well. Your well-being demands it.

Legal Considerations

Field Pronouncements. It has been well established that victims of blunt trauma who are pulseless on EMS arrival have virtually no chance of survival, and treatment efforts are almost always futile. Because of this, many EMS systems have established a policy whereby pulseless victims of blunt trauma are not treated or transported by EMS. Likewise, as more is learned about cardiac arrest resuscitation, it is apparent that there is virtually no benefit to be gained from hospital transport of patients who have received full advanced cardiac life support (ACLS) measures in the field but have not been resuscitated. There are always exceptions, such as pediatric cases and hypothermia. However, more and more paramedics will find themselves, in consultation with medical control, terminating resuscitative efforts in the field.

Field pronouncement can be a touchy situation. The general public is under the mistaken impression that patients are not dead until they arrive at a hospital and a physician pronounces them dead. When you make a field pronouncement, always let the family know that all appropriate measures were provided but failed. Also, let them know that the decision to terminate resuscitative efforts was made by a physician. Do not bring up such topics as "not transporting saves money" or not transporting "keeps the ambulance available for others," as most family members will not have the capacity to appreciate the benefit of these in their time of grief. The principal task in field pronouncements is to provide the family adequate information, help them with their grief to the extent possible, and activate their personal support system (e.g., friends, neighbors, clergy members).

Stress and Stress Management

Many aspects of EMS are stressful.[12] A time-honored definition of **stress**, according to stress researcher Hans Selye, is "the nonspecific response of the body to any demand."[13] The word *stress* also refers to a hardship or strain, or to a physical or emotional response to such a stimulus. Stress responses are natural reactions that help the organism adapt to a new environment or a sudden change in the usual environment. Stress results from the interaction of events and the capabilities of each individual to adjust to those events. A person's reactions to stressful events are individual and are affected by that person's previous exposure to the stress-causing event, perception of the event, general life experience, and personal coping skills. A stimulus that causes stress is known as a **stressor**.

Stress is both beneficial and detrimental. Stress is usually understood to generate a negative effect, or *distress*, in an individual. There is also "good" stress, which is called *eustress* (for example, seeing a lost loved one for the first time in years). Even eustress, however, generates physiological and psychological signs and symptoms.

Adapting to stress is a dynamic, evolving process. As a person adapts, he uses or develops any or all of the following:

- *Defensive strategies.* Though sometimes helpful for the short term, defensive strategies may deny or distort the reality of a stressful situation.

- *Coping.* This is an active process of confronting the stressful situation. By acknowledging the existence of stressors, the patient is able to gather information about them and then change or adjust as necessary. Coping may or may not serve as the best strategy for the long term, however.

- *Problem-solving skills.* These skills are regarded as the healthiest approach to everyday concerns. They involve problem analysis, which generates options for action, and determination of a course of action. Mastery—reflected in the ability to recognize multiple options and potential solutions for stressful situations—generally comes only as a result of extensive experience with similar situations.

EMS practice, of course, involves abundant stressors, which provide ample opportunities for the development of problem-solving skills. There are administrative stressors, such as waiting for calls, shift work, loud pagers, and inadequate pay. There are scene-related stressors, such as violent and abusive people, flying debris, vomit, loud noises, and chaos. There are emotional and physical stressors, such as fear, angry bystanders, abusive patients, frustration, exhaustion, hunger or thirst, and lifting heavy objects.

Environmental stress may be provided by siren noise, inclement weather, confined workspaces, and the frequent urgent need for rapid scene responses and life-or-death decisions. In addition, the often-difficult world of EMS can strain a paramedic's family relationships and may also lead to conflicts with supervisors and coworkers. Add this to some personality traits commonly found among paramedics, such as a strong need to be liked and often unrealistically high self-expectations, and the combination can lead to disturbing feelings of guilt or anxiety. All these stressors and stress responses take a toll on the paramedic.

To help you manage your own stress, you should learn these things:

- *Your personal stressors.* Each person has an individual list. What is stressful to you may be enjoyable to someone else. What was stressful to you last year may be replaced by new stressors this year.

- *The amount of stress you can take before it becomes a problem.* Stress occurs in a tornado-like continuum. It may start with a few breezes, but it can increase in force until it is whirling out of control. Stopping the "storm" early is key to your well-being. You need to know which stress responses are early indicators for you so you can deal with them at that point.

- *Stress management strategies that work for you.* Again, this is totally individual. Those who seek personal well-being must become well versed about personally appropriate stress management options.

Adapting to stressors is a dynamic process of receiving, processing, and dissipating stressors and their effects. You bring your life experience, temperament, emotional maturity, spiritual convictions, habits (good and bad), interpersonal skills, ability to be self-aware, gender, and recent activity to each moment of adapting to the world. If a person experiences a pile-on of stressor after stressor without regard for the consequences, the results are likely to be bad. In fact, the U.S. Surgeon General once estimated that stress-related diseases kill 80 percent of people who die of nontraumatic causes. Stress-related disease is avoidable if you make a habit of doing what is necessary to preserve your personal well-being. (Specific stress management techniques will be discussed later.)

Phases of Stress Response

There are three phases of a stress response: *alarm*, *resistance*, and *exhaustion*. At the end there may be a period of rest and recovery.

- *Stage I: Alarm.* The alarm phase is the "fight-or-flight" phenomenon. It occurs when the body physically and rapidly prepares to defend itself against a perceived threat. The pituitary gland begins by releasing adrenocorticotropic (stress) hormones. Hormones continue to flood the body via the autonomic nervous system, coordinated by the hypothalamus. Epinephrine and norepinephrine from the adrenal glands increase heart rate and blood pressure, dilate pupils, increase blood sugar, slow digestion, and relax the bronchial tree. These alarm-stage responses end when the event is recognized as not dangerous.

- *Stage II: Resistance.* This stage starts when the individual begins to cope with the stress. Over time, an individual may become desensitized or adapted to stressors. Physiological parameters, such as pulse and blood pressure, may then return to normal.

- *Stage III: Exhaustion.* Prolonged exposure to the same stressors leads to exhaustion of an individual's ability to resist and adapt. Resistance to all stressors declines. Susceptibility to physical and psychological ailments increases. A period of rest and recovery is necessary for a healthy outcome.

It would be great if we could manage each stressor to the point of recovery before the next one hits, but of course that is not how it works. Typically, people are still dealing with one stress (or the same ongoing one, such as the chronic stress of shift work) when additional stressors pile on, resulting in cumulative stress. If stress accumulates without intervention, the consequences can be serious.

Stress also helps us to function optimally. In fact, heightened stress levels improve our ability to function. You have surely experienced this phenomenon. For example, you are awakened from your sleep to respond to a motor vehicle collision. When you arrive on scene you find several critical patients. Although you may still be sleepy when you are first called to the scene, the stress responses heighten your alertness and your ability to perform the needed skills and procedures (Figure 4-12).

> **CONTENT REVIEW**
> - Phases of a Stress Response
>   - Alarm
>   - Resistance
>   - Exhaustion
> - Identify your own personal stressors and find out what stress management techniques work for you.

FIGURE 4-12 Phases of stress response.

(Adapted from J. Mitchell and G. Bray's Emergency Services Stress. Englewood Cliffs, NJ: Prentice Hall, 1990, p. 11)

Shift Work

There will always be shift work in EMS. Because EMS is a 24-hour, 7-days-a-week endeavor, someone must be functional at all times. But working odd hours is inherently stressful because of disruptions in the biorhythms of the body that are known as circadian rhythms and because of sleep deprivation.

Circadian rhythms are biological cycles that occur at approximately 24-hour intervals. These include hormonal and body temperature fluctuations, appetite and sleepiness cycles, and other bodily processes. When life patterns disrupt the circadian rhythms, such as with extensive travel between time zones, the biological effects can be stressful. Sleep deprivation is common among people who work at night. The inherent dangers to paramedics are clear. A recent study estimated that up to 20 percent of fatal crashes resulted from driver fatigue. The hours at which fatigue-related collisions most often occur are between 2:00 AM and 6:00 AM (early morning) and between 2:00 PM and 4:00 PM (midafternoon), when our circadian rhythm is at its lowest points. Males ages 18 to 30 are in the high-risk category. They tend to be overconfident about their driving ability and believe they can handle the situation. Women are less likely to be involved in fatigue-related crashes.[14]

If you work at night and have to sleep in the daytime, here are some tips to minimize the stress:

- Sleep in a cool, dark place that mimics the nighttime environment.
- Stick to sleeping at your **anchor time** (time you can rest without interruption), even on days off. Do not try to revert to a daytime lifestyle on days off. For example, if you work 9 PM to 5 AM and your anchor time is 8 AM to 12 noon, then go to bed "early" on days off and on workdays sleep from 8 AM to 3 PM.
- Unwind appropriately after a shift to rest well. Do not eat a heavy meal or exercise right before bedtime.
- Post a "day sleeper" sign on your front door, turn off your phone's ringer, and lower the volume of the answering machine.

Signs of Stress

A variety of factors can trigger a stress response. They include the loss of something valuable, injury or the threat of injury, poor health or nutrition, general frustration, and ineffective coping mechanisms. Remember, each individual is susceptible to different stressors and therefore has a different constellation of signs and symptoms.

However, the signs and symptoms of stress can be beneficial, because they are the body's way of warning that corrective stress management is needed. The warnings typically are mild at first, but if left uncorrected, they will build in intensity until you are forced to rest. If it means having a heart attack or collapsing, that is what the body will do. So pay attention early.

The signs and symptoms of excessive stress can be physical, emotional, cognitive, or behavioral (Table 4-5). They are unique to each person. Once again, an individual must perform a self-assessment. If you catch a warning sign of excessive stress early and manage it, there is no need to reach the extreme endpoint commonly referred to as **burnout**.

Table 4-5 Warning Signs of Excessive Stress

Physical	Cognitive	Emotional	Behavioral
Nausea/vomiting	Confusion	Anticipatory anxiety	Change in activity
Upset stomach	Lowered attention span	Denial	Hyperactivity, hypoactivity
Tremors (lips, hands)	Calculation difficulties	Fearfulness	Withdrawal
Feeling uncoordinated	Memory problems	Panic	Suspiciousness
Diaphoresis (profuse sweating), flushed skin	Poor concentration	Survivor guilt	Change in communications
Chills	Difficulty making decisions	Uncertainty of feelings	Change in interactions with others
Diarrhea	Disruption in logical thinking	Depression	Change in eating habits
Aching muscles and joints	Disorientation, decreased level of awareness	Grief	Increased or decreased food intake
Sleep disturbances	Seeing an event over and over	Hopelessness	Increased smoking
Fatigue	Distressing dreams	Feeling overwhelmed	Increased alcohol intake
Dry mouth	Blaming someone	Feeling lost	Increased intake of other drugs
Shakes		Feeling abandoned	Being overly vigilant to environment
Headache		Feeling worried	Excessive humor
Vision problems		Wishing to hide	Excessive silence
Difficult, rapid breathing		Wishing to die	Unusual behavior
Chest tightness or pain, heart palpitations, cardiac rhythm disturbances		Anger	Crying spells
		Feeling numb	
		Identifying with victim	

Common Techniques for Managing Stress

There are two main types of defense mechanisms and techniques for managing stress: beneficial and detrimental. Detrimental techniques may provide a temporary sense of relief, but they will not cure the problem. In fact, they make things worse. They include substance abuse (alcohol, nicotine, illegal and prescription drugs), overeating or other compulsive behaviors, chronic complaining, freezing out or cutting off others and the support they could give you, avoidance behaviors, and dishonesty about your actual state of well-being ("I'm just fine!").

It is far better for you to spend your energy on beneficial, or healthy, techniques that dissipate the accumulation of stress and promote actual recovery. When your stress response threatens your ability to handle the moment, try the following:

- *Use controlled breathing.* Focus attention on your breathing. Take in a deep breath through your nose. Then exhale forcefully but steadily through your mouth, so that you can hear the air rush out. Press all the air out of your lungs with your abdomen. Do this two or more times until you feel steadier. This technique helps to reduce your adrenaline levels and slow your heart rate, so you can do your job appropriately.

- *Reframe.* Mentally reframe interfering thoughts, such as "I can't do this" or "I'm scared." Consciously restate your negative thought in a positive way. For example, when you start to think "I can't do this," you might tell yourself, "I will do the best I can and ask another crew member or call medical direction if I need help." When you think, "I'm scared," you might replace that thought with "This is challenging, but I can get through it OK." Be sure to deal with the negative thoughts later, however, or they may continue to interfere with the performance of your duties.

- *Attend to the medical needs of the patient.* Even if you know the people involved, do not let those relationships interfere with your responsibilities as an EMS provider. Later, when it is appropriate to do so, address your stress about the call in some way, such as talking it over with family or fellow crew members or seeking spiritual solace or counseling.

For long-term well-being, one of the best stress management techniques is to simply to take care of *you*—physically, emotionally, and mentally. Remember that regular exercise does not have to be extreme. Do something that you enjoy and find relaxing. At stressful times, pay especially close attention to your diet. If you smoke, make it a goal to quit.

Create a non-EMS circle of friends, and renew old friendships or activities. Take a vacation or a few days off.

Say "no!" to the next offer of an overtime shift. Listen to music, meditate, and learn positive thinking. Try the soothing techniques of guided imagery and progressive relaxation. Some paramedics have even quit EMS for a while. In general, you have many choices. The key principle is to generate positive options for yourself, and keep choosing them until you have recovered.

Specific EMS Stresses

There are three clearly defined types of EMS stresses:

- *Daily stress.* Most EMS stress is unrelated to critical incidents and disasters. Instead, it is related to such things as pay, working conditions, dealing with the public, administrative matters, and other hassles of day-to-day living and working. To help deal with daily stress, all emergency personnel should develop personal stress management strategies, such as a personal support system made up of coworkers, family, clergy, and others.

- *Small incidents.* Incidents involving only one or two patients, including incidents that result in injuries or deaths of emergency workers, are best handled by competent mental health personnel in individual or small-group settings. Mental health professionals should be familiar with EMS and be ready to respond when needed. They should then continue to screen affected emergency workers for signs and symptoms of abnormal response to stress. If these are detected, they can refer these workers, as appropriate, to other competent mental health professionals who use accepted treatment methods.

- *Large incidents and disasters.* Most EMS personnel will never encounter a disaster situation. However, all must be ready in case such a catastrophe occurs. The stress of large-scale disasters can be mitigated by a well-coordinated and organized response. Use of the National Incident Management System (NIMS) or Incident Command System (ICS) in large incidents and disasters serves to appropriately direct responding personnel. It also provides for rotating personnel through rehabilitation and surveillance stations. Those who are showing signs of stress or fatigue are removed from duty, at least temporarily. Here, too, there is a role for competent mental health professionals, who should be readily available to provide psychological first aid.

Post-Traumatic Stress Disorder

In recent years, there has been an increased emphasis on the long-term effects of stress on EMS providers. One possible outcome of recurrent or unmitigated stress is the development of **post-traumatic stress disorder (PTSD)**.

PTSD is an anxiety disorder that develops following exposure to traumatic events. It was commonly seen in military personnel exposed to the horrors of war and has been recognized for years under various names (e.g., shell shock, combat exhaustion, survivor's guilt). Symptoms of PTSD include intrusive memories that may manifest, for example, in the following ways:

- Recurrent, unwanted distressing memories of the traumatic event(s)
- Reliving the traumatic event as if it were happening again (flashbacks)
- Recurring and unsettling dreams about the traumatic event(s)
- Severe emotional distress or physical reactions to something that reminds the person of the event

PTSD may also include avoidance of situations and places that can bring back thoughts and images of the traumatic event or events. Ultimately, PTSD can result in changes in how an individual reacts emotionally and can adversely affect the person's mood and thinking. PTSD, in some instances, can result in suicide or suicidal ideation.

The research is unclear as to whether there is an increased incidence of PTSD in EMS personnel. However, recurrent exposure to traumatic events in EMS is common. Even though not every person exposed to traumatic events will develop PTSD, it is definitely a risk.

Several strategies have evolved to help identify and prevent PTSD in EMS providers and other public safety personnel. One of these is the **Code Green Campaign**, founded in 2014 by a group of EMS professionals, which serves to raise awareness of mental health issues (e.g., PTSD, substance abuse, suicide) in first responders. It also provides education for responders on how to provide care for themselves and recognize issues in their peers. A similar organization in Canada is the **Tema Conter Memorial Trust**, which provides peer and psychological support for public safety personnel.

Mental Health Services

Mental health professionals can provide the information and education needed for rescuers to understand psychological or emotional trauma, what to expect, and where to get help, if needed. In addition, competent mental health personnel should be available at all major incidents to provide psychological first aid to rescuers and victims.

The basic principles of psychological first aid as may be practiced by mental health professionals are quite straightforward:

- *Contact and engagement.* Making contact with those in need of assistance; providing practical, instrumental assistance with compassion and care.

- *Safety and comfort.* Taking steps to provide as safe an environment as situations permit; providing as much comfort as circumstances allow.
- *Stabilization.* Attenuating anxiety, providing a calming presence, helping ground and orient the distraught, referring for emergency care where and when clearly indicated.
- *Information gathering (current needs and concerns).* Determining what the pressing needs are, *as seen by the person in need;* tailoring assistance efforts to address current needs while anticipating emerging situations.
- *Practical assistance.* Providing practical, instrumental help with identified needs; assisting with problem-solving strategies and access to helping resources.
- *Connection with social supports.* Helping those affected make contact with sources of social support important to them (e.g., friends, family, and community and spiritual resources); integrating their support into problem solving and recovery.
- *Information on coping.* Providing simple, practical, proven tips on managing stress and coping with demands of recovery—timed to match the situations and challenges at hand at any given juncture. Such tips can be useful and well received, especially when delivered in the context of practical assistance and social support.
- *Link to collaborative services.* Because many people may be unfamiliar with resources available to help with their various needs, providing assistance in navigating the resource network community can be particularly important.

Psychological first aid is not a treatment or packaged proprietary intervention technique. It is an attempt to provide practical palliative care and contact while respecting the wishes of those who may not be ready to deal with the possible onslaught of emotional responses in the early days following an incident. It entails providing comfort and information and meeting people's immediate practical and emotional needs.[15]

Disaster Mental Health Services

The emotional well-being of both rescuers and victims is an important concern in any multiple-casualty incident. In the past, Critical Incident Stress Management (CISM) was recommended for use in emergency services. However, evidence has clearly shown that CISM and Critical Incident Stress Debriefing (CISD) do not appear to mitigate the effects of traumatic stress and, in fact, may interfere with the normal grieving and healing process and should not be used. The American Psychological Association judges the status of psychological debriefing as "no research support/

treatment is potentially harmful."[16,17] Instead, mental health practitioners now recommend resiliency-based care. This program includes techniques and activities that promote emotional strength, while at the same time decreasing vulnerability to stress, adversity, and challenges.

However, an important role remains for competent mental health professionals in any multiple-casualty incident. Mental health personnel should be available on scene to provide psychological first aid (as already described) to all those affected by an incident—including EMS personnel. At the same time, they can survey rescuers and victims for the development of abnormal stress-related symptoms. In addition, mental health professionals should be available during the two months following a critical incident to screen and assist anyone who may be developing stress-related symptoms. Persons so affected may be referred for additional counseling or mental health care.[18]

General Safety Considerations

The topic of scene safety is vast and requires career-long attention. Considering the many problems that can occur, it is impressive how few injuries there are. Your risks include violent people, environmental hazards, structural collapse, motor vehicles, and infectious disease. Many of these hazards can be minimized with protective equipment, such as helmets, body armor, reflective tape for night visibility, footwear with ankle support, and Standard Precautions against infectious disease. You should use whatever protective equipment you have.

Interpersonal Relations

Safety issues that arise in out-of-hospital care often stem from poor interpersonal relations. Paramedics are public ambassadors of health care. Interpersonal safety begins with effective communication. If you can build a rapport with the strangers you have been sent to serve, you will gain their trust. Suspicious, angry, and upset people are far more likely to be defensive and inflict harm than those who see a reason to trust what you are doing.

Building rapport depends on the ability to put your personal prejudices aside. Everyone has prejudices, but as a representative of an institution far greater than yourself, you must never allow them to interfere with appropriate patient and bystander management. In fact, go beyond curbing prejudice and challenge yourself to treat every person you meet with dignity and respect.

You can begin by taking time to pay attention to the rich array of cultural diversity that exists in our nation and learning to see those differences as valuable and positive.

In particular, learn about the different cultural backgrounds of people in your area and how to work with them effectively. For example, although you may like a lot of eye contact, understand that it is regarded as more polite in several cultures to avoid eye contact. Therefore, someone showing you esteem might avoid eye contact with you. This is not wrong; it is just different. Listen well to the stories of other people and see what you can learn. When you learn to accept differences easily, it will become easier for you to work toward win–win situations on the streets.

Roadway Safety

Motor vehicle collisions are the greatest hazard for EMS personnel. The incidence of ambulance and emergency response vehicle collisions is increasing (Figure 4-13). Several factors seem to play a role in ambulance crashes. First, ambulances have become larger and more difficult to operate. Most modern ambulances are built on a commercial truck chassis. Many are built on a heavy truck chassis. With this increase in size come increased braking distances, less responsive steering systems, and slower acceleration (which decreases the ability to avoid certain collisions). Several ambulance types have a high center of gravity or are somewhat unstable. In addition, the person designated to drive the ambulance is often the person with the least training and the least experience. In many instances, an introductory emergency vehicle operator course (EVOC) is not provided or does not have an adequate session to practice driving and emergency techniques.[19]

Roadways are unsafe places. There are good books, classes, and mentors to help you become aware of the various roadway hazards. For all related emergency situations, acquire the necessary training for emergency rescue and

FIGURE 4-13 Ambulance collisions pose the greatest risk of injury or death for EMS providers.

(© Canandaigua Emergency Squad)

for the safe use of emergency rescue equipment. Learn the principles of:

- Safely following an emergency escort vehicle
- Intersection management, when traffic is moving in several directions
- Noting hazardous conditions, such as spilled hazardous materials (gasoline, industrial chemicals, and so on), downed power lines, and proximity to moving traffic. Also notice adverse environmental conditions.
- Evaluating the safest parking place when arriving at a roadway incident
- Safely approaching a vehicle in which someone is slumped over the wheel
- Patient compartment safety—in particular, bracing yourself against sudden deceleration or swerving to avoid roadway hazards; and making a habit of hanging on consistently, especially when changing positions. Restraint systems have been developed to help protect EMS personnel while riding in the patient compartment of the ambulance.
- Safely using emergency lights and siren

An ambulance escort can create additional hazards. Inexperienced ambulance operators often follow the escort vehicle too closely and are unable to stop when the escort does. Inexperienced operators also may assume that other drivers know that the ambulance is following an escort. In fact, other drivers frequently do not know that another emergency vehicle is coming and often pull out in front of the ambulance just after the escort vehicle passes.

Multiple-vehicle responses can be just as dangerous, especially when responding vehicles travel in the same direction close together. When two vehicles approach the same intersection at the same time, not only may they fail to yield, one to the other, but other drivers may also yield for the first vehicle only, not the second one. Extreme caution must be taken when approaching intersections.

Certain equipment is intended to promote your safety on roadways. For example, to be visible to oncoming drivers, who may have dirty, smeared, or pitted windshields and may not be sober, wear ANSI/ISEA compliant safety vests. In fact, you also may be issued other protective gear, especially if you are in the fire service. Using respiratory protection, gloves, boots, turnout coat and pants (or coveralls), and other specialty safety equipment is the mark of an aware, professional paramedic. Ask nonmedical personnel to set out flares or cones, if needed. Leave some emergency lights flashing, although you should be careful not to blind oncoming drivers.

To park safely at a roadway incident, make it a habit to scan each individual setting. Notice curves, hilltops, and the volume and speed of surrounding traffic. Ideally, you should park in the front of a crash site on the same side of the street. This facilitates access to the patient compartment and equipment, and it protects you from traffic coming from behind. However, when responding to an incident such as "person slumped behind wheel," maintain the defensive advantage by staying behind the vehicle, and use spotlights to "blind" the person until you know there are no hostile intentions. Walk to the vehicle with cautious alertness until you are sure it is not a trap.

The use of seat belts in the front of an ambulance should be an obvious habit, both for safety and for role modeling. Less obvious is the use of safety restraints in the patient compartment. An improper assumption is that the paramedic is too busy attending to the patient and passengers to wear a seat belt. However, buckling into a seat belt for a safer ride is, in fact, possible during much or most of ambulance transport times. Death and major disability is common when someone is in the patient compartment during a crash. For your well-being, wear a seat belt whenever possible, even "in back."[20]

Because ambulances represent help and hope, it is doubly tragic when a paramedic crew is involved in a motor-vehicle crash caused by the misuse of lights and siren. Lights and siren are tools, not toys. They are the paramedic's means for gaining quick access to people in dire need. Those who misuse the mandate to operate them chip away at the public's trust in EMS. Whether using lights and siren or not, the paramedic has a responsibility to drive with due regard for the safety of others. As a professional, you are obligated to study and use safe driving practices at all times.

Summary

The paramedic has the training and responsibility to manage the most complicated health problems posed by out-of-hospital citizens. This makes the paramedic a leader within the prehospital care community. Paramedics who attend to their own well-being are not only helping themselves, but they are also providing a positive role model for other EMS providers and the community at large.

Continuous assessment of personal lifestyle ranges from practices that affect the immediate future to practices that affect the paramedic in old age. They range from wearing PPE and parking safely at a crash site to managing stress daily, eating right, and exercising.

There are numerous elements to the topic of well-being, and the paramedic must strive continually to address each one. Take your knowledge beyond the introduction offered in this chapter. Be a lifelong student of well-being, and you are more likely to have a healthy long life. Your biggest challenge is this: Be well, so that you can help others be well, too.

You Make the Call

It's been a tough year for you on the paramedic squad. Lately, it just seems as if everything that can go wrong does. Arguing (again) with your spouse about paying the mortgage is not helping your irritation one bit. It is 2300 hours. You are tired, and all you ate all day was glazed doughnuts and fast food. Suddenly, the tone alert sounds: "Ambulance 44, respond to the corner of Fero and Bailey on a two-vehicle crash. Number of victims unknown."

You are the second EMS crew to arrive. You prefer the job of triage, and the paramedic who is doing it is too new to know much. Anyway, he has already triaged four patients. As you walk up to the scene, you notice the bumper sticker on one crash vehicle and realize it is your neighbor's daughter's car. You do not see her in the group of patients, and your heart leaps into your throat when you see the DOA covered with a sheet.

You are assigned two patients, one an unconscious teen with a crushed leg and the other an adult with a broken arm.

You take pride in your medical abilities, so handling the immobilization and other medical care is smooth. On the way to the hospital, the teen wakes up and presses you to tell him, "Is Debbie okay? Is she? Please! Tell me, is she all right?" Thus you find out that, indeed, the other person in your neighbor's car was Debbie, their daughter.

After delivering the patients to the hospital, you pop an antacid for your sour stomach and chew out your partner for his bumpy driving.

A couple of days later, you take on yet another overtime shift. Your mortgage payment is due, and besides, you can't face going to the funeral of your neighbor's daughter. You've seen enough death. Who needs another funeral anyway?

1. Are your stress levels inappropriately high? What are the indications?

2. Might it be a good idea for you to go to the funeral? Why or why not?

3. How can you improve stress management in the future?

See Suggested Responses at the back of this book.

Review Questions

1. Most paramedic injuries are caused by _____ and being in and around motor vehicles.

   a. falls

   b. stress

   c. lifting

   d. violence

2. Which of the following is *not* a benefit of achieving acceptable physical fitness?

   a. Increased muscle mass and metabolism

   b. Increased oxygen-carrying capacity

   c. Increased resting heart rate and blood pressure

   d. Increased resistance to illness and injury

3. According to the U. S. Department of Agriculture dietary guidelines, you should make _____ of the food on your plate fruits and vegetables.

   a. one-fourth

   b. one-third

   c. one-half

   d. two-thirds

4. Which of the following is *not* an important principle of lifting?

   a. Avoid twisting and turning whenever possible.

   b. Keep your palms up whenever possible.

   c. Move a load only if you can handle it safely.

   d. Position the load far away from your body and center of gravity.

5. A strict form of infection control that is based on the assumption that all blood and other body fluids are infectious, combining aspects of universal precautions and body substance isolation, is termed

   _____

   a. personal protective equipment.

   b. mode of transmission.

   c. incubation period.

   d. Standard Precautions.

6. _____ is the use of a chemical or a physical method, such as pressurized steam, to kill all microorganisms on an object.

   a. Cleaning   c. Sterilizing

   b. Disinfecting   d. Decontaminating

7. How many stages in the grief process have been identified by Elisabeth Kübler-Ross?

   a. 3   c. 7

   b. 5   d. 8

8. The most common initial stage of the grieving process, as identified by Elisabeth Kübler-Ross, is

   _____

   a. anger.

   b. denial.

   c. depression.

   d. bargaining.

9. What is an active process during which a person confronts the stressful situation?

   a. Coping

   b. Resistance

   c. Defensive strategies

   d. Problem-solving skills

10. For safety at a roadway incident it is appropriate to do all of the following *except*

    _____

    a. ask nonmedical personnel to set out flares or cones.

    b. wear reflective tape and an orange or lime-green vest.

    c. blind a slumped-over passenger with a spotlight as you approach.

    d. park on the opposite side of the street from the crashed vehicle.

See answers to Review Questions at the back of this book.

References

1. Maguire, B. J., K. L. Hunting, G. S. Smith, and N. R. Levick. "Occupational Fatalities in Emergency Medical Services: A Hidden Crisis." *Ann Emerg Med* (40) 2002: 625–632.

2. Boudreaux, E., C. Mandry, and P. J. Brantly. "Emergency Medical Technician Schedule Modification: Impact and Implications on Short- and Long-Term Follow-Up." *Acad Emerg Med* (5) 1998: 128–133.

3. Mitani, S., M. Fujita, and T. Shirakawa. "Circadian Variation on Cardiac Autonomic Nervous System Profile Is Affected in Japanese Men with a Working System of 24-H Shifts." *Int Arch Occup Environ Health* (79) 2006: 27–32.

4. Crill, M. T. and D. Hostler. "Back Strength and Flexibility of EMS Providers in Practicing Prehospital Providers." *J Occup Rehabil* (15) 2005: 105–111.

5. Studnek, J. R. and J. M. Crawford. "Factors Associated with Back Problems among Emergency Medical Technicians." *Am J Ind Med* (50) 2007: 464–469.

6. United States Department of Agriculture (USDA). *ChooseMyPlate.* (Available at http://www.choosemyplate.gov. For "10 Tips to a Great Plate," go to http://www.choosemyplate.gov/downloads/TenTips/DGTipsheet1ChooseMyPlate.pdf.)

7. Bledsoe, B. E., T. Dick, J. O. Page, and M. Taigman. "The Missing Drugs." *JEMS* (29) 2004: 30–36.

8. Friese, G. and K. Owsley. "Backbreaking Work: What You Need to Know about Lifting and Back Safety in EMS." *EMS Mag* (37) 2008: 63–72.

9. Centers for Disease Control and Prevention. *Standard Precautions.* (Available at http://www.cdc.gov/HAI/settings/outpatient/outpatient-care-gl-standard-precautions.html.)

10. Kübler-Ross, E. *On Death and Dying.* (Originally published 1969.) Scribner Classics reprint edition. New York: Simon & Schuster, 1997.

11. Olsen, J. C., M. L. Buenefe, and W. D. Falco. "Death in the Emergency Department." *Ann Emerg Med* (31) 1998: 758–765.

12. Boudreaux E., C. Mandry, and P. J. Brantley. "Stress, Job Satisfaction, Coping, and Psychological Distress among Emergency Medical Technicians." *Prehosp Disaster Med* (12) 1997: 242–249.

13. Selye, H. "A Syndrome Produced by Diverse Nocuous Agents." *Nature* (138) 1936: 32.

14. Cydulka, R. K., C. L. Emerman, B. Shade, and J. Kubincanek. "Stress Levels in EMS Personnel: A Longitudinal Study with Work-Schedule Modification." *Acad Emerg Med* (1) 1994: 240–246.

15. World Health Organization (WHO). Psychological First Aid: Guide for Field Workers. (Available at http://www.who.int/mental_health/publications/guide_field_workers/en/.)

16. Bledsoe, B. E. "Critical Incident Stress Management (CISM): Benefit or Rise for Emergency Services." *Prehosp Emerg Care* 7(2) 2003: 272–329.

17. McNally, R. J., R. A. Bryant, and A. Ehlers. "Does Early Psychological Intervention Promote Recovery from Posttraumatic Stress?" *Psych Sci Pub Int* (4) 2003: 45–79.

18. Devilley, G. J., R. Gist, and P. Cotton. "Ready! Fire! Aim! The Status of Psychological Debriefings and Therapeutic Interventions: In the Work Place and After Disasters." *Rev Gen Psych* 10(4) 2006: 318–345.

19. Ray, A. M. and D. F. Kupas. "Comparison of Rural and Urban Ambulance Crashes in Pennsylvania." *Prehosp Emerg Care* (11) 2007: 416–420.

20. Slattery, D. E. and A. Silver. "The Hazards of Providing Emergency Care in Emergency Vehicle: An Opportunity for Reform." *Prehosp Emerg Care* (13) 2009: 388–397.

Further Reading

Becknell, J. *Medic Life.* St. Louis: Mosby Lifeline, 1996.

Dernocoeur, K. B. *Streetsense: Communication, Safety, and Control.* 3rd ed. Redmond, WA: Laing Research Services, 1996.

Chapter 5
EMS Research

Bryan Bledsoe, DO, FACEP, FAAEM

Michael F. O'Keefe

STANDARD
Preparatory (Research)

COMPETENCY
Integrates comprehensive knowledge of EMS systems, the safety and well-being of the paramedic, and medical–legal and ethical issues, which is intended to improve the health of EMS personnel, patients, and the community.

 ## Learning Objectives

Terminal Performance Objective: After reading this chapter, you should be able to critically evaluate published reports of EMS research.

Enabling Objectives: To accomplish the terminal performance objective, you should be able to:

1. Define key terms introduced in this chapter.

2. Explain the relationship between EMS research and EMS practice.

3. Discuss how the National EMS Research Agenda and its recommendations could improve future EMS research and practice.

4. Describe each of the steps of the scientific method.

5. Differentiate among the types of research paradigms, including quantitative, qualitative, and mixed, and discuss the prospective and retrospective approaches to doing so.

6. Define the categories of experimental designs and discuss the various types of studies within these general categories.

7. Given a research proposal, identify the ethical considerations for human subjects that must be considered.

8. Discuss the proper use of various descriptive and inferential statistics in a research study.

9. Describe the purpose and intended content of each section of a research paper.

10. Describe what to look for and how to complete a review of published research.

11. Discuss the roles and responsibilities of the EMS provider who decides to participate in or undertake a research study.

KEY TERMS

abstract, p. 97

analysis of variance (ANOVA), p. 95

bench research, p. 93

bias, p. 89

case report, p. 92

case series, p. 92

chi square test, p. 95

cohort study, p. 91

confidence interval, p. 95

control group, p. 89

convenience sampling, p. 100

cross-sectional study, p. 92

data dredging, p. 100

data mining, p. 100

dependent variable, p. 89

descriptive statistics, p. 94

double blind study, p. 90

experiment, p. 87

experimental group, p. 89

experimental study, p. 89

external validity, p. 93

hypothesis, p. 87

in vitro, p. 93

in vivo, p. 93

independent variable, p. 89

inferential statistics, p. 94

institutional review board (IRB), p. 94

internal validity, p. 93

iterative process, p. 88

mean, p. 94

measures of central tendency, p. 94

median, p. 94

meta-analysis, p. 90

mixed research, p. 88

mode, p. 95

morbidity, p. 86

mortality, p. 86

National EMS Research Agenda, p. 86

nominal data, p. 95

nonrandomized controlled trial, p. 91

null hypothesis, p. 101

observational study, p. 90

odds ratio, p. 97

open access journals, p. 98

ordinal data, p. 95

outcomes-based research, p. 86

P value, p. 100

parameter, p. 95

peer review, p. 98

placebo, p. 91

population, p. 95

post hoc, p. 102

principal investigator (PI), p. 102

prospective study, p. 89

PubMed, p. 87

qualitative research, p. 88

qualitative statistics, p. 95

quality of life, p. 86

quantitative research, p. 88

quantitative statistics, p. 95

quasiexperimental study, p. 89

random sampling, p. 100

randomized controlled trial (RCT), p. 90

research, p. 86

retrospective study, p. 89

sampling error, p. 95

science, p. 87

scientific method, p. 87

single blind study, p. 90

standard deviation (SD or σ), p. 95

statistics, p. 94

systematic sampling, p. 100

t test, p. 95

time sampling, p. 100

treatment group, p. 89

validity, p. 93

variance, p. 95

Case Study

One slow day, two EMS crews were sitting in the station, and the conversation soon drifted back to "the way we used to do it." Robert, the most senior paramedic in the agency, had logged more than 30 years in the field. The younger crew members began to question Robert about the various antiquated practices that once were commonplace in EMS.

Robert said, "Well, one thing we routinely did was to give large doses of sodium bicarbonate to cardiac arrest victims." A young EMT piped in and asked, "Why did it stop?" Robert thought for a minute and said, "Well, it was one of those things that looked good on paper but did not

work in the field. The research showed that the outcomes from cardiac arrest were not any better for those who received sodium bicarbonate when compared to those who did not. So the American Heart Association took it out of their recommendations, and we stopped giving it."

Steve, a new EMT, said inquisitively, "What about MAST pants for shock or bleeding control?" Robert leaned back in the chair and said, "Ah, MAST pants. We used them all the time for trauma. I'll swear I've seen them work. But a research study from Houston found them ineffective, if not harmful, and they went the way of the covered wagon."

Robert went on, "We also used calcium chloride in cardiac arrests. I remember giving 100 milligrams of Decadron to head-injured patients—not sure why they had us do that. I have to admit that EMS has changed, and I think it has changed for the better."

"What do you mean?" asked Steve. Robert looked pensive and said, "In those days, we did what we did because it seemed like a good idea at the time. Now, EMS is more based on sound scientific principles developed through quality research. The goal has always been to do what was best for the patient. The problem was that we did not always know what was best for the patient. Many of the things that seemed so intuitive as an EMS practice have been proved through research to be ineffective. Even though I hate to see old practices go by the wayside, it is for the best, I guess. Research is what will drive EMS into the future, and I'm all for that."

The group sat quietly for a while, and finally the conversation took a different turn when Steve looked at his watch, jumped up, and said, "Hey, the Cowboys are playing. Turn on the TV."

Introduction

Scientific **research** has played a major role in the evolution of modern EMS. When EMS was developed more than 30 years ago, there were no scientific studies or objective evidence to guide development. Instead, various practices from other areas (e.g., hospital medicine, fire departments, the military) were applied to EMS. In many instances, these practices were based on expert opinions and rational conjecture. Now, as we have moved into the twenty-first century, many EMS practices have been examined through research methods. To the surprise of many, some EMS practices that were considered intuitive, such as endotracheal intubation and medical anti-shock trousers (MAST), have been found to be less effective than once thought.[1,2] One of the hallmarks of a profession, when compared to a trade, is the ability to change practices and procedures based on evolving research. Thus, a solid and objective research program is what should and will drive EMS practices in the coming years.

The importance of research to EMS cannot be overstated. To continue to receive the required funding and support, EMS must prove that the care and service it provides truly benefit the patients and the community and are cost effective. This is demonstrated primarily through **outcomes-based research**. Outcomes-based research can help determine whether a procedure, drug, treatment, or similar strategy actually improves patient outcomes (e.g., **mortality**, **morbidity**, and **quality of life**). If you can't prove it makes a difference, then why do you do it?

The **National EMS Research Agenda**, published in 2001 by the National Highway Traffic Safety Administration (NHTSA), provided a guide to future EMS research in the United States.[3] The document drew several conclusions about the need for EMS research and made several recommendations. These included:

- Develop a cadre of EMS researchers and support them early in their careers.

- Facilitate collaboration between EMS researchers and those from other disciplines (e.g., social scientists, economists, epidemiologists, and others).
- Establish a reliable funding stream for EMS research within government.
- Establish an alternate funding source for EMS research outside of government.
- Recognize the need for EMS research.
- View research as necessary for the improvement of patient care.
- Enhance ethical approaches to research.

They concluded that a national investment in EMS research infrastructure is necessary to overcome the obstacles that currently impede EMS research. Funding is needed to train new researchers and to establish their careers.

Increased financial support is necessary to develop effective treatments for the diseases that drive the design of the EMS system, including injury and sudden cardiac arrest. Innovative strategies to make EMS research easier to accomplish in emergency situations must be legitimized and implemented.

Researchers must have access to patient outcome information so that the impact of prehospital and out-of-hospital patient care can be evaluated and improved. Incorporating standard scientific methodology into the evaluation of biomedical and technical advances in prehospital and out-of-hospital care is crucial.

In summary, research is the key to maintaining an appropriate focus on improving the overall health of the community in a competitive and cost-conscious health care market. Most important, research is essential to ensure that the best possible patient care is provided in the prehospital and out-of-hospital setting.

This chapter will provide an overview of research and the scientific method. It will detail some of the research methodologies and provide insight to how EMS personnel should evaluate research studies. Hopefully, it will encourage you, as a paramedic, to venture into the world of research.

Research and the Scientific Method

The word **science** literally means "knowledge." However, science is generally defined as "knowledge attained through study or practice." Science is the state or fact of having knowledge that is derived through the scientific method (defined in the next paragraph). Use of the scientific method to study a given issue is known as *research*. Research is patient, careful, systematic study and investigation in some field of knowledge, undertaken to discover or establish facts or principles. In EMS, we use research to understand how EMS works and how it does not. However, as you will learn, paramedicine is a part of the discipline of medicine, and medicine is both an art and a science. The knowledge of EMS is science. How we apply that knowledge is art. Excellent paramedics know the science of EMS and use the art of EMS to apply the science.

The fundamental principle behind scientific research is the **scientific method**—a process by which scientists, collectively and over time, endeavor to construct an accurate representation of the world. This representation must be reliable, consistent, and nonarbitrary. The advantage of the scientific method is that it is unprejudiced if properly applied and reproducible.

The scientific method follows these distinct steps (Figure 5-1):

- *Observe and ask questions.* The first step in the scientific method is to observe something in the universe and ask a question. For example, you and your EMS colleagues have observed that calls for psychiatric patients are more common when the moon is full. Thus, you decide to determine whether this observation is true. You have made an observation and are now asking a question.
- *Conduct research, data collection, analysis, and synthesis.* The first step in answering your question is to do some background research. Today, this can be easily done through the Internet or through scientific databases such as **PubMed**, which is operated by the U.S. National Library of Medicine.[4] In your study about the effects of a full moon on psychiatric illness, you may find several prior studies and publications on the subject. You can also look at similar perceived

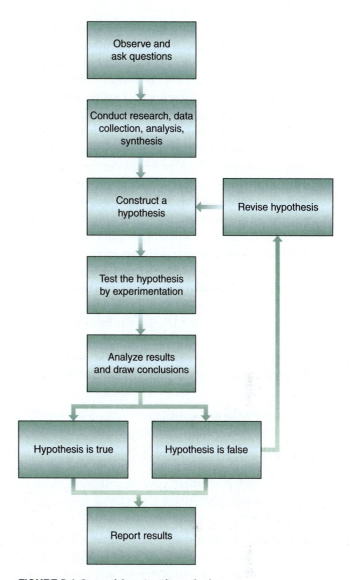

FIGURE 5-1 Steps of the scientific method.

phenomena, such as the rate of obstetrical deliveries when the moon is full. When embarking on a study, make it easier on yourself and see if your question or similar questions have already been addressed.

- *Construct a hypothesis.* In your background research you fail to find any study that has looked at whether there is an increase in psychiatric calls when the moon is full, so you decide to move forward with your research. The next step will be to construct a **hypothesis**. Your hypothesis is the specific question your study will answer. It must be something that can be clearly defined and measured. It must be constructed carefully so it will answer your original question. As you move forward with your psychiatric call study, a suitable hypothesis might be, "Psychiatric emergencies are more common when the lunar cycle is in a full moon phase."
- *Test the hypothesis by experimentation.* The next step is to set up an **experiment** to test your hypothesis to

CONTENT REVIEW

➤ Steps of the Scientific Method
  - Observe and ask questions.
  - Collect, analyze, and synthesize data.
  - Construct a hypothesis.
  - Test the hypothesis by experimentation.
  - Analyze results and draw conclusions.
  - Revise the hypothesis.
  - Report results.

determine whether it is true or false. The experiment must be a fair test and must be reproducible (that is, someone else could conduct the same test in the same way). You can conduct a fair test only by changing just one variable in your experiment at a time, while keeping all other conditions the same. In your investigation of psychiatric calls, you must clearly define the parameters of the experiment, which may not be as simple as it seems. First, you must define what constitutes a psychiatric call. It could be as easy as stating that a psychiatric call is any call that is marked on a patient run report as psychiatric. Next, you must define a full moon. Different people can look at the moon and have differing opinions about whether it is full. Thus, you might define a full moon as a five-day period that begins two days before the absolute day of the full moon, as stated in a reliable almanac or calendar, and two days after. During this five-day window, the moon will appear full to most people. Finally, you must define the time interval for the study, which might cover, say, three or six months of full-moon periods.

- *Analyze results and draw conclusions.* After you have completed your study, you must collect and analyze the results. This will typically involve some level of statistical analysis. Then, based on your analysis, you can determine whether your hypothesis is true or false. If, in fact, your hypothesis is found false, you can revise or construct a new hypothesis.

- *Revise the hypothesis.* If your hypothesis is found to be correct, you do not need to revise it. However, you might want to revise one parameter and run the experiment again. For example, you decide to change the definition of full moon to the single day of the lunar cycle when the moon is truly full, instead of the five-day definition you were initially using. Interestingly, in your study, you may actually find that psychiatric

emergencies are slightly less common during full moons, both when defined as a five-day period and when defined as only the day of the true full moon. So now you must revise your hypothesis again, to state "Psychiatric emergencies are not more common when the lunar cycle is in the full moon phase." Now your hypothesis is correct according to the data you collected.

- *Report results.* The practice in scientific research, especially medical research, is to share your findings regardless of whether your hypothesis was found to be true or false. In medicine, this primarily occurs through publishing the results in a peer-reviewed journal. The publishing of your data opens scientific discussion that will add further insight to your findings and hypothesis.

As you run your experiment or review the results, new information will often become available, causing you to stop and revise some of the steps in your experimental protocol. Stopping, backing up, and repeating a step in the scientific method is common and called an **iterative process**.

Types of Research

There are various types of research. Typically, research is described as quantitative, qualitative, or mixed. Stated simply, **quantitative research** describes phenomena in numbers, whereas **qualitative research** describes them in words. **Mixed research** is a combination of quantitative and qualitative research and uses both numbers and words to describe the phenomena being studied. These are totally different approaches and each has its strengths and weaknesses (Table 5-1). Most medical research is quantitative.

In addition, research is either retrospective or prospective. Retrospective research examines information that already exists, whereas prospective research involves

Table 5-1 Summary of Research Types

	Quantitative Research	Mixed Research	Qualitative Research
Scientific method	Researcher tests the hypothesis with data (deductive approach)	The researcher generates a hypothesis after collecting data (inductive approach)	Deductive and inductive
Focus	Narrow topic	Variable topic	Wide topic
Behavior	Studied under controlled conditions	Studied in more than one context	Studied in natural environment
Nature of reality	Objective	Commonsense (pragmatic)	Subjective
Nature of data	Numbers	Numbers and words	Words
Data analysis	Statistical	Statistical and words	Words
Results	Generalizable	May be generalizable	Nongeneralizable
Report	Statistical	Mixed	Narrative

study that starts now and examines what happens from this point forward (or to a predetermined ending date). Occasionally, some studies will have both prospective and retrospective components (e.g., a before-and-after study).

Quantitative versus Qualitative Research

Quantitative research is objective and specific. It is designed to determine the relationship between one thing (independent variable) and another (dependent or outcome variable) and describe it with numbers (statistics). The **independent variable** is the variable that affects the dependent variable under study. The **dependent variable** (or outcome variable) is the variable being affected or presumed affected by the independent variable. For example, a study that seeks to determine whether faster EMS response times affect patient survival would be considered quantitative research. The EMS response time would be the independent variable and mortality would be the dependent variable.

In addition to experimental quantitative research, as just described, one can find nonexperimental and survey-quantitative research. Nonexperimental quantitative research is often used when there are independent variables that cannot be manipulated for one reason or another (e.g., ethical concerns). Nonexperimental research measures primarily what naturally occurs or what has already occurred. Our study of psychiatric patients and the full moon is an example of nonexperimental quantitative research. Survey-quantitative research is a common strategy that is widely used outside medicine and the hard sciences. It is also considered a form of nonexperimental quantitative research. Typically, a survey (either a written questionnaire or an interview) will be performed in the target population. Then, the results will be analyzed and reported. Surveys are commonly used to reflect public opinion and for marketing and social science research.

Qualitative research primarily relies on collection of qualitative (nonnumeric) data. It primarily seeks the "why" and not the "how" of the phenomena being studied. Qualitative research primarily occurs in a natural setting. For example, many of the studies on stress in EMS have used qualitative methodologies. These studies often evaluate how an individual feels. Qualitative research has an important role in quality assurance. Customer surveys and patient satisfaction programs rely heavily on qualitative methods.

Prospective versus Retrospective Studies

A research project, regardless of whether it has a quantitative or a qualitative design, will be either a **retrospective study** or a **prospective study**. Retrospective studies look at existing data. For example, in our ongoing discussion of the psychiatric patients and full moon study, the design could either be retrospective or prospective. In a retrospective study, all EMS run sheets for a predetermined period of time (e.g., one year) would be carefully reviewed for psychiatric calls. When found, the date of the call and other necessary information would be recorded. In a prospective design, starting on a given day, all psychiatric calls would be flagged and the date recorded. The study would continue until a target date has been reached or a predetermined number of call records have been obtained. Generally speaking, prospective studies have greater validity than retrospective studies. There are several reasons for this. First, prospective studies use a research form or instrument specifically designed for the study. These tend to make the study more objective, accurate, and complete. When looking at historical data, it is often difficult to identify the specific data being sought. In addition, there is more chance for the introduction of **bias** in the data gathering for retrospective studies. Despite these problems, there are benefits to retrospective studies. First, the data already exist and are available immediately. Second, retrospective studies are generally less expensive than prospective methodologies.

Experimental Design

Not all studies are created equal. As a rule, the closer a study adheres to the scientific method, the more valid the study, and the more valid the study, the closer it is to the truth.

There are several types of experimental designs and these have varying degrees of validity. They include experimental studies, quasiexperimental studies, and observational studies. An **experimental study** will have both a **control group** (a group of subjects who do not have manipulation of the independent variable) and a **treatment group**, also called an **experimental group**. Subjects are randomly assigned to one of the groups. The researcher does not assign subjects or affect the assignment of subjects to the groups. The goal of randomization is to ensure that the demographics between the groups are similar. Experimental studies in which subjects are randomized into either the treatment group or the control group are considered among the most valid of studies.

A similar experimental design is the quasiexperimental study. A **quasiexperimental study** is one in which the scientist does not randomly assign subjects to the study groups. With quasiexperimental studies, there is a greater chance of having groups that are demographically different. Also, there is a greater chance of the introduction of bias (even subconsciously) into the study when subjects are not randomly assigned to the groups. Because of this, quasiexperimental studies are generally considered less valid than experimental studies. However, quasiexperimental studies are quite useful, because in some situations randomization is not possible or is unethical.

An **observational study** is one that does not have a control group. Instead, a single group or multiple groups are studied without comparison to a control. In an observational study, the scientist does not control the variables. Observational studies are considered less valid than experimental or quasiexperimental studies but have an important role in medicine. In many situations, it is unethical to withhold treatment from a group simply for the purposes of experimentation. For example, hydroxocobalamin has been found to be a safe antidote for cyanide poisoning, and failing to treat a victim of cyanide poisoning with a safe antidote might result in the victim's death. Because of this, it would be ethically and humanely impossible to study hydroxocobalamin in anything but an observational study. Observational studies are common in medicine.

Specific Study Types

Within the three general categories of scientific research just described (experimental, quasiexperimental, and observational), you will encounter various specific types of study in the medical literature. These are presented in a descending order of validity (Figure 5-2).

- *Meta-analysis of randomized controlled trials.* The advent of modern computing has made **meta-analysis** possible. In this study type, researchers locate all available appropriate randomized controlled trials (described next) of a particular area of study. Then,

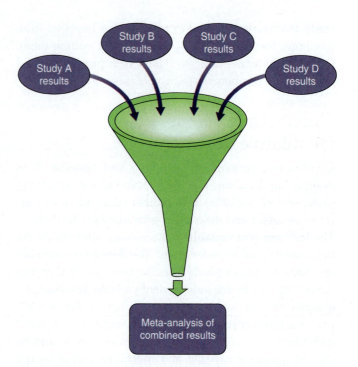

FIGURE 5-3 Meta-analysis is an analysis of the combined results of several prior studies.

they assimilate the raw data from all these studies into a single database. They subsequently analyze the data and draw conclusions. This is the most valid type of study because it represents a much larger part of the population and often represents a more diverse demographic than each individual study. It is possible to do a meta-analysis of observational studies, but these study types are not common. A meta-analysis is labor intensive and difficult to perform (Figure 5-3).

- *Randomized controlled trials (RCTs).* The **randomized controlled trial (RCT)** closely adheres to the scientific method and is extremely valid. Subjects are randomized into a treatment group (or groups) and a control group (Figure 5-4). The randomization can be achieved in different ways and the researchers cannot have a role in group assignment. One method of avoiding the introduction of bias into an RCT is to "blind" the scientist, the subject, or both. In a **single blind study**, the subjects do not know whether they are in the treatment group or the control group. This helps to prevent them from changing behavior during the experiment. In a **double blind study**, both the subjects and the experimenters are blinded as to who is in the control group and who is not (Figure 5-5). An example of a double blind study is one that was used to determine whether the administration of morphine affected subsequent emergency department assessment of patients with possible appendicitis. A pharmacist prepared identical-looking vials, one containing the morphine and the other containing normal saline. When ordered, neither

Levels of Validity

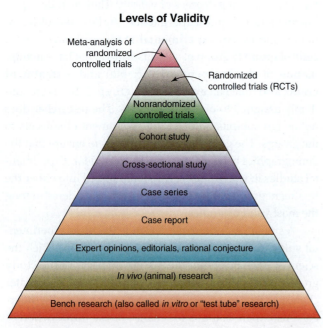

FIGURE 5-2 Hierarchy of validity of study types. The most valid type of study is at the top of the pyramid, the least valid at the bottom.

Randomized Controlled Trial (RCT)

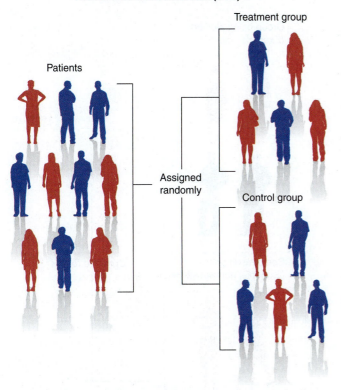

FIGURE 5-4 In a randomized controlled trial, a treatment group and a control group that is not receiving the treatment are being studied. The results of the two groups can be compared.

the doctor nor the patients knew whether they were getting the drug or the **placebo**. When the experiment was over the date were "unblinded," the analysis completed, and the hypothesis tested.

- *Nonrandomized controlled trials.* **Nonrandomized controlled trials**, also called quasiexperimental studies, as described earlier, have a control group and a treatment group—but assignment to these groups is not randomized (Figure 5-6). This type of study has less validity than an RCT, but it has utility in some circumstances. For example, two battalions of soldiers are going to be tested to determine whether a new IV access device is effective on the battlefield. One battalion serves as the control group and

does not receive the new device, whereas the other battalion receives the device. At a given point in time, the IV success rate between the groups will be analyzed and compared. The problem in this study design is that there is an increased chance that the two study groups will be different. For example, one battalion is from San Antonio and, incidentally, 25 percent of their soldiers had prior medical training. The other battalion is from Las Vegas and only 12 percent of their group had prior medical training. The prior experience of the San Antonio battalion could affect the results and not give a clear picture of the true effectiveness of the device.

- *Cohort study.* A **cohort study** is an observational study in which subjects who have a certain condition and/or who receive a particular treatment are followed over time and compared with another group who are not affected by the condition under investigation (Figure 5-7). For research purposes, a cohort is any group of individuals who are linked in some way or who have experienced the same significant life event within a given period. A commonly cited example of a cohort study is twin studies. When most twins reach adulthood, they typically go their separate ways. Scientists will look at behaviors or characteristics that are different in one twin (e.g., smoking, homosexuality) and compare them to the other twin (who is genetically identical or similar). This can help us to better understand what factors (genetic, social, environmental) are causing the differences.

Double Blind Study

Two kinds of pills:

Pill X

Pill Y

Only the trial manager knows what drug or nondrug is in each pill.

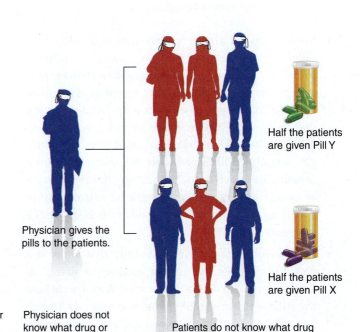

Half the patients are given Pill Y

Half the patients are given Pill X

Physician gives the pills to the patients.

Physician does not know what drug or nondrug is in each pill.

Patients do not know what drug or nondrug they are taking.

FIGURE 5-5 In the double blind study illustrated here, neither the experimenter nor the subjects know what drug they are taking. (The pills are not identified by drug name but only as "Pill A" and "Pill B.")

Nonrandomized Controlled Trial

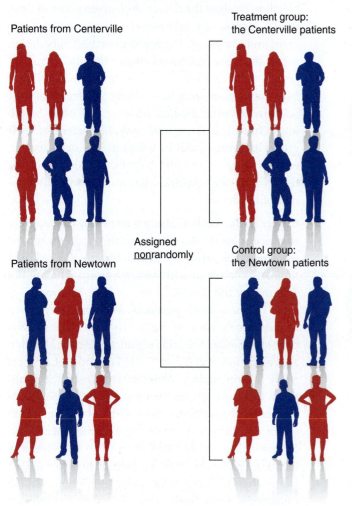

Patients from Centerville

Treatment group:
the Centerville patients

Assigned <u>non</u>randomly

Patients from Newtown

Control group:
the Newtown patients

Cohort Study

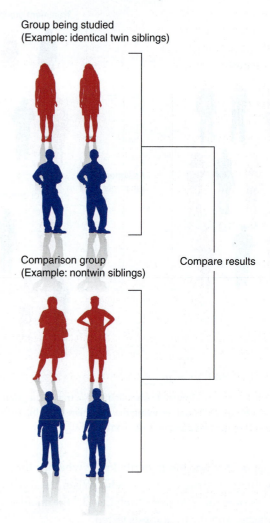

Group being studied
(Example: identical twin siblings)

Comparison group
(Example: nontwin siblings)

Compare results

FIGURE 5-6 In a randomized controlled trial, assignments to the treatment group and the control group are made at random. In a nonrandomized study, assignments to the two groups are, as the name indicates, not randomized.

FIGURE 5-7 A cohort is a group of subjects who share a certain characteristic. For example, all may be cancer patients. A cohort study observes and compares the cohort group with a group whose members do not have the cohort characteristic.

- *Cross-sectional study.* A **cross-sectional study**, also called a cross-sectional analysis, is an observational study and similar to a cohort study in that various groups are compared without a control. However, unlike a cohort study (which is a longitudinal study that looks at measurements over time), a cross-sectional study looks at a single point in time. For example, a study of EMS providers was completed on a certain date to determine the average number of years of formal education by training level existed within the group at that time. This would be an example of a cross-sectional study.

- *Case series.* A **case series** is a study that looks at a group of patients (typically a smaller number than found in an RCT) with a similar condition. This is how the AIDS epidemic in San Francisco was first identified. An epidemiologist noted a cluster of patients with similar disease findings (AIDS) and looked at the

similarities and differences between these patients in order to isolate a possible cause.

- *Case report.* A **case report** is a structured study of a single patient who is unique or interesting to the medical community in general. These are usually short reports and have limited scientific validity.

- *Expert opinions, editorials and rational conjecture.* When modern EMS was being planned, there was no identifiable body of knowledge to guide the development of the profession. Instead, physicians and other experts were consulted, and they provided their best opinion about needed practices and procedures. Although this strategy is suitable for use before scientific research is available or while scientific research is occurring, it can be problematic when research finally shows that the resulting practices are ineffective or harmful. Many modern EMS practices (e.g., spinal immobilization practices, critical incident stress debriefings) became established because an expert thought them appropriate or effective. However, as additional information has been revealed by the research process, these practices, or specific aspects of these practices, are now considered to be of questionable benefit.

- *Animal research.* Animal research, also called *in vivo* (within the living) research, is important in understanding how certain drugs and procedures affect biological systems. Humans are mammals, and there has certainly been some important information learned from animal research, especially research on other mammals. However, findings in one species do not necessarily apply to other species. Computer modeling is starting to replace some aspects of animal research.

- *Bench research.* **Bench research** is scientific research at its most basic level. This type of research, often called *in vitro* (within the glass) or "test tube" research, is extremely important in learning how the universe functions. Bench research is often the first step in a research strategy that ultimately leads to animal and human research.

When evaluating the quality of research supporting a clinical practice, reviewers will typically stratify the scientific evidence based on the type and validity of the experimental designs used (Figures 5-8 and 5-9).

Study Validity

Validity is an important part of scientific research. Validity concerns whether or how well the study supports the conclusions—that is, is the interpretation of the results appropriate? We often look at a study as having **external validity** and **internal validity**. External validity assures that the results can be generalized, or possess generalizability (i.e., the results will hold true for other persons at other places and in other times). Internal validity ensures that the results can be attributed to the cause (e.g, an increase in psychiatric calls can be attributed to the full moon) and not to other possible causes.

LEVELS OF EVIDENCE
Prospective randomized controlled trials
Natural randomized controlled trials
Prospective, nonrandomized controlled trials
Retrospective nonrandomized controlled trials
Case series (no control group)
Animal studies
Extrapolations
Rational conjecture

FIGURE 5-8 The American Heart Association levels of evidence.

LEVELS OF EVIDENCE	
Ia.	Meta-analysis of randomized controlled trials
Ib.	One randomized controlled trial
IIa.	Controlled trial without randomization
IIb.	Other type of quasiexperimental study
III.	Descriptive studies (e.g., comparative studies, correlation studies, and case-control studies)
IV.	Expert committee reports or opinions, or clinical experience of respected authorities, or both

FIGURE 5-9 Oxford Center for Evidence-Based Medicine levels of evidence.

Ethical Considerations in Human Research

Medical research is essential, but an overriding concern is the rights of those who serve as subjects in the studies. During the Nazi regime in Germany in the twentieth century, the physician Josef Mengele and others conducted experiments on prisoners, primarily Jews, in German concentration camps. All these studies were performed without the consent of the subjects and often ended in the death of the subject. Some of the experiments had devastating effects, such as when injection of chemicals into the eyes of children to change their eye color resulted in blindness.

After the Nazi experimental atrocities came to light, an international consensus developed that it was necessary to protect the rights of humans who participate in research studies. Following the postwar trials of key Nazis at Nuremburg, Germany, the trial verdict included a set of guidelines to protect human subjects in research. These guidelines, called the Nuremburg Code of 1947, were the first code to guide ethical practice in human research.[5]

The United States has not been free of unethical research, even after the Nuremburg guidelines were promulgated. As a notorious example, between 1928 and 1972 the U.S. Public Health Service and researchers from Tuskegee University in Alabama allowed African American men infected with syphilis to remain untreated in order to study the natural progression of the disease. The men were never told they were infected and little, if any, treatment was provided.[6]

Additional strategies and guidelines regarding protection of human subjects have been developed since the Nuremburg Code. These include the Helsinki

CONTENT REVIEW
➤ An overriding concern in medical research is the rights of those who serve as subjects.

Legal Considerations

The Law and Ethical Medical Research. The Nuremburg Code did not have the force of law, but it influenced laws and rules for the same purpose that were subsequently adopted in various countries, including regulations issued by the U.S. Department of Health and Human Services governing federally funded research in the United States.

Today, medical research in the United States is closely regulated. All studies must be approved by an independent review board and subjects must provide informed consent in order to participate. The study is continuously monitored and certain groups (e.g., prisoners) are not allowed to participate. Although there is a potential for harm in many studies, research overall is now a much safer endeavor and has provided many of the advancements in modern medical care—including many of those in prehospital care.

Declaration of 1964, developed by the World Medical Association, and amended in 1975, 1983, 1989, 2000, 2008, and 2013.[7] The fundamental principles of the Helsinki Declaration are respect for the individual, the ability of the subject to make an informed decision about participating in the research (initial and ongoing), and assurance by the researcher that the patient's safety will be protected. Partly as a result of the Tuskegee experiment, in 1979 the U.S. Department of Health, Education, and Welfare released the Belmont Report, which was formally titled *Ethical Principles and Guidelines for the Protection of Human Subjects of Research*.[8] In 1991, 14 other federal agencies joined what is now the Department of Health and Human Services (HHS) in adopting uniform rules for protection of human subjects. The Office for Human Research Protections (OHRP) was also established within HHS.

Institutional Review Boards

To ensure the protection of human subjects in research, institutions that perform these studies must have an **institutional review board (IRB)**. The IRB (sometimes called the ethical review board or independent ethics committee) is a committee that approves, monitors, and reviews human research.[9] The goal of the IRB is to protect human subjects. IRBs have the power to approve or disapprove a study before it begins. They also have the power to require researchers to modify or even terminate a study if they feel the subjects are at risk. Most journals will not consider a study for publication unless it has been formally approved by an IRB.

An Overview of Statistics

Statistics is the mathematics of collecting and analyzing data to draw conclusions and make predictions. It is an essential part of scientific study. There are two general categories of statistics: descriptive statistics and inferential statistics. **Descriptive statistics** are used to describe the basic features of the data obtained in a study. They provide a summary of the sample. Together with simple graphics analysis, they form the basis of virtually every quantitative analysis of data. **Inferential statistics** draw information from the sampled observations of a population and make conclusions about the population. Both kinds of statistics are important in research.[10]

Descriptive Statistics

Descriptive statistics describe the nature of a sample. The most common descriptive statistic you will encounter is the **mean**, or average. It is calculated by adding the values, and then dividing the sum by the number of values involved. This provides the average or typical value of a group of numbers or cases. The mean is especially useful when the data are what statisticians call "normally distributed." This means that if you graphed the data, they would form a shape similar to a bell curve—a symmetrical or nearly symmetrical curve with most data falling in the center of the graph and fewer data falling at the beginning and end. Height of individuals is an example of a normally distributed variable. Most people have a height close to the average, with a few very short and a few very tall people at each end of the graph.

When the data are not normally distributed, the **median** is a better way of finding a typical value. To compute the median, put the values into numerical order and find the middle value. This is the median, also known as the "fiftieth percentile." For example, if you have seven exam scores, to find the median, you put the scores in order and find the fourth highest (or fourth lowest, as this is the same).

Here is an example of how the median can be more useful than the mean in some situations: In many states, the number of emergency calls received by EMS agencies is not normally distributed. There are frequently a few very busy services in urban areas, a good number of moderately busy services, and a larger number of services in rural areas that receive a much smaller number of calls. If you were to compute the mean, or average number of calls, it would be skewed by the very busy services, even though there are only a few of them, because they receive such a high number. However, if you computed the median, you would get a smaller number that would better reflect the number of calls received by a typical service.

The mean and the median tell only one part of the story. They are called **measures of central tendency**, because they indicate the center of the group. A different but very important quality to know about a group is how spread out it is, or how dispersed the data are.

There are two closely related measures of dispersion that you are likely to see. The first is called the **variance**. To get it, we take each value and subtract the mean from it. We cannot take the average of these numbers and get anything useful, because the negative numbers will cancel out the positive numbers and we will get zero. To overcome this, we multiply each number by itself (square it) and add up the squared numbers. We then divide this sum by the number of values we started with. (For reasons statisticians can describe, when we are working with samples, we usually divide by one less than the number of values.) This is the variance.

To get the **standard deviation (SD or σ)**, the other common measure of dispersion, we take the square root of the variance. Figure 5-10 shows two examples of variance and standard deviation. The standard deviation gives us valuable information about the data. If two groups of data have the same mean, but the second has a standard deviation much larger than the first, the data in the second group are much more spread out than the data in the first group. The SD is also used in many statistical formulas.

Another way we can describe data is to give the **mode**. This is simply the most common value in a set of data. If you graph the data, with the data value on the horizontal axis and the frequency of occurrence on the vertical axis (also known as a frequency distribution), the mode is the value associated with the highest point on the graph.

Inferential Statistics

As noted earlier, the mean, median, variance, standard deviation, and mode are examples of descriptive statistics. They describe the nature of a sample of data taken from a **population**, a group we are interested in.

Descriptive statistics are related to, but quite different from, inferential statistics. Here, instead of describing the sample, we wish to draw inferences about the population the sample came from. In this case, we say we are estimating **parameters** of the population. For example, if the sample is of sufficient size and we make certain assumptions about the population and how the sample was selected, we can estimate the mean value of the population from which we drew our sample. Polling organizations commonly use these techniques in reporting results of their surveys. We must keep in mind, however, the phenomenon of **sampling error**. This is an estimation of the difference between the value obtained from the sample and the value that would be obtained from the entire population, stemming solely from the fact that only a sample of the population was included.

When researchers find that something occurs with a certain frequency, they usually report this proportion as a percentage. For example, survival from cardiac arrest caused by ventricular fibrillation (VF) may be 20 percent in a particular study. But since the study looked at a sample of patients in VF, this proportion is only an estimate and may, in reality, be higher or lower in the entire group with cardiac arrest. Investigators can calculate how much variability exists in this percentage based on the number of observations, the actual data, and how reliable they wish the estimate to be.

This variability (not the same as the variance) can then be added and subtracted to the original proportion to give what is called a **confidence interval**. For example, suppose the investigators calculated the variability in the previous example with 95 percent confidence and found it was 6 percent. Then we would have a 95 percent confidence interval of 20 percent, plus or minus 6 percent. This means that, assuming the hypothesis is true, we can be 95 percent confident that the actual rate of survival under the conditions studied was between 14 percent and 26 percent.

Confidence intervals are very important in interpreting the value of the research results. If the confidence interval for a proportion such as the previous one included zero, then there would be a real possibility that there is no actual difference between the study group outcome and the control group outcome. We would conclude that the results are not statistically significant and that there is insufficient reason to believe there is a difference between the two groups.

Quantitative and Qualitative Statistics

There are many tests for finding differences between groups. Statisticians frequently classify them into qualitative and quantitative tests. **Qualitative statistics** usually deal with data that are nonnumeric in nature (e.g., female, male) or that are nonnumeric in nature and have been assigned a number indicating ranking or ordering of importance or severity (stage I, II, and III of certain cancers, for example). These are sometimes called **nominal data** and **ordinal data**. Finding the mean of such data may be impossible or absurd since they are categorical in nature. **Quantitative statistics**, however, are numerical in nature, such as temperature measured in degrees on a thermometer or height of an individual measured in centimeters or inches. They are sometimes referred to as *continuous data*.

Other Types of Data

Commonly used tests you may see in research include *t test*, the **analysis of variance (ANOVA)**, and the **chi square test**. Which test is used depends to a great extent on the kind of data involved and the kinds of differences the investigators are looking for. We will not describe these tests here, but the interested reader can consult some of the sources listed at the end of this chapter.

Examples of Variance and Standard Deviation

To see how the variance and standard deviation can give valuable information about data, consider this example: Two different EMT-P classes take the same midterm exam. The classes are the same size (seven students each) and have the same mean (or average) score, 85%. If we did not look any further, we might think the two classes performed the same on the exam. By looking at the variance and standard deviation, though, we can see that they are actually quite different.

Class 1

	Score	Mean	Score − Mean	(Score − Mean)^2
	78	85	−7	49
	81	85	−4	16
	82	85	−3	9
	84	85	−1	1
	87	85	2	4
	89	85	4	16
	94	85	9	81
Sum	595		0	176

Recall that to get the variance we must find the mean, then find the differences between the scores and the mean, square these differences, add them up, and divide by one less than the number of scores. The mean is included in the second column to make it easier to calculate the difference between each score and the mean. The variance is then 176/6 = 29.3. The standard deviation is the square root of 29.3, which is 5.4.

Class 2

	Score	Mean	Score − Mean	(Score − Mean)^2
	82	85	−3	9
	83	85	−2	4
	84	85	−1	1
	85	85	0	0
	86	85	1	1
	87	85	2	4
	88	85	3	9
Sum	595		0	28

Again, to get the variance, we sum the squared differences in the last column and divide by one less than the number of scores: 28/6 = 4.7. The standard deviation is the square root of 4.7, or 2.2, less than half the standard deviation of the first class.

This implies that the scores in the first class are much more spread out than the scores in the second class. When we graph the scores, we can see that this is true:

FIGURE 5-10 Examples of variance and standard deviation.

Another test you may see is the **odds ratio**. This is used in case-control studies and consists of the odds of having a risk factor if the condition is present, divided by the odds of having the risk factor if the condition is not present. Simply put, the odds ratio describes how strong the association is between a risk factor and the condition with which it is associated. The larger the risk factor, the stronger is the association. When you see an odds ratio, look for the confidence interval. Because an odds ratio of 1 indicates that there is no risk associated with the risk factor, if the confidence interval includes 1, there is no statistically significant risk.

For example, suppose investigators survey paramedic students regarding how much education they had received before enrolling in their course. They wish to test the hypothesis that having at least a college degree is associated with passing the paramedic certification exam. After the course is over, they perform the proper calculations and determine that the odds ratio is 1.6. This means a student who passes is 1.6 times as likely to have at least a college degree compared with someone who does not pass the exam. The 95 percent confidence interval, though, is 0.8 to 2.4.

This means we are 95 percent confident that the true odds ratio lies between 0.8 and 2.4. Because this interval includes 1 (keep in mind that an odds ratio of 1 means that there is no association), we cannot be 95 percent confident that there really is an association, so we conclude that there is no statistically significant relationship between having at least a college degree and passing the paramedic exam in this group. However, if the 95 percent confidence interval had been 1.2 to 2.0, an interval that does not include 1, we would have concluded with 95 percent confidence that there is a statistically significant relationship and that a person who passes the paramedic exam is between 1.2 and 2.0 times as likely to have at least a college degree.

Many other statistical tests are used for different kinds of studies and different kinds of data. The References section at the end of this chapter lists several sources from which you can learn more about them.

Format of a Research Paper

When authors submit their findings to a journal, they structure their results in a standardized fashion that allows others to quickly understand what the researchers did and what they found (Table 5-2). The first thing to appear after the title and names of the authors is the **abstract**. This is a brief paragraph that summarizes the need for the study, the research methods used, and the results encountered. Many people use the abstract to determine whether the paper is one of interest to them and therefore worth reading.

Table 5-2 Research Paper Format for Some Emergency Medicine Journals

Prehospital Emergency Care	Annals of Emergency Medicine	Academic Emergency Medicine
Abstract	Abstract	Abstract
Introduction	Introduction	Introduction
Methods	Methods	Methods
Results	Results	Results
Discussion	Limitations	Discussion
Conclusions	Discussion	Limitations
References	References	Conclusions
		References

The *introduction* is the first section of the paper itself. This is a brief description of pertinent, previously published papers on the subject of the investigation. It should describe why the study was undertaken and what the purpose of the study was or what hypothesis the authors wanted to test.

Next comes the *methods* section. This describes exactly how the authors conducted the study, including what population they wished to study, how subjects were selected (and excluded), and what intervention was performed, if any. There should be enough information for interested readers to repeat the experiment should they so desire. The authors should also describe how they determined the sample size, how much statistical power there was to detect a difference, which statistical tests they used to analyze the data, and what level of significance they chose for their statistical tests.

The *results* come next. Here the researchers provide their data (or a summary of the data), frequently with tables, charts, and graphs to help make sense of the information they gathered. This section presents the data, but does not elaborate on them.

The *discussion* section is where the authors interpret their findings and describe their significance. There is usually a description of how this new information fits into the field of study and whether it supports or refutes previous research. There should also be a discussion of the limitations of the study, frequently followed by a call for further research to answer the questions raised by the study.

The *summary*, or conclusion, is a very brief (no more than a few sentences) recap of the main findings of the study.

How a Research Paper Is Published

Once the authors of a study have drafted their paper, they submit it to a scientific journal for publication. Each journal has its own rules, but all peer-reviewed journals follow the same general procedure. After receiving the paper, the editor sends it to one or more members of a review board—people who have significant expertise either in the field covered by the journal or in a related area, such as statistics or research methodology. Generally, the reviewers are blinded as to the names of the authors and the institution with which they are affiliated. This serves to ensure objectivity and minimize bias. The reviewers read the paper and evaluate it for its adherence to standards of research methods, its pertinence to the field, and the potential value it has for practitioners. The reviewers send their comments to the editor, who then decides whether to publish it, send it back for revisions, or reject it. A copy editor may review the paper to correct grammar, spelling, and syntax. Many papers submitted by researchers are not published, and some journals have reputations for being very selective.

A note here about the term "abstract": In the preceding section, we mentioned that the first part of a research paper is a brief summary paragraph called the abstract. The term *abstract* more commonly describes a brief form of a longer scientific research paper that is often published before the full research paper. The abstract may be presented at national peer meetings, and responses to the abstract may form the basis for adjustments to the full research paper that is subsequently published. Abstracts are also published and cited in peer review journals.

The **peer review** process has recently begun to receive greater attention than it has in the past. This has been the result, ironically, of several studies looking at the quality of published papers. A surprisingly large number of papers, when evaluated objectively for adherence to principles of research methodology, have been shown to be deficient. This has led at least one journal, *Annals of Emergency Medicine*, to review and revamp its review procedures.[11] Reviewers now get training in what to look for and how to evaluate papers, and closer attention will be paid to how statistics are used. This may be the beginning of a trend that should improve the quality of the research that is conducted and published.

Accessing the Scientific Literature

Medical school and university libraries have multiple floors containing stacks and stacks of scientific journals. In the past, accessing the scientific literature was a labor-intensive endeavor. Now, in the Internet age, a great deal of the scientific literature is readily available. For many years, journal publishers have archived their publications online. These can be downloaded as portable document files (PDF) or directly. Most journals require a subscription or library affiliation to access. Some are free and referred to as **open access journals** without financial, legal, or technical barriers. If you don't have access to a medical or university library, many community college and hospital libraries can access the papers for you.

In addition, the National Libraries of Medicine have long provided an accessible database of the medical and scientific literature called PubMed. It is free and allows users to enter various search terms to find the material needed (Figure 5-11). A page will open that lists all the references that are related to your search term (Figure 5-12). You can further refine your search by choosing all articles or review articles. When you find a reference that meets the needs of your research, you can click on the citation and the information about the article and the abstract for the article will open (Figure 5-13). You can then determine whether this is an article worthy of retrieving and reading. Because searching PubMed is a somewhat complex and specialized task, you may want to have a librarian help you with your search to ensure that you get exactly the information you are looking for. If you do not have access to a library, the National Libraries of Medicine operates a document retrieval service known as Loansome Doc. It can be accessed through the web.

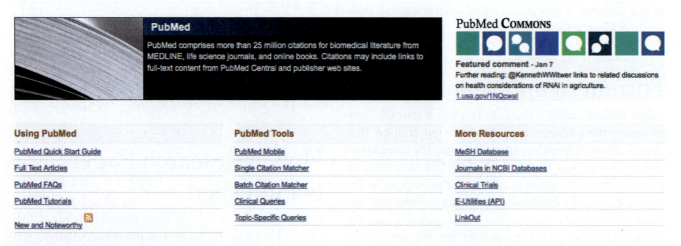

FIGURE 5-11 Opening screen of the PubMed database search engine.

(Source: NIH National Libraries of Medicine)

Search results

Items: 1 to 20 of 47295

<< First   < Prev   Page | 1 | of 2365   Next >   Last >>

☐ 1.   [Influence of EMS-physician presence on survival after out-of-hospital cardiopulmonary resuscitation: systematic review and meta-analysis.](#)
Böttiger BW, Bernhard M, Knapp J, Nagele P.
Crit Care. 2016 Jan 9;20(1):4.
PMID: 26747085   **Free PMC Article**
Similar articles

☐ 2.   [An environment for representing and using **medical** checklists on mobile devices.](#)
Losiouk E, Lanzola G, Visetti E, Quaglini S.
Conf Proc IEEE Eng Med Biol Soc. 2015 Aug;2015:7328-31. doi: 10.1109/EMBC.2015.7320084.
PMID: 26737984
Similar articles

☐ 3.   [[Traumatic Stress in **Emergency Medical Technicians**: Protective Role of Age and Education].](#)
Kılıç C, İnci F.
Turk Psikiyatri Derg. 2016 Winter;26(4):236-41. Turkish.
PMID: 26731020   **Free Article**
Similar articles

☐ 4.   [A modified Valsalva manoeuvre results in greater termination of supraventricular tachycardia than standard Valsalva manoeuvre.](#)
Smith GD.
Evid Based Med. 2016 Jan 4. pii: ebmed-2015-110357. doi: 10.1136/ebmed-2015-110357. [Epub ahead of print] No abstract available.
PMID: 26729773
Similar articles

☐ 5.   [Impact of a Novel Collaborative Long-Term Care -EMS Model: A Before-and-After Cohort Analysis of an Extended Care **Paramedic** Program.](#)
Jensen JL, Marshall EG, Carter AJ, Boudreau M, Burge F, Travers AH.
Prehosp Emerg Care. 2016 Jan-Feb;20(1):111-6. doi: 10.3109/10903127.2015.1051678. Epub 2015 Aug 17.
PMID: 26727341
Similar articles

FIGURE 5-12 Secondary scene of the PubMed database search engine after entering search term "paramedic."

Abstract ▾   Send to: ▾

Full text links

Prehosp Disaster Med. 2015 Feb;30(1):46-53. doi: 10.1017/S1049023X14001289. Epub 2014 Dec 9.

Glasgow Coma Scale Scoring is Often Inaccurate.

Bledsoe BE[1], Casey MJ[1], Feldman J[1], Johnson L[1], Diel S[2], Forred W[1], Gorman C[1].

⊕ Author Information

Save Items

☆ Add to Favorites ▾

Abstract
INTRODUCTION: The Glasgow Coma Scale (GCS) is widely applied in the emergency setting; it is used to guide trauma triage and for the application of essential interventions such as endotracheal intubation. However, inter-rater reliability of GCS scoring has been shown to be low for inexperienced users, especially for the motor component. Concerns regarding the accuracy and validity of GCS scoring between various types of emergency care providers have been expressed. Hypothesis/Problem The objective of this study was to determine the degree of accuracy of GCS scoring between various emergency care providers within a modern Emergency Medical Services (EMS) system.

METHODS: This was a prospective observational study of the accuracy of GCS scoring using a convenience sample of various types of emergency medical providers using standardized video vignettes. Ten video vignettes using adults were prepared and scored by two board-certified neurologists. Inter-rater reliability was excellent (Cohen's κ = 1). Subjects viewed the video and then scored each scenario. The scoring of subjects was compared to expert scoring of the two board-certified neurologists.

RESULTS: A total of 217 emergency providers watched 10 video vignettes and provided 2,084 observations of GCS scoring. Overall total GCS scoring accuracy was 33.1% (95% CI, 30.2-36.0). The highest accuracy was observed on the verbal component of the GCS (69.2%; 95% CI, 67.8-70.4). The eye-opening component was the second most accurate (61.2%; 95% CI, 59.5-62.9). The least accurate component was the motor component (59.8%; 95% CI, 58.1-61.5). A small number of subjects (9.2%) assigned GCS scores that do not exist in the GCS scoring system.

CONCLUSIONS: Glasgow Coma Scale scoring should not be considered accurate. A more simplified scoring system should be developed and validated.

KEYWORDS: EMS Emergency Medical Services; GCS Glasgow Coma Scale; SMS Simplified Motor Scale; SVS Simplified Verbal Scale; TBI traumatic brain injury; trauma care

Similar articles

Inter-rater reliability of the Full Outline of UnResponsiveness score and th [Crit Care. 2010]

The prehospital simplified motor score is as accurate as the prehospital [Emerg Med J. 2012]

Randomized controlled trial of a scoring aid to improve Glasgow Coma [Ann Emerg Med. 2015]

Review The use of Glasgow Coma Scale in injury assessment: a critical revie [Brain Inj. 2009]

Review A review of the predictive ability of Glasgow Coma Scale scc [J Neurosci Nurs. 2007]

See reviews...
See all...

PMID: 25489727 [PubMed - indexed for MEDLINE]

Cited by 1 PubMed Central article

Comparative Assessment of the Prognostic Value of Biomarkers in Trauma [PLoS One. 2015]

FIGURE 5-13 Individual citation screen of the PubMed database.

What to Look for When Reviewing a Study

Questions to ask when reviewing a study include the following (Table 5-3):

- *Was the research peer reviewed?* This is no guarantee of quality, but it at least indicates that experts have reviewed the study and found it to have some merit. Keep in mind that some journals will deliberately publish papers that they know to be of lower quality than usual in order to stir up debate about an important subject.

- *Was there a clear hypothesis or study purpose?* The paper should have a clear description of exactly what the investigators were evaluating and what their study hypothesis was. When a hypothesis is not clearly spelled out, it is very easy for the investigators to draw unjustified conclusions.

- *Was the study approved by an IRB, and was it conducted ethically?* An IRB is a group of people, usually at a hospital or university, who review study proposals to ensure that patients are protected when they participate in research as study subjects. Virtually all medical journals require IRB approval for research involving human subjects.

- *Was the study type appropriate?* Not every investigation lends itself to the format of the randomized controlled clinical trial. It may be necessary, for ethical or financial reasons, to use another format. Evaluate whether the questions the investigators asked were well suited to the type of study they conducted.

- *What population were the researchers studying?* Is the population similar to the one you see in your community and work?

Table 5-3 Questions to Ask When Reviewing a Study

- Was the research peer reviewed?
- Was there a clear hypothesis or study purpose?
- Was the study approved by an institutional review board (IRB), and was it conducted ethically?
- Was the study type appropriate?
- What population were the researchers studying?
- What inclusion and exclusion criteria did the researchers use?
- How did the investigators draw their sample?
- How many groups were patients divided into, and were patients assigned to control and study groups properly?
- Were the control and study groups the proper size?
- Were the effects of confounding variables taken into account?
- What kind of data did the investigators collect, and did they analyze the data with the proper statistical tests?
- Were the results reported properly?
- How likely is it that the study results would occur by chance alone?
- Are the authors' conclusions logical and based on the data?

- *What inclusion and exclusion criteria did the researchers use?* If the investigators excluded the patients most likely to have a condition or patients very similar to the ones you see, the study may have very little to tell you.

- *How did the investigators draw their sample?* Did they use true **random sampling**? **systematic sampling**? **time sampling**? **convenience sampling**?

- *How many groups were patients divided into, and were patients assigned to control and study groups properly?* The effects of bias and confounding must be taken into account for the study to yield worthwhile results. In particular, ask yourself:

  - For case-control and cohort studies, were selection bias and recall bias taken into account?

  - For randomized controlled studies, were randomization and blind assignment maintained?

- *Were the control and study groups the proper size?* Did the investigators describe the sample size necessary to produce sufficient power to avoid a type II error (a false negative)? What was the power of the study? (Was the study adequately performed to accurately test the hypothesis in question?)

- *Were the effects of confounding variables (other things that may have affected the study outcome) taken into account?* Did the investigators describe potential confounders and how they prevented them from interfering with the study?

- *What kind of data did the investigators collect, and did they analyze the data with the proper statistical tests?* There are many tests available and more than one may be appropriate for the conditions at hand. You may need to consult a statistician or researcher to determine whether the investigators used the right tests on the data. Did the investigators clearly determine before data collection took place which tests they were going to use, or was there **data mining**? When the data fail to provide statistically significant results, it is very tempting to perform more tests until one shows significant results. This kind of retrospective testing is called *data snooping* or **data dredging**. If one continues to perform statistical tests, eventually one will be significant just by chance alone. This inappropriate use of statistics is to be avoided.

- *Were the results reported properly?* When a paper includes a proportion or an odds ratio, is there also a 95 percent confidence interval?

- *How likely is it that the study results would occur by chance alone?* Remember that a *P* value reflects only the odds of seeing the results of a particular piece of research if the study hypothesis is true. A small *P* value may be very impressive, but it does not prove the study hypothesis. In addition, keep in mind the difference between association and causation. For example, it would be easy to show that the number of drownings increases with sales of ice cream. An inattentive reader might conclude that the sale of more ice cream causes more drownings to occur. In reality, this is an example of association, not causation. Ice cream sales go up when the weather gets warmer, which is also when more people go swimming and drown. This is also an example of confounding.

- *Are the author's conclusions logical and based on the data?* Occasionally a journal publishes a paper that goes against everything you know. It can then be difficult to determine whether you need to change your approach to a particular problem or consider the paper an aberration. After all, by chance alone, some studies will show statistically significant results that are the result of chance or coincidence. Sometimes, the prudent course is to see whether anyone else can replicate the experiment before changing your practice. This is a good example of how you should be very cautious in changing your practice based on just one study. If the conclusion is a real one and not spurious, someone else should be able to come up with it, too.

And here is one more consideration that is very important in EMS research:

- *How "good" was the EMS system in which the study was done?* This factor can have a profound effect on the validity of a study. As an extreme example, how valid would be the results of a study of the impact of AED use if the time from arrest to first responder arrival were 15 minutes? In this scenario, there would likely be no survivors, no matter what intervention was used!

Applying Study Results to Your Practice

Once you have evaluated a study, you will be in a better position to determine whether it should change your practice. Before you do so, though, you need to consider several factors. Rarely do clinicians make significant changes on the basis of just one study. Because no study can definitively prove a hypothesis, the reader must look at other studies and his own experience to construct an informed opinion. If every other study published on a particular topic comes to very different conclusions than the study at hand, the reader must wonder whether the study was poorly designed, subject to bias of some sort, affected by unknown confounding variables, or just the result of chance. One must evaluate the field and its knowledge base to make an informed decision about how to interpret a piece of research.

The clinical significance is another important piece of the puzzle to consider.

A P value with lots of zeroes (e.g., $P < 0.0001$) may be very impressive, but not very pertinent. Distinguish between the statistical significance and the clinical significance of the study. Was the difference found in the study large enough to make a real difference to patients?

When investigators conduct their experiments, they have the luxury of selecting patients who meet their criteria and excluding patients who do not. In the real world, things are not quite so tidy. Before we can apply the results of a piece of research to a particular patient, we must be sure the patient is similar enough to the study group to benefit from the intervention.

Finally, EMS providers do not function in a vacuum. Before implementing any significant changes in your practice, speak to the management of your organization, and especially to your medical director. You are responsible not only to your patients, but also to your bosses and your medical director. Including them in decision making of this nature is essential and will pay off in better patient care overall.

Participating in Research

Many EMS systems are not content to watch other people advance their field. They have decided to conduct research themselves. They have found that, by executing well-designed studies, they can not only improve care in their coverage areas, but also improve out-of-hospital care throughout the nation, sharpen the skills of their providers, and rekindle their providers' interest by doing something new and potentially groundbreaking.

Before you participate in such a study, there are certain things you should do and find out (Table 5-4). Usually, the first step is to ask a question. This should involve something of practical importance. Determining the value of a particular intervention (end-tidal CO_2 monitoring, for example) is clearly going to have more impact on EMS than finding out whether ambulances carry 24 four-by-four gauze pads or 48 four-by-four gauze pads.

Once you have focused on the issue and determined exactly what you wish to discover, you can go to the next step. This is where you generate your hypothesis, a statement of exactly what you are going to test. The **null hypothesis** is usually a statement that there is no difference between the

---

Table 5-4 What to Do When You Participate in a Study

- Determine the question.
- Prepare your hypotheses (null hypothesis and research hypothesis).
- Decide what you wish to measure and how you will do it.
- Define the population you are studying.
- Identify the limitations of your study.
- Get the approval of the proper authorities.
- Determine how you will get informed consent from study subjects.
- Gather data, perhaps after conducting pilot trials.
- Analyze the data.
- Determine what you will do with your results (publish, present at a conference, follow up with more studies).

Source: American College of Cardiology and the American Heart Association, Manual for ACC/AHA Guideline Writing Committees.

groups you are sampling from. The research hypothesis or alternate hypothesis is a statement that there is a difference between the groups. This is often, though not always, what you would like to show.

Once you know what you are evaluating, you need to decide what you want to measure and how you will do it. You also need to define the population you will be studying—that is, the group from which you draw your subjects and to which you plan to generalize your results.

Closely associated with this step is determining the limitations of your study. This might include limited ability to generalize your results because of the patient selection methods you used, even though you had little or no choice in the methods available to you. Similarly, the population you draw from might be significantly different from other populations.

For example, if you wished to test for improved survival in hypotensive trauma patients, some of whom received a large volume of IV fluids as treatment and some of whom did not, you would need to describe your EMS and trauma care system very carefully. You might have a primarily urban population with predominantly penetrating trauma, short transport times to Level I trauma centers, and experienced paramedics. Your results would have limited applicability to a rural population with predominantly blunt trauma, long transport times to small community hospitals, and less experienced Emergency Medical Responders and EMTs.

The best studies limit themselves to a single question or hypothesis. This is desirable because it allows you to focus better on the question at hand. The downside is that you may not find out everything you wanted to. This is usually considered an acceptable trade-off. No single study can answer every question.

The next step in conducting a study is usually to get approval from an IRB. This allows you to get an outside evaluation of your study methodology and reduces considerably the chance you will be accused of conducting an unethical study. One of the items the IRB will undoubtedly be interested in is the issue of informed consent (consent given by the patient based on full disclosure of information regarding the nature, risks, and benefits of the procedure or study).

Several reports in the media over the past few years have described unethical studies in which subjects were not given the opportunity to give or refuse consent because they were not informed of the risks and benefits of participating in the study. In some cases, subjects actually died because they did not receive standard treatment available at the time of the study. These stories have prompted an understandable reluctance on the part of many individuals to participate in research. The U.S. government even came out with standards for government-funded research that describe stringent requirements for informed consent. The IRB process will also determine what kind of consent will be required for your study.

A good **principal investigator (PI)**, the person who oversees the study, will be familiar with these requirements and will be able to guide you through them. The PI should also gain the approval of other appropriate agencies, including the medical director and the head of the service involved.

After you have determined how to gain informed consent, you need to gather your data. Sometimes a pilot trial is undertaken first so you can find unforeseen obstacles to data gathering. Seemingly trivial matters can become very important (such as whether busy EMS providers are reluctant to fill out any more forms). A good PI will meet with the EMS providers who are administering the study intervention and collecting the data. The PI should make sure they know how long the study is expected to last. This allows them to make plans and perhaps reschedule certain future activities they had anticipated. The providers collecting data need to know the name of the PI and how to contact him. The PI is usually, though not always, a physician. Many EMS physicians who conduct field research will recruit a field provider to coordinate and assist with data collection.

Other things to tell participants are the inclusion and exclusion criteria for enrolling patients in the study, the effect of the study on patient care in general, and the risks and potential benefits to patients in the study. Once everyone understands these factors, you will be prepared to go ahead with the study.

After you have collected the data and reached your predetermined sample size, it is time to analyze the data. Use the tests you described in your description of the methods for your study. Be very careful about performing additional tests, especially if your results do not show what you hoped or expected. Data snooping is a dangerous activity. If you perform enough statistical tests, you will eventually find one or more that give you "significant" results. Unfortunately, these results may very well be a product of chance rather than your intervention. When multiple statistical tests are planned for the same set of data, statisticians adjust for this with multiple testing procedures to avoid such false results. Similarly, *post hoc* analysis of subgroups that were not defined before the study can also be dangerous. This can be a good way of generating hypotheses for future studies, but it is not a good basis for drawing conclusions now.

Once you have finished your data analysis, you must decide what to do with your results. If you feel that your study addresses a pertinent timely issue, and you think your methods were well thought out and your study was carefully conducted, you should seriously consider submitting your results to a peer-reviewed journal. This is the best way to get such information out to the EMS community.

Alternatively, you may decide to present your findings at a conference. This usually involves summarizing your methods and results either orally or in the form of a poster, or both. This is less time consuming than writing up a paper for publication, but it can still get the word out about your results and stimulate others to investigate the same phenomenon.

Do not feel that a "negative" study is worthless. If your study shows no difference in outcomes between groups that did and did not receive an intervention, you may have reached important conclusions about the value, or lack of value, of an intervention.

A common result of a well-conducted study is more questions. This frequently stimulates the investigator and others to perform further studies. Once you get involved with researching the answers to questions, you may find yourself a little more skeptical about accepted, untested treatments and more interested in finding out what really works.

Evidence-Based Decision Making

In the past, traditional medical practices have been based on medical knowledge (often learned during initial education), intuition, and judgment. Although all of these are quite important, technology and science change. Thus, medical practice and the use of technology should focus on procedures and practices proven effective in improving patient outcomes. EMS is now at the point at which evidence-based decision making and practice are becoming standard. The use of "best practices" and "clinical pathways" that are based on the best available clinical and scientific evidence ensures that the care provided is safe, efficacious, and cost effective. The problem that remains, at least in the EMS setting, is that the available research is, at present, scant or of limited quality. Hopefully, as EMS evolves, this will change.

Evidence-based decision making involves first formulating a question about appropriate treatments. Then the medical literature is searched and organized for additional evaluation. Next, the scientific evidence is stratified based on validity and reliability (see Table 5-5 for the classification recommendations of the American College of Cardiology and the American Heart Association). Then, if the

Table 5-5 Applying Classification of Recommendations and Level of Evidence

		Size of Treatment Effect			
		Class I	**Class IIa**	**Class IIb**	**Class III**
		Benefit >>> Risk **Procedure/Treatment SHOULD be performed/administered**	Benefit >> Risk Additional studies with focused objectives needed **IT IS REASONABLE to perform procedure/administer treatment**	Benefit ≥ Risk Additional studies with broad objectives needed; Additional registry data would be helpful **IT IS NOT UNREASONABLE to perform procedure/administer treatment**	Risk ≥ Benefit No additional studies needed Procedure/Treatment should NOT be performed/administered SINCE IT IS NOT HELPFUL AND MAY BE HARMFUL
Estimate of Certainty (Precision) of Treatment Effect	**Level A** Multiple (3–5) population risk strata evaluated General consistency of direction and magnitude of effect	• Recommendation that procedure or treatment is useful/effective • Sufficient evidence from multiple randomized trials or meta-analyses	• Recommendation in favor of treatment or procedure being useful/effective • Some conflicting evidence from multiple randomized trials or meta-analyses	• Recommendation's usefulness/efficacy less well established • Greater conflicting evidence from multiple randomized trials or meta-analyses	• Recommendation that procedure or treatment not useful/effective and may be harmful • Sufficient evidence from multiple randomized trials or meta-analyses
	Level B Limited (2–3) population risk strata evaluated	• Recommendation that procedure or treatment is useful/effective • Limited evidence from single randomized trial or non-randomized studies	• Recommendation in favor of treatment or procedure being useful/effective • Some conflicting evidence from single randomized trial or non-randomized studies	• Recommendation's usefulness/efficacy less well established • Greater conflicting evidence from single randomized trial or non-randomized studies	• Recommendation that procedure or treatment not useful/effective and may be harmful • Limited evidence from single randomized trial or non-randomized studies
	Level C Very limited (1–2) population risk strata evaluated	• Recommendation that procedure or treatment is useful/effective • Only expert opinion, case studies, or standard of care	• Recommendation in favor of treatment or procedure being useful/effective • Only diverging expert opinion, case studies, or standard of care	• Recommendation's usefulness/efficacy less well established • Only diverging expert opinion, case studies, or standard of care	• Recommendation that procedure or treatment not useful/effective and may be harmful • Only expert opinion, case studies, or standard of care

Source: Circulation. http://circ.ahajournals.org/manual/manual_IIstep6.shtml

evidence supports a change in the practice, the change is made. However, the process does not end there. Once the practice has been changed, ongoing evaluation must be carried out to determine whether the practice is correctly applied to the proper group of patients. In addition, an ongoing outcomes study should occur to determine whether the change in practice is improving essential parameters such as mortality, morbidity, and costs.

Summary

The paramedic of the twenty-first century must have more than a passing knowledge of research. Solid, well-conducted scientific research is the key to improving prehospital care. It is also essential to prove that paramedics make a difference in terms of reducing mortality, morbidity, and pain and suffering. A side benefit to demonstrating the effectiveness of EMS will be an increased (and more appropriate) revenue stream. The future of EMS depends on an aggressive research program, and prehospital research depends on knowledgeable and engaged paramedics.

You Make the Call

One day, you and your partner are restocking the ambulance and notice that the crew that precedes you seems to be using a lot more naloxone (Narcan) than your crew. At a shift meeting you bring up the fact that some crews are using more naloxone than others. A discussion ensues, and the consensus is that there are not a great number of narcotic overdoses in the community, so the usage of naloxone might be a misapplication of a protocol. Because you and your partner brought up the issue, you have been asked to study the problem.

You and your partner decide to develop a research question. However, you feel that you really need to get a handle on the number of overdoses in the community that required naloxone. So you first do a retrospective study looking at all run reports over the last year. One of your fellow employees, who is on light duty following surgery, goes through all run reports for the prior year. He records the number of total runs, the number of times an opiate overdose was encountered, the number of times naloxone was given, the number of total doses of naloxone administered, and the ID number of the paramedic who administered the drug in each case. These data are placed into an Excel computerized database and analyzed.

When you analyze the data, you see that the incidence of narcotic overdoses requiring naloxone was 0.12 percent of all calls—a pretty low incidence. However, you note that two paramedics were responsible for 45 percent of all naloxone administrations during the study period.

You discuss your findings with your clinical manager and medical director. The medical director directs the clinical manager to provide a continuing education seminar on narcotic overdoses and the usage of naloxone to all paramedics in the system—including the part-timers.

For the next three months, you and your partner prospectively monitor the daily run reports and see whether any of the parameters in your initial study have changed. At three months, you find that the incidence of opiate overdoses requiring naloxone remains low, at 0.14 percent. The total amount of naloxone administered has diminished significantly, and statistical analysis finds that all paramedics in the system have been using the naloxone similarly. The medical director feels that the education program worked and thanks you and your partner for your efforts.

1. What is your study's hypothesis?

2. Did you prove or disprove your hypothesis?

3. What was the derived benefit from the study?

See Suggested Responses at the back of this book.

Review Questions

1. Proving that the care and service provided by EMS to the community is worthy of funding and support is demonstrated primarily through

   _____

   a. scientific research.
   b. outcomes-based research.
   c. the scientific method.
   d. quantitative research.

2. _____ research describes phenomena in numbers.
   a. Qualitative
   b. Quantitative
   c. Mixed
   d. Scientific

3. _____ research describes phenomena in words.
   a. Qualitative
   b. Quantitative
   c. Mixed
   d. Scientific

4. The variable that affects the dependent variable under study is the _____
   a. individual variable.
   b. independent variable.

   c. standard variable.
   d. quantitative variable.

5. A study that looks primarily at existing data is the

   _____

   a. retrospective study.
   b. prospective study.
   c. independent study.
   d. scientific study.

6. The closer a study adheres to _____, the more valid is the study.
   a. independent variables
   b. dependent variables
   c. the general hypothesis
   d. the scientific method

7. Which of the following is NOT a randomized controlled trial?
   a. Qualitative study
   b. Single blind study
   c. Double blind study
   d. Prospective study with randomization

See answers to Review Questions at the back of this book.

References

1. Wang, H. E. and D. M. Yealy. "Out-of-Hospital Endotracheal Intubation: Where Are We?" *Ann Emerg Med* 47 (2006): 532–541.
2. Lateef, F. and T. Kelvin. "Military anti-shock garment: Historical relic or a device with unrealized potential?" *J Emerg Trauma Shock* 1 (2008): 63–69.
3. Sayre, M. R., L. J. White, L. H. Brown, S. D. McHenry; National EMS Agenda Writing Team. "National EMS Research Agenda." *Prehosp Emerg Care* 6 (2002): S1–S43.
4. National Libraries of Medicine. PubMed. (Available at http://www.ncbi.nlm.nih.gov/pubmed/.)
5. National Institutes of Health. Directives for Human Experimentation. (Available at http://ohsr.od.nih.gov/guidelines/nuremberg.html.)
6. White, R. M. "Unraveling the Tuskegee Study of Untreated Syphilis." *Arch Int Med* 160 (2000): 585–598.
7. World Medical Association. WMA Declaration of Helsinki—Ethical Principles for Medical Research Involving Human Subjects. (Available at http://www.wma.net/en/30publications/10policies/b3/index.html.)
8. National Institutes of Health. The Belmont Report: Ethical Principles and Guidelines for the Protection of Human Subjects in Research. (Available at http://ohsr.od.nih.gov/guidelines/belmont.html.)
9. Mann, H. "Research Ethics Committees and Public Dissemination of Clinical Trial Results." *Lancet* 360 (2002): 406–408.
10. Goodacre, S. "Critical Appraisal in Emergency Medicine 2: Statistics." *Emerg Med J* 394 (2008): 1–6.
11. Waeckerle, J. F. and M. L. Callaham. "Medical Journals and the Science of Peer Reviewing: Raising the 'Standard.'" *Ann Emerg Med* 28 (1996): 75–77.

Further Reading

Brown, L. H., E. L. Criss, and N. H. Prasad. *An Introduction to EMS Research.* Upper Saddle River, NJ: Pearson/Brady, 2002.
Rumsey, D. *Statistics for Dummies.* Hoboken, NJ: Wiley, 2003.
Wiersma, W. *Research Methods in Education: An Introduction.* 7th ed. Boston, MA: Allyn and Bacon, 2000.

Chapter 6
Public Health

Bryan Bledsoe, DO, FACEP, FAAEM

STANDARD
Public Health

COMPETENCY
Applies fundamental knowledge of principles of public health and epidemiology, including public health emergencies, health promotion, and illness and injury prevention.

 ## Learning Objectives

Terminal Performance Objective: After reading this chapter, you should be able to apply principles of public health in your role as a paramedic.

Enabling Objectives: To accomplish the terminal performance objective, you should be able to:

1. Define key terms introduced in this chapter.

2. Identify EMS roles that are within the domain of public health, and components that must be in place for EMS and public health to work together.

3. Define the three categories of public health laws and discuss public health efforts that have improved the quality of life.

4. Explain basic concepts of epidemiology.

5. Give examples of how EMS providers can be involved in public health strategies.

6. Describe the roles of EMS organizations and EMS providers in the prevention of EMS provider illness and injury.

7. Identify areas of need for prevention programs in the community.

KEY TERMS

Case Study

It's a hot July day and Timmy is spending it with John, whose family has an in-ground pool. At approximately 9:00 AM, John's mom receives a phone call. The two boys, who had been watching cartoons in the living room, run out to the patio, grab the large inflatable alligator raft, and head for the water. Timmy pronounces himself "king of the alligator killers" as he jumps on the raft. John says he is the "true king" and plops himself down on top of Timmy. In the resulting tussle, Timmy rolls off the raft and into the water. He tries, but is unable, to get a good enough grasp on the edge of the concrete pool. John watches his friend struggle and, terrified, runs to the side of the house to hide. All this takes about 7 minutes.

At approximately 9:10 AM, John's mom hangs up the phone. As she steps out onto the patio, she sees Timmy's small form floating face down in the pool. She races to the pool, jumps in, and pulls Timmy out. She checks to see whether he is breathing, but he is not. She starts for the phone, but stops short. Where is John? It takes her another minute to find him and another 30 seconds to get to the phone to dial 911.

It takes you and your partner 6 minutes to respond. While waiting, John's mother stays with Timmy, turning him on his side to let the water drain from his mouth and lungs and pleads with him softly to "hang in there." When you arrive on scene, you perform a scene size-up and a primary assessment and start CPR. Timmy begins to breathe in about a minute, but he does not regain consciousness. You rush him to the hospital emergency department. There, the staff praises your actions and tell you, "You did the best you could."

Almost a year later, Timmy has still not regained consciousness. The costs for Timmy's care so far have reached more than $650,000. It is difficult to predict the total cost. With good medical care, Timmy could live for many years. This unfortunate situation could have been prevented through the use of relatively inexpensive alarms and locks on doors leading to the swimming pool, as well as a pool alarm that detects changes in water displacement when an object falls into the pool.

Introduction

Many EMS providers are first drawn to emergency medical services because of the opportunity to make a dramatic contribution to society and those in need. We respond to countless scenes of crisis and tragedy and feel genuine excitement when the critically ill or injured patient improves after receiving emergency medical care. Beyond the excitement of the moment, however, is a sobering reality. How often do EMS crews respond to incidents that could easily have been prevented? How often have you thought to yourself, "What a shame" or "I wish there was something I could have done" in the wake of senseless circumstances surrounding an accidental injury or illness?

Such thoughts are all too common after an incident. But what if EMS providers, leaders, and administrators asked these questions *before* an incident occurred? How many injuries could be prevented? How many lives could be saved? This chapter focuses on these questions and discusses the interaction between paramedicine and public health.

Basic Principles of Public Health

Public health is defined as the science and practice of protecting and improving the health of a community through the use of preventive medicine, health education, control of communicable diseases, application of sanitary measures, and monitoring of environmental hazards. Public health measures have played a significant role in improving the safety and quality of life of humankind. The primary tenet of public health is to identify and prevent injury and illness—that is, to take steps to remedy a situation *before* it results in an injury or an illness. The roles of public health in modern society are diverse and extremely important (Figure 6-1). As EMS has evolved, it has become clear that EMS has some roles and responsibilities that are clearly within the domain of public health (Figure 6-2). In fact, some communities are working to closely link their EMS and public health systems. To achieve this, a community must have the following:

- Strong medical oversight of both public health and EMS
- A desire and an effort to educate both emergency care and public health providers about the others' roles
- Recognition of the role of and a commitment to developing and maintaining relationships among leaders of the component groups through regular meetings, team-building exercises, and planning
- Bringing community stakeholders (businesses, clinics, universities, and others) into the planning process
- Creating disaster plans that are developed locally, involve public health and emergency care, and are repeatedly drilled
- Aggressively pursuing and securing funding

Public Health Functions

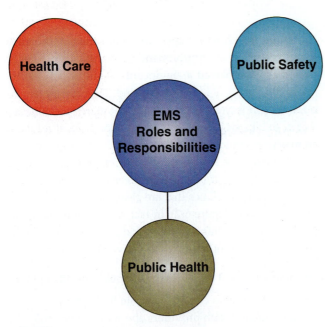

FIGURE 6-1 An overview of public health.
(Source: Centers for Disease Control and Prevention)

FIGURE 6-2 Much of the role of EMS falls within the domain of public health.

Accomplishments in Public Health

Public health has improved both the quality of life and the lifespan of humankind. These improvements have occurred through research, epidemiology, surveillance, prevention, and other strategies. Some of the most important public

Table 6-1 Public Health Accomplishments (United States)

Public Health Accomplishments (United States)
Vaccination
Motor vehicle safety
Safer workplaces
Control of infectious diseases
Decline in deaths from coronary artery disease and stroke
Safer and healthier foods
Healthier mothers and babies
Family planning
Fluoridation of drinking water
Recognition of tobacco as a health hazard

health accomplishments of the past century are detailed in Table 6-1.

Public Health Laws

Public health laws—laws that affect public health practice and strategies—are generally divided into three categories:

- *Illness and prevention.* These laws give public health officials the necessary legal tools to perform their jobs.
- *Police powers for public health agencies.* These laws allow public health entities to act in the general interest of the public, when necessary. Sometimes these actions are in conflict with individual civil liberties. However, in certain situations, such as epidemics and disasters, the needs of the public as a whole generally outweigh the needs of the individual.
- *Epidemiological tools.* These laws give public health agencies the power to use epidemiological tools to analyze legal issues related to public health practice and enforcement.

In 2009, the Public Health Law Research Program (PHLRP) was established at Temple University in Philadelphia. This program, funded by the Robert Wood Johnson Foundation, aids public health entities in promoting effective regulatory and legal solutions to public health problems.[1]

Epidemiology

Epidemiology is the branch of medicine that deals with the incidence and prevalence of disease in large populations. It also works to detect the source and cause of epidemics of infectious disease and other health events. Epidemiology is concerned primarily with the frequency and pattern of health events that occur in a population.

A number of concepts and terms are used in epidemiology. One such concept is **years of productive life**, a calculation made by subtracting the age at death from 65. (For example, in a liability lawsuit concerning the death of a 45-year-old, a jury might assess damages based on the deceased's loss of 20 years as a wage earner.) Another concept is **injury**, which refers to the intentional or unintentional damage to a person resulting from acute exposure to thermal, mechanical, electrical, or chemical energy or from the absence of such essentials as heat and oxygen. An accident is an *unintentional injury*, but an injury that is purposefully inflicted either on oneself (e.g., suicide) or on another person (e.g., homicide) is an *intentional injury*. Intentional injuries make up about a third of all injury deaths. Other categories of intentional injury include rape, assault, and domestic, elder, and child abuse.

Another concept related to epidemiology is **injury risk**, which is a hazardous or potentially hazardous situation that puts people in danger of sustaining injury. As medical professionals, EMS providers should assess every scene and situation for injury risk and maintain statistics as part of an **injury surveillance program**, which is the ongoing systematic collection, analysis, and interpretation of injury data essential to the planning, implementation, and evaluation of public health practice.

An injury surveillance program must also include a component for the timely dissemination of data to those who need to know. The final link in the injury surveillance chain is the application of these data to prevention and control. "Teachable moments" occur shortly after an injury, when the patient and observers remain acutely aware of what has happened and may be more receptive to learning about how a similar injury or illness could be prevented in the future.

By becoming involved in injury prevention, EMS providers can focus on **primary prevention**, or keeping an injury from ever occurring.[2] Medical care and rehabilitation activities that help to prevent further problems from occurring are referred to, respectively, as **secondary prevention** and **tertiary prevention**.

Epidemiology has six major roles in public health practice:

- *Public health surveillance.* Public health surveillance is the ongoing and systematic collection, analysis, interpretation, and dissemination of health data to aid the public and to aid in health care decision making and action.
- *Field investigation.* Following detection of a health concern through public health surveillance, a field investigation is typically begun. This investigation may be limited to a simple phone call or may involve fieldwork to identify the extent and cause of the health problem in question.

- *Analytic studies.* In most situations, surveillance and field investigations can identify the causes, modes of transmission, and appropriate control and prevention measures for most public health problems. However, when the health problem is more complex (e.g., epidemic), analytic methods are often employed. An example of this was the investigation and detection of AIDS (acquired immunodeficiency syndrome) in 1981. Researchers in both New York and California began to see an unusual form of skin cancer (Kaposi's sarcoma) and an unusual form of pneumonia (*Pneumocystis* pneumonia) among gay men in their communities. This resulted in significant public health efforts to identify the disease and its cause and required the use of analytic methods. In 1983, researchers at the Pasteur Institute in France isolated the human immunodeficiency virus (HIV) that was believed to be the causative agent of what is now called HIV/AIDS. Researchers subsequently backtracked the cases of AIDS that were known at the time and found that a Canadian flight attendant, who was nicknamed "patient zero," was the most likely source for introducing the HIV virus into the general population. By 1985, a test kit for HIV was available and approved by the FDA. In 1987, treatment regimens were developed for HIV. Today, although HIV/AIDS remains a serious infection, the incidence has declined and people with the disease are living almost-normal lifespans.[3]
- *Evaluation.* Evaluation, from an epidemiological standpoint, is an ongoing process that determines the effectiveness, efficiency, and impact of activities related to public health initiatives. In other words, it is a system to verify that public health policies are doing what they were intended to do and are cost effective.
- *Linkage.* A true public health system requires interaction among various agencies and other entities. As public health policies have been refined, there has been a push to integrate other disciplines, such as emergency medical services, into public health efforts. Interactions include developing preestablished protocols and agreements, memoranda of understanding, and the sharing of information between organizations. These strategies tie in to the interoperability agreements recommended by the Department of Homeland Security (DHS) and the National Incident Management System (NIMS).
- *Policy development.* In many situations, epidemiologists and other public health professionals have the needed expertise to assist in development of policies, rules, and regulations that have a positive impact on the health and welfare of the population.

EMS Public Health Strategies

Although there are clear differences between EMS practice and public health, at its most fundamental level, EMS is a public health system. Over the past few years, based on the *EMS Agenda for the Future*, there has been a concerted effort to integrate EMS into public health, and vice versa.[4]

The numerous roles for EMS in the public health arena include the following:

• *Health promotion.* EMS personnel can play several important roles in public health. These include such primary prevention strategies as providing health care screenings and vaccinations. With these services, there is an educational component, an opportunity for EMS personnel to inform the public about injury and illness prevention. This can be taken a step further to target high-risk populations in an effort to ensure that they are receiving needed medical care. Many elderly, homeless, and destitute individuals avoid seeking health care because of cost or transportation issues. Many EMS systems, usually in conjunction with social service organizations, periodically assist in helping these high-risk communities.

• *Disease surveillance.* EMS is often the first to encounter an evolving public health emergency such as an epidemic or terrorist activity. By its nature, the EMS system can be an effective monitor of the community. An increase in EMS calls for certain medical conditions or injuries is often an indicator of an evolving larger issue. Several programs provide real-time surveillance. For example, FirstWatch® provides ongoing, live analysis of data to identify patterns and trends as they emerge. This early detection allows actions to be taken quickly, hopefully saving lives and protecting property. When a threat is detected, FirstWatch automatically sends alerts to authorized, appropriate personnel via e-mail, pager, SMS (short message service) text messaging, or fax. Alerts can contain summary reports, charts, graphs, maps, and other important or mission-critical information (Figure 6-3).

• *Disaster management.* The EMS system is at the core of disaster response. As disasters play out, the mission changes from rescue to recovery. Although EMS personnel are well prepared for rescue and emergency

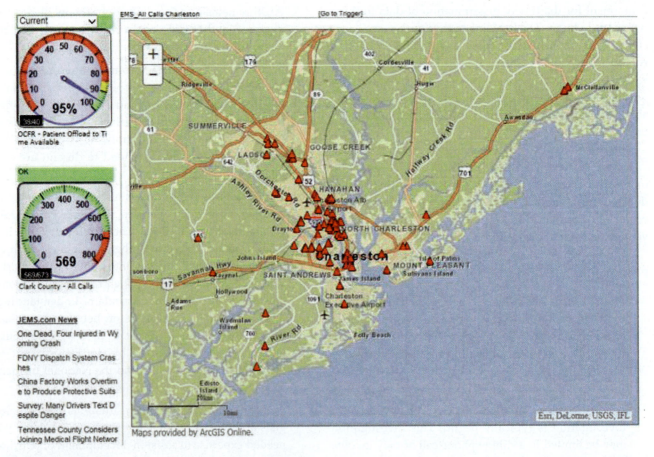

Maps provided by ArcGIS Online.

FIGURE 6-3 EMS is often a harbinger for public health events. Early warning systems, such as that provided by FirstWatch, are now more commonplace.

(www.FirstWatch.net)

medical care endeavors, they are less prepared for recovery efforts. From a medical standpoint, recovery efforts include prevention of disease and further injury and definitive care of injuries that may have been stabilized during the initial hours and days after the onset of the disaster. EMS personnel may be called on to assist in recovery and need the knowledge and skills required to achieve these tasks.

- *Injury prevention.* Although many people believe that injuries "just happen," evidence shows that injuries often result from interaction with identifiable potential hazards in the environment. Thus, it has been suggested that motor vehicle accidents (MVAs) should be called motor vehicle collisions (MVCs), because driving drunk or at 80 mph and crashing is no accident. In other words, many injuries may be predictable and, thus, preventable. EMS can play an important role in injury prevention. Common strategies include child safety seat classes, bicycle safety training, drunk driving education programs, smoking prevention, and swimming pool safety programs.[5]

Public Health and EMS

Other than the victims or survivors and their families, no one experiences the aftermath of illness and trauma more directly than EMS providers. Every day, paramedics witness the tragic effects of preventable injuries and illnesses. Even armed with the best equipment and technology, they cannot save every life. However, by being first on the scene of emergencies, EMS personnel have become prime candidates to be advocates of injury prevention.

EMS providers perform CPR and other life-saving procedures as part of an everyday routine. In addition, as partners in public health and safety, members of the EMS community must go beyond their normal daily routine and work cooperatively with members of the public to prevent avoidable illness and injury.[6]

EMS providers are widely distributed in the population, often reflecting the composition of their communities. They are often considered to be champions of the health care consumer and are welcome in schools and other community institutions. Medical personnel are high-profile role models and, as such, can have a significant impact on the reduction of injury rates in this country. In rural areas, EMS providers may be the most medically educated individuals, and are often looked to for advice and direction. Essentially, the more than 600,000 EMS providers in the United States comprise a great arsenal in the war to prevent injury and disease.

Organizational Commitment

EMS organizational commitment is vital to the development of any prevention activities. As a member of the EMS community, you should become familiar with available resources and your responsibilities in preventing illness and injury.

- *Protection of EMS providers.* The leadership of EMS agencies must ensure that policies are in place to promote response, scene, and transport safety. The appropriate Standard Precautions and personal protective equipment (PPE) should be issued to protect against exposure to bloodborne and airborne pathogens, as well as environmental hazards. An overall commitment to safety and wellness should be emphasized and supported.

- *Education of EMS providers.* EMS personnel must understand the need for involvement in prevention activities. A "buy-in" from employees at every level is key to the success of any prevention program. EMS managers have the responsibility of instructing their personnel in the fundamentals of primary prevention during initial training and in continuing education courses. Public and private sector specialty groups may be called on for specific EMS education and training. EMS providers should also have the skills and training necessary to defend against violent patients or other hostile attackers. Classes in on-scene survival techniques should be commonplace in every EMS agency.

- *Data collection.* Monitoring and maintaining records of patient illnesses and injuries is essential in determining trends and in developing and measuring the success of prevention programs. Each agency should contribute data to local, regional, state, and national systems that track such information.

- *Financial support.* An agency's internal budget should reflect support for prevention strategies as a priority. If necessary, support must be sought from outside the organization. Large corporations are often willing to donate funds in exchange for stand-by coverage at an event or company function. State highway safety offices can offer funding for traffic-related projects, such as those involving child safety seats, seat belts, and drunk driving. Advertising agencies may contribute billboards for safety messages and public service announcements (Figure 6-4). Partnerships with local hospitals can result in advertising safety messages in newsletters and flyers. Community groups such as Mothers against Drunk Driving (MADD) and junior auxiliaries also are great resources for initiating community and school programs.

- *Empowerment of EMS providers.* The ultimate factor in achieving success in a prevention program lies in the hands of the frontline personnel. Managers should identify, encourage, and foster employee interest, support, and involvement. Likewise, such involvement should be recognized and rewarded from top management. It is also recommended that managers rotate assignment to prevention programs and provide salary for off-duty injury prevention activities.

FIGURE 6-4 EMS in the United States needs to be proactive in public education programs.

(Dr. Bryan E. Bledsoe)

EMS Provider Commitment

Illness and injury prevention should begin at home and be carried over into the workplace.[7] The priority for EMS providers is to protect themselves from harm. Employers have an obligation to provide a safe working environment. Written guidelines and policies should promote wellness and safety among employees. (See the chapter "Workforce Safety and Wellness" for more information on the points discussed in the following sections.)

Standard Precautions

Under the guidelines of the Occupational Safety and Health Administration (OSHA), employers and employees share responsibility for ensuring that Standard Precautions are used to assist in preventing contamination from blood and other bodily fluids. PPE, such as gloves and eyewear, plays a major role in EMS operations and is one of the provider's basic lines of defense (Figure 6-5).

Physical Fitness

The often hectic and chaotic lifestyle of a paramedic may often interfere with your normal, healthy daily routine. Therefore, you must make an extra effort to consistently incorporate exercise, fitness, and a health-minded attitude into your life to minimize the risk of injury and to improve your overall quality of life. Encourage your partner, crew members, and other coworkers to do the same. A wellness program that includes a proper diet, cardiovascular fitness, and strength training can increase energy levels, boost immune systems, and help fend off disease and injury.

Note that although lifting and moving techniques and back safety programs have become routine for prehospital staff, back injuries remain a leading cause of disability among EMS workers. Make a solid effort to follow proper lifting techniques in order to prevent bodily injury, strain, and pain.

Stress Management

Members of today's workforce, particularly EMS providers, must learn to control, or at least handle, the stress in their lives. It is often difficult for even the healthiest individual to balance personal, family, and work life. Know your limits and take time out when necessary. Take time to relax. Pick a pastime or hobby that alleviates stress. If work becomes too stressful, speak with a supervisor to prevent burnout or future conflicts. Balance your life with exercise, good nutrition, and healthy activities to keep stress in check.

Seeking Professional Care

EMS providers should not be ashamed of needing or asking for professional counseling. Paramedics are called in to assess and treat people during the worst times of their lives. Facing tragedy, disease, death, and despair are part of the daily routine for EMS personnel. Do not forget that paramedics are vulnerable to the same stressors, emotions, illnesses, and injuries as everyone else. If your job or life becomes overwhelming, you may choose to seek counseling from a trained professional.

Many employers will offer employee assistance programs that include counseling, stress management, nutrition, healthy lifestyle inventories, and general wellness. It is often a great benefit for employees to take advantage of these opportunities to help themselves through a crisis or stressful time.

Driving Safety

Safe driving is an essential part of EMS response. As an emergency vehicle operator, be familiar with traffic laws and obey them. Never drink and drive. Always fasten your seat belt. In addition, you must be able to understand the capabilities and limitations of your emergency vehicle, handle weather and road conditions with precision, and accurately respond to all traffic conditions quickly. Safe emergency operation of EMS vehicles can be achieved only when proper use of warning devices is coupled with sound emergency and defensive driving practices.

FIGURE 6-6 Every paramedic should have the appropriate safety equipment readily available and in good repair.

(© Ken Kerr)

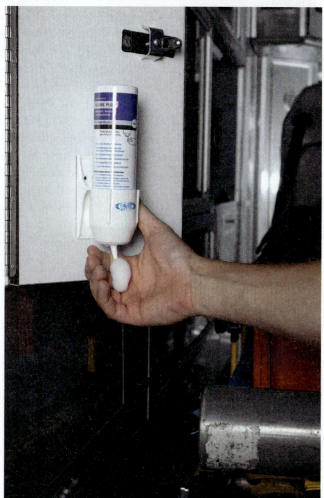

FIGURE 6-5 Disease prevention starts with health care workers.

(Top Photo: Dr. Bryan E. Bledsoe)

Scene Safety

Safety is always your first priority. Once your unit is dispatched to a call, evaluate the dispatch information prior to arrival. Focus your attention on the response and equipment that will be needed (Figure 6-6). Do not approach potentially dangerous scenes until law enforcement has arrived and deemed the scene safe for EMS to enter. On arrival, park the unit in the safest and most convenient place to load the patient as well as to leave the scene. Consider traffic, road conditions, and all other possible hazards. Directing traffic is primarily the responsibility of local law enforcement agencies. The safest method for traffic control at serious vehicle collisions is to stop all traffic and reroute it to different roads. This is for the safety of patients, bystanders, and rescue personnel.

If you are called to an area with potential health hazards, such as an industrial park or a chemical plant or an area with high crime rates, approach the scene with caution. Be sure to protect yourself appropriately. If you do not have adequate protection or are not specifically trained to control the specific hazards, never enter a hazardous scene. Call in specialized teams, such as a hazardous materials crew, if necessary. Law enforcement agencies should be contacted for any violent, potentially violent, or dangerous scene, including those involving domestic abuse or other crimes.

If the scene is safe to enter, be sure to wear reflective clothing to provide added protection on the scene. With Standard Precautions in place, approach patients with your own safety in mind. Determine the mechanisms of injury (forces that caused injury) or the nature of illness. Treat the patient according to protocol.

After patient care is addressed and a transport decision is made, make sure your unit is secure before departure. Have your partner check the outside of the unit to make certain that all doors are secured. The patient should be secured on an ambulance stretcher with at least three straps, as well as shoulder straps if available. If a family member is allowed to accompany the patient, that person should be placed in the passenger seat in the front compartment with vehicle restraints in place. All crew members, including those caring for the patient, should be adequately restrained while the ambulance is in motion.

Prevention in the Community

As a component of health care, EMS has a responsibility not only to prevent injury and illness among EMS workers, but also to promote prevention among the members of the public. EMS providers can be an appropriate and effective means of prevention in several situations.

Areas of Need

Infants and Children

Each year, nearly 290,000 infants are born weighing less than 5.5 pounds (2,500 grams), often as a result of inadequate prenatal care. Low birth weight is a key indicator of poor health at the time of birth. Babies born too small or too soon are far more likely to die in the first year of life. Annually, more than 4,000 die of low birth weight and prematurity. Among those who survive, an estimated 2 to 5 percent have a disability, and one-quarter of the smallest survivors (born weighing less than 1,500 grams) have serious disabilities such as mental retardation, cerebral palsy, seizure disorders, or blindness.[8]

One of every three deaths among children in the United States results from an injury. The number of injuries, of course, far exceeds the number of deaths. The most common causes of fatal injuries in children include motor vehicle collisions, pedestrian or bicycle injuries, burns, falls, and firearms. Injuries generally can be classified into intentional events (such as shootings and assaults), unintentional events (such as motor vehicle collisions), and alleged unintentional events (such as suspicious injury patterns that suggest possible abuse).

In motor vehicle collisions, young children are easily thrown on impact. Because a young child's head is large in proportion to the body, unrestrained children tend to fly head first into the windshield or out of the car when a collision occurs. The back seat is the best seat for children 12 years old or younger. In this location, a properly restrained child is least likely to sustain injuries in a crash. Car safety seats, booster seats (for older children), and seat belts can prevent most severe injuries to passengers of all ages if they are used correctly. Air bags are designed to save people's lives when used with seat belts, and they can protect drivers and passengers who are correctly buckled.

Cars backing up in driveways or parking lots commonly injure infants and toddlers. Children between the ages of 5 and 9 who are struck by cars typically have darted out in front of traffic. Children riding bicycles can be injured when they collide with cars or other fixed objects or when they are thrown from the bicycle. The most serious bicycle-related injuries are head injuries, which can cause death or permanent brain damage. Bicycle safety programs, which promote helmet use and safe riding, can help attenuate this problem.

Falls are the most frequent cause of injury to children younger than 6 years old. About 200 children die from falls each year. Fire and burn injuries occur in the highest numbers in the very young. Most are caused by scalding from a hot liquid, as when children grab pot handles and spill the contents.

In this modern age of media and the Internet, children and young adults are bombarded with an incredible amount of information and are often faced with some of the same stressors as adults. Sometimes those stressors become overwhelming.

One of the most troubling recent trends is the increased number of violent acts among young people, occurring in the form of self-destructive behavior, gang violence, and assaults. In addition, firearm injury is becoming more common as a result of the accessibility of handguns to children. An increasing number of injuries and deaths occur when children and adolescents take guns to school. The number of firearm deaths has doubled since 1953. About 15 percent of all firearm-related deaths are unintentional, often resulting from improper handling and lack of safety mechanisms.

Motor Vehicle Collisions

For years, the EMS industry and law enforcement have referred to collisions among trucks and automobiles as motor vehicle accidents (MVAs). However, that term does not accurately reflect the circumstances of the incident. The term *motor vehicle collision* (MVC) more accurately reflects the fact that few collisions are accidents: Something caused the crash to occur. Such crashes are responsible for more than half of all deaths from unintentional injuries. Alcohol use is a factor in about half of all motor vehicle fatalities.

Geriatric Patients

Falls account for the largest number of preventable injuries for persons over 75 years of age. As a result of slower reflexes, failing eyesight and hearing, and arthritis, the elderly are at increased risk of injury from falls. Falls frequently result in fractures, as the bones become weaker and more brittle with age. Because the aging brain begins to shrink and stretch the vessels connected to the inner skull, falls in which the head strikes the floor or other object are more likely to cause dangerous bleeding inside the cranium in an elderly person than in a younger person.

CONTENT REVIEW

➤ Areas Where EMS Can Be Active in Prevention
- Infants and children
- Motor vehicle collisions
- Geriatric patients
- Work and recreation hazards
- Medications
- Early discharge

Most geriatric patients are coherent, although some may suffer from some degree of dementia. Alzheimer's disease is merely one example of the conditions that can affect the elderly. The associated confusion can contribute to dangerous behaviors such as wandering away from home or into a roadway, which places these patients at greater risk of injury.

Work and Recreation Hazards

In the workplace, back injuries account for 22 percent of all disabling injuries. Injuries to the eyes, hands, and fingers are responsible for another 22 percent. Even the quietest office setting can be hazardous. Never underestimate the potential dangers in an area that appears to be safe. Many areas and aspects of the work environment are potentially dangerous, including copy machines, electrical cords, faulty wiring, and shoddy building construction, among others.

Sports injuries are commonly seen in persons of all ages as a result of the increased popularity and participation in outdoor recreational activities. Football, soccer, and baseball, as well as running, hiking, and biking, are among popular sports that can result in fractures, dislocations, sprains, and strains.

Medications

When an illness or injury occurs and treatment is sought, medications are often part of the treatment regimen. These medications are occasionally taken improperly (too much or not enough or in dangerous combinations), or they are taken by others, sometimes causing serious medical problems. Medications of any kind should be taken only by those for whom they are prescribed. They should be stored according to label directions. They should also be continued until the prescription is completed. Following the physician's, the pharmacist's, and the label directions is imperative.

Early Discharge

Managed care organizations, such as HMOs and insurance companies, often mandate shorter hospital stays and early discharges from hospitals, urgent care centers, and other outpatient facilities. Such policies often result in more patients being at home sooner with illnesses that are less completely treated. These patients may call 911 for supportive care and intervention.

Cultural Considerations

Elderly and Impoverished Populations. Studies have shown that the incidence of EMS calls is higher in areas where there is poverty or where there are many elderly people. EMS personnel must recognize that this will be a significant part of the job.

Implementation of Prevention Strategies

The following is a list of prevention strategies that you should be able to implement:

- *Preserve the safety of the response team.* Always remember that your first priority is your safety and the safety of your fellow crew members. (If you and other crew members are ill or injured, you cannot help others.) The next priorities are the patient and, finally, bystanders. Do what you can and what is within your training to maintain a safe and secure working area. If there is a chance of risk or further danger on scene, act quickly and appropriately to correct the situation. Do not hesitate to contact backup units and law enforcement personnel, if necessary.

- *Recognize scene hazards.* To prevent illness or injury to EMS personnel and further illness or injury to patients, size up the scene for potential risks or dangers before entering. Be aware of your surroundings. Is there anyone or anything that could cause harm to you, your crew, or the patient? Does the mechanism that injured the patient still pose a threat to the rescuers? Are there any hazardous materials in the area? Has any crime been committed? Are there structural risks? Are there temperature extremes for which you are unprepared? If the scene is not safe and there is an immediate and imminent danger, retreat immediately and call for the appropriate assistance.

- *Document findings.* Document your patient care findings at the end of every call. EMS patient forms often can be designed to include specific data on injury prevention, to benefit researchers and implement future prevention programs. Such a form should include scene conditions at the time of EMS arrival, which may play a major role in determining intentional and unintentional injuries, and the mechanism of injury, which is the best determinant of patient care on scene. It should also include a place where you can describe any risks that were overcome. If protective devices were used (or not used) during the emergency, these should also be documented (Figure 6-7).

- *Engage in on-scene education.* Taking advantage of a teachable moment is a chance to decrease future emergency responses.

CONTENT REVIEW

➤ Prevention Strategies for EMS Personnel
- Preserve response team safety
- Recognize scene hazards
- Document findings
- Conduct on-scene education
- Know your community resources
- Assess community needs

FIGURE 6-7 Example of documentation of primary and secondary injury prevention.

Remember that to communicate effectively, you must gain your listeners' trust. Remain objective, nonjudgmental, and nonthreatening. Inform them of how they can prevent the recurrence of a similar emergency and, if needed, instruct them on the use of protective devices.

• *Know your community resources.* Treating the medical needs of a patient is often not enough. You must also seek to identify and meet the psychosocial needs of your patient. At times, you may find it appropriate to consider your patient a "customer." Determine what his needs are and how you may assist him. Your patient may require a referral to an outside agency such as a prenatal clinic; a social service organization that offers food, shelter, clothing, mental health resources or counseling; or other services. Your system may also allow for referral or transportation to a clinic, urgent care center, or alternative form of health care. Be aware of the presence of both licensed and unlicensed child care centers in your area. Encourage parents to provide preexisting consent for treatment and transport in case of illness or injury at a child care facility. Be sure to follow local protocols and report suspected abuse situations to the appropriate child protective agency. Consider developing a social service resource guide for your organization to determine solutions and ideas for these and other situations.

Cultural Considerations

Immunizing At-Risk Populations. Many illnesses can be prevented through immunization of at-risk populations. The Centers for Disease Control and Prevention (CDC) and other organizations frequently update and publish a list of recommended immunizations for children and persons at increased risk of contracting a preventable disease. However, for various reasons, some patients are hesitant to obtain these life-saving immunizations. This is especially true in communities with a large number of illegal immigrants. People who are in the country illegally often will not seek health care for fear that their presence in the country will be revealed to immigration authorities and they will be deported. As a result, this population is at increased risk of developing diseases that could be prevented through proper immunization.

In several areas, paramedics have been called on to provide immunizations as a community service. In these situations, it has been demonstrated that persons unlikely to go to a standard health clinic for immunizations are more likely to attend an immunization session provided by EMS. Thus, by using the trustworthy image of EMS, paramedics can help target populations for preventive immunizations who might not obtain them by traditional means.

It is important to remember that, for many conditions, the best treatment is prevention.

- *Conduct a community needs assessment.* Each community should determine its own specific approaches to prevention. Conducting a formal needs assessment will assist in identifying priorities. Consider the following that your community may already have or may need to develop:

  - Childhood and flu immunizations[9]
  - Prenatal and well-baby clinics
  - Elder-care clinics
  - Defensive driving classes

- Workplace safety courses
- Health clinics (cosponsored by local hospitals or health care organizations)
- Prevention information on your agency's website

These are just a few of the ideas that may be appropriate for your organization. The population served and its ethnic, cultural, and religious makeup may affect the needs and approaches that are most appropriate. Also consider community members who are learning disabled or physically challenged.

Summary

Each member of EMS shares the responsibility of promoting wellness and preventing illness and injury among coworkers and the community. EMS services have gone beyond the traditional treatment-and-transport-only and have followed the steps of the fire service by adding prevention to their repertoire. It is commonplace for EMS services to offer programs to the public such as first aid and CPR classes, infectious disease prevention classes, safe driving classes, child safety seat classes, and even swimming lessons. You should begin to partner with members of your community in new and innovative ways to make everyone more aware of how to prevent avoidable illness and injury. If we can prevent one injury, one disabling disease, or one avoidable death, it will have been more than worth the effort.

You Make the Call

As you walk into work on a sunny, warm Saturday morning, your supervisor greets you at the door. He is beaming with excitement as he tells you, "The boss just approved our budget for EMS Week. And he and I agree that you are just the person to coordinate this year's effort." He continues by insisting that the organization must become "more active" in injury and illness prevention, and EMS Week is the perfect platform to begin such a campaign. You agree to the concept and accept the assignment. The supervisor responds, "Here is the budget overview and the planning kit for last year and this one. I would like a preliminary plan from you by the end of today's shift," and wanders back into his office. You briefly scan the packet and proceed to prepare for your shift.

Later, during an hour or so of downtime, you and your partner decide to brainstorm ideas on how best to prepare for the event. Your partner mentions that he thinks "this whole idea of us doing prevention is hokey and ridiculous." He continues by saying, "That stuff is for the public health people. I'm a paramedic. I don't have time to be working on prevention." Another paramedic, fresh out of medic school, joins in the conversation and adds, "Yeah. If we prevented all the injuries and illnesses, we would be out of a job. I don't want that after all I went through to get my certification." You slump slightly into your chair as you begin to discover how difficult this task might become.

1. How will you counter the arguments the two paramedics made?

2. Why is prevention an important responsibility of being a paramedic?

3. List ten ideas for an illness and injury prevention program that may be appropriate in your area.

See Suggested Responses at the back of this book.

Review Questions

1. The study of the factors that influence the frequency, distribution, and causes of injury, disease, and other health-related events in a population is called
   _____

   a. logistics.

   b. census gathering.

   c. epidemiology.

   d. pathophysiology.

2. Intentional injuries make up about _____ of all injury deaths.

   a. 1/4   c. 2/3

   b. 1/3   d. 1/2

3. Rehabilitation after an injury or illness that helps to prevent further problems from occurring is referred to as _____

   a. primary prevention.

   b. tertiary prevention.

   c. secondary prevention.

   d. teachable moments.

4. Under the guidelines of _____, employers and employees share responsibility for Standard Precautions.

   a. DOT   c. OSHA

   b. FEMA   d. HIPAA

5. What has been found to still be a leading cause of disability among EMS workers?

   a. Fall injuries

   b. Back injuries

   c. Head injuries

   d. Extremity injuries

6. What have public health studies found to be the type of accidental injury that is the most common preventable injury in people over 75 years of age?

   a. Burns

   b. Falls

   c. MVCs

   d. Head injuries

See answers to Review Questions at the back of this book.

References

1. Public Health Law Research Program. *Public Health Law Research.* (Available at http://www.publichealthlawresearch.org.)

2. Jaslow, D., J. Ufberg, and R. Marsh. "Primary Injury Prevention in an Urban EMS System." *J Emerg Med* 25 (2003): 167–170.

3. Shilts, R. *And the Band Played On: Politics, People, and the AIDS Epidemic.* New York: Stonewall Inn Editions/St. Martins Press, 2000.

4. National Highway Traffic Safety Administration. *Emergency Medical Services: Agenda for the Future.* (Available at http://www.nhtsa.dot.gov/people/injury/ems/agenda/.)

5. Yancey, A. H., 2nd, R. Martinez, and A. L. Kellermann. "Injury Prevention and Emergency Medical Services: The 'Accidents Aren't' Program." *Prehosp Emerg Care* 6 (2002): 204–209.

6. Weiss, S. J., R. Chong, M. Ong, A. A. Ernst, and M. Balash. "Emergency Medical Services Screening of Elderly Falls in the Home." *Prehosp Emerg Care* 7 (2003): 79–84.

7. Maguire, B. J., K. L. Hunting, G. S. Smith, and N. R. Levick. "Occupational Fatalities in Emergency Medical Services: A Hidden Crisis." *Ann Emerg Med* 40 (2002): 625–632.

8. Streger, M. "Keeping Kids Safe: Injury Prevention Programs in EMS." *Emerg Med Serv* 36 (2002): 24.

9. Mosesso, V. N., Jr, C. R. Packer, J. McMahon, T. E. Auble, and P. M. Paris. "Influenza Immunizations Provided by EMS Agencies: The MEDICVAX Project." *Prehosp Emerg Care* 7 (2003): 74–78.

Further Reading

Angle, J. S. *Occupational Safety and Health in the Emergency Services,* 2nd ed. Florence, KY: Delmar/Cengage Learning, 2004.

Sachs, G. M. *The Fire and EMS Department Safety Officer.* Upper Saddle River, NJ: Pearson/Prentice Hall, 2001.

Chapter 7
Medical–Legal Aspects of Out-of-Hospital Care

Bryan Bledsoe, DO, FACEP, FAAEM

Wes Ogilvie, MPA, JD, LP

STANDARD
Preparatory (Medical–Legal and Ethics)

COMPETENCY
Integrates comprehensive knowledge of EMS systems, the safety and well-being of the paramedic, and medical–legal and ethical issues, which is intended to improve the health of EMS personnel, patients, and the community.

 ## Learning Objectives

Terminal Performance Objective: After reading this chapter, you should be able to recognize and appropriately respond to medical–legal issues in the practice of paramedicine.

Enabling Objectives: To accomplish the terminal performance objective, you should be able to:

1. Define key terms introduced in this chapter.

2. Describe the four primary sources of law.

3. Differentiate between the categories of law—civil and criminal—and how they relate to the paramedic.

4. Outline the events that occur in a civil lawsuit in which a paramedic may be involved.

5. Discuss the application of legal concepts such as scope of practice, licensure and certification, motor vehicle laws, mandatory reporting, and others that are pertinent to paramedic practice.

6. Discuss the four components that must be present in a negligence claim.

7. Name and describe the defenses that can be used by the paramedic against a claim of negligence.

8. Describe the special liability situations encountered in the prehospital environment.

9. Take measures to protect patients' confidentiality and privacy and comply with HIPAA.

10. Discuss the various ways that defamation of the patient could occur, and how the paramedic can avoid these occurrences.

11. List and describe the levels of patient consent that can be employed by the paramedic, and how to properly handle refusal of consent.

12. Define how professional boundaries pertain to the paramedic, and identify ways in which the paramedic can maintain these boundaries.

13. Define and identify situations that could lead to claims of abandonment, assault, battery, false imprisonment, and excessive force.

14. Identify and discuss the various forms of advanced directives that the paramedic is likely to encounter in the prehospital environment.

15. Take appropriate actions to avoid destroying evidence at potential crime scenes.

16. Discuss what the paramedic typically has a duty to report, and explain the elements of excellent documentation.

17. Discuss employment laws as they pertain to the paramedic and his or her employer.

KEY TERMS

abandonment, p. 134

actual damages, p. 126

advance directive, p. 136

assault, p. 134

battery, p. 134

breach of duty, p. 125

civil law, p. 122

civil rights, p. 128

common law, p. 122

competent, p. 130

confidentiality, p. 128

consent, p. 130

constitutional law, p. 122

criminal law, p. 122

defamation, p. 129

Do Not Resuscitate (DNR) order, p. 136

duty to act, p. 125

emancipated minor, p. 131

employment laws, p. 141

excited delirium syndrome (ExDS), p. 128

expressed consent, p. 130

false imprisonment, p. 135

Good Samaritan laws, p. 124

Health Insurance Portability and Accountability Act (HIPAA), p. 129

immunity, p. 124

implied consent, p. 131

informed consent, p. 130

intentional tort, p. 125

invasion of privacy, p. 130

involuntary consent, p. 131

liability, p. 121

libel, p. 129

living will, p. 136

malfeasance, p. 126

minor, p. 131

misfeasance, p. 126

negligence, p. 125

negligence *per se*, p. 126

nonfeasance, p. 126

physician orders for life-sustaining treatment (POLST), p. 138

positional asphyxia, p. 128

professional boundaries, p. 134

proximate cause, p. 126

reasonable force, p. 135

regulatory law, p. 122

res ipsa loquitur, p. 126

restraint asphyxia, p. 128

scope of practice, p. 123

slander, p. 129

standard of care, p. 126

statuatory law, p. 122

tort law, p. 122

Case Study

A police officer has pulled a 27-year-old female driver off to the side of the road at the intersection of Quincy Place and Route 122. Because of the dangerous driving he witnessed and the driver's erratic behavior, unsteady gait, and slurred speech, the officer suspects that the driver is intoxicated. To be safe, the officer requests immediate EMS backup.

EMS 117 paramedics arrive on scene in 2 minutes and find a young woman arguing with the police officer.

As the paramedics are assessing scene safety, they see the patient turn and lunge at the officer. The officer subdues the patient, who thrashes around briefly before losing consciousness.

At the officer's signal, the paramedics run in to do their jobs. They perform a primary assessment, quickly determining that the patient's airway is clear and breathing and circulation are adequate. They do not detect any immediate life threats, and they begin to review possible causes of the altered mental status. To rule out hypoglycemia, they perform a rapid glucose determination using a glucometer. Then, while one paramedic conducts a physical exam of the patient, the other notes that her blood sugar is 22 mg/dL. Per approved standing orders, an IV is established and 50 mL of 50 percent dextrose is administered. The patient responds quickly, becomes fully oriented, and thanks the paramedics for their help. She then mentions that she has been ill for a few days and has not been eating well.

The paramedics urge the patient to go to the hospital for additional evaluation. She declines, stating that she has recently scheduled a physician's appointment and that she is late for a meeting. The paramedics advise the patient of the risks of refusing care. Nevertheless, she continues to refuse assistance. The paramedics assure themselves that the patient is fully conscious, oriented, and capable of refusing consent. They instruct the patient to go immediately to the mini-mart across the street to get something to eat, and she agrees. They then aseptically discontinue the IV and have the patient sign a release-from-liability form, which is witnessed by the police officer. They return their equipment to the ambulance, and notify the dispatcher that they are back in service.

Introduction

To practice competent prehospital care today, paramedics must become familiar with the legal issues they are likely to encounter in the field. As a paramedic, you must be prepared to make the best medical decisions and the most appropriate legal decisions. This chapter addresses general legal principles in addition to specific laws and legal concepts that affect the paramedic's daily practice.

Note that because laws vary from state to state, and protocols can vary from county to county, the information contained in this chapter cannot be used as a substitute for competent legal advice. Just as with the practice of medicine, the practice of law involves some art and some science, and is always heavily dependent on the unique facts present in each situation. If you are faced with a specific legal question, you must rely on the advice of your attorney.

Legal Duties and Ethical Responsibilities

As a paramedic, you have specific legal duties to your patient, crew, medical director, and the public (Figure 7-1). These duties are based on generally accepted standards and are often set by statutes and regulations. The failure of a paramedic to perform his or her job appropriately can result in civil or criminal liability. Your best protection from **liability** (legal responsibility) is to perform a systematic patient assessment, provide the appropriate medical care, and maintain accurate and complete documentation of all incidents.

A paramedic also is responsible for meeting the ethical standards expected of a professional emergency medical care provider. (See the chapter "Ethics in Paramedicine" for a detailed discussion.) Ethical standards are not laws. They are principles that identify desirable conduct by

FIGURE 7-1 Each EMS response has the potential of involving paramedics in the legal system.

members of a particular group. Your ethical responsibilities include the following:

- Respond promptly to both the physical and emotional needs of every patient.
- Treat all patients and their families with courtesy and respect.
- Maintain mastery of your skills and medical knowledge.
- Participate in continuing education programs, seminars, and refresher training.
- Critically review your performance, and constantly seek improvement.
- Report honestly and with respect for patient confidentiality.
- Work cooperatively with and respect other emergency professionals.

In addition to the legal and ethical duties, the paramedic will encounter moral issues on a day-to-day basis. Morality, unlike legal obligations, is the principle of right and wrong as governed by individual conscience. Remember, always strive to meet the highest legal, ethical, and moral standards when providing patient care.[1]

The Legal System

Sources of Law

In the United States, there are four primary sources of law: constitutional law, common law, legislative (or statutory) law, and administrative (or regulatory) law.

Constitutional law is based on the Constitution of the United States. The U.S. Constitution sets forth our basic governmental structures, which include the executive branch (the president), legislative branch (Congress), and judicial branch (the Supreme Court). Constitutional law also protects people against governmental abuse. For example, the Fourth Amendment to the Constitution protects people from unreasonable searches and seizures by the government.[2]

Common law, which also is referred to as "case law" or "judge-made law," originated with the English legal system and was adopted by Americans in the 1700s. It was derived from society's acceptance of customs and norms over time. Common law changes and grows over the years as established principles are tested and adapted to meet new situations. It is a fundamental principle of our legal system that precedents set by the courts should be followed by other courts. This means that cases with similar facts should be decided in the same way.

For example, the U.S. Supreme Court issued a decision in the case of *Miranda v. Arizona* in 1966. In *Miranda*, the Court said that a person who is taken into police custody must be informed prior to interrogation that (1) he has the right to remain silent, (2) anything he says can be used against him in court, (3) he has the right to the presence of an attorney, and (4) if he cannot afford an attorney, one will be appointed to him if he so desires. In 2000, the Supreme Court upheld the rules set forth in *Miranda*, affirming that a confession will not be admissible at trial if it is found that the defendant was not advised of his rights before making his statement.[3]

Statuatory law (or legislative law) does not come from court decisions; it is created by lawmaking or legislative bodies. Statutes are enacted at the federal, state, and local levels by the legislative branches of government. Examples of legislative bodies include the U.S. Congress, state assemblies, city councils, and district boards. Legislative law is written in a very clear and concise manner and takes precedence over common-law decisions.

Regulatory law (or administrative law) is enacted by an administrative or governmental agency at either the federal or state level. Administrative agencies, such as the Occupational Safety and Health Administration (OSHA), will produce rules and regulations necessary to implement a statute enacted by a legislative body. The agency is given the authority to make regulations based on that statute; enforce rules, regulations, and statutes under its authority; and hold administrative hearings to carry out penalties for any violations of its rules.

Categories of Law

The United States has two general categories of law: civil law and criminal law. **Criminal law** deals with crime and punishment. It is an area of law in which the federal, state, or local government will prosecute an individual on behalf of society for violating laws meant to protect society. Homicide, rape, and burglary are examples of criminal wrongs. Violations of criminal laws are punished by imprisonment, a fine, or a combination of the two.

Civil law deals with noncriminal issues, such as personal injury, contract disputes, and matrimonial issues. In civil litigation, which involves conflicts between two or more parties, the *plaintiff* (person initiating the litigation) will seek to recover damages from the *defendant* (person against whom the complaint is made). **Tort law**, which is a branch of civil law, deals with civil wrongs committed by one individual against another (rather than against society). Tort law claims include negligence, medical malpractice, assault, battery, and slander.

The United States has a *federal court system* and a *state court system*. The federal court system was created by the U.S. Constitution. Generally, only cases that involve a question of federal law or cases in which the parties are citizens of different states will be heard in a federal court. The state court system is the location for most of the cases in which a paramedic may become involved. Note that each state has its own sets of laws, each of which only apply to matters within that particular state. Thus, the decisions of another state's court system another state's statutes or regulations are unlikely to impact an EMS provider in a different state.

In *trial courts,* a judge or jury determines the outcome of individual cases. *Appellate courts* hear appeals of decisions by trial courts or other appeals courts. The decisions of appellate courts may set precedents for later cases.

Anatomy of a Civil Lawsuit

If you have ever been served with legal papers, you know that being sued or even being called to testify at a trial can be very unsettling. A basic understanding of the legal system can help. The following is a brief description of the components of a civil lawsuit:

- *Incident.* For example, a person is driving on a road and fails to see a stop sign. When he passes through the intersection, he hits another car and that driver sustains several injuries.

- *Investigation.* The injured driver's attorney makes a preliminary inquiry into the facts and circumstances surrounding the incident to determine if the case has merit.

- *Filing of the complaint.* The injured driver (now called the plaintiff) commences the lawsuit by filing a complaint with the court. In some states, the complaint may also be called a *petition.* The complaint contains information such as the names of the parties, the legal basis for the claim, and the damages sought by the plaintiff. A copy of the complaint is served on the defendant. In some locations, law enforcement, particularly a sheriff's office, may be responsible for serving the complaint on the defendant.

- *Answering the complaint.* The defendant's attorney then prepares an answer, which addresses each allegation made in the complaint. The answer is then filed with the court, and a copy is given to the plaintiff's attorney.

- *Discovery.* Before any lawsuit appears in front of a judge or jury, both parties to an action participate in pretrial discovery. In this stage of the lawsuit, all relevant information about the incident is shared so the parties can prepare their trial strategies. Discovery may include:

  - *An examination before trial,* which is also called a "deposition," allows a witness to answer questions under oath with a court stenographer present.

  - *An interrogatory,* used by either side, is a set of written questions that requires written responses.

  - *Requests for document production* entitle each side to request relevant documents, including the patient care report, records of the receiving hospital, any subsequent medical records, police records, and other records necessary to help prove or defend the lawsuit.

- *Trial.* A trial will be commenced at the appropriate level of trial court. (Some states have different trial courts depending on the type of case and/or amount of money involved.) At the trial, each side will be given the opportunity to present all relevant evidence and testimony from witnesses.

- *Decision.* After deliberations, the judge or jury determines the guilt or liability of the defendant and then

decides the amount of damages to award the plaintiff, if any.

- *Appeal.* After the jury's decision is entered by the court, either party may be entitled to an appeal. Generally, grounds for an appeal are limited to errors of law made by the court. Appeals are typically heard by an appellate court.

- *Settlement.* This can occur at any stage of the lawsuit. Generally, the defendant will offer the plaintiff an amount of money that is less than the amount for which he is being sued. The plaintiff may then agree to accept the reduced amount on the condition, for example, that he will no longer pursue the case.

Laws Affecting EMS and the Paramedic

Most of the laws that affect EMS and paramedics are state laws. Although these laws vary from state to state, they share common principles.

Scope of Practice

The range of duties and skills paramedics are allowed and expected to perform is called the **scope of practice**. Usually, the scope of practice is set by state law or regulation and/or by local medical direction. Often, a state will have a general "medical practice act" that governs the practice of medicine and all health care professionals. These acts prescribe how and to what extent a physician may delegate authority to a paramedic. As you learned in the chapter "Roles and Responsibilities of the Paramedic," paramedics may function only under the direct supervision of a licensed physician through a delegation of authority. Generally, paramedics should follow orders given by on-line and off-line medical direction. However, you should not blindly follow orders that you know are medically inappropriate.

Circumstances in which an order from medical direction may be legitimately refused include when you are ordered to provide a treatment that is beyond the scope of your training or inconsistent with established protocols or procedures, and when you are ordered to administer a treatment that you reasonably believe would be harmful to the patient. If you are confronted with a situation in which an ordered treatment might possibly harm your patient, you should take appropriate action. First, raise the concern with the physician. If the physician still insists, you should refuse to follow the order and document the incident thoroughly on the patient care report.

In addition, every EMS system should have a policy in place to guide paramedics in dealing with intervener physicians (on-scene physicians who are professionally unrelated to the patient and who are attempting to assist with patient care). Generally, such a policy requires that certain conditions be met before the paramedic should allow the intervener physician to assume control of patient care. That is, the physician must be properly identified to the paramedic, licensed to practice medicine in the state, willing to accept the responsibility of continuing medical care until the patient reaches the hospital, and willing to document the intervention as required by the local EMS system.

Licensure and Certification

Other laws that directly affect the paramedic's ability to practice relate to certification and licensure requirements. *Certification* refers to the recognition granted to an individual who has met predetermined qualifications to participate in a certain activity. It is usually given by a certifying agency (not necessarily a government agency) or professional association. For example, after completing an approved paramedic program in New York State, a student who passes an approved written and practical examination will become a certified New York State paramedic.

Licensure is a process used to regulate occupations. Generally, a governmental agency, such as a state medical board, grants permission to an individual who meets established qualifications to engage in a particular profession or occupation. Certification or licensure, or perhaps both, may be required by your state or local authorities for you to practice as a paramedic.

Most states have laws that govern paramedic practice and set forth the requirements for certification, licensure, recertification, and relicensure. It is your responsibility to understand fully the EMS laws and regulations in your state. Again, it should be noted that the EMS laws and regulations of various states differ. In some cases, the relevant regulations may differ even among cities or counties in one state.

Motor Vehicle Laws

As with other EMS-related laws, motor vehicle laws vary from state to state. Generally, there are special motor vehicle laws that govern the operation of emergency vehicles and the equipment they carry. These laws apply to areas such as vehicle maintenance and use of the siren and emergency lights. It is important that you become familiar with the laws of your state. Keep up to date with local regulations, too.

Many states and local jurisdictions have enacted laws and ordinances governing the use of mobile devices such as phones, tablets, and GPS devices. These may or may not apply when operating an emergency vehicle.

Reporting Requirements

Each state enacts different laws designed to protect the public. For example, most states have laws that require a health care worker to report to local authorities any suspected spousal abuse, child abuse and neglect, or abuse of the elderly. In many states, violent crimes—such as sexual assault, gunshot wounds, and stab wounds—must be reported to law enforcement. Emergencies that threaten public health, such as animal bites and communicable diseases, also must be reported to the proper authorities. The content of such reports and to whom they must be made is set by law, regulation, or policy. Become familiar with the circumstances under which you are required to make a report. If you fail to make a required report, you may be criminally and civilly liable for your inaction. In addition, such inaction may place your licensure or certification in jeopardy.

CONTENT REVIEW

➤ Commonly Mandated Reports
- Spouse abuse
- Child abuse and neglect
- Elder abuse
- Sexual assault
- Gunshot or stab wound
- Animal bite
- Communicable disease

Legal Protection for the Paramedic

In addition to the laws that protect patients, legislative bodies have enacted laws to protect paramedics. For example, some jurisdictions have enacted laws that criminally punish a person who commits assault or battery against a paramedic while he is providing medical care. Others have laws prohibiting the obstruction of paramedic activity.[4]

Immunity, or exemption from legal liability, is another form of protection. Governmental immunity is a judicial doctrine that prohibits a person from bringing a lawsuit against a government without its consent. This type of liability protection, even if allowed under law, generally serves to protect only the government agency, not the individual paramedic, although the specific protections vary from state to state. Therefore, you should not rely on governmental immunity to protect you from claims of negligence. Additionally, governmental immunity would not typically protect a paramedic working for a nongovernment employer. It should be noted that, even with immunity, a plaintiff may still file a lawsuit, which will typically require the paramedic to hire an attorney to defend the claim.

Virtually every state has **Good Samaritan laws**, which provide immunity to people who assist at the scene of a medical emergency. Although these laws vary from state to state, they generally protect a person from liability if that person acts in good faith, is not negligent (most states will cover acts of simple negligence but not ones of gross negligence), acts within his scope of practice, and does not accept payment for services. The Good Samaritan laws of many states have been expanded to protect both paid and volunteer prehospital personnel.[5]

As a paramedic, you should also become familiar with local laws and regulations governing the use of physical restraints for dangerous or violent patients. There also may be regulations governing entry into restricted areas, such as military installations, nuclear power plants, and sites with hazardous materials. Because the laws affecting paramedic practice vary from state to state, your agency should obtain the advice of an attorney in order to minimize potential exposure to liability.

Other laws are designed to protect the paramedic in the event of exposure to bloodborne or airborne pathogens. For example, the Ryan White Comprehensive AIDS Resources Emergency Act (Ryan White CARE Act) requires hospitals and EMS agencies to create a notification system to provide information and assist the paramedic when an exposure occurs. This law allows the paramedic who has been exposed to certain diseases (such as hepatitis B, AIDS, and tuberculosis) access to medical records to determine whether the patient has tested positive for, or is exhibiting signs and symptoms of, an infectious disease. The Ryan White CARE Act is a federal law, but many states have enacted similar or even more comprehensive laws to protect paramedics who may have been exposed to infectious diseases. It is important for each agency to appoint an infection control officer and for this individual to implement protocols and an appropriate infection control plan.

Legal Accountability of the Paramedic

As a paramedic, you are required to provide a level of care to your patients that is consistent with your education and training and equal to that of any other competent paramedic with equivalent training. You also are expected to perform your duties in a reasonable and prudent manner, as any other paramedic would in a similar situation. Any deviation from this standard might open you to allegations of negligence and liability for any resulting damages.

Most civil claims against EMS providers center around claims for negligence, but some are based on intentional torts. An **intentional tort** is a civil wrong committed by one person against another based on a willful act. Most forms of immunity do not provide protection when the claim is based on an intentional tort.

Negligence and Medical Liability

Negligence is defined as a deviation from accepted standards of care recognized by law for the protection of others against the unreasonable risk of harm. It can result in legal accountability and liability. In the health care professions, negligence is synonymous with malpractice (Table 7-1).

CONTENT REVIEW

➤ The Four Elements of Negligence
- Duty to act
- Breach of that duty
- Actual damages
- Proximate cause

Table 7-1 EMS Liability Claims

Summary of 275 EMS Liability Claims from a Large National EMS Insurer for a Two-Year Period

Cause	Percentage
Patient handling	45%
Emergency vehicle movement or collision	31%
Medical management	11%
EMS response or transport	8%
Lack or failure of equipment	4%
Other Causes	9%

Components of a Negligence Claim

To prevail in a negligence claim against a paramedic, the plaintiff must establish and prove four particular elements: a duty to act, a breach of that duty, actual damages to the patient or other individual, and proximate cause (causation of damages).

First, the plaintiff must establish that the paramedic had a **duty to act**. That is, he must prove that the paramedic had a formal contractual or informal legal obligation to provide care. Note that the act of voluntarily assuming care of a patient may imply that there was a duty to act, which creates a continuing duty to act. For example, in some states, if an off-duty paramedic witnesses a person choking, he may be under no legal duty to act. However, if that paramedic initiates care, then he has a duty to continue care. The rationale behind this rule is that if bystanders see that a victim is being helped, they may walk away. If the paramedic rendering assistance walks away after initiating treatment, but not completing it, the patient may actually be left in a worse condition than if the paramedic never tried to help.

Duties that are expected of the paramedic include:

- Duty to respond to the scene and render care to ill or injured patients
- Duty to obey federal, state, and local laws and regulations
- Duty to operate the emergency vehicle reasonably and prudently
- Duty to provide care and transportation to the expected standard of care
- Duty to provide care and transportation consistent with the paramedic's scope of practice and local medical protocols
- Duty to continue care and transportation through to appropriate conclusions

Second, the plaintiff must prove there was a **breach of duty** by the paramedic. A paramedic always must exercise the degree of care, skill, and judgment that would be expected under like circumstances by a similarly trained, reasonable paramedic in the same community. The **standard of care** specific to the paramedic's practice is generally established by court testimony and referenced to published codes, standards, criteria, and guidelines applicable to the situation. In a civil lawsuit, the trier of fact (most often, the jury) decides what the standard of care is. A breach of duty may occur by **malfeasance, misfeasance**, or **nonfeasance**:

- *Malfeasance* is the performance of a wrongful or unlawful act by the paramedic. For example, a paramedic commits malfeasance if he assaults a patient.

- *Misfeasance* is the performance of a legal act in a manner that is harmful or injurious. For example, a paramedic commits misfeasance when he inadvertently intubates a patient's esophagus, fails to confirm tube placement, and leaves the tube in place.

- *Nonfeasance* is the failure to perform a required act or duty. For example, it would be an act of nonfeasance to fail to properly secure a patient to the stretcher and in the ambulance prior to transport.

In some cases, negligence may be so obvious that it does not require extensive proof. Unlike criminal cases, which require proof "beyond a reasonable doubt," civil cases require only a proof of guilt by a "preponderance of evidence." In most cases, the burden of proving negligence rests on the plaintiff. As a result, when it is difficult to do so, a plaintiff may sometimes invoke the doctrine of *res ipsa loquitur*, which is Latin for "the thing speaks for itself."

To support a claim of *res ipsa loquitur*, the complainant must prove that the damages would not have occurred in the absence of someone's negligence, the instruments causing the damages were under the defendant's control at all times, and the patient did nothing to contribute to his own injury. After the doctrine of *res ipsa loquitur* is invoked in court, the burden of proof shifts from the plaintiff to the defendant.

For example, a classic situation in which *res ipsa loquitur* might be used occurs when a patient has an appendectomy and wakes to find that a surgical instrument has been left inside his abdomen. To prove negligence in this case, the plaintiff's attorney would show that the damage would not have occurred without the physician's negligence, that the surgical instrument was under the physician's control at all relevant times, and that the patient did not contribute to the injury. Many cases involving incorrect intubations or airway management have a *res ipsa loquitur* claim. Many cases in which *res ipsa loquitur* would be successful are settled out of court.

Another situation in which little proof is required occurs when the paramedic violates a statute and injury to a plaintiff results. Some laws state that if a statute is violated and an injury results, a person will be liable under the theory of **negligence** *per se*, or automatic negligence. For example, if a paramedic who is driving in nonemergency mode fails to stop at a red light and hits a pedestrian, the paramedic's negligence is obvious. He violated vehicle and traffic statutes that prohibit a vehicle from running a red light, and he is therefore guilty of negligence *per se*.

After a duty to act and a breach of that duty have been proven, **actual damages** is the third required element of proof in a negligence claim. That is, the plaintiff must prove that he was actually harmed in a way that can be compensated by the award of damages. This is an essential component. A lawsuit cannot be won if the paramedic's action caused no ill effects. The plaintiff must prove that he suffered compensable physical, psychological, or financial damage, such as medical expenses, lost wages, lost future earnings, conscious pain and suffering, or wrongful death.

In addition, the plaintiff may seek punitive (punishing) damages. These are awarded only when a defendant commits an act of gross negligence or willful and wanton misconduct. An act of ordinary negligence, such as accidentally allowing an IV to infiltrate, will not support an award of punitive damages. If punitive damages are awarded to the plaintiff, most insurance policies will not cover them. Therefore, the paramedic may become personally liable for any punitive damages awarded to the plaintiff.

Finally, to prove negligence, the plaintiff must show that the paramedic's action or inaction was the **proximate cause** of the damages; that is, the action or inaction of the paramedic immediately caused or worsened the damage suffered by the plaintiff. For example, a cardiac patient who breaks his arm during an ambulance collision while en route to the hospital will likely be able to prove that his injuries resulted from the incident; that is, the collision was the proximate cause of his injuries. However, a patient with a sprained wrist who happens to suffer a stroke while in the ambulance would have difficulty proving that the ambulance ride was the proximate cause of the stroke.

Proximate cause may also be thought of in terms of "foreseeability." To show the existence of proximate cause, the plaintiff needs to prove that the damage to the patient was reasonably foreseeable by the paramedic. This is usually established by expert testimony. For example, imagine that a paramedic negligently crashes into a telephone pole with the ambulance. As a result, two people are injured—the patient who was in the back of the ambulance and, two blocks away, a baby who was dropped by his mother when the loud crash startled her. It should be easy for the patient to prove proximate cause, because it was reasonably foreseeable that an ambulance crash could hurt passengers. However, if the woman who dropped her baby sued the paramedic, she probably would not be able to establish proximate cause. Although the crash was the reason her baby was injured, it was not a foreseeable injury resulting from the ambulance crash.

Defenses to Charges of Negligence

If you are accused of negligence, you may be able to avoid liability if you can establish a defense to the plaintiff's claim. The following is a list of potential defenses to negligence:

- *Good Samaritan laws.* If the paramedic can establish that his actions were protected by a Good Samaritan law, liability may be avoided. Note that such laws generally do not protect providers from acts of gross negligence, reckless disregard, or willful or wanton conduct (such as an intentional tort), and they do not prohibit the filing of lawsuits.

- *Governmental immunity.* In many states, these laws do not offer much protection for the individual paramedic accused of negligence. The breadth of governmental immunity established varies from state to state. You may want to become familiar with the governmental immunity law in the state where you practice.

- *Statute of limitations.* This is a law that sets the maximum time period during which certain actions can be brought in court. After the time limit is reached, no legal action can be brought regardless of whether or not a negligent act occurred. Statutes of limitations vary from state to state, so review the laws in your state carefully. Note that they may vary for different negligent acts and for cases involving children.

- *Contributory or comparative negligence.* Some state laws will reduce or eliminate a plaintiff's award of damages if the plaintiff is found to have caused or worsened his own injury. For example, imagine that a patient involved in a car crash complained of neck pain but refused to let the paramedics properly immobilize his spine. The paramedics explained the risks of refusing treatment, but the patient signed a release-from-liability form anyway. Later, the patient learns that he has permanent spinal cord damage and sues the paramedics for negligence. Many courts will find that the paramedics were not negligent because, by refusing necessary treatment, the patient contributed to the exacerbation of his own injury.

To protect yourself against claims of negligence, you should receive appropriate education, training, and continuing education; receive appropriate medical direction, both on-line and off-line; always prepare accurate, thorough documentation; have a professional attitude and demeanor at all times; always act in good faith; and use your own common sense. In addition, several studies have shown that health care providers who have a positive, pleasant attitude are less likely to be the subjects of complaints or lawsuits.

It is essential for every paramedic to be covered by medical liability insurance. Liability insurance contains a "duty to defend" clause that provides the insured party with legal counsel to represent them during litigation. Although many agencies have liability insurance that covers their employees, there are two drawbacks to relying on it. First, your agency's coverage may be inadequate. Additionally, you and your employer may not have the same interests. For these reasons, paramedics should consider obtaining their own liability insurance coverage.

Special Liability Concerns

Medical Direction

If a paramedic makes a mistake in the field and is sued by the injured patient, it is possible that the patient will also sue the paramedic's medical director and the on-line physician. The on-line physician may be liable to a patient for giving the paramedic medically incorrect orders or advice, for the refusal to authorize the administration of a medically necessary medication, or for directing an ambulance to take a patient to an inappropriate medical facility.

A paramedic's medical director may be liable to the patient for the negligent supervision of the paramedic. For the patient to be successful in this type of claim, he would have to prove that the physician breached a duty to supervise the paramedic and that breach was the proximate cause of the patient's injuries. Examples include the medical director's failure to establish medication protocols or standing orders consistent with the current standards of medical practice for the paramedic to use in the field; the medical director observing but failing to correct a paramedic's poor intubation technique; or the medical director receiving complaints of inappropriate care by a paramedic and then failing to effectively investigate and resolve the problem.[6]

Borrowed Servant Doctrine

As a paramedic, you may find yourself in the position of supervising other emergency care providers, such as EMTs or AEMTs. When doing so, it will be your responsibility to make sure they perform their duties in a professional and medically appropriate manner. Depending on the degree of supervision and the amount of control you have, you may be liable for any negligent act they commit. This is called the "borrowed servant" doctrine. For it to apply, the paramedic accused of negligence must have taken the employees of another employer under his control and exercised supervisory powers over them.

Civil Rights

In addition to suing you for negligence, a patient may be able to sue you under certain circumstances for violating his **civil rights** if you fail to render care for a discriminatory reason. As a paramedic, you may not withhold medical care for reasons such as race, creed, color, gender, sexual orientation, national origin, or, in some cases, ability to pay. Also, all patients should be provided with appropriate care regardless of their status, condition, or disease (including AIDS/HIV, tuberculosis, and other communicable diseases).

Off-Duty Paramedics

Liability may also arise in a situation in which an off-duty paramedic renders assistance at the scene of an illness or injury.[7] Generally, any person who provides basic emergency first aid to another person would be protected from liability under a Good Samaritan law. Again, it should be noted that few states have established a legal duty for a paramedic to provide care in an off-duty capacity, regardless of the paramedic's personal moral or ethical beliefs. However, when the off-duty paramedic provides advanced life support, a problem may arise. In many states and in many EMS systems, paramedics cannot practice advanced skills unless they are practicing within an EMS system. To perform paramedic skills and procedures that require delegation from a physician while off duty may constitute the crime of practicing medicine without a license. Learn the law in your jurisdiction as well as your EMS system's definition of what constitutes being "on duty."

Airway Issues

Issues related to airway management have always been problematic.[8] Failure to secure an airway or failure to recognize that an airway has been improperly placed can result in devastating or fatal injuries for the patient. Numerous lawsuits and settlements have been filed related to airway management, especially failure to recognize that an endotracheal tube has been improperly placed. The topic of intubation has been further complicated by several studies that question the overall benefit of prehospital endotracheal intubation.

Paramedics must know that intubation is a high-risk procedure and ensure that it is performed properly, that placement is verified by objective measures (e.g., capnography), and that the procedure is properly documented.

Restraint Issues

Almost inevitably, as a paramedic, you will eventually encounter a patient who must be physically or chemically restrained because the patient's behavior is a direct threat to his own health and safety and/or that of others. The cause may be a medical condition, a psychiatric condition, substance abuse, or any combination of these.

Over recent decades, several phenomena have been identified that place restraint patients at risk. **Excited delirium syndrome (ExDS)** is most commonly seen in conjunction with abuse of stimulant drugs. It typically presents as a triad of delirium, psychomotor agitation, and physiological excitation. It has been estimated that approximately 8 to 14 percent of people with ExDS die. An associated phenomenon is called **restraint asphyxia** or **positional asphyxia**. This type of asphyxia may occur alone or in the presence of ExDS. During the process of being restrained, for the reasons just cited or for other reasons, some patients may sustain injury or death. Some studies indicate that restraint maneuvers may impair respiratory excursion. Other studies indicate that the cause is multifactorial. Positional asphyxia often occurs in patients who have used CNS depressants (e.g., alcohol, opiates) and results from the patient being in a physical position that interferes with his airway or with ventilation.[9]

There has been an increase in negligence suits against EMS and law enforcement personnel related to deaths and injuries that occur during restraint. Paramedics must understand and practice safe restraint techniques. The use of medications, especially in ExDS, can help to minimize problems. Paramedics must understand that medical restraint is a high-risk issue and ensure that it is performed safely (for all involved, both patient and rescuers), the restrained patient is carefully monitored, and that the circumstances of the call are documented in exquisite detail. (See the section "Reasonable Force" later in this chapter, as well as the chapter "Psychiatric and Behavioral Disorders," for additional information on patient restraint.)

Paramedic–Patient Relationships

The relationship you establish with your patient is a very important one. Not only must you provide the best medical care, but you also have legal and ethical duties to protect the patient's privacy and treat him with honesty, respect, and compassion.

Confidentiality

All records related to the emergency care rendered to a patient must be kept strictly confidential. Keeping patient **confidentiality** means that any medical or personal information about a patient—including medical history, assessment findings, and treatment—will not be released to a third party without the express permission of the patient or legal guardian. However, there are specific circumstances under which a patient's confidential information may be released:

- *Patient consents to the release of his records.* A patient may request a copy of his medical records for any reason. If the patient is a child, consent for release of medical records must be obtained from the child's parent or other legal guardian. The request should be accepted only if it is in writing, specifically authorizes the agency to release the records, and contains the patient's signature (or other authorized signature). If the request so directs, it is permissible to forward the records to the patient's physician, insurance company, attorney, or any other party the patient specifies. Be sure your agency retains a copy of the consent document.

- *Other medical care providers have a need to know.* For example, it is not a breach of patient confidentiality to discuss the patient's condition with on-line medical direction or to give a patient report to an emergency department nurse on arrival at the hospital. This is permitted because it allows medical care appropriate for the patient to be continued. It is not acceptable, however, to discuss confidential patient information with medical providers who have no responsibility for the patient's care.

- *EMS is required by law to release a patient's medical records.* Records may be requested by a court order that is signed by a judge, or they may be requested by *subpoena* (a command to appear at a certain time and place to give testimony). When an agency receives a court order or subpoena, it is good practice to consult with an attorney to make sure that the order is valid and for assistance with compliance. Failure to comply with a court order or subpoena may result in severe penalties.

- *There are third-party billing requirements.* For EMS agencies that bill patients for services, it is generally necessary to release certain confidential information to receive reimbursement from private insurance companies, Medicaid, or Medicare. If possible, the agency should obtain patient authorization for this purpose.

The law provides penalties for the breach of confidentiality. The improper release of information may result in a lawsuit against the paramedic for defamation (libel or slander), breach of confidentiality, or invasion of privacy. If found guilty, the paramedic may be made responsible for paying monetary damages to the patient.

Health Insurance Portability and Accountability Act

The **Health Insurance Portability and Accountability Act of 1996 (HIPAA)** changed the methods EMS providers use to file for insurance and Medicare payments. It also adds important new layers of privacy protection for EMS patients. The privacy protections provide, among other things, that all EMS employees be trained in HIPAA compliance. Furthermore, EMS providers must develop administrative, electronic, and physical barriers to unauthorized disclosure of patients' protected health information. Disclosures of information—except for purposes of treatment, obtaining payment for services, health care operations, and disclosures mandated or permitted by law—must be pre-authorized in writing. HIPAA requires providers to post notices in prominent places advising patients of their privacy rights and provides both civil and serious criminal penalties for violations of privacy.[10]

Patients are given the right to inspect and copy their health records, restrict use and disclosure of their individually identifiable health information, amend their health records, require a provider to communicate with them confidentially, and account for disclosures of their protected health information except for treatment, payment, health care operations, and legally required reporting purposes. The requirements of HIPAA are detailed and every EMS provider must become familiar with them.

Defamation

Defamation occurs when a person makes an intentional false communication that injures another person's reputation or good name. A patient may sue a paramedic for defamation if the paramedic communicates an untrue statement about a patient's character or reputation without legal privilege or consent. Defamation can occur in written form or through verbal statements.

Libel is the act of injuring a person's character, name, or reputation by false statements made in writing or through the mass media with malicious intent or reckless disregard for the falsity of those statements. Allegations of libel can be avoided by completing an accurate, professional, and confidential patient care report. Do not use slang and value-loaded words or phrases in your report (for example, do not refer to a patient as "stupid" or use any derogatory race-based terms). Because many states consider the patient care report part of the public record, never write anything on it that could be considered libelous.

Slander is the act of injuring a person's character, name, or reputation by false or malicious statements spoken with malicious intent or reckless disregard for the falsity of those statements. An allegation of slander can be avoided by limiting oral reporting of a patient's condition to appropriate personnel only. Note that many EMS systems record ambulance–hospital radio transmissions. In addition, scanners, which give the public access to EMS transmissions, are common in the United States. Therefore, information transmitted over the radio should be limited to essential matters of patient care. In most cases, the patient's name and insurance status should not be transmitted over the radio.

Invasion of Privacy

A paramedic may be accused of **invasion of privacy** for the release of confidential information, without legal justification, regarding a patient's private life, which might reasonably expose the patient to ridicule, notoriety, or embarrassment. That includes, for example, the release of information regarding HIV status, other sensitive medical information, or even a potentially embarrassing set of circumstances in which the patient was found. The fact that released information is true is not a defense to an action for invasion of privacy.

Invasion of privacy has taken on a new level of importance with the rise of cell phone cameras and social media. Paramedics should never allow social media or networking to interfere with a patient's privacy. Many EMS employers have social media policies that govern the use of social media when on duty or representing the employer. Violating these policies may lead to loss of one's job. Particularly in the case of non-government employers, First Amendment free speech protections are unlikely to apply (Figure 7-2).

Consent

By law, you must get a patient's consent before you can provide medical care or transport. **Consent** is the granting of permission to treat. More accurately, it is the granting of

FIGURE 7-2 The use of social media can pose risks if protected patient information or employment information is distributed.

permission to touch. It is based on the concept that every adult human being of sound mind has the right to determine what should be done with his own body. Touching a patient without appropriate consent may subject you to charges of assault and battery.[11]

A patient must be **competent** to give or withhold consent. A competent adult is one who is lucid and able to make an informed decision about medical care. He understands your questions and recommendations, and he understands the implications of his decisions made about medical care. Although there is no absolute test for determining competency, keep the following factors in mind when making a determination: the patient's mental status, the patient's ability to respond to questions, statements regarding the patient's competency from family or friends, evidence of impairment from drugs or alcohol, or indications of shock or hypoxia.

Informed Consent

Conscious, competent patients have the right to decide what medical care to accept. However, for consent to be legally valid, it must be **informed consent**, or consent given based on full disclosure of information. That is, a patient must understand the nature, risks, and benefits of any procedures to be performed. Therefore, before providing medical care, you must explain the following to the patient in a manner he can understand:

- Nature of the illness or injury
- Nature of the recommended treatments
- Risks, dangers, and benefits of those treatments
- Alternative treatment possibilities, if any, and the related risks, dangers, and benefits of accepting each one
- Dangers of refusing treatment and/or transport

Informed consent must be obtained from every competent adult before treatment may be initiated. Conscious, competent patients may revoke consent at any time during care and transport. In most states, a patient must be 18 years of age or older in order to give or withhold consent. Generally, a child's parent or legal guardian must give informed consent before treatment of the child can begin.

Expressed, Implied, and Involuntary Consent

There are three more types of consent: expressed, implied, and involuntary. **Expressed consent** is the most common. It occurs when a person directly grants permission to treat—verbally, nonverbally, or in writing. Often, the act of a patient requesting an ambulance is considered an expression of a desire to be treated. However, just because the patient consents to a ride to the hospital does not mean he has consented to all types of treatment (such as the initiation of an IV and/or the administration of medications). You must obtain consent for each treatment you plan to provide. Consent from the patient does not always need to be granted verbally. It may be expressed by allowing care to be rendered.

Unconscious patients cannot grant consent. When treating them or any patient who requires emergency intervention but is mentally, physically, or emotionally unable to grant consent, treatment depends on **implied consent** (sometimes called "emergency doctrine"). That is, it is assumed that the patient would want lifesaving treatment if he were able to give informed consent. Implied consent is effective only until the patient no longer requires emergency care or until the patient regains competence.

Occasionally, a court will order patients to undergo treatment, even though they may not want it. This is called **involuntary consent**. It is most commonly encountered with patients who must be held for mental health evaluation or as directed by law enforcement personnel who have the patient under arrest. It also is used on occasion to force patients to undergo treatment for a disease that threatens the community at large (tuberculosis, for example). Law enforcement personnel often will accompany patients who are undergoing court-ordered treatment.

Consent issues also can arise when a paramedic is called by law enforcement officials to treat a sick or injured prisoner or arrestee. The officers may tell you that they have the legal authority to give consent to treatment for the patient simply because the patient is in police custody. However, a competent adult in police custody does not necessarily lose the right to make medical decisions for himself. In fact, many prisoners have successfully sued health care providers for rendering treatment without consent. Generally, forced treatment is limited to emergency treatment necessary to save life or limb, or treatment ordered by the court. Be sure that you are familiar with your local protocols and laws on this issue.

Special Consent Situations

In the case of a **minor** (depending on state law, this is usually a person under the age of 18), consent should be obtained from a parent, legal guardian, or court-appointed custodian. The same is true of a mentally incompetent adult. If a responsible person cannot be located, and if the child or mentally incompetent adult is suffering from an apparent life-threatening injury or illness, treatment may be rendered under the doctrine of implied consent.

Generally, an **emancipated minor** is considered an adult. This is a person under 18 years of age who is married, pregnant, a parent, a member of the armed forces, or financially independent and living away from home. As an adult, an emancipated minor may legally give informed consent. Anyone else under the age of 18 may not grant informed consent.

Withdrawal of Consent

A competent adult may withdraw consent for any treatment at any time. However, refusal must be informed. That is, the patient must understand the risks of not continuing treatment or transport to the hospital in terms he can fully understand. A common example of a patient withdrawing consent occurs after a hypoglycemic patient regains full consciousness with the administration of dextrose. The patient should be encouraged—*but may not be forced*—to go to the emergency department. If he is competent, the patient may refuse transport. In such cases, advanced life support measures, such as IV fluids, which were initiated when the patient was unconscious should be discontinued. The patient also should complete a release-from-liability form (Figure 7-3).

REFUSAL OF TREATMENT AND TRANSPORTATION

I, THE UNDERSIGNED, HAVE BEEN ADVISED THAT MEDICAL ASSISTANCE ON MY BEHALF IS NECESSARY AND THAT REFUSAL OF SAID ASSISTANCE AND TRANSPORTATION MAY RESULT IN DEATH, OR IMPERIL MY HEALTH. NEVERTHELESS, I REFUSE TO ACCEPT TREATMENT OR TRANSPORT AND ASSUME ALL RISKS AND CONSEQUENCES OF MY DECISION AND RELEASE GOLD CROSS AMBULANCE COMPANY AND ITS EMPLOYEES FROM ANY LIABILITY ARISING FROM MY REFUSAL.

_____
SIGNATURE OF PATIENT

_____
WITNESSED BY

_____
DATE SIGNED

FIGURE 7-3 Example of a "release-from-liability" form.

Cultural Considerations

Religious and Cultural Beliefs. Religious and cultural beliefs affect a patient's health care decisions. Some, such as Christian Scientists, prefer to use prayer instead of traditional health care and may refuse treatment on religious grounds. Similarly, Jehovah's Witnesses believe that blood transfusions are prohibited by biblical teachings.

Sometimes patients choose to accept one recommended treatment, but refuse others. For example, a patient involved in a motor vehicle crash may refuse to be fully immobilized but ask to be transported to the hospital. It is very important for you to do everything in your power to be sure he understands why spinal precautions are necessary and what may happen if they are not taken. If a competent adult continues to refuse care, be sure to thoroughly document his reason for refusal and your attempts to convince him to change his mind. Have the patient and a witness sign a release-from-liability form.

Refusal of Service

Not every EMS run results in the transportation of a patient to a hospital. Emergency care should always be offered to a patient, no matter how minor the injury or illness may be. However, often, the patient will refuse. If this occurs, you must:

- Be sure that the patient is legally permitted to refuse care; that is, the patient must be a competent adult.
- Make multiple and sincere attempts to convince the patient to accept care.
- Enlist the help of others, such as the patient's family or friends, to convince the patient to accept care.
- Make certain that the patient is fully informed about the implications of his decision and the potential risks of refusing care.
- Consult with on-line medical direction.
- Have the patient and a disinterested witness, such as a police officer, sign a release-from-liability form.
- Advise the patient that he may call you again for help, if necessary.
- Attempt to get the patient's family or friends to stay with the patient.
- Document the entire situation thoroughly on your patient care report.[12]

Remember, the refusal of care must be informed. That is, the patient must be told of and understand all possible risks of refusal. Decisions not to transport should involve medical direction. It is a good idea to put the patient directly on the phone with the on-line physician. If all efforts fail, be sure to thoroughly document the reasons for refusal and your efforts to change the patient's mind. If an on-line physician was involved, it is a good idea to obtain his signature on your patient care report. (See Figure 7-4 for an example of an EMS patient refusal checklist.)

Problem Patients

As a paramedic, you will occasionally encounter a "problem patient"—one who is violent, a victim of a drug overdose, an intoxicated adult or minor, or an ill or injured minor with no adult available to provide consent for medical treatment. Such a patient can present you with a medical–legal dilemma. For example, consider the patient who has allegedly taken an overdose of medication. Concerned family members may panic and activate the EMS system. However, on your arrival at the scene, you find the patient alert, oriented, denying that he has taken any medication, and refusing to give consent for treatment or transport.

In a case such as this, attempt to develop trust and some rapport with the patient. If he continues to refuse, and remains alert and oriented, a refusal form should be completed and witnessed by a police officer. If the patient will not sign the form, have a police officer or family member sign it, indicating that the patient verbally refused care. If, however, the situation becomes dangerous, or you have reason to suspect the patient has tried to injure himself, police officers or family members should consider legal measures to force the patient to receive treatment.

The intoxicated person who refuses treatment and transport also poses a problem for the paramedic. Every effort should be made to encourage the patient to accept care and transport to the hospital. If the patient refuses, explain to him in a calm and detailed manner the implications of refusal. However, if you determine that the patient cannot understand the nature of his illness or the consequences of his refusal, then he may not refuse treatment because he is not competent to do so. Involve law enforcement at this point. If the patient is competent to make such a decision, then have him sign a refusal form. Your conversation with the patient and his refusal should be witnessed by a disinterested third party, such as a police officer.

Regardless of the type of problem patient, always document the encounter in detail. Your records should include a description of the patient, the results of any physical examination (or reasons for the lack of one), important statements made by the patient and other persons at the scene, and the names and addresses of any witnesses. If you are going to include an important statement from the patient or witnesses in your patient care report, put the exact statement in quotation marks.

Ideally, a police officer should respond to the scene of all problem patients and should either sign the patient care report as a witness or, if the paramedic's safety is at risk, accompany the patient and paramedic to the emergency department.

EMS PATIENT REFUSAL CHECKLIST

PATIENT'S NAME:_____ AGE: _____

LOCATION OF CALL: _____ DATE: _____

AGENCY INCIDENT #: _____ AGENCY CODE: _____

NAME OF PERSON FILLING OUT FORM: _____

I. ASSESSMENT OF PATIENT (Check appropriate response for each item)

1. Oriented to: Person? ☐ Yes ☐ No
   Place? ☐ Yes ☐ No
   Time? ☐ Yes ☐ No
   Situation? ☐ Yes ☐ No

2. Altered level of consciousness? ☐ Yes ☐ No

3. Head injury? ☐ Yes ☐ No

4. Alcohol or drug ingestion by exam or history? ☐ Yes ☐ No

II. PATIENT INFORMED (Check appropriate response for each item)

☐ Yes ☐ No   Medical treatment/evaluation needed

☐ Yes ☐ No   Ambulance transport needed

☐ Yes ☐ No   Further harm could result without medical treatment/evaluation

☐ Yes ☐ No   Transport by means other than ambulance could be hazardous in light of patient's illness/injury

☐ Yes ☐ No   Patient provided with Refusal Information Sheet

☐ Yes ☐ No   Patient accepted Refusal Information Sheet

III. DISPOSITION

☐ Refused all EMS assistance

☐ Refused field treatment, but accepted transport

☐ Refused transport, but accepted field treatment

☐ Refused transport to recommended facility

☐ Patient transported by private vehicle to_____

☐ Released in care or custody of self

☐ Released in care or custody of relative or friend

Name: _____ Relationship:_____

☐ Released in custody of law enforcement agency

Agency: _____ Officer: _____

☐ Released in custody of other agency

Agency: _____ Officer: _____

IV. COMMENTS: _____
_____
_____
_____

FIGURE 7-4 Some EMS systems have checklists for procedures to follow when a patient refuses care and/or transport.

Boundary Issues

There are ethical and societal limits to the interactions between paramedics or other health care personnel and the patients they serve. These are called **professional boundaries** and serve to protect both the paramedic and the patient. EMS professionals have certain legal and ethical responsibilities to their patients, themselves, and the EMS system. Crossing professional boundaries can result in breaching these responsibilities. Danger zones for boundary crossing include being tired, being seduced, and being unprepared.

- *Being tired.* Fatigue can lead to problems such as medication errors, poor decision making, vehicle crashes, and more. EMS must be provided 24 hours a day, and long shifts and a heavy workload are common. You owe it to yourself and your patients to see to it that you are well rested and clear-headed.

- *Being seduced.* In modern society "being seduced" is generally thought of as being enticed into some sort of sexual liaison. However, by definition, "being seduced" means being led away from one's principles, ethics, faith, or allegiance. Certainly, a sexual relationship between a health care provider and a patient is unethical and must be avoided at all costs. There are other temptations, though—such as money, food, items of value, and drugs—that may cause some to stray from honorable and appropriate behavior. The physical and mental demands of EMS work, including the isolation, can sometimes lead to addictive behavior and lapses in judgment.

- *Being unprepared.* The motto of the Boy Scouts is "Be Prepared," and preparation is also a fundamental tenet of EMS. At some point in your EMS career you will encounter a situation for which your education and experience has not prepared you. Unfortunately, when we don't have the time and opportunity to think through a situation, we make errors. For example, several years ago, two paramedics encountered a pregnant woman who was killed in a motor vehicle collision. The death was sudden, and their response time was short. They decided to attempt to save the life of the baby through a postmortem Caesarean section. This was a procedure that their education and experience had not prepared them for, and it was met with sanctions from the state and the local medical director.

Boundary issues can be avoided by adhering to one's personal ethics and integrity and to the ethics expected of the profession.[13] Try to look down the road and see whether any of your thoughts, actions, or circumstances could cause problems in the future. Generally, signs of potential trouble will be obvious. Keep in mind that loneliness and isolation can lead to boundary crossings. Always maintain a healthy lifestyle and have a life and circle of friends outside EMS. Keep your priorities straight and maintain high standards and ethics. As Ralph Waldo Emerson said, "Character is higher than intellect."

Legal Complications Related to Consent

There are many legal complications related to consent to treatment. If the paramedic does not obtain the proper consent to treat or fails to continue appropriate treatment, he may be liable for damages based on a tort cause of action, such as abandonment, assault, battery, or false imprisonment.

Abandonment

Abandonment is the termination of the paramedic–patient relationship without providing for the appropriate continuation of care while it is still needed and desired by the patient. You cannot initiate patient care and then discontinue it without sufficient reason. You cannot turn the care of a patient over to personnel who have less training than you without creating potential liability for an abandonment action. For example, a paramedic who has initiated advanced life support should not turn the patient over to an EMT or an AEMT for transport.

Abandonment can occur at any point during patient contact, including in the field or in the hospital emergency department. Physically leaving a patient unattended, even for a short time, may also be grounds for a charge of abandonment. If, for example, you leave a patient at a hospital without properly turning over his care to a physician or nurse, you may be liable for abandonment. It is always a good idea to have the nurse or physician to whom you have passed responsibility for patient care sign your patient care report.

Assault and Battery

Failure to obtain appropriate consent before treatment could leave the paramedic open to allegations of assault and battery. **Assault** is defined as unlawfully placing a person in apprehension of immediate bodily harm without his consent. For example, your patient states that he is scared of needles and refuses to let you start an IV. If you then show him an IV catheter and bring it toward his arm as if to start an IV, you may be liable for assault.

Battery is the unlawful touching of another individual without his consent. It would be battery to actually start an IV on a patient who does not consent to such treatment. A paramedic can be sued for assault and battery in both criminal and civil contexts.

False Imprisonment

False imprisonment may be charged by a patient who is transported without consent or who is restrained without proper justification or authority. It is defined as intentional and unjustifiable detention of a person without his consent or other legal authority, and may result in civil or criminal liability. Like assault and battery, a charge of false imprisonment can be avoided by obtaining appropriate consent.

This is a particular problem with psychiatric patients. In most cases, you can avoid allegations of false imprisonment by having a law enforcement officer apprehend the patient and accompany you to the hospital. If no officer is available, you should attempt to consult with medical direction and carefully judge the risks of false imprisonment against the benefits of detaining and treating the patient. You should determine whether medical treatment is immediately necessary and whether the patient poses a threat to himself or to the public when you are making your decision to treat or transport.

Reasonable Force

If it is safe to do so, you may use a reasonable amount of force to control an unruly or violent patient. **Reasonable force** is the minimum amount of force necessary to ensure that the patient does not cause injury to himself, you, or others. Use of excessive force can result in liability for the paramedic. Force used as punishment will be considered assault and battery, for which the patient may be able to recover damages, and the paramedic may face criminal charges.

The use of restraints may be indicated for a combative patient. Restraints must conform to your local protocols. Restraining devices typically used by EMS providers include straps, jackets, and restraining blankets. Paramedics should take special care to prevent positional asphyxia in restrained patients. As discussed under the section "Restraint Issues" earlier in this chapter, positional asphyxia occurs when a patient's position prevents him from being able to breathe or to breathe adequately. In some EMS systems, paramedics are authorized to use chemical restraints, such as benzodiazepines and antipsychotics, in lieu of or in addition to physical restraints. In most EMS systems, paramedics are not authorized to apply law enforcement restraints such as handcuffs or leg irons. If a paramedic accompanies a patient who is handcuffed, it is imperative that a law enforcement officer also accompany the patient in case the restraints need to be removed.

For the combative patient, an EMS team's goal is to use the least amount of force necessary to safely control the patient while causing him the least amount of discomfort. Whenever the use of force and/or the use of restraints is

FIGURE 7-5 Patient restraint is a high-risk endeavor. The safety of personnel and the patient should be the highest priority.

indicated, involve law enforcement officials (Figure 7-5). For more information on the use of restraints, see the "Psychiatric and Behavioral Disorders" chapter.

Patient Transportation

The transportation of patients to a health care facility is an integral part of the patient care continuum. During transportation to a health care facility, be sure to maintain the same level of care as was initiated at the scene. This means that if you, as a paramedic, initiate advanced emergency care procedures, you must either ride with the patient to the hospital or ensure that another paramedic will accompany the patient. If you fail to do so, and the patient is harmed as a result, you may be liable for abandonment.

One of the greatest areas of potential liability for paramedics is emergency vehicle operations. It is essential that you become familiar with your state and local laws. The laws that provide exceptions from driving rules and regulations may allow you, for example, to drive at a rate of speed in excess of a posted speed limit, but if you are negligent at any time during the operation of your vehicle, you will not be protected from liability.

Another issue that will arise is patient choice of destination. If you work in a small area with only one hospital, you are not likely to encounter difficulties. However, many paramedics work in areas that have many hospitals and medical centers to choose from. Over the past few years, increasing numbers of lawsuits involving facility selection have been brought by patients. Some have sued paramedics themselves, claiming negligence based on the failure to transport to the nearest or most appropriate hospital.

CONTENT REVIEW
➤ Advance Directives
- Living wills
- Durable powers of attorney for health care
- DNR orders
- POLST orders
- Organ donor cards or directives (such as found on a driver's license)

An additional issue you may need to address involves the patient's insurance company protocols. In some situations, it may be appropriate to respect a patient's choice of facility based on his insurance company's facility-choice protocols. Local restrictions by insurance companies and health maintenance organizations may determine under what conditions and to what facilities patient transport may be authorized and paid for. Although most areas are not yet being confronted with restrictions on service provision, it may be only a matter of time. However, never put patient care in jeopardy by transporting to a less-appropriate facility because of insurance concerns.

In general, facility selection should be based on patient request, patient need, and facility capability. Local written protocols, the paramedic, on-line medical direction, and the patient should all play a role in facility selection. The patient's preference should be honored unless the situation or the patient's condition dictates otherwise. Become familiar with your system's protocols regarding hospital destinations as well as the capabilities of specialty care facilities such as trauma centers or stroke centers.

Resuscitation Issues

Advances in medical technology have saved and prolonged thousands of lives. However, in some instances, the use of sophisticated medical technology may only prolong pain, suffering, and death. When a person is seriously injured or gravely ill, family members must make difficult decisions regarding the intensity of medical care to be provided, including the use or withdrawal of life-support systems.

Generally, you are under obligation to begin resuscitative efforts when summoned to the scene of a patient who is unresponsive, pulseless, and apneic (not breathing). There are times, however, when you will determine that resuscitation is not indicated. This occurs with patients who have a valid **Do Not Resuscitate (DNR) order**, with patients who are obviously dead (decapitated, for example), with patients with obvious tissue decomposition or extreme dependent lividity (gravitational pooling of blood in dependent areas of the body), or with a patient who is at a scene that is too hazardous to enter.

As more is learned about resuscitation, it is now becoming common practice, in selected cases, either not to begin resuscitation or to terminate resuscitative efforts in the field. For example, pulseless victims of blunt trauma have virtually no chance of survival. Because of this, many EMS systems now have protocols in place whereby resuscitation of pulseless blunt trauma victims is not attempted. Likewise, resuscitation research has shown that patients who are not resuscitated from standard ALS measures in the prehospital setting will not benefit from transportation to the hospital. In this circumstance too, many EMS systems

have established protocols for termination of resuscitation efforts in the field.

Always follow your state laws, local protocols, and medical direction. The role of medical direction should be clearly delineated and included in your agency's protocols. If you are authorized to determine that resuscitative efforts are not indicated, be sure to thoroughly document your decision and the criteria on which it was based.

Advance Directives

To improve communication among patients, their family members, and physicians regarding such matters, the federal government enacted the Patient Self-Determination Act of 1990. This act requires hospitals and physicians to provide patients and their families with sufficient information to make informed decisions about medical treatment and the use of life support measures, including cardiopulmonary resuscitation (CPR), artificial ventilation, nutrition, hydration, and blood transfusions.

Patients and their families are therefore more likely than ever to have prepared a written statement of the patient's own preference for future medical care, or an **advance directive**. An advance directive is a document created to ensure that certain treatment choices are honored when a patient is unconscious or otherwise unable to express his choice of treatments. Advance directives come in a variety of forms. The most common encountered in the field are living wills, durable powers of attorney for health care, Do Not Resuscitate orders, and organ donor cards.

The types of advance directives recognized in each state are governed by state law and local protocols. Medical direction must establish and implement policies for dealing with advance directives in the field. Those policies should clearly define the obligations of a paramedic who is caring for a patient with an advance directive. They should also provide for reasonable measures of comfort to the patient and emotional support to the patient's family and loved ones. Some states do not allow paramedics to honor living wills in the field but do allow them to honor valid Do Not Resuscitate orders. Be sure you are familiar with your state law and local policies.

Living Will

A **living will** is a legal document that allows a person to specify the kinds of medical treatment he wishes to receive, should the need arise (Figure 7-6). For example, many states allow patients to include in living wills their wishes concerning dying in a hospital or at home, receiving CPR, and donation of their organs and other body parts. In addition, patients with prolonged illnesses sometimes invoke the right to choose a person who may make health care decisions for them in the event that their mental functions become impaired. They might formalize this decision by way of a special notation in a living will. (They may also do

LIVING WILL

I, _____ _____ , make the following Living Will declaration to my family, physicians, hospitals, and other health care providers and any Court or Judge:

After thoughtful consideration and while I am of sound mind, I make this statement as an expression of my settled and firm wishes if the time comes when I can no longer take part in decisions about my own future health.

My Wishes. If at any time I have a terminal condition, and in the opinion of my attending or treating physician there is no reasonable probability that I will recover and the condition can be expected to cause my death within a relatively short time if medical procedures which serve only to prolong the process of dying are not used, or if I am in a persistent vegetative state in which I have no voluntary action or cognitive behavior and cannot communicate or interact purposefully and which is a permanent and irreversible condition of unconsciousness, **I request that I be allowed to die naturally and not be kept alive by artificial means.** I ask that all life-prolonging procedures, including medical assistance to eat and drink when it is highly unlikely that I will regain the capacity to eat and drink without medical assistance, be withheld or withdrawn in such a situation.

Resuscitation. It is my further wish that no cardiopulmonary resuscitation shall thereafter be administered to me if I sustain a cardiac or respiratory arrest. In those circumstances I consent to an order not to resuscitate, and direct that such an order be placed in my medical record.

I direct that these decisions shall be carried into effect even if I am unable to personally reconfirm or communicate them, without seeking judicial approval or authority.

I recognize that there may be instances besides those described above for which life-sustaining treatment should be withheld or withdrawn and this instrument shall not be construed as an exclusive enumeration of these circumstances.

Revocation and Responsibility. This instrument and its instructions may be revoked by me at any time and in any manner. However, no physician, hospital, or other health care provider who withholds or withdraws life-sustaining treatment in reliance upon this Living Will or upon my personally communicated instructions shall have any liability or responsibility to me, my estate, or any other persons for having withheld or withdrawn treatment.

I intend this declaration to be accepted in the circumstances described as an exercise of my legal right to refuse medical treatment even if I am unable to personally reconfirm or communicate that. It is made in the presence of the witnesses who have signed below.

Signed on (date): _____

Signature: _____

Witness: _____

Witness: _____

FIGURE 7-6 Example of a living will.

this through execution of a document called a "durable power of attorney for health care" or "health care proxy.") Living wills, once signed and witnessed, are effective until they are revoked by the patient.

Be sure you know your local protocols concerning living wills. If any question arises on scene, contact medical direction for instructions.

Do Not Resuscitate Orders

A Do Not Resuscitate (DNR) order is a common type of advance directive (Figure 7-7). Usually signed by the patient and his physician, the DNR order is a legal document that indicates to medical personnel which, if any, life-sustaining measures should be taken when the patient's heart and respiratory functions have ceased.

PREHOSPITAL DO NOT RESUSCITATE ORDERS

ATTENDING PHYSICIAN

In completing this prehospital DNR form, please check Part A if no intervention by prehospital personnel is indicated. Please check Part A and options from Part B if specific interventions by prehospital personnel are indicated. To give a valid prehospital DNR order, this form must be completed by the patient's attending physician and must be provided to prehospital personnel.

A) _____ **Do Not Resuscitate (DNR):**
No Cardiopulmonary Resuscitation or Advanced Cardiac Life Support to be performed by prehospital personnel

B) _____ **Modified Support:**
Prehospital personnel administer the following checked options:
_____Oxygen administration
_____Full airway support: intubation, airways, bag-valve mask
_____Venipuncture: IV crystalloids and/or blood draw
_____External cardiac pacing
_____Cardiopulmonary resuscitation
_____Cardiac defibrillator
_____Pneumatic anti-shock garment
_____Ventilator
_____ACLS meds
_____Other interventions/medications (physician specify)
_____

Prehospital personnel are informed that (print patient name)_____
should receive no resuscitation (DNR) or should receive Modified Support as indicated. This directive is medically appropriate and is further documented by a physician's order and a progress note on the patient's permanent medical record. Informed consent from the capacitated patient or the incapacitated patient's legitimate surrogate is documented on the patient's permanent medical record. The DNR order is in full force and effect as of the date indicated below.

_____   _____

Attending Physician's Signature

_____   _____

Print Attending Physician's Name   Print Patient's Name and Location
                                             (Home Address or Health Care Facility)

_____

Attending Physician's Telephone

_____   _____

Date   Expiration Date (6 Mos from Signature)

FIGURE 7-7 Example of an EMS Do Not Resuscitate (DNR) order.

DNR orders generally direct EMS personnel to withhold CPR in the event of a cardiac arrest. When you honor a DNR order, do not simply pack up your equipment and leave the scene. You still may have the patient's family and loved ones to attend to. Provide emotional support as appropriate.

DNR orders pose a particular problem in the field. Paramedics are often called to nursing homes or residences where they find a patient in cardiac arrest and in need of resuscitation. As a rule, you are legally obligated to attempt resuscitation. If a physician has written a specific order to avoid it, the paramedics should not have

been summoned. Even so, people tend to panic and will call for help. Valid DNR orders should be honored as your protocols allow. Note, however, that if there is any doubt as to the patient's wishes, resuscitation should be initiated.

Physician Orders for Life-Sustaining Treatment

A newly emerging paradigm in end-of-life directives is **physician orders for life-sustaining treatment (POLST)**. POLST orders are designed for terminally ill patients. In the POLST paradigm, the terminally ill patient and the physician have an opportunity to consult on the patient's wishes and incorporate these wishes into a set of specific orders as to the patient's care, signed by the physician, to be honored by health care providers who deal with that patient during a medical crisis.

Although not all states have adopted POLST, some states have already enacted a version of POLST as state law. States that do have POLST laws usually allow for the POLST order to be honored and followed throughout the health care system, from prehospital care to inpatient and hospice care.

Potential Organ Donation

Over the past few years, advances in medicine have led to an increased number of organ transplants and a higher survival rate of transplant patients. Because organs and tissues are in very high demand and short supply, many EMS systems are now becoming a vital link in the organ procurement and transplant process. Some have developed protocols that specifically address organ viability after a patient's death. These include providing circulatory support through IV fluids and CPR and ventilatory support via endotracheal tube. Whether or not your EMS has protocols in place for potential organ donation, it is important for you to consult with on-line medical direction when you have identified a patient as a potential donor (Figure 7-8).

Death in the Field

Whether you arrive at the scene of a patient who has died prior to your arrival or you make an authorized decision to terminate resuscitative efforts, a death in the field must be appropriately dealt with and thoroughly documented. Paramedics should carefully follow state and local protocols. It is also important for the paramedic to contact on-line medical direction for guidance.

FIGURE 7-8 Transporting organs for transplantation.
(© LifeGift Organ Donation, Houston, TX)

Crime and Accident Scenes

Because it may be your duty as a paramedic to treat a patient found at a crime scene, you should be aware of crime-scene preservation issues. However, you must not sacrifice patient care to preserve evidence or to become involved in detective work. You can best assist investigating officers by properly treating the patient and by doing your best to avoid destroying any potential evidence. As a paramedic, your responsibilities at a crime scene include the following:

- If you believe a crime may have been committed on scene, immediately contact law enforcement if they are not already involved.

- Protect yourself and the safety of other EMS personnel. This should always be your primary consideration. You will not be held liable for failing to act if a scene is not safe to enter.

- Once a crime scene has been deemed safe, initiate patient contact and medical care.

- Do not move or touch anything at a crime scene unless it is necessary to do so for patient care. Observe and document the original placement of any items moved by your crew. If the patient's clothing has holes made by a gunshot or a stabbing, leave them intact, if possible. If the patient has an obvious mortal wound, such as decapitation, try not to touch the body at all. Do your best to protect any potential evidence.

- If you need to remove items from the scene, such as an impaled weapon or bottle of medication, be sure to document your actions and notify investigating officers.

You should treat the scene of an accident in the same way. Your goals are to ensure your own safety and the safety of your crew and to treat your patients as medically indicated. Use the resources available to you, and be prepared to summon additional personnel and rescue equipment as necessary.

Duty to Report

As a paramedic, you have an ethical duty to protect those at risk—especially the more vulnerable among us. During the course of your work, you may encounter patients who may have been abused or neglected. When abuse or neglect is suspected, you must balance the need to protect patient confidentiality against the need to notify the proper authorities. As a rule, you should always act with the patient's best interest in mind.

Abuse of the elderly, children, and invalids is all too common. Many states have rules that require EMS personnel to report suspected abuse to the proper authorities. If abuse or neglect is suspected, you should report your concerns to the proper authority in an objective and timely manner. You should not confront the abuser. It is not necessary for you to prove that abuse or neglect occurred before reporting. As a rule, you will be doing the proper thing if you report acting in the patient's best interest. You should learn and review the rules and requirements for reporting abuse and neglect in your state. Often, the failure to report abuse or neglect is a bigger liability than reporting.

Documentation

The importance of developing and maintaining superior documentation skills and habits cannot be overemphasized. As a paramedic, you must recognize that the treatment of your patient does not end until you have properly documented the entire incident, from initial response to the transfer of patient care to the hospital emergency department staff.

A complete, well-written patient care report is your best protection in a malpractice action. In fact, a well-written report may actually discourage a plaintiff from filing a malpractice case in the first place. In general, a plaintiff's attorney will request copies of all medical records, including the paramedic's report, before filing a lawsuit. If the paramedic's report is sloppy, incomplete, or otherwise not well written, this may encourage the plaintiff to sue, even if the paramedic's conduct was not negligent.

A well-documented patient care report has the following characteristics:

- *It is completed promptly after patient contact.* It should be made in the course of business, not long after the event. Any delay could cause you to forget important observations or treatments. If possible, a copy of the completed report should be left with the emergency department staff before you leave the hospital. This copy will become part of the patient's permanent medical records. Proper documentation is so important that some EMS systems now require paramedics to dictate their reports, which are later transcribed and placed in the patient's permanent records. Some systems use template-driven electronic records (Figure 7-9).

  Note: Never delay patient care to attend to a patient care report.

- *It is thorough.* The report should paint a clear and complete picture of the patient's condition and the care that was provided. Its main purpose is not simply to record patient data, but also to support the diagnosis and treatment that you provided to the patient. All actions, procedures, and administered medications should be documented as well. Remember this saying: "If you didn't write it down, you didn't do it."

FIGURE 7-9 Template-driven electronic patient records are becoming more common in modern EMS.

- *It is objective.* Avoid the use of emotional and value-loaded words. Not only are they irrelevant to patient care, but they also may be the cause of a libel suit against you.

- *It is accurate.* Be as precise as possible, avoiding the use of abbreviations and jargon that are not commonly understood or are approved within your EMS system. Also try to limit your report to information that you have personally seen or heard. If you need to document something of which you do not have personal knowledge, be sure to indicate the source of your information. Document your observations, not your assumptions, and do not draw a medical conclusion that you are not competent to make. For example, you are unlikely to conclusively diagnose a patient as having pneumonia. You can, however, report your suspicion of pneumonia and document findings that are consistent with this condition.

- *It maintains patient confidentiality.* Your agency should have well-defined policies regarding the release of patient information. Whenever possible, patient consent should be obtained prior to release of information.

The medical record should never be altered. An intentional alteration amounts to an admission of guilt by the paramedic. If a patient care report is found to be incomplete or inaccurate, a written amendment should be attached to the report. The date and time the amendment was written, not the date of the original report, should be noted on the addendum. Also, be sure to send a copy of the addendum to the receiving hospital so it will become a part of the patient's medical records. For computerized medical records, amendments and corrections are generally automatically flagged and dated as such.

Medical records need to be maintained for a period of time that is prescribed by state law. For example, in New York State patient care reports must be maintained by an EMS agency for a period of six years, or for three years after the patient reaches the age of 18, whichever is longer. Be sure to become familiar with the record retention requirements in your state.

Employment Laws

Employment laws are laws that address employee–employer relationships. Even volunteer agencies fall under the jurisdiction of many of these laws. Employment law can be complex; you should consult an attorney with expertise in this area of law should a problem arise. There are several employment laws that paramedics should be familiar with. Many states have employment laws that parallel federal laws. Some state laws may even expand employees' rights beyond those provided under federal law.

- *Americans with Disabilities Act.* The Americans with Disabilities Act (ADA), enacted in 1990, prohibits private employers, state and local governments, employment agencies, and labor unions from discriminating against qualified individuals with disabilities in job application procedures, hiring, firing, advancement, compensation, job training, and other terms, conditions, and privileges of employment. The ADA covers employers with 15 or more employees, including state and local governments. It also applies to employment agencies and to labor organizations. The ADA's non-discrimination standards apply to federal employees as well. An employer is required to make a reasonable accommodation to the known disability of a qualified applicant or employee if it would not impose an "undue hardship" on the operation of the employer's business. Reasonable accommodations are adjustments or modifications provided by an employer to enable people with disabilities to enjoy equal employment opportunities. EMS agencies should abide by the ADA, both for employees and for those patients requesting accommodations under the ADA.

- *Title VII.* A federal law that prohibits workplace harassment and discrimination, Title VII is a part of the Civil Rights Act of 1964. It covers all private employers, state and local governments, and educational institutions with more than 15 employees. It prohibits discrimination against employees on the basis of race, color, national origin, religion, and gender. It has been extended to protect against discrimination on the basis of pregnancy, sex stereotyping, and sexual harassment. EMS agencies, regardless of the type, should have well-established policies and procedures to address the requirements of Title VII.

- *Amendments to Title VII.* The Civil Rights Act of 1964 has been amended several times. The Equal Employment Opportunity Act of 1972 made discrimination in employment illegal. Equal Employment Opportunity programs include affirmative action for employment as well as processing of and remedies for discrimination complaints. All employees, including supervisors, managers, former employees, and applicants for employment, regardless of grade level or position, are covered under this legislation. The Age Discrimination and Employment Act of 1967 (ADEA) and the Age Discrimination Act of 1975 prohibit discrimination on the basis of age and protect individuals who are 40 years of age or older from employment discrimination based on age.

- *Family Medical Leave Act.* The Family and Medical Leave Act of 1993 (FMLA) allows eligible employees to take off for up to 12 workweeks in any 12-month period for the birth or adoption of a child, to care for a family member, or if the employees themselves have a serious health condition. This act was amended in 2008 to permit a spouse, son, daughter, parent, or next of kin to take up to 26 workweeks of leave to care for a member of the Armed Forces.

- *Fair Labor Standards Act.* The Fair Labor Standards Act of 1938 (FLSA) was enacted following the Great Depression and established certain standards with regard to employment. It has been amended multiple times over the years. FLSA establishes the minimum wage, overtime pay, record keeping, and child labor standards. It applies to both full-time and part-time workers in the private sector as well as those employed in federal, state, and local government.

- *Occupational Safety and Health Act.* The Occupational Safety and Health Act was signed into law in 1970. The purpose of OSHA was to ensure that employers provide employees with an environment that is healthy and safe. The act also established the Occupational Safety and Health Administration (OSHA) to oversee workforce safety, and the National Institute for Occupational Safety and Health (NIOSH) to guide occupational health and safety research.

- *The Ryan White CARE Act.* The Ryan White Comprehensive AIDS Resources Emergency (CARE) Act was enacted in 1990 and was designed to fund programs to improve the availability of health care for victims of AIDS and their families. The act also mandated that EMS personnel learn whether they have been exposed to life-threatening diseases while providing emergency care. The Ryan White act was set to expire on September 30, 2009, but the Ryan White HIV/AIDS Treatment Extension Act of 2009 extended the benefits for an additional four years. August 18, 2015 marked the 25th anniversary of the act. Although it has not been extended, lawmakers have continued to fund it through annual appropriations, and it provides assistance to over 500,000 Americans living with HIV.

Summary

The very nature of a paramedic's job requires interaction with law enforcement authorities and frequent involvement in situations that can give rise to litigation. For example, not only will police be called to the same emergencies to which paramedics are called, such as motor vehicle collisions or scenes where violence caused injuries, but paramedics also may become material witnesses to crimes or domestic disputes. It is therefore in your best interest to learn and follow all state laws and local protocols related to your practice as a paramedic.

In addition, be sure to receive good training and keep current by attending continuing medical education programs and conferences, reading industry journals, and obtaining recertification or relicensure as required by state law.

Remember, a paramedic is not immune from allegations of negligence or malpractice. However, the potential for liability may be limited or avoided by adhering to the following guidelines:

- Always obtain informed consent before initiating treatment and/or transport.
- Practice only the skills and procedures that a reasonable and prudent paramedic would, given the same or similar circumstances.
- Practice only procedures that you are trained to perform and are directly authorized to perform by a medical-control physician or by approved local standing orders.
- Prepare accurate, legible, and complete medical records that thoroughly document the entire EMS incident, from initial response to the transfer of patient care to hospital emergency department staff.
- Discuss patient information only with those who need to know. Limit writings and oral reports to information essential to patient care.
- Purchase and maintain malpractice insurance, and see that your employer does the same.
- Be nice to your patients and their families.

Always act in good faith and use your common sense. High-quality patient care and high-quality documentation are always your best protection from liability.

You Make the Call

You and the rest of the crew of EMS Unit 116 receive a call to assist an unconscious 5-year-old girl. On arriving at the scene, you are met by the child's babysitter, who states that for the past hour the child had been acting "strangely," after which she fell asleep and would not wake up. The babysitter also tells you that the child had been playing in her bedroom alone all afternoon. You ask the babysitter to call the child's parents immediately. She tells you that they are unreachable but are expected home in approximately 20 minutes.

While your partner searches the child's room, you assess the patient and note the following physical findings: respiratory depression, hypotension, bradycardia, and constricted pupils. Quickly searching, your partner finds an empty bottle of Darvocet under the child's bed. You now suspect a narcotic overdose and determine that the child needs immediate medical intervention and transport to an appropriate medical facility. You prepare to start an IV, when the babysitter tells you that she will not consent to treatment and tells you to wait for the parents to return home. A neighbor arrives on scene and insists that the child's parents would want only the family physician to treat her, and begs you to drive her to the physician's office.

1. You believe that the child needs emergency care, but the child's parents are unavailable. What should you do?

2. If you decide to treat the child without consent, can you be sued for doing so?

3. What would you do if the parents returned home and refused to grant permission for treatment?

See Suggested Responses at the back of this book.

Review Questions

1. _____ _____ originated with the English legal system and was adopted by Americans in the 1700s.
   a. Common law
   b. Civil law
   c. Criminal law
   d. Constitutional law

2. _____ _____ is enacted by an administrative or governmental agency at either the federal or state level.
   a. Civil law
   b. Criminal law
   c. Legislative law
   d. Administrative law

3. The _____ _____ is the location of most of the cases in which a paramedic may become involved.
   a. appellate court system
   b. state court system
   c. federal court system
   d. supreme court system

4. On-scene licensed physicians who are professionally unrelated to the patient and who are attempting to assist with patient care are called _____.
   a. intervener physicians.
   b. direct control physicians.
   c. on-line medical control.
   d. indirect control physicians.

5. Legislative statutes that generally protect the person who provides care at no charge at the scene of a medical emergency are called _____.
   a. medical practice laws.
   b. scope of practice laws.
   c. Good Samaritan laws.
   d. standard of care laws.

6. In a negligence claim against a paramedic, the plaintiff must establish and prove four particular elements to prevail. Which of the following is *not* one of those elements?
   a. Proximate cause
   b. Duty to act
   c. Level of compensation
   d. Breach of the duty to act

7. The law provides penalties for the breach of confidentiality. The improper release of information may result in a lawsuit against the paramedic for _____
   a. defamation.
   b. invasion of privacy.
   c. breach of confidentiality.
   d. all of the above.

8. Which court-ordered type of consent is most commonly encountered with patients who must be held for mental-health evaluation or as directed by law enforcement personnel who have the patient under arrest?
   a. Implied
   b. Expressed
   c. Involuntary
   d. Guardianship

9. _____ is the termination of the paramedic–patient relationship without providing for the appropriate continuation of care while it is still needed and desired by the patient.
   a. Libel
   b. Slander
   c. Neglect
   d. Abandonment

10. A well-documented patient care report is _____
    a. accurate.
    b. objective.
    c. thorough.
    d. all of the above.

See Suggested Responses at the back of this book.

References

1. Sine, D. M. and N. Northcutt. "A Qualitative Analysis of the Central Values of Professional Paramedics." *Am J Disaster Med* 3 (2008): 335–343.

2. United States of America. *Constitution of the United States.* (Available at http://www.archives.gov/exhibits/charters/constitution.html.)

3. *Miranda v. Arizona,* 384 U.S. 436 (1966).

4. Hoffman, S., R. A. Goodman, and D. D. Stier. "Law, Liability and Public Health Emergencies." *Disaster Med Public Health Prep* 3 (2009): 117–125.

5. Nagorka, F. W. and C. Becker. "Immunity Statutes: How State Laws Protect EMS Providers." *Emerg Med Serv* 36 (2005): 47–52.

6. Hall, S.A. "Potential Liabilities of Medical Directors for Actions of EMTs." *Prehosp Emerg Care* 2 (1998): 76–80.

7. Erich, J. "Where Duty Ends: The Perils and Pitfalls of the Off-Duty Response." *Emerg Med Serv* 33 (2004): 49–52.

8. Wang, H. E. and D. M. Yealy. "Out-of-Hospital Endotracheal Intubation: Where Are We?" *Ann Emerg Med* 47 (2006): 532–541.

9. Chan, T. C., G. M. Vilke, and T. Neuman. "Reexamination of Custody Restraint Position and Positional Asphyxia." *Am J Forensic Med Pathol* 19 (1998): 201–205.

10. Department of Health and Human Services. *Health Information Privacy Act.* (Available at http://www.hhs.gov/ocr/privacy/.)

11. Ayres, R. J., Jr. "Legal Considerations in Prehospital Care." *Emerg Med Clin North Am* 11 (1993): 853–867.

12. Graham, D. H. "Documentation of Patient Refusals." *Emerg Med Serv* 30 (2001): 56–60.

13. Maggiore, W. A. "Professional Boundaries: Where They Are & Why We Cross Them." *JEMS* 32(12): 68–76, 2007. (This article is available online at http://www.jems.com. Click on "JEMS/issues" to locate a PDF of this article in Vol. 32, No. 12, December 2007.)

Further Reading

The Ambulance Service Guide to HIPAA Compliance. Mechanicsburg, PA: Page, Wolfberg, & Wirth, 2003.

Cohn, B. M. and A. J. Azzara. *Legal Aspects of Emergency Medical Services.* Philadelphia: W. B. Saunders, 1998.

Lee, N. G. *Legal Concepts and Issues in Emergency Care.* Philadelphia: W. B. Saunders, 2001.

Louisell, D. and H. Williams. *Medical Malpractice.* New York: Matthew Bender, 1995.

Page, J. O. "Anatomy of a Lawsuit." *JEMS* 1989: 14.

Schneid, Thomas D. *Fire and Emergency Law Case Book.* Albany, NY: Delmar Publishing, 1997.

Wang, H. E., R. J. Fairbanks, M. N. Shah, and D. M. Yealey. "Tort Claims from Adverse Events in Emergency Medical Services." *Prehosp Emerg Care* 11 (2007): 96–97.

Chapter 8
Ethics in Paramedicine

Bryan Bledsoe, DO, FACEP, FAAEM

STANDARD
Preparatory (Medical–Legal and Ethics)

COMPETENCY
Integrates comprehensive knowledge of EMS systems, the safety and well-being of the paramedic, and medical–legal and ethical issues, which is intended to improve the health of EMS personnel, patients, and the community.

 ## Learning Objectives

Terminal Performance Objective: After reading this chapter, you should be able to apply the ethical principles of paramedicine to your work as a paramedic.

Enabling Objectives: To accomplish the terminal performance objective, you should be able to:

1. Define key terms introduced in this chapter.

2. Describe the relationship between ethics and morals, laws, and religion.

3. Compare and contrast different approaches to ethical decision making.

4. Identify codes of ethics that serve to guide health care professionals, including EMS providers.

5. Explain the fundamental principles of ethics—beneficence, maleficence, autonomy, and justice.

6. Given a variety of scenarios involving ethical dilemmas, take actions you can defend on the basis of ethical principles of paramedicine and tests of ethical decisions.

KEY TERMS

autonomy, p. 149	ethics, p. 146	morals, p. 146
beneficence, p. 149	justice, p. 149	nonmaleficence, p. 149

Case Study

Mrs. Weinberg has fractured her hip. Her right lower extremity is obviously shortened and externally rotated. Fortunately, she has no apparent life-threatening injuries. As you and your partner tend to her, you notice that she seems more anxious than other patients you have seen with a similar problem. When your partner goes to the ambulance to retrieve additional pillows, she whispers to you, "I would really prefer if you took care of me."

"Why?" you ask.

She rolls up her sleeve and shows you a tattoo of a number on her left forearm. "This is why," she says. "When I was a little girl back in Germany, I was in a Nazi concentration camp. Your partner reminds me of the men who worked there. They killed my family, and they almost killed me. Could you take care of me on the way to the hospital?"

You do not have much time to think about this question, but you promise to help. Before you leave the scene, you approach your partner discreetly. "Heinz," you say to him, "this patient is a concentration camp survivor. Apparently your blond hair, blue eyes, and German accent remind her of the men who killed her family. Would you mind driving to the hospital on this call? I realize you enrolled in an exchange program to gain experience in patient care here in the United States, but there will be other calls." Heinz has no objection, so he drives to the hospital, and you take care of Mrs. Weinberg in the back of the ambulance.

After the call, the two of you discuss what happened. "Boy," you say, "I've never had a patient make a request like that. I think it was really great of you to accommodate her. Did it make you uncomfortable?" "No," he says, "but it surprised me. The Holocaust was long before my time. It remains an embarrassment for all of us in my country." You agree that the best way to make Mrs. Weinberg comfortable was to switch places. You also agree that the two of you handled a difficult situation gracefully.

Later, when you think about the call a little more, you realize that this situation was truly a first for you. Is it right, you wonder, to accommodate a request like this? Heinz was not going to harm her. Were you assuaging her fears or validating her prejudices? What if the patient had been an elderly white man who asked you to switch places with your black partner? Would the patient's ignorance have been enough of a reason to accommodate him? What if the patient had been a neo-Nazi skinhead who insisted on having a white person care for him?

Was the situation just a matter of being courteous, as you first thought? After all, no one was hurt, and it was only a minor inconvenience for you and your partner to switch positions. Or was it actually a matter of ethics? You realize you are not quite sure how to determine the best thing to do under circumstances like these. It is time, you realize, to brush up on your ethics.

Introduction

Consider the following: A physician administers 15 milligrams of intravenous morphine to a dying patient to alleviate pain and suffering. Another physician administers 15 milligrams of intravenous morphine to a dying patient to end the patient's life. What's the difference? Although the question is seemingly simple, it is actually quite complex. Is there a moral difference between these two actions?

When asked what the most difficult part of the job is, most paramedics do not say "ethics." Nonetheless, in one recent survey almost 15 percent of ALS calls in an urban EMS system generated some ethical conflict.[1] In another survey, EMS providers responded that they frequently have ethical problems related to patients refusing care, conflicts regarding hospital destination, and difficulties with advance directives.[2] Other aspects of prehospital care present potential ethical problems. These include patient confidentiality, consent, the obligation to provide care, and research.

Although ethical problems often have a legal aspect, most ethical problems are solved in the field and not in a courtroom. However, there are times when ethical problems spill over into the legal arena and become the subject of legislation or regulations. The federal government, for instance, recently instituted rules to protect patients who are unable to consent to emergency care.

Ethical issues often begin with specific circumstances and lead to broad general rules or principles for behavior. This chapter examines how the most common principles and approaches are applied to common prehospital situations.

Overview of Ethics

Ethics and morals are closely related concepts. **Morals** are generally considered to be social, religious, or personal standards of right and wrong. **Ethics**, also known as *moral philosophy*, is a branch of philosophy that addresses questions about morality. Generally speaking, ethics more often refers to the rules or standards that govern the conduct of members of a particular group or profession and how our institutions should function. Both ethics and morals address a question Socrates asked: "How should one live?"

Relationship of Ethics to Law and Religion

Ethics and the law have a great deal in common, but they are distinctly separate disciplines (Figure 8-1). Although ethical discussions have an unfortunate tendency to degenerate into arguments about what is legal and who might be liable, ethics is not the same as law. In general, laws have a much narrower focus than ethics. Laws frequently describe what is wrong in the eyes of society. Ethics goes beyond examining what is wrong. It also looks at what is right, or good, behavior. As a result, the law frequently has little or nothing to say about ethical problems. In fact, laws themselves can be unethical. For example, for many years, laws existed and were enforced that perpetuated racial segregation in the United States. These were ethically wrong and, ultimately, made legally wrong.

Even though ethics and the law are different, ethical discussions can sometimes benefit from techniques developed by the law over the centuries. In particular, the law emphasizes impartiality, consistent procedures, and methods to identify and balance conflicting interests.

Just as ethics differs from the law, it also differs from religion. In a pluralistic society such as ours, ethics must be understood by and applied to people who hold a broad

Relationship of Ethical and Legal Issues with Medicine

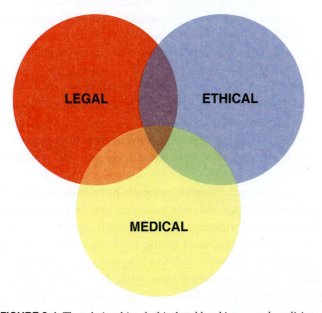

FIGURE 8-1 The relationship of ethical and legal issues and medicine.

Cultural Considerations

The population of North America has certainly become a cultural blend. You can see it in the different ways people respond to serious illness or injury. Some may look at an illness as a disease process with predictable results. Others may look at it as destiny. Others will simply attribute an illness to God's will. In some cultures, certain illnesses and injuries are believed to be the work of the devil or a result of witchcraft, curses, or spells. To those who believe, such interpretations are as real and as plausible as any other. For them, the only successful treatment possible may involve countering the effects of the curse or spell in question. Thus, they may not have much confidence that your skilled prehospital care will make much of a difference.

Paramedics must recognize that people of different cultural backgrounds respond to illnesses and injuries in different ways. Never criticize or chastise patients for beliefs that differ from yours. These beliefs are so culturally ingrained that a single contact with an EMS provider is unlikely to change them. It is important to acknowledge such beliefs and never to ridicule those who hold them.

range of religious beliefs, or no religious beliefs at all. Thus, ethics cannot derive from a single religion. It is true, however, that religion can enhance and enrich one's ethical principles and values.

Making Ethical Decisions

There are many different approaches one can use to determine how a medical professional should behave under different circumstances. One approach is to say that each person must decide how to behave and whatever decision that person makes is okay. This approach is known as *ethical relativism*. People sometimes say that they believe in ethical relativism. However, when questioned, they typically admit they do not find it satisfactory. For example, no reasonable person would say that it was acceptable for the Nazis, especially Nazi physicians, to behave as they did.

A similar approach is to say, "Just do what is right." This sounds fine, but in reality it does not answer the question of how a health care professional should act. This occurs because different people have different beliefs about what is "right." Ethics and morality overlap, but professional ethics go beyond what one individual thinks is right or wrong. Even the Golden Rule—"Do unto others as you would have them do unto you"—is not a sufficient guideline. What happens when the person making the decision has desires and values that are radically different from the patient's? It becomes clear that reason and logic must be used and emotion must be excluded as much as possible from the decision-making process.

Another approach is to say that people should just fulfill their duties. This is known as the *deontological method*.

A very simple example of this approach is someone who says, "Just follow the Ten Commandments." Unfortunately, although the Ten Commandments provide useful instruction, they do not provide enough guidance for medical professionals who must make difficult ethical decisions in health care situations.

A very different approach is *consequentialism*. Followers of this school of thought believe that actions can be judged as good or bad only after we know the consequences of those actions. Utilitarians, who believe that the purpose of an action should be to bring the greatest happiness to the greatest number of people, are consequentialists. One difficulty with the utilitarians' approach is determining what constitutes happiness. Another challenge arises when the happiness of one person is in conflict with the happiness of another person. Utilitarianism offers a "bankbook" approach to resolving these conflicts, asking the decision maker to weigh relative "amounts" of happiness.

Codes of Ethics

Over the years, a number of organizations have drafted codes of ethics for the members of their organizations. The American Medical Association and the American Osteopathic Association have codes of ethics for physicians. The American College of Emergency Physicians has a code of ethics specifically for emergency physicians.[3] The American Nurses Association and Emergency Nurses Association both have codes for practitioners in their fields. The National Association of EMTs adopted a code of ethics for EMTs in 1978 (see the chapter "Roles and Responsibilities of the Paramedic"). Most codes of ethics address broad humanitarian concerns and professional etiquette. Few, however, provide solid guidance on the kind of ethical problems commonly faced by practitioners.

Ethical codes often address the following areas:

- Honesty
- Objectivity
- Integrity
- Carefulness
- Openness
- Legality
- Confidentiality
- Responsible publication
- Responsible mentoring
- Respect for colleagues
- Social responsibility
- Nondiscrimination
- Competence

- Respect for intellectual property
- Human subjects protection

Many of the areas listed above have direct application to EMS.[4]

Impact of Ethics on Individual Practice

Only by consistently displaying ethical behavior will paramedics gain and maintain the respect of their colleagues and their patients. It is vital that individual paramedics exemplify the principles and values of their profession. Paramedics must understand and agree to abide by the responsibilities, both implicit and explicit, of their profession. Occasionally, this can be a problem. A paramedic is expected to work, for example, in an uncontrolled environment that is sometimes dangerous. A person who is unwilling to enter a scene until every risk has been totally eliminated is not acting in accordance with the expectations of the profession. Conversely, a paramedic is expected to refrain from entering a hazardous area until the risks have been made manageable. Common sense should help in resolving conflicts such as these.

The Fundamental Questions

The single most important question a paramedic must answer when faced with an ethical challenge is "What is in the patient's best interest?" Most of the time the answer to this question is obvious: The patient wants reassurance, relief from pain, and prompt, safe transport to a hospital emergency department. However, sometimes the answer to this question is not so obvious. For example, what is in the best interest of a terminally ill patient who goes into cardiac arrest? Is it to resuscitate him? Or is it to not start resuscitation in order to prevent further suffering?

Under ideal circumstances, a written statement describing the patient's desires will be available. In many states, such a statement (which meets other specified state and local requirements) is, in fact, required before a paramedic may elect not to start resuscitation efforts. In less extreme circumstances, the patient may state verbally what he wishes you to do and not do. As long as the patient is competent and the desires are consistent with good practice, the paramedic is obligated to respect the patient's desires.

Traditionally, family members have been an important source of information for physicians in determining the wishes of a patient. This approach, however, is not necessarily appropriate in the field. In the hospital or especially in the years before a hospital admission, physicians are able to spend time with the patient and the patient's family and develop a relationship with them. In the field, paramedics typically do not know the patient or the family. There is usually not enough time for a paramedic to develop the same kind of relationship that physicians do in their practices. Additionally, the family is under a great deal of stress when the paramedic encounters them.

For these reasons and others, a paramedic must be very cautious in accepting a family's description of what a patient desires. The paramedic must also take into consideration the state and local laws regarding patient resuscitation desires and documentation of those desires.

It may sometimes be difficult for a paramedic to agree with a patient's wishes, but it is important that he respect them. Only by demonstrating "good faith" in following a patient's wishes does a paramedic show respect for the patient. A paramedic must also realize that the family may not agree with the patient's desires. This may lead family members to substitute their own desires for the patient's. This is another reason that the paramedic should not necessarily accept a family's description of a patient's desires at face value.

Fundamental Principles

A common approach to resolving problems in bioethics today is to employ four fundamental principles or values. These principles are beneficence, nonmaleficence, autonomy, and justice.

Beneficence is related to a more familiar term, *benevolence*. Both come from Latin and concern doing good. However, *benevolence* means the *desire* to do good (usually the main reason people become paramedics), whereas *beneficence* means actually *doing* good (the paramedic's obligation to the patient).

Maleficence means doing harm, the opposite of *beneficence*. **Nonmaleficence** means *not* doing harm. Few medical interventions are without risk of harm. Under the principle of nonmaleficence, however, the paramedic is obligated to minimize that risk as much as possible. This includes, for example, making the scene safe and protecting the patient from impaired or unqualified health care providers. The Latin phrase *primum non nocere*, which means "first, do no harm," sums up nonmaleficence very well.

Autonomy refers to a competent adult patient's right to determine what happens to his own body, including treatment for medical illnesses and injuries. The paramedic has an obligation to respect this right of self-determination. Under ordinary conditions, a patient must give consent before the paramedic can begin treatment. There are, of course, exceptions to this, including the patient who is not competent and for whom the doctrine of implied consent applies. However, the competent patient must receive accurate information to make an informed decision. This implies that the paramedic must be truthful in describing to the patient his condition and the risks and benefits of treatment for it. It also implies respect for the patient's privacy.

Justice refers to the paramedic's obligation to treat all patients fairly. For example, the paramedic should provide necessary emergency care to all patients without regard to sex, race, ability to pay, or cultural background, among other conditions.

Resolving Ethical Conflicts

Even if everyone agreed on the same principles and procedures for resolving ethical difficulties, there would still be disagreements in specific situations. These disagreements can be resolved at different levels. Even the government sometimes takes action when issues become very important to the public. For example, there are now laws to protect the rights of hospitalized patients and members of managed care organizations. Many states have implemented laws or regulations that allow for the use of advance directives. The federal government has instituted rules to protect the rights of patients in emergency research when they are unable to consent.

The health care community has also responded to the challenge. Long before the federal government instituted rules regarding consent in emergency research, hospitals and universities set up institutional review boards (IRBs). These groups serve to protect the rights of subjects participating in research projects. Hospitals throughout the world have had ethics committees for many years to assist in clarifying patients' desires and in weighing competing interests in ethically challenging situations.

The paramedic, however, cannot depend on these institutions to assist in the field. He needs to have a system for resolving these conflicts, one that will allow him to weigh the various factors, including all relevant facts, principles, and values, that lead to responsible, defensible actions. One such system or method of resolving ethical issues before or after they arise is illustrated in the following scenario:

> You are the official representative of your service to the regional EMS coordinating agency. At the most recent meeting, the head nurse for the emergency department (ED) of the largest hospital in the county mentioned how recent cutbacks in support staff had led to more difficulty retrieving patients' medical records in a timely manner. This has led to a number of difficulties in treating patients. As a result, the ED was considering asking incoming ambulances to give patients' names and dates of birth on the radio. This would give the ED staff additional time to search for the patient's medical records.
>
> After the meeting, you consider the issue's ethical aspects. First, you identify the problem, which in this case is: Is it justifiable to breach patient confidentiality

to expedite the retrieval of medical records? Second, you list the possible actions that might be taken in this situation. Possibilities include:

- Provide all patients' names and dates of birth on the radio.
- Continue the current policy of identifying patients only by age and sex.
- Provide selected patients' names and dates of birth on the radio.

To reason out an ethical problem, first state the action in a universal form. Then list the implications or consequences of the action. Finally, compare them to relevant values (Figure 8-2). The application of this method to the scenario described would be as follows:

To state an action in a universal form, describe what should be done, who should do it, and under what conditions. For example, EMS (who) will volunteer names and dates of birth for all patients (what) on the radio (condition).

The immediate implications are that the ED will be able to get records sooner for patients who have records at that hospital. There will be no change for most patients because hospital records are often irrelevant to emergency care. The ED admitting staff may be able to admit patients more quickly. However, patients' names and dates of birth will be broadcast to thousands of people listening with scanners. The long-term consequences are that people with scanners will learn more about patients who go to the hospital via EMS. Because private information may be broadcast, patients may become reluctant to call EMS. Conceivably, there may be more burglaries at homes of patients who use EMS.

Finally, compare those consequences to values that are relevant. A list of values that pertain to this case might include beneficence, nonmaleficence, autonomy, and confidentiality. That is, if EMS provided names and dates of birth for all patients on the radio, what would be the benefit to the patient (beneficence)? A few patients might be cared for sooner because their records arrived sooner. Most patients will see no benefit because they have no records at

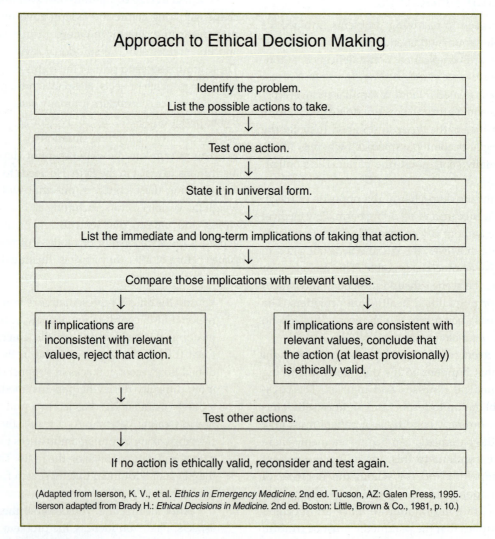

FIGURE 8-2 An approach to ethical decision making.

that hospital or time is not a significant issue (such as for a laceration that requires sutures). Furthermore, from a legal standpoint, such a practice would probably violate patient confidentiality laws such as HIPAA.

Autonomy suffers under this arrangement because the patient is not given the opportunity to consent (or decline). The patient's name and date of birth go out over the air without his permission. And, in this case, nonmaleficence and confidentiality are intertwined. There is potential for harm to the patient and to future patients who lose faith in the EMS system's ability to maintain privacy.

Therefore, because the possible consequences of providing all patients' names and dates of birth on the radio are not compatible with the values we consider important and relevant, you must go back and test another action using this same method.

When you evaluate the choice of continuing the current policy of identifying all patients over the radio only by age and sex, you may find the following consequences: People listening to scanners can learn facts about patients EMS is transporting, but no more than they have in the past; a few patients may get care that is delayed or less than optimal because their hospital records do not arrive quickly enough; and the ED staff are still stressed because they cannot get records in a timely manner. A comparison with relevant values reveals that patient confidentiality and patient confidence in EMS are unchanged, but the patients who might benefit from earlier arrival of their records may be suffering.

Continue to evaluate any other options you listed. In this case, the third and final one is: Provide selected patients' names and dates of birth on the radio. A comparison with relevant values shows that there is some potential benefit

for selected patients, a breach of confidentiality for patients who might benefit, and no breach of confidentiality for patients who would not benefit. Therefore, the scenario may conclude as follows:

CONTENT REVIEW

➤ Quick Ways to Test Ethics
  • Impartiality test
  • Universalizability test
  • Interpersonal justifiability test

The third option sounds closer to being acceptable, but you might wonder if there is a way to further limit loss of confidentiality. You revise your rule to read, "EMS broadcasts the initials and dates of birth of selected patients who meet predetermined criteria when there is no other private means of communication available." This strictly limits the loss of confidentiality to patients who may benefit from it and encourages both EMS and the ED to find other less public means of identifying patients. For example, paramedics could broadcast a patient's age, sex, and hospital card number or, if the patient does not have a hospital identification card available and time allows, someone at the scene could telephone the ED to relay the patient's name and date of birth privately.

The method just described is useful when you come upon a new ethical problem and time is not an issue. In situations where time is limited, an abbreviated method can sometimes be used (Figure 8-3). First, ask yourself whether the current problem is similar to other problems for which you have already formulated a rule. Then, if the answer is yes, follow that rule. If the answer is no, determine whether you can do something to buy time. Finally, if you can find a reasonable way to postpone dealing with

Quick Approach to New Ethical Problems

Consider the ethical problem.

*Do you already have a rule for dealing with this problem?

*Or, can you reasonably extend a rule to apply to the situation?

If yes to either of the above, follow the rule.

If no to the above,

*Can you buy time to consider a solution without causing significant risk to the patient?

*If you cannot, then apply the impartiality test, the universalizability test, or the interpersonal justifiability test.

(Based on Iserson, K. V., et al. *Ethics in Emergency Medicine.* 2nd ed. Tucson, AZ: Galen Press, 1995.)

FIGURE 8-3 A quick approach to new ethical problems.

the issue for a while, do so. If you cannot, analyze the best rule you have against three tests suggested by Iserson: the *impartiality test*, the *universalizability test*, and the *interpersonal justifiability test*:

- *Impartiality test*—asks whether you would be willing to undergo this procedure or action if you were in the patient's place. This is really a version of the Golden Rule (do unto others as you would have them do unto you), which helps to reduce the possibility of bias.

- *Universalizability test*—asks whether you would want this action performed in all relevantly similar circumstances, which helps the paramedic to avoid shortsightedness.

- *Interpersonal justifiability test*—asks whether you can defend or justify your actions to others. It helps to ensure that an action is appropriate by asking the paramedic to consider whether other people would think the action reasonable.[5]

When there is little time to consider a new ethical problem, these three questions can help a paramedic navigate murky waters, allowing him to find an acceptable solution in a short time.

Ethical Issues in Contemporary Paramedic Practice

The first part of the chapter built a foundation for ethical decision making by describing and demonstrating methods for dealing with these types of issues. The following discussion is meant to help you apply those principles to several commonly encountered situations. It also describes some of the ethical considerations to take into account in less common situations you may face.

Resuscitation Attempts

Consider the following scenario:

You are leaving the ED in your ambulance when an approximately 50-year-old woman jumps out of a window on the third floor of the hospital and lands on the road in front of you. Your partner stops the vehicle, and you get your equipment to begin assessment and management of the patient. As you reach her, a breathless aide runs out the door and says, "Don't do anything! She's got a DNR order!" How does this affect the care you administer?

You have virtually no time to think about what to do for this woman, who is bleeding on the street and appears unresponsive. Your instincts say, treat her now and let the hospital sort things out later if she survives.

In this case, your instincts are probably steering you in the right direction for a number of reasons. First, every state that has laws or rules regarding Do Not Resuscitate (DNR) orders requires that you see the order and verify its legitimacy in some manner. In this case, the order is not available for you to see, so you are under no legal obligation to withhold care.

Second, if the patient is alive (as she appears to be), even a valid DNR order would not prevent you from assessing the patient and administering basic care, including comfort care.

Third, the principle of nonmaleficence says do no harm. Refraining from helping her might cause irreversible harm, including perhaps death. The principles of beneficence and nonmaleficence both urge you to help the patient. The potential conflict arises when you consider autonomy. The competent patient of legal age has a right to determine what happens to her body. You have some reason to believe she has determined that she does not wish resuscitation efforts if her heart stops but, in this case, the accuracy of this information cannot be verified.

The conclusion of the scenario is as follows:

Considering the lack of verifiable information and the severe time limitations you are facing, you and your partner go ahead and assess the patient. You find that she responds to verbal stimuli by moaning, her airway is open, ventilations are adequate, and she has several lacerations and apparent fractures. Because you are literally in front of the hospital, you limit your interventions to quick immobilization on a spine board with bleeding control and oxygen by mask. You rapidly move her to the ED and turn her over to the team there.

Later, you discover that she had originally been admitted for evaluation of new-onset seizures. When the doctors told her that she might have a brain tumor, she signed a DNR form. Fortunately, no tumor was found and her prognosis is actually quite good. The trauma team finds no life-threatening injuries from her fall and expects her to be able to begin psychiatric treatment before she leaves the hospital. This additional information makes you very glad you decided to go ahead with treatment.

More states are passing laws or regulations allowing prehospital personnel to withhold certain treatment when the patient has a DNR order. A valid order consists of a written statement describing interventions a particular patient does not wish to have that is recognized by the authorities of that state. Before following a DNR order, the paramedic must be aware of several things.

First, the order must meet state and local requirements regarding wording and witnesses (a standardized form is usually available). Also, there may be a time limit on how long a DNR order is valid in certain jurisdictions. A patient with a valid prehospital DNR order may be required to wear or have nearby a particular means of identification, such as a bracelet with a special symbol. There should be a clear description of which interventions are to be withheld and under which circumstances. And finally, every patient is still entitled to reasonable measures intended to make the patient more comfortable (comfort care). Similarly, the family and loved ones are entitled to emotional support from EMS providers. (See the chapter "Medical/Legal Aspects of Preshospital Care" for legal aspects of DNR orders.)

Paramedics spend a great deal of time and energy learning how to assess and treat patients with life-threatening problems. It becomes difficult, then, for a paramedic to watch someone die without doing something to try to stop it. You must nonetheless respect the patient's wishes when a competent patient has clearly communicated what he really wants. DNR orders make this easier because they typically must be signed or approved by a physician, increasing the likelihood that the decision was thoroughly thought through.

When there is no such order, however, it becomes more difficult for the paramedic to determine what the patient's wishes truly are. Family members may be able to describe the patient's desires, but they can have conflicts of interest that make their statements less credible. For example, the patient may have accepted his impending death before his family has. They may want you to attempt resuscitation when that was clearly against the patient's expressed wishes. A less common situation is one in which the patient wishes all resuscitation efforts, but the family does not because they do not wish to prolong their own suffering or they have other, less noble, motivations.

The general principle for paramedics to follow in cases such as these is: "When in doubt, resuscitate." This usually satisfies the principles of beneficence and nonmaleficence, admittedly perhaps at the expense of autonomy, but one of the biggest advantages to this approach is that, unlike the alternative, it is not irreversible. If you refrain from attempting resuscitation, it is certain that the patient will die. If you attempt resuscitation, there is no guarantee that the patient will survive, but the patient can be removed from life-sustaining equipment later if that is deemed appropriate. Another advantage is that there will be more time later to sort out competing interests.

What about not attempting resuscitation when the situation appears futile? This option may appear attractive at first glance. After a little investigation, though, the issue becomes much more complex. How would a reasonable person or society define "futile"? This is an issue that has

received a good deal of attention and the conclusion is that, except at the extreme ends of the spectrum, there is no consensus on what constitutes a futile attempt at resuscitation.

In addition, there is the issue of who would actually make the decision that a resuscitation attempt is futile in a particular case. Is it the experienced paramedic who has seen very few lives saved under similar circumstances or the new paramedic who is still excited about the prospect of saving lives every day? How can it be fair to have such wide disparities in such an important decision? Clearly, the concept of futility does not provide a useful guide for whether or not to attempt resuscitation.

Another related topic is what to do when an advance directive is presented to you after you have begun resuscitation. Once you have verified the validity of the order and the identity of the patient, you are obligated ethically (and perhaps legally, depending on your state) to cease resuscitation efforts. This can be a very difficult situation for you emotionally, but you have an obligation to respect the patient's autonomy and stop doing something to him that he did not want. Follow your local protocols regarding procedures for cessation of resuscitation efforts.

Confidentiality

Consider this scenario:

You are called at one o'clock in the morning to a local hotel for a man reported to be unresponsive (but breathing) at the front desk. When you arrive, one of the guests at the hotel meets you at the front door. He tells you that he tried to call the front desk from his room to request a wake-up call but got no answer. When he went to the front desk, he found the clerk slumped over in his chair, apparently unconscious, with what smelled like alcohol on his breath.

When you approach the patient, you see an approximately 25-year-old male who appears to be unresponsive. His skin appears normal, and he is moving air well. He does not respond when you call him by the name on his name plate, which is Howard. He has a strong, regular radial pulse that is within normal limits. You do not smell anything except for a faint minty odor. When you shake his shoulder and call his name again, he moans. Further shaking and shouting eventually bring him to the point where his eyes are open, he is looking around, and he asks, "Who are you?"

You explain to Howard that you were called by a concerned guest who could not wake him up. Howard says he is fine now and does not want to go to a hospital. He is alert and oriented to person, place, and time. He denies any complaints, takes no medications, and has no past medical history. His vital signs are within normal limits. He denies any alcohol intake or use of any other drugs. The physical exam is unremarkable.

By your protocols and standard operating procedures, you have no reason to attempt to force the patient to go to a hospital. You complete the appropriate documentation for a refusal of transport and are leaving the lobby when the guest who called 911 stops you. "Aren't you going to take him to the hospital?" he asks. No, you reply, he does not want to go. "But what if there's a fire in the hotel and he's passed out and unable to help guests evacuate?"

This makes you stop and think, and you begin to weigh the rights of the hotel guests against the rights of your patient.

Your obligation to the patient is to maintain as confidential the information you obtained as a result of your participation in this medical situation. Clearly, the most beneficial thing you can do for his privacy is not to notify anyone about his condition. Additionally, there are questions regarding what you could accurately report. The patient denies alcohol and drug intake, and you could find no objective signs to dispute his claim. He might just be a heavy sleeper. Reporting that he is or may be under the influence of alcohol or drugs might lead to the loss of his job and to legal trouble for you.

However, what if there is an emergency in which the desk clerk's assistance is needed and he is unable to provide it? That is an unlikely, though certainly a conceivable, possibility. However, there is no clear and present danger that would require you to report. In fact, depending on the state you're in, you may have a legal obligation to maintain confidentiality under circumstances such as these.

There are a number of reasons to respect confidentiality in general. In an emergency, a patient typically has little choice about who is going to come to his aid. He is assuming that he can be honest with these strangers who have come to help him because they will protect his privacy. If that trust was routinely violated without sufficient cause, patients might very well be embarrassed or humiliated. This would undermine the public's trust in EMS and any particular patient's trust in the paramedics and others coming into his home. If word got around that private information was being made public, patients might not be forthcoming in giving their medical histories, potentially leading to disastrous consequences. For example, a man who had recently taken sildenafil (Viagra) for erectile dysfunction might deny taking it before you give him nitroglycerin. This drug interaction is potentially serious, possibly even fatal.

There are, nonetheless, times when it is appropriate and necessary to breach confidentiality. Every state has laws requiring the reporting of certain health facts such as births, deaths, particular infectious diseases, child neglect and abuse, and elder neglect and abuse. These last requirements have the most applicability to EMS. They are considered justifiable reasons to breach confidentiality because, in the eyes of society, the benefit to someone who is defenseless (protection from harm and perhaps even death) and to the public (a safer environment for children) outweighs the right to privacy of a particular person. A valid court order is also considered a reasonable justification for breaching confidentiality. So is a clear threat by a patient to a specific person, as well as informing other health care professionals who will care for the patient.

Clearly, patient confidentiality is an important principle, but not an inviolable one. When determining whether it is appropriate to breach confidentiality, take into account the probability of harm, the magnitude of the expected harm, and alternative methods of avoiding harm that do not require encroaching on confidentiality.

In the previous scenario, factors do not justify breaching confidentiality. The person who called 911 for emergency assistance, however, is under no such obligation. The scenario comes to an end as follows:

When you inform the guest that you are unable to discuss the case with anyone because of confidentiality, he replies, "Well, you may not be able to do anything about it, but I can. I'm calling the manager!"

Consent

Consider this scenario:

Bob, a 58-year-old male, has been having crushing substernal pain radiating to his left arm for several hours. He also is pale, sweaty, and nauseated. He denies shortness of breath. His condition remains unchanged after you give him oxygen and nitroglycerin. When you ask Bob which hospital he wants to go to, he tells you, "I'm not going to any hospital." Surprised, you find it difficult to understand why someone in this much pain would not want to go to a hospital. You try to enlist the help of relatives over the telephone (Bob lives alone), but they are unable to persuade the patient. He has no regular physician, so that option is not available to you. Finally, you decide to try on-line medical direction. While you are waiting for the physician to come to the phone, you wonder: If the patient continues to refuse, can you force him to go? How can you act in the best interest of a patient who refuses to accept what you feel certain is best for him?

A competent patient of legal age has the fundamental right to decide what health care he will receive and will not receive. This is at the core of patient autonomy. To exercise this right, a patient must have the information necessary to make an informed decision, the mental faculties to weigh the risks and benefits of various treatment options, and the freedom from restraints that might hamper his ability to exercise his options (such as threats).

It is sometimes appropriate to use the doctrine of implied consent to force the patient to go to the hospital. For the paramedic to use this approach, the patient must be unable to give consent. Typically, the doctrine is invoked when the patient is unable to communicate, but it also can be employed when the patient is incapacitated because of drugs, illness, or injury. In this scenario, however, the patient shows no signs of being incapacitated. He is alert; oriented to person, place, and time; aware of his surroundings; and making judgments and answering questions in a manner completely compatible with competence. The fact that the patient refuses something you recommend does not, in itself, necessarily indicate that he is incompetent.

Before you leave the patient, you must not only do the things you need to do to protect yourself legally, but you must also assure yourself that the patient truly understands the issues at hand and is able to make an informed decision. As difficult as it may be for the paramedic, if the patient is able to do these things, the paramedic may have to accept the patient's desires and leave him.

Allocation of Resources

Paramedics do not usually think of themselves as guardians of finite resources, but occasionally they are. The most obvious example of this is when there are more patients present than the paramedic is able to manage, such as in a multiple-casualty incident (MCI). While learning how to provide emergency medical care for multiple patients at the same scene, you might ask: What are the ethics of triage?

There are several possible approaches to consider in parceling out scarce resources. Patients could all receive the same amount of attention and resources (true parity). They could receive resources based on need. Or they could receive what someone has determined they've earned.

The civilian method of triage, in which the most seriously injured patients receive the most care, is based on need. This is intended to produce the most good for the most people. However, other methods of triage are in use. Military triage, for example, has traditionally concentrated on helping the least seriously injured because this approach produces the greatest number of soldiers who can return to duty. When the president or vice president visits a town or city, there is typically an ambulance dedicated for the dignitary's use, if needed. The ambulance is not to be used for anyone else. Because these officials are so important and because so many others need them, the typical order of care is changed.

A controversy exists in emergency medicine as to whether or not celebrities should be treated ahead of others. The argument for doing so typically emphasizes the disorder brought to the ED by the presence of a celebrity and the need to get the person out of the ED as quickly as possible to restore normal operation. The argument against takes the position that giving preferential treatment to a celebrity is an affront to justice and fairness.

All these methods have their proponents for different situations. The key to resolving the issue of allocation of scarce resources is to examine the competing theories in light of the circumstances at hand.

Obligation to Provide Care

By virtue of membership in a profession, a paramedic takes on a responsibility to help others. The public, through the government, grants certain privileges to professionals in return for the expectation of professional behavior. As a practitioner of paramedicine, the paramedic has even greater responsibilities. Those who provide emergency care have a special obligation to help all those in need. Many other health care professionals are free to pick and choose their patients, accepting only those who have health insurance or who can themselves pay for the services delivered by the health care professional. This is not the case in emergency medicine.

Paramedics, like other emergency professionals, are obligated to provide medical care for those in need without regard to ability to pay. They also have an ethical obligation to prevent and report instances of patient "dumping," where those without insurance are transferred against their will to public or charity hospitals.

A particular issue arises regarding the patient who is a member of a managed-care organization such as a health maintenance organization (HMO). The HMO may insist that the patient be treated at a particular facility with which the HMO has a contract. This must not be allowed to interfere with the patient's emergency care. The paramedic, like every other member of the EMS system, has an obligation to act in the patient's best interest, even when that goes against the HMO's economic interests.

A very different aspect of providing care has to do with offering assistance when off duty. Although only two states require paramedics, among others, to stop and render help when they come upon someone in need of emergency care, there is still a strong ethical obligation to do so. This does not extend to situations in which the paramedic would put himself in danger (such as getting into a car

Legal Considerations

Intervening Outside Your EMS System.   The paramedic functions under the auspices of the EMS medical director as detailed in system protocols and standing orders. Providing ALS skills or interventions outside your EMS system can lead to possible legal problems and litigation.

teetering on the edge of a cliff), if assisting would interfere with important duties owed to others (such as leaving young children unattended in a car), or when someone else is already providing assistance. In return, society offers limited liability in the form of Good Samaritan statutes in every state in the United States.

Teaching

Many paramedics act as preceptors or mentors in their EMS systems. Two issues raised by this role are whether or not patients should be informed that a student is working on them, and how many attempts a student should be allowed to have in performing critical interventions before the preceptor steps in.

When patients call for EMS, they generally expect to receive care from individuals who have finished their education and who hold credentials qualifying them to work. If a system decides not to inform patients of the presence of students, the system runs the risk of being accused of concealing important information from patients.

To avoid this problem, EMS systems with students working in them should make sure students are clearly identified as such by the uniform they wear. The preceptor should also, when appropriate, inform patients of the presence of a student and request the patient's consent before the student performs a procedure. This sounds more cumbersome than it actually is. Patients who are unable to consent obviously do not fall into this category; implied consent is invoked in this case. And patients who are able to consent are frequently very understanding of the student's need for experience. As long as the preceptor stresses that he is overseeing the student, the vast majority of patients usually give their consent.

Another issue related to students is how many attempts they should be allowed in order to perform procedures such as intravenous placement and endotracheal intubation before the preceptor steps in. Factors to consider include the student's skill level (as determined by classroom practice on mannequins and previous field experience), the anticipated difficulty of the procedure (some patients are obviously going to be more difficult to intubate or start an IV on), and the relative importance of the procedure (not all IVs are equally important). It is important to have a limit, at least initially, for the number of times a student will be allowed to attempt a procedure. Such a number will need to be decided by each system in consultation with the medical director.

Professional Relations

As a health care professional, the paramedic answers to the patient. As a physician extender, the paramedic answers to a physician medical director. As an employee (or volunteer), the paramedic answers to the EMS system. These competing interests can sometimes make life difficult. Each can lead to ethical challenges.

In general, there are three potential sources of conflict between paramedics and physicians. One possibility is a case in which a physician orders something the paramedic believes is contraindicated. For example, suppose a physician ordered a paramedic to transport a critical blunt-trauma patient without attempting any intravenous access, either at the scene or en route during the anticipated 45-minute transport. This order runs counter to standard medical practice. The patient will have spent more than an hour since the trauma without receiving any intravenous fluid or intravenous access.

A different situation arises when the physician orders something the paramedic believes is medically acceptable but not in the patient's best interests. For example, imagine you are transporting a patient with stable vital signs who is complaining of abdominal pain. In accordance with your protocols, you and your partner have each tried twice to start an IV line without success. The patient's veins are some of the worst you have ever seen, and you have no expectation that you will be successful on further attempts. The patient experienced considerable pain with each attempt and is now crying, asking you not to try anymore. The physician, however, insists that you continue attempts to gain access.

A third potential source of conflict is the situation in which the physician orders something the paramedic believes is medically acceptable, but morally wrong. For example, say you are ordered to stop CPR on a young male patient found in cardiac arrest after blunt trauma. His initial rhythm of asystole has remained unchanged, and you know it is almost always associated with death. Nonetheless, although there is a very slim chance of recovery for the patient if you continue your resuscitation efforts, you would not be able to live with yourself if you did not at least try.

In each of the three cases, it is certainly appropriate for the paramedic to start by confirming the order and asking the physician to repeat it. If the order is confirmed, the medic would be prudent to ask the physician for an explanation, given the controversial nature of the orders in the first two situations (in the third, the physician's thoughts and goals are fairly clear). The next steps will depend on the physician's explanation, the patient's condition, the need for the intervention in the judgment of the paramedic, the feasibility of performing the intervention (like gaining IV access), and the amount of time available to discuss the issue.

Ultimately, the paramedic must determine for himself how the patient's interests are best served. This typically does not lead to conflict, but on occasion the paramedic may run into situations similar to the ones previously described. In these cases, the medic must consider the competing interests of beneficence, nonmaleficence, autonomy, and justice; the roles of the physician and the paramedic; the relative confidence (or lack thereof) the paramedic has in his own medical and ethical judgment; how far the paramedic is willing to go as an advocate for his patient; and the degree of risk acceptable to the paramedic in contravening physician orders.

It is important for the paramedic to understand that no matter what decision he makes, he will have to defend it. The explanation that he was just following the doctor's orders (or, conversely, just doing what he felt was right) will not be sufficient in and of itself. A paramedic is expected to be more than a robot. He or she is expected to simultaneously be a physician extender, working under a physician's license, and a clinician with the ability and independence to recognize and question inappropriate orders. The paramedic should also understand that he is not expected to act in ways he feels are immoral. However, if the individual's morals are significantly out of step with the expectations of the profession, he needs to reconsider his profession.

Disagreements with physician orders happen rarely. Usually they are the result of poor communication (such as saying one thing while meaning another or static interfering with the radio transmission) or lack of sufficient information. Conflicts with physicians that reach the level in the previous examples are fortunately rare. When they happen, the paramedic must be willing to be an advocate for the patient and act in the patient's best interests.

Research

EMS research is relatively new but absolutely important for the profession to advance. Research is the foundation on which all scientific endeavors, including medicine, are built. Research will help introduce new innovations that improve patient outcomes and remove those that do not. As this occurs, paramedics will become instrumental in implementing research protocols and gathering data. It is essential that a paramedic participating in a research project understand the importance of gaining expressed patient consent or following federal, state, and local regulations regarding implied consent.

The goal of patient care is to improve the patient's condition. The goal of research, however, is to help future patients by gaining knowledge about a specific intervention. The two goals are not the same, so patients must be protected from untoward outcomes as much as possible.

One very important way of protecting the patient is by gaining the patient's expressed consent. There are several difficulties with this. One is the concern that a patient experiencing an emergency may not be able to truly consent because of the emotional pressures he is feeling. This pressure may occur in spite of the paramedic's best efforts to explain matters calmly and impartially.

Another concern is with the patient who is unable to consent. An excellent example of this occurs in cardiac arrest research. By the very nature of the problem being studied, the investigators will be unable to gather consent from the patient. In this case, the federal government has strict rules—for example, about community notification before the study begins and gaining consent from the patient or an appropriate family member as soon as possible after a patient is entered into the study. A paramedic participating in such a study needs to be familiar with these rules and their implications.

Although many interventions have been tested and found to be life saving, there are unfortunately documented instances of patients denied treatment for life-threatening conditions in the name of research in the United States (e.g., the Tuskegee syphilis research project). The paramedic has an obligation to prevent such things from happening in EMS research.

Summary

Should you start CPR or withhold it? Do you allow the patient to refuse essential care or not? These are some of the most challenging and most common ethical challenges seen in EMS.

As a paramedic, you must learn to make ethical decisions that will have an effect on you, your patient, or others. Your decision-making process should always be based on the patient's best interest. Keep in mind that the patient's best interest includes more than lifesaving procedures. Cultural sensitivity should also be included in the decision and respected, even if it is against your personal beliefs. Remember, the patient has autonomy; that is, he has a right to determine what happens to his own body and can legally dictate that. Remember there is a clear distinction between ethics, religion, and law even though there is common ground between them.

At some point in your career you may be called on to defend a decision you made. The best defense results from being able to state that your actions were legal and within your scope of practice (justice), helpful (beneficence), not harmful (nonmaleficence), and the direct wishes of the patient (autonomy). As long as you can defend your decision using these staples of ethics, your decision is correct.

You Make the Call

You are transporting a 32-year-old male patient, Phil Cornock, who has a long history of kidney stones and has all the classic signs of having another one now. He is in severe pain and is unable to find a comfortable position. You know that although this condition can be excruciating, it is not generally life threatening. He is allergic to the only narcotic analgesic you can administer for pain. He asks you, "Can't you use the lights and sirens to get to the hospital faster?" Your service's policy regarding the use of lights and sirens restricts their use to cases in which the paramedic believes there is a significant threat to life or limb. This patient's condition does not qualify. You wonder, though, whether you should use the lights and sirens to speed up transport since the patient is in severe pain.

1. What potential benefits are there in yielding to the patient's request (beneficence)?
2. What potential harm is there in yielding to the patient's request (nonmaleficence)?
3. How does justice come into play in this situation?
4. How should paramedics in general respond when a patient requests an intervention that is not medically indicated?

See Suggested Responses at the back of this book.

Review Questions

1. _____ are generally considered to be one's personal social, religious, or other standards of right and wrong.
   a. Ethics
   b. Morals
   c. Standards
   d. Principles

2. What is the Latin-derived term used in medicine for not doing harm to the patient?
   a. Autonomy
   b. Maleficence
   c. Nonmaleficence
   d. Beneficence

3. Which groups serve to protect the rights of subjects participating in research projects?
   a. IRBs
   b. HMOs
   c. EMS
   d. CQI

4. Which quick way to test ethics asks whether you would be willing to undergo a particular procedure or action if you were in the patient's place?
   a. Impartiality test
   b. Navigation test
   c. Universalizability test
   d. Interpersonal justifiability test

5. Every state has laws requiring the reporting of certain health facts, such as

   _____

   a. births.
   b. deaths.
   c. child neglect and abuse.
   d. all of the above.

See answers to Review Questions at the back of this book.

References

1. Adams, J. G., R. Arnold, L. Siminoff, and A. M. Wolfson. "Ethical Conflicts in the Prehospital Setting." *Ann Emerg Med* 21 (1992): 1259–1265.
2. Hilicser, B., C. Stocking, and M. Siegler. "Ethical Dilemmas in Emergency Medical Services: The Perspective of the Emergency Medical Technician." *Ann Emerg Med* 27 (1996): 239–243.
3. American College of Emergency Physicians. "Code of Ethics for Emergency Physicians." *Ann Emerg Med* 52 (2008): 581–590.
4. Touchstone, M. "Part 3: How to Adhere to a Code of Ethics in EMS." *EMS Magazine* 39 (2010): 75–76.
5. Iserson, K. V., et al. *Ethics in Emergency Medicine.* 2nd ed. Tucson, AZ: Galen Press, 1995.

Further Reading

Hope, T. *Medical Ethics: A Very Short Introduction.* Oxford, New York: Oxford University Press, 2004.

Larkin, G. L. and R. L. Fowler. "Essential Ethics for EMS: Cardinal Virtues and Core Principles." *Emerg Med Clin North Am* 20 (2002): 887–911.

Chapter 9
EMS System Communications

Bryan Bledsoe, DO, FACEP, FAAEM

Kevin McGinnis, MPS, EMT-P

STANDARD
Preparatory (EMS System Communication)

COMPETENCY
Integrates comprehensive knowledge of EMS systems, the safety and well-being of the paramedic, and medical–legal and ethical issues, which is intended to improve the health of EMS personnel, patients, and the community.

 Learning Objectives

Terminal Performance Objective: After reading this chapter, you should be able to use technology and knowledge of EMS communications systems and skills to communicate effectively in carrying out your responsibilities as a paramedic.

Enabling Objectives: To accomplish the terminal performance objective, you should be able to:

1. Define key terms introduced in this chapter.

2. Identify the parties with whom you must communicate in the course of an EMS response and what you must communicate with each.

3. Explain how the basic communication model applies to EMS communications.

4. Follow standard reporting procedures and format when communicating in the EMS system.

5. Identify the uses of written communication in EMS, particularly those of the patient care report (PCR).

6. Depict the sequence of communications in an EMS response.

7. List and describe emerging technologies designed to enhance communication to and within EMS.

8. Describe the typical equipment, including advantages and disadvantages, and types of frequencies used in EMS system communication.

9. Discuss the regulation of public safety communications.

10. Explain the importance of the ability to communicate effortlessly between multiple agencies and jurisdictions.

KEY TERMS

accelerometers, p. 168

ad hoc database, p. 172

advanced automatic crash notification (AACN), p. 168

automatic crash notification (ACN), p. 167

automatic location information (ALI), p. 167

automatic number identification (ANI), p. 167

bandwidth, p. 177

call routing, p. 167

cells, p. 175

cellular telephone system, p. 175

cognitive radio, p. 177

common operating picture (COP), p. 171

communication, p. 163

communication protocols, p. 164

data dictionary, p. 165

dead spot, p. 171

digital communications, p. 174

duplex, p. 173

echo procedure, p. 165

emergency medical dispatcher (EMD), p. 169

Federal Communications Commission (FCC), p. 180

geographic information system (GIS), p. 172

global positioning systems (GPS), p. 167

hand-off, p. 170

hotspot, p. 175

information communications technology (ICT), p. 172

mission-critical communications, p. 175

mobile data unit (MDU), p. 175

multiband radio, p. 177

multiplex, p. 174

National Emergency Medical Services Information System (NEMSIS), p. 165

prearrival instructions, p. 169

prehospital care report (PCR), p. 165

priority dispatching, p. 169

public safety answering point (PSAP), p. 167

radio band, p. 172

radio frequency, p. 172

repeaters, p. 172

SafeCom, p. 163

semantic, p. 163

simplex, p. 173

situational awareness (SA), p. 171

smart phone, p. 175

10-code, p. 163

terrestrial-based triangulation, p. 167

trunking, p. 174

ultrahigh frequency (UHF), p. 173

very high frequency (VHF), p. 173

voice over Internet protocol (VOIP), p. 168

Case Study

TODAY

On a dry, warm Sunday afternoon, a 31-year-old man loses control of his car at 50 miles per hour and strikes a bridge abutment. No one witnesses the incident, as it is on a remote stretch of secondary roadway. The first motorist happens on the crash 20 minutes later and dials 911 on his mobile phone. Emergency medical dispatcher Vern Holland takes the necessary information and dispatches a basic life support engine company and an advanced life support ambulance. As Holland dispatches the emergency units, his partner, paramedic dispatcher Fred Hughes, instructs the caller in basic emergency care.

The units receive the call via a computer printout of essential information. They arrive at the scene 20 minutes later, initiate the appropriate care, and call for a medical helicopter. Because the patient has a severe head injury, the paramedic performs only a limited assessment and immediately initiates transport to a preplanned remote landing site, where the

helicopter will land in 20 minutes. As the ambulance departs, he relays the following by radio to Dr. Doyle, the medical direction physician at the regional trauma center:

Paramedic: Depew Ambulance to Mercy Hospital.

Dr. Doyle: Go ahead, Depew.

Paramedic: We are leaving the scene of a car accident on Route 17 in Mount Vernon. We have one patient, a male in his thirties, the driver of a car that went off the roadway and struck a bridge abutment. He responds to pain only, with obvious facial and chest trauma. There is a large laceration above the right eye with an exposed skull fracture. There is also blood draining from the right ear. Vital signs are blood pressure 110/60, pulse 110 and regular, respirations 10 and labored. Pupils are dilated and minimally reactive, yet equal. Palpation of the cervical spine does not reveal any obvious deformity. There is no tracheal deviation. Breath sounds are symmetrical, yet diminished. There is subcutaneous emphysema on the right side of his chest and several palpable rib fractures. The abdomen is soft, and the pelvis appears stable. There may be some lower extremity fractures. A rigid C-collar is in place.. An endotracheal tube has been placed. Respirations are being assisted with a BVM using supplemental oxygen. We will attempt an IV en route to the remote landing site where LifeFlight 2 is 15 minutes out. The patient's ETA to your facility is 40 minutes.

Dr. Doyle: We copy, Depew. Attempt an IV, but expedite transport and notify us of any further problems.

Paramedic: We copy. Attempt an IV and we will notify you with any changes.

Dr. Doyle: The trauma team will be in the ED awaiting the patient's arrival.

Paramedic: Copy that, Mercy. Depew clear.

A rapid transfer to the helicopter and exchange of information with its crew is accomplished. On arrival at the trauma center, the trauma team and a neurosurgeon meet the patient. The time interval from injury to surgical intervention is 1 hour and 40 minutes. Despite comprehensive care, the patient dies as a result of his head injury. At the family's request, the patient's organs are harvested. They are sent to cities more than 1,500 miles away and used in two transplant operations.

THE NOT-TOO-DISTANT FUTURE

On a dry, warm Sunday afternoon, a 31-year-old man loses control of his car at 50 miles per hour and strikes a bridge abutment. No one witnesses the incident, as it is on a remote stretch of secondary roadway. The vehicle's advanced automatic crash notification (AACN) device immediately sends a data burst to the AACN call center, where the data message is identified as a crash and is automatically forwarded to the public safety answering point (PSAP) for the global positioning system (GPS)-identified jurisdiction of the crash. Voice and video links are also patched to the PSAP.

The emergency medical dispatcher, Vern Holland, tries the voice and video links, with no voice response or useful pictures from the crashed car, while he reviews the data from the vehicle. He knows, within a minute of

the crash, the type of vehicle, its location, speed, and direction of impact. Seeing a "potential major injury" warning displayed, he initiates a response protocol keyed to that warning. He dispatches a heavy rescue/extrication truck, a support engine company, and an advanced life support ambulance. Simultaneously, he requests LifeFlight 2 to launch and puts the Mercy Hospital Trauma Center on alert. The responding vehicle crews have all the AACN data on their mobile data units (MDUs) as they leave their quarters (location data are automatically fed to the onboard GPS and a best route provided by a local transportation authority hourly update). The extrication crew en route views on their MDU a "just in time training" review of the hazards and best entry and cutting points for the identified crash vehicle. The helicopter and trauma center staffs receive the AACN information as well.

The ground units arrive at the scene 20 minutes later. The paramedic performs a primary survey and simultaneously speaks his patient findings into a throat microphone (same report as given in the first, "today," version of the case study), activates the video camera on his safety glasses, and places a wireless multi–vital-sign monitor with probes on the patient's chest. He inserts a flash memory card, the size of thumbnail and worn by the patient, into his public safety communications device (PSCD—a combined very smart phone and push-to-talk radio device) and downloads the patient's pertinent medical history. The paramedic's patient report is translated to a text file and stored on his PSCD and sent to the ambulance MDU, as are the patient video, multi–vital-sign data, and medical history. Immediately, the MDU sends a signal to dispatcher Holland, who notifies LifeFlight 2 and Mercy Hospital of the patient data feed availability. Dr. Doyle taps into the four data feeds from his electronic tablet and sends a message confirming the IV order. The helicopter medical crew reviews the patient feeds and doctor's order, then messages the ground paramedic of their three-minute estimated time of arrival (ETA) and willingness to get the IV going in the air if not already established.

A rapid transfer to the helicopter and exchange of information with its crew are accomplished. On its arrival at the trauma center, the trauma team and a neurosurgeon meet the patient. The time interval from injury to surgical intervention is 50 minutes. The patient leaves the hospital alive with months of intensive rehabilitation ahead but a bright prognosis.

(AACN systems, PSAPs, GPS, smart phones, and MDUs will be discussed in more detail later in the chapter.)

Introduction

The way people communicate has changed radically in the past 40 years. Coincidentally, this is also the period during which modern EMS went from birth to maturity. Unfortunately, in that same time span, the way we communicate in EMS has remained largely unchanged.

In society, person-to-person communication has evolved from face-to-face, telephoned, telegraphed, radioed, and postal dialogue to face-to-face, telephoned, mobile-phoned, radioed, e-mailed, texted, and social-network-messaging dialogue. In EMS, person-to-person communication has typically been face to face, telephone, and voice radio dialogue; cycles of telemetry data use; and handwritten records. Mobile phones and other voice radio systems (e.g., trunked systems) have augmented these methods, but, EMS, by and large, still communicates as it did in the 1970s.

This lag in the development of EMS communications technology has resulted in two impacts on current paramedic practice. First, for the near future, face-to-face, written records (whether handwritten or electronic records), and voice radio or wireless telephone will continue to be the prime methods of communication in EMS. The first part of this chapter focuses on effective verbal and written communications and the sequence of communications on a typical EMS call as they take place today.

Second, the availability of increasingly sophisticated diagnostic and treatment technology and the busier environments in which paramedics, medical direction physicians, and other EMS team members work will soon force changes in the information communications technology used in EMS. The last part of this chapter discusses those changes.

Effective Communications

Knowledge of communications plays an important role in your paramedic training. All aspects of prehospital care require effective, efficient communications. During a routine transfer or a life-threatening emergency run, you will communicate with a wide variety of people, including the following:

- *The emergency medical dispatcher (EMD),* whose job it is to manage an entire system of EMS response and readiness, not just your call. You will transmit administrative information such as "responding," "arrived," "transporting," and "back in service." The EMD must know the location of all his resources to manage the system effectively. On a serious emergency call, the EMD can be your best ally by securing for you the resources you need to manage your incident.

- *Your patient, his family, bystanders, and others* who may, at times, not understand what you are doing and become obstructive. Quite often, people misconstrue your actions and words. You must try to keep them well informed.

- *Personnel from other responding agencies,* such as the police department, fire department, or mutual aid ambulances who may not share your priorities at the scene. You must communicate effectively with other responders to coordinate and implement your treatment plan. You will accomplish this face to face, via the radio, and through data messages and other data transmission. These communications require you to exhibit confidence and authority.

- *Health care staff* from physicians' offices, health care facilities, and nursing homes that frequently do not understand the extent of your training or abilities. Often, uninformed staff may think you are just "ambulance drivers." In these cases, you must exhibit professionalism and a calm demeanor while you ask pertinent questions and discuss the case intelligently.

- *The medical direction physician* who teams with you to interpret patient findings and make medical decisions that will best benefit your patient. The physician's expertise and advice can be a tremendous resource for you during the call. You will need to communicate patient information and scene assessment effectively to him.

  The medical direction physician can prepare for your arrival if you have communicated to him the needs of your patient. For example, you are transporting a patient with a serious head injury who exhibits a decreasing level of consciousness. By reporting this information, the emergency department can arrange for the trauma team, including a neurosurgeon, to meet you in the ED on arrival. In such cases, good communication results in good patient care.

You must interact effectively with everyone involved in the call to coordinate a unified effort resulting in top-quality patient care. EMS is the ultimate team endeavor. Your performance as a paramedic is just one component in a series of interactions that ensure continuous first-rate care. From the call taker to the rehabilitation specialist, all the players in this continuum are equally important—only their specific roles differ.

Communication is not merely one aspect of an EMS response; it is the key link in the chain that results in the best possible patient outcome. Effective communication optimizes patient care during every phase of the EMS response.

Basic Communication Model

Communication is the process of exchanging information between individuals. It begins when you have an idea or message you would like to convey to someone else. You then encode that information in the language best suited for the situation. The language you use might include words, numbers, symbols, or special codes. For instance, if you wanted to describe a patient's condition to the medical direction physician, you would ideally choose medical terminology that is precise and takes less time to convey than a description using nonmedical terms. In some systems, we communicate using codes. For example, a "Code Blue" might mean a cardiac arrest.

In addition to encoding your message, you must select the medium for sending it. You can speak face to face, send a fax, leave a voice message, send a letter or electronic mail (email), or speak directly by telephone or radio. You might send your encoded message via a paging system that posts words or numbers; some pagers allow you to speak your message. Next, your intended receiver must decode and understand your message. Finally, that person must give you feedback to confirm that he received your message and understood it. You might then confirm his reply and conclude the communication. Consider the following example of an effective radio communication:

Dispatcher: Control to Unit 192, respond high priority to 483 County Route 22, cross street Canfield Road, on a possible heart.

Unit 192: Control, Unit 192 copy, responding high priority to 483 County Route 22.

Dispatcher: Unit 192 responding, 1228 hours.

In this simple example, the sender (dispatcher) encodes his message in a language that he knows the receiver (Unit 192) will understand. Unit 192 receives the message and acknowledges by repeating the key data. Finally, the sender confirms and concludes the communication (Figure 9-1).

Verbal Communication

Factors that can enhance or impede effective communication may be **semantic** (the meaning of words) or technical (communications hardware). Communication requires a mutual language. For example, a city unit and a county unit that use different **10-code** systems will find it difficult to communicate effectively. A "10-10" may mean a working fire in one system and a cardiac emergency in another. Therefore, many EMS systems have stopped using 10-codes and changed to plain English. In fact, it is now a standard, embraced by all major public safety associations in an effort through U.S. Department of Homeland Security's **SafeCom** Program, to use plain English emergency radio communications.[1] Although regional variations in the use of plain English terminology exist, stopping the practice of enshrouding messages in coded substitutions for plain English is a reasonable start at clarifying communications in an emergency environment.

When reporting your patient's condition to the medical direction physician, you should use terminology that is widely accepted by both the medical and emergency services communities. Telling the medical direction physician that you have a victim of a "MAC 10 drive-by" or "Signal G" (by which you mean "assault with a gun") may be meaningless. Conversely, if the medical direction physician asks you for your pregnant patient's EDC (due date) or her LMP (last menstrual period) and you do not know those

FIGURE 9-1 Communication occurs when individuals exchange information through an encoded message.

abbreviations, you have failed to communicate. The receiver must be able to decode the sender's message.

Reporting Procedures

As a paramedic, you must effectively relay all relevant medical information to the receiving hospital staff. Initially, you might do this over the radio or by mobile phone. Later, when you deliver your patient to the emergency department, you can give additional information in person to the appropriate receiving hospital personnel.

One of your most important skills will be gathering essential patient information, organizing it, and relaying it to the medical direction physician. The medical direction physician will then issue appropriate orders for patient care. The amount and type of information you relay to the medical direction physician will depend on the type of technology you use, your patient's priority, and your local **communication protocols**. For example, if communications in your region are not secure (private), you must limit the type of information you can communicate without breaching patient confidentiality. The acuteness of your patient's clinical status and the amount of local radio traffic also may determine the length of your report. For a critical patient, you may give a brief report while you tend to your patient's medical needs. For a complicated medical emergency, you may wish to communicate a greater share of the results of your history and physical exam to the medical direction physician.

Standard Format

Communicating patient information to the hospital or to the medical direction physician is a crucial function. Verbal communications by radio or phone give the hospital enough information on your patient's condition so its staff can prepare for his care. These communications also should elicit the medical orders you need to treat your patient in the field.

A standard format for transmitting patient assessment information helps to achieve those goals in several ways. First, it is efficient. Second, it helps the physician assimilate information about the patient's condition quickly. Third, it ensures that medical information is complete.

In general, your verbal reports to medical direction should include the following information:

- Identification of unit and provider
- Description of scene
- Patient's age, sex, and approximate weight (for drug orders)
- Patient's chief complaint and severity
- Brief, pertinent history of the present illness or injury
- Pertinent past medical history, medications, and allergies

- Pertinent physical exam findings
- Treatment given so far/request for orders
- Estimated time of arrival at the hospital
- Other pertinent information

The formats and contents of reports for medical patients and for trauma patients differ to include only the information relevant to either type of emergency. Reports for medical patients emphasize the history in the beginning of the report; reports for trauma patients emphasize the injuries and the physical exam.

After transmitting your report, you will wait for further questions and orders from the medical direction physician. On arrival, your spoken report will give essential patient information to the provider who is assuming care. It should include a brief history, pertinent physical findings, treatment you have provided, and the patient's responses to that treatment.

General Radio Procedures

All radio transmissions must be clear and crisp, with concise, professional content (Figure 9-2). Always follow these guidelines for effective radio use:

1. Listen to the channel before transmitting to ensure that it is not in use.
2. Press the transmit button for one second before speaking.
3. Speak at close range, approximately 2 to 3 inches, directly into, or across the face of, the microphone.

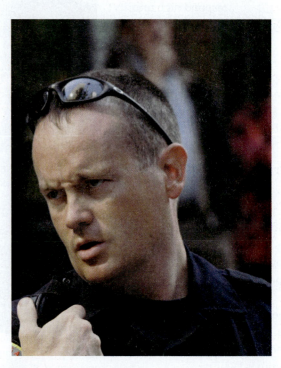

FIGURE 9-2 The professionalism of your communications reflects on the professionalism of your patient care.

(© Kevin Link)

4. Speak slowly and clearly. Pronounce each word distinctly, avoiding words that are difficult to understand.

5. Speak in a normal pitch, keeping your voice free of emotion.

6. Be brief. Know what you are going to say before you press the transmit button.

7. Avoid codes unless they are part of your EMS system (if they are, work to change to plain English).

8. Do not waste airtime with unnecessary information.

9. Protect your patient's privacy. When appropriate:

   • Use the telephone rather than a radio.

   • Turn off the external speaker.

   • Do not use your patient's name; doing so violates FCC regulations (unless your system is considered a closed system by the FCC).

10. Use proper unit or hospital numbers and correct names or titles.

11. Do not use slang or profanity.

12. Use standard formats for transmission.

13. Be concise, to hold the attention of the person receiving your radio report.

14. Use the **echo procedure** when receiving directions from the dispatcher or orders from the physician. Immediately repeating each statement will confirm accurate reception and understanding.

15. Always write down addresses, important dispatch communications, and physician orders.

16. When completing a transmission, obtain confirmation that your message was received and understood.

Occasionally, communications equipment will not function properly. Even a weak battery can disrupt clear communication. If you are far from the base station, particularly if you have a portable radio, try to broadcast from higher terrain. Structures that contain steel and concrete can interfere with radio transmission. Simply moving outside the building or standing near a window may improve communications. If that does not work, try a telephone.

Written Communication

Written records are another important aspect of EMS communications. Your **prehospital care report (PCR)** (also called patient care report) is a written or an electronic, keyboard/mouse-entered record of events. The written report includes administrative information such as times, location, agency, and crew, as well as medical information. Hospital staff, agency administrators, system quality assurance/improvement committees, insurance and billing departments, researchers, educators, and lawyers will

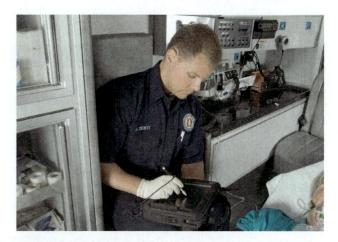

FIGURE 9-3 The prehospital care report is as important as the run itself. Complete it promptly and legibly.

use it. The data collected from your PCR can help to monitor and improve patient care through medical audits, research, education, and system policy changes. Furthermore, your written documentation becomes a legal record of the incident and may become part of your patient's permanent medical record. All legal rules regarding confidentiality and disclosure pertain to your PCR.

Most of the same factors that influence verbal communication also affect written communication. Be objective, write legibly (the written version of speaking clearly), thoroughly document your patient's assessment and care, and use terminology that is widely accepted in the medical community (Figure 9-3). Finally, your PCR illustrates your professionalism. A sloppy, incomplete PCR suggests sloppy, inefficient care. The chapter "Documentation" deals with PCRs and other written communications in much greater detail.

The data elements that are collected on the PCR and how they are interpreted are usually defined in a **data dictionary**. All states and territories have agreed to adopt, as soon as is practical for each, the **National Emergency Medical Services Information System (NEMSIS)** data dictionary and to participate in reporting some data to a NEMSIS national database.[2] This will, for the first time, allow national EMS performance to be assessed.

Terminology

Every industry develops its own terminology. Doing so makes communication within the industry more clear, concise, and unambiguous for those within that industry. The airline industry, for example, uses the term *payload* to describe the total weight of everything (passengers, fuel, luggage, and other items) on an airplane. Musical composers and arrangers use terms like *allegro, fortissimo,* or *a cappella* to describe a specific tempo or style.

The medical field also uses an extensive list of terms, acronyms, and abbreviations that allow quick, accurate

Table 9-1 Common Radio Terminology

Term	Meaning
Copy, 10-4, roger	I understand
Affirmative	Yes
Negative	No
Stand by	Please wait
Repeat	Please repeat what you said
Landline	Telephone communications
Rendezvous	Meet with
LZ	Landing zone (helicopter)
ETA	Estimated time of arrival
Over	I am finished with my transmission
Mobile status	On the air, driving around
Stage	Wait before entering a scene
Clear	End of transmission
Unfounded	We cannot find the incident/patient
Be advised	Listen carefully to this

communication of complex information. (The chapter "Documentation" includes an extensive table of standard charting abbreviations.) An emergency physician may request a CBC (complete blood count), ABGs (arterial blood gases), or a CMP (comprehensive metabolic panel)—common terms describing diagnostic tests run on patients.

The emergency services industry has developed its own terms for radio communication (Table 9-1). These words or phrases shorten airtime and transmit thoughts and ideas quickly. For example, "copy" means "I heard you and I understand what you said." Using industry terminology appropriately is an important part of effective communication, providing a commonly understood means of communicating with other emergency care professionals. Terminology is considered to be plain English within the discipline in which it is used; its use is not considered to be the same as coded substitutions for plain English (such as 10-codes), which were discussed earlier, and are discouraged.

The Importance of Communications in EMS Response

Your ability to communicate effectively during a stressful EMS response is very likely to determine the success or failure of your efforts. A brilliant assessment and management plan will be futile if you cannot communicate it to others.

Dealing effectively with your patient and bystanders requires a variety of communication skills, such as empathy, confidence, self-control, authority, and patience. Your clinical experience will suggest which skills to use in any particular situation. For example, you might display confidence and use an authoritative posture when dealing with unruly bystanders. On the other hand, you would need to be gentle and empathetic with a child or an elderly grandmother. If you were in charge of an incident, you would have to communicate authoritatively within the structure of the emergency scene to providers from other responding agencies. Delegating tasks, listening to initial reports, and coordinating the scene require effective communication and interpersonal skills.

Sequence of Communications in an EMS Response

The sequence of an EMS response illustrates the importance of communications in prehospital care. A typical EMS response includes the chain of events described next.

Detection and Citizen Access

To begin the response to any emergency, someone must detect the problem and summon EMS (Figure 9-4). Any citizen with an urgent medical need should have a simple and reliable mechanism for accessing the EMS system. In the United States, most people access EMS by telephone; thus, a well-publicized universal telephone number such

CONTENT REVIEW

➤ Sequence of Communications in EMS Response
- Detection and citizen access
- 911
- Advanced automatic crash notification
- Emergency medical dispatch
- Discussion with medical direction
- Transfer communications

FIGURE 9-4 The EMS response begins when someone detects an emergency and summons EMS assistance.

as 911 provides direct citizen access to the communications center.

The 911 system has been available since the late 1960s. The first 911 system simply provided the common, easy-to-remember access number and allowed 911 centers to automatically "ring back" a caller's phone if there was a disconnect. At newer Enhanced 911 (E911) communication centers, a computer also displays the caller's telephone number (a feature called **automatic number identification, [ANI]**) and location (a feature called **automatic location information [ALI]**).

911

Currently, 99 percent of the population in the United States and 96 percent of the nation's geographic area have a 911 system. Of the geography covered by 911 systems, 93 percent has E911 service. Highway 911 call boxes, citizens band (CB) radio, and amateur radio all provide alternative means of accessing emergency help in some regions.

Increasingly, manual and automatic alerting systems are used by the elderly and those who are incapacitated, such as "Help, I've fallen and I can't get up" devices. Other types of patient home monitoring devices may have automatic alarms as well. Typically, all these types of devices alert a monitoring center, which, in turn, calls 911, rather than sending a message directly from the device to 911. **Automatic crash notification (ACN)** is another type of automatic event alerting system that may result in EMS dispatch.[3] (A more sophisticated version of ACN—advanced notification [AACN]—will be discussed later.)

Most 911 centers are now called **public safety answering points (PSAPs)**. The PSAP routes the 911 call to the appropriate agency for dispatch and response if it does not also do the dispatching itself. In some systems, the PSAP call taker will elicit the information, determine the nature of the needed response, and dispatch the appropriate responding agencies. In others, the call taker will simply answer with the question "Is this a police, fire, or medical emergency?" and transfer the caller to the appropriate dispatcher, who will then elicit specific information. Many systems use computerized technology at the PSAP to connect the caller automatically with the appropriate agency. Some even provide language translation.

E911 technology has always worked well with landline systems in which there is a wired connection all the way from the caller's phone to the PSAP. The landline connection also allows ANI and ALI (which identify the phone number and location of the caller) to work because of the unique, direct-wired connection to a telephone associated with a physical address to which EMS could respond. This automatic provision of ANI and ALI allows dispatch of an emergency response even while emergency medical dispatch (EMD) prearrival instructions are being given. Few EMS providers would disagree that E911 in connection with landline telephone service saves many lives each year.

By 2010, however, a full third of the 240 million annual 911 calls in the United States (half or more in some communities) have come from wireless/mobile phones. Without a direct-wired connection to a physical location, ANI and ALI did not work with the early wireless phone systems. An emergency dispatcher who received a call from a cell phone had to rely on the caller's ability to state his location and phone number. In many cases, the caller, who was traveling in an unfamiliar area or had an altered level of consciousness or was incapacitated, could not provide his location and number and could not be found. These cases were often associated with bad patient outcomes.

Further complicating the problem has been the issue of **call routing**. Typically, wire-line 911 calls are routed via a trunk line and a specialized address database to the nearest 911 center. Wireless 911 calls that do not carry address database data with them cannot be automatically routed to the nearest 911 center. Thus, emergency calls from early wireless telephone systems were often routed out of the caller's location to the location associated with the wireless service provider—which may have been a different city, county, state, region, or even country.

In many cases, the caller is simply too excited to provide the emergency dispatcher with the correct information. One such case involved a 19-year-old girl in a rural New York State community who called 911 to report an oven fire. She was cooking dinner at her grandmother's home when the fire began. She helped her grandmother out of the home and dialed 911 on her wireless phone. When the dispatcher asked her for her address, she gave her own home address, not the address of her grandmother's home. The resulting confusion over the location of the emergency was responsible for total loss of the structure. Cases like this are still not unheard of, even with the increasingly widespread installation of sophisticated E911 systems that can determine the location of a wireless or mobile phone (using triangulation or GPS technology, as will be described next). This event happened not that long ago—in 2002.

Recognizing the rapidly expanding popularity of cell phones in the last decades of the twentieth century, the Federal Communications Commission (FCC) began phased implementation of rules requiring wireless providers to enable ANI and one of two versions of an ALI application. PSAPs would also be required to accommodate the data to enable them to display and use this number and location identification data.

Wireless phones can now be located by **terrestrial-based triangulation**, by **global positioning systems (GPS)**, or by a combination of the two. Triangulation of a wireless signal involves the use of three mobile phone towers. Based on the strength of telephone signal and time of signal arrival at each of the towers, the signal location can be calculated to within several meters. This calculated location is identified as a longitude/latitude that is then translated to a map location and street address in a specialized database. Because the call is recognized as having come from a phone with a unique identifier, another specialized database assigns the correct callback number associated with that specific phone. This packet of information—a phone call with a 911 prefix, ALI data, and ANI data—is then transmitted digitally through selective routers and trunk lines to the closest PSAP.

Geographic regions, such as individual counties, have had to decide to which PSAP they prefer to have these calls sent. Systems that use global positioning location data require that the individual phones be fitted with hardware and software that allow them access to the GPS system. Emergency 911 calls originating from such phones are still routed in the same manner and require access to the ANI database but not to an ALI database. Location information is transmitted automatically with the packet of data that comes from the phone when a 911 prefix is associated with the call. The data from these phones are transmitted to the appropriate PSAP.

Call takers and dispatchers see the data from wireless/mobile phones in the same format as they see for landline E911 calls. In other words, the method of data transmission is inconsequential to the dispatch personnel, because data are provided in identical formats with both methods, ANI/ALI or landline. Putting these new communications technologies in place ensures the reliability of Enhanced 911 as cellular communications continue to increase.

A more recent 911 phenomenon has been the emergency access issue created by **voice over Internet protocol (VOIP)** technology which, like cellular technology, has rapidly gained in popularity. VOIP uses both wired and wireless Internet access technology (e.g., cable, fiber-optics, wireless air card, wireless hotspot) through a computer or mobile Internet access device to provide voice communications that are increasingly of comparable quality to other forms of telephony. Low calling costs through VOIP have helped drive its popularity. Unfortunately, as with early cell phone systems, VOIP was not designed with ANI, ALI, or best-routing-to-closest-PSAP capabilities. Technology has become available to alleviate these issues, however, and organizations such as the National Emergency Number Association (NENA)[4] and the Association of Public Safety Communications Officials-International (APCO)[5] are working to incorporate the capabilities required.

The challenges of new technology with 911 center implications do not end with cell and VOIP phones. The ability to send photos, video, or text messages from a handheld device to a 911 number or to access or interact with social networking systems presents similar issues. As a result, an initiative called Next Generation 911 (NG-911) is under way,

spearheaded by NENA, APCO, and the EMS Office in the National Highway Traffic Safety Administration (NHTSA), which has federal responsibility for the program.[6]

Advanced Automatic Crash Notification

The 2009 Centers for Disease Control and Prevention (CDC) report, *Recommendations from the Expert Panel: Advanced Automatic Collision Notification and Triage of the Injured Patient*,[7] found that **advanced automatic crash notification (AACN)** can improve outcomes among seriously injured patients by:

- Predicting the likelihood of serious injury among vehicle occupants.

- Decreasing response times by prehospital care providers.

- Assisting with field triage destination and transportation decisions.

- Decreasing the time it takes for patients to receive definitive trauma care.

It further found that systems like AACN may be especially important in rural or isolated areas, where there may not be a passerby to report a crash and a Level I trauma center is too far away to treat the kind of injuries sustained in severe crashes. The Case Study at the beginning of this chapter illustrates just this kind of situation.

AACN systems are data collection and transmission mechanisms that may change the way we assess and treat victims of car crashes. As the name implies, AACN systems can automatically contact a national call center or local PSAP and transmit crash-specific data.

For example, imagine a car with a driver and one passenger traveling at 45 miles per hour along a highway. The driver loses control of the vehicle, leaves the roadway, rolls over, and comes to rest against a tree. Because the AACN system in the vehicle contains special sensors called **accelerometers**, it can measure the change in total velocity ("change in velocity" is written as delta V or ΔV), the forces that were applied to the vehicle, the direction in which they were applied, whether or not the car rolled over, whether or not air bags were deployed, and the car's final resting position. The sensor also has a GPS-enabled chip that can transmit the exact location of the vehicle. In the future, other data available from the system may contribute to the determination of whether a severe injury was likely to have occurred.

As in the second Case Study at the beginning of this chapter, protocols can be established for the automatic notification and routing of AACN data to responders and hospitals likely to be involved and for the automatic dispatch of resources, rather than waiting for a responder to arrive at the scene and make that determination. In rural responses, this can save minutes to hours in the time required for definitive surgical intervention.

Emergency Medical Dispatch

Once a 911 call is received at a PSAP and determined to have emergency medical consequences, it should be managed from then on by a dispatcher with the special training and resources to do so. This is the **emergency medical dispatcher (EMD)**, who is the public's first contact with the EMS system and who plays a crucial role in every EMS response.

In a coordinated system known as **priority dispatching**, emergency medical dispatchers interrogate a distressed caller using a set of medically approved questions to elicit essential information about the chief complaint (Figure 9-5). Then, the dispatcher follows established guidelines to determine the appropriate level of response (Figure 9-6).

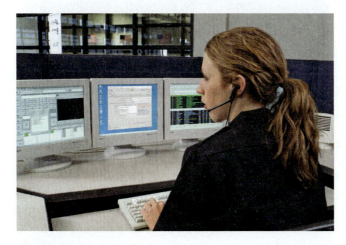

FIGURE 9-5 Priority dispatching and prearrival medical instructions are commonly used in EMS.

(From Advanced MPDS v13.0 © 1979–2015 International Academies of Emergency Dispatch and ProQA Paramount v5.1 © 2007–2015 Priority Dispatch Corp. All Rights Reserved. Used by permission.)

FIGURE 9-6 The dispatcher determines the appropriate level of response according to established guidelines.

These predetermined guidelines are based on criteria approved by the medical director. For example, an elderly man with a history of heart problems who is complaining of chest pain radiating to his left arm may indicate a high-priority response (life-threatening emergency, lights and siren). In some systems, the appropriate response may include a fire department basic life support first responding unit, a paramedic engine company, and a transporting ambulance. Other systems may require only a paramedic ambulance. Another type of call may result in a nonemergency response, and another call may be transferred to a consulting-nurse advice line because it would not be an appropriate use of EMS resources to respond.

This form of call screening, when done appropriately, saves time and money, because only the necessary resources are sent. It also limits the liability associated with a lights-and-siren response to possible life-threatening incidents by authorizing such responses only when necessary. Because these systems make decisions that may result in a nonemergency response or in no EMS response, they must be undertaken cautiously, using only priority dispatch systems that have been proven to support these decisions effectively. Many private and public EMS systems throughout the United States use the priority dispatching system.[8]

PREARRIVAL INSTRUCTIONS Many EMS systems provide **prearrival instructions**, a service that is considered the standard of care. Prearrival instructions complement the call-screening process in a priority dispatch system and are an essential part of the EMD function. As the dispatcher sends the appropriate response, the caller remains on the line and receives instructions for suitable emergency measures to carry out while waiting for the emergency responders to arrive, such as cardiopulmonary resuscitation or hemorrhage control.

During prearrival instructions, the dispatcher also can obtain further information for the responding units. In the case of cardiac arrest, the dispatcher can relay information concerning the presence of a living will, a Do Not Resuscitate (DNR) form, or other advance directives. In another case, paramedics en route to help a baby who had stopped breathing could reduce their response speed if they learned that the child had now started breathing and was conscious.

Prearrival instructions have saved many lives. They also are useful for comforting a distressed caller or providing emotional support to bystanders, family members, or the patient himself.[9]

CALL COORDINATION AND INCIDENT RECORDING After sending the appropriate response and providing prearrival instructions, the EMD's main duties are support and coordination. He will provide the responding units with any additional resources needed and will record information about the call, such as times, locations, and

FIGURE 9-7 You may occasionally need to discuss a case with a physician to guide further care.

units involved. Your dispatcher can be your best friend. He can assign the resources you need to manage an incident, such as additional medical personnel to help with a cardiac arrest or the fire department to provide specialized rescue. He also may facilitate communication with other agencies, hospitals, communication centers, and support services.

Discussion with the Medical Direction Physician

After conducting your assessment and initiating care as outlined by your local protocols, you will contact the medical direction physician to discuss the case. Following consultation, he may give you further orders for interventions such as medications or other medical procedures. The many ways to conduct this communication today include radio, telephone, and mobile phone. Taping these communications for use later is advisable. For example, if a discrepancy arose as to what your orders had been, you could always refer to the tape, which never lies.

After consulting the medical direction physician, you will continue treatment and prepare your patient for transport. You will then contact your dispatcher, who will record the time when you leave the scene and the time when you arrive at your destination.

Your professional relationship with medical direction physicians must be based on trust. Transmission of clear, concise, controlled reports will encourage your medical direction physicians to accept your assessments and on-scene treatment plans. Your ability to communicate effectively on the

radio will secure a large part of your professional reputation. The general radio procedures and standard format sections given earlier in this chapter offer guidelines for communicating with the medical direction physician and transmitting patient information (Figure 9-7).[10]

Transfer Communications

As you transfer care of your patient to the receiving facility staff, you must give the receiving nurse or physician a formal verbal briefing (Figure 9-8). This report, commonly called the **hand-off**, should include your patient's vital information, chief complaint and history, physical exam findings, and any treatments that have been rendered.[11]

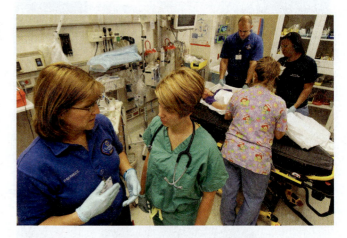

FIGURE 9-8 The patient hand-off is an essential aspect of emergency care and ensures continuity of care between the prehospital and hospital environments.

Do not assume that the receiving nurse heard your radio report and knows about your patient or that this information has been given to the physician you may first encounter. Some systems require the receiving nurse to sign the PCR to verify and document the transfer of care. Many systems also require the medical direction physician to sign the PCR for any medications administered by paramedics, especially if they included controlled substances such as morphine or diazepam.

Never leave your patient until you have completed some type of formal transfer of care; otherwise, you may be charged with abandonment. In all cases, end your PCR documentation with information about the transfer of care. It may also be appropriate to have a parting chat with your patient, particularly if the patient is not receiving immediate care and has questions or anxiety.

Information and Communications Technology

Modern EMS is approximately 40 years old. Prior to the EMS systems we know today, ambulances were, by and large, "horizontal taxicabs" capable of little more than transportation. Communications from the scene of the injury or illness, or during transport to the receiving hospital, did not exist.

In the early era of modern EMS, radios were installed in ambulances and hospital emergency departments. The 1970s brought the practice of notifying a receiving hospital of an ambulance's impending arrival. The 1970s also saw the widespread development of medical direction systems and the advance of field capabilities. Crews would send voice descriptions of patient condition by VHF radio, and in some cases could send telemetry ECG data by UHF radio, and in exchange receive real-time review and medical orders from an emergency physician. These developments constituted the birth of field medical intervention.

Unfortunately, the majority of EMS communications systems have not kept pace with the blooming sophistication of EMS in general—nor have they kept pace with concurrent rapid developments in communications technology. With some notable exceptions, often in a pilot project or other experimental form, the methods by which EMS providers are dispatched, communicate with resources as needed for response and patient care, and communicate with hospital medical supervisors and staff are the same as they were 35 to 40 years ago.

If one asks average paramedics whether their communications system adequately supports them, their fast answer often will be "yes." They may describe **dead spots** (where communications transmission and reception are poor), but aside from that they can talk to their dispatcher, can talk with other resources (either directly or through a dispatcher), and can talk to the hospital staff as needed.

However, press those same average paramedics to think about whether they could use additional pieces of information that would benefit their next response and patient if they could have that information earlier or more easily, and the answer also would probably be "yes." When EMS providers really think about it, they know they are often frustrated by the lack of information they passively "wonder about" as they make their way through an emergency call.

How often do we know how serious the call is only when we get there, and only then are able to call for additional resources (which may or may not be available)? How often do we wonder, en route to a call 20 minutes away, if a resource will be available if the call turns out to be a "bad one," then take the initiative to ask for it, only to have that resource become unavailable by the time we reach the destination? With the voice, data, and video technology available today, "wondering" should become increasingly unnecessary.

Situational awareness (SA) and **common operating picture (COP)** are important considerations in EMS. These are concepts that address how prepared a paramedic and his team are to perform their jobs effectively at any given moment, particularly when time is a factor. Both awareness and operating procedure are improved by having just the right amount of updated information exactly when it is needed—information about resources the team can bring to bear and events that may affect their current situation (Figure 9-9).

As EMS emergency call volumes continue to grow and medical direction physicians become busier with ED overcrowding, the opportunity for the paramedic in the field and the ED physician providing medical direction to

FIGURE 9-9 Situational awareness on the part of EMS providers helps ensure efficient patient care as well as provider and patient safety.

communicate becomes increasingly constrained. The likelihood is rapidly diminishing that paramedic and physician are going to be available to talk at the same time. Voice communications then become a bottleneck to the emergency patient care process.

Further, there are no generally available systems through which EMS providers can access real-time information concerning events and resource status that may affect their work. For example, an EMS crew may have no information on the number and severity of the patients to whom they are responding until they arrive at the scene, no information about the availability of air medical or extrication resources until they actually call for them, and no information about the availability of the hospital to which they want to transport until they call that hospital.

In the future, it will be necessary to develop networks of databases that contain information about events and resources updated in real time and accessible through a user-friendly **geographic information system (GIS)** capable of interface with smart phone/electronic tablet/communication devices carried by responders and physicians, mobile data units in EMS vehicles, and desktop units at responders' bases of operations, dispatch centers, and hospitals.

A GIS-based interface screen would show a rough depiction of an ambulance service's relevant operations area. It would represent the jurisdictions and catchment areas of the user; list information about neighboring services, hospitals, and other resources with which it commonly operates; and detail events occurring within those areas. Selecting an icon and opening a second screen would access information not readily available on the initial screen.

This array of databases (e.g., the status of hospitals, ambulances, helicopter services, and EMS calls in current operation) might be called an EMS Resource and Event Monitoring System (EMREMS). It would be one information communications network that is linked with similar networks for fire, police, departments of transportation, and other responder colleagues. Although such a system may now seem a thing of dreams, its concept has been repeatedly described in EMS and emergency planning literature as a necessary next step to ensure SA and COP in the paramedic's everyday work.

In the new "EMREMS" systems to be developed, an **ad hoc database** will be created each time a patient is encountered. Multiple vital signs, video, electronic health record, and voice-to-text translation of medic findings will be pushed to those databases and parked until the intended recipient (e.g., an incoming air medical crew or a medical direction physician in the hospital) is available to review them. These recipients can then pull down those data to their own screen and push queries or orders back to the EMS crew for consumption and response when they are available. When an emergency dictates, either party could

break into the other's process and revert to voice and data communication as needed.

Some of the capabilities described have been employed in the military. Hospital- and health-care-system–based electronic medical-records–sharing networks are being established in many states. These systems allow emergency department and primary care physicians to access the records of patients in the system who present for care. Such systems would have application for providing pertinent medical history information to EMS providers in real time during calls. At least one EMS system, one based in Indiana, has already implemented this capability.

Modern EMS communications needed to provide adequate SA and COP require both voice and data communications support. This becomes a blending of two systems and sets of professional skills: (1) traditional communications technology, which generally involves telecommunications engineers and (2) data systems technology, which involves hardware and software development professionals. **Information communications technology (ICT)** is the new concept that blends traditional communications technology (CT) systems and information technology (IT) systems.

Technology Today

Depending on where you practice as a paramedic, you may be living in a communications world of 1970s technology (a VHF simplex voice radio system—with or without access to a UHF duplex system with biotelemetry capability), or with hints of the 1990s technology (trunked 800 MHz with lots of channels and talk groups; cell phones used routinely and perhaps transmitting 12-lead ECGs) or hints of future technology (mobile data unit—a hardened laptop—that uses air-card access to wireless phone providers and/or hotspot access to the Internet and beyond; video transmission connection to the ED; and multi-vital–sign transmission from your monitors to the ED using one of these connections).

Regardless, your communication network must consist of reliable equipment designed to afford clear communication among all agencies within the system. This becomes a challenge in systems that cover large geographical areas or where terrain interferes with transmission and reception. If you want to communicate with a unit clear across the county but your radio is not powerful enough to transmit that far, communication will be difficult, if not impossible. A system that covers a large geographical expanse can place **repeaters** strategically throughout its service area. These devices receive transmissions from a low-powered source and rebroadcast them at a higher power (Figure 9-10).

Your regional EMS system may consist of many agencies that have conducted business for decades on different **radio bands** and **radio frequencies**. City units may transmit

FIGURE 9-10 Example of EMS repeater system.

on **ultrahigh frequency (UHF)** radio waves because they penetrate concrete and steel well and are less susceptible to interference. Rural and suburban units may use a lower band frequency—**very high frequency (VHF)**—because those waves travel farther and better over varied terrain. In any event, communicating among agencies will be difficult unless all units share a common frequency. This is rarely the case. Again, the spectrum of communications equipment currently ranges from antiquated radios to mobile data units mounted inside emergency vehicles.

Geographically integrating communications networks would enable routine and reliable communication among EMS, fire, law enforcement, and other public safety agencies. This would, in turn, facilitate coordinated responses during both routine and large-scale operations. Developing the necessary hardware (equipment and network) and software (language) will be essential to improving emergency communications.

See further discussion in the Public Safety Communications System Planning and Funding section near the end of this chapter.

Radio Communication

Many types of radio transmission are possible, with new technologies being developed every day. Usage may vary from system to system. This section discusses some of the more common technologies in use today.

SIMPLEX The most basic communications systems use **simplex** transmissions. These systems transmit and receive on the same frequency and thus cannot do both simultaneously (Figure 9-11). After you transmit a message, you must release the transmit button and wait for a response. This slows communication because you have to wait for all traffic to stop before you can speak. It also makes the system more formal and prevents open discussion. Simplex communication systems are most effective on the scene, when the incident commander or EMS dispatcher must transmit orders or directions without interruption. Most dispatch systems and on-scene communications use simplex transmissions.

DUPLEX **Duplex** transmissions allow simultaneous two-way communications by using two frequencies for each

> **CONTENT REVIEW**
>
> ➤ Types of Radio Communication
> • Simplex
> • Duplex
> • Multiplex
> • Trunked
> • Digital

FIGURE 9-11 Simplex communications systems transmit and receive on the same frequency.

FIGURE 9-12 Duplex communications systems use two frequencies for each channel.

channel (Figure 9-12). Each radio must be able to transmit and receive on each channel. For example, on a UHF radio, a hospital base station might transmit on 468.000 megahertz (MHz) and receive on 478.000 MHz. Field radios would then transmit on 478.000 MHz and receive on 468.000 MHz—just the opposite. Either party could then transmit and receive on the same channel simultaneously.

Duplex systems work like telephone communications. Many areas use them for communications between the field paramedic and the medical direction physician. The duplex system's major advantage is that one party does not have to wait to speak until the other party finishes his transmission. This allows for a much freer discussion and consultation between physician and paramedic. For example, the medical direction physician can interrupt your report with an important question or concern. On the other hand, this ability to interrupt can be a disadvantage if abused.

All duplex systems allow you to transmit either voice messages or data such as ECG strips.

MULTIPLEX **Multiplex** systems are duplex systems with the additional capability of transmitting voice and data simultaneously (Figure 9-13). This enables you to carry on a conversation with the medical direction physician while you are transmitting an ECG strip. Speaking while you are transmitting the ECG strip, however, causes much interference on the ECG strip.

TRUNKING Many communications systems operating in the 800-MHz range use **trunking** to hasten communica-

tions. Trunked systems pool all frequencies. When a radio transmission comes in, a computer routes it to the first available frequency. The computer routes the next transmission to the next available frequency, and so on. When a transmission terminates, that frequency becomes available and reenters the pool of unused frequencies. Trunking thus frees the dispatcher or field unit from having to search for an available frequency.

Trunked 800-MHz systems have been developed over the past 20 years, usually by one sponsoring state system user (e.g., police, transportation). When states began to suffer financial setbacks in the 1990s and more recently, these systems became forced to seek other users, generally at a "per device per month" or "per year" cost. Trunked systems appeal to potential fire and EMS users because they offer more channels to use and the ability to configure special "talk groups" (a preselected set of users who can be instantly keyed up and addressed as a group with no others participating).

EMS users now using VHF and UHF systems should be aware of the need to plan, engineer, and coordinate system development if they expect to change to a trunked system. A city jurisdiction that switches to this system and includes all hospitals may create problems for rural EMS units that occasionally transfer patients into those hospitals and use only VHF or UHF frequencies. Suburban and rural users may find that the cost of new antennas needs to be factored in, because transmission distances and coverage will be less with 800-MHz equipment than with UHF and VHF systems. Buyers beware!

DIGITAL COMMUNICATIONS Voice transmission can be time consuming and difficult to understand. The trend toward combining radio technology with computer technology (ICT) has encouraged a shift from analog to **digital communications**. Digital radio equipment is becoming increasingly popular in emergency services communication systems. This technology translates, or encodes, sounds into digital code for broadcast. Digital transmission is much faster and much more accurate than analog transmission. Because the messages are transmitted in condensed form, they help to ease the overcrowding of radio frequencies. Mobile phone companies now use digital transmissions. Issues remain with

FIGURE 9-13 Multiplex systems can transmit voice and data at the same time.

the use of digital communications in certain noise environments, such as fire grounds, that cause distortion of voice transmissions. This may be alleviated with changes in radio technology but may also constrain the abandonment of analog voice communications altogether.

The **mobile data unit (MDU)** in many emergency vehicles (typically a "ruggedized" or "hardened" laptop computer) is a robust form of digital communications. MDUs are mounted in the vehicle cab or patient compartment (depending on use) and wired to the radio, a wireless **hotspot** modem (in urban settings), or through a wireless provider air card. These are replacing mobile data terminals that are radio-based devices (more often used in law enforcement) that have limited applications because they have no broadband capacity. MDUs, however, may be used for receiving dispatch and other information and sending status information such as "en route," "arrived," or "transporting to the hospital," but may also be used to send electronic PCR data to the hospital or back to quarters for processing.

It is a positive step forward to begin to use data communications on a daily basis in EMS. These cutting-edge applications are increasingly widespread, and gaining experience with them is instructive for all of us. Dependence on commercial cellular and other wireless providers (air cards and hotspots) and on unlicensed, municipal hotspot/"mesh" technology (2.4-GHz systems) for **mission-critical communications** (e.g., when the information must get through without fail because a patient's well-being depends on it) is not recommended. These systems are not built to public safety reliability, security, or infrastructure hardening standards. Furthermore, they are shared with the general public whose use is rapidly increasing, and offer no higher priority of use for EMS. If mission-critical data communications are required, explore the public safety licensed option of 4.9 GHz in urban areas or teaming with transportation colleagues for use of 5.9 GHz intelligent transportation systems (ITS) channels. Another, better solution is under development—the FCC's proposed national public safety broadband network at 700 MHz. This solution promises broadband coverage in areas beyond urban centers.

Although means of digital communication are developing rapidly, it is important to remember that voice communications will always have a place in emergency services. Crews will always need to speak to one another, to physicians and nurses, or to dispatchers.

CELL PHONES AND MOBILE BROADBAND Many EMS systems have found that a **cellular telephone system** provides a cost-effective way to transmit essential patient information to the hospital (Figure 9-14). Cellular technology is available in even the most remote areas of the country, though availability is wireless provider dependent. A cell phone service is divided into regions called **cells**. These cells are radio base stations that communicate with mobile

FIGURE 9-14 Modern mobile phones have amazing capabilities and are becoming increasingly more sophisticated.

telephones. When the transmission leaves one cell's range, another cell picks it up immediately, without interruption. Agreements among wireless providers now allow seamless roaming across cell regions and states, coast to coast. Limitations in any one provider's roaming arrangements, however, can limit access in certain areas of the country.

Handheld cell phone devices still exist with capabilities that do not extend beyond simple voice communications. These can also send limited data such as ECGs when connected to a heart monitor that is set up for this operation. However, these devices are "narrowband" and, like the VHF/UHF/800-MHz radio systems we commonly use today (which are also narrowband—and with the VHF/UHF systems, as discussed earlier, getting even narrower), they support limited data transmission. In fact, they send data more slowly than the first dial-up Internet connections 20 years ago and only about 20 percent as fast as basic dial-up connections today.

More common today are **smart phone** devices, in which the voice capability of a basic cell phone is joined by the ability to perform a variety of data messaging functions, such as taking and sending photos and video, sending and receiving e-mail and text messages, and connecting with the Internet and its variety of communications options (e.g., using the handheld as a wireless hotspot VOIP device to save cell phone call charges).

Smart phones incorporate broadband data capability to be able to accomplish these functions by, essentially, widening the "pipe" through which data flow, allowing more data to flow faster and increasingly supporting data- and bandwidth-hungry operations (e.g., gaming with multiple players and sophisticated, highly responsive graphics in real time; and the sending of video and higher quality photos in social networking environments while texting/instant messaging among recipients).

Broadband data capabilities are rapidly expanding and becoming more sophisticated as technology moves from second to third and, now, fourth generations ("2G",

"3G", "4G") of development. The popularity of smart phones, smart pads/tablets, and netbook devices, added to the data transmission demands of laptop and desktop computer users, creates a real issue of "pipe availability" to send data. It is not uncommon, particularly in urban and suburban environments, to see commercial wireless data sending and receiving rates fluctuate greatly with time of day and day of week. Occasional system "crashes" leave users of some wireless providers without data communications for varying periods of time. As with older-generation, narrowband cell phones, availability of newer generations of data communications varies with the commercial wireless provider company and the area of the country (with large urban areas usually the first to be upgraded).

Like duplex radio transmissions, cell and smart phones make communication less formal, promote discussion, and reduce on-line times. They further allow the medical direction physician to speak directly with the patient and offer the additional advantages of being widely available and highly reliable. The telephones themselves are inexpensive, but commercial wireless providers charge a monthly fee for their use, generally with additional charges for data services and specific data applications.

As with data communications, even simple voice communications are not always reliable in commercial wireless systems. Their major disadvantage is that each cell can handle only a limited number of calls. Geography can interfere with the cell phone's signals, and in large metropolitan areas the cells often fill up and become unavailable, especially during peak hours. Cell congestion occurs frequently in times of disaster when many local, state, and federal response agencies, news media, and citizens all require communications.[12] The National Communications System in the U.S. Department of Homeland Security, however, has programs that local and state EMS agencies can subscribe to that provide priority access to wire line and wireless communications services in emergencies.

Further, although some commercial wireless providers offer a "push to talk" (PTT) feature that resembles that of your mobile EMS radio, no cell or smart phone is capable of communicating directly with another phone even if the callers are standing next to one another. All calls must go through the cell system network. In addition, these phones are not capable of "one-to-many" communications, as radios are. If a caller wants to get a voice message to several responders, the caller would have to call each individually.

Despite their limitations, commercial wireless phones have become a popular medium for on-scene and medical direction communications. When using wireless phones for on-line medical direction, it is important to contact the base station physician on a recorded line. On-line medical direction recordings have been used as powerful allies in cases of litigation. Be sure to find out how to do this in your system.

Because of all the limitations just described, no paramedic or EMS provider agency should ever rely solely on commercial wireless communications for mission-critical voice communications. This is also true of municipal or other 2.4-GHz unlicensed hotspot systems that are common in urban areas to provide Internet access to residents (4.9-GHz public safety licensed systems are another matter; they have limitations for voice communications, and have good potential for urban hotspot and "mesh"—interconnected hotspot antennae to make citywide or area-wide network operations).

EXPANDING COMPUTER USES Computers have entered every aspect of our daily lives. In emergency services communications, they have revolutionized system management and incident data collection. Most dispatchers no longer enter data by pen and pencil, time-stamping machines, or typewriters. They can make a permanent record of any incident's events in real time. Virtually all new PCR systems are no longer paper based, but rely on the electronic input of patient and call data into ruggedized mobile laptops and/or computers at the ED or EMS quarters.

It is increasingly commonplace for an EMS unit to "dump" its electronic PCR data for recent calls to a central database at its quarters, using an air card in the computer and a commercial wireless provider's network. Crews in the field will be able to use their smart phones, tablets, or laptops to access regional health care system medical record depositories for medical history data on their current patient in real time. (The first well-publicized system of this kind is in Indiana, but such regional and statewide record systems are in development virtually everywhere, following the federal push for universal electronic health records use.)

Computers also make research faster and easier. For example, if you wanted to determine the day of the week when most cardiac calls happen, or what time of day is busiest, or which area of a city needs more coverage, you could retrieve the pertinent data from your computerized records immediately. You can program your system to provide whatever type of data you want, in whatever format you desire. It also eliminates the need to enter retrospective data when conducting research. For example, the times, locations, and particulars of a call will already be in the computer files for immediate retrieval during a research project.

SOFTWARE-DEFINED RADIO In many areas of the country, it is not unusual for ambulances to have multiple communications devices. These may be required to talk with other response agencies that use other bands (e.g., VHF versus 800 MHz), to overcome areas of bad reception, or for other reasons. In rural services, it would not be unusual to find a VHF radio (to talk locally), a cell phone, an 800-MHz trunked radio (to talk with hospitals in "the big city"), and a satellite phone for areas that are totally "dead" for other forms of communications. The trick is knowing which device to use at any given moment in the middle of an emergency.

Now imagine a communications device that combines all these bandwidths, is smart enough to "sniff" the airwaves covered for strong signals and no competing transmissions, and then obeys a protocol programmed into it for connecting the user with the desired target, say "Hospital A." The feature of combining a wide range of radio bands is called **multiband radio**. The feature of "sniffing" the airwaves for signal strength and clear channels among the bands in the device is called **cognitive radio**. Like trunked radios, it can pick an open, strong frequency without the user knowing which one was selected (they just know they are talking to Hospital A). Finally, the ability to combine all these features and then program them with additional operational protocols (e.g., "select satellite transmission only if all other options are unreliable"—because satellite use can be relatively expensive).

Multiband radios are now available that cross bands from high frequency to VHF, UHF, and 800 MHz in one device. These radios can be programmed to jump from channels in one band to another very quickly and to scan channels throughout. Devices that combine the new public safety broadband capability and satellite capability are expected to be produced to give universal public safety interoperable broadband coverage. Cognitive and software-defined radios are widely available and beginning to make inroads in the public safety arena.

New Technology

When planning got under way for a nationwide public safety broadband system, between 2005 and 2010, planners watched popular commercial applications such as the Apple iPhone cause a boom in broadband use that began eating up an increasing share of available **bandwidth**. Consequently, public safety communications planners in the FCC and the emergency services began to investigate how much bandwidth they were going to require.

One of the earliest efforts in this vein was sponsored by the National Public Safety Telecommunications Council (NPSTC), the National Association of State EMS Officials (NASEMSO), and the National Association of EMS Physicians (NAEMSP), and was funded by the federal government. An expert panel was created that produced a report in 2010. The panel was asked to consider: "What potential diagnostic and treatment technologies may possibly be used in the next 10 years that have implications for voice and data communications technology and bandwidth use?" The panel's report affirmed some national consensus work by the Intelligent Transportation Society of America (ITSA) in 2008 and the U.S. Department of Homeland

Security's SafeCom in its document *Public Safety Communications Statement of Requirements*" in 2006.

The following sections describe some of the new technologies that the expert panel and others have predicted. These predicted technologies are being used by researchers, the FCC, and others to develop various projections of bandwidth that will be needed for a public safety broadband system.

One conclusion is clear: If any of these technologies become used to any great degree by multiple EMS provider agencies in any given area, broadband access will be mandatory. Current communications capabilities in the narrowband frequencies EMS has traditionally used, and continues to use, cannot support these patient care operations.

Medical Quality Video and Imaging

The use of video to send patient images from the scene or ambulance to a physician consultant/medical director is being used currently in Texas, Arizona, and Louisiana.[13] Although the utility of video in EMS remains an open question in the national EMS community, it is more likely to have a role in rural settings than in urban settings for two reasons: a lesser call volume and the emerging concept of community paramedicine in rural areas.

CALL VOLUME First, urban systems have high call volumes, and can afford highly trained EMS personnel (paramedics) who have a high level of patient interaction experience. The combination in urban systems of a large call volume, short transport times to hospitals, and the training and experience of personnel means that true emergencies are dealt with effectively and that subtleties in signs and symptoms that may become a treatment factor later can be managed by a physician in the ED after a few minutes' transport.

Rural areas often do not have the call volume to be able to afford the cost of paramedic-level personnel or to provide sufficient experience to maintain an effective emergency practice. Transport times are relatively long, and subtle signs and symptoms that may not be appreciated by personnel with a lesser amount of training and experience may become a treatment factor before arrival at the hospital.

Therefore, in urban areas, injecting the expense and process of video transmission may not be as value-added as it could be in rural areas. In the rural areas, the interpretive eye of an emergency physician able to view the patient, see portable CT images (e.g., to determine the type of stroke a patient is suffering), or review portable ultrasound video/images of the patient (e.g., to determine the presence of internal bleeding) may make a critical difference in treatment and how and where the patient is transported.

Today, satellite-based and wired broadband audio/video/imaging systems operate in military and civilian applications to link remote and rural medical facilities with specialists in urban centers to provide intensive care monitoring and treatment and "tele-trauma" consultation. The public safety broadband network, including satellite backup and node links to telemedicine and other fiber networks, could wirelessly provide these capabilities to ambulance and rural hospital/clinic personnel to effectively intervene in life-threatening situations that they would otherwise not be adequately trained or experienced to accomplish.

COMMUNITY PARAMEDICINE   Second, an emerging concept in rural EMS and health care is community paramedicine. Under a widely discussed "medical home" concept of implementation and financing, paramedics and other EMTs could become affordable in rural communities because they not only provide advanced life support services, but also help to fill gaps in primary health care services. Working in and out of rural clinics and hospitals, paramedics and other EMTs could provide preventive care services in the community and other primary care and follow-up services in patient homes. They would be responsible for patient remote monitoring and for visiting patients in their homes, thereby reducing the need for clinic visits and catching incipient problems before they necessitate an ambulance call or a clinic or ED visit.

Paramedics would be able to respond to some emergency calls and be able to address the patient's needs without transport to a hospital. (One study suggests that transports could be reduced by 15 percent with such a system in an urban setting.)[14] Because it would not be cost effective to train these EMS providers at a level to make them independent practitioners, the ability to conduct wireless video consults with physicians and mid-level practitioners in rural clinics and hospitals will become crucial for the benefits of community paramedicine to be robustly realized.

This concept projects a need for ongoing and frequent broadband use by EMS in rural areas in years to come.

Other EMS Applications

The following are other technology applications with broadband implications that the national EMS communications initiatives have suggested:

- *Patient Multi-Vital–Signs Monitoring.* The ability to attach one or more micro-monitors to a patient to wirelessly receive and transmit electrocardiograph, capnography, blood pressure, and other vital signs packaged for display in a database.

- *Responder Multi-Vital–Signs Monitoring.* Similar to the patient multi-vital–sign monitoring but intended for use by EMS responders monitoring fire, police, and other responders in hazardous circumstances (e.g., firefighters inside a burning building, SWAT team members inside a building in a hostage-taking scenario).

This could also be used to detect chemicals, gases, radioactivity, and other hazards being encountered by monitored responders.

- *Stand-Off Vital-Signs Monitoring.* The ability to wirelessly detect, receive, and wirelessly transmit multiple vital signs to a database without physically touching the patient.

- *Infrared Crowd Disease Detection.* The ability to wirelessly scan, receive, and transmit to a database the body temperatures (and body area temperatures) of individuals in crowds that suggest illness.

- *Wireless Speech-to-Text Translation.* The ability to speak into a microphone in a noisy emergency scene environment and have that speech translated and wirelessly transmitted into an ad hoc patient-event database for real-time review by others on the scene, coming to the scene, or in a hospital ED supervising care at the scene.

- *Receipt of Electronic Patient Records in Real Time.* The ability of on-scene EMS staff to receive and potentially manipulate (to focus on pertinent records only) medical history for their patients, either wirelessly from a regional health care medical record system or by patient-carried data records.

- *Creation of Ad Hoc Multi-Component Patient Databases.* This is simply transmission of electronic PCRs to hospitals before the patient arrives, augmented by separate transmissions of 12-lead electrocardiography and simple vital sign transmission. Using technologies already described, this system would have the ability to create, in a single-user interface window, data sent wirelessly from the scene that includes video, multi-vital signs, voice-to-text translated patient notes, and pertinent patient history components. This database could be made available in real time to authorized responders (e.g., incoming air-medical crews who will transport the patient), specialists guiding care remotely (e.g., trauma surgeons directing a specialized procedure in the field), and emergency physicians routinely supervising EMS calls.

- *EMS-Mediated Remote Patient-Monitoring Systems and "Just in Time" Patient Warning and Reference Guidance.* In community paramedicine and other settings, patients with post-hospital discharge and/or chronic health-monitoring needs can be remotely followed through the use of multi-vital–signs monitors (as described earlier), video, or specialized monitors appropriate to their condition. These could be monitored at EMS dispatch and/or nurse advice service centers and would have alarms should the vital signs monitored go outside a preset range.

Although this kind of monitoring could be done by wireline service in most settings, though less so in rural areas, the ability to rebroadcast the monitoring device transmissions to responding EMS crews would need to be wireless. In addition, based on the patient history and current monitoring results, care warnings pertinent to the particular patient and condition, along with other relevant reference or medical protocol guidance, could automatically be sent to EMS responders in real time. In a similar fashion, "I've fallen and I can't get up" emergency alerting systems, currently wireline dependent and plaguing responders as a common source of false alarms, could be set up with audio–video and vital-signs–monitoring interfaces with not only wireline support but also wireless retransmission to responding EMS crews.

- *Advanced Automatic Crash Notification (AACN) Data Rebroadcasting and "Just in Time" Training and Reference Material Rebroadcasting.* AACN has the potential to significantly reduce death and disability in rural car crashes by eliminating the time now required to "discover" that the crash has occurred, the time required to determine the physical location of the crash, and the time now required to respond to a crash and determine whether specialty response (e.g., extrication, special resources) is needed.

To take optimum advantage of these potential time savings, the AACN data should be transmitted simultaneously to all potential responders and to hospital and specialty care facilities that have requested to be notified of crashes exceeding a certain severity in a specific geographic area. In addition, certain crash data need to be automatically assessed and resulting information transmitted to responders and facilities based on the assessment. For example, speed/rollover/impact-vector data may be among data used to determine the severity of the crash and result in automatic dispatch of airmedical and other specialty responders and notification of trauma centers.

Other vehicle data such as vehicle type and year/speed/rollover/impact vector could be used to send an electronic vehicle access manual to responding extrication crews with diagrams and methods for best accessing patients and avoiding hazards in that vehicle.

- *Closed Circuit Television (CCTV) Scene Transmission.* Wireless receipt of live video feeds of an emergency scene from traffic, police, homeland security, and other public monitoring CCTV systems by responding crews will help plan approach and vehicle staging at the scene.

- *Robotic Remote Hazard Suppression and Patient Extrication.* The use of remotely controlled robots to defuse/suppress hazards and remove patients from hazardous settings. This application requires audio, video, and robot-control data transmission.

- *Wireless Vehicle Systems, Equipment and Supply Monitoring.* The ability now exists to monitor virtually every critical system of a public safety vehicle. Radio frequency identification (RFID) and other tagging device technology make it possible to track the inventory of equipment and supplies in a vehicle. Wirelessly transmitting this information to the vehicle operator's communications unit, with event-linked special warnings (e.g., sending a "leaving scene to transport to hospital" message while a critical patient care device is registered as not having been returned to the vehicle; transmitting an "en route to scene" message with a critically low air pressure in a tire or low inventory of a critical supply) would reduce delays in restocking and inventorying vehicles and medical errors caused by missing equipment or supplies.

- *Syndromic Surveillance and Quick Alerting to Specific Populations.* Real-time transmission of dispatch and ePCR data to monitoring systems that assess for specific patterns of patient complaints, signs, and symptoms in specific geographic areas. Transmission of these assessments to EMS responders and public health authorities when specific outbreak or hazardous event occurrence is predicted.

Legal Considerations

Keeping It Private. Many modern EMS communication systems use encryption or similar technologies to ensure privacy and security. However, people can monitor certain EMS communications, including some cell phone communications, with scanners or similar devices, which are becoming as sophisticated as the radios and phones themselves. It was once thought that radio communication was secure, but in fact it may not be. Furthermore, in many emergency departments, EMS radios are within earshot of patients, staff, and visitors. Thus, you should always assume that someone other than the intended recipient might hear any EMS radio communication. Because of this, you must carefully limit any information that might identify a particular patient. This includes such things as name, race, financial (insurance) status, and similar descriptors. Transmission of such information does not enhance patient care and may actually violate patient confidentiality laws, including the Health Insurance Portability and Accountability Act and similar statutes. Always carefully plan your radio communications—especially when they deal with a particular patient.

Public Safety Communications System Planning and Funding

Since 9/11, the need for statewide systems with nationwide capability for interoperability has changed the ways public safety communications systems are planned and implemented. No longer can EMS communications systems be planned as a "stovepipe" activity. Today, they must be part of larger local, regional, statewide, and national interoperable public safety and health care communications systems. To that end, and because EMS has a poor track record of participating in and benefiting from federal and state planning and funding initiatives compared with the success of fire and law enforcement, today's paramedic and agency officials should be aware of opportunities to be a part of communications system planning and funding initiatives.

Under the auspices of the U.S. Department of Homeland Security's Office of Emergency Communications (OEC), much progress has been made in ensuring well-planned development of interoperable public safety communications systems on the national, state, regional, and local levels. In 2009, for the first time ever, a National Emergency Communications Plan (NECP) was developed by OEC. Also, for the first time ever, virtually every state and territory developed a statewide communications interoperability plan (SCIP) under the leadership of a statewide, multidisciplinary public safety committee (generically referred to as a statewide interoperability executive committee [SIEC] but given different names in various states). States are now developing statewide interoperability coordinator (SWIC) positions as a single point of responsibility for system development and funding disbursement. All states are encouraged by OEC, and by grant incentives, to have SCIPs,

SIECs, and SWICs. (The funding initiatives through which OEC provides funding generally require the states to pass 80 percent of the funds to local agency providers.) It is up to local paramedics and agencies to take advantage of these opportunities to be heard and to have projects funded.

Public Safety Communications Regulation

The **Federal Communications Commission (FCC)** controls and regulates all nongovernmental communications in the United States. This includes AM and FM radio, television, aircraft, marine, and mobile land-frequency ranges. The FCC has designated frequencies within each radio band for special use. They include public safety frequencies in all bandwidths. In 2008, the FCC established a new office to handle public safety issues, the Public Safety and Homeland Security Bureau. The FCC's primary functions include:

- Licensing and allocating radio frequencies
- Establishing technical standards for radio equipment
- Licensing and regulating the technical personnel who repair and operate radio equipment
- Monitoring frequencies to ensure appropriate usage
- Spot-checking base stations and dispatch centers for appropriate licenses and records

The FCC requires all EMS communications systems to follow appropriate governmental regulations and laws. In licensing activities, the FCC requires public safety agencies to use frequency coordinators. For EMS, this is the International Municipal Signal Association (IMSA). You must stay abreast of and obey any FCC regulations that apply to your communications.

Summary

This is an extremely exciting time to be involved in EMS. Advances in communications technology are dramatically improving the communications among patients, paramedics, and physicians. As systems improve and technology becomes more affordable, paramedics will be able to arrive on scene of an injury within just a few minutes and, with the click of a button, obtain all the necessary medical information from the patient. As they load and transport the patient, the satellite communications system will link streaming video and audio with the emergency room doctor.

As one of the fundamental aspects of prehospital care, accurate and effective communications help ensure an EMS system's efficiency and improve a patient's survivability. Communications includes not only your radio traffic, but also your spoken and nonspoken (body language) messages. All your communications must be concise, professional, and complete and must conform to national and local protocols. As communications systems and technology continue to advance, so will patient care and survival rates. The paramedic will be able to quickly gain access to the appropriate facility and medical direction, allowing for a much quicker and more seamless treatment plan through discharge at the hospital.

You Make the Call

A call comes into your unit for a "possible heart attack" on State Route 11. You and your partner climb into Palermo Rescue, a nontransport first-response vehicle. Your response time is about 10 minutes. On arrival, a family member meets you. He leads you into the den of a small farmhouse. Here, you see your patient sitting in an overstuffed chair. You note that your patient is a 69-year-old man in obvious distress.

You begin questioning your patient to develop a history. As he speaks, you immediately notice that he has difficulty breathing. He complains of severe chest pain, which began about 30 minutes ago. With his hand, he indicates that the pain is pressure-like and substernal. He also indicates that it radiates to his left arm and jaw. He describes a history of heart disease, including two prior heart attacks. Three years ago, he had cardiac bypass surgery. He currently takes Lanoxin, Lasix, Capoten, and an aspirin a day. He is allergic to Mellaril.

You and your partner complete your assessment. Your patient says he weighs about 250 pounds. He is alert, but anxious. He exhibits jugular venous distention and bibasilar crackles. His abdomen is nontender. His distal pulses are good. Vital signs include blood pressure 210/110 mmHg, pulse of 70 per minute and regular, and respirations of 20 breaths per minute and mildly labored. Pulse oximetry is 93 percent on supplemental oxygen. During your assessment, your patient becomes progressively more dyspneic. The transporting ambulance arrives and the paramedic asks you to give a radio report to the receiving hospital based on your assessment while she prepares her patient for transport.

- Based on the information above, organize and prepare your radio report to inform the receiving hospital of your patient's condition.

See Suggested Responses at the back of this book.

Review Questions

1. The process of exchanging information from one individual to another is _____.
   a. encoding.
   b. decoding.
   c. communication.
   d. communion.

2. General radio procedures include all of the following except:
   a. Listen for radio traffic before speaking.
   b. Depress the PTT button for 1 second before speaking.
   c. Speak slowly and clearly.
   d. Describe in detail your needs and the situations before releasing the transmit button.

3. When receiving orders from a dispatcher or physician you should _____
   a. use the echo procedure.
   b. confirm the order.
   c. write the order down.
   d. none of the above.

4. A recent report titled "Recommendations from the Expert Panel: Advanced Automatic Collision Notification and Triage of the Injured Patient" discusses that _____ shows promise in improving outcomes among severely injured crash patients.
   a. ACANN
   b. AACN
   c. ANCCA
   d. NCAS

5. A recent report titled "Recommendations from the Expert Panel: Advanced Automatic Collision Notification and Triage of the Injured Patient" found that Advanced Collision Notification can improve outcomes among seriously injured patients by providing all of the following except _____
   a. predicting the likelihood of serious injury among vehicle occupants.
   b. decreasing response times by prehospital care providers.
   c. assisting with field triage destination and transportation decisions.
   d. notifying the receiving hospitals that they will be getting a trauma patient.

6. Which radio frequencies may be used by cities and municipalities for their ability to better transmit through concrete and steel?
   a. UHF
   b. VHF
   c. 800-mHz
   d. none of the above

7. Which frequency band is typically used by county and suburban agencies due to its ability to transmit over various terrains and longer distances?
   a. UHF
   b. VHF
   c. 800-mHz
   d. none of the above

8. What is the name of the basic communications system that uses the same frequency to both transmit and receive?
   a. Multiplex
   b. Duplex
   c. Simplex
   d. Complex

9. A communications system that uses a different transmit and receive frequency allowing for simultaneous communications between two parties is called _____
   a. multiplex.
   b. duplex.
   c. simplex.
   d. complex.

10. _____ communications systems are capable of transmitting both voice and electronic patient data simultaneously.
   a. Multiplex
   b. Duplex
   c. Simplex
   d. Complex

See answers to Review Questions at the back of this book.

References

1. Department of Homeland Security. SAFECOM. (Available at http://www.dhs.gov/safecom/)
2. National EMS Information System (NEMSIS). The NEMSIS Technical Assistance Center (TAC). (Available at http://www.nemsis.org//.)
3. American College of Emergency Physicians (ACEP). "Automatic Crash Notification and Intelligent Transportation Systems." *Ann Emerg Med* 55 (2010): 397.
4. National Emergency Number Association (NENA). National Emergency Number Association. (Available at: http://www.nena.org)
5. Association of Public-Safety Communications Officials (APCO). [Available at: http://www.apco911.org/]
6. Department of Transportation, Research and Innovative Technology Administration. Next Generation 911. (Available at: http://www.its.dot.gov/ng911/.)
7. Centers for Disease Control and Prevention. Recommendations from the Expert Panel: Advanced Automatic Collision Notification and Triage of the Injured Patient. (See NHTSA summary at http://www.nhtsa.gov/Research/Biomechanics+&+Trauma/Advanced+Automatic+Collision+Notification+-+AACN)
8. Wilson, S., M. Cooke, R. Morrell et al. "A Systematic Review of the Evidence Supporting the Use of Priority Dispatch of Emergency Ambulances." *Prehosp Emerg Care* 6 (2002): 42–29.
9. Billittier, A. J., 4th, E. B. Lerner, W. Tucker, and J. Lee. "The Lay Public's Expectations of Prearrival Instructions When Dialing 911." *Prehosp Emerg Care* 4 (2000): 234–237.
10. Munk, M. D., S. D. White, M. L. Perry, et al. "Physician Medical Direction and Clinical Performance at an Established Emergency Medical Services System." *Prehosp Emerg Care* 13 (2009): 185–192.
11. Cheung, D. S., J. J. Kelly, C. Beach, et al. "Improving Handoffs in the Emergency Department." *Ann Emerg Med* 55 (2010): 171–180.
12. Chan, T. C., J. Killeen, W. Griswold, and L. Lenert. "Information Technology and Emergency Medical Care during Disasters." *Acad Emerg Med* 11 (2004): 1229–1236.
13. DREAMS Ambulance Project. (See article at: https://www.ems1.com/ems-products/technology/articles/1183110-DREAMS-revolutionizes-communication-between-ER-and-ambulance/.)
14. Haskins, P. A., D. G. Ellis, and J. Mayrose. "Predicted Utilization of Emergency Medical Services Telemedicine in Decreasing Ambulance Transports." *Prehosp Emerg Care* 6 (2002): 445–448.

Further Reading

Bass, R., J. Potter, K. McGinnis, and T. Miyahara. "Surveying Emerging Trends in Emergency-related Information Delivery for the EMS Profession." *Topics in Emergency Medicine* 26 (April–June 2004): 2, 93–102.
Fitch, J. "Benchmarking Your Comm Center." *JEMS* 2006: 98–112.
McGinnis, K. K. "The Future of Emergency Medical Services Communications Systems: Time for a Change." *N C Med J* 68 (2007): 283–285.
McGinnis, K. K. *Future EMS Technologies: Predicting Communications Implications.* National Public Safety Telecommunications Council, National Association of State EMS Officials, National Association of EMS Physicians, June, 2010.
McGinnis, K. K. "The Future Is Now: Emergency Medical Services (EMS) Communications Advances Can Be as Important as Medical Treatment Advances When It Comes to Saving Lives." *Interoperability Today* (SafeCom, U.S. Department of Homeland Security), Volume 3, 2005.
McGinnis, K. K. *Rural and Frontier Emergency Medical Services Agenda for the Future.* National Rural Health Association Press: October 2004.

Chapter 10
Documentation

Bryan Bledsoe, DO, FACEP, FAAEM

Jeff Brosious, EMT-P

STANDARD
Preparatory (Documentation)

COMPETENCY
Integrates comprehensive knowledge of EMS systems, the safety and well-being of the paramedic, and medical–legal and ethical issues, which is intended to improve the health of EMS personnel, patients, and the community.

 ## Learning Objectives

Terminal Performance Objective: After reading this chapter, you should be able to create complete, well-written patient care reports.

Enabling Objectives: To accomplish the terminal performance objective, you should be able to:

1. Define key terms introduced in this chapter.

2. Explain the purposes and goals of the patient care report in EMS.

3. Explain the importance of proper spelling, terminology, abbreviations, and acronyms (or as an alternative, plain English) in written documentation.

4. Given a series of patient care reports, identify the elements of good documentation.

5. Identify the main sections of narrative writing on a patient care report and discuss the acronyms suggested to help ensure completeness of documentation.

6. Discuss the differences in documentation for special situations such as refusals of care and mass casualty incidents.

7. Predict the consequences of inappropriate documentation.

8. Discuss the benefits and drawbacks of electronic patient care reports as compared to paper patient care reports.

KEY TERMS

Case Study

Tom Brewster is nervous. He has never been to a deposition before, and even though everyone has assured him that he is not the target of any legal action, he has to wonder what the lawyers want from him.

   As he sits outside the conference room, he goes over the call in his head. It was about 2:30 in the morning. He and Eric Billings, his partner, had just finished cleaning up from a GI bleeder when they were dispatched to the single-vehicle crash. The driver had gone off the left side of the road, crossed a ditch, and smashed into a tree. He had been lucky. He was out of the car, standing on the side of the road, and did not seem to have any serious injuries. He told Tom and Eric, "I think I'm fine, I just fell asleep and ran off the road." Still, they had performed a primary assessment followed by a rapid trauma assessment, immobilized the man, administered oxygen, and transported him to the emergency department. Tom rode in the back with the patient. On the way to the hospital he checked the patient's glucose level, started an IV as a precaution, and applied a cardiac monitor.

   "Everything was normal," Tom now thinks. "What did I miss?" He has reread his prehospital care report a hundred times. Even though it has been three years, he now remembers almost every detail of the call. Until two weeks ago, however, he had almost completely forgotten about it.

   All too soon, the lawyers call Tom into the conference room, introduce themselves, and swear him to honesty. One of the lawyers begins. "Do you recall the crash that occurred on the evening in question?"

   "Yes, I do," Tom replies. He recounts that on their arrival at the scene, the driver was out of the vehicle. Tom states that they managed him like any other trauma patient, and he had no obvious injuries or indications of illness.

   "Did the gentleman tell you he is diabetic?"

   "No," Tom answers, "but we checked his blood sugar, and it was normal."

   "Did he tell you he has heart problems?"

   "No," Tom says again, "but we did put him on the heart monitor, and his rhythm was normal."

   "Did he tell you he ran off the road because he passed out?"

   "No, he told me he fell asleep." Tom feels better. He has the answer to every question, and he has the PCR to back him up.

   After a few more questions, the lawyers dismiss Tom and allow him to leave. He has no idea what they were getting at, but he does know that he answered every question honestly. He wonders if he would have had all the answers if the case had been from six or eight years ago. He has really worked on his documentation in the past few years, and he knows he would have never remembered all those details without the help of his PCR.

   Six weeks later Tom gets a letter from the lawyer thanking him for his testimony. It turned out that the patient was suing his private doctor for not "recognizing his obvious diabetes and heart problems. He claimed these illnesses caused him to be involved in the motor vehicle accident, and it resulted in serious injury." Tom's testimony—and his PCR—have been pivotal in getting the case dismissed.

Introduction

The **prehospital care report (PCR)** is a factual record of events that occur during an EMS call or other patient contact. When written correctly, it accurately describes your assessment and care throughout the emergency call. It documents exactly what you did, when you did it, and the effects of your interventions. It can be your best friend—or your worst enemy—in a court proceeding.

   Your PCR is your sole permanent, complete written record of events during the ambulance call. The dispatch center may have a record of the call times and audiotapes of radio transmissions, and your patient will have his memory of the call. You and other responders also may have some recollections about the call—but your PCR will always be considered the most comprehensive and reliable record of the event. In addition, it reflects your professionalism. A well-written, thorough PCR suggests a thorough, efficient assessment and quality care. A sloppy, incomplete PCR suggests sloppy, inefficient care.

You will often be the first member of the health care system with whom the patient interacts. At the very least, the results of patients' interactions with you and other EMS personnel will affect their opinion of the health care system in general. EMS is a profession in which you can make a difference. Every call and every patient interaction can literally mean the difference between life and death for the patient. Few professions carry such awesome responsibility.

The PCR has three major goals:

- *To provide information to subsequent health care professionals about the patient and treatments provided in the prehospital setting.* This information helps the nursing staff, emergency physicians, and even physicians who will be caring for the patient in the hospital.

- *To provide essential information for proper billing of the patient.* There is a direct correlation between the detail of the report and the level of reimbursement subsequently provided for care and transport of the patient.

- *To provide a legal record of the call's circumstances.* There have been many cases in which poor documentation was a factor in EMS personnel losing a lawsuit and many cases in which good documentation has resulted in EMS personnel winning a lawsuit—or, more likely, not being sued in the first place.

Uses for Documentation

Your PCR will be a valuable resource for a variety of people. They include medical professionals, EMS administrators, researchers, and occasionally, lawyers.

Medical

Hospital staff (nurses and physicians) may need more information from you than they can get before you have to take another call. For example, they may want a chronological account of your patient's mental status from the time you arrived on the scene. Your PCR can tell the emergency department staff of your patient's condition before he arrived at the hospital. It serves

as a baseline for comparing assessment findings and detecting trends that indicate improvement or deterioration. The surgical staff will want to know the mechanism of injury and other pertinent findings during your primary assessment of your patient and the scene.

If your patient is admitted to the hospital, the floor or intensive care unit staff may need more information about his original condition than he can remember. In addition, your PCR provides them with information from people at the scene to whom they might not have access—family, bystanders, first responders, or other witnesses. Knowing about the circumstances that led to the event or the mechanism of injury may also help rehabilitation specialists to provide better therapy. Your PCR becomes an important document that helps ensure your patient's continuous effective care (Figure 10-1).

Administrative

EMS administrators must gather information for quality improvement and system management. Information regarding **response times**, call location, the use of lights and siren, and date and time is vital to evaluating your system's readiness to respond to life-threatening emergencies. It also is essential to providing information about community needs. The quality improvement or quality assurance committee will use PCRs to identify problems with individual paramedics or with the EMS system. In some agencies, the billing department will need to determine which services are billable. Insurance carriers may need to know more about the illness or injury to process the claim. Some states will use your PCR data to allocate funding for regional systems.

> **CONTENT REVIEW**
>
> ➤ Uses for PCRs
>   - Medical
>   - Administrative
>   - Research
>   - Legal

Prehospital Care Report

Agency Name	ARLINGTON RESCUE

MILEAGE
END 2 4 4 9 6
BEGIN 2 4 4 7 6
TOTAL 0 0 0 2 0

Dispatch Information: CARDIAC

Call Location: 124 CYPRUS ST 2nd FLOOR

CHECK ONE: ☑ Residence ☐ Health Facility ☐ Farm ☐ Indus. Facility ☐ Other Work Loc. ☐ Roadway ☐ Recreational ☐ Other

LOCATION CODE: 0 1 2 4

CALL TYPE AS REC'D
☑ Emergency
☐ Non-Emergency
☐ Stand-by

MECHANISM OF INJURY
☐ MVA (✓ seat belt used) N/A
☐ Fall of _____ feet
☐ Unarmed assault
☐ GSW
☐ Knife
☐ Machinery
☐ _____

USE MILITARY TIMES
CALL REC'D 0 7 0 5
ENROUTE 0 7 0 7
ARRIVED AT SCENE 0 7 1 9
FROM SCENE 0 7 3 8
AT DESTIN 0 7 5 4
IN SERVICE 0 8 1 0
IN QUARTERS 0 8 3 2

FIGURE 10-1 The run data in a prehospital care report is vital to your agency's efforts to improve patient care.

(© Kevin Link/Science Source)

FIGURE 10-2 The handheld electronic clipboard enables you to enter your prehospital care report directly into a computer.

(Source: Kevin Link/Science Source)

Research

Your PCR may give researchers useful data about many aspects of the EMS call. For example, they may analyze your recorded data to determine the efficacy of certain medical devices or interventions such as drugs and invasive procedures. They also may use the data to cut costs, alter staffing, and shorten response times. Some systems use computerized or electronic PCRs and a computerized database to analyze the data (Figure 10-2). Regardless of the method you use, your written documentation provides the basis for continuously improving patient care in your EMS system.

Legal

Your PCR becomes a permanent part of your patient's medical record. Lawyers may refer to it when preparing court actions, and in a legal proceeding it might be your sole source of information about the case. You may be called on to testify in a case in which your PCR becomes the central piece of evidence in your testimony. Or your PCR may serve as evidence in a criminal case and help determine the accused's innocence or guilt. Each state has its own laws regarding the length of time the hospital must keep its records.

Always write your PCR as if you know you will have to refer to it someday in a court proceeding. Describe your patient's condition when you arrived and during your care, and note his status on arrival at the hospital. Always document his condition before and after any interventions, and avoid writing any subjective opinions such as "the patient is intoxicated, obnoxious, and looks like a crack addict." After your PCR is written, ask your partner to review it for completeness and accuracy. A complete, accurate, and objective account of the emergency call may be your best and only defense against a plaintiff's attorney who will try to find inconsistencies and ambiguities in your account.

Assessment Pearls

Don't Write Patient Data on Your Gloves. Many EMS providers write vital signs and other essential information on their medical exam gloves. There are several problems with this. First, unless the gloves are properly disposed of, you could be cited for a HIPAA violation. More important, if you are involved in direct contact with a patient, you should take off your gloves or change gloves before using such personal objects as a clipboard or a pen. Leaving the gloves on (or laying them on an ED countertop) to read the information you wrote can contaminate your personal materials.

Instead, use a whiteboard or piece of tape to record your information. If you use a whiteboard, use the pen only during patient care and clean it often. If you use a piece of tape or something similar, have a dedicated pen that you use only during the patient encounter (not the one you might stick in your mouth when contemplating where you'll eat later). Always remember to wipe the whiteboard or properly dispose of the tape after each call.

General Considerations

Every EMS system has its own specific requirements for documentation. The type of call record used also varies from system to system. Some systems use reports with check boxes, some use **bubble sheets**, computer-scannable reports on which to record patient information by filling in boxes or "bubbles" (Figure 10-3). Still others may use computerized documentation. The particular type of operational data collected, such as time intervals, will also differ among systems. For example, proprietary EMS agencies may require more billing information than community-based volunteer agencies. The general characteristics of a well-written PCR, though, remain constant among all agencies and systems.

Medical Terminology

An essential component of good documentation is the appropriate use of medical terminology. Medical terms, though sometimes difficult to spell, transform your report into a universally accepted medical document. Learning the meanings and correct spellings of the medical terms that you will use in your PCRs is essential. Misused or misspelled words reflect

CONTENT REVIEW

➤ Characteristics of a Well-Written PCR
  - Appropriate medical terminology
  - Correct abbreviations and acronyms
  - Accurate, consistent times
  - Thoroughly documented communications
  - Pertinent negatives
  - Relevant oral statements of witnesses, bystanders, and patient
  - Complete identification of all additional resources and personnel

FIGURE 10-3 This prehospital care report's format can be scanned into a computer.

(Scannable paper PCR form. Copyright © by EMS Data Systems, Inc. Used by permission EMS Data Systems, Inc.)

poorly on your professionalism and may confuse the report's readers.

If you do not know how to spell a word, look it up or use another word. Many paramedics carry pocket-size medical dictionaries in their ambulances for this purpose. Using "plain English" is acceptable when you do not know the appropriate medical term or its correct spelling. *Chest* is just as accurate as *thorax* and better than "thoracks." *Belly* is not as professional as *abdomen*, but it is still better than "abodemin."

Abbreviations and Acronyms

Both abbreviations and acronyms are formed from the initial letters of the words they stand for. An acronym, however, is an abbreviation you can pronounce as a word. For example, *CPR*, for *cardiopulmonary resuscitation*, is an abbreviation. *AIDS*, for *acquired immune deficiency syndrome*, is an acronym.

Medical abbreviations and acronyms allow you to increase the amount of information you can write quickly on your report (Table 10-1). They also pose problems, however, because they can have multiple meanings. For instance, their meanings can vary in different areas of medicine. Is *CP* chest pain, cardiovascular perfusion, or cerebral palsy? Is *CO* cardiac output or carbon monoxide? Is *BLS* basic life support or burns, lacerations, and swelling? These are all common abbreviations with more than one accepted meaning. Furthermore, many abbreviations are specific to one community. You must be familiar with those used in your local EMS system.

Abbreviations and acronyms can cause considerable confusion when someone unfamiliar with the call reads your report. Health care professionals who are not familiar with local customs or with emergency medicine might not understand them. One way to clarify the meaning of a new abbreviation or acronym is to write it out the first time you use it, followed by the abbreviation or acronym in parentheses. After that, you can use the abbreviation alone throughout the report. The following examples illustrate how abbreviations and acronyms can shorten your narratives. In standard English the report might be written as follows:

> The patient is a 54-year-old conscious and alert male who complains of sudden onset of chest pain and shortness of breath that started 20 minutes ago. He has taken two nitroglycerin with no relief. He denies any nausea, vomiting, or dizziness. He has a past history of coronary artery disease, a heart attack three years ago, and high blood pressure. He takes nitroglycerin as needed, Procardia XL, hydrochlorothiazide, and potassium. He has no known drug allergies.

Using abbreviations and acronyms, the same report might be written this way:

> Pt. is 54 y/o CAO male c/o sudden onset CP/SOB × 20 min. Pt took NTG × 2 Ø relief. n/v, dizziness. PH: CAD, AMI × 3y, HTN. Meds: NTG prn, Procardia XL, HCTZ and K$^+$; NKDA.

Times

Incident times are another important but perilous part of the PCR. The times you record on your PCR are considered the official times of the incident. For medical and legal purposes, you must ensure their accuracy.[1]

The PCR typically has spaces for the time the call was received, the dispatch time, the time of arrival at the scene, time of departure from the scene, time of arrival at the hospital, and time back in service (refer to Figure 10-1). Other time intervals are important, as well. The time you and your crew arrived at the patient's side is often very different from the time the ambulance arrived at the scene—when your patient is on the fourth floor of a building without an elevator, for example, or in a field several hundred yards from the road. Whatever the reason, document in your report any significant discrepancies between your arrival at the scene and your arrival at the patient. The times of vital signs assessment, medication administration, certain medical procedures as local protocols require, and changes in patient condition are also important and require accurate documentation.

One common problem with documenting times is inconsistencies among the dispatch center clock, the ambulance clock, and your watch. Imagine a report that documents that the ambulance arrived on scene at 20:32 according to the dispatch time, that CPR was started at 20:29 according to your watch, and the first defibrillation was administered at 20:43 according to the defibrillator's internal clock. Even though we may recognize this phenomenon and tend to discount the accuracy of the recorded times, they are nonetheless the official, legal times. Whenever possible, therefore, record all times from the same clock. When that is not possible, be sure that all the clocks and watches you use are synchronized. If they cannot be synchronized and the documented times seem to conflict with each other, explain this in your narrative. A simple statement such as the following will suffice: "All time intervals on the scene were documented using my watch; all other times are those reported by the dispatch center."

Communications

Your communications with the hospital are another important item to document. Your system may make voice recordings of those communications, but the recordings are usually not kept indefinitely. Again, the PCR will likely

Table 10-1 Standard Charting Abbreviations

Patient Information/Categories

Asian	A	Medications	Med
Black	B	Newborn	NB
Chief complaint	CC	Occupational history	OH
Complains of	c/o	Past history	PH
Current health status	CHS	Patient	Pt
Date of birth	DOB	Physical exam	PE
Differential diagnosis	DD	Private medical doctor	PMD
Estimated date of confinement	EDC	Review of systems	ROS
Family history	FH	Signs and symptoms	S/S
Female	♀	Social history	SH
Hispanic	H	Visual acuity	VA
History	Hx	Vital signs	VS
History and physical	H&P	Weight	Wt
History of present illness	HPI	White	W
Impression	IMP	Year-old	y/o
Male	♂		

Body Systems

Abdomen	Abd	Gynecological	GYN
Cardiovascular	CV	Head, eyes, ears, nose, and throat	HEENT
Central nervous system	CNS	Musculoskeletal	M/S
Ear, nose, and throat	ENT	Obstetric	OB
Gastrointestinal	GI	Peripheral nervous system	PNS
Genitourinary	GU	Respiratory	Resp

Common Complaints

Abdominal pain	abd pn	Lower back pain	LBP
Chest pain	CP	Nausea/vomiting	n/v
Dyspnea on exertion	DOE	No apparent distress	NAD
Fever of unknown origin	FUO	Pain	pn
Gunshot wound	GSW	Shortness of breath	SOB
Headache	H/A	Substernal chest pain	Sscp

Diagnoses

Abdominal aortic aneurysm	AAA	Chronic obstructive pulmonary disease	COPD
Abortion	Ab	Chronic renal failure	CRF
Acute myocardial infarction	AMI	Congestive heart failure	CHF
Adult respiratory distress syndrome	ARDS	Coronary artery bypass graft	CABG
Alcohol	ETOH	Coronary artery disease	CAD
Atherosclerotic heart disease	ASHD	Cystic fibrosis	CF

(Continued)

Table 10-1 Standard Charting Abbreviations *Continued*

Diagnoses			
Dead on arrival	DOA	Multiple sclerosis	MS
Deep vein thrombosis	DVT	Non-insulin-dependent diabetes mellitus	NIDDM
Delirium tremens	DTs	Organic brain syndrome	OBS
Diabetes mellitus	DM	Otitis media	OM
Dilation and curettage	D&C	Overdose	OD
Duodenal ulcer	DU	Paroxysmal nocturnal dyspnea	PND
End-stage renal failure	ESRF	Pelvic inflammatory disease	PID
Epstein-Barr virus	EBV	Peptic ulcer disease	PUD
Foreign body obstruction	FBO	Pregnancies/births (gravida/para)	G/P
Hepatitis B virus	HBV	Pregnancy-induced hypertension	PIH
Hiatal hernia	HH	Pulmonary embolism	PE
Hypertension	HTN	Rheumatic heart disease	RHD
Infectious disease	ID	Sexually transmitted disease	STD
Inferior wall myocardial infarction	IWMI	Transient ischemic attack	TIA
Insulin-dependent diabetes mellitus	IDDM	Tuberculosis	TB
Intracranial pressure	ICP	Upper respiratory infection	URI
Mass casualty incident	MCI	Urinary tract infection	UTI
Mitral valve prolapse	MVP	Venereal disease	VD
Motor vehicle crash	MVC	Wolff-Parkinson-White syndrome (disease)	WPW

Medications			
Angiotensin-converting enzyme	ACE	Lactated Ringer's, Ringer's lactate	LR, RL
Aspirin	ASA	Magnesium sulfate	$MgSO_4$
Bicarbonate	HCO_3^-	Morphine sulfate	MS
Birth control pills	BCP	Nitroglycerin	NTG
Calcium	Ca^{2+}	Nonsteroidal anti-inflammatory agent	NSAID
Calcium channel blocker	CCB	Normal saline	NS
Calcium chloride	$CaCl_2$	Penicillin	PCN
Chloride	Cl^-	Phenobarbital	PB
Digoxin	Dig	Potassium	K^+
Dilantin (phenytoin sodium)	DPH	Sodium bicarbonate	$NaHCO_3$
Diphendydramine	DPHM	Sodium chloride	NaCl
Diphtheria-pertussis-tetanus	DPT	Tylenol	APAP
Hydrochlorothiazide	HCTZ		

Anatomy/Landmarks			
Abdomen	Abd	Anterior-posterior	A/P
Antecubital	AC	Distal interphalangeal (joint)	DIP
Anterior axillary line	AAL	Dorsalis pedis (pulse)	DP
Anterior cruciate ligament	ACL	Gallbladder	GB

Table 10-1 Standard Charting Abbreviations *Continued*

Anatomy/Landmarks

Intercostal space	ICS	Midaxillary line	MAL
Lateral collateral ligament	LCL	Posterior axillary line	PAL
Left lower lobe	LLL	Posterior cruciate ligament	PCL
Left lower quadrant	LLQ	Proximal interphalangeal (joint)	PIP
Left upper lobe	LUL	Right lower lobe	RLL
Left upper quadrant	LUQ	Right lower quadrant	RLQ
Left ventricle	LV	Right middle lobe	RML
Liver, spleen, and kidneys	LSK	Right upper lobe	RUL
Lymph node	LN	Right upper quadrant	RUQ
Medial collateral ligament	MCL	Temporomandibular joint	TMJ
Metacarpophalangeal (joint)	MCP	Tympanic membrane	TM
Metatarsophalangeal (joint)	MTP		

Physical Exam/Findings

Arterial blood gas	ABG	Heel-to-shin (cerebellar test)	H → S
Bilateral breath sounds	BBS	Hemoglobin	Hgb
Blood sugar	BS	Inspiratory	Insp
Breath sounds	BS	Jugular venous distention	JVD
Cardiac injury profile	CIP	Laceration	Lac
Central venous pressure	CVP	Level of consciousness	LOC
Cerebrospinal fluid	CSF	Moves all extremities (well)	MAEW
Chest X-ray	CXR	Nontender	NT
Complete blood count	CBC	Normal range of motion	NROM
Computerized tomography	CT	Palpation	Palp
Conscious, alert, and oriented	CAO	Passive range of motion	PROM
Costovertebral angle	CVA	Point of maximal impulse	PMI
Deep tendon reflexes	DTR	Posterior tibial (pulse)	PT
Dorsalis pedis (pulse)	DP	Pulse	P
Electrocardiogram	EKG, ECG	Pupils equal and reactive to light	PEARL
Electroencephalogram	EEG	Pupils equal, round, reactive to light and accommodation	PERRLA
Expiratory	Exp	Range of motion	ROM
Extraocular movements (intact)	EOMI	Respirations	R
Fetal heart tones	FHT	Tactile vocal fremitus	TVF
Full range of motion	FROM	Temperature	T
Full-term normal delivery	FTND	Unconscious	Unc
Heart rate	HR	Urinary incontinence	UI
Heart sounds	HS		

(Continued)

Table 10-1 Standard Charting Abbreviations *Continued*

Miscellaneous Descriptors			
After (post-)	p̄	Not applicable	n/a
After eating	pc	Number	No or #
Alert and oriented	A/O	Occasional	Occ
Anterior	ant.	Pack years	pk/yrs, p/y
Approximate	≈	Per	/
As needed	prn	Positive	+
Before (ante-)	ā	Posterior	post.
Before eating (*ante cibum*, before meal)	a.c.	Postoperative	PO
Body surface area (%)	BSA	Prior to arrival	PTA
Celsius	C	Radiates to	→
Change	Δ	Right	R
Decreased	↓	Rule out	R/O
Equal	=	Secondary to	2°
Fahrenheit	F	Superior	sup.
Immediately	stat	Times (for 3 hours)	× (×3h)
Increased	↑	Unequal	≠
Inferior	inf.	Warm and dry	W/D
Left	L	While awake	WA
Less than	<	With (*cum*)	c̄
Moderate	mod.	Within normal limits	WNL
More than	>	Without (*sine*)	s̄
Negative	−	Zero	0
No, not, none	Ø		

Treatments/Dispositions			
Advanced cardiac life support	ACLS	Intermittent positive-pressure ventilation	IPPV
Advanced life support	ALS	Long spine board	LSB
Against medical advice	AMA	Nasal cannula	NC
Automated external defibrillator	AED	Nasogastric	NG
Bag-valve mask	BVM	Nasopharyngeal airway	NPA
Basic life support	BLS	No transport—refusal	NTR
Cardiopulmonary resuscitation	CPR	Nonrebreather mask	NRM
Carotid sinus massage	CSM	Nothing by mouth	NPO
Continuous positive airway pressure	CPAP	Occupational therapy	OT
Do not resuscitate	DNR	Oropharyngeal airway	OPA
Endotracheal tube	ETT	Oxygen	O_2
Estimated time of arrival	ETA	Per square inch	psi
External cardiac pacing	ECP	Physical therapy	PT

Table 10-1 Standard Charting Abbreviations *Continued*

Treatments/Dispositions			
Positive end-expiratory pressure	PEEP	Treatment	Tx
Short spine board	SSB	Turned over to	TOT
Therapy	Rx	Verbal order	VO

Medication Administration/Metrics			
Centimeter	cm	Keep vein open	KVO
Cubic centimeter	cc	Kilogram	kg
Deciliter	dL	Liter	L
Drop(s)	gtt(s)	Liters per minute	Lpm, L/min, liters/min
Drops per minute	gtts/min	Microgram	mcg
Every	Q	Milliequivalent	mEq
Grain	gr	Milligram	mg
Gram	g, gm	Milliliter	mL
Hour	h, hr, or °	Millimeter	mm
Hydrogen-ion concentration	pH	Millimeters of mercury	mmHg
Intracardiac	IC	Minute	min
Intramuscular	IM	Orally	PO
Intraosseous	IO	Subcutaneous	SC, SQ
Intravenous	IV	Sublingual	SL
Intravenous push	IVP	To keep open	TKO
Joules	J		

Cardiology			
Atrial fibrillation	AF	Paroxysmal atrial tachycardia	PAT
Atrial tachycardia	AT	Paroxysmal supraventricular tachycardia	PSVT
Atrioventricular	AV	Premature atrial contraction	PAC
Bundle branch block	BBB	Premature junctional contraction	PJC
Complete heart block	CHB	Premature ventricular contraction	PVC
Electromechanical dissociation	EMD	Pulseless electrical activity	PEA
Idioventricular rhythm	IVR	Supraventricular tachycardia	SVT
Junctional rhythm	JR	Ventricular fibrillation	VF
Modified chest lead	MCL	Ventricular tachycardia	VT
Normal sinus rhythm	NSR	Wandering atrial pacemaker	WAP

be the only permanent record of your discussion with the medical direction physician. Specifically, you should document any medical advice or orders you receive and the results of implementing that advice and those orders. In some situations, you might need to document what you reported to the physician and/or discussed with him, so the reader will be able to understand the decision-making process. Finally, always document the physician's name on your PCR and, if possible, have him sign it to verify your treatments.

Pertinent Negatives

The patient assessment and medical interventions are the essence of the EMS event and become the core of your PCR. We will discuss specific approaches to documenting assessment and interventions later in this chapter, but some general rules apply regardless of the method.

Document all findings of your assessment, even those that are normal. Although the positive findings are usually of most interest, some negative findings—known as *pertinent negatives*—are also important. For example, if your respiratory distress patient does not have swollen ankles or crackles, that helps rule out a field diagnosis of congestive heart failure. Or if your patient with a broken leg does not have loss of sensory or motor function, it suggests he has no serious neurologic injury. You should include such information in your report.

The pertinent negatives vary for each chief complaint. In general, if a positive assessment finding for any given chief complaint would be important, a negative finding probably is pertinent. Even though these findings do not warrant medical care or intervention, your seeking them demonstrates the thoroughness of your examination and history of the event.

Oral Statements

Also essential to every PCR, regardless of approach, are the statements of witnesses, bystanders, and your patient. They help to document the mechanism of injury, your patient's behavior, the events leading up to the emergency, and any first aid or medical care others rendered before you arrived. They also may include information regarding the disposition of personal items such as wallets or purses. At crime scenes, document safety-related information such as weapons disposition. Your PCR may be the only written report of what happened to a murder weapon. Other details such as where you first saw a victim, what position he was in, and the time you arrived on the scene may someday be crucial evidence in a criminal proceeding.

Whenever possible, quote the patient—or other source of information—directly. Clearly identify the quotation with quotation marks, and identify its source. For example:

> Bystanders state the patient was "acting bizarre and threatening to jump in front of the next passing car."

Additional Resources

Document all the resources involved in the event. If an air medical service transported your patient, your documentation should include your assessment and all interventions up to the point when you transferred care. Identify the air medical service and your patient's ultimate destination, if you know it. If other EMS, fire, rescue/extrication, or law enforcement agencies were involved in the call, document their roles. This can be particularly important in mutual aid calls, when many different agencies cooperate in your patient's care. Also include information about personnel from law enforcement and

the coroner's or medical examiner's office for dead-on-arrival (DOA) scenes.

If a physician stops to help, identify him by name and document his qualifying credentials. If one of your medical direction physicians is on the scene and directs care, document his activities. Likewise document the names, credentials, and activities of any other medically qualified personnel present who offer to help. Your clinical experience and local protocols will determine how you integrate qualified health care workers into your emergency scene. Document that integration carefully.

Elements of Good Documentation

A well-written PCR is accurate, legible, timely, unaltered, and professional. Each of these traits is essential.

Completeness and Accuracy

The accurate PCR should be precise but comprehensive.[2] Include all the relevant information that anyone might be expected to want later, and exclude superfluous information. For example, if your patient's foot was run over by a lawn mower, reporting that his great toe on that foot had been amputated six years ago would be important; documenting that he had his tonsils removed when he was three years old probably would not. That you applied direct pressure to the bleeding foot is pertinent; that the lawn mower was a John Deere model 6354 is not.

Many PCRs provide check boxes and a space for written narratives (Figure 10-4). You should complete both the narrative and check-box sections of every PCR. All check-box sections of a document must show that you attended to them, even if you did not use a given section on a call. The check boxes can help to ensure that routine, common information is recorded for every call, but no PCR has a check box for every possible chief complaint, assessment finding, or intervention.

The narrative is the core of the documentation. Even if you document something in a check box, repeating that information in the narrative might be worthwhile. By doing so, you can expand on the yes-or-no limitations of the check box to explain the timing, the assessment findings, the circumstances, or the changes in patient condition associated with

CONTENT REVIEW
➤ Elements of Good Documentation
- Complete
- Accurate
- Legible
- Timely
- Without alterations
- Professional
➤ Document exactly what you did, when you did it, and the effects of your interventions.

Prehospital Care Report

FOR BLS FR USE ONLY

M	D	Y				RUN NO.					AGENCY CODE			VEH. ID.

DATE OF CALL   RUN NO.   AGENCY CODE   VEH. ID.

Name

Address

Ph #

Agency Name	MILEAGE		USE MILITARY TIMES
Dispatch Information	END		CALL REC'D
Call Location	BEGIN		ENROUTE
	TOTAL		ARRIVED AT SCENE

CHECK ONE: ☐ Residence ☐ Health Facility ☐ Farm ☐ Indus. Facility ☐ Other Work Loc. ☐ Roadway ☐ Recreational ☐ Other

LOCATION CODE

FROM SCENE

AGE ☐☐☐ DOB M ☐☐ D ☐☐ Y ☐☐ SEX M☐ F☐

Physician

CALL TYPE AS REC'D.
☐ Emergency
☐ Non-Emergency
☐ Stand-by

COMPLETE FOR TRANSFERS ONLY
Transferred from ☐☐☐
☐ No Previous PCR
☐ Unknown if Previous PCR
Previous PCR Number ☐ - ☐☐☐☐☐

AT DESTIN
IN SERVICE
IN QUARTERS

CARE IN PROGRESS ON ARRIVAL:
☐ None   ☐ Citizen   ☐ PD/FD/Other First Responder   ☐ Other EMS

MECHANISM OF INJURY
☐ MVA (✓ seat belt used →)   ☐ Fall of ___ feet   ☐ GSW   ☐ Machinery
☐ Struck by vehicle   ☐ Unarmed assault   ☐ Knife   ☐ _____

☐ Extrication required _____ minutes

Seat belt used?
☐ Yes ☐ No ☐ Unknown

Seat Belt Use Reported By
☐ Crew ☐ Patient
☐ Police ☐ Other

CHIEF COMPLAINT   **SUBJECTIVE ASSESSMENT**

PRESENTING PROBLEM
If more than one checked, circle primary

☐ Airway Obstruction
☐ Respiratory Arrest
☐ Respiratory Distress
☐ Cardiac Related (Potential)
☐ Cardiac Arrest

☐ Allergic Reaction
☐ Syncope
☐ Stroke/CVA
☐ General Illness/Malaise
☐ Gastro-Intestinal Distress
☐ Diabetic Related (Potential)
☐ Pain

☐ Unconscious/Unresp.
☐ Seizure
☐ Behavioral Disorder
☐ Substance Abuse (Potential)
☐ Poisoning (Accidental)

☐ Shock
☐ Head Injury
☐ Spinal Injury
☐ Fracture/Dislocation
☐ Amputation

☐ Other _____

☐ Major Trauma
☐ Trauma-Blunt
☐ Trauma-Penetrating
☐ Soft Tissue Injury
☐ Bleeding/Hemorrhage

☐ OB/GYN
☐ Burns
Environmental
☐ Heat
☐ Cold
☐ Hazardous Materials
☐ Obvious Death

PAST MEDICAL HISTORY		TIME	RESP	PULSE	B.P.	LEVEL OF CONSCIOUSNESS	GCS	R	PUPILS	L	SKIN	STATUS
☐ None ☐ Allergy to ___ ☐ Hypertension ☐ Stroke ☐ Seizures ☐ Diabetes ☐ COPD ☐ Cardiac ☐ Other (List) ☐ Asthma Current Medications (List)	V I T A L S I G N S		Rate: ☐ Regular ☐ Shallow ☐ Labored	Rate: ☐ Regular ☐ Irregular		☐ Alert ☐ Voice ☐ Pain ☐ Unresp.			Normal Dilated Constricted Sluggish No-Reaction		☐ Unremarkable ☐ Cool ☐ Pale ☐ Warm ☐ Cyanotic ☐ Moist ☐ Flushed ☐ Dry ☐ Jaundiced	C U P S
			Rate: ☐ Regular ☐ Shallow ☐ Labored	Rate: ☐ Regular ☐ Irregular		☐ Alert ☐ Voice ☐ Pain ☐ Unresp.			Normal Dilated Constricted Sluggish No-Reaction		☐ Unremarkable ☐ Cool ☐ Pale ☐ Warm ☐ Cyanotic ☐ Moist ☐ Flushed ☐ Dry ☐ Jaundiced	C U P S
			Rate: ☐ Regular ☐ Shallow ☐ Labored	Rate: ☐ Regular ☐ Irregular		☐ Alert ☐ Voice ☐ Pain ☐ Unresp.			Normal Dilated Constricted Sluggish No-Reaction		☐ Unremarkable ☐ Cool ☐ Pale ☐ Warm ☐ Cyanotic ☐ Moist ☐ Flushed ☐ Dry ☐ Jaundiced	C U P S

OBJECTIVE PHYSICAL ASSESSMENT

COMMENTS

TREATMENT GIVEN
☐ Moved to ambulance on stretcher/backboard
☐ Moved to ambulance on stair chair
☐ Walked to ambulance
☐ Airway Cleared
☐ Oral/Nasal Airway
☐ Esophageal Obturator Airway/Esophageal Gastric Tube Airway (EOA/EGTA)
☐ EndoTracheal Tube (E/T)
☐ Oxygen Administered @ ___ L.P.M., Method _____
☐ Suction Used
☐ Artificial Ventilation Method _____
☐ C.P.R. in progress on arrival by: ☐ Citizen ☐ PD/FD/Other First Responder ☐ Other
☐ C.P.R. Started @ Time ▶ _____
Time from Arrest Until C.P.R. ▶ ___ Minutes
☐ EKG Monitored (Attach Tracing) [Rhythm(s) _____]
☐ Defibrillation/Cardioversion No. Times ___ ☐ Manual ☐ Semi-automatic

☐ Medication Administered (Use Continuation Form)
☐ IV Established Fluid _____ Cath. Gauge ☐☐
☐ Mast Inflated @ Time _____)
☐ Bleeding/Hemorrhage Controlled (Method Used: _____)
☐ Spinal Immobilization Neck and Back
☐ Limb Immobilized by ☐ Fixation ☐ Traction
☐ (Heat) or (Cold) Applied
☐ Vomiting Induced @ Time ___ Method _____
☐ Restraints Applied, Type _____
☐ Baby Delivered @ Time ___ In County _____
        ☐ Alive   ☐ Stillborn   ☐ Male   ☐ Female
☐ Transported in Trendelenburg position
☐ Transported in left lateral recumbent position
☐ Transported with head elevated
☐ Other _____

DISPOSITION (See list)

DISP. CODE ☐☐☐

CONTINUATION FORM USED YES ←

CREW	IN CHARGE	DRIVER'S NAME	NAME	NAME
	☐ EMT ☐ AEMT #	☐ CFR ☐ EMT ☐ AEMT #	☐ CFR ☐ EMT ☐ AEMT #	☐ CFR ☐ EMT ☐ AEMT #

AGENCY COPY/WHITE

EMS 100 (11/86) provided by NYS-EMS PROGRAM
DOH 3822 (6/94)

FIGURE 10-4 Complete both the narrative and check-box sections of every PCR.

(PCR with narrative and check-box sections. Copyright © by NYS Department of Health Bureau of EMS. Used by permission of NYS Department of Health Bureau of EMS.)

the indicated action. Always make sure that the information in your checked boxes and in your narrative are consistent. Inconsistencies will be extremely difficult to explain later on, especially in front of a jury.

Remember that proper spelling, approved abbreviations, and proper acronyms also affect your PCR's accuracy. Misspelled words lose their meaning; many abbreviations are not universally recognized; and several acronyms have more than one meaning. Make sure that the meaning of any abbreviation or acronym is clear.

Legibility

Poor penmanship and illegible reports lead to poor documentation. Some EMS providers say, "I wrote it, and I can read it. That's all that matters." This is simply not true. The PCR does not exist solely for its author's reference. It is a permanent record that many different people use. Your handwriting must be neat enough that other people can read and understand the report, especially the narrative. It must also be neat enough that you can read and understand it yourself many years from now, long after the event has faded from your memory. Your writing must be heavy enough to transfer to any carbon copies. Using a ballpoint pen whenever possible makes carbon copies more legible and makes it difficult for someone to tamper with the document. Clearly mark the check boxes to eliminate any doubt that a check mark is not just a meaningless scratch. Always remember that other members of the health care team may use the report for medical information, research, or quality improvement.

Timeliness

As a rule, you should avoid writing your report in the ambulance during transport of your patient for two reasons. First, the bumpy ride makes it difficult to write neatly. More importantly, your time is better spent communicating with your patient and conducting ongoing assessments. Most hospitals have an area where you can sit and complete your paperwork once patient care has been transferred.

Ideally, you should complete your report immediately after you complete the emergency call, when the information is fresh in your mind and you can check with your partner or patient if you have any questions about the events. At times you may be too busy to complete the entire documentation immediately following a call. If so, make notes on scratch paper and write enough of the report that you will be able to finish it completely and accurately later. The sooner you finish it, the more details you are likely to recall and the better the report will be.

Absence of Alterations

Mistakes happen. During a busy shift or in the middle of the night you will check the wrong box, misspell a word, or omit important information. You will be thinking of one medication and write another's name on your report. If you make a mistake writing your report, simply cross through the error with one line and initial it (Figure 10-5). Some systems may expect you to date the correction as well. Do not scribble over or blacken out any area of the call report. Never try to hide an error. Such foolish tactics only raise the reader's curiosity about what you wrote originally. After crossing out the error, continue with the correct information. If you find the error after you've already written several more sentences, submit an **addendum**.

Whenever possible, have everyone involved in the call read or reread the PCR before you submit it. Make all corrections before you submit the report to the hospital or to the EMS administrative offices. Do not make changes on the original report after you have submitted it. If for any reason you need to make corrections after you have submitted the report, or some portion of it, place an addendum. Simply note on the original report, "See addendum," and attach the addendum to the original report. Write the addendum on a separate sheet of paper or on an official form if one exists. Likewise, if more information comes to your attention after you have submitted the report, write a supplemental narrative on a separate report form.

Write any addendum to your report as soon as you realize that you made an error or that additional information is needed. Note the purpose of the revision and why the information did not appear on your original report. The addendum should document the date and time that it was written, the reason it was written, and the pertinent information. Only the original author of a report should attach an addendum, as it is part of the official call record. Agencies should have separate forms for other EMS personnel, supervisors, or citizens who, for some reason, want to contribute to the documentation.

FIGURE 10-5 The proper way to correct a PCR is to draw a single line through the error, write the correct information beside it, and initial the change.

The ~~left~~ *JM* right pupil was fixed and dilated

Professionalism

Write your report in a professional manner. Remember that someday it may be scrutinized by hospital staff, quality improvement committees, supervisors, lawyers, and the news media. Your patient's family may request, and is entitled to, a copy of your report from your agency. Write cautiously and avoid any remarks that might be construed as derogatory. **Jargon** can be confusing and does little to enhance your image. Do not describe a patient well known to EMS providers as a "frequent flyer." Never include slang, biased statements, or irrelevant opinions. Include only objective information. "The patient smelled of beer and had slurred speech and difficulty walking" are factual statements. "The patient was very drunk" is an inference; even if accurate, it is still just your opinion. **Libel** and **slander** are, respectively, writing or speaking false and malicious words intended to damage a person's character. Always write and speak carefully. A seemingly innocent phrase or comment can come back to haunt you.

Narrative Writing

The narrative is the part of the written report in which you depict the call at length. Less structured than the check-box or fill-in sections of your report, the narrative allows you the freedom to describe your assessment findings in detail. When other people read your report, they usually will rely on your written narrative for the most relevant information. For example, as you transfer care to the emergency nurse, the nurse will usually scan your PCR for information concerning your patient's history, vital signs, and physical exam.

Narrative Sections

Any patient documentation includes three sections of importance: the subjective narrative, the objective narrative, and the assessment/management plan.

Subjective Narrative

The subjective part of your narrative typically comprises any information that you elicit during your patient's history. This includes the chief complaint (CC), the history of present illness (HPI), the past history (PH), the current health status (CHS), and the review of systems (ROS). In trauma, this also includes the mechanism of injury (MOI), as told to you by your patient or bystanders. The following is a typical subjective narrative on a patient complaining of shortness of breath:

CC:	The patient is a 74-year-old conscious black female who complains, "I can't catch my breath."

HPI	Gradual onset of severe shortness of breath for the past 3 hours; began while sitting in living room watching television; nothing provokes or relieves the dyspnea; her son states this is worse than usual for her. She has had a three-day history of some vague chest discomfort. She denies any chest pressure, nausea, or dizziness.
PH	She has a five-year history of heart problems and congestive heart failure; hospitalized for this problem three times in the past five years; no surgeries.
CHS	Meds: Isosorbide, nitroglycerin, furosemide, digoxin, potassium; no known drug allergies; 50 pack/year smoker; nondrinker; non-drug abuser.
ROS	Resp: Unproductive cough for one day; audible wheezing; no hx of COPD or asthma; last chest X-ray one year ago. Card: no palpitations, pressure, or pain; + orthopnea; + paroxysmal nocturnal dyspnea; + edema for past few days; past ECG one year ago. GU: No changes in urinary patterns. Per. Vasc: + pitting edema for few days; cold feet.

Objective Narrative

The objective part of your narrative usually includes your general impression and any data that you derive through inspection, palpation, auscultation, percussion, and diagnostic testing. This includes vital signs, physical exam, and tests such as cardiac monitoring, pulse oximetry, and blood glucose determination.

To document your physical exam, you can use either of two approaches: head-to-toe or body systems. Although the medical community accepts both extensively, emergency medical services more often use the head-to-toe approach.

HEAD-TO-TOE APPROACH The head-to-toe approach is well suited for any call when you perform an entire physical exam, because you document your findings in the same order in which you conducted the exam—from head to toe. However, even though you may have conducted your pediatric assessment from toe to head, you should document it in head-to-toe order. This style encourages you to be systematic and thorough. It is appropriate for major trauma and serious medical emergencies, when you examine every body area and system. Include all circulatory and

CONTENT REVIEW

➤ Physical Exam Documentation Approaches
- Head-to-toe approach
- Body systems approach

neurologic findings within the body area you are documenting. For example, when recording findings in the extremities, include distal neurovascular function. When documenting the head, include the results of cranial nerve testing. The following illustrates the head-to-toe approach for a patient who has been in a collision:

General	The patient presents in the front seat of the car, in moderate distress with bruises to his forehead and some facial lacerations. Pt. is alert and oriented to self, time, and place.
Vital signs	Pulse—100 strong, regular radial; BP—110/88; resp—24 nonlabored; skin pale and cool.
HEENT	Depression to right frontal bone, minor bleeding controlled prior to arrival; no drainage from ears, nose. No periorbital ecchymosis or Battle's sign; pupils equal and reactive to light; extraocular movements intact, cranial nerves II–XII intact.
Neck	Trachea midline; no jugular vein distention; + cervical spine tenderness.
Chest	Equal expansion; bruises across the chest wall; no deformities; equal bilateral breath sounds.
Abdomen	Soft, nontender, nondistended.
Pelvis	Unstable pelvic ring; pain on palpation.
Extremities	+ Circulation, sensory, and motor function in all four extremities; no deformities noted.
Posterior	No obvious injuries noted.
Labs	Sinus tachycardia, no ectopy, pulse oximetry 97% on supplemental oxygen.

BODY SYSTEMS APPROACH The body systems approach, as the name indicates, focuses on body systems instead of body areas. It is best suited to screening and preadmission exams in which you conduct a comprehensive exam involving all body systems. Each body system has different key components that you should assess and document.

When you use the body systems approach in emergency medicine, you usually will focus only on the system, or systems, involved in the current illness or injury. For example, a patient having an asthma attack would require an in-depth evaluation of the respiratory system. Another patient with lower abdominal pain would need a close examination of the gastrointestinal system. Neither patient would require a full head-to-toe physical exam but, instead,

would need intensive documentation of the affected body system or systems. The body systems approach can be one of the most comprehensive approaches to documentation. The following illustrates a body systems approach for a patient with chest pain and shortness of breath:

General	Patient is a healthy-looking female who presents sitting upright in her chair, able to speak in phrases only.
Vital Signs	Pulse—irregular, 90; BP—170/80; resp—28 labored; skin—warm and diaphoretic.
HEENT	+ Lip cyanosis and pursing; some nasal flaring; pink, frothy sputum; jugular veins distended.
Respiratory	Labored respiratory effort; accessory neck muscle use; trachea midline; + intercostal, supraclavicular, suprasternal retractions; = chest expansion; diffuse crackles and wheezing in all lung fields, decreased breath sounds.
Per. Vasc.	+ Ascites fluid wave; + 2 pitting edema in lower extremities; strong peripheral pulses.
Labs	Sinus tachycardia with occasional unifocal premature ventricular contractions. Pulse oximetry—92% room air; 97% on supplemental oxygen.

Assessment/Management Plan

In the assessment/management section, you document what you believe to be your patient's problem. This is also known as your **field diagnosis**, or impression. For example, your field diagnosis for a patient with chest pain may be "possible angina or rule out myocardial infarction." You do not have to make an exact diagnosis. When you are not sure, simply document what you suspect is the general problem. Sometimes, for instance, your field impression might be "rule out acute abdomen, or seizures." *Rule out* identifies possible diagnoses that you believe the emergency physician should evaluate.

Record your complete management plan from start to finish. This includes how you packaged and moved your patient to the ambulance. Did you carry him on a stair-chair or on a backboard fully immobilized, or did he walk? List any interventions you completed before contacting your medical control physician. For example, did you control bleeding with direct pressure? Did you start an IV? Then describe any orders from the medical control physician, and always include his name. Describe how you transported your patient and the effects of any interventions such as drug administration or other invasive procedures. Include the results of ongoing assessments and any changes in your patient's condition. Finally, describe your patient's condition when you transferred care to the emergency staff. The following example is a management plan for a trauma patient with a pelvic fracture whose condition deteriorates en route to the hospital:

On-Scene

Extrication	Rapid extrication from vehicle, placed supine on backboard
Airway	Airway cleared with suctioning, nasopharyngeal airway inserted
Breathing	Oxygen @ 15 liters/min via nonrebreather mask
Circulation	Foot of stretcher raised 30°; bleeding from arm laceration controlled with dry sterile dressing and direct pressure; PASG applied; IV—16 ga. left antecubital area—normal saline run KVO per Dr. Johnson.

Transport

Transported by ground ambulance to University Hospital with full body immobilization supine on long spine board; ETA 10 minutes.

Ongoing	Patient becomes restless and anxious; VS: pulse—120 weak carotid only, BP—50 palpated, resp—28, skin: cool, pale, clammy with some mottling; PASG inflated; initial IV run wide open; second IV 16 ga. right antecubital normal saline—run wide open.

Arrival

Patient transferred to ED staff; restless; VS: pulse 120, BP—80 palpated, resp—26, skin—mottled and cool.

General Formats

The acronyms SOAP and CHART are memory aids that identify two common patterns for organizing a narrative report. These acronyms provide templates that can be used for most medical and trauma reports. They help you to arrange your history, physical exam, and management plan into a logical, readable structure. They are widely used

because they group information in categories that differentiate between subjective and objective information. For example, someone wanting only to determine your patient's medications can find that list easily in history or current health status segments of either the SOAP or the CHART format. Either pattern is acceptable and effective when used consistently.

SOAP Format

SOAP stands for *S*ubjective, *O*bjective, *A*ssessment, and *P*lan. The detailed SOAP format includes:

Subjective	• Chief complaint • History of present illness • Past history • Current health status • Family history • Psychosocial history • Review of systems
Objective	• Vital signs • General impression • Physical exam • Diagnostic tests
Assessment	• Field diagnosis
Plan	• Standing orders • Physician orders • Effects of interventions • Mode of transportation • Ongoing assessment

CHART Format

CHART stands for *C*hief complaint, *H*istory, *A*ssessment, *R*x (treatment), and *T*ransport. The detailed CHART format includes:

Chief complaint	• Primary problem or complaint
History	• History of present illness • Past history • Current health status • Review of systems
Assessment	• Vital signs • General impression • Physical exam • Diagnostic tests • Field diagnosis

Rx	• Standing orders
	• Physician orders
Transport	• Effects of interventions
	• Mode of transportation
	• Ongoing assessment

Other Formats

Like patient assessment itself, documentation is not "one size fits all." No one narrative format is ideal for all situations. Two additional formats—patient management and call incident—are appropriate in certain circumstances.

PATIENT MANAGEMENT The patient management format is preferred for some critical patients, such as those in cardiac arrest, when you focus on immediately managing a variety of patient problems and not on conducting a thorough history and physical exam. This format is a chronological account from the time you arrived on the scene until you transferred care to someone else. It emphasizes your assessment and management of the conditions you found. Simply begin your chart with a description of the event and any other pertinent information and then document your management, starting with your airway, breathing, and circulation (ABC) assessment. Record everything in real time and in absolute chronological order, and always include the results of your interventions. A patient management chart would look like this:

Patient is an 89-year-old Hispanic male who was found by his wife unconscious on the floor immediately after collapsing. He presents pulseless and apneic.

Time	Intervention
1320	Immediate CPR while monitor applied.
1322	Quick look—ventricular fibrillation.
1322	Defibrillation @ 200 joules—no change.
1323	CPR resumed; IV access 18 gauge left antecubital area—normal saline KVO; epinephrine 1:10,000 1 mg IVP.
1325	Defibrillation @ 200 joules—no change;
1326	CPR resumed; amiodarone 300 mg IVP.
1328	Defibrillation @ 260 joules—patient converts to normal sinus rhythm rate of 72 with strong peripheral pulses, BP—110/76, no spontaneous respirations. ET tube inserted. + lung sounds bilaterally with BVM.
1330	Ventilation continued @ 12/min via BVM;
1332	Patient transferred to ambulance on stretcher—transported to University Hospital.

Time	Intervention
1335	Patient has spontaneous respirations @ 20/min, + bilateral breath sounds; becoming more awake; HR—72, BP—120/76.
1340	Arrived at UH—Patient is conscious, alert, and oriented with retrograde amnesia.

CALL INCIDENT The call incident approach simply emphasizes the mechanism of injury, the surrounding circumstances, and how the incident occurred. Use this approach to begin documenting a trauma call with a significant mechanism of injury. It is most suitable when the events surrounding the call might be significant. It would be inappropriate for a man sitting in his living room with chest pain or for someone who simply cut his finger with a carving knife. You may use this style in both the subjective and objective sections of your PCR. The following example shows call incident documentation for a motor vehicle crash:

Subjective	The patient is a 46-year-old conscious and alert white male who was an unrestrained driver in a low-speed, head-on, two-car motor vehicle crash, moderate front-end damage, no passenger compartment intrusion, deformity to windshield, dashboard, and steering wheel. Patient states he "reached for cigarette on floor and when he looked up, there was another vehicle in front of him." He denies any loss of consciousness and can recall all details prior to and immediately following the crash. Patient complains of pain to the head, neck, chest, and hip from being thrown against the dashboard and windshield.
Objective	The patient presents in the front seat of the car, appears in moderate distress with bruises to his forehead, facial lacerations, and a deformed left leg. His left leg is pinned underneath the dashboard with his left foot hooked around the brake pedal. On arrival, fire department rescue personnel were holding manual stabilization of his head and neck and stabilizing the vehicle.

These are not the only systems of documentation. Indeed, you may use some combination of these systems or develop a unique format for your regional system. The important thing is for your documentation to be complete, accurate, and consistent. By using the same system to document every call, you will be less likely to accidentally overlook or omit something.

Special Considerations

Some circumstances create special problems for EMS documentation. Patient refusals, calls when transport is unnecessary, multiple patients, and mass casualties are among the more common examples. In these and other unusual circumstances, take extra care to document everything that happened during the call.

Patient Refusals

Two types of patients might refuse care. The first type is the person who is not seriously ill or injured and simply does not want to go to the hospital. For example, the belted driver in a minor automobile crash has an abrasion on his knee from striking the dashboard. He is alert and oriented, has no other injuries, and claims he will seek medical attention if it bothers him later. This type of patient usually signs your PCR in a special place marked "Refusal of Care," and you return to service.[3]

The second type of patient is more worrisome. This patient refuses care even though you feel he needs it. This is known as **against medical advice (AMA)**. Some legal experts regard AMA as your failure to convince your patient to accept necessary treatment and transport. Such patient refusals are particularly troublesome because they have the most potential to end badly. Still, patients retain the right to refuse treatment or transportation if they are competent to make that decision and are not actively suicidal.

Although you cannot make a legal determination of competence (sometimes it takes a court decision), document that you believe your patient was competent to refuse care. Although specific laws vary from state to state, your patient will demonstrate competence by his understanding of the circumstances and the risks associated with refusing care and by accepting those risks and the responsibility for refusing care. Assess your patient as thoroughly as possible, with special emphasis on his mental status and behavior. Pay extra attention to any patient suspected of being under the influence of drugs or alcohol. Clearly document that your patient has an adequate mental status and understands your field diagnosis, alternative treatments, and the consequences of refusing care. In addition, record his reason for refusing care (Table 10-2).

Even after you document your patient's competence, most patient refusals require more thorough documentation than the typical EMS run because the opportunity for and consequences of abandonment charges are tremendous. Simply having your patient sign your PCR is not sufficient. Again, document that you described your patient's injuries to him and that he understood the risks of refusing treatment and transport. Inform him of potential complications from injuries that might not be obvious. Discuss those associated risks as well, and document this discussion.

Table 10-2 Refusal of Care Documentation Checklist

- Thorough patient assessment
- Competency of patient
- Your recommendation for care and transport
- Explanation to the patient about possible consequences of refusing care, including possibility of death, if appropriate
- Other suggestions for accessing care
- Willingness to return if patient changes mind
- Patient's understanding of statements and suggestions and apparent competence to refuse care based on that understanding

Also document any involvement of the patient's family or friends.

Because ruling out serious injury is all but impossible in the field, you may need to make clear the possibility of your patient's dying. Although this might seem extreme, it plainly conveys that the risks are serious. A patient who was informed that he was at risk of dying, refused care, and subsequently had his leg amputated because of an infection would have a hard time convincing a jury that he did not think the risks were serious.

In many systems, you must contact the medical direction physician before allowing a patient to refuse transport. If you confer with a physician, document any information, advice, or orders that the physician gives you. If your patient speaks directly to the physician, document that as well. Once more, document that your patient understands the circumstances and the risks and still chooses to refuse transport. Note that you instructed him to call an ambulance or go to the emergency department if his condition worsened, or if he just changed his mind. You can ask a bystander or law enforcement officer to witness the patient refusal, although this is not always required.[4]

Your documentation also should include a complete narrative with quotations and statements from others on the scene. For example, if your patient's wife and son plead with him to go to the hospital, include their comments in your report. If your system uses a specific form for patient refusals, complete that paperwork as well (Figure 10-6). The additional form, however, is not a substitute for a complete documentation of the circumstances.

Services Not Needed

Some systems allow you to determine that your patient does not need ambulance transport. Although such policies help to reduce ambulance utilization rates, the risks of denying transport are even greater than those of patient refusals. In these cases, the documentation must clearly demonstrate that transport was unnecessary. As with patient refusals, document any discussion you have with

---

RELEASE FROM RESPONSIBILITY

DATE _____ 19 _____ TIME _____ a.m.
                                               p.m.

This is to certify that _____

is refusing   ☐ TREATMENT   ☐ TRANSPORTATION

against the advice of the attending Emergency Medical Technician and of the Phoenix Fire Department, and when applicable, the base hospital and the base hospital physician.

I acknowledge that I have been informed of the following:

1. The nature and potential of the illness or injuries.
2. The potential risks of delaying treatment and transportation, up to and including death.
3. The availability of ambulance transportation to a hospital for treatment.

Nevertheless, I assume all risks and consequences of my decision, including further physical deterioration, loss of limb, paralysis, and even death, and hereby release the attending Emergency Medical Technician and the Phoenix Fire Department, and when applicable, the base hospital and the base hospital physician from any ill effects which may result from my refusal.

Witness _____   Signed: **X** _____

Witness _____   Relationship to Patient _____

Refusal must be signed by the patient; or by the nearest relative or legal guardian in the case of a minor, or when patient is physically or mentally incompetent.

☐ Patient refuses to sign release despite efforts of attending Emergency Medical Technician to obtain such signature after informing patient of concerns listed in numbers 1, 2, and 3 above.

GUIDELINES — Patient Refusal Documentation

In addition to those items normally documented (chief complaint, history of present illness, mechanism of injury, physical assessment, etc.) the following items should be recorded, regardless of patient's cooperation:

● Mental Status (orientation, speech, etc.)

● Suspected presence of alcohol or drugs

● Patient's exact words (as much as possible) in the refusal of care OR the signing of the release form

● Circumstances or reasons (including exact words of patient, if possible) for INCOMPLETE ADVISEMENT (risk of injury, abusiveness, unruliness, risk of injury other than from patient, etc.)

● Advice given to patients' guardian(s)

FIGURE 10-6 One example of a refusal of care form.

the emergency physician and any advice you give to your patient.

Transportation may not be needed for other reasons, as well. Ambulances are often called to minor accidents where no injuries have occurred. When this happens, first responders such as the fire department rescue unit or a police agency might cancel the ambulance. If the ambulance is canceled en route, document the canceling authority and the time of notification. If you arrive on the scene and find no patients, document that. If, when you arrive, you are canceled by on-scene personnel, document that you made no patient contact and record the person and agency that canceled you. The difference between "no patients found" and "only minor injuries, patients refusing transport" is considerable. Although they might refuse transport, evaluate people with even the most minor injuries. Consider them patients and document them accurately.

Multiple Casualty Incidents

Multiple patients, mass casualties, and disasters all present special documentation problems. The number of patients needing care and transport during such situations may overwhelm you. Often, more than one ambulance crew cares for the many patients. Some EMS personnel may fill only support roles and never actually provide patient care. Obtaining complete patient information might be impossible, and completing documentation for one patient before going on to care for others might be impractical.[5]

In these situations, you must weigh your patients' needs against the demand for complete documentation. Document as much as possible—as quickly as possible—on your PCR. You can complete the documentation later as an addendum. If you cannot remember the particulars of a specific patient or transport, do not guess. Document only what you know to be factual and accurate. A simple note at the end of the documentation explaining the circumstances will account for any missing information.

Some EMS agencies use special forms for multiple patient events, and most provide a general incident report form or record that anyone connected with the call may complete. You should become familiar with local policies and procedures for documenting these situations. Many systems use **triage tags** to record vital information on each patient quickly (Figure 10-7). A triage tag has just enough room for your patient's vital information—name, major

FRONT

BACK

FIGURE 10-7 A triage tag offers a quick way to record vital information.

(Triage Tag front and back. Copyright © by The American Civil Defense Association. Used by permission of The American Civil Defense Association.)

injuries, vital signs, treatment, and priority (urgent, nonurgent). You affix it to your patient, and it remains there throughout the event; you can transfer its information to your PCR later. Whatever your local policies, document as completely and accurately as possible without detracting from patient care.

Consequences of Inappropriate Documentation

Inappropriate documentation can have both medical and legal consequences.[6] The medical consequences of inadequate documentation are potentially the most serious. Health care providers across several disciplines may refer to your PCR in planning their care for a patient. Do not

guess about your patient's medical problems if you are not certain. An inaccurate or incomplete report can affect patient care for many hours, or even days, after the ambulance call ends. Failing to document a medication allergy or documenting an incorrect medical history could have grave effects. If no one can read your sloppy report, it is useless despite the importance of its information. Good documentation now enables good care later.[7]

The potential legal consequences of inadequate

CONTENT REVIEW

➤ Consequences of Poor or Good Documentation
  • Medical:
    • Poor documentation can result in poor care; good documentation contributes to good care.
  • Legal:
    • Poor documentation encourages frivolous lawsuits; good documentation discourages them.

documentation are enormous. If poor documentation results in inappropriate care, you may be held responsible. Or if the documentation does not make it clear that you informed a patient of the risks when he refused transport, you may be legally accountable for any harmful consequences. If the documentation does not explicitly say the patient in ventricular fibrillation was defibrillated immediately, you might be accused of providing inadequate care. Even though you did everything appropriately, poor, incomplete, or inaccurate documentation will encourage anyone who is pursuing a frivolous lawsuit. Good documentation discourages such actions. Always remember that if it is not documented, you did not do it.

Inaccurate, incomplete, illegible documentation also reflects poorly on the EMS provider writing the report. Missing information, misspelled words, and poor penmanship give the impression of a sloppy, incompetent provider. Good documentation, on the other hand, enhances the EMS provider's professional stature.

Electronic Patient Care Records

A growing trend in EMS is the use of computerized patient record-keeping software, also known as electronic patient care records, or ePCRs.[8] A number of ePCR systems are available. These platforms offer some advantages over the traditional paper chart; however, they also carry some drawbacks.[9]

The benefits of ePCR systems are numerous. The following is a partial list:

- *Greater ease of data collection and analysis.* These systems are built on a database platform, which makes data analysis and reporting significantly faster than trying to read through hundreds of paper charts, looking for a specific key word.

- *A consistent, uniform, easily read patient chart,* which can be a benefit to hospitals, nurses, and physicians.

- *The reduction of poor penmanship and spelling errors* common to handwritten charts.

- *The opportunity for an EMS administrator to configure and alter the software* to best suit that service's particular operational model, needs, and requirements. Because different states use different mandatory data sets for reporting, different fields may be required.

- *Integration with dispatch software, billing services, and regulatory agencies.*

- *Interface with medical devices.* For example, cardiac monitor data can be uploaded into the ePCR software.

- *Better quality assurance processes, chart reviews, and feedback to the EMT or paramedic.*

Data within the ePCR software can be collected in several different ways. Some fields may include a simple "pick from" list, on which acceptable values are presented and the EMT can select the appropriate item or items from the list (Figure 10-8).

Other parts of the ePCR software may include a graphic interface. For example, patient body surveys are often collected using a picture of a person and a list of clinical findings. To record the proper findings, the EMT would select the body part and then the appropriate finding: "right lower leg—amputation," as an example (Figure 10-9).

Another means for entering data is manual entry, in which the EMT types in the correct value. This is most commonly seen in the "Vital Signs" or "Times" sections, where most values are numeric (Figure 10-10).

There are many benefits to implementation and use of an ePCR system, as already noted, but there are drawbacks as well. First, and most obvious, is the cost. Such programs vary in price, but all of them have a price tag that some EMS agencies might find prohibitive. Once past the initial cost, there may be yearly fees for technical support, upgrades,

FIGURE 10-8 A sample screen snap from ePCR.

(© ESO Solutions)

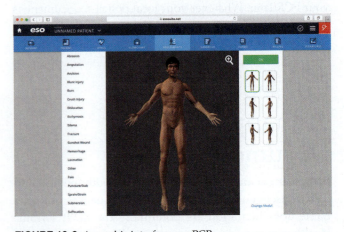

FIGURE 10-9 A graphic interface on ePCR.

(© ESO Solutions)

FIGURE 10-10 Example of an ePCR manual entry screen.

(© ESO Solutions)

and continued support from the software vendor. Additionally, as with any advanced software program, ePCR systems require that one or more people within the organization are technically savvy enough to administer and deal with any day-to-day issues. Finally, there is often an institutional reluctance or push-back from the field crews, who may be resistant to change: "We've always done paper charts, so why do we need to change now?" or "We're too busy to take time to get used to some new system." The positives, negatives, costs, and benefits of ePCR software must be evaluated individually by each EMS operation.

Closing

As a paramedic, you will assume responsibility for your documentation. Although documentation is often a begrudged task, it is one of the most important parts of an EMS call. Ensuring that your documentation is complete, accurate, legible, and appropriate is one of your professional responsibilities. As a professional, you should recognize this responsibility and set a positive example for others as you fulfill it.

Your report's confidentiality cannot be overemphasized. Confidentiality is your patient's legal right. Do not discuss your report with anyone not medically connected directly with the case. Generally, you are allowed to share patient information with another health care provider who will continue care, with third-party billing companies, with the police if it is relevant to a criminal investigation, and with the court if it issues a subpoena. Your report also may be used for quality assurance or research. In these cases, block out the patient's name.

Electronic charting will certainly become common in the future. Several systems now on the market allow you to enter data electronically, transmit that information to the receiving facility, and immediately receive a printed report. When you use such systems, remember that the principles of effective documentation still apply.

Legal Considerations

The PCR: Your Best Friend or Your Worst Enemy. It is often difficult to sit and write a PCR after a long and difficult call. However, the importance of this record cannot be overemphasized. Years later, when the call is nothing but a distant memory, the PCR will be there to provide the facts and details of the patient encounter. Thus, for accuracy and clarity, the PCR must be completed as soon as possible after the call when all the facts are known. Waiting even a few hours may result in a PCR that is less than complete or is inaccurate.

The PCR is a valuable document. Not only does it provide medical personnel with the details of care provided in the prehospital setting, but it can also protect prehospital providers from negligence claims and malpractice allegations. In a court of law, it has been said, what is not documented in the patient record was not performed. Although this may not always be the case, it is difficult to prove that a certain prehospital procedure was performed if it was not documented in the PCR.

Although still relatively uncommon, malpractice suits against EMS personnel are on the rise. Most claims of negligence include such allegations as failure to secure and maintain an airway, failure to follow accepted protocols, failure to transport when care was necessary, and failure to properly restrain a combative or dangerous patient. You should be aware of the various aspects of EMS practice that can result in allegations of negligence and document these accurately. For example, proper placement of an endotracheal tube should be verified by at least three methods and documented in the PCR. In addition, you should document that the tube remained in proper position by repeated patient evaluations and through use of monitoring systems such as capnography and pulse oximetry. You must also document care to show that you followed appropriate protocols and standing orders. If you deviated from these, you must document in detail why this occurred and whether medical direction was contacted.

Patient refusal is a difficult area for EMS. Competent patients have the right to refuse medical care, even when the failure to obtain medical care may result in harm. However, paramedics cannot adequately determine which patients are competent and which are not (competency is a finding of law). Thus, when faced with a nontransport situation, document the circumstances well and obtain a statement from a third-party witness to the refusal.

Patient restraint poses a significant risk for both the patient and rescuers. Always follow local protocols regarding patient restraint and document that these were followed. Try to involve law enforcement personnel in any situation in which restraint may be needed.

If you are sued for negligence, the PCR can be either your best friend or your worst enemy. If you prepared it well and documented details of the call, then you have little to worry about. If you prepared it sloppily or incompletely, then be prepared to answer a lot of difficult questions. Always take the time to prepare an accurate patient report—you will not regret it when it is needed.

Summary

Regardless of the system you use for documentation, all EMS records should possess the same basic attributes. Appropriate terminology, proper spelling, accepted abbreviations and acronyms, and accurate times are essential. A description of the patient assessment and interventions, including pertinent negatives and communications with on-line physicians, is equally important. Finally, all the personnel and resources involved in a call must be documented. The record must be accurate and precise, free of jargon, and neatly written. Corrections should be made properly, including the use of an addendum when appropriate.

Prehospital care providers may use many systems of documentation, including the CHART and SOAP formats. Whatever system you use, it is best if you use the same one consistently. This results in more reliable, complete documentation and reduces the chances of omitting important information. Any of the existing documentation systems can incorporate a head-to-toe assessment of the patient. Special situations, such as multiple patients and refusals of transportation, require extra attention. They are often the most difficult calls to document, yet they are also the calls for which good documentation can be most valuable. A complete narrative—in addition to any check boxes—is the best way to ensure that all the necessary information is documented.

Although EMS providers frequently dislike documentation, it is one of the most important parts of the EMS call. Ensuring that the documentation is complete, accurate, legible, and appropriate is one of an EMS provider's professional responsibilities. Your PCR, whether written or electronic, is the only permanent record of the ambulance call and the only permanent reflection of your professionalism.

You Make the Call

While helping the quality assurance officer in your agency, you come across the following narrative: "We were dispatched to a 10-48, coroner Main/Spice. Vehicle is upside down. PMD on scene reports no serious injuries. Patient is nasty and abusive. Looks like a drug abuser. Is walking around acting abnoctious. Minor injuries identified and treated per protocol. Police arrested patient. EMS transport not needed."

1. What is wrong with this narrative? (You should be able to identify at least ten faults.)

2. What will you do to make sure your documentation is better than this?

See Suggested Responses at the back of this book.

Review Questions

1. Your prehospital care report will be a valuable resource for _____
   a. medical professionals.
   c. researchers.
   b. EMS administrators.
   d. all of the above.

2. You should always attempt to complete your PCR _____
   a. at the scene.
   b. en route to the hospital.
   c. immediately after the call.
   d. at the end of your duty shift.

3. The proper way to correct an error in your handwritten prehospital care report is to

   _____

   a. completely and immediately blacken out the error.
   b. draw a single line through the error, correct, and initial.
   c. highlight the error and place quotation marks around it.
   d. erase the error completely and enter the correct information.

4. The call incident approach to documentation emphasizes _____

  a. the mechanisms of injury.

  b. all the information you provided to the hospital during your field report.

  c. patient assessment findings.

  d. the patient's response to treatment.

5. If your patient refuses transport and care, simply having him sign your PCR is not sufficient.

  a. True

  b. False

6. Of the following abbreviations, which one means "drops"?

  a. Gtts

  c. Drps

  b. Dps

  d. Gms

7. The medical abbreviation that means "hypertension" is _____.

  a. HBV

  b. HPTN

  c. HPI

  d. HTN

8. The medical abbreviation that means that your patient has difficulty breathing during physical effort is _____.

  a. CHF

  b. MOI

  c. DOE

  d. DOA

See Answers to Review Questions at the back of this book.

References

1. Frisch, A. N., M. W. Dailey, D. Heeren, and M. Stern. "Precision of Time Devices Used by Prehospital Providers." *Prehosp Emerg Care* 13 (2009): 247–250.

2. Brice, J. H., K. D. Friend, and T. R. Delbridge. "Accuracy of EMS-Recorded Patient Demographic Data." *Prehosp Emerg Care* 12 (2008): 470–478.

3. Graham, D. H. "Documenting Patient Refusals." *Emerg Med Serv* 30 (2001): 56–60.

4. Weaver, J., K. H. Brinsfield, and D. Dalphond. "Prehospital Refusal-of-Transport Policies: Adequate Legal Protection?" *Prehosp Emerg Care* 4 (2000): 53–56.

5. Barnhart, S., P. M. Cody, and D. E. Hogan. "Multiple Information Sources in the Analysis of Disaster." *Am J Disaster Med* 4 (2009): 41–47.

6. Wesley, K. "Write It Right: Keeping Your PCR Clinical and Factual." *JEMS* 24 (2008): 190–196.

7. Laudermilch, D. J., M. A. Schiff, A. B. Nathens, and M. R. Rosengart. "Lack of Emergency Medical Services Documentation Is Associated with Poor Patient Outcomes: A Validation of Audit Filters for Prehospital Trauma Care." *J Am Coll Surg* 210 (2010): 220–227.

8. Taigman, M. "Ending the Paper Trail. Electronic Documentation in EMS." *Emerg Med Serv* 31 (2002): 65–68.

9. Kuisma, M., T. Varynen, T. Hiltunen, K. Porthan, and J. Aaltonen. "Effect of Introduction of Electronic Patient Reporting on the Duration of Ambulance Calls." *Am J Emerg Med* 27 (2009): 948–955.

Further Reading

Snyder, J. *EMS Documentation.* Upper Saddle River, NJ: Pearson/Brady, 2007.

Chapter 11
Human Life Span Development

Bryan Bledsoe, DO, FACEP, FAAEM

STANDARD
Life Span Development

COMPETENCY
Integrates comprehensive knowledge of life span development.

 ## Learning Objectives

Terminal Performance Objective: After reading this chapter, you should be able to anticipate and respond to the physical, physiologic, and psychosocial needs of patients across the life span.

Enabling Objectives: To accomplish the terminal performance objective, you should be able to:

1. Define key terms introduced in this chapter.

2. Describe the physiologic/psychosocial development and characteristics of infants.

3. Describe the physiologic/psychosocial development and characteristics of toddlers and preschoolers.

4. Describe the physiologic/psychosocial development and characteristics of school age children.

5. Describe the physiologic/psychosocial development and characteristics of adolescents.

6. Describe the physiologic/psychosocial development and characteristics of early adulthood and middle adulthood.

7. Describe the physiologic/psychosocial development and characteristics of aging and late adulthood.

KEY TERMS

Case Study

You and your partner respond to an early morning call and find several people upset and milling around. As you announce yourselves as paramedics, a woman sticks her head out of a doorway down the hallway and beckons you into a room. There you find a woman in her early 20s who is lying in bed and seems very uncomfortable. A young man, visibly pale, is sitting on the edge of the bed, holding her hand.

The first woman tells you that the patient is in her final month of pregnancy and that she has been experiencing mild contractions for about 12 hours. She spoke with her doctor several hours ago and was told to go to the hospital when her contractions were approximately 5 minutes apart. "Unfortunately, her water broke, and since that time the contractions have been really close together; about 3 minutes apart," the woman tells you. They were afraid to attempt the drive to the hospital, so they decided to call the paramedics.

After asking some pertinent questions, you prepare to examine the patient for crowning. Having done so, you realize it will be necessary to allow the child to be delivered at home. Preparations are made, and within a short time, a beautiful baby girl is wrapped in warm blankets and snuggled in her mother's arms. You explain that you will now prepare the mother and baby to be transported to the hospital where they can be examined to be sure there are no problems.

As you leave the room to get your stretcher, the first woman, who is the grandmother of the new baby, is spreading the happy news to the rest of the family. By the time you return to the room, several family members are gathered around a rocking chair where an elderly woman sits, holding her new great-grandchild in her arms. You think to yourself: "Four generations. Wow." Truly a beautiful family event, which you have been privileged to attend.

Introduction

Even though human anatomy and physiology basically stay the same, people do change over the span of a lifetime (Figure 11-1). Besides the obvious changes in size and appearance, there are also changes in vital signs, body systems, and psychosocial development. Some of those changes make it necessary for you to adjust your treatment of patients. For example, the amount of medication a patient receives is based on body size, weight, and the ability of the patient to process it. A child, therefore, usually requires a smaller dosage than a full-grown adult does. Many of the changes experienced over a lifetime can be identified in developmental stages. Those discussed in this chapter are:

- *Infancy*—birth to 12 months
- *Toddler*—12 to 36 months

FIGURE 11-1 People change over the span of a lifetime.

- *Preschool age*—3 to 5 years
- *School age*—6 to 12 years
- *Adolescence*—13 to 18 years
- *Early adulthood*—19 to 40 years
- *Middle adulthood*—41 to 60 years
- *Late adulthood*—61 years and older

Infancy
Physiologic Development
Vital Signs

The greatest changes in the range of vital signs are in the pediatric patient (Table 11-1). The younger the child, the more rapid are the pulse and respiratory rates. At birth, the heart rate ranges from 100 to 180 beats per minute during the first 30 minutes of life and usually settles to around 120 beats per minute after that. The initial respiratory rate is from 30 to 60 breaths per minute but tends to drop to 30 to 40 breaths per minute after the first few minutes of life. Tidal volume is 6 to 8 mL/kg initially and increases to 10 to 15 mL/kg by 12 months of age.

As with the other vital signs, the normal range for blood pressure is related to the age and weight of the infant, tending to increase with age. The average systolic blood pressure increases from a range of 60 to 90 at birth to a range of 87 to 105 at 12 months.

FIGURE 11-2 Infants double their weight by 4 to 6 months old and triple it by 9 to 12 months.

(Source: Michal Heron)

fluid in the first week of life, the infant's weight usually drops by 5 percent to 10 percent; however, infants usually exceed their birth weight by the second week. During the first month, infants grow at approximately 30 grams per day, and they should double their birth weight by 4 to 6 months and triple it at 9 to 12 months (Figure 11-2). The infant's head is equal to 25 percent of total body weight.

Growth charts are good for comparing physical development to the norm, but parents and health care providers should keep in mind that every child develops at his own rate.

Cardiovascular System

As newborns make the transition from fetal to pulmonary circulation in the first few days of life, several important

Weight

Normal birth weight of an infant usually is between 3.0 and 3.5 kg. Because of the excretion of extracellular

> **CONTENT REVIEW**
>
> ➤ The younger the child, the more rapid are the pulse and respiratory rates.

Table 11-1 Normal Vital Signs

	Pulse (Beats per Minute)	Respiration (Breaths per Minute)	Blood Pressure (Average mmHg)	Temperature	
Infancy:					
At birth:	100–180	30–60	60–90 systolic	98–100°F	36.7–37.8°C
At 1 year:	100–160	30–60	87–105 systolic	98–100°F	36.7–37.8°C
Toddler (12 to 36 months)	80–110	24–40	95–105 systolic	96.8–99.6°F	36.0–37.5°C
Preschool age (3 to 5 years)	70–110	22–34	95–110 systolic	96.8–99.6°F	36.0–37.5°C
School-age (6 to 12 years)	65–110	18–30	97–112 systolic	98.6°F	37°C
Adolescence (13 to 18 years)	60–90	12–26	112–128 systolic	98.6°F	37°C
Early adulthood (19 to 40 years)	60–100	12–20	120/80	98.6°F	37°C
Middle adulthood (41 to 60 years)	60–100	12–20	120/80	98.6°F	37°C
Late adulthood (61 years and older)	*	*	*	98.6°F	37°C

*Depends on the individual's physical health status.

changes occur. Shortly after birth, the *ductus venosus,* a blood vessel that connects the umbilical vein and the inferior vena cava in the fetus, constricts. As a result, blood pressure changes and the *foramen ovale,* an opening in the interatrial septum of the fetal heart, closes. The *ductus arteriosus,* a blood vessel that connects the pulmonary artery and the aorta in the fetus, also constricts after birth. Once it is closed, blood can no longer bypass the lungs by moving from the pulmonary trunk directly into the aorta.

These changes lead to an immediate increase in systemic vascular resistance and a decrease in pulmonary vascular resistance. Although the constriction of the ductus arteriosus may be functionally complete within 15 minutes, the permanent closure of the foramen ovale may take from 30 days to 1 year. The left ventricle of the heart will strengthen throughout the first year.

(You may wish to note that in an adult, the ductus venosus becomes a fibrous cord called the *ligamentum venosum,* which is superficially embedded in the wall of the liver. Also, in an adult, the site of the foramen ovale is marked by a depression called the *fossa ovalis,* and the ductus arteriosus is represented by a cord called the *ligamentum arteriosum.*)

Pulmonary System

The first breath an infant takes must be forceful, because until that moment the lungs have been collapsed. Fortunately, the lungs of a full-term fetus continuously secrete surfactant. *Surfactant* is a chemical that reduces the surface tension that tends to hold the moist membranes of the lungs together. After the first powerful breath begins to expand the lungs, breathing becomes easier.

In general, an infant's airway is shorter, narrower, less stable, and more easily obstructed than at any other stage in life. The infant is primarily a "nose breather" until at least 4 weeks of age; therefore, it is important for the nasal passages to stay clear. A common complaint in infants less than 6 months of age is nasal congestion. This occurs because, as mentioned, young infants are obligate nasal breathers. Even a mild nasal obstruction, as occurs with a viral upper respiratory infection, can cause difficulty breathing, especially during feeding.

An infant's lung tissue is fragile and prone to *barotrauma* (an injury caused by a change in atmospheric pressure). Because of this, prehospital personnel must be careful when applying mechanical ventilation with a bag-valve-mask unit. There are fewer alveoli with decreased collateral ventilation. In addition, the accessory muscles for breathing are immature and susceptible to early fatigue, so they cannot sustain a rapid respiratory rate over a long period of time. Breathing becomes ineffective at rates higher than 60 breaths per minute because air moves only in the upper airway, never reaching the lungs. Rapid respiratory rates also lead to rapid heat and fluid loss.

The chest wall of the infant is less rigid than an adult's, and the ribs are positioned horizontally, causing diaphragmatic breathing. Therefore, when you assess respiratory rate and effort in an infant, it is important to observe the abdomen rise and fall. An infant needs less pressure and a lower volume of air for ventilation than an adult does, but the infant has a higher metabolic rate and a higher oxygen consumption rate than an adult.

Renal System
Usually, the newborn's kidneys are not able to produce concentrated urine, so the baby excretes a relatively dilute fluid with a specific gravity that rarely exceeds 1.0. (Specific gravity is the weight of a substance compared to an equal amount of water. For comparison, water is considered to have a specific gravity of 1.0.) For this reason, the newborn can easily become dehydrated and develop a water and electrolyte imbalance.

Immune System
During pregnancy, certain antibodies pass from the maternal blood into the fetal bloodstream. As a result, the fetus acquires some of the mother's active immunities against pathogens. Thus, the fetus is said to have naturally acquired passive immunities, which may remain effective for six months to a year after birth. A breast-fed baby also receives antibodies through the breast milk to many of the diseases the mother has had.

Nervous System
Sensation is present in all portions of the body at birth, so a young infant feels pain but lacks the ability to localize it and isolate a response to it. As nerve connections develop, the response to pain becomes much more localized. In addition, motor and sensory development are most advanced in the cranial nerves at birth, because of their life-sustaining function and protective reflexes. Because the cranial nerves control such things as blinking, sucking, and swallowing, the infant has strong, coordinated sucking and gag reflexes. The infant also will have well-flexed extremities, which move equally when the infant is stimulated.

REFLEXES The infant has several reflexes that disappear over time. These include the Moro, palmar, rooting, and sucking reflexes. The **Moro reflex**, which is sometimes referred to as the "startle reflex," is the characteristic reflex of newborns. When the baby is startled, he throws his arms wide, spreading his fingers and then grabbing instinctively with the arms and fingers. The reflex should be brisk and

CONTENT REVIEW
➤ An infant's airway is shorter, narrower, less stable, and more easily obstructed than at any other stage in life.

symmetrical. An asymmetric Moro reflex (in which one arm does not respond exactly like the other) may imply a paralysis or weakness on one side of the body.

The **palmar grasp** is a strong reflex in the full-term newborn. It is elicited by placing a finger firmly in the infant's palm. The palmar grasp weakens as the hand becomes less continuously fisted. Sometime after 2 months, it merges into the voluntary ability to release an object held in the hand.

The **rooting reflex** causes the hungry infant to turn his head to the right or left when a hand or cloth touches his cheek. If the mother's nipple touches either side of the infant's face, above or below the mouth, the infant's lips and tongue tend to follow in that direction. Stroking the infant's lips causes a sucking movement, or the **sucking reflex**, in the infant. Both the rooting and sucking reflexes should be present in all full-term babies and are most easily elicited before a feeding. They usually last until the infant is 3 or 4 months old; however, the rooting reflex may persist during sleep for 7 or 8 months.

FONTANELLES Fontanelles allow for compression of the head during childbirth and for rapid growth of the brain during early life. They are diamond-shaped soft spots of fibrous tissue at the top of the infant's skull where three or four bones will eventually fuse together. The fibrous tissue is strong and, generally, can protect the brain adequately from injury. The posterior fontanelle usually closes in 2 or 3 months, and the anterior one closes between 9 and 18 months. You may wish to note that the fontanelles, especially the anterior one, may be used to provide an indirect estimate of hydration. Normally, the anterior fontanelle is level with the surface of the skull, or slightly sunken. With dehydration, the anterior fontanelle may fall below the level of the skull and appear sunken.

SLEEP A newborn usually sleeps for 16 to 18 hours daily, with periods of sleep and wakefulness distributed evenly over a 24-hour period. Sleep time will gradually decrease to 14 to 16 hours per day, with a 9- to 10-hour period at night. Infants usually begin to sleep through the night within two to four months. The normal infant is easily aroused from sleep.

Musculoskeletal System

The developing infant's extremities grow in length from growth plates, which are located on each end of the long bones. The infant also has *epiphyseal plates,* or secondary bone-forming centers that are separated by cartilage from larger (or parent) bones. As each epiphysis grows, it becomes part of the larger bone. Bones grow in thickness by way of deposition of new bone on existing bone. Factors affecting bone development and growth include nutrition, exposure to sunlight, growth hormone, thyroid hormone, genetic factors, and general health. Muscle weight in infants is about 25 percent of the entire musculoskeletal system.

Other Developmental Characteristics

Expect rapid changes during an infant's first year of life. At about 2 months of age, he is able to track objects with his eyes and recognize familiar faces. At about 3 months of age, he can move objects to his mouth with his hands and display primary emotions with distinct facial expressions (such as a smile or a frown). At 4 months of age, he drools without swallowing and begins to reach out to people. By 5 months, he should be sleeping through the night without waking for a feeding, and he should be able to discriminate between family and strangers. Teeth begin to appear between 5 and 7 months of age.

At 6 months, the baby can sit upright in a high chair and begin to make one-syllable sounds, such as "ma," "mu," "da," and "di." At 7 months, he has a fear of strangers and his moods can quickly shift from crying to laughing. At 8 months, the infant begins to respond to the word "no," he can sit alone, and he can play "peek-a-boo." At 9 months, he responds to adult anger.

At about 9 months old, the baby begins to pull himself up to a standing position, and explores objects by mouthing, sucking, chewing, and biting them. At 10 months, he pays attention to his name and crawls well. At 11 months, he attempts to walk without assistance and begins to show frustration about restrictions. By 12 months, he can walk with help, and he knows his own name.

Psychosocial Development

Family Processes and Reciprocal Socialization

The psychosocial development of an individual begins at birth and develops as a result of instincts, drives, capacities, and interactions with the environment. A key component of that environment is the family. The interactions babies have with their families help them to grow and change and help their families do the same. This is called "reciprocal socialization," a model that recognizes the child's active role in his own development.

Raising a baby requires a lot of hard work, but studies show that healthy, happy, and self-reliant children are the products of stable homes in which parents give a great deal of time and attention to their children.

CRYING A newborn's only means of communication is through crying. Although every cry may seem the same to a stranger, most mothers quickly learn to notice the differences among a basic cry, an anger cry, and a pain cry.

ATTACHMENT Infants have their own unique timetables and paths to becoming attached to their parents. **Bonding** is initially based on **secure attachment**, or an infant's sense that his needs will be met by his caregivers. Secure attachment is consistent with healthy development, and leads to a child who is bold in his explorations of the world and competent in dealing with it. It is important for this sense of security to develop within the first 6 months of an infant's life.

When an infant is uncertain about whether or not his caregivers will be responsive or helpful when needed, another type of attachment develops. It is called **anxious resistant attachment**. It leads to a child who is always prone to separation anxiety, causing him to be clinging and anxious about exploring the world.

A third type of attachment is called **anxious avoidant attachment**. It occurs when the infant has no confidence that he will be responded to helpfully when he seeks care. In fact, the infant expects to be rebuffed. This causes him to attempt to live without the love and support of others. The most extreme cases result from repeated rejection or prolonged institutionalization and can lead to a variety of personality disorders, from compulsive self-sufficiency to persistent delinquency.

TRUST VS. MISTRUST Some psychologists believe that human life progresses through a series of stages, each marked by a crisis that needs to be resolved. Each of the crises involves a conflict between two opposing characteristics. From birth to approximately 1½ years of age, the infant goes through the stage called **trust vs. mistrust**. According to psychologists, the infant wants the world to be an orderly, predictable place where causes and effects can be anticipated. When this is true, the infant develops trust based on consistent parental care. When an infant begins life with irregular and inadequate care, he develops anxiety and insecurity, which have a negative effect on family and other relationships important to the development of trust. This may lead to feelings of mistrust and hostility, which may in turn develop into antisocial or even criminal behavior.

Scaffolding

Infants learn in many ways from their parents and others around them. One way they learn—from infancy and throughout their school years—is through **scaffolding**, or building on what they already know. For example, parents or caregivers usually talk to infants as a natural part of caring for them. With scaffolding, the dialogue is maintained just above the level at which the child can perform activities independently. As the baby learns, the parent or caregiver changes the nature of the dialogues so that they continue to support the baby but also give him responsibility for the task. In this way, infants continue to build on what they know.

Temperament

An infant may be classified as an easy child, a difficult child, or a slow-to-warm-up child. An **easy child** is characterized by regularity of bodily functions, low or moderate intensity of reactions, and acceptance of new situations. A **difficult child** is characterized by irregularity of bodily functions, intense reactions, and withdrawal from new situations. A **slow-to-warm-up child** is characterized by a low intensity of reactions and a somewhat negative mood.

Situational Crisis and Parental-Separation Reactions

Infants who have good relationships with their parents usually follow a predictable sequence of behaviors when they experience a situational crisis (a crisis caused by a particular set of circumstances), such as being separated from parents. The first stage of parental-separation reaction is protest, the second stage is despair, and the last is detachment or withdrawal.

Protest may begin immediately on separation and continue for about one week. Loud crying, restlessness, and rejection of all adults show how distressed the infant is. In the second stage, despair, the infant's behavior suggests growing hopelessness marked by monotonous crying, inactivity, and steady withdrawal. In the final stage, detachment or withdrawal, the infant displays renewed interest in its surroundings, even though it is usually a remote, distant kind of interest. This phase is apathetic and may persist even if the parent reappears.

Toddler and Preschool Age
Physiologic Development

Vital signs for toddlers (12 to 36 months, Figure 11-3) and preschool-age children (3 to 5 years old, Figure 11-4) are not the same as an infant's. The heart rate for toddlers

FIGURE 11-3 A toddler beginning to stand and walk on his own.

FIGURE 11-4 In the preschool-age child, exploratory behavior accelerates.

(© Dr. Bryan E. Bledsoe)

ranges from 80 to 110 beats per minute. Respiratory rate ranges from 24 to 40 breaths per minute. Systolic blood pressure ranges from 95 to 105 mmHg. For preschoolers, heart rate ranges from 70 to 110 beats per minute, respiratory rate from 22 to 34 breaths per minute, and systolic blood pressure from 75 to 110 mmHg. Normal temperature for both ranges from 96.8 to 99.6°F (36.3 to 37.9°C). In addition, the rate of weight gain is slowing dramatically. The average toddler or preschooler gains approximately 2.0 kg per year.

Changes in body systems include the following:

- *Cardiovascular system.* The capillary beds are now better developed and assist in thermoregulation of the body more efficiently. Hemoglobin levels approach normal adult levels at this point.

- *Pulmonary system.* The terminal airways continue to branch off from the bronchioles and alveoli increase in number, providing more surfaces for gas exchange to take place in the lungs. It is still important to remember that children have immature chest muscles and cannot sustain an excessively rapid respiratory rate for long. They will tire quickly and their respiratory rate will decrease, indicating the onset of ventilatory failure.

- *Renal system.* The kidneys are well developed by the toddler years. Specific gravity and other characteristics of urine are similar to those that would be found in an adult.

- *Immune system.* By this point in life, the passive immunity born with the infant is lost, and the child becomes more susceptible to minor respiratory and gastrointestinal infections. This occurs at the same time the child is being exposed to the infections of other children in child care and preschool. Fortunately, the toddler and preschooler will develop their own immunities to common pathogens as they are exposed to them.

- *Nervous system.* The brain is now at 90 percent of adult weight. Myelination (the development of the covering of nerves) has increased, which allows for effortless walking as well as other basic skills. Fine motor skills, including the use of hands and fingers in grasping and manipulating objects, begin developing at this stage.

- *Musculoskeletal system.* Both muscle mass and bone density increase during this period.

- *Dental system.* All the primary teeth have erupted by the age of 36 months.

- *Senses.* Visual acuity is at 20/30 during the toddler years. Hearing reaches maturity at 3 to 4 years of age.

In addition, though children are physiologically capable of being toilet trained by the age of 12 to 15 months, they are not psychologically ready until 18 to 30 months of age. Therefore, it is important not to rush toilet training. Children will let their parents know when they are ready. The average age for completion of toilet training is 28 months.

Psychosocial Development

Cognition

Children begin to use actual words at about 10 months, but they do not begin to grasp that words "mean" something until they are about 1 year of age. Usually, by the time they are 3 or 4 years old, they have mastered the basics of language, which they will continue to refine throughout their childhood. Between 18 and 24 months, they begin to understand cause and effect. Between the ages of 18 and 24 months, they develop separation anxiety, becoming clinging and crying when a parent leaves. Between 24 and 36 months, they begin to develop "magical thinking" and engage in play-acting, such as playing house and similar activities.

Play

Exploratory behavior accelerates at this stage. The child is able to play simple games and follow basic rules, and he begins to display signs of competitiveness. Play provides an emotional release for youngsters, because it lacks the right-or-wrong, life-and-death feelings that may accompany interactions with adults. Therefore, observations of children at play may uncover frustrations otherwise unexpressed.

Sibling Relationships

There are many positive aspects to growing up with siblings, but there also may be negative ones, which can lead to sibling rivalry. The first-born child often finds it very difficult to share the attention of his parents with a younger sibling. If the older child must also help care for the younger ones, he may become even more frustrated. Although first-born children usually maintain a special relationship with parents, they also are expected to exercise more self-control and show more responsibility when interacting with younger siblings. Younger children often see only the apparent privileges extended to the older children, such as later bedtimes and more freedom to come and go. Still, when asked if they would be happier if their siblings did not exist, most prefer to keep them around.

Peer-Group Functions

Peers, or youngsters who are similar in age (within 12 months of each other), are very important to the development of toddler and school-age children. In fact, peer groups actually become more important as childhood progresses. Peers provide a source of information about other families and the outside world. Interaction with peers offers opportunities for learning skills, comparing oneself to others, and feeling part of a group.

Parenting Styles and Their Effects

There are three basic styles of parenting: authoritarian, authoritative, and permissive.

- **Authoritarian** parents are demanding and desire instant obedience from a child. No consideration is given to the child's view, and no attempt is made to explain why. Frequently, the child is punished for even asking the reason for some decision or directive. This parenting style often leads to children with low self-esteem and low competence. Boys are often hostile, and girls are often shy.

- **Authoritative** parents respond to the needs and wishes of their children. They believe in parental control, but they attempt to explain their reasons to the child. They expect mature behavior and will enforce rules, but they still encourage independence and actualization of potential. These parents believe that both they and children have rights and try to maintain a happy balance between the two. This parenting style usually leads to children who are self-assertive, independent, friendly, and cooperative.

- **Permissive** parents take a tolerant, accepting view of their children's behavior, including aggressive behavior

and sexual behavior. They rarely punish or make demands of their children, allowing them to make almost all of their own decisions. They may be either "permissive-indifferent" or "permissive-indulgent" parents, but it is very difficult to make the distinction. This parenting style may lead to impulsive, aggressive children who have low self-reliance, low self-control, and low maturity, and lack responsible behavior.

Divorce and Child Development

Nearly half of today's marriages end in divorce. As a result of divorce, a child's physical way of life often changes (a new home, for example, or a reduced standard of living). The child's psychological life is also touched. The effects on the child's development, however, depend greatly on the child's age, his cognitive and social competencies, the amount of dependency on his parents, how the parents interact with each other and the child, and even the type of child care. Toddlers and preschoolers commonly express feelings of shock, depression, and a fear that their parents no longer love them. They may feel they are being abandoned. They are unable to see the divorce from their parents' perspective, and therefore believe the divorce centers on them. The parent's ability to respond to a child's needs greatly influences the ultimate effects of divorce on the child.

Television and Video Games

Virtually every family has at least one television in the home, and many have video game players of one kind or another. Most children watch television and/or play video games for several hours each day—many with few, if any, parental restrictions. Television violence increases levels of aggression in toddlers and preschoolers, and it increases passive acceptance of the use of aggression by others. Parental screening of the television programs children watch may be effective in avoiding these outcomes. Some video games also feature violent scenarios that parents may do well to monitor.

Modeling

Toddlers and preschool-age children begin to recognize sexual differences, and, through **modeling**, they begin to incorporate gender-specific behaviors they observe in parents, siblings, and peers.[1,2]

School Age
Physiologic Development

Between the ages of 6 and 12 years, a child's heart rate is between 65 and 110 beats per minute, respiratory rate is between 18 and 30 breaths per minute, and systolic blood pressure ranges from 97 to 112 mmHg. Body temperature

CONTENT REVIEW

➤ Vital signs in most children reach adult levels during the school-age years.

is approximately 98.6°F (37°C). The average child of this age gains 3 kg per year and grows 6 cm per year. In most children, vital signs reach adult levels during this period of time, but their lymph tissues are proportionately larger than those of an adult. In addition, brain function increases in both hemispheres, and primary teeth are being replaced by permanent ones.

Psychosocial Development

School-age children (Figure 11-5) have developed decision-making skills, and usually are allowed more self-regulation, with parents providing general supervision. Parents spend less time with school-age children than they do with toddlers and preschoolers.

The development of a self-concept occurs at this age. School-age children have more interaction with both adults and other children, and they tend to compare themselves to others. They are beginning to develop self-esteem, which tends to be higher during the early years of school than in the later years. Often, self-esteem is based on external characteristics and may be affected by popularity with peers, rejection, emotional support, and neglect. Negative self-esteem can be very damaging to further development.

As children mature, moral development begins when they are rewarded for what their parents believe to be

FIGURE 11-5 School-age children are allowed more self-regulation and independence as they grow older.

right and punished for what their parents believe to be wrong. With cognitive growth, moral reasoning appears and the control of the child's behavior gradually shifts from external sources to internal self-control. According to one theory, there are three levels of moral development: **preconventional reasoning**, **conventional reasoning**, and **postconventional reasoning**, with each level having two stages.

- *Preconventional reasoning.* Stage one is punishment and obedience; that is, children obey rules in order to avoid punishment. There is no concern about morals. Stage two is individualism and purpose: Children obey the rules, but only for pure self-interest. They are aware of fairness to others, but only as it pertains to their own satisfaction.

- *Conventional reasoning.* In stage three, children are concerned with interpersonal norms, seeking the approval of others and developing the "good boy" or "good girl" mentality. They begin to judge behavior by intention. In stage four, they develop the social system's morality, becoming concerned with authority and maintaining the social order. They realize that correct behavior is "doing one's duty."

- *Postconventional reasoning.* Stage five is concerned with community rights as opposed to individual rights. Children at this level believe that the best values are those supported by law because they have been accepted by the whole society. They believe that if there is a conflict between human need and the law, individuals should work to change the law. Stage six is concerned with universal ethical principles, such as that an informed conscience defines what is right, or people act not because of fear, approval, or law, but from their own standards of what is right or wrong.

According to this theory, individuals will move through the levels and stages of moral development throughout school age and young adulthood at their own rates.

Adolescence
Physiologic Development

Vital signs in adolescents (13 to 18 years old) are as follows: heart rate is between 60 and 90 beats per minute, respiratory rate is between 12 and 26 breaths per minute, and systolic blood pressure is between 112 and 128 mmHg. Body temperature is approximately 98.6°F (37°C). In addition, the adolescent usually experiences a rapid 2- to 3-year growth spurt, beginning distally with enlargement of the feet and hands followed by enlargement of the arms and legs. The chest and trunk enlarge in the final stage of growth. Girls are usually finished growing by the age of 16

FIGURE 11-6 Children reach reproductive maturity during adolescence.

and boys by the age of 18. In late adolescence, the average male is taller and stronger than the average female. At this age, both males and females reach reproductive maturity (Figure 11-6). Secondary sexual development occurs, with noticeable development of the external sexual organs. Pubic and axillary hairs appear and, mostly in males, vocal quality changes. In females, menstruation has begun, breasts and the ductal system of the mammary glands develop, and there is increased deposition of adipose tissue in the subcutaneous layer of the breasts, thighs, and buttocks. In addition, in the female, endocrine system changes include the release of *follicle-stimulating hormone (FSH)*, *luteinizing hormone (LH)*, and *gonadotropin*, which promotes estrogen and progesterone production. In the male, gonadotropin promotes testosterone production.

Muscle mass and bone growth are nearly complete at this stage. Body fat decreases in early adolescence and increases later. Females require 18 to 20 percent body fat in order for menarche, or the first menstruation, to occur. Blood chemistry is nearly equal to that of an adult, and skin toughens through sebaceous gland activity. (You may wish to note that a disorder of the sebaceous glands is responsible for acne, which is common in adolescence. In acne, the glands become overactive and inflamed, ducts become plugged, and small red elevations containing blackheads or pimples appear.)

Psychosocial Development

Family

Adolescence can be a time of serious family conflicts as the adolescent strives for autonomy and parents strive for continued control. The many biological changes that occur at this stage cause inner conflict in both adolescents and their parents. Privacy becomes extremely important at this stage of life and, because of modesty, the adolescent prefers that parents not be present during physical examinations. It also is likely that when a patient history is being taken, questions asked in the presence of parents or guardians may not be answered honestly.

Children experience an increase in idealism during adolescence. They believe that adults should be able to live up to their expectations, which of course they cannot always do, which leads to disappointment.

Development of Identity

At this age, adolescents are trying to achieve more independence. They take "time out" to experiment with a variety of identities, knowing that they do not have to assume responsibility for the consequences of those identities. As they attempt to develop their own identity, self-consciousness and peer pressure increase. They become interested in others in a sexual way, and they find this somewhat embarrassing. They really do not know how to handle this increased interest. They want to be treated like adults and do not know how to achieve this.

How well and how fast adolescents progress through the various stages of identity development depends on how well they are able to handle crises. Minority adolescents tend to have more identity crises than others. In general, antisocial behavior usually peaks at around the eighth or ninth grade.

Body image is a great concern at this point in life. Peers continually make comparisons, and certainly the media lead to unrealistic ideas of what the "perfect" body should look like. This is a time when eating disorders are common. It also is a time when self-destructive behaviors begin, such as use of tobacco, alcohol, and illicit drugs. Depression and suicide are more common at this age group than in any other.

Ethical Development

As adolescents develop their capacity for logical, analytical, and abstract thinking, they begin to develop a personal code of ethics. Just as they get disappointed when adults do not live up to their expectations, they tend to get disappointed in anyone who does not meet their personal code of ethics.

Early Adulthood

Between the ages of 19 and 40 years, heart rate averages 70 beats per minute, respiratory rate averages between 12 and 20 breaths per minute, blood pressure averages 120/80 mmHg, and body temperature averages 98.6°F (37°C). This is the period of life during which adults develop lifelong habits and routines.

Peak physical condition occurs between the ages of 19 and 26 years of age, when all body systems are at optimal performance levels. At the end of this period, the body begins its slowing process. Spinal disks settle, leading to a decrease in height. Fatty tissue increases, leading to weight gain. Muscle strength decreases, and reaction times level off and stabilize. Accidents are a leading cause of death in this age group.

The highest levels of job stress occur at this point in life, the time in which the young adult strives to find his place in the world. Love develops, both romantic and affectionate. Childbirth is most common in this age group, with new families providing new challenges and stress (Figure 11-7). In spite of all this, this period is not associated with psychological problems related to well-being.

> **CONTENT REVIEW**
> ➤ Peak physical condition is reached in early adulthood; accidents rather than disease are a leading cause of death.

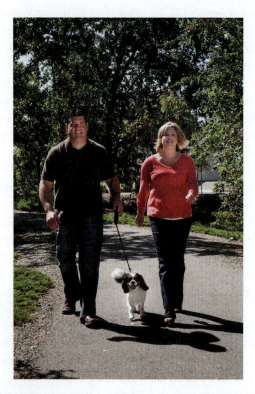

FIGURE 11-7 Peak physical conditions occur in early adulthood.

Middle Adulthood

Between the ages of 41 and 60 years, average vital signs are as follows: heart rate, 70 beats per minute; respiratory rate between 12 and 20 breaths per minute; blood pressure averages 120/80 mmHg; and body temperature averages 98.6°F (37°C).

The body still functions at a high level with varying degrees of degradation based on the individual (Figure 11-8). There are usually some vision and hearing changes during this period. Cardiovascular health becomes a concern, with cardiac output decreasing and cholesterol levels increasing. Cancer often strikes this age group, weight control becomes more difficult, and, for women in the late 40s to early 50s, menopause commences.

Adults in this age group are more concerned with the "social clock" and become more task oriented as they see the time for accomplishing their lifetime goals recede. Still, they tend to approach problems more as challenges than as threats. This is also the time of life for "empty-nest syndrome," or the time after the last offspring has left home. Some women feel depression or a sense of loss and purposelessness at this time, feelings that are made worse by aging and menopause. Sometimes a father also becomes depressed, but the syndrome seems to affect mothers to a greater extent. Many parents, however, view the period after children have left home as a time of increased freedom and opportunity for self-fulfillment. Unfortunately, adults in this age group often find themselves burdened by financial commitments for elderly parents, as well as for young adult children.

> **CONTENT REVIEW**
> ➤ Cardiovascular health becomes a concern during middle adulthood.

FIGURE 11-8 People in middle adulthood still function at a high level.

Late Adulthood

Maximum life span is the theoretical, species-specific, longest duration of life, excluding premature or "unnatural" death. For human beings, maximum life span is approximately 120 years. **Life expectancy**, which is based on the year of birth, is defined as the average number of additional years of life expected for a member of a population. Human beings almost always die of disease or accident before they reach their biological limit.

Physiologic Development

Vital Signs

At 61 years of age and older, vital signs—heart rate, respiratory rate, and blood pressure—depend on the individual's physical health status. Body temperature still averages 98.6°F (37°C).

Cardiovascular System

During late adulthood, the cardiovascular system changes in ways that affect its overall function. The walls of the blood vessels thicken, causing increased peripheral vascular resistance and reduced blood flow to organs. There is decreased baroreceptor sensitivity and, by 80 years of age, there is approximately a 50 percent decrease in vessel elasticity.

In addition, the heart tends to show disease in the heart muscle, heart valves, and coronary arteries. Increased workload causes cardiomegaly (enlargement), mitral and aortic valve changes, and decreased myocardial elasticity.

Patho Pearls

Life Span and Disease. The life span of individuals in most countries in the industrialized world continues to increase. This is due to many factors, which include better health care, widespread availability of vaccinations, safer agricultural and manufacturing equipment, safer automobiles, the absence of major wars, and many others. With an extended life span, we are starting to commonly see diseases that were once uncommon. For example, only in the past 20 to 30 years have we started to see an increase in cases of Alzheimer's disease. But is the incidence of Alzheimer's disease now more common, or is it just that people are now living long enough for the disease to manifest itself? Although it will take structured research to determine this for sure, the latter part of the statement is surely true. Typically, approximately 10 percent of people age 65 show signs of the disease, whereas 50 percent of persons age 85 have symptoms of Alzheimer's. The proportion of persons with Alzheimer's begins to decrease after age 85 because of the increased mortality caused by the disease, and relatively few people over the age of 100 have the disease. Thus, the increased incidence of Alzheimer's disease may simply be due to the fact that people are living longer.

The myocardium is less able to respond to exercise, and the SA node and other cells responsible for producing heartbeats become infiltrated with fibrous connective tissue and fat. Pacemaker cells diminish, resulting in arrhythmia. Because of prolonged contraction time, decreased response to various medications that would ordinarily stimulate the heart, and increased resistance to electrical stimulation, the heart also becomes less able to contract. Tachycardia (abnormally rapid heart action) is not well tolerated.

Functional blood volume decreases in late adulthood. Decreases also can be expected in platelet count and the number of red blood cells (RBCs), which can lead to poor iron levels.

Respiratory System

The trachea and large airways increase in diameter in late adulthood, and enlargement of the end units of the airway results in a decreased surface area of the lungs. Decreased elasticity of the lungs leads to an increase in lung volume and to a reduction in surface area. The decreased elasticity also causes the chest to expand and the diaphragm to descend. The ends of the ribs calcify to the breastbone, producing stiffening of the chest wall, which increases the workload of the respiratory muscles.

These changes lead to an increased likelihood for older adults to develop lung disease and progressive declines in lung function. Metabolic changes also may lead to decreased lung function, and because of lifelong exposure to pollutants, diffusion through alveoli is diminished. Coughing also becomes ineffective because of a weakened chest wall and bone structure. Of all the factors that influence lung function, smoking continues to produce the greatest amount of disability.

Endocrine System

During this stage of life, there is a decrease in glucose metabolism and insulin production. The thyroid shows some diminished triiodothyronine (T3) production, cortisol (from the adrenal cortex) is diminished by 25 percent, the pituitary gland is 20 percent less effective, and reproductive organs atrophy in women.

Gastrointestinal System

One way the gastrointestinal system is affected at this stage of life is by way of tooth loss. Age-related dental changes do not necessarily lead to loss of teeth. Usually tooth loss is caused by cavities or periodontal disease, both of which may be prevented by good dental hygiene. With age, the location of cavities in teeth changes and an increasing amount of root cavities and cavities around existing sites of previous dental work are seen. Tooth loss can lead to changes in diet, an increased chance of malnutrition, and serious vitamin and mineral deficiencies.

This is also true when the individual has false teeth, which do not completely restore normal chewing ability and can reduce taste sensation. In addition, alterations in swallowing are more common in older people without teeth because they tend to swallow larger pieces of food. Swallowing takes 50 to 100 percent longer, probably because of subtle changes in the swallowing mechanism. Peristalsis is decreased and the esophageal sphincter is less effective.

In general, the gastrointestinal system shows less age-associated change in function than other body systems. Stomach contractions appear to be normal, but it does take longer to empty liquids from the stomach. The amount of stomach acid secretions decreases, probably because of the loss of the cells that produce gastric acid. There is usually a small amount of atrophy to the lining of the small intestine. In the large intestine, expect to see atrophy of the lining, changes in the muscle layer, and blood vessel abnormalities. Approximately one of every three people over 60 has diverticula, or outpouchings, in the lining of the large intestine resulting from increased pressure inside the intestine. Weakness in the bowel wall also may be a contributing factor.

The number of some opiate receptors increases with aging, which may lead to significant constipation when narcotics are ingested. Changes may occur in the metabolism and in absorption of some sugars, calcium, and iron. Highly fat-soluble compounds such as vitamin A appear to be absorbed faster with age. The activity of some enzymes such as lactase—which aids in the digestion of some sugars, particularly those found in dairy products—appears to decrease. The absorption of fat also may change, and the metabolism of specific compounds, including drugs, can be significantly prolonged in elderly people.

Renal System
With aging, there is a 25 to 30 percent decrease in kidney mass. About 50 percent of nephrons are lost and abnormal glomeruli are more common. Reduced kidney function leads to a decreased clearance of some drugs and decreased elimination. The kidneys' hormonal response to dehydration is reduced as is the ability to retain salt under conditions when it should be conserved. The ability of the kidneys to modify vitamin D to a more active form may also lessen.

The Senses
Taste buds diminish during this stage of life, which leads to a loss of taste sensation. Smell declines rapidly after the age of 50 and the parts of the brain involved in smell degenerate significantly so that by age 80, the detection of smell is almost 50 percent poorer than it was at its peak. Because taste and smell work together to make enjoyment of food possible, appetite often declines. Response to painful stimuli is diminished, as is kinesthetic sense, or the ability to sense movement.

Visual acuity and reaction time are diminished, and there are actual changes in the organs of hearing. The ear canal atrophies, the eardrum thickens, and there may be degenerative and even arthritic changes in the small joints connecting the bones in the middle ear. Significant changes take place in the inner ear. These changes in structure significantly affect hearing. Hearing loss for pure tones, which increases with age in men and women, is called "presbycusis." With presbycusis, higher frequencies become less audible than lower frequencies. Pitch discrimination plays an important role in speech perception so, with age, speech discrimination declines. When exposed to loud background noise or indistinct speech, older people hear less, but at the same time, they may be very sensitive to loud sounds.

Nervous System
With aging, there is a decrease of neurotransmitters and a loss of neurons in the cerebellum, which controls coordination, and the hippocampus, which is involved in some aspects of memory function. The sleep–wake cycle also is disrupted, causing older adults to have sleep problems.

Psychosocial Development
Even though disease may reduce physical and mental capabilities, the ability to learn and adjust continues throughout life, and is greatly influenced by interests, activity, motivation, health, and income (Figure 11-9). However, the **terminal-drop hypothesis** asserts that there is a decrease in cognitive functioning over a five-year period prior to death. The individual may or may not be aware of diffuse changes in mood, mental functioning, or the way his body responds to various stimuli.

Housing
Although most older adults would rather stay in their own homes, it is not always possible because home-care services are not affordably available in all communities as a viable alternative to nursing homes. Home-care services usually provide assistance with household chores such as preparing meals, cleaning and laundry, and performing personal care tasks such as feeding and bathing. Health care services in the home are provided by nurses and physical or speech therapists. To be eligible for these services under Medicare, the patient must be home-bound, need an intensive level of services, and be expected to

FIGURE 11-9 The ability to learn and adjust continues throughout life.

benefit from such services over a reasonable amount of time. Home-care services are usually time-limited.

An alternative to home-care services is "assisted living," or living in a facility that offers a combination of home care and nursing home facilities. There is a greater sense of control, independence, and privacy in these facilities because the older adult has more choices while still being in an institutional setting. Bedrooms and bathrooms can be locked by residents, but dining and recreational facilities are usually shared.

About 95 percent of older adults live in communities, from simple groupings of homes where mostly older adults live to a relatively new type of living arrangement called the "continuing-care retirement community." The appeal of these communities is that future health care needs are covered in a setting that is an attractive residential campus where cultural and recreational activities are available. Entrance fees to this type of community are often rather expensive.

Challenges

One of the major challenges for the older adult is maintaining a sense of self-worth. Senior citizens are commonly seen as "over the hill," less intelligent than younger adults, and certainly less able to care for themselves. Many older adults are forced into retirement because they are seen as less productive. In reality, although older workers may have slowed down a bit, they are often more concerned with producing quality work than younger workers are. Another problem older adults face at this stage of life is a feeling of declining well-being. It is not until adults reach the age of 40 that ill health—as opposed to accidents, homicide, and suicide—becomes the major cause of death. Arteriosclerotic heart disease is the major killer after the age of 40 in all age, sex, and racial groups.

Financial Burdens

The duration of each stage in the life cycle, and the ages of family members for each stage, will vary from family to family. Obviously, this will have an effect on the financial status of families. For example, a couple who completes their family while in their early adult years will have a different lifestyle when their last child leaves home than a couple with a "change-of-life" child. Late children can cause serious economic problems for retirees on fixed incomes who are trying to meet the staggering costs of education.

Retirement brings about changes for both spouses, but it seems to be particularly stressful for wives who are not prepared emotionally or financially. Retirement usually means a decrease in income and in the standard of living, which can be very difficult to handle.

A decreasing level of interest in work is natural as one grows older, but it has a severe impact on the income of older people. Almost 22 percent of all older people live in households below the poverty level. More than 50 percent of all single women above age 60 live at or below the poverty level. Older women in the United States make up the single poorest group in our society.[3–6]

Dying Companions or Impending Death

Whether it is the death of a companion or one's own impending death, fear and grief seem to have a great deal in common. Grief not only follows death, but when there is advance warning, grief may well precede death. Frequently, the death or impending death of a companion leads us to fear for our own lives. Psychiatrist Elisabeth Kübler-Ross believes that regardless of whether it is one's own death or the death of a companion, everyone must go through certain emotions. Although the five stages in her theory may sometimes overlap, everyone must deal with each of the stages of death before the grieving process ends. (Review the chapter "Workforce Safety and Wellness" for Kübler-Ross's five stages.)

Note: Human physiologic and psychosocial development will be discussed in more detail in the chapters on patient assessment, medical emergencies, and trauma emergencies, and especially in the chapters "Neonatology," "Pediatrics," "Geriatrics," and "The Challenged Patient."

Summary

The changes that take place during the span of a lifetime are innumerable. At some stages, especially birth through preschool, the changes seem to occur almost daily. The stages of infant through adolescent constitute our pediatric population. By knowing the typical developmental characteristics of each age group, you will be better prepared to evaluate a sick or injured pediatric patient. This is especially important when a caregiver may not be readily available. You can compare the child's current state to an established norm and determine whether there is a significant difference. Remember, however, that not every person develops at the same rate and in the same way, and established norms are only guidelines that should never take the place of a thorough assessment and history obtained from someone who is intimately familiar with the patient.

Only through experience with patients at all the various stages of life—adult as well as pediatric—will you come to feel comfortable dealing with patients at each of these stages. Remember that no matter what the stage of development, a thorough assessment, patience, and a sincere desire to help will guide you to make the right emergency care decisions for each patient.

You Make the Call

You are dispatched to respond to a patient who is complaining of abdominal pain. When you arrive at the scene, you are met at the door by a middle-aged man who tells you that the patient is his daughter. She is upstairs in her bedroom, and her mother is with her. You climb the stairs, followed closely by the father. When you enter the bedroom, you find a 16-year-old female lying on the bed. Her mother is sitting beside her, holding a damp cloth to her forehead. A younger sister is hovering around, trying to help.

The mother tells you that the patient woke about an hour ago, crying that her stomach hurt. The pain has gotten progressively worse over the last hour, and the patient has been complaining of nausea as well.

You begin your assessment of the patient, but she will not allow you to examine her abdomen. When you attempt to ask questions about what led up to this pain, the date of her last menstrual period, and whether or not she could possibly be pregnant, she refuses to answer you, shifting her eyes toward her parents and sister, who are still in the room. Her mother tells her to please answer your questions, but the patient just begins to cry.

1. Do you believe that this is normal behavior for a patient of this age and in this particular situation?
2. What is a likely reason for this behavior?
3. What might you do to make this patient more cooperative?

See Suggested Responses to "You Make the Call" at the end of this book.

Review Questions

1. At birth, the heart rate ranges from _____ beats per minute during the first 30 minutes of life.
   - a. 90 to 120
   - b. 100 to 120
   - c. 100 to 180
   - d. 160 to 240

2. The infant's head is equal to _____ percent of total body weight.
   - a. 10
   - b. 15
   - c. 20
   - d. 25

3. The _____, a blood vessel that connects the pulmonary artery and the aorta in the fetus, constricts after birth.
   - a. ductus venosus
   - b. foramen ovale
   - c. ductus arteriosus
   - d. ligamentum venosum

4. The _____, which is sometimes referred to as the "startle reflex," is the characteristic reflex of newborns.

   a. Moro reflex
   b. rooting reflex
   c. sucking grasp
   d. palmar grasp

5. Parents who are _____ encourage independence but will enforce rules.

   a. dismissive
   b. permissive
   c. authoritative
   d. authoritarian

6. In this stage of moral development, children are concerned with interpersonal norms, seeking the approval of others, and developing the "good boy" or "good girl" mentality.

   a. permissive reasoning
   b. conventional reasoning
   c. preconventional reasoning
   d. postconventional reasoning

7. The theoretical, species-specific, longest duration of life, excluding premature or "unnatural" death, is called the _____

   a. life expectancy.
   b. total age duration.
   c. maximum life span.
   d. maximum age.

8. As adults reach the age of _____, ill health—as opposed to accidents, homicide, and suicide—becomes the major cause of death.

   a. 25
   b. 30
   c. 40
   d. 60

9. Which of the following would be an expected set of vital signs for a patient who is 35 years old, without any illness or injury?

   a. Blood pressure of 124/80, heart rate of 72/min, and respirations of 14/min
   b. Blood pressure of 98/60, heart rate of 84/min, and respirations of 16/min
   c. Blood pressure of 166/76, heart rate of 82/min, and respirations of 10/min
   d. Blood pressure of 220/180, heart rate of 70/min, and respirations of 12/min

10. What is the age range for someone in "middle adulthood"?

   a. 21 to 45 years of age
   b. 32 to 55 years of age
   c. 41 to 60 years of age
   d. 48 to 65 years of age

See Answers to Review Questions at the end of this book.

References

1. American Academy of Pediatrics Section on Orthopaedics, American Academy of Pediatrics Committee on Pediatric Emergency Medicine, American Academy of Pediatrics Section on Critical Care, et al. "Management of Pediatric Trauma." *Pediatrics* 121 (2008): 849-854.

2. American College of Surgeons Committee on Trauma, American College of Emergency Physicians, National Association of EMS Physicians, Pediatric Equipment Guidelines Committee-Emergency Medical Services for Children (EMSC) Partnership for Children Stakeholder Group, and American Academy of Pediatrics. "Policy Statement—Equipment for Ambulances." *Pediatrics* 124 (2009): e166–e171.

3. Peterson, L. K., R. J. Fairbanks, A. Z. Hettinger, and M. N. Shah. "Emergency Medical Service Attitudes toward Geriatric Prehospital Care and Continuing Medical Education in Geriatrics." *J Am Geriatr Soc* 57 (2009): 530–535.

4. Shah, M. N., J. J. Bazarian, E. B. Lerner, et al. "The Epidemiology of Emergency Medical Services Use by Older Adults: An Analysis of the National Hospital Ambulatory Medical Care Survey." *Acad Emerg Med* 14 (2007): 441–447.

5. Shah, M. N., T. V. Caprio, P. Swanson, et al. "A Novel Emergency Medical Services-Based Program to Identify and Assist Older Adults in a Rural Community." *J Am Geriatr Soc* 58 (2010): 2205–2211.

6. Weiss, S. J., R. Chong, M. Ong, A. A. Ernst, and M. Balash. "Emergency Medical Services Screening of Elderly Falls in the Home." *Prehosp Emerg Care* 7 (2003): 79–84.

Further Reading

Craig, G. J. and W. L. Dunn. *Understanding Human Development.* 2nd ed. Upper Saddle River, NJ: Pearson, 2010.

Kall, R. V. and J. C. Cavanaugh. *Human Development: A Life-Span View.* Florence, KY: Wadsworth Publishing, 2008.

Chapter 12
Pathophysiology

Bryan Bledsoe, DO, FACEP, FAAEM

STANDARD
Pathophysiology

COMPETENCY
Integrates comprehensive knowledge of pathophysiology of major human systems.

 ## Learning Objectives

Terminal Performance Objective: After reading this chapter, you should be able to describe the pathophysiology of common patient disorders encountered by paramedics in the out-of-hospital setting.

Enabling Objectives: To accomplish the terminal performance objective, you should be able to:

1. Define key terms introduced in this chapter.

2. Explain the hierarchical structure of the body from cells to the biosphere.

3. Explain how the predisposing factors of age, gender, genetics, lifestyle, and environment affect the development of disease.

4. List and describe each of the classifications of diseases by cause.

5. Differentiate among covalent, ionic, and hydrogen bonds.

6. Recognize the six major chemical elements and four major chemical compounds that make up the human body.

7. Describe the nature and roles of carbohydrates, proteins, nucleic acids, lipids, and water in the body.

8. Explain acid–base production, mechanisms to manage acid, and common acid–base imbalances.

9. Explain the basic structure and function of a typical human cell and the components of a cell.

10. Explain the movement of water and solutes into and out of cells under various mechanisms, such as osmosis, diffusion, facilitated diffusion, active transport, endocytosis, and exocytosis.

11. Describe the fluid and electrolyte composition of the cellular environment, and discuss imbalances of these.

12. Describe the composition and function of blood, including both plasma and formed elements.

13. Predict the physiologic effects of infusing various types of intravenous fluids.

14. Explain the processes of cellular respiration and energy production.

15. Describe the different cellular responses to stress, cell injury, and cell death.

16. Describe the embryonic origins of body tissues and discuss the basic structure and function of epithelial, connective, muscle, and nervous tissues.

17. Describe the process of neoplasia, including factors associated with cancer.

18. Discuss the risk factors and basic pathophysiology of common disorders seen by the out-of-hospital care provider.

19. Describe the physiology of perfusion, the pathophysiology of hypoperfusion, and compensatory mechanisms employed by the body during periods of hypoperfusion.

20. Differentiate among cardiogenic, hypovolemic, neurogenic, anaphylactic, and septic shock and discuss basic treatment goals for each.

21. Describe the pathophysiology of multiple organ dysfunction syndrome (MODS).

22. Describe the basic characteristics of bacteria, viruses, fungi, parasites, and prions that act as human pathogens.

23. Describe the body's three lines of defense against pathogens.

24. Explain the structure and function of the immune system.

25. Discuss the process of inflammation in the body.

26. Describe variances in immunity and inflammation.

27. Describe the stress response and how this can contribute to disease states.

KEY TERMS

13. Predict the physiologic effects of infusing various types of intravenous fluids.

14. Explain the processes of cellular respiration and energy production.

15. Describe the different cellular responses to stress, cell injury, and cell death.

16. Describe the embryonic origins of body tissues and discuss the basic structure and function of epithelial, connective, muscle, and nervous tissues.

17. Describe the process of neoplasia, including factors associated with cancer.

18. Discuss the risk factors and basic pathophysiology of common disorders seen by the out-of-hospital care provider.

19. Describe the physiology of perfusion, the pathophysiology of hypoperfusion, and compensatory mechanisms employed by the body during periods of hypoperfusion.

20. Differentiate among cardiogenic, hypovolemic, neurogenic, anaphylactic, and septic shock and discuss basic treatment goals for each.

21. Describe the pathophysiology of multiple organ dysfunction syndrome (MODS).

22. Describe the basic characteristics of bacteria, viruses, fungi, parasites, and prions that act as human pathogens.

23. Describe the body's three lines of defense against pathogens.

24. Explain the structure and function of the immune system.

25. Discuss the process of inflammation in the body.

26. Describe variances in immunity and inflammation.

27. Describe the stress response and how this can contribute to disease states.

KEY TERMS

ABO blood groups, p. 320
acid–base reaction, p. 249
acidosis, p. 252
acids, p. 249
acquired immunity, p. 317
active transport, p. 259
acute, p. 232
adenosine triphosphate (ATP), p. 245
adipocytes, p. 289
adipose tissue, p. 289
aerobic metabolism, p. 303
afterload, p. 300
AIDS (acquired immunodeficiency syndrome), p. 340
albumin, p. 270
alkalosis, p. 252
allergy, p. 336
amino acids, p. 241
amylopectin, p. 240
amylose, p. 240

anabolism, p. 247
anaerobic metabolism, p. 303
anaphylaxis, p. 310
anion, p. 238
antibiotic, p. 314
antibody, p. 317
antigen, p. 317
antigen–antibody complexes, p. 322
antigen-presenting cells (APCs), p. 325
antigen processing, p. 325
apoptosis, p. 281
atom, p. 235
atomic number, p. 235
atrophy, p. 281
autoimmune disease, p. 232
autoimmunity, p. 336
B lymphocytes, p. 317
bacteria (singular, bacterium), p. 314
basement membrane, p. 286

bases, p. 249
basophils, p. 333
benign, p. 233
buffer, p. 250
carcinogenesis, p. 294
cardiac contractile force, p. 300
cardiac output, p. 300
cardiogenic shock, p. 307
carrier proteins, p. 258
cartilage, p. 290
cascade, p. 330
catecholamines, p. 300
cation, p. 238
cell, p. 254
cell-mediated immunity, p. 318
cell membrane, p. 255
cellular adaptation, p. 280
cellular respiration, p. 276
cellulose, p. 241
centrioles, p. 275
chemoreceptors, p. 252

Case Study

Medic 14 is dispatched to 1514 Houston on the outskirts of downtown. Paramedics quickly recognize the address as the Union Gospel Mission. It is a shelter for the homeless and the location of many EMS calls. On arrival, the crew is met by Reverend Williams, the aged gentleman who has operated the shelter for as long as anyone can remember. He recognizes Armando, the senior paramedic, and tells him, "It's Bill Jamison again. He looks bad this time." Paramedics roll the stretcher to the elevator, only to learn that it is again broken. They grab the essential bags and climb four flights of stairs to reach Bill's room.

Bill is a chronic inebriate well known to virtually all EMS providers in the city. He is a former wrecker driver who used to interact with paramedics on accident scenes. However, his disease, alcoholism, eventually took his job, his family, his home, and now his health. EMS providers and the local county hospital have watched Bill's steady and predictable decline to his current condition. Bill is found prone on the floor in a dirty sleeping bag. He is unresponsive with snoring respirations. Paramedics know that Bill has type 2 diabetes and is often noncompliant with his medications. He is often found to be hypoglycemic—as a result of either his alcoholism or his medication.

They gently roll Bill to a supine position, and he moans slightly. His airway, though, is patent and his vitals are stable. They notice multiple bruises and a nosebleed. Bill has virtually all the stigmata of alcoholism and is now jaundiced. Armando says, "I'll bet he is hypoglycemic again." Armando's partner and rookie paramedic, Sam, begins to look for a vein. Reverend Williams holds a flashlight to help illuminate the dark and odorous room. No vein is identifiable. Armando switches places with Sam and takes a look. He, too, sees no veins. They then begin to discuss whether to give glucagon intramuscularly or place an intraosseous (IO) line. Armando decides on the IO. The line is placed without incident, and Bill awakens after receiving half an amp of $D_{50}W$. Bill is transported to University Hospital without incident.

On the way back from the hospital, Sam asks Armando why he chose the IO instead of the intramuscular glucagon. Armando explains, "Glucagon is a hormone that stimulates the release of glucose from carbohydrate storage sites, such as glycogen in the liver.

Because of Bill's liver disease and poor diet, he has little, if any, glycogen stores and glucagon is unlikely to work. Besides, I've tried it in the past and it never has worked." Sam pondered the statement for a minute and asked, "What was the bleeding from?" Armando answers, "Not sure really. I could not see a source. But it is probably a bleeding disorder." "What do you mean?" inquires Sam. Armando responds, "Many of the clotting factors, especially prothrombin, are made and stored in the liver. As the liver fails, as is the case with Bill, his body loses its ability to properly clot, and he is prone to bleeding. Actually, the bleeding points to severe, or even end-stage, liver disease." Sam thinks for a minute and states, "Wow. You can learn something from every call—even at the Union Gospel Mission." Armando smiles and nods gently.

Introduction

The human body normally maintains its internal environment in a steady state of balance that is termed **homeostasis**. A significant disruption in homeostasis often leads to disease. **Disease** is an abnormal structural or functional change within the body. The study of disease is called **pathophysiology** and can be defined as the functional changes that occur within living cells and tissues that are associated with, or result from, disease or injury. **Pathology** is the medical science that deals with all aspects of disease. There is an emphasis on the essential nature, causes, and development of abnormal conditions, as well as with the structural and functional changes that result from disease processes. A physician who specializes in pathology is called a **pathologist**.

Before embarking on the study of pathophysiology, it is essential that you first master the related normal anatomy and physiology. Only through understanding how the body is normally structured and works can one understand abnormal processes. To be an effective health care professional, the paramedic must understand the basic principles of pathophysiology so you can properly assess and treat the disease and injury processes that affect humankind.

This chapter is divided into six parts:

Part 1: Disease

Part 2: Disease at the Chemical Level

Part 3: Disease at the Cellular Level

Part 4: Disease at the Tissue Level

Part 5: Disease at the Organ Level

Part 6: The Body's Defenses against Disease and Injury

Hierarchical Structure of the Body

We start with the concept that all living things that share this big blue-and-green planet known as Earth interact with each other at some point and on some level. Scientists have organized Earth's biological life into levels.

In this chapter we examine the disease processes that arise from the human body's cells, tissues, organs, organ systems, and, ultimately, the organism (body) itself.

Cells, the smallest unit of life, are made up of chemical *molecules* (which are made up of individual *atoms*). A group of similar cells that performs a common function is known as a *tissue*. A group of tissues working together to perform a similar function is called an *organ*. A group of organs working together to perform a common or similar function is referred to as an *organ system*. Finally, a group of organ systems functioning together is called an *organism*. A human being is an organism. Humans have 11 different organ systems.

The organism, or individual, is the unit of life that is capable of surviving and reproducing in the environment. Humans, like many other "higher" animals, are social creatures. That is, we tend to associate with others of our kind. Humans are unique in that we also use other organisms for work and companionship.

Life can also be organized and stratified beyond the individual. For example, all the organisms of the same species residing in a distinct geographic area (e.g., continent, city) are called a *population*. A *community* is the sum total of all living organisms occupying a defined geographic area. A community and its physical environment are referred to as an *ecosystem*. An ecosystem can vary in size, based on the construct being studied, but is self-contained. Any number of ecosystems may exist within a *biome*. A

CONTENT REVIEW

➤ Hierarchy of the Body
- Cells
  ↓
- Tissues
  ↓
- Organs
  ↓
- Organ systems
  ↓
- Organism

CONTENT REVIEW

➤ Levels of Life beyond the Individual
- Individual organism
  ↓
- Population
  ↓
- Community
  ↓
- Ecosystem
  ↓
- Biome
  ↓
- Biosphere

biome is a geographic area with similar climatic conditions, such as a desert biome, a forest biome, a grasslands biome, or a marine biome. Finally, all ecosystems, biomes, and by definition all living organisms, form a *biosphere*. A biosphere is the portion of Earth where life is found. Our biosphere extends from the depths of the deepest oceans (where life can be found) to approximately seven miles above sea level.

PART 1: Disease

All cells and tissues are vulnerable to the effects of disease or injury, which can adversely affect the biology of the cells or tissues in question. **Predisposing factors** may lead to disease. These factors tend to increase the body's vulnerability to a specific disease. For example, it has been demonstrated that prolonged exposure to cigarette smoke changes the cellular structure of the respiratory tract. Sometimes these changes can result in abnormal cell function and cancer. Thus, cigarette smoking is a predisposing factor to the development of lung cancer.

Predisposing Factors to Disease

Factors that lead to the development of disease include age, gender, genetics, lifestyle, and environment.

- *Age.* A factor that leads to the development of disease is age. Humans at both ends of the age spectrum are especially vulnerable to disease. Infants, for example, are vulnerable because their immune systems are immature and they have not developed the necessary defenses. We augment these defenses by providing timely immunizations to enhance the infant's immune system. As we age, there is a decline in immune function that places us at increased risk for disease in our later years. This is due to a general decline in homeostatic function.

- *Gender.* Gender also plays a role in disease development. For example, men tend to develop heart disease at a younger age than women. Women are predisposed to certain diseases, such as osteoporosis, as they age. Often, these differences in disease development are due to the effects of the sex hormones.

- *Genetics.* A major factor in the development of disease is genetics. Only in recent years has the human genetic code

been mapped through the Human Genome Project. Researchers are finding, with increasing frequency, that many diseases are due to expression of specific genes.

Certain diseases are more common in certain families. For example, one family may have a history of atherosclerotic heart disease that routinely kills male members in the fifth or sixth decade of life. Other families may routinely develop diabetes mellitus.

Because our ethnicity and race are also genetically encoded, certain diseases are common in certain races. For example, people of African and Mediterranean descent tend to develop sickle cell disease. People of Native American and Mexican descent tend to develop diabetes mellitus. Ashkenazi Jews (Jews of central European descent) are vulnerable to many diseases, such as cystic fibrosis and Tay-Sachs disease, among others. This is thought to be due to significant intermarriage within the group, resulting in a small gene pool. A small gene pool from intermarriage can result in expression of disease-causing genes that would likely not be expressed if the gene pool were more varied. In fact, genetic testing has shown that 40 percent of the current Ashkenazi population is descended from just four women.[1]

- *Lifestyle.* Another major factor in the development of disease is lifestyle. This is particularly evident in today's society. A century ago, people ate primarily unprocessed foods. Today, foods are processed, removing many of the healthful ingredients that protected our ancestors from some of the diseases that are common today. Heart disease was much less common in the nineteenth century when compared to the latter half of the twentieth and the first part of the twenty-first century.

- In addition, the modern population obtains considerably less exercise than earlier generations because of the availability of cars and other forms of mechanized transportation and the fact that many farm and industry jobs that demanded intense physical labor have been replaced by more sedentary occupations. When you combine a lack of exercise with a diet that is devoid of quality calories (but rather is high in fats and carbohydrates), you end up with obesity. Obesity is one of the biggest health problems in the United States and is quickly becoming as great a problem in other developed countries, such as the United Kingdom, Australia, and Canada.

- *Environment.* Finally, our environment can predispose us to disease. Native Americans have long believed that an individual's health and the health of the community are directly related to the environment. We now know that numerous environmental factors are associated with the development of disease. For example, exposure to asbestos has been directly linked to

CONTENT REVIEW

➤ Predisposing Factors to Disease
- Age
- Gender
- Genetics
- Lifestyle
- Environment

the development of an uncommon lung cancer called mesothelioma.[2] Pollutants have been linked to the development of significant birth defects (such as anencephaly, lack of parts of the brain or skull, in babies born to Mexican mothers in the lower Rio Grande river valley in south Texas, presumably caused by chemicals dumped into the river upstream.[3] In Ukraine, the incidence of cancers—specifically, thyroid cancer—has increased dramatically following the nuclear disaster in 1986 at Chernobyl.[4] Cumulative exposure to toxic substances also plays a role in disease development.

Any of these factors, or a combination of them, can lead to the development of disease. The effects of these factors can sometimes be cumulative. For example, an older person who smokes and also has a family history of lung cancer may be at a risk of developing the disease that is significantly increased over a person who has just one of those risk factors—age, or smoking, or family history—but not two or three of them.

Risk Analysis

It is important to point out that some predisposing factors can be modified, whereas others cannot. Although we cannot control our genetics, gender, or age, we can certainly control our lifestyle and, to a lesser degree, our environment. Minimizing some of these predisposing factors can also slow the effects of age. In the near future, genetic engineering may allow us to manipulate genes to prevent their expression and subsequent disease development.

We also know that there is a kind of cross-pollination of pathophysiologic factors, where risk factors figure in more than one kind of disease, and diseases become risk factors for other diseases. For example, various studies have identified as risk factors for cardiovascular disease such things as smoking, elevated blood pressure, cholesterol levels ("good" cholesterol versus "bad" cholesterol), diet, family history, age, gender, weight, level of exercise, obesity, diabetes, kidney disease, and lung disease (Figure 12-1).

Using data from large-population studies, one can actually predict, with some degree of accuracy, whether a given person will develop any particular disease and how rapidly he will develop it. These data can, therefore, be used to modify the risk factors that can be modified, thus holding off disease development. For example, a 34-year-old male paramedic is 30 pounds overweight, gets little exercise, routinely eats fast food, smokes half a pack of cigarettes a day, has a moderate family history of heart disease, and has mild hypertension. Although he cannot modify his gender or genetics, he can increase his exercise and decrease his fast food intake. This will allow him to lose weight and improve the ratio of bad to good cholesterol. Concurrently, the weight loss can lead to reduction in his

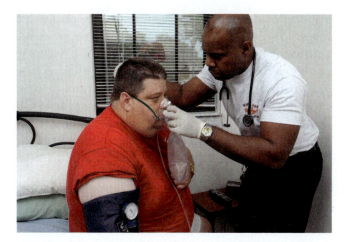

FIGURE 12-1 Obesity is one of many risk factors for cardiovascular disease.

blood pressure. Abandonment of cigarette use further significantly decreases his risks for early development of heart disease. Together, these can modify or attenuate the development of cardiovascular disease, even though he is genetically predisposed to it. As he ages, he should stay abreast of practices that continue to minimize his risk for developing heart disease. For example, when he turns 50, he may be advised to begin taking an aspirin a day.

Risk analysis can now be used to look at a person's whole life. There are programs that can actually predict one's life expectancy. These take into consideration health factors such as have been presented here, but they also take into consideration environmental and lifestyle practices. High-risk behaviors such as scuba diving, skydiving, piloting single-engine aircraft, and rock climbing can statistically decrease projected life expectancy. Other more common behavioral practices that are risk factors include driving long distances, not wearing seatbelts, carrying a handgun, practicing unsafe sex, illicit drug or significant alcohol use, and so on. Minimizing any of these risks can increase life expectancy and, in some instances, also enhance the quality of life.

Disease

Disease is an abnormal structural or functional change within the body. There is normally a defined sequence of events that leads to development of a disease. This is referred to as the **pathogenesis** of the disease. As already noted, a number of factors can be identified that predispose a person to certain diseases. In some instances, predisposing factors cannot be identified. In that case, we say the disease is **idiopathic**.

The study of disease causes is termed **etiology**. Etiology comprises the occurrences, reasons, and variables of a disease. Etiology is often defined as consisting of *causality*, *contribution*, and *correlation*. Again using the example of smoking and lung cancer, we know that various factors are involved in the development of the disease. In some patients, the cause may be repeated exposure to cigarette smoke, whereas in others it may be due to genetic expression. In the person who develops lung cancer from genetic expression, genetics is the cause but cigarette smoking and age may be contributing factors. It has been suggested, but not proven, that secondhand smoke may contribute to the development of lung cancer. In the example we have been using, secondhand smoke exposure in a lung cancer patient who had never smoked might be simply correlated to the condition. That is, it is a suspected factor but cannot be proven to either cause or contribute to the condition.

The manifestation of a disease is known as the **clinical presentation**. The clinical presentation includes both signs and symptoms of the disease. A **symptom** is what the patient tells you about the disease—a subjective complaint. Symptoms are often detailed when you obtain the patient's history. An objective finding that you can identify through physical examination is referred to as a **sign**. Some diseases have a specific constellation of commonly found signs and symptoms. These are referred to as a **syndrome**. However, some signs and symptoms are common among a variety of diseases and are referred to as being nonspecific symptoms or generalized symptoms.

The process of identifying and assigning a name to a disease in an individual patient or a group of patients with similar signs and symptoms is termed **diagnosis**. A diagnosis is a generalization and an assumption that a disease will follow a prescribed course. However, just as people are different, all diseases are different, and each follows its own course. Some diseases have a sudden onset and are referred to as **acute**, whereas others have a much slower onset and are referred to as **chronic** or **insidious**. The symptoms of a chronic disease are often milder and more difficult to initially identify.

When a disease such as diabetes mellitus is first identified, the primary problem is impaired glucose **metabolism**. However, as the disease progresses, other body systems can be affected. With diabetes, the eyes and kidneys can be adversely affected, causing both blindness and renal failure. Such abnormalities that result from the original problem are referred to as **complications**. When these resulting complications are common, or even expected, they are referred to as **sequelae** of the disease.

Many diseases are fairly well understood, and so we can predict their outcome. This expected outcome is referred to as the **prognosis**. For example, we know that hepatitis A has an incubation period of approximately 28 days and the disease lasts from two weeks to three months with relatively mild symptoms. Whenever the disease varies from the expected prognosis, it is important to reevaluate the patient to ensure that the diagnosis was correct and that complications are not occurring.

Classifications of Disease

There are various ways to classify diseases. The most common is by disease cause. On this basis, the following system of disease classification will be used in this text:

- **Infectious.** Infectious diseases are those that result from invasion of the body and colonization by a pathogenic organism. Most of these are microorganisms such as prions, viruses, bacteria, and fungi. Others are larger multicelled pathogenic organisms such as tapeworms and liver flukes.

- **Immunologic.** Overreactions of the immune system, commonly called allergies or hypersensitivity, can cause diseases such as anaphylaxis. Sometimes the immune system fails to recognize certain tissues as belonging to the host and mounts an immune response as if the tissues were foreign. This phenomenon, referred to as **autoimmune disease**, is responsible for such conditions as rheumatic heart disease and rheumatoid arthritis. Inadequate immune system function makes the human more susceptible to pathogenic organisms and can result in overwhelming infection, such as that seen with acquired immune deficiency syndrome (AIDS).

- **Inflammatory.** Inflammatory diseases are those that result from the body's response to another disease process (primary disease). For example, pelvic inflammatory disease (PID) in a female is secondary to a bacterial infection in the reproductive tract—often gonorrhea or chlamydia. The infection causes inflammation of the organs and supporting structures in the pelvis.

- **Ischemic.** Many diseases are due to diminished blood supply. Thus, the affected tissues may be deprived of oxygen and essential energy substrates, which can lead to cell death. Common examples of ischemic diseases include acute coronary syndrome (ACS), ischemic stroke, and ischemic bowel disease.

- **Metabolic.** Metabolic diseases result when there is a disturbance in the biochemical and metabolic processes within the body. Examples include diabetes mellitus, which results from decreased insulin secretion from the endocrine pancreas, and thyrotoxicosis that results from abnormally elevated

---

CONTENT REVIEW

➤ Disease Classified by Cause
  - Infectious
  - Immunologic
  - Inflammatory
  - Ischemic
  - Metabolic
  - Nutritional
  - Genetic
  - Congenital
  - Neoplastic
  - Trauma
  - Physical agents
  - Iatrogenic
  - Idiopathic

FIGURE 12-2 Down syndrome is a congenital disease.

(© Daniel Limmer)

levels of thyroid hormones that can markedly increase the basal metabolic rate, causing significant signs and symptoms.

- *Nutritional.* Nutritional diseases primarily result from a deficiency in one or all of the major nutritional sources (carbohydrates, proteins, fats). Vitamin deficiencies can also lead to nutritional diseases, because vitamins are required for normal metabolic processes. Examples of nutritional diseases are malnutrition and diseases that result from vitamin deficiency, such as scurvy and rickets.

- *Genetic.* Genetic diseases are those that are coded for in a person's genetic material and thus are passed from parent to child. Examples of genetic diseases are hemophilia, Huntington's disease, and color blindness.

- *Congenital.* Certain diseases can result from problems that occur during fetal development. Most fetal development occurs during the first trimester of life. It is during this period that the fetus is most susceptible to external factors that can adversely affect development (**teratogens**). However, many cases of congenital disease never have an identifiable cause. Examples of congenital diseases are cleft lip and palate, congenital heart disease, and Down syndrome (Figure 12-2).

- *Neoplastic.* On occasion, certain cells will begin abnormal or uncontrolled cell growth. This process is referred to as **neoplasia**. The result is a tumor, or **neoplasm** (Figure 12-3). A neoplasm can be **benign** (not cancerous, not able to spread to other tissues) or **malignant** (cancerous, able to spread), depending on the changes present in the cell line. Often, the body's immune system is successful in removing cells that begin abnormal growth. However, when the cell growth is rapid, or if the cell is particularly resistant to removal by the body's defenses, the disease progresses and can eventually kill the patient. Fibroid tumors in the uterus, more accurately called uterine leiomyomas, are an example of a benign neoplastic process. Breast cancer (which usually arises from the breast ducts) is an example of a malignant neoplastic process.

- *Trauma.* External physical forces can mechanically change or disrupt the structure of the body and, as a result, affect body function. These external forces are referred to as **trauma**. An example might be blunt trauma to a kidney that fractures the kidney into multiple portions. This can cause the kidney to totally fail or to significantly decrease its ability to function.

- *Physical agents.* Myriad physical agents can adversely affect body structure and function. These include chemicals, poisons, ionizing radiation, extremes in temperature, changes in atmospheric pressure, and electrical shock. Examples of diseases caused by physical agents include transitional-cell bladder cancer, caused by exposure to chemicals such as ink, and ultraviolet keratitis (welder's flash) that results from looking at a welding arc that is producing ultraviolet radiation.

- *Iatrogenic.* Medical treatments for a disease can sometimes result in the development of other diseases or problems. A disease that occurs in this way is referred to as an **iatrogenic disease**. For example, a subclavian central intravenous line is placed into a patient to administer intravenous nutrition following a severe burn. During the line insertion, the dome of the lung is inadvertently punctured, resulting in a pneumothorax. This would then be termed an iatrogenic pneumothorax.

  Some procedures or treatments are so complicated or harsh that iatrogenic effects may be expected. The chances of developing iatrogenic complications are

Neoplasia

FIGURE 12-3 How cancers grow. Factors such as genetic predisposition, smoking, pollution, and exposure to radiation or the sun's ultraviolet rays can trigger abnormal cell growth.

Abnormal or uncontrolled cell growth results in a tumor, or neoplasm.

weighed against the perceived benefit of the treatment. An example is vaginal candidiasis following antibiotic therapy. The vagina normally has microorganisms present on its surface. These include both bacteria and fungi. The bacteria usually keep the fungi concentration low. However, if the patient is placed on potent antibiotics, the antibiotics can kill the normal vaginal bacteria (flora), which allows the fungus to proliferate, resulting in candidiasis. The disease is iatrogenic in that it resulted directly from medical treatment.

Patho Pearls

The practice of medicine has become so complex that many patients actually die from the very treatments that are supposed to help them. It has been estimated that almost 200,000 patients a year suffer in-hospital deaths that are possibly preventable. Little is known about preventable out-of-hospital deaths. Further, a recent medical study found that medical errors caused up to 98,000 deaths annually and should be considered a national epidemic. Many of us forget that the primary dictum of medicine is *primum non nocere* (first, do no harm). We owe it to our patients, present and future, to ensure that our practices do not violate this dictum and bring them harm when they are seeking our help.

- *Idiopathic.* In many instances, as noted earlier, the specific cause of a disease is unknown. In this case, the disease is classified as idiopathic. Sometimes, a cause may be identified later. However, in many cases a specific cause is never found.

PART 2: Disease at the Chemical Level

To fully understand and appreciate anatomy, physiology, and pathophysiology, as a paramedic you must understand some basic chemistry and biochemistry as discussed in this chapter. Virtually every medical condition involves or affects biochemical mechanisms.

When did human life begin? This question has been a subject of discussion for thousands of years. In the sixth century B.C.E., pre-Socratic Greek philosophers spent a great deal of time discussing the possible origins of life. Although the true answer may never be known, the prevailing theory is that the universe was created almost 15 million years ago in a phenomenon referred to as the "Big Bang." The Big Bang theory (Figure 12-4) was first put forth in 1927 by Belgian priest Georges Lemaître. He proposed that the universe began with the explosion of a primeval atom. Years later, the noted astronomer Edwin Hubble found experimental evidence to help validate Lemaître's theory. He found that distant galaxies in every direction were moving away from us at speeds proportional to their distance.

The theory of a Big Bang explained why distant galaxies were traveling away from the earth at great speeds. The theory also predicted the existence of cosmic background radiation (the energy left over from the explosion itself). The Big Bang theory received its strongest confirmation when, in fact, cosmic radiation was discovered in 1964 by

The Big Bang Theory

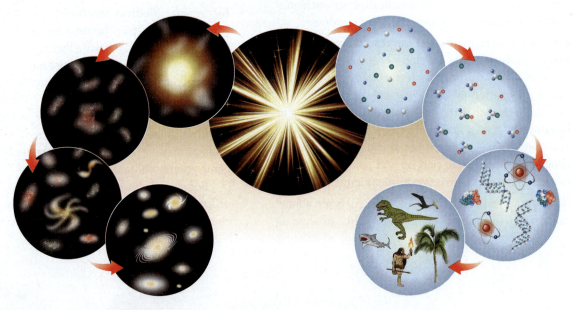

The Big Bang theory proposes that the universe began with the explosion of a primeval atom—resulting in both the formation of galaxies in a still-expanding universe and the origin of life from simple chemicals.

FIGURE 12-4 Development of the universe originating from a rapid expansion (explosion) of hot, dense primeval material is known as the "Big Bang theory."

Arno Penzias and Robert Wilson, who later won the Nobel Prize for this discovery. In 2006, a distant NASA space probe detected the light released just after the Big Bang. This cosmic afterglow, known as microwave background, is further support for the Big Bang theory. It is the oldest radiation ever detected, still traveling almost 14 billion years after it was emitted.

A related component to the origin of the universe is the origin of life as we know it. The prevailing scientific theory is that simple chemicals present in the primordial atmosphere and ocean combined to form larger, more complex chemicals. This theory is referred to as *chemical evolution*. Powered by the energy of the sun and other sources, the chemistry of the atmosphere and oceans changed over time. This ultimately led to the formation of complex chemicals that were able to *self-replicate* (produce identical copies of themselves). The ability of a chemical to self-replicate marked the transition from chemical evolution to *biological evolution*. Once biological evolution began, *natural selection* began. (Natural selection is the tendency of traits that help a species to adapt and survive to become common in a population by being passed down to succeeding generations.) As these chemicals replicated and multiplied, they became more complex. The self-replicating chemical soon became surrounded by a membrane and cellular life began.

The Chemical Basis of Life

As stated previously, to understand pathophysiology, you must first understand normal anatomy and physiology. To understand normal anatomy and physiology, you must understand the chemical basis for life. In this section of the chapter, we will summarize the basics of chemistry as they apply to pathophysiology. Then, we will detail the biochemical processes that are affected by injury and illness.

The fundamental chemical unit is the **atom**. Within the atom are particles, referred to as subatomic particles, which include electrons, protons, and neutrons. **Protons** and **neutrons** exist within the nucleus of the atom. **Electrons** are considerably smaller particles and orbit the nucleus (Figure 12-5). Protons (p^+) have a positive electrical charge, neutrons (n) are electrically neutral, and electrons (e^-) have a negative electrical charge. Opposite charges attract and like charges repel. When the number of protons and the number of electrons are the same, the atomic charge is electrically neutral.

An **element** is a substance that cannot be separated into simpler substances. The number of protons in the nucleus of an atom (the **atomic number**) defines the element. Elements are usually classified by their atomic number in a scheme known as the *periodic table of elements* (Figure 12-6).

Elements cannot be reduced to simpler substances by normal chemical means. That is, naturally occurring processes cannot break them down into more elemental structures. While each element contains a characteristic number of protons, the number of neutrons can vary. Elements that have the same number of protons but vary in the number of neutrons are referred to as **isotopes**, or variants of the same element. Some elements, such as uranium, can have multiple isotopes. The number of protons in an atom's nucleus is referred to as the atomic number, and the total number of neutrons and protons in an atom is referred to as the **mass number**.

Electrons spin in shells around the nucleus.

Electron shell

Electron (−)

Proton (+)

Nucleus

Neutron (no charge)

2p
2n

8p
8n

Helium (He)

Helium (He)

Oxygen (O)

(a) A three-dimensional representation of an atom of helium, showing protons and neutrons in the nucleus and electrons occupying a region around the nucleus.

(b) A two-dimensional representation of an atom of helium.

(c) A two-dimensional representation of an atom of oxygen.

FIGURE 12-5 Atoms can be represented in various ways.

(Goodenough, Judith and Betty A. McGuire, Biology of Humans: Concepts, Applications, and Issues, *3rd Edition, © 2010. Reprinted by permission of Pearson Education, Inc. Upper Saddle River, NJ.)*

FIGURE 12-6 A portion of the periodic table of elements. Each element has an atomic number (the number of protons), a mass number (the total number of neutrons and protons), and a one- or two-letter symbol.

(Freeman, Scott, Biological Science, 4th Edition, © 2011. Reprinted by permission of Pearson Education, Inc., Upper Saddle River, NJ.)

Some combinations of neutrons and protons make the nucleus that contains them inherently unstable. These atoms are called **radioactive isotopes** because their nuclei break down and emit radiation, or alpha, beta, and gamma rays, until the atom regains stability. This process is referred to as **radioactive decay**. The initial isotope is referred to as the parent and the resulting isotope is the daughter. The rate of radioactive decay is constant and specific for a given isotope. The rate of decay is usually measured in a unit called a half-life. A **half-life** is the time it takes for the parent isotope to decrease by one-half (Figure 12-7).

Electrons rotate around the nucleus of the atom in a specific region referred to as an **orbital**. Each orbital has a specific shape and can hold two or more electrons. Orbitals occupy

Clinical Note

There are numerous medical uses of radiation. These include the diagnosis of disease, radiation therapy, and many aspects of research. Many of the diagnostic modalities that use radiation range from fairly routine X-rays to complex computed tomography (CT) scans and the injections of radioactive material for nuclear medicine imaging. In general, radiation therapy involves delivering a large dose of radiation to a small area of the body. Therapy is directed primarily to the killing of tumor cells as part of the treatment of cancer. Radiation is also used in research to find new ways to diagnose and treat disease.

(a)	Number of half-lives elapsed	Fraction remaining	Percentage remaining
	0	$1/1$	100
	1	$1/2$	50
	2	$1/4$	25
	3	$1/8$	12.5
	4	$1/16$	6.25
	5	$1/32$	3.125
	6	$1/64$	1.563
	7	$1/128$	0.781

(b) **Half-Lives of Isotopes of Americium**

- Am241— 432.2 years
- Am242— 16.02 hours
- Am243— 7,380 years

FIGURE 12-7 The half-life of a radioactive isotope is the time it takes for half the atoms of that substance to disintegrate into another form. The half-life of any radioactive isotope is unique to that isotope, so that a substance can be identified by discovering its half-life. (a) As half-lives elapse, smaller and smaller fractions of the original substance remain. (b) Half-lives can range from fractions of a second to billions of years. For example, the element americium has many isotopes with vastly different half-lives, three of which—americium 241, 242, and 243—are listed here.

levels that are defined based on their distance from the nucleus. These levels are referred to as **electron shells** and are numbered starting with the closest shell to the nucleus. Electrons first fill the electron shells closest to the nucleus and then progressively fill the more distant shells. The filling order of the more distant shells is complicated. The first shell can hold two electrons, and the second shell can hold eight electrons. The number of electrons a shell can hold increases with each level (2, 8, 18, 32, 50) (Figure 12-8). The outermost shell of an atom is referred to as the **valence shell**. The electrons found in that shell are referred to as **valence electrons**. An atom is most stable when the valence shell is full. The only elements that have a full valence shell are the six that are

Hydrogen atom (atomic number = 1)

Carbon atom (atomic number = 6)

Oxygen atom (atomic number = 8)

The shell closest to the nucleus can hold up to 2 electrons.

The next shell out can hold up to 8 electrons (the shell shown here has 6). Atoms with more than 10 electrons have additional shells.

FIGURE 12-8 Hydrogen, carbon, and oxygen atoms. Each concentric circle around the nucleus represents an electron shell.

(Goodenough, Judith and Betty A. McGuire, Biology of Humans: Concepts, Applications, and Issues, 3rd Edition, © 2010. Reprinted by permission of Pearson Education, Inc., Upper Saddle River, NJ.)

called the noble gases: helium, neon, argon, krypton, xenon, and radon. Because their valence shells are full, the noble gases are extremely stable.

Chemical Bonding

Most atoms become stable by bonding to other atoms. For example, the simplest atom is hydrogen. Hydrogen contains only one electron. However, the first orbital shell can hold two electrons. Thus, to attain stability, hydrogen must find a second electron to fill the first shell. When two

hydrogen atoms approach each other, they begin to share their two electrons, and then both atoms fill their valence shell and become stable.

Covalent Bonds

The equal sharing of electrons results in what is called a **covalent bond**, which tends to hold the atoms together. A substance made up of atoms held together by one or more covalent bonds is referred to as a **molecule** (Figure 12-9). Covalent bonds are the strongest of the three types of chemical bonds.

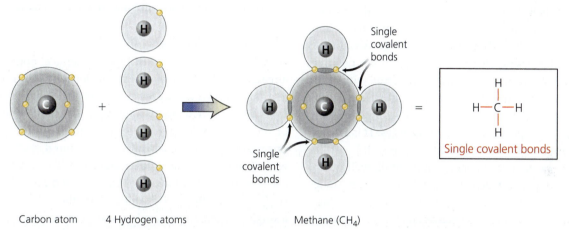

Carbon atom   4 Hydrogen atoms   Methane (CH_4)

(a) The molecule methane (CH_4) is formed by the sharing of electrons between one carbon atom and four hydrogen atoms. Because in each case one pair of electrons is shared, the bonds formed are single covalent bonds.

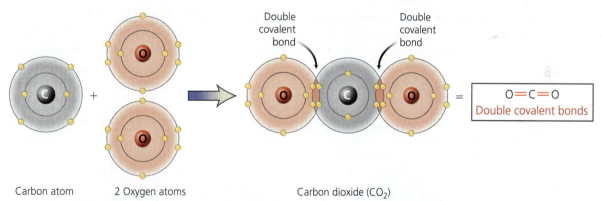

Carbon atom   2 Oxygen atoms   Carbon dioxide (CO_2)

(b) The oxygen atoms in a molecule of carbon dioxide (CO_2) form double covalent bonds with the carbon atom. In double bonds, two pairs of electrons are shared.

Nitrogen atom   Nitrogen atom   Nitrogen gas (N_2)

(c) The nitrogen atoms in nitrogen gas (N_2) form a triple covalent bond in which three pairs of electrons are shared.

FIGURE 12-9 Covalent bonds are formed when electrons are shared between atoms. Shown here are examples of single, double, and triple covalent bonds. The structural formula of each is shown at the far right.

(Goodenough, Judith and Betty A. McGuire, Biology of Humans: Concepts, Applications, and Issues, *3rd Edition,* © 2010. *Reprinted by permission of Pearson Education, Inc., Upper Saddle River, NJ.)*

Ionic Bonds

In addition to covalent bonds, atoms can be held together when atoms with an electrical charge are attracted to each other. An atom or molecule that has acquired an electrical charge by either gaining or losing one or more electrons is referred to as an **ion**. Neutral atoms have an equal number of protons and electrons. When an atom or molecule loses one or more electrons, the number of protons exceeds the number of electrons, thus giving the atom or molecule a net positive charge. (Remember that a proton has a positive charge, whereas an electron has a negative charge.) Conversely, when an atom or molecule gains one or more electrons, there are then more electrons than protons and the atom or molecule has a net negative charge. An atom or molecule with missing electrons and thus a net positive charge is called a **cation**. An atom or molecule with extra electrons and a net negative charge is called an **anion**. Because opposite charges attract, bonds form between atoms of opposite (positive/negative) charges. This kind of bond is referred to as an **ionic bond** (Figure 12-10).

As with covalent bonds, ions will try to fill their outermost shell in order to reach stability. Thus, certain atoms tend to interact with other atoms to fill their outermost shell. Elements that are classified as **metallic elements** tend to lose electrons. Likewise, elements that are described as **nonmetallic elements** tend to gain electrons. Thus, most ionic bonds are between a metal and a nonmetal. The prototypical example of this is the ionic bonding of the atoms sodium (a metal) and chlorine (a nonmetal). Sodium is extremely reactive and occurs only in compounds in nature. Chlorine is also quite reactive and usually exists as a salt in nature. Sodium has one electron in its outer shell and chlorine has seven electrons in its outer shell. Thus, sodium (Na) must lose an electron to reach stability, and chlorine (Cl) must gain an electron to reach stability. When the two atoms come into close proximity, the sodium atom loses an electron to the chlorine atom, thus becoming a positively charged cation (abbreviated as Na^+). The chlorine atom, gaining an electron, becomes a negatively charged anion (abbreviated as Cl^-). The opposite ions are then attracted to each other, thus forming an ionic bond and becoming sodium chloride (NaCl), a salt (the main ingredient in common table salt).

Hydrogen Bonds

A hydrogen bond is the last type of chemical bonding. As already noted, the equal sharing of electrons forms a covalent bond. However, in selected cases, the sharing of electrons between two atoms is unequal. Thus, different parts of the same molecule can have an unequal charge. An unequal covalent bond is called a **polar bond**, and the molecule is referred to as a **polar molecule**. This relationship can be explained by looking at the water molecule. In water (H_2O), two hydrogen (H) atoms share their electrons with a single oxygen (O) molecule, but the electrons spend more time orbiting the oxygen atom compared to the hydrogen atoms. Thus, the oxygen atom has a slightly negative charge and each hydrogen ion has a slight positive charge, thereby making the entire water molecule polar. In nature, the hydrogen ions of a water molecule, because they have a slight positive charge, are attracted to the oxygen atoms of

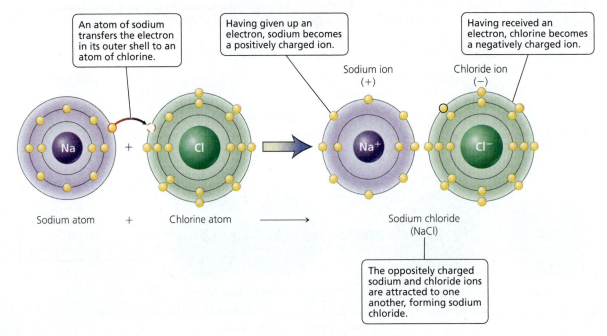

An atom of sodium transfers the electron in its outer shell to an atom of chlorine.

Having given up an electron, sodium becomes a positively charged ion.

Having received an electron, chlorine becomes a negatively charged ion.

Sodium ion (+)

Chloride ion (−)

Na   +   Cl   Na⁺   Cl⁻

Sodium atom   +   Chlorine atom   ⟶   Sodium chloride (NaCl)

The oppositely charged sodium and chloride ions are attracted to one another, forming sodium chloride.

FIGURE 12-10 An ionic bond involves the transfer of electrons between atoms. Such a transfer creates oppositely charged ions that are attracted to each other.

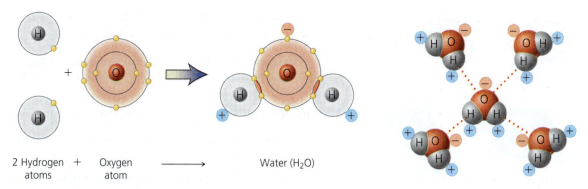

(a) Water is formed when an oxygen atom covalently bonds (shares electrons) with two hydrogen atoms. Due to unequal sharing of electrons, oxygen carries a slight negative charge and the hydrogen atoms carry a slight positive charge.

(b) The hydrogen atoms from one water molecule are attracted to the oxygen atoms of other water molecules. This relatively weak attraction (shown by dotted lines) is called a hydrogen bond.

FIGURE 12-11 The hydrogen bonds of water. (a) Shown at left, water is formed when an oxygen atom covalently bonds with two hydrogen atoms. Because of unequal sharing of electrons, the oxygen atom has a slight negative charge and the hydrogen atoms have a slight positive charge. (b) Shown at right, the hydrogen atoms of one water molecule are attracted to the oxygen atoms of other water molecules. This relatively weak attraction (shown by dotted lines) is called a hydrogen bond.

(Goodenough, Judith and Betty A. McGuire, Biology of Humans: Concepts, Applications, and Issues, 3rd Edition, © 2010. Reprinted by permission of Pearson Education, Inc., Upper Saddle River, NJ.)

other water molecules (because they have a slight negative charge). This attraction between a slightly positively charged hydrogen atom and a slightly negatively charged oxygen atom is referred to as a **hydrogen bond**. Hydrogen bonds are much weaker than either covalent bonds or ionic bonds. Collectively, they are important in that they give water its special physical properties (Figure 12-11).

Inorganic and Organic Chemicals

In general chemistry, chemicals are usually classified as organic or inorganic. **Inorganic chemicals** are chemicals that do not contain the element carbon. **Organic chemicals** are all the chemicals that do contain the element carbon. More than 90 percent of all known chemicals are organic, and most chemicals found in plants and animals are organic. Six elements (carbon, hydrogen, nitrogen, oxygen, phosphorus, and sulfur) make up approximately 98 percent of the body weight of most living organisms. Of these, the four major elements of living systems are carbon (C), hydrogen (H), oxygen (O), and nitrogen (N).

A **compound** is the chemical union of two or more elements. The four major compounds of living systems are carbohydrates, proteins, nucleic acids, and lipids. Molecules of these compounds are composed mostly of atoms from the four major elements, plus some additional elements, such as phosphorus (P), sulfur (S), iron (Fe), magnesium (Mg), sodium (Na), chlorine (Cl), potassium (K), iodine (I), and calcium (Ca) (Figure 12-12).

Because of the diversity of the world of biochemistry, we will limit this discussion primarily to animals. Plants have very unique biochemical processes, but these are not pertinent, for the most part, to the study of human pathophysiology.

Classes of Biological Chemicals

There are four major classes of biological chemicals. These are the four major compounds already mentioned: carbohydrates, proteins, nucleic acids, and lipids (fats). Water, as well, plays an extremely important role in biological chemistry.

FIGURE 12-12 Common table salt (sodium chloride, NaCl) is a compound of sodium and chlorine. Sodium is a silver-colored solid metal; chlorine is a yellow gas. Table salt is, obviously, neither a silvery metal nor a yellow gas, but a grainy white compound that is quite different from its elements.

CONTENT REVIEW

➤ Classes of Biological Chemicals
 • Carbohydrates
 • Proteins
 • Nucleic acids (DNA, RNA)
 • Lipids (fats)

FIGURE 12-13 Glucose is a monosaccharide, a six-carbon sugar that is the principal energy source for the human body.

(Goodenough, Judith and Betty A. McGuire, Biology of Humans: Concepts, Applications, and Issues, 3rd Edition, © 2010. Reprinted by permission of Pearson Education, Inc., Upper Saddle River, NJ.)

Carbohydrates

Carbohydrates are compounds that contain the elements carbon (C), hydrogen (H), and oxygen (O). Typically, the hydrogen and oxygen atoms occur in a 2:1 ratio. Carbohydrates provide the majority of calories in most diets. They are typically divided into the sugars and the polysaccharides.

SUGARS   The **sugars** can be classified as either simple sugars (monosaccharides) or complex sugars (disaccharides).

Monosaccharides   The **monosaccharides** are simple sugars. Examples of monosaccharides are glucose, fructose, and galactose.

- **Glucose** is a six-carbon sugar and the principal energy source for the human body (Figure 12-13).
- **Fructose** is a five-carbon sugar that is found in many plants and vegetables as well as honey.
- **Galactose**, also a six-carbon sugar, is primarily found in dairy products.

Sugars are the most important sources of energy for most cells. They are soluble in water.

Disaccharides   The **disaccharides** are complex sugars. They are combinations of the simple sugars joined together by a glycosidic bond to form a double-sugar molecule. Examples of disaccharides are sucrose, lactose, and maltose.

- **Sucrose** is common table sugar. It is a combination of glucose and fructose (Figure 12-14).
- **Lactose** is the principal sugar in milk. It is a combination of glucose and galactose.
- **Maltose** is a breakdown product of starch. It is a combination of two glucose molecules.

Sucrose and maltose are frequently encountered in the diet. As noted, maltose results from the degradation of starch.

POLYSACCHARIDES   Polysaccharides are the second type of carbohydrates. Major polysaccharides are the starches, cellulose, and glycogen. Plants store glucose in the form of starches or cellulose. Animals store glucose in the form of glycogen. Starches and cellulose are major parts of the human diet.

Starches   **Starches** are polymers of glucose. A **polymer** is a large organic molecule formed by combining many smaller molecules (**monomers**) in a regular pattern. In the case of starch, the smaller molecule is glucose. Thus, starches are long chains of glucose molecules connected by glycosidic bonds. Unlike the monosaccharides, starches are insoluble in water. This allows them to serve as storage reservoirs for glucose.

There are two types of starches:

- **Amylose** is a linear, unbranched chain of several hundred glucose molecules. (Portions of larger molecules, such as the glucose molecules that make up amylose, are called *residues*.)
- **Amylopectin** differs from amylose in that it is highly branched, not linear like amylose. The glucose residues in a molecule of amylopectin number several thousand.

FIGURE 12-14 Sucrose is a disaccharide made when two monosaccharides, glucose and fructose, combine.

(Goodenough, Judith and Betty A. McGuire, Biology of Humans: Concepts, Applications, and Issues, 3rd Edition, © 2010. Reprinted by permission of Pearson Education, Inc., Upper Saddle River, NJ.)

Cellulose   Like starch, **cellulose** is a polysaccharide polymer with glucose as its monomer. However, cellulose differs significantly from starch in its chemical properties. Cellulose is the most abundant organic molecule in the world and the major structural material of plants. For example, wood is largely cellulose, and cotton and paper are almost pure cellulose. Humans do not have the enzyme necessary to digest cellulose; thus, it passes through our gastrointestinal systems undigested. However, the fiber that cellulose provides is important in creating bulk and moving fecal matter through the large intestine.

Glycogen   In terms of human pathophysiology, glycogen is certainly the most important polysaccharide. **Glycogen** (Figure 12-15) is a glucose polymer much like amylopectin except that the branches tend to be shorter and less frequent. Glycogen is stored primarily in the liver and skeletal muscle. When needed, it is broken down to glucose in a process called **glycogenolysis**. Glycogenolysis is controlled by the hormones glucagon and epinephrine. In persons with liver disease, such as chronic alcoholics, glycogen stores may be scant, and thus administration of glucagon is often ineffective in elevating the blood glucose level in hypoglycemia.

Proteins

Proteins, which are nitrogen-based complex compounds, are the basic building blocks of cells. Proteins are essential for the growth and repair of living tissues. They are the most abundant class of biological chemicals in the body (Table 12-1). Proteins consist of smaller building blocks called **amino acids**.

Glycogen

FIGURE 12-15 Glycogen is the storage polysaccharide in animals. It is stored primarily in the liver and in skeletal muscle.

Clinical Note

It is common practice in EMS to administer glucagon to patients with hypoglycemia. Glucagon elevates the blood glucose indirectly by stimulating glycogenolysis. Although this is usually effective, many patients, such as chronic alcoholics, have limited stores of glycogen because of their liver disease and associated malnutrition; thus, glucagon may be ineffective in this population. Decreased glycogen stores are also associated with increased physical activity, as is seen with endurance events (e.g., marathon races, football matches). Decreased glycogen stores are also often present in patients with malnutrition. In neonates it is important to remember that liver glycogen stores become rapidly depleted within hours of birth. When you suspect that your patient might have inadequate glycogen stores, administer glucose (orally or intravenously) to increase blood glucose levels (Figure 12-16).

FIGURE 12-16 Glucagon administration may be ineffective in patients with limited stores of glycogen, such as alcoholics because of liver disease and malnutrition. If you suspect your patient may have limited glycogen stores, administer glucose to increase blood glucose levels.

Table 12-1 Protein Functions

Protein Type	Function
Antibodies and complement protein	Defense (destruction of disease-causing agents)
Contractile and motor proteins	Movement
Enzymes	Catalyze chemical reactions
Peptide hormones	Signal and control the activities of cells
Receptor proteins	Receive chemical signals from outside of the cell and initiate cellular response
Structural proteins	Support cells and tissues; major factor in various body structures
Transport proteins	Move substrates across cell membranes and throughout the body

Polypeptide chain

FIGURE 12-17 Amino acid monomers combine to form polymers consisting of long chains called polypeptides.

(Freeman, Scott, Biological Science, 4th Edition, © 2011. Reprinted by permission of Pearson Education, Inc., Upper Saddle River, NJ.)

The amino acids are held together in proteins by **peptide bonds**. These bonds occur when two amino acid molecules join and a molecule of water is released. The shape and other properties of each protein are dictated by the precise sequence of amino acids it contains. Proteins consist of one or more unbranched chains of amino acids. Thus, like the polysaccharides already discussed, proteins are polymers. There are 20 types of amino acids (monomers) that are synthesized in protein polymers.

The typical protein will contain 200–300 amino acid molecules. A protein chain containing less than 10 amino acids is often called a **peptide** and a chain of greater than 10 amino acids is called a **polypeptide**. Some proteins are extremely large, consisting of more than 20,000 amino acid monomers (Figure 12-17).

Proteins have four levels of structure: primary, secondary, tertiary, and quaternary. The precise sequence of amino acids in a protein is referred to as the primary structure. This sequence of amino acids in a protein is determined by the person's genes. The secondary structure of a protein results from bending and folding of the amino acid chain. The shape results from hydrogen bonding between parts of the chain. The overall three-dimensional shape of a protein is called the tertiary structure. Covalent, ionic, and hydrogen bonds all play a role in a protein's tertiary structure. Finally, some proteins will have more than one polypeptide chain. Each chain forms a subunit of the protein. The forces that hold the subunits together are the charges present on the side-chains. This level of protein structure is referred to as the quaternary structure (Table 12-2).

Table 12-2 Protein Structure

Level	Description	Stabilized by	Example: Hemoglobin
Primary	The sequence of amino acids in a polypeptide	Peptide bonds	Gly — Ser — Asp — Cys
Secondary	Formation of alpha helices and beta-pleated sheets in a polypeptide	Hydrogen bonding between groups along the peptide-bonded backbone; thus, depends on primary structure	One α-helix
Tertiary	Overall three-dimensional shape of a polypeptide (includes contribution from secondary structures)	Bonds and other interactions between side chains or between side chains and the peptide-bonded backbone; thus, depends on primary structure	One of hemoglobin's subunits
Quaternary	Shape produced by combinations of polypeptides (thus, combinations of tertiary structures)	Bonds and other interactions between side chains, and between peptide backbones of different polypeptides; thus, depends on primary structure	Hemoglobin, which consists of four polypeptide subunits

Changes in the environment of a protein can result in the protein losing its three-dimensional shape. Various factors can cause this, including heat, chemicals, and pH. These usually affect the secondary and tertiary structure, although they can also affect the primary structure. The loss of a protein's three-dimensional shape is called **denaturation**. The classic example of this is the act of cooking an egg. The egg white is primarily protein. When heat is applied, the proteins in the egg white denature and lose their shape. This causes the egg white to change from a translucent substance to the white cooked egg.

Patho Pearls

Congenital Metabolic Diseases. There are a large number of congenital genetic diseases that affect aspects of metabolism. Formerly referred to as *inborn errors of metabolism*, they are now more accurately referred to as **congenital metabolic diseases**. These diseases can affect carbohydrate, protein, and lipid metabolism, as well as other metabolic processes. Examples of these diseases include glycogen storage disease, phenylketonuria, acute intermittent porphyria, congenital adrenal hyperplasia, and many others. At present, treatment is extremely limited and many conditions are ultimately fatal. The use of gene therapy, when refined, holds great promise for these conditions.

ENZYMES Most enzymes are proteins. **Enzymes** are substances that speed up chemical reactions. They accomplish this without being consumed in the process. Most chemical reactions that occur in the body occur too slowly to meet the needs of the body. Thus, we have multiple enzyme systems that speed these necessary chemical reactions—sometimes by as much as 10,000 to 1,000,000 times the rate at which such reactions would occur without the aid of the enzyme.

The substance an enzyme works on is called a **substrate**. The substrate binds to the enzyme, forming the **enzyme–substrate complex**. The substrate is then converted to the end product, the enzyme then binds to another substrate, and the process begins again (Figure 12-18). Some enzyme systems require **cofactors** to function. Cofactors are nonprotein substances that aid in the conversion of substrate to end product. Some cofactors are found in inorganic substances, whereas others, such as vitamins, are organic. Organic cofactors are usually referred to as **coenzymes**.

Patho Pearls

Free Radicals, a Side-Effect of Aging. The effects of age are manifested throughout the body. Numerous metabolic processes, including metabolism as a whole, slow with age. This is due to multiple factors, including a loss in muscle tissue, but is also due to hormonal and neurologic changes.

One of the side-effects of aging is the development of **free radicals**. Free radicals are highly reactive molecules or atoms

Step 1: The cycle begins when the active site of the enzyme is unoccupied and the substrate is present.

Step 2: The substrate binds to the active site of the enzyme, forming an enzyme–substrate complex.

Step 3: The substrate is converted to products that are released from the active site, and the cycle can begin again.

Substrate

Products

Enzyme   Enzyme–substrate complex   Enzyme

(a) A decomposition reaction involving an enzyme

Substrates   Product

Enzyme   Enzyme–substrate complex   Enzyme

(b) A synthesis reaction involving an enzyme

FIGURE 12-18 The working cycle of an enzyme.

(Goodenough, Judith and Betty A. McGuire, Biology of Humans: Concepts, Applications, and Issues, *3rd Edition, © 2010. Reprinted by permission of Pearson Education, Inc., Upper Saddle River, NJ.)*

that have an unpaired electron in an outer orbital that is not contributing to molecular bonding (and is thus free). Atoms or small molecules that are free radicals tend to be the most unstable. The free-radical theory of aging (FRTA), advanced by Denham Harman more than 50 years ago, posits the following: *Cells continuously produce free radicals, and constant radical damage eventually kills the cell. When radicals kill or damage enough cells in an organism, the organism ages.*[5] Aging occurs when energy-producing cells die, either when the mitochondria begin to die out because of free radical damage or when less functional mitochondria remain within these cells. (Free radicals are also discussed in the chapter "Airway Management and Ventilation.")

The body contains compounds called *antioxidants* that are molecules that eliminate radicals. Thus, elevated levels of antioxidants prevent much of the damage done by radicals. There are numerous antioxidant molecules found in the body, including superoxide dismutase, catalase, glutathione, and others. It has been postulated that administration of antioxidant substances can help delay the effects of aging. Vitamins A, C, and E, as well as several cofactors and minerals, have antioxidant properties. Although the theory seems appropriate, clinical studies have failed to show any

FIGURE 12-19 Colorful fruits and vegetables (other than green) are rich in antioxidants, although, contrary to popular belief, research has not shown that increasing their consumption has any cancer-preventing benefit.

(Source: Michal Heron)

significant benefit on aging from the dietary addition of antioxidants (Figure 12-19).

Nucleic Acids

The class of molecules known as nucleic acids has two members: deoxyribonucleic acid (DNA) and ribonucleic acid (RNA). Adenosine triphosphate (ATP) is an important monomer of RNA.

DNA AND RNA **Deoxyribonucleic acid (DNA)** is the nucleic acid that contains the genetic instructions for life.

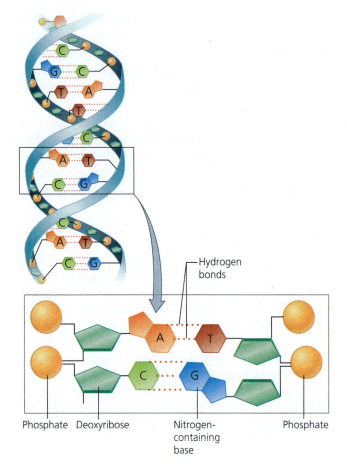

FIGURE 12-20 DNA is a nucleic acid in which two chains of nucleotides twist around one another to form a double helix (spiral). The two chains are held together by hydrogen bonds between the nitrogen-containing bases. Each nucleotide of DNA contains the five-carbon sugar deoxyribose a phosphate group, and one of four nitrogen-containing nucleobases: adenine (A), thymine (T), cytosine (C), and guanine (G).

(Goodenough, Judith and Betty A. McGuire, Biology of Humans: Concepts, Applications, and Issues, *3rd Edition, © 2010. Reprinted by permission of Pearson Education, Inc., Upper Saddle River, NJ.)*

Clinical Note

The ability to repair or replace abnormal genes will forever change the practice of medicine. Genes, which are carried on chromosomes, contain the basic physical and functional units of heredity. Genes are specific sequences of bases that encode instructions to make proteins. The proteins perform most life functions and even make up the majority of cellular structures. When genes are altered so that the encoded proteins are unable to carry out their normal functions, genetic disorders can result.

Gene therapy is a technique for correcting defective genes responsible for disease development. Researchers may use one of several approaches for correcting faulty genes. These include inserting a normal gene into a nonspecific location within the genome to replace a nonfunctional gene. This approach is most common. In addition, an abnormal gene could be repaired through selective reverse mutation, which returns the gene to its normal function. Finally, the regulation (the degree to which a gene is turned on or off) of a particular gene could be altered. In most gene therapy studies, a "normal" gene is inserted into the genome to replace an "abnormal," disease-causing, gene. A carrier molecule, called a vector, must be used to deliver the therapeutic gene to the patient's target cells. Currently, the most common vector is a virus that has been genetically altered to carry normal human DNA.

It is composed of two long polymers called nucleotides that are joined by paired substances called nucleobases. There are four nucleobases in DNA, and the sequence of these encodes information known as the genetic code (Figure 12-20). DNA contains segments referred to as genes that code for the specific amino acid sequence that makes up a specific protein. DNA is further organized into chromosomes. The number of chromosomes present in the cell nucleus varies with the type of organism (e.g., humans have 46, dogs have 78).

The other member of the class of nucleic acids is **ribonucleic acid (RNA)**, a chemical that is similar to DNA (Figure 12-21). RNA plays a major role in protein synthesis, serving as a template for protein synthesis.

The fundamental building blocks of the nucleic acids, DNA and RNA, are **nucleotides**. Nucleotides are five-carbon sugar molecules that are bound to a nitrogen base and a phosphate group (Figure 12-22). They form a long chain-like molecule. There are only five nitrogen bases: adenine,

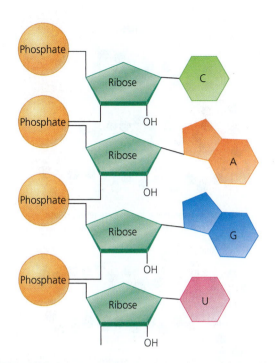

FIGURE 12-21 RNA is a single-stranded nucleic acid formed by the linking together of nucleotides composed of the five-carbon sugar ribose, a phosphate group, and one of four nitrogen-containing nucleobases: cytosine (C), adenine (A), guanine (G), and uracil (U).

(Goodenough, Judith and Betty A. McGuire, Biology of Humans: Concepts, Applications, and Issues, *3rd Edition, © 2010. Reprinted by permission of Pearson Education, Inc., Upper Saddle River, NJ.)*

FIGURE 12-22 Nucleotides consist of a five-carbon (pentose) sugar bonded to a phosphate molecule and one of five nitrogen-containing bases: adenine, cytosine, guanine, thymine, and uracil. Nucleotides are the building blocks of the nucleic acids DNA and RNA.

(Goodenough, Judith and Betty A. McGuire, Biology of Humans: Concepts, Applications, and Issues, *3rd Edition, © 2010. Reprinted by permission of Pearson Education, Inc., Upper Saddle River, NJ.)*

cytosine, guanine, thymine (found only in DNA), and uracil (found only in RNA). It is the sequence of these bases in both DNA and RNA that subsequently determines the sequence of amino acids in a protein.

DNA is a double-stranded helical chain, whereas RNA is single-stranded. In DNA, the five-carbon sugar is deoxyribose; in RNA, the five-carbon sugar is ribose. RNA does not use the nitrogen base thymine, and DNA does not use the nitrogen base uracil. DNA has the capacity for self-replication (Table 12-3).

Table 12-3 RNA and DNA Structural Differences

Characteristic	RNA	DNA
Sugar	Ribose	Deoxyribose
Bases	Adenine, guanine, cytosine, uracil	Adenine, guanine, cytosine, thymine
Number of strands	One	Two, twisted to form a double helix

ATP Adenosine triphosphate (ATP) is a nucleotide that is one of the monomers of RNA. ATP is the principal source of energy for most of the energy-using activities of the cells. Often called the "energy currency" of the cells, ATP consists of the base adenine, the sugar ribose, and three phosphate groups. Energy is stored in ATP when an energy-requiring chemical reaction adds an inorganic phosphate molecule, through covalent bonding, to adenosine diphosphate (ADP), forming ATP.

The phosphate bonds in ATP are highly unstable. Thus, when cells require energy, the phosphate bond is broken, liberating the stored energy, and the ATP then returns to ADP and an inorganic phosphate (Figure 12-23). The liberated energy can then be used for chemical reactions occurring within the cell.

In humans, ATP also acts outside the cell. It is released from damaged cells and elicits pain. It is also released from the stretched wall of the urinary bladder and signals when the bladder needs to be emptied.

Lipids

The final major category of biological chemicals is the lipids. **Lipids** are chemicals that do not dissolve in water. Lipids are nonpolar, whereas water is polar. Thus, water is not attracted to lipids, and lipids are not attracted to water.

In the human, lipids function in the long-term storage of biochemical energy, insulation, structure, and control. The lipids that pertain to human pathophysiology are triglycerides, phospholipids, and steroids (Figure 12-24).

TRIGLYCERIDES Triglycerides are rich sources of energy for the body. In fact, they provide approximately twice as much energy per gram as do proteins or carbohydrates. Triglycerides consist of one molecule of glycerol and three fatty acid molecules (Figure 12-25). Fatty acids are long chains of carbon and hydrogen with an acid (carboxyl) group at one end.

Triglycerides can be classified as saturated or unsaturated. A **saturated fatty acid** has a single bond between each pair of carbon atoms, leaving room on the atom for two hydrogen atoms. Thus, the chemical is said to be saturated. When a double bond exists between carbon atoms, there is space for only one hydrogen atom, and

FIGURE 12-23 The nucleotide adenosine triphosphate (ATP) consists of the sugar ribose, the base adenine, and three phosphate groups. The phosphate bonds of ATP are unstable. When cells need energy, the last phosphate bond is broken, yielding adenosine diphosphate (ADP), a phosphate molecule, and energy.

(Goodenough, Judith and Betty A. McGuire, Biology of Humans: Concepts, Applications, and Issues, 3rd Edition, © 2010. Reprinted by permission of Pearson Education, Inc., Upper Saddle River, NJ).

Lipids

Triglycerides have three fatty acid chains attached to a molecule of glycerol

Phospholipids have two fatty acid chains attached to glycerol and phosphate

Steroids have a unique shape consisting of four carbon rings

FIGURE 12-24 The lipids that pertain to human pathophysiology are triglycerides, phospholipids, and steroids.

thus the molecule is said to be an **unsaturated fatty acid**. Double bonds produce a bend in the fatty acid molecule and give it a different physical property (Figure 12-26). Molecules with many of these bends cannot be packed as closely together as straight molecules, so these fats are less dense. As a result, triglycerides composed of unsaturated fatty acids melt at lower temperatures than those with saturated fatty acids. For example, margarine contains more saturated fat than corn oil. At room temperature it is solid, whereas corn oil remains liquid.

PHOSPHOLIPIDS Another important lipid class is the **phospholipids**. These are extremely important in biological systems, as they form the membrane that surrounds the cells. Structurally, phospholipids are similar to triglycerides in that they contain a glycerol base. Instead of three fatty acid chains, they contain two fatty acid chains

FIGURE 12-25 A triglyceride consists of a molecule of glycerol linked to three fatty acids.

(Freeman, Scott, Biological Science, 4th Edition, © 2011. Reprinted by permission of Pearson Education, Inc., Upper Saddle River, NJ.)

(a) A fatty acid bonds to glycerol through dehydration synthesis.

(b) This triglyceride contains one unsaturated fatty acid (note the presence of a double bond between the carbon atoms) and two saturated fatty acids (note the absence of any double bonds between the carbon atoms).

FIGURE 12-26 The triglyceride shown here contains one unsaturated fatty acid (note the double bond between the carbon atoms) and two saturated fatty acids (note the absence of any double bonds between the carbon atoms).

(Goodenough, Judith and Betty A. McGuire, Biology of Humans: Concepts, Applications, and Issues, *3rd Edition, © 2010. Reprinted by permission of Pearson Education, Inc., Upper Saddle River, NJ.)*

and a phosphate group that has a negative charge. Other smaller variable molecules are linked to the phosphate group. Thus, phospholipids have two distinct regions with different physical characteristics. The region with the two fatty acid chains, essentially the tail, is nonpolar and rejects water (hydrophobic). The phosphate region, essentially the head, is polar and thus attracts water (hydrophilic). This feature is what makes phospholipids an important part of biological membranes (Figure 12-27). Two layers of phospholipids form the membrane. The hydrophobic tails are oriented to the inside of the membrane, and the hydrophilic heads are on the outside

(Figure 12-28). The tails form a protective region and hold the membrane together.

STEROIDS   The last major class of biological lipids is the **steroids**. Steroids have a unique shape. That is, they have a four-carbon ring as the backbone of their structure (Figure 12-29). The basic unit is cholesterol, which is a component of plasma membranes and the base for synthesis of most of the steroid class of hormones (i.e., estrogen, testosterone, cortisol, and aldosterone). The synthesis of steroid compounds by the body is termed **anabolism**. Steroids became a part of the human diet

A phospholipid

Polar head
(hydrophilic)

Nonpolar tail
(hydrophobic)

FIGURE 12-27 The phospholipid has a nonpolar (hydrophobic) "tail" consisting of two fatty acids and a polar (hydrophilic) "head" consisting of a phosphate region.

(Freeman, Scott, Biological Science, 4th Edition, © 2011. Reprinted by permission of Pearson Education, Inc., Upper Saddle River, NJ.)

when the species went from a vegetarian to a carnivorous diet.

Water

Water has been called the "universal solvent." It is abundant in the body and plays a significant role in numerous biological processes. In fact, the physical properties of water are essential for life as we know it. As discussed earlier, water is a polar molecule and has the tendency to create hydrogen bonds, which causes water molecules to adhere to each other (Figure 12-30). This gives water its liquid property. However, hydrogen bonds are the weakest of the chemical bond types. Consequently, the hydrogen bonds of water are frequently broken and re-formed.

Its polarity makes water an excellent solvent that can dissolve both polar and charged substances. Water also plays a major role in the transport of substances throughout the body and plays a significant role in maintaining a constant body temperature. Water has a high heat capacity, and therefore it can absorb a large amount of heat energy before the temperature elevates. This property plays a major role in keeping the body cool. In addition to a high heat capacity, water has a high heat of vaporization, meaning that it takes a great deal of heat energy to make water

FIGURE 12-28 Two layers of phospholipids form a biological membrane, with hydrophobic tails oriented to the inside of the membrane and hydrophilic heads oriented to the outside.

(Goodenough, Judith and Betty A. McGuire, Biology of Humans: Concepts, Applications, and Issues, 3rd Edition, © 2010. Reprinted by permission of Pearson Education, Inc., Upper Saddle River, NJ.)

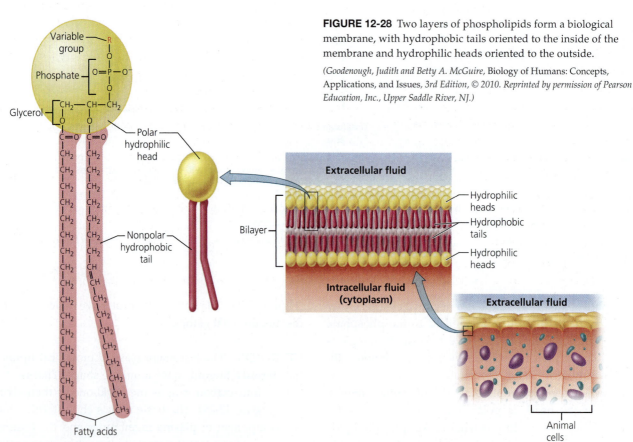

(a) A phospholipid consists of a variable group designated by the letter R, a phosphate, a glycerol, and two fatty acids. Because the variable group is often polar and the fatty acids nonpolar, phospholipids have a polar hydrophilic (water-loving) head and a nonpolar hydrophobic (water-fearing) tail.

(b) Within the phospholipid bilayer of the plasma membrane, the hydrophobic tails point inward and help hold the membrane together. The outward-pointing hydrophilic heads mix with the watery environments inside and outside the cell.

FIGURE 12-29 All steroids have a structure consisting of four carbon rings. Steroids such as cholesterol, estrogen, and testosterone differ in the groups that are attached to the four carbon rings.

(Goodenough, Judith and Betty A. McGuire, Biology of Humans: Concepts, Applications, and Issues, *3rd Edition, © 2010. Reprinted by permission of Pearson Education, Inc., Upper Saddle River, NJ.)*

(a) Water is polar.

Electrons are pulled toward oxygen

(b) Hydrogen bonds form between water molecules.

FIGURE 12-30 Water is polar and participates in hydrogen bonds.

(Freeman, Scott, Biological Science, *4th Edition, © 2011. Reprinted by permission of Pearson Education, Inc., Upper Saddle River, NJ.)*

vaporize. When water vaporizes, it carries away a significant amount of heat, thus cooling the body.

Acids and Bases

In solution, water has a tendency to break up into ions. That is, the water molecule is not a completely stable molecule. A water molecule, which is made up of hydrogen and oxygen atoms, can break apart into ions. This is a **dissociation reaction**. (A dissociation reaction is any reaction in which a compound or a molecule breaks apart into separate components.) This is reflected in the following equation:

$$H_2O \leftrightarrow H^+ + OH^-$$

This equation indicates that water dissociates into a hydrogen ion (H^+) and a hydroxide ion (OH^-). A hydrogen ion is a molecule that has lost its lone electron and is simply a proton. Substances that give up protons during chemical reactions are called **acids**. Likewise, substances that acquire protons during a chemical reaction are called **bases**. Any chemical reaction that results in the transfer of protons is referred to as an **acid–base reaction**.

Protons do not exist by themselves. In water, they actually associate with another water molecule to form a hydronium ion (H_3O^+). One of the water molecules gives up a proton and acts as an acid. The other water molecule accepts the proton and acts as a base. This process is reflected in the following equation:

$$H_2O + H_2O \leftrightarrow H_3O^+ + OH^-$$

By acting as a proton donor or proton acceptor, water has the unique ability to act as either an acid or a base. Most chemicals that are acids act only as acids, and most chemicals that are bases act only as bases. Acid–base reactions occur because of the number of protons present in the water solution at any given time.

The actual concentration of protons in water has been scientifically measured. In a sample of pure water at 25°C (77°F), the number of protons (in the form of H^+) is 1.0×10^{-7} M. (*M* represents **molarity**, or moles of solute per liter of solution. A **mole** is a measure of mass or weight used in chemistry. Mole is sometimes defined as "molecular weight.") Because the actual number of protons is so small, it is best to use a logarithmic representation. (A **logarithm** is a base number that is raised to a certain power. A common example is $2^3 = 8$. In other words, 2 to the third power—$2 \times 2 \times 2$—equals 8. In that example, 2^3 is a logarithm. With a positive exponent, like the ^{3} in 2^3, a logarithm simplifies working with very large numbers. With a negative exponent, like the $^{-7}$ in 1.0×1.0^{-7}, a logarithm simplifies working with very small numbers.)

The accepted convention to express the degree of acidity or basicity (alkalinity) of a substance is to use the logarithmic **pH scale**. (A logarithmic scale is based on exponents or powers that raise the value of the base number rather than the base number itself.) The term pH comes from the French term *puissance d'hydrogène*, which literally means "power of hydrogen." In the pH scale, the greater the number of hydrogen ions, the higher the acidity.

The pH of a solution is the negative of the base-10 logarithm (log) of the hydrogen ion **concentration** [H^+] and can be expressed in the following formula:

$$pH = -\log [H^+]$$

It can also be written as:

$$pH = \log \frac{1}{[H^+]}$$

The pH scale ranges from 0 to 14. A drop in the pH scale of 1 unit indicates a 10-fold increase in the hydrogen ion concentration, whereas a 2-unit drop indicates a 100-fold increase in the number of hydrogen ions, and so on.

Table 12-4 The pH Scale and Hydrogen Ion Concentrations

pH		Example	Hydrogen Ion Concentration	
Acidic	0	Hydrochloric acid	10^{-0}	(1.0)
	1	Stomach secretions	10^{-1}	(0.1)
	2	Lemon juice	10^{-2}	(0.01)
	3	Cola drinks	10^{-3}	(0.001)
	4	White wine	10^{-4}	(0.0001)
	5	Tomato juice	10^{-5}	(0.00001)
	6	Coffee, urine, saliva	10^{-6}	(0.000001)
Neutral	7	Distilled water	10^{-7}	(0.0000001)
Basic	8	Blood, semen	10^{-8}	(0.00000001)
	9	Bile	10^{-9}	(0.000000001)

Pure water has a pH of 7.0 (1.0×10^{-7} M). Thus, a solution with a pH of 7.0 has an equal number of hydrogen ions and hydroxide ions. Substances with a pH of <7.0 are acidic, whereas substances with a pH >7.0 are basic. The normal pH of arterial blood is slightly basic, ranging from 7.35 to 7.45 (Table 12-4).

Just as there is a pH scale, there is also a **pOH scale**, although that scale is infrequently used in medicine. The pOH scale represents the number of hydroxide ions present in a solution. The pOH is the opposite of pH.

$$pH + pOH = 14$$

The pOH of water is equal to the pH (7.0). When the pH goes up, the pOH comes down, and vice versa.

Buffer Systems

Free hydrogen ions are being constantly produced by the body, primarily from *glycolysis*, and result in the formation of carbon dioxide. These free hydrogen ions determine the body's pH. It is important to understand that all of the body's metabolic processes operate properly only when the pH is normal. In addition, all chemical reactions that depend on enzymes are susceptible to changes in pH. In fact, significant changes in pH can destroy these needed enzymes. Thus, biological systems function properly only within a very limited pH range.

Buffers are needed to counter the body's normal production of acids and to prevent significant variations in the body's pH. A **buffer** is a substance dissolved in water that counteracts changes in pH. When the hydrogen ion concentration increases, buffers remove excess hydrogen ions from the solution. Conversely, when the hydrogen ion concentration falls, buffers add hydrogen ions to the solution. The body has three major buffer systems:

- *Carbonic acid–bicarbonate buffer system.* The carbonic acid–bicarbonate buffer system is the most important buffer system in the extracellular fluid (ECF), including the blood. It is also the most rapidly acting of the three buffer systems.

- *Protein buffer system.* The protein buffer system works by way of selective amino acid monomers accepting or releasing hydrogen ions. This system plays a major role in pH regulation in both the ECF and intracellular fluid (ICF) compartments. It interacts significantly with the other buffer systems.

- *Phosphate buffer system.* The phosphate buffer system plays a role in buffering the pH of the ICF and the urine.

CARBONIC ACID–BICARBONATE BUFFER SYSTEM

The pH of the blood is primarily regulated by the carbonic acid–bicarbonate buffer system. The primary role of this system is to buffer changes in pH caused by organic acids and fixed acids in the ECF. When carbon dioxide (CO_2) is added to water (H_2O), it forms carbonic acid (H_2CO_3). Carbonic acid, in turn, quickly dissociates into hydrogen ions (H^+) and bicarbonate ions (HCO_3^-). Carbonic acid is a volatile acid in that it will readily leave a solution and enter the atmosphere. In the lungs, carbonic acid breaks down into carbon dioxide and water. The carbon dioxide diffuses into the alveoli and is expelled with ventilation. In the peripheral tissues, carbon dioxide, a waste product of metabolism, combines with water to form carbonic acid. Carbonic acid then dissociates to release hydrogen ions and bicarbonate ions. This can be represented by the following equation:

$$CO_2 + H_2O \leftrightarrow H_2CO_3 \leftrightarrow H^+ + HCO_3^-$$

Water plays a significant role in the carbonic acid–bicarbonate system and is better represented by the following equation:

$$H_3O^+ + HCO_3^- \leftrightarrow H_2CO_3 + H_2O \leftrightarrow 2\,H_2O + CO_2$$

This reaction occurs spontaneously in body fluids. However, it occurs much faster in the presence of the enzyme *carbonic anhydrase*. Carbonic anhydrase is found in red blood cells, the liver, kidneys, stomach, and other structures. Carbonic anhydrase promotes the rapid formation of water and carbon dioxide, thus making the reaction significantly faster.

$$CO_2 + H_2O \xleftarrow{\text{Carbonic anhydrase}} H_2CO_3 \leftrightarrow H^+ + HCO_3^-$$

The carbonic acid–bicarbonate buffer system has several important limitations. First, it does not effectively protect the extracellular fluid from changes in pH that are due to changes in carbon dioxide levels. Because carbon

---

CONTENT REVIEW

➤ Major Acid–Base Buffer Systems
- Carbonic acid–bicarbonate buffer system
- Protein buffer system
- Phosphate buffer system

dioxide is the weak acid in the carbonic acid–bicarbonate system, the system cannot protect against changes in the concentrations of one of its constituents (carbon dioxide). If this were to occur, elevated levels of carbon dioxide would mix with water, forming carbonic acid, thus generating hydrogen ions (driving the equation to the right). This would be harmful, in that hydrogen ions would reduce the pH of the plasma.

Second, despite what has just been described, the carbonic acid–bicarbonate system can function only when the respiratory system and respiratory control centers are functioning normally. When the carbonic acid–bicarbonate buffer system buffers an organic or fixed acid, carbon dioxide is produced. This then elevates the partial pressure of carbon dioxide in the blood ($PaCO_2$). The respiratory centers in the brain must detect this increase and increase respirations accordingly to remove the excess carbon dioxide by exhaling it from the body. If this increase in respirations cannot occur, for whatever reason, the carbonic acid–bicarbonate system becomes considerably less effective. Stated another way, the buffer system cannot remove the hydrogen ions efficiently unless the respiratory system is functioning properly.

Third, the ability to buffer acids is limited by the amount of available bicarbonate ions. Every time a hydrogen ion is removed from the blood, it takes a bicarbonate ion with it. However, the body normally has an extremely large supply of bicarbonate ions, known as the *bicarbonate reserve*.

The normal pH of the blood can be calculated with the *Henderson-Hasselbalch equation*, which states:

$$pH = 6.1 + \log\frac{Base}{Acid}$$

$$pH = 6.1 + \log\frac{HCO_3^-}{H_2CO_3} \quad \text{or} \quad pH = 6.1 \log\frac{HCO_3^-}{\alpha^2 PaCO_2}$$

$$pH = 6.1 + \log\frac{20}{1}$$

$$pH = 6.1 + 1.3$$

$$pH = 7.4$$

[Note: In this equation, 6.1 is the pK_a of this system (the negative log of the ionization constant) and α is the solubility coefficient of 0.226 mM/kPa. The equation is based on the fact that the normal ratio of base to acid is 20:1.]

PROTEIN BUFFER SYSTEM   Protein buffers depend on the ability of select amino acids in the protein chain to react to changes in pH by accepting or releasing hydrogen ions. Proteins in the plasma play an important role in buffering pH changes in the blood. Similarly, protein fragments and amino acids play a role in buffering the pH of the interstitial fluid.

An important part of the protein buffer system is the *hemoglobin buffer system*. Red blood cells contain large quantities of hemoglobin and the enzyme carbonic anhydrase. Thus, they can have a significant effect on the pH of ECF. Carbon dioxide readily and rapidly diffuses into red blood cells that take in carbon dioxide from the plasma. There, they are rapidly converted into carbonic acid. When the carbonic acid dissociates, bicarbonate ions are excreted into the plasma (in exchange for chloride) in a phenomenon called the *chloride shift*. The remaining hydrogen ions are then buffered by the hemoglobin molecules present in the red blood cells. Overall, the hemoglobin buffer system plays a major role in preventing significant changes in ECF pH when the $PaCO_2$ is either rising or falling.

PHOSPHATE BUFFER SYSTEM   The last major buffer system is the phosphate buffer system, which is somewhat similar to the carbonic acid–bicarbonate buffer system. The phosphate buffer system uses the anion dihydrogen phosphate ($H_2PO_4^-$), which is actually a weak acid. Dihydrogen phosphate (a weak acid) combines with hydrogen ion to form monohydrogen phosphate (HPO_4^{2-}). Monohydrogen phosphate is an anion and can be represented by the following equation:

$$H_2PO_4^- \leftrightarrow H^+ + HPO_4^{2-}$$

The phosphate buffer system can be represented by the following equation:

$$pH = 6.8 + \log\frac{Base}{Acid}$$

$$pH = 6.8 + \log\frac{HPO_4^{2-}}{H_2PO_4}$$

[Note: In this equation, 6.8 is the pK_a of this system (the negative log of the ionization constant).]

The phosphate buffer system is limited in the ECF but plays a major role in stabilizing the pH of urine.

Acid–Base Balance

As just presented, the acid–base balance must be tightly controlled. Even though the buffer systems described are effective in binding acids and rendering them harmless, these acids must then be removed from the body. Thus, excess hydrogen ions must be bound to water molecules and removed through the exhalation of carbon dioxide from the lungs or be removed from the body via secretion by the kidneys. The maintenance of body pH is a constant balance between gains and losses of hydrogen ion that is achieved through the use of the buffer system, the respiratory system, and the kidneys. These systems secrete or absorb hydrogen ions, control the excretion of acids and bases, or create additional buffers when needed.

Whenever a change in pH occurs, the buffer systems react fastest. However, soon the respiratory system will be activated to help correct the problem through its direct effect on the carbonic acid–bicarbonate buffer system. This occurs primarily through a change in respiratory rate. **Chemoreceptors** in the carotid and aortic bodies sense changes in the PCO_2 in the circulating blood. Similar chemoreceptors are present in the medulla oblongata of the brain. When these receptors are stimulated, the respiratory rate increases, which leads to increased CO_2 loss through the lungs, which then increases the pH. Increasing or decreasing the respiratory rate will affect the PCO_2 that, in turn, affects the pH.

When the PCO_2 rises, the pH will fall, and the carbonic acid–bicarbonate equation will be driven to the right:

$$\uparrow H^+ + HCO_3^- \rightarrow H_2CO_3 \rightarrow \uparrow CO_2 + H_2O$$

Once enough carbon dioxide is lost to the environment, the respiratory rate returns to normal.

Conversely, when the PCO_2 of the blood falls, the chemoreceptors are inhibited, and the respiratory rate falls, thus causing a return of the PCO_2 to normal levels.

The renal system also plays a major role in acid–base balance. However, it tends to work more slowly than the other body systems. The renal effect is referred to as *renal compensation* and is due to the selective secretion or reabsorption of hydrogen ions or bicarbonate ions in response to changes in the plasma pH. In this way the kidneys effectively assist the lungs in maintenance of acid–base balance. When the pH falls, the kidneys respond by increasing the levels of bicarbonate to supply the carbonic acid–bicarbonate buffer system with adequate amounts of buffer. When the pH rises, bicarbonate ions are excreted from the body, thus removing the excess base. When the bicarbonate is lost from carbonic acid, hydrogen ions are liberated, thus further lowering the pH.

The pH can also be affected by movement of electrolytes from the inside of cells to the ECF. That is, sodium (Na^+) and potassium (K^+) ions can be exchanged for hydrogen ions (H^+) in the ECF, thereby moving the acid. Thus, potassium levels and hydrogen ion levels are a major aspect of pH (Table 12-5).

Table 12-5 Maintenance of Acid–Base Balance

System	Mechanism	Rate of Action
Buffer pairs • Carbonic acid–bicarbonate • Proteins/ hemoglobin • Phosphate	Releases or absorbs hydrogen ions	Immediate
Respiratory system	Retain or remove CO_2 (H_2CO_3)	Minutes to hours
Electrolyte shifts	Exchange Na^+ and/or K^+ for H^+ in ECF	Minutes to hours
Renal system	Secretion or absorption of H^+ and/or HCO_3^-, phosphate, and ammonia buffering	Hours to days

Table 12-6 pH as a Function of Metabolism and Respiration

$$pH = \frac{Base}{Acid} \text{ thus } pH = \frac{Bicarbonate (HCO_3^-)}{Carbonic\ Acid\ (H_2CO_3)\ or\ Carbon\ Dioxide\ (CO_2)}$$

$$pH = \frac{Metabolic\ Function}{Respiratory\ Function}$$

$$pH = \frac{Renal\ Compensation}{Respiratory\ Compensation}$$

Acid–Base Disorders

Any significant deviation of pH outside the normal operating parameters (7.35–7.45) can be classified as an acid–base disorder (Table 12-6). The two major body systems involved in acid–base balance are the respiratory system and the renal system.

There are two classes of acid–base disorders: respiratory acid–base disorders and metabolic acid–base disorders. Of these, there are two types. **Acidosis** is an excess of acids in the body, and **alkalosis** is an excess of bases in the body. **Respiratory acid–base disorders** result from an inequality in carbon dioxide generation in the peripheral tissues and carbon dioxide elimination in the respiratory system. The hallmark of respiratory acid–base disorders is a change in the $PaCO_2$. Respiratory acid–base disorders can be classified as:

- Respiratory acidosis
- Respiratory alkalosis

The second class of acid–base disorders is the **metabolic acid–base disorders**. These result from the production of either organic or fixed acids or by conditions that affect the levels of bicarbonate in the ECF. Metabolic acid–base disorders can be classified as:

- Metabolic acidosis
- Metabolic alkalosis

Respiratory Acidosis

Respiratory acidosis occurs when the respiratory system cannot effectively eliminate all the carbon dioxide generated through metabolic activities in the peripheral tissues. Normally, the respiratory system reacts rapidly and corrects changes in carbon dioxide levels before the ECF pH is affected. However, in respiratory acidosis, the respiratory system cannot maintain the pH within accepted values. With respiratory acidosis, there is an increase in PCO_2 and a decrease in pH. An elevation in the plasma CO_2 level is referred to as **hypercapnia**. The usual cause is **hypoventilation**. Hypoventilation can occur

> **CONTENT REVIEW**
>
> ➤ Acid–Base Disorders
> - Respiratory acidosis
> - Respiratory alkalosis
> - Metabolic acidosis
> - Metabolic alkalosis

In the prehospital setting, acid–base disorders are detected primarily by physical exam techniques. The introduction of capnography, which measures end-tidal carbon dioxide (CO_2) levels, provides additional important information. Initially, these devices detected only end-tidal CO_2 ($ETCO_2$) levels. Modern capnography measures the exhaled CO_2 level throughout the respiratory cycle. CO_2 can be displayed as the partial pressure or maximal concentration of carbon dioxide at the end of an exhaled breath and is expressed as a percentage of CO_2 or partial pressure of CO_2 in mmHg. Normal levels are 5–6 percent or 35–45 mmHg. When the value is expressed as a partial pressure of CO_2 in mmHg, it is normally called the $PETCO_2$. For example, you might state, "The patient had a $PETCO_2$ of 22."

During normal circulatory and respiratory function, the alveolar carbon dioxide partial pressure ($PACO_2$) is closely comparable to arterial carbon dioxide partial pressure ($PaCO_2$) and thus to exhaled CO_2. Therefore, $PaCO_2$ is equivalent to exhaled CO_2. The difference between $PaCO_2$ and exhaled CO_2 is known as the CO_2 gradient. Normally, $PETCO_2$ is about 38 mmHg at 760 mmHg of atmospheric pressure, and thus less than a 6-mmHg gradient between $PaCO_2$ and exhaled carbon dioxide. Thus, for most conditions, except extremely low-flow states, capnography can aid in the diagnosis of respiratory acid–base disorders (Figure 12-31).

FIGURE 12-31 A capnogram associated with an acid–base disorder resulting from hypoventilation.

when the minute volume falls. The **minute volume** is the amount of air moved into and out of the respiratory tract in one minute. It is reflected in the following formula:

$$V_{min} = V_t \times \text{Respiratory Rate}$$

where V_{min} equals minute volume and V_t equals tidal volume (the amount of air moved through the respiratory system with each breath). Thus, a decrease in respiratory rate, tidal volume, or a combination of the two can cause respiratory acidosis.

Respiratory Alkalosis

Respiratory alkalosis occurs when the respiratory system eliminates too much carbon dioxide through hyperventilation, resulting in **hypocapnia**. **Hyperventilation** can result from emotional situations, metabolic disorders, medical conditions, environmental factors, or a combination of these. For example, anxiety, fear, or hysteria stimulates the respiratory centers in the brain, resulting in what is referred to as **hyperventilation syndrome**. This results in excessive CO_2 elimination and thus a respiratory alkalosis. Fever and hyperthyroidism can cause respiratory alkalosis. These conditions increase the body's metabolic rate, resulting in increased CO_2 elimination. Medical conditions such as congestive heart failure (CHF) and liver failure can cause increased CO_2 elimination. CHF can cause a respiratory alkalosis because of hypoxia-induced hyperventilation. Liver failure results in the accumulation of ammonia in the blood. Increased levels of ammonia can stimulate the respiratory center, causing hyperventilation with resultant metabolic alkalosis. Ascension to a high altitude can cause hyperventilation. At higher elevations, oxygen levels are markedly decreased and the victim must increase respirations to ensure adequate oxygen levels until becoming acclimated to the altitude or descending to lower levels.

Metabolic Acidosis

Metabolic acidosis is a deficiency of bicarbonate (HCO_3^-) in the body. It usually results from an increase in metabolic acids—primarily through anaerobic metabolism. When oxygen stores are low, energy production switches from aerobic metabolism to anaerobic metabolism. Anaerobic metabolism results in the production of pyruvic acid, which is rapidly converted to lactic acid.

The kidney plays a major role in maintaining stable pH levels. The kidney can retain acids and excrete HCO_3^- as needed to maintain pH. Typically, bicarbonate levels in the body are stable. Thus, when there is an increase in metabolic acids, HCO_3^- buffers the excessive acid, keeping the pH neutral. This results in a relative decrease in HCO_3^- because body stores remain stable—they are just bound to metabolic acids. Likewise, when the kidney retains acids, the total amount of acids increases while bicarbonate levels remain the same. This mechanism also results in a relative decrease in HCO_3^- levels. True HCO_3^- deficits result when the kidney excretes bicarbonate. Metabolic acidosis is a common problem and can be caused by disease processes such as diabetes, kidney disease, and similar conditions.

Metabolic Alkalosis

Metabolic alkalosis is relatively uncommon and is due to an increase in HCO_3^- levels or a decrease in circulating acids. Metabolic alkalosis results from an abnormal loss of hydrogen ions (H^+), an increase in HCO_3^- levels, or a decrease in extracellular fluid levels. Vomiting (or nasogastric suctioning) is the most common cause of metabolic alkalosis. Stomach secretions are highly acidic—primarily hydrochloric acid (HCl). Vomiting or suctioning removes the HCl, leaving a deficit in both H^+ and chloride ions (Cl^-). When this occurs, the bicarbonate anion shifts from the ICF to the ECF to replace the lost Cl^- ions, causing an increase in ECF HCO_3^- levels and thus a metabolic alkalosis. Several other conditions can cause metabolic alkalosis, all of which involve either the loss of H^+ or variations in circulating HCO_3^- levels.

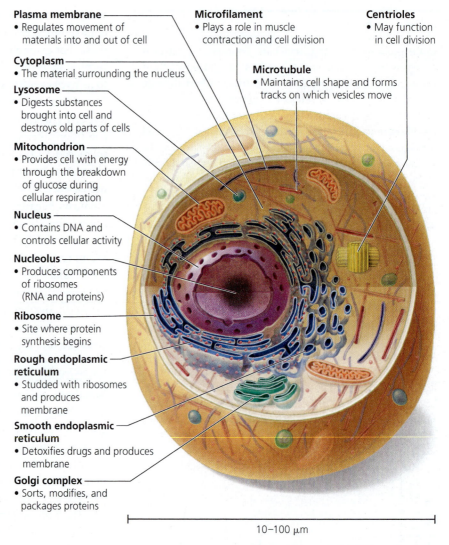

Plasma membrane
• Regulates movement of materials into and out of cell

Cytoplasm
• The material surrounding the nucleus

Lysosome
• Digests substances brought into cell and destroys old parts of cells

Mitochondrion
• Provides cell with energy through the breakdown of glucose during cellular respiration

Nucleus
• Contains DNA and controls cellular activity

Nucleolus
• Produces components of ribosomes (RNA and proteins)

Ribosome
• Site where protein synthesis begins

Rough endoplasmic reticulum
• Studded with ribosomes and produces membrane

Smooth endoplasmic reticulum
• Detoxifies drugs and produces membrane

Golgi complex
• Sorts, modifies, and packages proteins

Microfilament
• Plays a role in muscle contraction and cell division

Microtubule
• Maintains cell shape and forms tracks on which vesicles move

Centrioles
• May function in cell division

10–100 μm

FIGURE 12-32 Eukaryotic cells, such as the generalized animal cell shown here, have internal membrane-bound organelles.

(Goodenough, Judith and Betty A. McGuire, Biology of Humans: Concepts, Applications, and Issues, *3rd Edition, © 2010. Reprinted by permission of Pearson Education, Inc., Upper Saddle River, NJ.)*

This discussion of acid–base disorders is simply an overview of these conditions from a biochemical standpoint. They will be discussed in considerable detail in the respiratory and renal chapters of this text.

PART 3: Disease at the Cellular Level

The Cell

The **cell** is the basic unit of all living organisms. The cell is capable of independent functioning and can typically be divided into two types: eukaryotic cells and prokaryotic cells. Distinction between the two is based on whether or not the cell has internal compartments—a nucleus and organelles—that are enclosed by membranes. The **nucleus** is the central portion of a cell that contains organelles and other components. **Organelles** are structures within the nucleus that carry out necessary biological processes. **Prokaryotic cells** do not contain a nucleus and do not contain organelles. Most prokaryotic cells are surrounded by a rigid cell wall. Many of the single-celled organisms, such as bacteria, are prokaryotes. **Eukaryotic cells** contain a nucleus and organelles. The cells of most multicellular organisms, including humans, are eukaryotes (Figure 12-32).

The Plasma Membrane and Cytoplasm

Cells are so small that they can be visualized only with a microscope. Their small size is necessary because they need a small surface-area-to-volume ratio that will allow movement of substances into and out of the cell.

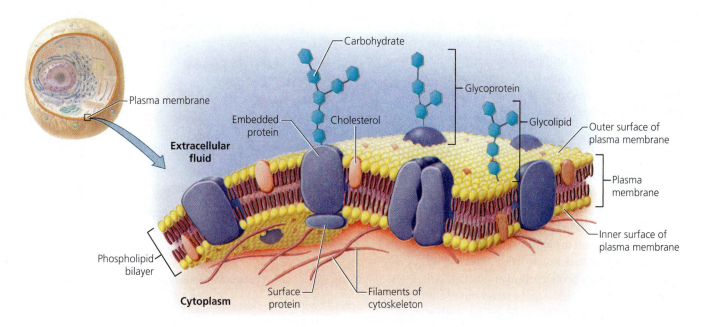

FIGURE 12-33 The hydrophilic heads of the phospholipid molecules on the outer layer of the plasma membrane are in contact with extracellular fluid. The hydrophilic heads of the phospholipid molecules on the inner layer of the plasma membrane are in contact with the cytoplasm.

(*Goodenough, Judith and Betty A. McGuire,* Biology of Humans: Concepts, Applications, and Issues, *3rd Edition, © 2010. Reprinted by permission of Pearson Education, Inc., Upper Saddle River, NJ.*)

Cells are surrounded by a **plasma membrane**. This membrane consists of several chemicals, of which the phospholipids are among the more important.

As discussed earlier, phospholipid molecules have two distinct regions with different physical characteristics. The region with the two fatty acid chains, essentially the tail of the molecule, is nonpolar and rejects water (is hydrophobic). The phosphate region, essentially the head of the molecule, is polar and attracts water (is hydrophilic). Two layers of phospholipids, referred to as a **lipid bilayer**, form the **cell membrane**. Some of the hydrophilic heads face outward toward the environment outside the cells. Other hydrophilic heads face inward toward the inner contents of the cell. In the middle of the membrane, the hydrophobic tails of outward- and inward-facing phospholipids face each other and hold the layers of the membrane together.

The hydrophilic heads of the phospholipid molecules on the outer layer of the plasma membrane are in contact with *extracellular fluid*. The hydrophilic heads of the phospholipid molecules on the inner layer of the plasma membrane are in contact with the **cytoplasm** (Figure 12-33). Cytoplasm, also called *cytosol*, fills the inside of cells and consists of water, salts, organic molecules, and many enzymes that catalyze numerous biochemical reactions. The water component of the cytoplasm is referred to as *intracellular fluid*.

Throughout the lipid bilayer are proteins that serve numerous purposes. Some of these proteins span the entire membrane (*integral proteins*), whereas others may be embedded on the membrane surface (*peripheral membrane proteins*). The membrane proteins and their functions (Figure 12-34) include the following:

- *Linkers.* Some membrane proteins attach the membrane to the cytoskeleton of the cell, thus allowing the cell to maintain its shape and to secure the membrane in a certain place when needed.

- *Enzymes.* Some proteins function as enzymes and carry out the different steps of the metabolic reactions that take place near the cell membrane.

- *Receptors.* Some membrane proteins act as receptor sites for messenger molecules that signal the cell to start or stop a specific metabolic activity.

- *Transporters.* These proteins make the membrane **semipermeable**, also called *selectively permeable*, thus controlling the movement of substances into and out of the cell.

Membrane Proteins

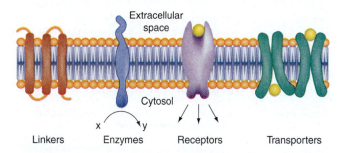

FIGURE 12-34 Membrane proteins include linkers, enzymes, receptors, and transporters.

These varied membrane proteins give the cell membrane a mosaic quality. Yet even with the presence of proteins in the plasma membrane, the membrane still maintains a fluid quality. Therefore, the structure of the membrane is referred to as a *fluid mosaic*.

Plasma Membrane Functions

The plasma membrane has several functions in addition to the obvious function of separating the extracellular from the intracellular environment (Table 12-7). First, the plasma membrane plays a major role in the ability of cells to adhere to one another, or stick together. This is achieved primarily through proteins (linkers) called *cell adhesion molecules (CAMs)* that extend out of the plasma membrane. CAMs hold cells together and play a role in cellular movement, tissue development, and healing (Figure 12-35).

The plasma membrane helps with *cell–cell recognition*, the ability of a cell to distinguish one type of cell from another. Peripheral membrane proteins, often glycoproteins, differ from cell to cell and from species to species. Cell–cell recognition allows the body to recognize foreign cells, including cells that may cause infection or even cancer.

The plasma membrane maintains the structural integrity of the cell. It provides anchor sites for the interior cytoskeleton, which is both a muscle and a skeleton and is responsible for cell movement and the organization of the organelles within the cell. (The cytoskeleton will be described in more detail later.)

The plasma membrane also plays a major role in communications between cells. Certain substances, such as

Cell Adhesion Molecules

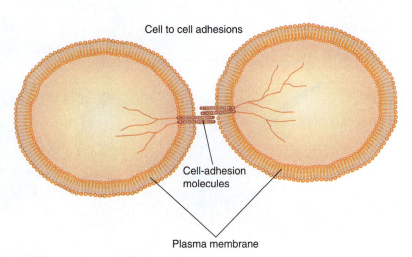

Cell to cell adhesions

Cell-adhesion molecules

Plasma membrane

FIGURE 12-35 Cell adhesion molecules (CAMs) extend out of the plasma membrane to bind cells to each other.

hormones, will bind to the receptor proteins in the plasma membrane. The plasma membrane protein then relays the message of the bound substance to the interior of the cell, where it is transmitted to nearby molecules. Through a series of biochemical reactions, the message ultimately initiates the desired response by the cell.

Finally, the cell membrane regulates the movement of substances into and out of the cell. A large number of substances are routinely moved across the plasma membrane, but these are highly regulated by the cell. Because of this, the plasma membrane is said to be *semipermeable*.

Simple Diffusion

Substances will move across a membrane from an area of higher concentration on one side to an area of lower concentration on the other side until the concentration of the substance is equal in both areas (a state of equilibrium) (Figure 12-36). Even after the concentrations reach equilibrium, because of random movement, the substance continues to move back and forth across the membrane. However, the net rate of movement in each direction now remains the same. This process of passive movement across a membrane is called **simple diffusion**.

The plasma membrane essentially creates an intracellular environment separate from the extracellular environment. Thus, the concentration of substances inside the plasma membrane is often different from those outside the membrane. Smaller molecules, such as water, carbon dioxide, oxygen, ethanol, and urea,

Table 12-7 Mechanism of Transport across the Plasma Membrane

Mechanism	Description
Simple diffusion	Random movement from region of high to region of low concentration
Facilitated diffusion	Movement from region of high to region of low concentration with the aid of a carrier or channel protein
Osmosis	Movement of water from a region of high water concentration (low solute concentration) to a region of low water concentration (high solute concentration)
Active transport	Movement from region of high to region of low concentration with the aid of a carrier or channel protein and energy, usually from ATP
Endocytosis	Materials engulfed by the plasma membrane and drawn into the cell in a vesicle
Exocytosis	Membrane-bound vesicle from inside the cell fuses with the plasma membrane and spills contents outside the cell

CONTENT REVIEW

➤ Types of Movement through a Cell Membrane
- Simple diffusion
- Osmosis
- Facilitated diffusion
- Active transport
- Endocytosis
- Exocytosis

FIGURE 12-36 Simple diffusion is the random movement of molecules from a region of higher concentration to a region of lower concentration. Solutes diffuse across the membrane until equilibrium is reached on both sides.

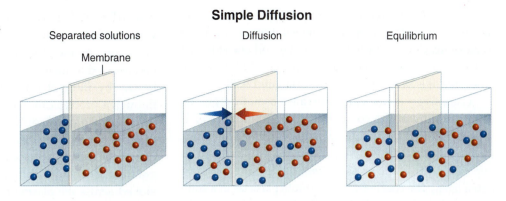

Simple Diffusion

Separated solutions | Diffusion | Equilibrium

Membrane

readily move across the plasma membrane. They pass either directly through the lipid bilayer or through pores created by certain integral proteins. The rate of transport for a particular molecule is proportional to the lipid solubility or hydrophobicity of the molecule in question. (Hydrophobicity is the tendency of a molecule to be repelled by water. An example is molecules of fat or oil that do not mix with water.) Oxygen, carbon dioxide, and ethanol are highly lipid soluble and therefore diffuse across the bilayer membrane almost as if it were not there.

On the other hand, molecules that are large or contain a charge (are ionized) do not pass readily through the membrane and, in many cases, are repelled. The rate of diffusion is generally proportional to the **concentration gradient** across the membrane. (The concentration gradient is the difference in the number of molecules or ions of the substance on one side of the membrane from the number of molecules on the other.) The greater the concentration gradient, the more rapid is the rate of diffusion. **Osmotic gradient** is a similar term but applies specifically to the movement of water across a semipermeable membrane. Another example of concentration gradient is the movement of oxygen. For example, oxygen concentrations are always higher outside a cell when compared to those inside a cell. Therefore, oxygen diffuses down its concentration gradient (from higher to lower concentration) into the cell. Carbon dioxide, on the other hand, typically is at a higher concentration inside the cell and tends to diffuse out of the cell.

Osmosis

Osmosis is a specific type of diffusion. It is the movement of water molecules from an area of high water concentration to an area of low water concentration (Figure 12-37). Semipermeable membranes, such as the cell membrane, allow the unrestricted movement of water across the membrane, at the same time restricting the movement of **solute** molecules and ions. It has been estimated that an amount of water roughly equivalent to 250 times the volume of the cell diffuses across the red blood cell membrane every

second. Despite this large movement of water molecules, the cell does not lose or gain water, because equal amounts go in and out.

The concentration of water on different sides of a semipermeable membrane is a result more of the solutes present than of the amount of water present. That is, different concentrations of solute molecules on different sides of the membrane result in different concentrations of molecules of **free water** (water that is free of solute) on either side of the membrane. On the side of the membrane with higher free water concentration (which contains a lower solute concentration), more water molecules will strike the pores in the membrane in a given interval of time. The more membrane strikes there are, the more molecules pass through the pores. This then results in a net diffusion of water from the compartment with high concentration of free water to that with a low concentration of free water. Looking at it a different way, water molecules will diffuse from an area of lower *solute* concentration to an area of greater *solute* concentration.

Water is the universal *solvent* and necessary for many biochemical processes.

When the concentrations of solutions on both sides of a semipermeable membrane are equal, they are said to be **isotonic**. When a solution on one side of the membrane is

Osmosis (Water Movement)

Unequal concentrations across a membrane | Water movement

Osmosis

FIGURE 12-37 Osmosis is a specific type of diffusion in which water molecules move from an area of high water concentration to an area of low water concentration.

more concentrated (has a greater quantity of solute) than the solution on the other side, the solution is said to be **hypertonic**. Conversely, when a solution on one side of a membrane is less concentrated than the solution on the other side, it is said to be **hypotonic** (Figure 12-38).

Osmosis generates a pressure called **osmotic pressure**. If the pressure in the compartment into which water is flowing is raised to the equivalent of the osmotic pressure, movement of water will stop. (Osmotic pressure and its opposite, hydrostatic pressure, will be described in more detail later.) The concentration of solute particles in a solution is called the **osmolarity**. A similar measurement, the **osmolality**, is used to measure the concentration of particles in body fluids such as plasma and urine. The body's osmolality increases with dehydration and decreases with overhydration. Normal human osmolality ranges from 280 to 300 mOsm/kg.

Facilitated Diffusion

Water-soluble molecules and ionized molecules cannot move through the plasma membrane by simple diffusion. Because of this, their transport must be assisted, or "facilitated," by integral proteins in the plasma membrane through a process called **facilitated diffusion**. Facilitated diffusion, like simple diffusion, does not require an expenditure of metabolic energy. The force driving facilitated diffusion, as with simple diffusion, is the concentration gradient. There are many important substances that are moved across the plasma membrane by facilitated diffusion, including glucose, sodium ions, and chloride ions. Glucose is water soluble; sodium and potassium are ionized and are thus classified *as lipid-bilayer-excluded substances* (Figure 12-39). That is, they cannot pass through the lipid bilayer by simple diffusion but rather, as just described, their passage across the plasma membrane must be assisted, or facilitated.

There are two major groups of integral membrane proteins involved in the process of facilitated diffusion:

- *Carrier proteins.* **Carrier proteins**, also called transporters, bind a specific type of solute and are induced to undergo a series of conformational changes that effectively carries the solute to the other side of the membrane. The carrier protein then releases the solute and, through another conformational change, is restored in the membrane to its original state. Typically, a given carrier will transport only a small group of related molecules.

Tonicity

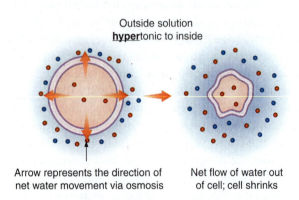

Outside solution **hyper**tonic to inside

Arrow represents the direction of net water movement via osmosis

Net flow of water out of cell; cell shrinks

Outside solution **hypo**tonic to inside

Net flow of water into cell; cell swells or even bursts

Isotonic solutions

No change

FIGURE 12-38 Osmosis can shrink or burst a membrane-bound vesicle as water moves out of the vesicle to dilute a hypertonic outside solution or into the vesicle to concentrate an outside solution, always seeking to achieve isotonicity inside and outside the vesicle.

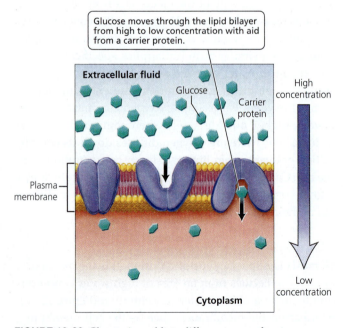

Glucose moves through the lipid bilayer from high to low concentration with aid from a carrier protein.

Extracellular fluid

Glucose

Carrier protein

High concentration

Plasma membrane

Low concentration

Cytoplasm

FIGURE 12-39 Glucose is unable to diffuse across a plasma membrane by itself but can be moved across by a carrier protein embedded in the membrane, a process known as facilitated diffusion.

(Goodenough, Judith and Betty A. McGuire, Biology of Humans: Concepts, Applications, and Issues, 3rd Edition, © 2010. Reprinted by permission of Pearson Education, Inc., Upper Saddle River, NJ.)

Ion Channels

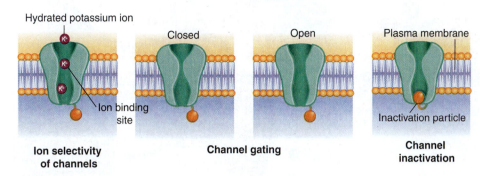

Hydrated potassium ion

Ion binding site

Closed

Open

Plasma membrane

Inactivation particle

Ion selectivity of channels

Channel gating

Channel inactivation

FIGURE 12-40 The function of a voltage-gated ion channel. (a) Several ways a channel can select for different ions are shown: (1) Negative charges at the opening of the channel repel anions and attract cations. (2) The pore diameter restricts the size of ions that can pass. (3) Ion-selective binding strips off water molecules so ions can pass through. (b) Channel gating occurs when a portion of the channel changes conformation when the membrane potential changes, effectively swinging the gate open or shut. (c) Inactivation of the sodium channel occurs when an inactivating particle blocks the pore.

- *Ion channels.* **Ion channels** are essentially hydrophilic pores through the membrane that open and allow certain types of solutes, usually inorganic ions, to pass through. (Note that the term **hydrophilic**, meaning attracted to water, is the opposite of the term **hydrophobic**, meaning repellent to water.) Typically, these ion channels are quite specific for a particular type of solute. Transport through ion channels is considerably faster than transport by carrier proteins. In addition, many ion channels are gated, which in effect controls the channel's permeability. When the gate is open, the ion channel transports the desired substance. When the gate is closed, no transport occurs. Ion channel gates can be controlled either by voltage across the membrane (voltage-gated channels) or by having a binding site for a *ligand* (a molecule that will bind to a site) that, when bound, causes the channels to open

(ligand-gated channels). Ion channels are particularly important in excitable cells, such as neurons and muscle cells, because they allow current flow to occur across the membrane (Figure 12-40).

Active Transport

Sometimes it is necessary for a cell to move a solute across the plasma membrane against the concentration gradient. As with facilitated diffusion, this process, called **active transport**, uses a carrier protein but also uses energy in the form of ATP (Figure 12-41). Thus, with active transport substances are moved from areas of lower solute concentration to those with higher solute concentration. This is especially important in regard to sodium and potassium ions. The concentration of sodium ions outside the cell membrane is much higher than inside the membrane. Conversely, the concentration of potassium ions is much higher inside the cell membrane than outside. The transport of sodium ions out of the cell and potassium ions into the cell, against the concentration gradient, is achieved by the **sodium–potassium pump**. The sodium–potassium pump is an enzyme (Na^+-K^+-ATPase) in the plasma membrane and is powered with ATP. Each of these enzymes binds three sodium ions on the inside of the cell membrane and transports them to the outside of the cell membrane. ATP is used in this step. Following that, two potassium ions are bound on the outside of the cell and transported to the inside of the cell. During this part of the process, ATP rebinds to the pump and is ready for another cycle. (Figure 12-42).

Extracellular fluid

Plasma membrane

A substance moves through the lipid bilayer from low to high concentration with the aid of a carrier protein and energy.

Carrier protein

ATP

ADP

Cytoplasm

Extracellular fluid

Low concentration

High concentration

Cytoplasm

FIGURE 12-41 Active transport moves a solute across the plasma membrane with the help of a carrier protein and energy in the form of ATP.

Sodium-Potassium Pump

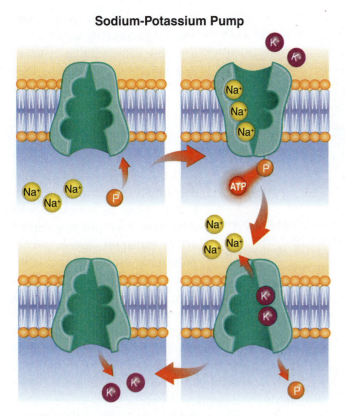

FIGURE 12-42 The sodium–potassium pump.

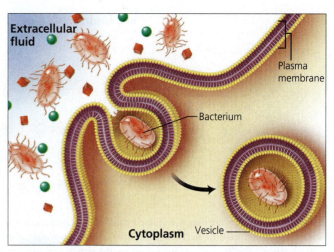

FIGURE 12-43 Phagocytosis. The cell engulfs large particles or bacteria.

(Goodenough, Judith and Betty A. McGuire, Biology of Humans: Concepts, Applications, and Issues, *3rd Edition, © 2010. Reprinted by permission of Pearson Education, Inc., Upper Saddle River, NJ.)*

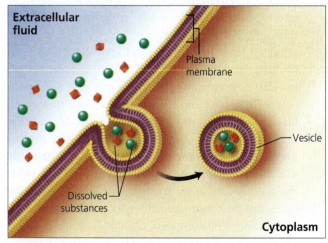

FIGURE 12-44 Pinocytosis. The cell engulfs droplets of extracellular fluid.

(Goodenough, Judith and Betty A. McGuire, Biology of Humans: Concepts, Applications, and Issues, *3rd Edition, © 2010. Reprinted by permission of Pearson Education, Inc., Upper Saddle River, NJ.)*

Endocytosis

Substances can also enter the cell through a process called **endocytosis**. With endocytosis, large molecules, single-celled organisms (bacteria), and fluid containing dissolved substances can enter the cell. During endocytosis, a section of the plasma membrane encircles the substance to be ingested. Once the substance is completely encircled, the membrane portion is pinched off from the cell membrane, resulting in a sac-like structure called a *vesicle*. When separated from the cell membrane, the vesicle is released into the cell.

Endocytosis is often divided into two categories: phagocytosis and pinocytosis. **Phagocytosis** is the process whereby the cell engulfs large particles or bacteria (Figure 12-43). **Pinocytosis** is the process by which the cell engulfs droplets of fluid carrying dissolved substances (Figure 12-44). Both mechanisms are necessary for cell survival.

Exocytosis

It is sometimes necessary for large molecules to leave the cells. For example, hormones are often large molecules that cannot readily pass through the cell membrane. As with endocytosis, large molecules can leave the cell by becoming encircled in a membrane vesicle. This process, called **exocytosis**, occurs in a fashion opposite to that of endocytosis. The membrane-bound vesicle containing the substance to be released from the cell approaches the cell membrane. There, it fuses with the cell membrane, and its contents are released outside the cell (Figure 12-45).

The Cellular Environment: Fluids and Electrolytes

Many pathological conditions, both medical and traumatic, adversely affect the fluid and electrolyte balance of the body. Certain disease processes, such as diabetic ketoacidosis and heat emergencies, are associated with certain electrolyte abnormalities. Severe derangements in fluid and electrolyte status can result in death. For this reason, as a paramedic, you need to have a good understanding of the fluids and electrolytes present in the human body.

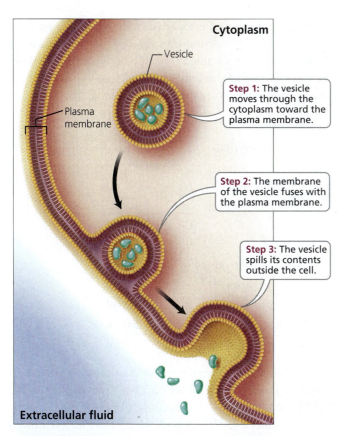

Cytoplasm

Vesicle

Plasma membrane

Step 1: The vesicle moves through the cytoplasm toward the plasma membrane.

Step 2: The membrane of the vesicle fuses with the plasma membrane.

Step 3: The vesicle spills its contents outside the cell.

Extracellular fluid

FIGURE 12-45 Exocytosis. A membrane-bound vesicle is taken into the cell membrane and its contents are released to the exterior.

(Goodenough, Judith and Betty A. McGuire, Biology of Humans: Concepts, Applications, and Issues, *3rd Edition, © 2010. Reprinted by permission of Pearson Education, Inc., Upper Saddle River, NJ.)*

compartment contains the remaining 30 percent of all body water. It contains the **extracellular fluid (ECF)**, all the fluid found outside the body cells.

There are two divisions within the extracellular compartment. The first contains the **intravascular fluid**—the fluid found outside cells and within the circulatory system. It is essentially the same as the blood plasma and accounts for about 5 percent of body water. The remaining compartment contains the **interstitial fluid**—all the fluid found outside the cell membranes, yet not within

> **CONTENT REVIEW**
>
> ➤ Distribution of Fluid among Body Compartments
> - Intracellular fluid (ICF)
> - Extracellular fluid (ECF)
>   - Intravascular fluid
>   - Interstitial fluid

Table 12-8 Body Fluid Compartments

Compartment	Percentage of Total Body Water	Volume in 70-kg Adult (42 L total body water)
Intracellular fluid	70.0 percent	29.40 L
Extracellular fluid	30.0 percent	12.60 L
Interstitial fluid	25.0 percent	10.50 L
Intravascular fluid	5.0 percent	2.10 L

Water

Water is the most abundant substance in the human body. In fact, water accounts for approximately 60 percent of total body weight (the average for all ages). The total amount of water in the body at any given time is referred to as the **total body water (TBW)**. In an adult weighing 70 kilograms (154 pounds), total body water would be approximately 42 liters (11 gallons) (Figure 12-46).

Water is distributed among various compartments of the body (Table 12-8). These compartments are separated by cell membranes. The largest compartment is the *intracellular compartment.* This compartment contains the **intracellular fluid (ICF)**, which is all the fluid found inside body cells. Approximately 70 percent of all body water is found within this compartment. The *extracellular*

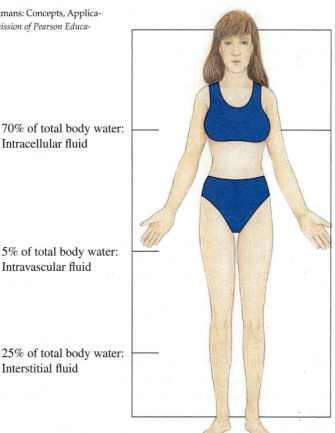

70% of total body water: Intracellular fluid

5% of total body water: Intravascular fluid

25% of total body water: Interstitial fluid

60% of body weight: Total body water

FIGURE 12-46 Water comprises approximately 60 percent of body weight. The water is distributed into three spaces: intracellular, intravascular, and interstitial.

the circulatory system, making up about 25 percent of body water. For example, minute amounts of fluid are found in the synovial fluid that lubricates the joints; the aqueous humor of the eye; secretions including saliva, gastric juices, and bile; and so on.

Total body water and its distribution vary with age and physiologic condition. At birth, an infant's TBW is about 75 to 80 percent of its body weight, compared to the 65 percent TBW of the average adult. Infants have a higher TBW for two reasons. First, infants have less fat than adults. (Fat does not absorb water, so the less fat in the body, the more water.) Second, water is essential for the high rates of metabolism that are necessary to promote growth in the infant. The TBW slowly decreases to approximately 70 to 75 percent by age 1. Diarrhea is especially worrisome in the infant, because it can mean the loss of a significant percentage of TBW. In addition, body systems that compensate for fluid loss are still immature, so infants can rapidly become dangerously dehydrated and subject to electrolyte imbalances. By late childhood, the TBW decreases to 65 to 70 percent.

By early adulthood, the TBW of males and females begins to differ. In adult males, TBW constitutes approximately 65 to 70 percent of the body weight, whereas in adult females, the average TBW is 60 to 65 percent. The gender difference is the result of hormonal differences that result in the male's greater muscle mass and the female's greater percentage of body fat.

As the human body ages, the loss of muscle mass, increased percentage of fat, and the body's decreasing ability to regulate fluid levels lowers the TBW to around 45 to 55 percent. As a result of a decreasing ability to regulate electrolytes and fluid levels, the elderly, like the very young, are at high risk for dehydration and disorders related to electrolyte imbalances.

Hydration

Water is the universal **solvent**. That is, most substances dissolve in water. When they do, chemical changes take place. For this reason, the water content of the body is crucial to virtually all of the body's biochemical processes. Normally, the total volume of water in the body, as well as the distribution of fluid in the three body compartments, remains relatively constant. This occurs despite wide fluctuations in the amount of

---

CONTENT REVIEW

➤ Factors That May Cause Dehydration
- Gastrointestinal losses (vomiting, diarrhea, malabsorption)
- Increased insensible loss (perspiration, water vapor, saliva)
- Increased sweating (diaphoresis)
- Internal losses ("thirdspace" losses to the interstitial space)
- Plasma losses (from burns, drains, fistulas, open wounds)

---

water that enters and is excreted from the body on a daily basis. The water coming into the body is referred to as *intake*. The water excreted from the body is referred to as output. To maintain relative homeostasis, the intake must equal the output, as shown in the following text.

Intake

digestive system:

liquids	1,000 mL
food (solids)	1,200 mL
metabolic sources:	300 mL
TOTAL:	2,500 mL

Output

lungs (water vapor):	400 mL
kidneys (urine):	1,500 mL
skin (perspiration):	400 mL
intestines (feces):	200 mL
TOTAL:	2,500 mL

Several mechanisms work to maintain a relative balance between input and output. For example, when the fluid volume drops, the pituitary gland secretes antidiuretic hormone (ADH), which causes the kidney tubules to reabsorb more water into the blood and to excrete less urine. This process helps to restore the fluid volume to normal values.

Thirst also regulates fluid intake. The sensation of thirst normally occurs when body fluids decrease, stimulating the person to take in more fluids orally. Conversely, when too many fluids enter the body, the kidneys are activated and more urine is excreted, thus eliminating excess fluid.

The body also maintains fluid balance by shifting water from one body space to another.

DEHYDRATION   **Dehydration**, an abnormal decrease in the TBW, can result from several factors:

- *Gastrointestinal losses* result from prolonged vomiting, diarrhea, or malabsorption disorders.

- *Increased insensible loss* is loss of water through normal mechanisms that is difficult to detect or measure (e.g., perspiration, water vapor from the lungs, saliva). These can be increased in fever states, during hyperventilation, or with high environmental temperatures.

- *Increased sweating* (also called perspiration or diaphoresis) can result in significant fluid loss. Although sweating is a form of insensible water loss, it is a significant concern with many medical conditions or high environmental temperatures.

- *Internal losses* are commonly called "third-space" losses because fluid is lost from intravascular or intracellular spaces into the interstitial space. With dehydration, fluid is typically lost from the intravascular compartment into the interstitial compartment, which effectively takes it out of the circulating volume. This can occur with peritonitis, pancreatitis, or bowel obstruction. It can also occur in poor nutritional states in which there is not enough protein in the vascular system to retain water.

- *Plasma losses* occur from burns, surgical drains and fistulas, and open wounds.

Dehydration rarely involves only the loss of water. More commonly, there is also a loss of electrolytes. At the hospital, fluid replacement will be based on both fluid and electrolyte deficits once the patient's electrolyte abnormalities are determined through laboratory testing.

Clinically, the dehydrated patient will exhibit dry mucous membranes and poor skin **turgor**. There often is excessive thirst. As it becomes more severe, dehydration will be accompanied by an increased pulse rate, decreased blood pressure, and orthostatic hypotension (increased pulse and decreased blood pressure on rising from a supine position). In infants, the anterior fontanelle may be sunken and the diaper may be dry or reveal the presence of highly concentrated (dark yellow, strong-smelling) urine. The absence of tears in a crying infant, a capillary refill time greater than 2 seconds, dry mucosa, and a decrease in urinary output are signs that indicate severe dehydration. The treatment for dehydration is replacement of fluid.

OVERHYDRATION **Overhydration** can occur as well. The major sign of overhydration is edema. Patients with heart disease may manifest overhydration much earlier than patients without heart disease. In severe cases of overhydration, overt heart failure may be present. Treatment is directed at removing the excessive fluid.

Electrolytes

How to Read Chemical Notation

To describe chemical substances and reactions, scientists use chemical notation, a kind of "shorthand." Every chemical element has a one- or two-letter abbreviation. Just four elements—hydrogen, oxygen, carbon, and nitrogen—make up more than 99 percent of the body's atoms. These are called the "major elements." Nine "trace elements" account for the remaining less than 1 percent.

Major Element	Symbol	Percent	Trace Element	Symbol
Hydrogen	H	62.0%	Calcium	Ca
Oxygen	O	26.0%	Chlorine	Cl
Carbon	C	10.0%	Iodine	I
Nitrogen	N	1.5%	Iron	Fe
			Magnesium	Mg
			Phosphorus	Ph
			Potassium	K
			Sodium	Na
			Sulfur	S

An atom is the smallest particle of an element. A molecule is a combination of atoms. The notation for a molecule combines the notations of the included elements. A subscript number after an element indicates the number of atoms of that element. If there is just one atom, there is no number. For example:

NaCl (Sodium chloride, or table salt. A sodium chloride molecule has 1 sodium atom and 1 chlorine atom.)

H_2O (Water. A water molecule has 2 hydrogen atoms and 1 oxygen atom.)

H_2CO_3 (Carbonic acid. A carbonic acid molecule has 2 hydrogen, 1 carbon, and 3 oxygen atoms.)

Ions

Each atom is made up of even smaller particles: electrons (that have a negative electrical charge), protons (that have a positive electrical charge), and neutrons (that are uncharged). Protons and neutrons are in the inner core, or nucleus, of the atom, and electrons occupy outer orbits around the nucleus. Sometimes an atom of an element can lose one or more of its outer electrons or can capture one or more extra electrons from another element.

An *ion* is an atom that has lost one or more negatively charged electrons and now has a positive charge, or an atom that has gained one or more electrons and now has a negative charge. A superscript plus ($^+$) indicates a positively charged cation. A superscript minus ($^-$) indicates a negatively charged anion. For example:

Na^+ (A sodium ion has lost an electron and has a positive charge.)

Ca^{++} (A calcium ion has lost two electrons and has a double positive charge.)

Cl^- (A chloride ion has gained an electron and has a negative charge.)

Electrolytes are substances that form ions when they break down, or dissociate, in water. Remember that the body and its blood are mostly water. The ions formed by dissociation of electrolytes in the body's fluids are a major factor in body metabolism.

Chemical Reactions

Notations for chemical reactions use a plus sign (+) to indicate substances that are combined and an arrow ($\rightarrow$) to show the direction of the reaction. The reactants are usually on the left, with the product of the reaction on the right.

$$2H + O \rightarrow H_2O$$

(2 hydrogen atoms + 1 oxygen atom = 1 water molecule)

In some circumstances, a reaction may be reversible. That is, separate elements may synthesize (combine), or the synthesized substance may dissociate (break down) into separate components. A two-directional arrow ($\leftrightarrow$) shows that a reaction is reversible and can be read in either direction.

$$CO_2 + H_2O \leftrightarrow H_2CO_3$$

Read as: (carbon dioxide + water = carbonic acid) or (carbonic acid = water + carbon dioxide).

Notice that no atoms are gained or lost in a chemical reaction. In the previous example, the two oxygen atoms in CO_2 and the single oxygen atom in H_2O combine to equal the three oxygen atoms in H_2CO_3. The hydrogen and carbon atoms are also equal on both sides of the reaction.

Up and down arrows ($\uparrow\downarrow$) are used to indicate an increase or decrease in the substance that follows the arrows. For example:

$\uparrow H^+$ (an increase in hydrogen ions)

$\downarrow CO_2$ (a decrease in carbon dioxide)

Types of Electrolytes: Cations and Anions

The chemical substances present throughout the body can be classified as either electrolytes or nonelectrolytes. **Electrolytes** are substances that **dissociate** into electrically charged particles when placed into water. The charged particles are referred to as *ions*. Ions with a positive charge are called cations; ions with a negative charge are called anions.

An example of this would be the dissociation of the drug sodium bicarbonate when it is placed into water. Sodium bicarbonate is a neutral salt. When placed into water, it dissociates into two charged particles, as shown here.

$$NaHCO_3 \rightarrow Na^+ + HCO_3^-$$

Sodium bicarbonate $\rightarrow$ sodium cation
+ bicarbonate anion neutral salt $\rightarrow$ cation + anion

Sodium bicarbonate is an example of an electrolyte that is taken into the body as a medication. However, there are many naturally occurring electrolytes present in the body.

The most frequently occurring cations include the following:

- *Sodium (Na^+).* Sodium is the most prevalent cation in the extracellular fluid. It plays a major role in regulating the distribution of water because water is attracted to and moves with sodium. In fact, it is often said that "water follows sodium." Sodium is also important in the transmission of nervous impulses. An abnormal increase in the relative amount of sodium in the body is called *hypernatremia,* whereas an abnormal decrease is referred to as *hyponatremia.*

- *Potassium (K^+).* Potassium is the most prevalent cation in the intracellular fluid. It is also important in the transmission of electrical impulses. An abnormally high potassium level is called *hyperkalemia,* whereas an abnormally low potassium level is referred to as *hypokalemia.*

- *Calcium (Ca⁺⁺).* Calcium has many physiologic functions. It plays a major role in muscle contraction as well as nervous impulse transmission. An abnormally increased calcium level is called *hypercalcemia,* whereas an abnormally decreased calcium level is called *hypocalcemia.*

- *Magnesium (Mg⁺⁺).* Magnesium is necessary for several biochemical processes that occur in the body and is closely associated with phosphate in many processes. An abnormally increased magnesium level is called *hypermagnesemia;* an abnormally decreased magnesium level is called *hypomagnesemia.*

The most frequently occurring anions include the following:

- *Chloride (Cl⁻).* Chloride is an important anion. Its negative charge balances the positive charge associated with the cations. It also plays a major role in fluid balance and renal function. Chloride has a close association with sodium.

- *Bicarbonate.* Bicarbonate is the principal buffer of the body. This means that it neutralizes the highly acidic hydrogen ion (H⁺) and other organic acids. (Buffering will be discussed in more detail later in this chapter.)

- *Phosphate.* Phosphate is important in body energy stores. It is closely associated with magnesium in renal function. It also acts as a buffer, primarily in the intracellular space, in much the same manner as bicarbonate.

Many other compounds carry negative charges. Among these are some of the proteins, certain organic acids, and other compounds. Electrolytes are usually measured in milliequivalents per liter (mEq/L). A milliequivalent is one thousandth (10^{-3}) of the relative weight of an element that has the same combining capacity as a given weight of another element (e.g., element, molecule, ion).

Nonelectrolytes are molecules that do not dissociate into electrically charged particles. These include glucose, urea, proteins, and similar substances.

Transport of Water and Electrolytes

In this section, we will review the concepts of diffusion, osmosis, active transport, and facilitated diffusion across a membrane—discussed earlier under "Plasma Membrane Functions"—as they concern the movement of water and electrolytes.

As noted earlier, the body's fluid compartments are separated by cell membranes. These membranes are called semipermeable or selectively permeable, meaning that they allow the easy passage of certain materials while restricting the passage of others. Compounds with small molecules, such as water (H_2O), pass readily through the membrane; larger compounds, such as proteins, are restricted. The movement of fluids through a membrane is enabled by the presence of pores (openings) in the membrane. Electrolytes do not pass through the membrane as readily as water. This is due not so much to the size of electrolyte molecules as to their electrical charge.

When solutions on opposite sides of a semipermeable membrane are equal in concentration, the relationship is said to be *isotonic.* When the concentration of a given solute (dissolved substance) is greater on one side of the membrane than on the other, it is said to be *hypertonic.* When the concentration is less on one side of the cell membrane, as compared to the other, it is referred to as *hypotonic.* This difference in concentration is known as the *osmotic gradient.*

The natural tendency of the body is to keep the balance of electrolytes and water equal on both sides of the cell membrane. This is an example of *homeostasis,* the body's normal tendency to maintain its internal environment in a steady state of balance. If one side of a cell membrane has an increased quantity of a given electrolyte (is hypertonic), there will be a shift of the electrolyte from that side and a shift of water from the other side to restore a balance in concentration—the balanced state.

The tendency of molecules to move from an area of higher concentration to an area of lower concentration is referred to as *diffusion* (or *simple diffusion*), a passive process that does not require energy (Figure 12-47). The diffusion of a solute (usually an electrolyte) across a cell membrane from the area of higher concentration to the area of lower concentration continues until balance is attained. This movement from an area of higher concentration to an area of lower concentration is termed a movement *with the osmotic gradient.*

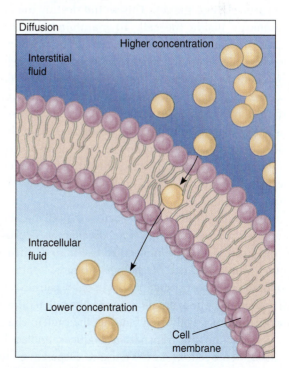

FIGURE 12-47 Diffusion is the movement of a substance from an area of great concentration to an area of lesser concentration.

Water also moves across the cell membrane so as to dilute the area of increased electrolyte concentration. The movement of water is more rapid than the movement of electrolytes. This form of diffusion (the passage of any solvent, usually water, through a membrane) is referred to as *osmosis* (Figure 12-48). It occurs in the direction opposite to the direction of solute movement. For example, if a semipermeable membrane separates solutions of water and sodium, and if the concentration of sodium is two times higher on one side of the membrane than on the other, then two things will occur: Sodium will diffuse from the area of higher concentration (the hypertonic side) to the area of lesser concentration (the hypotonic side). Concurrently, water will diffuse in the opposite direction. That is, water will leave the hypotonic side and diffuse across the membrane to the hypertonic side. These actions will continue until the concentration of water and sodium on both sides has equalized.

In addition to diffusion, two other mechanisms—active transport and facilitated diffusion—can transport substances across cell membranes. *Active transport* is the movement of a substance across the cell membrane *against the osmotic gradient* (that is, toward the side that already has more of the substance). For example, the body requires cells of the myocardium to be negatively charged on the inside of the cells as compared to the outside. However sodium, with its positive charge, tends to diffuse passively into the cell. This would destroy the negative charge inside the cell. To maintain the desired negative charge, sodium ions are actively pumped out of the cell, while potassium ions are pumped into the cell, by a mechanism known as the *sodium–potassium pump*. (Sodium and potassium ions are both positive, but more sodium ions are pumped out of the cell than potassium ions are pumped in, creating the desired negative charge inside the cell.) Active transport is faster than diffusion, but it requires the expenditure of energy, which diffusion does not. Proteins are moved across the cell membrane in a similar fashion.

Certain molecules can move across the cell membrane by another process known as *facilitated diffusion*. Glucose is an example of such a molecule. Facilitated diffusion requires the assistance of "helper proteins," parts of a membrane transport system that exist on the surface of the cell membrane. These proteins, once activated, bind to the glucose molecule. Following binding, the protein changes its configuration and transports the glucose molecule to the inside of the cell, where it is released. Depending on the substance that is being transported, facilitated diffusion may or may not require energy.

FIGURE 12-48 Osmosis is the movement of water from an area of higher water concentration to an area of lesser water concentration. Because water is a solvent, it moves from an area of lower solute concentration to an area of higher solute concentration.

Water Movement between Intracellular and Extracellular Compartments

The mechanisms by which water and solutes move across cell membranes ensure that the *osmolality* of body water (the concentration of particles within the water) inside and outside the cells is normally in equilibrium. Sodium, the most abundant ion in the extracellular fluid, is responsible for the osmotic balance of the extracellular space. Potassium plays the same role in the intracellular space.

Generally, the osmolality of intracellular fluid does not change very rapidly. However, when there is a change in the osmolality of extracellular fluid, water will move from the intracellular to the extracellular compartment, or vice versa, until osmotic equilibrium is regained.

Water Movement between Intravascular and Interstitial Compartments

Within the extracellular compartment, movement of water between the plasma in the intravascular space and the interstitial space is primarily a function of forces at play in the capillary beds.

In general, the movement of water and solutes across a cell membrane is governed by *osmotic pressure*. Osmotic pressure is the pressure exerted by the concentration of solutes on one side of a semipermeable membrane, such as a cell membrane or the thin wall of a capillary. Osmotic pressure can be thought of as a "pull" rather than a "push," because a hypertonic concentration of solutes tends to pull water from the other side of the membrane until the osmotic pressure on both sides is equal.

Generally, as already described, this is a two-way street as solutes move out of a space while water moves into the space to balance the concentration of solutes and the osmotic pressure on both sides of the membrane. However, there is a somewhat different osmotic mechanism that operates between the plasma inside a capillary and the interstitial space outside the capillary. Blood plasma generates **oncotic force**, which is sometimes called *colloid osmotic pressure.* Plasma proteins are colloids—large particles that do not readily move across the capillary membrane. They tend to remain within the capillary. At the same time, there is very little water in the interstitial space. The small amount of water that does get into the interstitial space is usually taken up by the lymphatic system. Therefore, because there is little water outside the capillary, and because plasma proteins do not readily move outside the capillary, the forces governing movement of water between the capillary and the interstitial space are almost all on one side, governed by the plasma on the inside of the capillary.

Another force inside the capillaries is **hydrostatic pressure**, which is the blood pressure, or force against the vessel walls, created by contractions of the heart. Hydrostatic pressure does tend to force some water out of the plasma and across the capillary wall into the interstitial space, a process that is called **filtration**. Hydrostatic pressure (a force that favors filtration, pushing water out of the capillary) and oncotic force (a force opposing filtration, pulling water into the capillary) together are responsible for **net filtration**, which is described in *Starling's hypothesis:*

Net filtration = (Forces favoring filtration) − (Forces opposing filtration)

Net filtration in a capillary is normally zero. It works this way: As plasma enters the capillary at the arterial end, hydrostatic pressure forces water to cross the capillary membrane into the interstitial space. This loss of water increases the relative concentration of plasma proteins. By the time the plasma reaches the venous end of the capillary, the oncotic force exerted by the increased concentration of plasma proteins is great enough to pull the water from the interstitial space back into the capillary. The outcome is that water is retained in the intravascular space and does not remain in the interstitial space.

Edema

Edema is the accumulation of water in the interstitial space. It occurs when there is a disruption in the forces and mechanisms that normally keep net filtration at zero (retaining water in the vascular system as plasma flows through the capillaries, according to Starling's hypothesis, previously described) or a disruption in the forces that would normally remove water from the interstitial space.

The mechanisms that most commonly result in accumulation of water in the interstitial space are a decrease in plasma oncotic force, an increase in hydrostatic pressure, increased permeability of the capillary membrane, and lymphatic obstruction.

- *A decrease in plasma oncotic force* may result from a loss or decrease in production of plasma proteins (albumins, globulins, and clotting factors). Plasma proteins are synthesized in the liver, so a liver disorder may be responsible for decreased production. Plasma loss from open wounds, hemorrhage, and burns may also cause a loss of plasma proteins. The result is that oncotic force is reduced to the point that some of the water lost through hydrostatic pressure is not regained.

- *An increase in hydrostatic pressure* can result from venous obstruction, salt and water retention, thrombophlebitis, liver obstruction, tight clothing at the extremities, or prolonged standing. The increase in hydrostatic pressure forces more water into the interstitial space than the oncotic force can recover.

- *Increased capillary permeability* generally results from the mechanisms of inflammation and immune response. These can result from allergic reactions, burns, trauma, or cancer. The greater permeability allows plasma proteins to escape from the capillaries, permitting water to remain in the interstitial space through the osmotic pressure of increased interstitial proteins and the reduction of oncotic force within the capillaries.

- *Lymphatic channel obstruction* can result from infection. Lymphatic channels are also sometimes removed through surgery. The loss of lymphatic channels interferes with the normal absorption of interstitial fluid by the lymphatic system. For example, removal of axillary lymph nodes in the treatment of breast cancer can result in edema of the arm.

Edema can be localized or generalized. Local swelling may appear at the site of an injury (e.g., a sprained ankle) or within a certain organ system such as the brain (cerebral edema), lungs (pulmonary edema), heart (pericardial effusion), or abdomen (ascites). A generalized edema may present as dependent edema, in which gravity pulls water to the lowest areas (e.g., in the feet and ankles when standing or in the sacral area when supine). You can identify dependent edema by pressing a finger over a bony prominence. A pit may remain after you remove your finger (*pitting edema*).

Edema is not only a sign of an underlying disease or problem; edema itself causes problems. It interferes with the movement of nutrients and wastes between tissues and capillaries. It may diminish capillary blood flow, depriving tissues of oxygen. In turn, this may slow the healing of wounds, promote infection, and facilitate formation of pressure sores. Edema affecting organs such as the brain, lung, heart, or larynx may be life threatening.

Body water that is retained in the interstitial spaces is body water that is not available for metabolic processes in the cells. Therefore, even though the total body water is normal, edema can cause a relative condition of dehydration.

The body has regulatory mechanisms that help to maintain homeostasis by controlling total body water and water distribution. Antidiuretic hormone (ADH), also known as *vasopressin*, is the chief regulator of water retention and distribution. Throughout the body, a network of sensors detects fluctuations in fluid and changes in the osmolar concentration of plasma. Osmoreceptors are located in the anterior hypothalamus. If there is an increase of 1 to 2 percent in osmolality—that is, if there is relatively less fluid in the plasma—the osmoreceptors will stimulate the release of ADH in an attempt to retain more fluid. Another type of receptor, baroreceptors, will detect both high and low pressure levels. Baroreceptors located in the carotid sinus, aortic arch, and kidney detect increases and decreases in pressure. Signals from the baroreceptors are relayed to the hypothalamus, which, again, will stimulate release of ADH as needed.

Definitive treatment of edema requires treatment of the underlying cause. Supportive care may include applying compression stockings, restricting salt intake, improving nutritional status, avoiding prolonged standing, and taking diuretics. Little can be done in the prehospital setting except elevation of edematous limbs.

Intravenous Therapy

Intravenous (IV) therapy is the introduction of fluids and other substances into the venous side of the circulatory system. It is used to replace blood lost through hemorrhage, for electrolyte or fluid replacement, and for introduction of medications directly into the vascular system.

Blood and Blood Components

To understand IV therapy, it is necessary to understand the function of blood and its components. The blood is the fluid of the cardiovascular system. An adequate amount of blood is required for the transport of nutrients, oxygen, hormones, and heat. Blood consists of the liquid portion, or plasma, and the formed elements, or blood cells (Figure 12-49).

PLASMA   Plasma is made up of approximately 92 percent water, 6 to 7 percent proteins, and a small portion consisting of electrolytes, lipids, enzymes, clotting factors, glucose, and other dissolved substances.

FORMED ELEMENTS   The formed elements include the red blood cells, or **erythrocytes**; the white blood cells, or **leukocytes**; and the platelets, or **thrombocytes**. More than 99 percent of the blood cells are erythrocytes. Erythrocytes contain hemoglobin and are responsible for transporting oxygen to the body's peripheral cells. **Hemoglobin** is an

FIGURE 12-49 Blood components.

Plasma: 54%

White cells: 1%

Red cells: 45%

Hematocrit

FIGURE 12-50 The percentage of the blood occupied by the red blood cells is termed the hematocrit.

iron-based compound that binds with oxygen in the pulmonary (lung) capillaries and transports the oxygen to the peripheral tissues, where it can be unloaded and taken into the cells. Factors such as pH (discussed later in this chapter) and oxygen concentration affect the amount of oxygen that can be transported by hemoglobin.

The leukocytes are responsible for immunity and fighting infection. The thrombocytes play a major role in blood clotting. The viscosity (thickness) of the blood is determined by the ratio of plasma to formed elements. The greater the proportion of formed elements within the plasma, the greater the viscosity.

The plasma can be separated from the formed elements by centrifugation. That is, blood can be placed in a test tube inside a centrifuge and spun at high speed. The heavier cells—the erythrocytes—will be forced to the bottom of the tube, leaving the plasma portion at the top. Usually, the erythrocytes will account for approximately 45 percent of the blood volume. The percentage of blood occupied by erythrocytes is referred to as the **hematocrit** (Figure 12-50).

Fluid Replacement

The most desirable fluid for blood loss replacement is whole blood. There are several reasons for this. First, blood contains hemoglobin, which can transport oxygen. In addition, it is the most natural replacement. However, even in the hospital setting, the routine use of whole blood is not practical (Table 12-9). Blood is a precious commodity, and it must be conserved so it can benefit the most people. Because of this, blood is often fractionated, or separated into parts. The red cells are packaged separately as packed red blood cells. The white cells are used for other purposes. Plasma is packaged as fresh frozen plasma for use when plasma or clotting factors are needed. Thus, with the exception of true hemorrhagic shock (resulting from blood loss), where whole blood is the fluid of first choice, packed red blood cells are now more frequently used than whole blood.

Before blood, or blood products, can be administered to a patient, they must be typed and cross-matched to prevent a severe allergic reaction. The exception to this is fresh frozen plasma, which does not require cross-matching. If there is not adequate time for typing and cross-matching, O-negative blood (type O, Rh negative), the universal donor, can be administered.

Transfusion Reaction

Blood and blood products are rarely used in the field. However, on occasion, you may be called on to transport a patient with blood infusing. Because of this, you must be able to recognize the signs and symptoms of a transfusion reaction. Transfusion reactions occur when there is a discrepancy between the blood type of the patient and the blood type of the blood being transfused. In addition to the ABO and Rh types, there are many minor types that can cause a transfusion reaction. Common signs and symptoms of a transfusion reaction include fever, chills, hives, hypotension, palpitations, tachycardia, flushing of the skin, headaches, loss of consciousness, nausea, vomiting, or shortness of breath.

Table 12-9   Resuscitation Fluids

	Resuscitation Fluid Used			
Diagnosis	1st Choice	2nd Choice	3rd Choice	4th Choice
Hemorrhagic shock	Whole blood	Packed RBCs	Plasma or plasma substitute	Lactated Ringer's or normal saline
Shock due to plasma loss (burns)	Plasma	Plasma substitute	Lactated Ringer's or normal saline	—
Dehydration	Lactated Ringer's or normal saline	—	—	—

Intravenous Fluids

Intravenous fluids are the most common products used in prehospital care for fluid and electrolyte therapy. Intravenous fluids occur in two standard forms—colloids and crystalloids.

COLLOIDS A **colloid** contains proteins or other high-molecular-weight molecules that tend to remain in the intravascular space for an extended period of time. In addition, as described earlier, colloids have oncotic force (colloid osmotic pressure), which means that they tend to attract water into the intravascular space from the interstitial space and the intracellular space. Thus, a small amount of a colloid can be administered to a patient with a greater-than-expected increase in intravascular volume. The following are examples of colloids:

- *Plasma protein fraction (Plasmanate)* is a protein-containing colloid. The principal protein present is **albumin**, which is suspended along with other proteins in a saline solvent.

- *Salt-poor albumin* contains only human albumin. Each gram of albumin holds approximately 18 milliliters of water in the bloodstream.

- *Dextran* is not a protein, but a large sugar molecule with osmotic properties similar to albumin. It comes in two molecular weights: 40,000 and 70,000 Daltons. Dextran 40 has 2 to 2.5 times the colloid osmotic pressure of albumin.

- *Hetastarch (Hespan)*, like dextran, is a sugar molecule with osmotic properties similar to protein. It does not appear to share many of dextran's side effects. Colloid replacement therapy, at present, does not have a significant role in prehospital care except under rare circumstances. The colloid products are expensive and have a short shelf life.

CRYSTALLOIDS **Crystalloids** are the primary compounds used in prehospital intravenous fluid therapy. There are multiple fluid preparations. It is often helpful to classify them according to their **tonicity** relative to plasma:

- *Isotonic solutions* have electrolyte composition similar to the blood plasma. When placed into a normally hydrated patient, they will not cause a significant fluid or electrolyte shift. Examples include normal saline (0.9 percent sodium chloride, also written as 0.9 percent NaCl) and lactated Ringer's.

- *Hypertonic solutions* have a higher solute concentration than the cells. These fluids will tend to cause a fluid shift out of the interstitial space and intracellular compartment into the intravascular space when administered to a normally hydrated patient. Later, there will be a diffusion of solute in the opposite direction. An example is 7.5 percent sodium chloride solution.

- *Hypotonic solutions* have a lower solute concentration than the cells. When administered to a normally hydrated patient, they will cause a movement of fluid from the intravascular space into the interstitial space and intracellular compartment. Later, solutes will move in an opposite direction. An example is 5 percent dextrose in water (D_5W).

Intravenous replacement fluids should be chosen based on the needs of the patient and the patient's underlying problem. This is typically guided by laboratory studies obtained in the hospital. However, these studies are not available in the prehospital setting. Hemorrhage occurs so fast that there is usually not time for a significant fluid shift to occur between the intravascular space and interstitial/intracellular spaces. Because of this, isotonic replacement fluids, such as lactated Ringer's and normal saline, should be used (Figure 12-51).

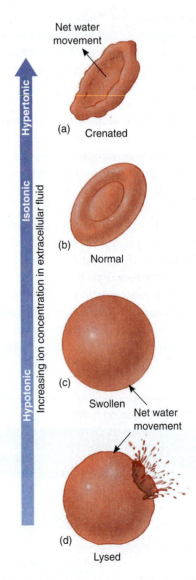

FIGURE 12-51 The effects of hypertonic, isotonic, and hypotonic solutions on red blood cells.

Certain conditions, such as gastroenteritis (characterized by diarrhea, vomiting, and fever), can cause a patient to lose water more rapidly than sodium. These patients will have a deficit in TBW due to reduced water intake, excessive water loss, or a combination of both. When water is lost in this manner, the level of sodium in the serum can increase, resulting in hypernatremia (elevated sodium levels). Patients with hypernatremia primarily need water. Because of this, hypotonic intravenous solutions, such as 0.45 percent sodium chloride (half-normal saline), are often chosen, because they provide the needed water with less sodium. However, it is important to point out that, even in cases of hypernatremia, initial fluid replacement therapy should consist of an isotonic solution until adequate blood pressure and adequate tissue perfusion have been restored.

Some replacement fluids contain a single element, such as sodium chloride or dextrose, whereas others contain multiple elements. Solutions such as lactated Ringer's are designed so that the concentration of electrolytes is very similar to that of the plasma. As a result, these solutions are referred to as *balanced salt solutions*.

The most commonly used solutions in prehospital care are lactated Ringer's solution, 0.9 percent sodium chloride (normal saline), and 5 percent dextrose in water (D_5W).

- *Lactated Ringer's* is an isotonic electrolyte solution of sodium chloride, potassium chloride, calcium chloride, and sodium lactate in water.

- *Normal saline* is an electrolyte solution of sodium chloride in water. It is isotonic with the extracellular fluid.

- *D_5W* is a hypotonic glucose solution used to keep a vein open and to supply calories necessary for cell metabolism. It will have an initial effect of increasing the circulatory volume, but glucose molecules rapidly diffuse across the vascular membrane. Water follows the glucose into the interstitial space, resulting in an increase in interstitial water.

Both lactated Ringer's solution and normal saline are used for fluid replacement, because their administration causes an immediate expansion of the circulatory volume. However, as was noted earlier, due to the movement of electrolytes and water, two-thirds of either of these solutions is lost into the interstitial space within 1 hour.

The Internal Cell

Earlier in this chapter, we discussed the basic structure of the cell, its plasma membrane, and cytoplasm. Within the cell are numerous specialized structures called organelles, as well as a permeating structure called the cytoskeleton, which will be described next.

Organelles and Their Functions

As discussed previously, eukaryotic cells contain specialized internal compartments, enclosed by membranes, called organelles. Various biochemical processes that are necessary to cell survival and reproduction occur within the organelles. This is a much more efficient system than that seen in prokaryotic cells, because, in eukaryotic cells, molecules that perform a similar task are situated together for efficiency.

The roles and functions of the organelles are diverse. The following sections describe the major intracellular organelles and their functions.

Nucleus

The *nucleus* is among the largest organelles and contains all of the cell's genetic information (Figure 12-52). Genetic information is encoded by base sequences on the DNA

> **CONTENT REVIEW**
> ➤ Organelles within Cells
> - Nucleus
> - Ribosomes
> - Endoplasmic reticulum
> - Golgi apparatus
> - Lysosomes
> - Vacuoles
> - Peroxisomes
> - Mitochondria

In some areas, the nuclear membrane is continuous with the endoplasmic reticulum.

Nucleus — Rough endoplasmic reticulum — Nucleus — Nucleolus — Nucleoplasm — Nuclear envelope — Chromatin (DNA and its associated proteins) — Nuclear pore

Diagram of the nucleus.

FIGURE 12-52 Diagram of the nucleus.

(Goodenough, Judith and Betty A. McGuire, Biology of Humans: Concepts, Applications, and Issues, 3rd Edition, © 2010. Reprinted by permission of Pearson Education, Inc., Upper Saddle River, NJ.)

Chromosomes

FIGURE 12-53 Chromosomes are composed of DNA and associated proteins. During cell division, as shown here, chromosomes shorten and condense.

molecule. DNA controls cell functions and the production of specific proteins. All cells in an organism contain precisely the same information. However, some cells will express certain parts of the genetic information, whereas others express other parts.

The genetic information is carried on threadlike structures called **chromosomes** made up of DNA and other proteins (Figure 12-53). The number of chromosomes varies from species to species. Humans have 46 chromosomes (23 pairs), with one pair being the chromosomes that determine sex. Typically, chromosomes are visible (with a light microscope) only during the phase when cell division is occurring. During the process of division, chromosomes shorten and condense. The remainder of the time they are extended and are not visible. During this extended phase, before shortening and condensation, the genetic material is called **chromatin**.

A double membrane encases the nucleus and is referred to as the **nuclear envelope.** The nuclear envelope contains the chromatin and the other materials inside the nucleus that are collectively referred to as **nucleoplasm**. Communications between the inside of the nucleus and the surrounding cytoplasm occurs through openings in the nuclear envelope called **nuclear pores**.

There is a specialized region within the nucleus referred to as the **nucleolus.** As with the chromosomes, the nucleolus is visible only during certain cell phases. The nucleolus is not surrounded by a membrane. The nucleolus is a region of the DNA that is active in the production of a specialized type of RNA called ribosomal RNA (rRNA). The rRNA leaves the nucleus of the cell and joins with messenger RNA (mRNA) to form a ribosome. Ribosomes then manufacture the protein coded for by the RNA.

Ribosomes

Ribosomes are spherical structures that can account for up to 25 percent of the dry weight of a cell (Figure 12-54). The primary role of the ribosomes is the synthesis of polypeptides and proteins. The ribosome consists of two subunits, each consisting of rRNA and protein. These subunits leave the cell nucleus, bind with mRNA, and become a functional ribosome in the cytoplasm. The ribosomes interpret the information from mRNA and translate it into an amino acid sequence until the desired protein is formed. The necessary conformational changes will occur (bending, folding) to make the protein fully functional.

Endoplasmic Reticulum

The **endoplasmic reticulum** is a network of tubules, vesicles, and sacs that interconnect with the plasma membrane, nuclear envelope, and many of the other organelles in the cell. Certain parts of the endoplasmic reticulum contain ribosomes during protein synthesis and are referred to as **rough endoplasmic reticulum (RER).** The RER sends the proteins to the Golgi apparatus in vesicles called cisternae or, if they are membrane proteins, insert them into the plasma membrane. (The Golgi apparatus and cisternae will be described next.)

The portion of the endoplasmic reticulum without ribosomes is called **smooth endoplasmic reticulum (SER)**. SER has multiple functions, depending on the cell type. The vast network of SER provides an increased surface area for the action or storage of key enzymes and the products of these enzymes. For example, SER in muscle

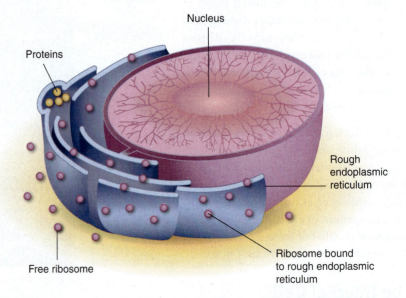

FIGURE 12-54 Ribosomes are spherical structures within the cell that function in the synthesis of polypeptides and proteins. Some ribosomes are suspended in the cytoplasm (free ribosomes); other ribosomes are attached to the endoplasmic reticulum (bound ribosomes).

FIGURE 12-55 The endoplasmic reticulum has rough and smooth portions. Rough endoplasmic reticulum (RER) has ribosomes attached during protein synthesis. Smooth endoplasmic reticulum (SER) has no attached ribosomes and serves various functions, depending on the cell type.

(Goodenough, Judith and Betty A. McGuire, Biology of Humans: Concepts, Applications, and Issues, 3rd Edition, © 2010. Reprinted by permission of Pearson Education, Inc., Upper Saddle River, NJ.)

cells serves as a store of calcium that is released as one step in the contraction process. Calcium pumps move the calcium.

The endoplasmic reticulum also plays a major role in replenishment and maintenance of the plasma membrane. The protein components of the plasma membrane come from the RER, whereas the lipid components come from the SER (Figure 12-55).

Golgi Apparatus

The **Golgi apparatus**, also called the *Golgi complex*, is an important organelle whose function is to process proteins for the cell membrane and other cell organelles. The Golgi apparatus serves as a sort of "post office" for the cell, as it is essentially a protein-processing and packaging center. The transport vesicles (**cisternae**) from the endoplasmic reticulum fuse with the face of the Golgi apparatus and empty their protein content into the lumen of the Golgi apparatus. The proteins are then transported to the opposite side of the Golgi apparatus and are modified along the way. They are labeled with a sequence of molecules according to their final destination. Some proteins, such as those bound for the plasma membrane, are packaged in vesicles (Figure 12-56). Other proteins are packaged in lysosomes (described next).

FIGURE 12-56 The route by which protein-filled vesicles from the rough endoplasmic reticulum travel to the Golgi complex for processing and then move on to the plasma membrane for release.

(Goodenough, Judith and Betty A. McGuire, Biology of Humans: Concepts, Applications, and Issues, 3rd Edition, © 2010. Reprinted by permission of Pearson Education, Inc., Upper Saddle River, NJ.)

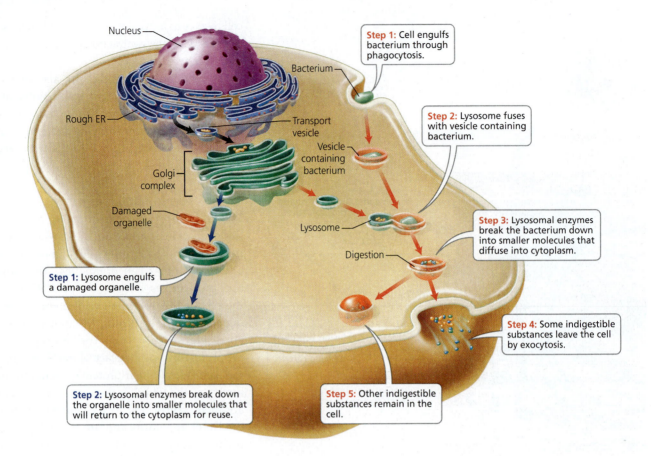

Nucleus

Bacterium

Step 1: Cell engulfs bacterium through phagocytosis.

Rough ER

Transport vesicle

Step 2: Lysosome fuses with vesicle containing bacterium.

Golgi complex

Vesicle containing bacterium

Damaged organelle

Lysosome

Digestion

Step 3: Lysosomal enzymes break the bacterium down into smaller molecules that diffuse into cytoplasm.

Step 1: Lysosome engulfs a damaged organelle.

Step 4: Some indigestible substances leave the cell by exocytosis.

Step 2: Lysosomal enzymes break down the organelle into smaller molecules that will return to the cytoplasm for reuse.

Step 5: Other indigestible substances remain in the cell.

FIGURE 12-57 Lysosome formation and function in intracellular digestion. Lysosomes released from the Golgi complex digest a bacterium engulfed by the cell (pathway shown on right). Lysosomes also digest obsolete parts of the cell itself (pathway shown on left).

(Goodenough, Judith and Betty A. McGuire, Biology of Humans: Concepts, Applications, and Issues, *3rd Edition, © 2010. Reprinted by permission of Pearson Education, Inc., Upper Saddle River, NJ.)*

Lysosomes

Lysosomes serve as the "garbage disposal system" of the cells. That is, they degrade and remove products of ingestion (the process called *phagocytosis*) and worn out parts from the cell. They also play a role in converting complex nutritional molecules to simple nutritional molecules. Lysosomes are spherical in shape and surrounded by a single membrane. Each lysosome can contain up to 40 digestive enzymes and has an extremely low pH (pH 4.8). The enzymes and membranes of lysosomes are manufactured by the RER and sent to the Golgi apparatus for packaging. Ultimately, a lysosome that contains all the necessary digestive enzymes surrounded by a plasma membrane will bud from the Golgi apparatus into the cytoplasm (Figure 12-57).

One of the major functions of lysosomes is to break down foreign substances and invaders, such as a bacterium. Once a bacterium is isolated through the process of phagocytosis, it is enclosed in a large vesicle called a vacuole. (Vacuoles will be described next.) Soon, vesicles containing lysosomal enzymes (primary lysosomes) will fuse with the vesicle. The pH of the newly formed complex then becomes more acidic, and this activates the digestive

enzymes. The vacuole thus becomes a secondary lysosome and degrades the bacterium. Lysosomes also degrade worn-out organelles such as mitochondria. The remnants of the process are either reprocessed for use again or released from the cell through exocytosis.

Lysosomes also process the macromolecule products needed for cell energy production. The macromolecule ultimately winds up in food vacuoles. These vacuoles then fuse with primary lysosomes, where digestive enzymes break down the macromolecules into simple molecules that diffuse out of the vesicle into the cytoplasm for use as energy substrates for the cell.

Vacuoles

Vacuoles are membrane-bound organelles used for temporary storage or transport of substances such as food sources. The lysosome can fuse with the vacuole membrane and place digestive enzymes into the food vacuole to break down the food source within.

Peroxisomes

Peroxisomes are similar to lysosomes in size and the lack of obvious internal structure. Peroxisomes have the ability

Clinical Note

Pediatric

Tay-Sachs disease (pronounced tay-SACKS) is a genetic disorder that can result in paralysis, blindness, convulsions, mental retardation, and death. It was first described in 1881, and in 1887 was found to be more prevalent in Ashkenazi Jews (Jews of Central European descent). It is also seen, although on a more limited basis, in French Canadians of southeastern Quebec and in Cajuns of southern Louisiana. These populations all tend to marry within their population, leading to less genetic diversity and increased expression of mutations. Tay-Sachs disease is quite rare in families of other ethnic backgrounds.

It has been determined that a mutation on chromosome 15 causes the absence of the lysosomal enzyme hexosamidase (Hex A), which is responsible for breaking down lipids in nerve cells. Without Hex A, nerve cells swell with undigested lipids which ultimately causes a progressive and irreversible deterioration in nervous system functioning.

Tay-Sachs disease normally becomes noticeable around the age of six months. Prior to that, the baby acts normally. However, once the symptoms of Tay-Sachs begin to appear, several noticeable changes occur. First, the baby will become listless and will stop interacting with other people and will often develop a staring gaze. Even normal levels of noise tend to startle the baby to an abnormal degree. Eventually, the baby will develop dementia, mental retardation, decreased muscle tone, seizures, and death. There is no treatment, and the disease is 100 percent fatal—usually by age 4 to 5.

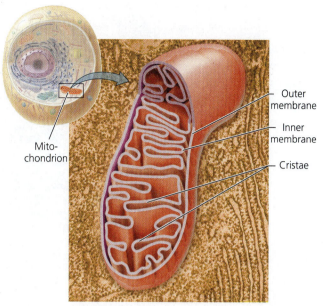

Diagram of a mitochondrion showing the double membrane that creates two compartments.

FIGURE 12-58 Mitochondria are sites of energy conversion in the cell.

(Goodenough, Judith and Betty A. McGuire, Biology of Humans: Concepts, Applications, and Issues, *3rd Edition, © 2010. Reprinted by permission of Pearson Education, Inc., Upper Saddle River, NJ.)*

to generate and degrade hydrogen peroxide (H_2O_2). Hydrogen peroxide is highly toxic to cells. However, it can be degraded to water and oxygen by the enzyme catalase. Because of its toxicity, eukaryotic cells protect themselves by placing the biochemical pathways that generate and degrade H_2O_2 into the isolated compartment called a peroxisome.

Peroxisomes are found in virtually all cell types but are more prevalent in the liver and kidneys. They play an important role in detoxifying harmful substances such as alcohols and formaldehyde. Peroxisomes are also important in the breakdown of fatty acids. Because they can produce oxygen, peroxisomes play a role in the regulation of oxygen tension within the cell.

Mitochondria

The **mitochondria** are the "powerhouses" of the cells in that they provide the energy needed for all of a cell's biochemical processes. Cellular respiration, which is the conversion of food to energy, occurs primarily in the mitochondria. Cellular respiration is a three-phase process that first begins in the cytoplasm and continues in the mitochondria. (Cellular respiration will be described in more detail later.)

The number of mitochondria present varies from cell to cell, depending on the specialized function of the cell. Mitochondria, like the nucleus, are surrounded by a double membrane forming two separate compartments. The inner membrane folds form shelves within the mitochondria, referred to as **cristae**, where the last phases of cellular respiration occur. The mitochondria also can contain some ribosomes and some of the cell's genetic material (Figure 12-58).

The Cytoskeleton and Other Internal Cell Structures

Within eukaryotic cells is a complex system of filaments, microtubules, and intermediate filaments referred to as the **cytoskeleton**.

Microtubules are long, hollow rods made of the protein *tubulin*. Microfilaments are made from the protein *actin*. Intermediate filaments are made up of different proteins, depending on the cell type. Near the cell nucleus are two structures called **centrioles**, cylindrical structures composed of groups of microtubules arranged in a ring pattern that are thought to play an important role in cell division (Figure 12-59).

The cytoskeleton forms a dynamic three-dimensional structure that fills the cytoplasm and serves as a skeleton

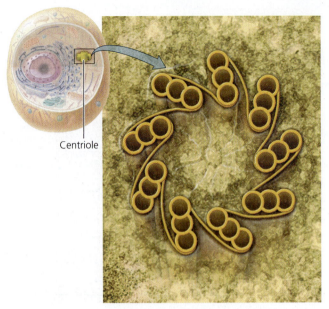

Centriole

Diagram of a centriole. Each centriole is composed of nine sets of triplet microtubules arranged in a ring.

FIGURE 12-59 Centrioles are thought to play an important role in cell division.

(Goodenough, Judith and Betty A. McGuire, Biology of Humans: Concepts, Applications, and Issues, *3rd Edition, © 2010. Reprinted by permission of Pearson Education, Inc., Upper Saddle River, NJ.)*

for cell stability and as a muscle for cell movement. In addition to stability, the cytoskeleton plays an important role in both intracellular transport and cellular division.

Two structures important in cell movement, cilia and flagella, are made up of microtubules. **Cilia** are numerous hairlike structures that move in a back-and-forth motion. This motion can sweep debris away from the cell and play an important role in protection of the respiratory system and in the reproductive system (Figure 12-60). **Flagella** are much longer than cilia and move in an undulating, wavelike manner. Human sperm move via the undulations of flagella.

Cilium

FIGURE 12-60 Cilia are short hairlike structures on the surfaces of cells, such as those that line the respiratory tract, where they sweep away debris trapped in mucus.

Cellular Respiration and Energy Production

The cell needs a constant supply of energy. We get the energy our body needs through nutrients in our diet. Our digestive system breaks down the three major classes of nutrients—carbohydrates, proteins, and lipids—into simpler compounds, typically simple sugars and amino acids, that can enter the cell and be converted to energy. Some of the energy is used to manufacture ATP and some is given off as heat. Once nutrients reach the cells, they will enter a metabolic pathway—either cellular respiration or fermentation. Cellular respiration is aerobic and requires oxygen. Fermentation is anaerobic and does not require oxygen.

When nutrients are converted to energy by the cells, there is a transport of electrons from one molecule to another. The loss of electrons from one atom to another is called **oxidation**. The gain of electrons by one atom from another is called **reduction**. In cellular respiration, glucose is oxidized to simpler compounds, producing energy in the process.

Cellular Respiration

A glucose molecule must pass through three distinct biochemical processes to produce energy through **cellular respiration**: glycolysis, the citric acid cycle, and electron transport (Figure 12-61). Glycolysis occurs in the cytoplasm, whereas the citric acid cycle and electron transport occur in the mitochondria. The complete breakdown of glucose yields water, carbon dioxide, and energy in the form of ATP. This relationship is illustrated by the following equation:

$$C_6H_{12}O_6 \;+\; 6O_2 \;\rightarrow\; 6CO_2 \;+\; 6H_2O \;+\; \approx 36ATP$$

Glucose *Oxygen* *Carbon Dioxide* *Water* *Energy*

Glycolysis

The first step in the breakdown of the six-carbon sugar glucose is called **glycolysis** and occurs in the cytoplasm. In glycolysis, one molecule of glucose is oxidized through several steps to two molecules of pyruvic acid. The process of glycolysis is anaerobic—that is, it does not require oxygen.

There are two phases of glycolysis: the energy-using phase and the energy-yielding phase. During the first phase, two molecules of ATP are used to prepare the glucose molecule for splitting into two three-carbon subunits. During the second phase, the two three-carbon molecules are broken down to pyruvic acid (the anion of pyruvic acid is pyruvate). During this phase, four molecules of ATP are produced, giving a net yield of two molecules of ATP per

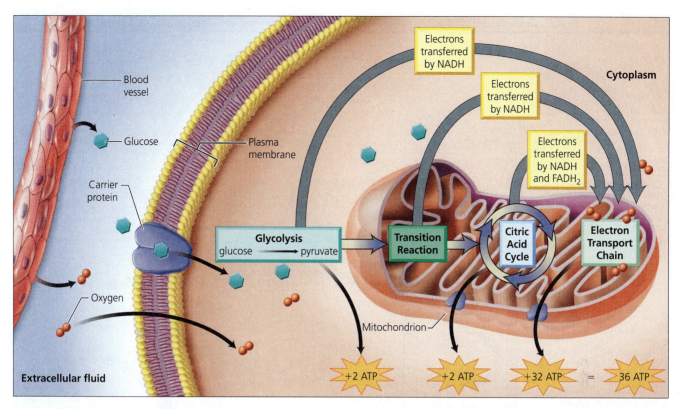

FIGURE 12-61 Summary of cellular respiration in which a glucose molecule undergoes glycolysis, the citric acid cycle, and transport to produce energy.

(Goodenough, Judith and Betty A. McGuire, Biology of Humans: Concepts, Applications, and Issues, *3rd Edition, © 2010. Reprinted by permission of Pearson Education, Inc., Upper Saddle River, NJ.)*

molecule of glucose. The two molecules of pyruvic acid then move from the cytoplasm into the liquid matrix of the mitochondria, where the citric acid cycle occurs. Glycolysis also produces two molecules of *nicotine adenine dinucleotide (NADH)*, which carry energy to the electron transport chain (Figure 12-62).

Citric Acid Cycle

Once the two molecules of pyruvic acid have entered the mitochondria, they enter the second phase of glucose metabolism, called the **citric acid cycle**. The citric acid cycle, also called the *Krebs cycle* or the *tricarboxylic acid (TCA) cycle*, requires oxygen. In the first step, called the transition reaction, the pyruvic acid molecule reacts with a substance called coenzyme A (CoA) (Figure 12-63). This removes a carbon atom (in the form of carbon dioxide) from the pyruvic acid molecule. The resulting two-carbon molecule (called an acetyl group) binds to the CoA molecule and becomes acetyl CoA. Acetyl CoA then formally enters the citric acid cycle. In an eight-step process, the citric acid cycle completely oxidizes the remainder of the glucose molecule. On the completion of glucose oxidation, the citric acid cycle yields two molecules of ATP and releases carbon dioxide as waste (Figure 12-64). It also yields several molecules of two other compounds: NADH

and flavin adenine nucleotide ($FADH_2$). NADH and $FADH_2$ carry high-energy electrons into the final part of cellular metabolism—the electron transport chain.

Electron Transport

NADH and $FADH_2$ derived from glycolysis and the citric acid cycle donate their electrons to carrier proteins known as the electron transport chain. The **electron transport chain** consists of five types of carriers. (All the carriers except one are proteins.) These proteins are embedded on the cristae in the inner membrane of the mitochondria. When electrons are transferred from one molecule to the next, energy is released. This energy is then used to create ATP for use as an energy source by the cells. The electrons are ultimately passed to oxygen, which is the ultimate *electron acceptor*. On accepting the electron, oxygen combines with two molecules of hydrogen to form a molecule of water. If there is insufficient oxygen, electrons begin to accumulate on the carrier proteins, and this will ultimately stop the citric acid cycle.

The electron transport chain, when functioning optimally, can produce 32 molecules of ATP. Together, cellular respiration produces approximately 36 molecules of ATP (2 ATP from glycolysis, 2 ATP from the citric acid cycle, and 32 ATP from electron transport). The actual number

Glycolysis (in cytoplasm)

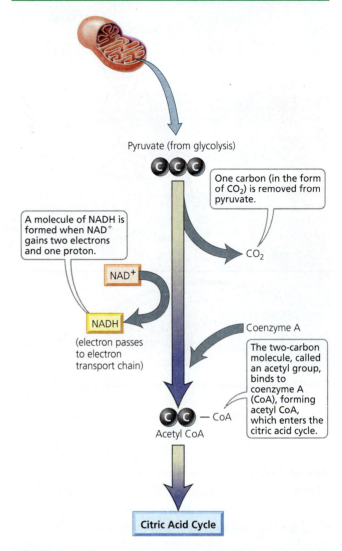

Cytoplasm

During the first steps, two molecules of ATP are *consumed* in preparing glucose for splitting.

Glucose

Energy-investment phase

2 ATP

2 ADP

During the remaining steps, four molecules of ATP are *produced*.

4 ADP

4 ATP

2 NAD$^+$

Energy-yielding phase

2 NADH

The two molecules of pyruvate then diffuse from the cytoplasm into the inner compartment of the mitochondrion, where they pass through a few preparatory steps (the transition reaction) before entering the citric acid cycle.

2 Pyruvate

Two molecules of nicotine adenine dinucleotide (NADH), a carrier of high-energy electrons, also are produced.

FIGURE 12-62 Glycolysis is a sequence of reactions in the cytoplasm in which glucose, a six-carbon sugar, is split into two three-carbon molecules of pyruvate.

(Goodenough, Judith and Betty A. McGuire, Biology of Humans: Concepts, Applications, and Issues, 3rd Edition, © 2010. Reprinted by permission of Pearson Education, Inc., Upper Saddle River, NJ.)

Transition Reaction (in mitochondrion)

Pyruvate (from glycolysis)

One carbon (in the form of CO_2) is removed from pyruvate.

A molecule of NADH is formed when NAD$^+$ gains two electrons and one proton.

CO_2

NAD$^+$

NADH

(electron passes to electron transport chain)

Coenzyme A

Acetyl CoA — CoA

The two-carbon molecule, called an acetyl group, binds to coenzyme A (CoA), forming acetyl CoA, which enters the citric acid cycle.

Citric Acid Cycle

FIGURE 12-63 The transition reaction is the link between glycolysis and the citric acid cycle.

(Goodenough, Judith and Betty A. McGuire, Biology of Humans: Concepts, Applications, and Issues, 3rd Edition, © 2010. Reprinted by permission of Pearson Education, Inc., Upper Saddle River, NJ.)

produced at any given time varies and is dependent on numerous factors (Figure 12-65).

Fermentation

An alternative pathway to energy production is available during times when oxygen is unavailable. The breakdown of glucose without oxygen is called **fermentation**.

In fermentation, the glucose molecule proceeds through glycolysis, as it does in cellular respiration, as glycolysis does not require oxygen. This results in the creation of two molecules each of pyruvate, NADH, and ATP. During fermentation, the chemical reactions continue in the cytoplasm instead of entering the mitochondria. In fermentation, the final electron acceptor is pyruvate, not oxygen. Electrons are transferred from the NADH molecule to pyruvate, which generates NAD$^+$. This helps generate ATP through glycolysis. Fermentation is very inefficient and produces only 2 ATP, compared to 36 ATP from cellular respiration.

Two types of fermentation can occur in humans: lactic acid fermentation and alcohol fermentation. As just discussed, NADH passes electrons directly to pyruvate.

Citric Acid Cycle (in mitochondrion)

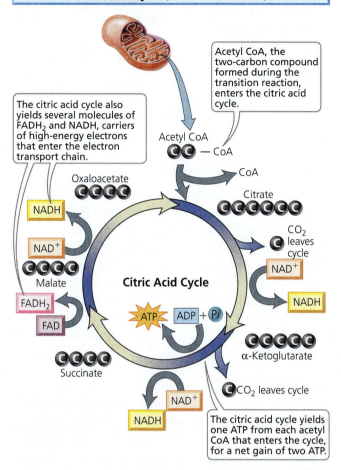

FIGURE 12-64 The citric acid cycle is a series of reactions that yields two molecules of ATP and several molecules of NADH and FADH$_2$ and releases carbon dioxide as waste.

(Goodenough, Judith and Betty A. McGuire, Biology of Humans: Concepts, Applications, and Issues, *3rd Edition, © 2010. Reprinted by permission of Pearson Education, Inc., Upper Saddle River, NJ.)*

Electron Transport Chain (inner membrane of mitochondrion)

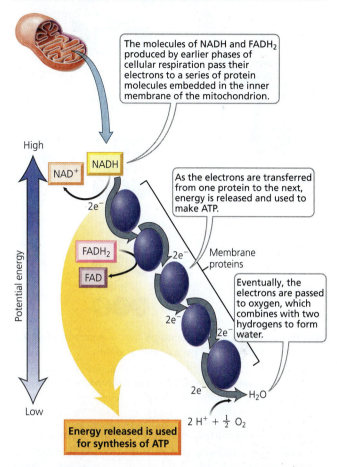

FIGURE 12-65 The electron transport chain is the final phase of cellular respiration. This phase releases up to 32 molecules of ATP per molecule of glucose.

(Goodenough, Judith and Betty A. McGuire, Biology of Humans: Concepts, Applications, and Issues, *3rd Edition, © 2010. Reprinted by permission of Pearson Education, Inc., Upper Saddle River, NJ.)*

Clinical Note

Hydrogen cyanide gas and cyanide salts are among the most rapidly acting of all known poisons. Even small concentrations are extremely hazardous. Cyanide is a byproduct of the combustion of burning rubber and plastic and is often found in smoke from fires. Cyanide binds to the iron in the enzyme of the fourth complex in the electron transport chain (cytochrome oxidase). This deactivates the enzyme, thereby preventing the final transport of electrons from cytochrome oxidase to oxygen. Thus, the electron transport chain is disrupted, and the cell can no longer produce ATP aerobically for energy. Recent research has shown that carbon monoxide (CO) acts on cytochrome oxidase in a similar fashion, but to a lesser degree.

The signs and symptoms of cyanide intoxication are dose dependent. Low to intermediate levels of exposure produce vague and nonspecific symptoms such as headache, vertigo, nausea, and vomiting. Higher levels of exposure can result in altered mental status, seizures, and increased respirations. Very high levels of exposure result in an abrupt loss of consciousness, respiratory depression, and cardiac arrest.

An antidote, called hydroxocobalamin, is effective in the treatment of cyanide poisoning if given early enough. Hydroxocobalamin is a precursor to cyanocobalamin (vitamin B$_{12}$). When administered, it removes the cyanide molecule, the cytochrome oxidase (forming harmless vitamin B$_{12}$), thus allowing the cell to resume normal metabolic processes.

Pyruvate is converted by an enzyme called lactate dehydrogenase (LDH) into the waste product known as lactate or lactic acid (lactate is the anion of lactic acid). During periods of extreme stress or exercise, oxygen levels in muscle tissue become low. In this case, muscle tissues may use lactic acid fermentation to generate ATP (Figure 12-66).

FIGURE 12-66 Lactic acid fermentation does not require oxygen and yields two molecules of ATP per molecule of glucose.

(Goodenough, Judith and Betty A. McGuire, Biology of Humans: Concepts, Applications, and Issues, 3rd Edition, © 2010. Reprinted by permission of Pearson Education, Inc., Upper Saddle River, NJ.)

Alcohol fermentation is more complex. In alcohol fermentation, a molecule of carbon dioxide is removed from pyruvate, leaving a two-carbon molecule called acetaldehyde. With alcohol fermentation, electrons are not passed to pyruvate. Instead, NADH passes electrons to acetaldehyde, forming ethanol (ethyl alcohol).

Cellular Response to Stress

The cell normally functions within a stable environment. It can react to changes in its environment through homeostasis, the tendency of the body to initiate whatever processes are necessary to restore stability when it is disrupted. Severe stresses and pathological conditions may require the cell itself to change. Such physiologic and structural changes to the cell, in response to change or stress, are referred to as **cellular adaptation**.

Cellular Adaptation

There are several possible cellular responses to an increase in stress. Some cellular responses can come in the form of normal growth, whereas others involve abnormal changes in size or function. There are two types of normal-growth responses to cellular stress: an increase in the number of cells (hyperplasia) and an increase in the size of the cells (hypertrophy). Other types of responses to stress may involve a decrease in the size and function of the cell (atrophy) or a change from one cell type to another (metaplasia) (Figure 12-67).

Hyperplasia

An increase in the number of cells in a tissue or organ is termed **hyperplasia**. This usually results in the tissue or organ in question increasing in size. Hyperplasia can be divided into two functional categories: hormonal hyperplasia and compensatory hyperplasia. Hormonal hyperplasia results from stimulation by hormones. Examples of hormonal hyperplasia are the development of the breasts during puberty and enlargement of the breasts during pregnancy. Compensatory hyperplasia is an increase in tissue mass following tissue injury or loss. An example of compensatory hyperplasia is regeneration of the liver following partial hepatic lobectomy.

Sometimes hyperplasia is pathological. That is, if the hyperplasia is not compensatory and is not due to hormonal stimulation (or does not revert to normal after hormonal stimulation is removed), the process may be pathological and a possible precursor of cancer.

Hypertrophy

An increase in the size of cells in a tissue or organ is referred to as **hypertrophy**. Hypertrophy is not due to the cells swelling. Instead, it is due to the creation of more structural components (i.e., organelles) within the cell. An organ that is hypertrophied does not contain

Cellular Adaptation

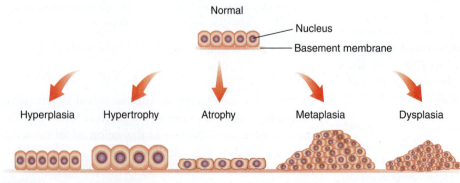

FIGURE 12-67 Abnormal cell responses to stress include hypertrophy, hyperplasia, atrophy, metaplasia, and dysplasia.

more cells (as would be the case with hyperplasia). Instead, the cells that are present have simply enlarged. If the cell is capable of dividing in response to stress, both hyperplasia and hypertrophy may develop. Some cells, such as cardiac muscle cells, do not divide but simply hypertrophy in response to stress.

Hypertrophy can be classified as physiologic or pathological. Physiologic hypertrophy usually results from increased physical demand. For example, say a person begins a vigorous exercise program. Because the cells of the heart cannot increase in number, the cells that are there increase in size to handle the added demand. Enlargement of the uterus during pregnancy is due to both physiologic hypertrophy and hormonal hyperplasia. The uterus returns to normal once the stress of pregnancy and the hormonal influence are removed.

Pathological hypertrophy results from abnormal stress, in contrast to physiologic hypertrophy, which is associated with pregnancy or exercise. There is an observable difference in the two types of cardiac hypertrophy. With physiologic hypertrophy, the cardiac septum (vertical wall between halves of the heart) enlarges and so do the sizes of the cardiac chambers. With pathological hypertrophy, the septum thickens while the chambers decrease in size.

Atrophy

A decrease in the size of a cell is termed **atrophy**. Atrophy can result from several factors, including a decreased workload, decreased blood supply, loss of nervous control, inadequate nutritional intake, lack of endocrine stimulation, and aging. As with hypertrophy, atrophy may be either physiologic or pathological. For example, during the reproductive years, the vagina is soft and well lubricated. This is principally due to the effect of hormones (primarily estrogen), an excellent blood supply, and periodic use. As a woman ages, the vagina atrophies. The tissues of the vagina become thin and friable, and the overall size decreases. This is due primarily to a combination of the loss of hormonal stimulation, aging, and decreased use. Some of the effects of vaginal atrophy can be delayed through the use of hormonal therapy (topical and oral estrogen). Vaginal atrophy with aging is an example of physiologic atrophy.

Pathological atrophy is a result of disease or injury. For example, a person who has sustained a spinal cord injury will eventually develop atrophy in the muscles affected by the injury. This results from a combination of the loss of nervous control, a decreased workload, and, in some instances, a change in blood supply.

Metaplasia

In certain situations, a cell can change from one adult cell type to another adult cell type. This process is called **metaplasia** and is reversible. Metaplasia is an adaptive response

that serves to protect the organism from stress. For example, portions of the respiratory tract are lined with columnar epithelial cells. These cells contain cilia that help to move mucus and foreign materials up the airway to the pharynx, from which they can be swallowed or expelled by sneezing or coughing. This action serves to protect the airway. With exposure to a chronic irritant, such as cigarette smoke, the ciliated columnar epithelial cells can transition to stratified squamous epithelial cells, thereby replacing delicate cells with hardier ones better able to withstand the irritant. When this occurs, the benefits of ciliary motion are lost.

By itself, metaplasia is not harmful and does not lead to cancer. When the irritant is removed (e.g., the person stops smoking), the cells return to their normal state as ciliated columnar epithelial cells. However, when the irritant continues to be present, the metaplastic cells may eventually become cancerous. Thus, although metaplasia can be beneficial and protective for the organism, the precursors that cause metaplasia, if not corrected, can induce malignant cell transformation.

Cell Injury and Cell Death

When cells are stressed to the point at which that they can no longer adapt, or when they are exposed to toxic agents, cell injury can result. If cell injury is persistent or severe, cell death may ultimately occur.

Cell injury may be classified as reversible or irreversible. If the cell injury is irreversible, cell death will occur. Irreversibly damaged cells will undergo either necrosis or apoptosis. If there is damage to the plasma membranes of the cell, enzymes released from the lysosomes will digest the contents of the cell, resulting in cellular **necrosis**, or cell death caused by outside forces such as infection that attack the cell membrane. Necrosis is sometimes called "cell murder."

However, cell death occurs as a normal process of keeping the body healthy by sloughing off old or damaged cells and making room for new, healthy cells. This preprogrammed form of cell death occurs normally and is called **apoptosis**. To distinguish it from necrosis, apoptosis is sometimes called "cell suicide." In apoptosis, if toxic substances damage the DNA of the cell, the nucleus will dissolve, yet the membranes of the cell will remain intact. Necrosis is always a pathological process, whereas apoptosis is normally physiologic but may also have a pathological cause.

Numerous factors can cause cell injury and, possibly, cell death. These include hypoxia, physical

> **CONTENT REVIEW**
> ➤ Cellular Injury
> • Ischemic and hypoxic injury
> • Oxidative stress
> • Chemical injury
> • Apoptosis
> • Dysplasia

agents, chemical agents, infection, immune reactions, genetic problems, and problems with nutrition. In some cases, a single agent is all that is involved. In most cases, cell death has a combination of causes. Overall, the way the cell responds to injury depends on the type of injury, the duration of injury, and the severity of the injury. The response also depends on the cell type, current state of the cell, and the cell's ability to adapt to the injury.

Ischemic and Hypoxic Injury

The most common type of cellular injury is that due to ischemia and hypoxia. **Ischemia** results from diminished blood flow, whereas **hypoxia** is due to a decreased availability of oxygen. When cells face ischemia or hypoxia, cellular respiration is usually impaired, and energy production is usually limited to glycolysis. The beneficial effects of glycolysis stop after all the pyruvate stores have been depleted, ATP is unavailable for the first step, or metabolic products that would normally be removed begin to accumulate. Because of this, ischemia tends to injure cells and tissues faster than does hypoxia (Figure 12-68).

The extent of injury resulting from ischemia depends on several factors. First, up to a certain point, cellular injury from ischemia is reversible if the cell has not been significantly damaged before blood flow is restored. However, if the damage is not reversed, the cell eventually reaches a point of no return at which cellular damage is so massive that the cell cannot overcome it and survive. With ischemic cell injury, the oxygen concentration of the blood falls. Because oxygen is the ultimate electron acceptor, this stops the action of the electron transport chain and that, in turn, stops the citric acid cycle. This causes a markedly decreased supply of ATP. The lack of ATP causes failure of the sodium–potassium pump. This allows sodium to diffuse into the cell and potassium to diffuse out. Because water follows sodium readily across the plasma membrane, the cell will begin to swell until it lyses (splits open), causing cell death.

Oxidative Stress

Even when the blood supply and oxygen are restored to cells previously inadequately perfused, these cells still may die. Generally, cells that are reversibly injured may survive, whereas those that are irreversibly injured will not.

However, some cells that are reversibly injured will die even after blood flow resumes—either by necrosis or by apoptosis. With the introduction of reperfusion, some tissues that were reversibly damaged may become irreversibly damaged. This can be the result of new damage from oxygen free radicals, increased permeability of the mitochondria, and inflammation.

Oxygen free radicals (oxygen atoms with unpaired electrons in the outer shell) steal electrons from other compounds and generate new species of free radicals. This process can continue until the components of the cell are used up. Increased mitochondrial permeability results in the entry of macromolecules into the mitochondria, resulting in mitochondrial swelling and rupture and eventually leading to cell death. The infiltration of cells of the immune system, in the process of inflammation, also can cause secondary ischemic injury and cell death.

Chemical Injury

Various chemicals, including drugs, can cause injury to a cell. This occurs through two mechanisms: direct action on cells or through the creation of chemical precursors that are converted to a **cytotoxic** metabolite. (*Cytotoxic* means "poisonous to cells.") Numerous toxins are capable of cellular injury. In addition, some substances used routinely in medicine, such as acetaminophen, can cause cellular toxicity (mainly to the liver) if an overdose occurs.

Apoptosis

Apoptosis occurs when a cellular program is activated that causes the release of enzymes that destroy the

Area of infarct

FIGURE 12-68 Prolonged ischemia resulting from reduced flow of arterial blood to the heart muscle is the chief cause of myocardial infarction (death of heart muscle).

Apoptosis

Cell shrinkage

Cell disintegration

Apoptotic body

Phagocytic cell

FIGURE 12-69 The process of apoptosis. Once the cell is dead, fragments called apoptotic bodies are cleared by scavenger cells (phagocytosis).

genetic material within the nucleus of the cell and selected proteins in the cytoplasm. Fragments of the dead cell (apoptotic bodies) are then cleared by scavenger cells before the toxic contents leak out and cause inflammation (Figure 12-69).

Apoptosis can be physiologic or pathological. Causes of physiologic apoptosis include the programmed destruction of the cell just described, involution of the cell following removal of a hormonal stimulus, normal cell deletion in areas where there is a proliferating cell population, cells that have served their purpose, elimination of cells that are potentially harmful to the organism, and through a defensive mechanism in which cytotoxic cells of the immune system cause the cell death.

Pathological apoptosis results from cell death secondary to cell injury, cell death from viral infections, cell death from atrophy after destruction or blockage of a duct, and cell death in tumors. Even in cells that die by necrosis, there may be a component of apoptosis present to help minimize the possibility of an inflammatory response.

Dysplasia

Abnormal or disordered growth in a cell is referred to as **dysplasia**. Dysplasia is more common in cells that reproduce rapidly, such as epithelial cells, and is often a precursor to the development of cancer. With dysplasia, there is a loss in the uniformity of the cells present, as well as in their architectural orientation. In addition, the nucleus of dysplastic cells tends to be abnormally large and abnormally dense. When an entire cell layer contains dysplastic cells, it is considered to be a preinvasive neoplasm and is referred to as *carcinoma in situ.* Although dysplasia is often associated with cancer, it does not necessarily progress to cancer.

Clinical Note

Cervical dysplasia is the presence of abnormal, precancerous cells on the surface of the cervix or its canal (Figure 12-70). Cervical cells are epithelial cells that turn over fairly rapidly and thus grow rapidly. The interior of the cervix consists of columnar epithelial cells, whereas the outer part of the cervix consists of squamous epithelial cells. The demarcation between these two cell types is called the *squamocolumnar junction.* Distal to the squamocolumnar junction is an area of

Cervical Dysplasia

Normal cervix

Normal cervical cells

Cervical dysplasia

Cancerous or pre-cancerous cells

FIGURE 12-70 Cervical dysplasia is the presence of abnormal, precancerous cells on the surface of the cervix or its canal.

immature squamous metaplastic epithelial cells. Trauma, chronic irritation, and cervical infections play a role in the development and maturation of the squamous epithelium of the cervix. The squamocolumnar junction is the point at which cervical dysplasia often arises and should be monitored yearly through a sampling called a Pap smear (more frequently if there is a history of cervical dysplasia).

It has been established that there is a relationship between the human papillomavirus (HPV) and cervical dysplasia and cancer. In fact, more than 90 percent of women with cervical cancer carry HPV. HPV is the virus that causes genital warts and is quite common, affecting more than 24 million Americans. The warts are sometimes hard to detect, as they can be skin colored or occur only in the vagina.

The risk of cervical dysplasia is increased in women who have multiple sex partners, who had unprotected sex at a young age (under 18) or with partners who have had multiple partners, who have a history of sexually transmitted diseases, or who smoke cigarettes.

Cervical dysplasia, carcinoma *in situ*, and cervical cancer can be successfully treated if detected early enough. A vaccine is now available that can protect women against HPV infection, which helps to mitigate the chances of cervical cancer.

PART 4: Disease at the Tissue Level

Tissues

A group of cells that serve a common purpose is called a **tissue**. There are four general categories of tissue: epithelial, connective, muscle, and nervous. The study of tissues is called **histology**. The study of abnormal or diseased tissue is called **histopathology**.

In this section we describe the types of tissue as they apply to emergency care. In addition, we discuss the development of cancerous tissues and factors that contribute to the process.

Origin of Body Tissues

All the tissues of the body are derived from three distinct cell lines seen during early embryonic development. About two weeks after conception, the cells of the embryo start to differentiate into three layers (Figure 12-71). These cell layers are referred to as **germ layers** and consist of primitive cell types that differentiate into the various

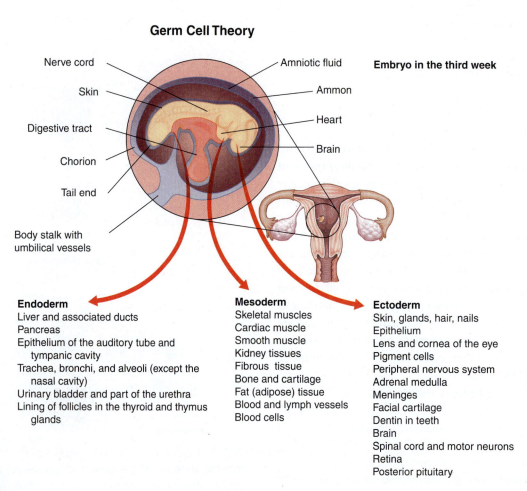

Germ Cell Theory

Nerve cord
Skin
Digestive tract
Chorion
Tail end
Body stalk with umbilical vessels

Amniotic fluid
Ammon
Heart
Brain

Embryo in the third week

Endoderm
Liver and associated ducts
Pancreas
Epithelium of the auditory tube and tympanic cavity
Trachea, bronchi, and alveoli (except the nasal cavity)
Urinary bladder and part of the urethra
Lining of follicles in the thyroid and thymus glands

Mesoderm
Skeletal muscles
Cardiac muscle
Smooth muscle
Kidney tissues
Fibrous tissue
Bone and cartilage
Fat (adipose) tissue
Blood and lymph vessels
Blood cells

Ectoderm
Skin, glands, hair, nails
Epithelium
Lens and cornea of the eye
Pigment cells
Peripheral nervous system
Adrenal medulla
Meninges
Facial cartilage
Dentin in teeth
Brain
Spinal cord and motor neurons
Retina
Posterior pituitary

FIGURE 12-71 Embryonic germ layers: endoderm, mesoderm, and ectoderm.

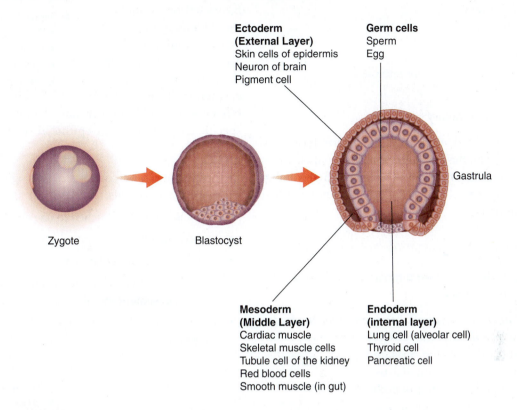

Germ Cell Differentiation

**Ectoderm
(External Layer)**
Skin cells of epidermis
Neuron of brain
Pigment cell

Germ cells
Sperm
Egg

Gastrula

Zygote

Blastocyst

**Mesoderm
(Middle Layer)**
Cardiac muscle
Skeletal muscle cells
Tubule cell of the kidney
Red blood cells
Smooth muscle (in gut)

**Endoderm
(internal layer)**
Lung cell (alveolar cell)
Thyroid cell
Pancreatic cell

FIGURE 12-72 The germ layers give rise to the various differentiated tissues of the body.

tissues and organs of the body. There are three germ layers (Figure 12-72):

- *Endoderm.* The **endoderm** is the innermost germ cell layer and gives rise to epithelial tissue, most of which is glandular epithelium. The endoderm is the first germ layer to develop. Cells from the endoderm eventually form the entire epithelial lining of the digestive tract with the exception of a portion of the mouth and a portion of the rectum. In addition to the digestive tract, the endoderm gives rise to the epithelial cells that line all the exocrine glands and structures that open into the digestive tract. These include:
  - Liver and associated ducts
  - Pancreas
  - Epithelium of the auditory tube and tympanic cavity
  - Trachea, bronchi, and alveoli (except the nasal cavity)
  - Urinary bladder and part of the urethra
  - Lining of follicles in the thyroid and thymus glands
- *Mesoderm.* The middle germ layer, or **mesoderm**, gives rise to numerous body tissues. These include:
  - Skeletal muscle
  - Cardiac muscle

- Smooth muscle
- Kidney tissue
- Fibrous tissue
- Bone and cartilage
- Fat (adipose) tissue
- Blood and lymph vessels
- Blood cells

- *Ectoderm.* The **ectoderm** is the outermost germ layer and gives rise to all the tissues that cover the body surfaces as well as the nervous system. The ectoderm has three parts, each resulting in different tissues:
  - External ectoderm
    - Skin (along with glands, hair, nails)
    - Epithelium of the mouth and nasal cavity
    - Lens and cornea of the eye
  - Neural crest
    - Melanocytes (cells that produce melanin, or pigment)
    - Peripheral nervous system
    - Adrenal medulla
    - Meninges

- Facial cartilage
- Dentin (in teeth)
- Neural tube
  - Brain
  - Spinal cord and motor neurons
  - Retina
  - Posterior pituitary

Epithelium is derived from all three germ layers. In summary, cells from the endoderm form the epithelial lining inside viscera, cells from the mesoderm form the lining outside viscera, and cells from the ectoderm become the epithelium in skin.

Tissue Types

The germ layers just described ultimately differentiate into four primary tissue types:

- *Epithelial tissue.* **Epithelial tissues** cover the body surfaces. In addition, they line all passageways that communicate with the outside. Distribution of the epithelial tissues includes the interior of body cavities, the lining of organs and blood vessels, the outer layers of skin, and others.

- *Connective tissue.* **Connective tissues** provide a framework on which epithelial tissue rests and within which nerve tissue and muscle tissue are embedded. Blood vessels and nerves travel through connective tissue. Connective tissue not only functions as a mechanical support for other tissues but also provides an avenue for communication and transport among other tissues. Connective tissues play a major role in protecting the body through immunity and inflammation.

- *Muscle tissue.* **Muscle tissues** are responsible for the movement of the organism and for movement of substances through the organism.

- *Nervous tissue.* **Nerve tissues** coordinate the activities of the body. They are capable of conducting electrical impulses from one region of the body to another. Most nervous tissue is found within the brain and the spinal cord.

Epithelial Tissue

Epithelial tissue includes the *epithelia* (plural of *epithelium*) and the glands associated with the epithelia (Figure 12-73). The epithelium forms a barrier between the organism and the environment. The specific characteristics of epithelial tissues include the following:

- Epithelial tissue covers surfaces with an uninterrupted layer of cells.
- Epithelial cells are attached to one another.
- Intercellular spaces in epithelia are small.
- Epithelial cells are polarized.
- Epithelial cells are separated from the underlying tissue by a **basement membrane**.
- There is an absence of blood vessels within epithelial tissue.

CONTENT REVIEW
➤ Tissue Types
- Epithelial tissue
- Connective tissue
- Muscle tissue
- Nervous tissue

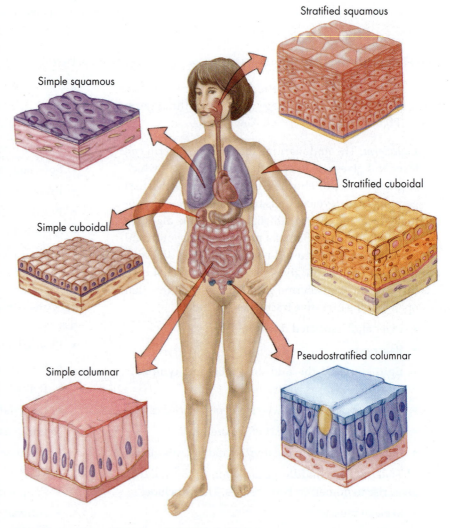

FIGURE 12-73 Types and locations of epithelial tissue.

Epithelial tissue covers both external and internal body surfaces and lines any passageways that communicate with the outside. The functions of epithelial tissue are either protective or metabolic in nature. Specifically, they include the following:

- *Provides physical protection.* Epithelial tissue efficiently protects both the external and internal surfaces from injury, infection, and water loss.

- *Controls permeability.* Epithelial tissue is a selective barrier in that it allows the passage of certain substances, such as proteins, but is impermeable to other substances.

- *Provides special senses.* Specialized epithelial cells provide information to the nervous system regarding changes in the environment.

- *Produces specialized secretions.* Some types of epithelial tissue contain glands that produce secretions. These secretions are classified by the mode of secretion: exocrine or endocrine. **Exocrine secretions** are deposited on the surface of the skin or another epithelial surface through ducts. There are three types of exocrine secretions:

  - *Serous*—watery secretions that contain enzymes (e.g., digestive secretions)

  - *Mucous*—thick, slippery secretions (e.g., nasal mucus)

  - *Mixed*—contains secretions from more than one type of cell (e.g., salivary glands)

  Endocrine secretions are released into the bloodstream or surrounding tissues and occur without the aid of ducts.

CLASSES OF EPITHELIUM   As epithelial tissue arises from embryonic germ layers, it becomes differentiated and specialized. Each type of epithelium has a special purpose in the organism. Epithelial tissues are usually classified according to the number of cell layers present and the shape of the exposed cells.

Epithelial tissues can be classified as *simple epithelium* or *stratified epithelium*. Simple epithelium is a single cell layer thick and provides limited protection. Thus, it is found primarily in internal body surfaces. Stratified epithelium is several layers thick and provides a greater degree of protection.

The shape of the cell is also used to describe and classify epithelial tissues. Tissues with thin and flat cells are called *squamous epithelium*. Cells that have a cubelike or square shape are called *cuboidal epithelium*. Finally, cells that are tall and more slender are called *columnar epithelium*.

Using this classification system there are several types of epithelial tissue, each with a different appearance and function. These include (Table 12-10):

- *Simple squamous epithelia*—found in areas where absorption occurs or when friction reduction is necessary, such as the renal tubules, the alveoli, the lining of body cavities, the lining of blood vessels, and the lining of the heart.

- *Simple cuboidal epithelia*—found in areas where secretion or absorption is occurring. Simple cuboidal epithelium secretes enzymes and buffers in the pancreas and salivary glands and lines the ducts of these glands. It is also found in portions of the kidney tubules.

- *Simple columnar epithelia*—found in areas where secretion and absorption occur but where additional protection is needed, such as the lining of the stomach and digestive tract as well as in many excretory ducts.

- *Pseudostratified epithelia*—found in areas where there is a mixture of cell types. Pseudostratified epithelium is not really stratified, although it appears to be. In pseudostratified epithelia, all cells are in contact with the basement membrane. This tissue type will often have cilia. It is found in the respiratory tract (nasal cavity, trachea, bronchi) and portions of the male reproductive tract.

Table 12-10 Types of Epithelial Tissue

Shape	Number of Layers	Example Locations	Functions
Squamous (flat, scale-like cells)	Simple (single layer)	Linings of heart and blood vessels; air sacs of lungs	Allows passage of materials by diffusion
	Striated (multilayers)	Linings of mouth, esophagus, vagina; outer layer of skin	Protects underlying areas
Cuboidal (cube-shaped cells)	Simple	Kidney tubules; secretary portions of glands and ducts	Secretion; absorption
	Striated	Ducts of sweat glands, mammary glands, salivary glands	Protects underlying areas
Columnar	Simple	Most of digestive tract; bronchi; excretory ducts of some glands; uterus	Absorbs; secretes mucus, enzymes, and other substances
	Striated	Rare: urethra; junction of esophagus and stomach	Protects underlying areas; secretes mucus

Exocrine Secretions

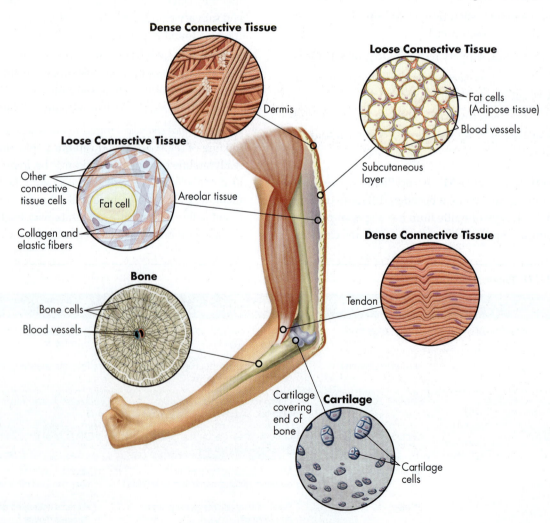

Merocrine   Apocrine   Holocrine

Multicellular exocrine gland	Method of Secretion	Examples
1. Merocrine	Watery serous fluid or mucus secreted through the cell membrane.	• salivary glands • pancreatic glands • some sweat glands
2. Apocrine	The part of the cell containing the secretion "pinches" off and then releases its contents.	• some sweat glands • mammary glands
3. Holocrine	Cells fill up with secretion and then burst, releasing their product.	• sebaceous glands

FIGURE 12-74 Multicellular exocrine glands and their methods of secretion.

- *Transitional epithelia*—found in areas where there is a need for protection and where there are significant changes in volume that can give rise to changes in physical factors such as pressure. Transitional cells are found in the ureters and urinary bladder.

- *Stratified squamous epithelia*—found in areas where mechanical stresses are severe. These include the surface of the skin and the lining of the mouth, tongue, esophagus, vagina, and anus.

- *Glandular epithelia*—selected types of epithelia produce exocrine secretions. These are secreted by one of three methods (Figure 12-74):

  - *Merocrine secretion*—the secretion is released through exocytosis (the most common method).

  - *Apocrine secretion*—the part of the cell containing the secretion "pinches" off and then releases the secretion.

  - *Holocrine secretion*—the entire cell is packed with secretions and then bursts apart and dies in the process.

Connective Tissue

Connective tissues are deep tissues that are never exposed to the external environment (Figure 12-75). They bind

FIGURE 12-75 Types and locations of connective tissues.

together and support the tissues of the body. Unlike epithelial tissue, which consists primarily of cells, connective tissue consists primarily of a substance called the *extracellular matrix*. Specific characteristics of connective tissue include the following:

- Connective tissue consists of individual cells scattered within an extracellular matrix consisting of protein fiber and a noncellular material called *ground substance*. There are three types of protein fibers:

  - *Collagen fibers*—are strong and have great tensile strength such as seen in ligaments and tendons.

  - *Elastic fibers*—are randomly coiled and thus capable of stretch. They are common in the skin, lungs, and blood vessels.

  - *Reticular fibers*—are thin strands of **collagen** that form interconnective networks that help support other tissues.

  Ground substance can be solid (as in bone), liquid (as in blood), or flexible (as in cartilage). In ordinary connective tissue, the ground substance consists of water stabilized by proteins and glycoproteins. In bone, the ground substance includes minerals. In blood, the ground substance is liquid (plasma).

- Cells of connective tissue are not directly attached to one another (unlike epithelial cells).

- Individual connective tissue cells are normally separated from one another by varying amounts of extracellular matrix.

- Connective tissue is derived from the embryonic mesoderm (unlike most epithelial tissue, which is derived from ectoderm and endoderm).

There are several cell types found in connective tissues. These include:

- *Fibroblasts.* **Fibroblasts** are the most abundant cell type found in connective tissue and are responsible for the production of connective tissue fibers and ground substance.

- *Macrophages.* **Macrophages** are scattered throughout the connective tissues and engulf damaged cells or pathogens.

- *Adipocytes.* **Adipocytes**, or fat cells, contain large amounts of lipids and serve as energy stores.

- *Mast cells.* **Mast cells** are small mobile cells that are found in the connective tissues—often near blood vessels. They release chemicals as part of the body's defense system.

- *Other cells.* Occasionally other cells can be found in connective tissue such as white blood cells reacting to injury or infection.

CLASSES OF CONNECTIVE TISSUE Connective tissue is classified by the physical properties of the ground substance. It is often classified as connective tissue proper and specialized connective tissue.

Connective tissue proper includes (Table 12-11):

- *Loose connective tissue.* Loose connective tissue, also called *areolar tissue*, contains more cells and fewer fibers than dense connective tissue. Loose connective tissue forms the layer that separates the skin from underlying muscle.

  - *Adipose tissue.* **Adipose tissue**, or fat, is a form of loose connective tissue that contains a large number of fat cells (adipocytes).

Table 12-11 Types of Connective Tissue

Type	Example Locations	Functions
Connective Tissue Proper		
Loose, areolar	Between muscles, surround glands, wrapping small blood vessels and nerves	Wraps and cushions organs
Loose, adipose (fat)	Under skin, around kidneys and heart	Stores energy, insulates, cushions organs
Dense	Tendons, ligaments	Attaches bone to bone (ligaments) or bone to muscle (tendons)
Specialized Connective Tissue		
Cartilage (semisolid)	Nose (tip); rings in respiratory air tubules; external ear	Provides support and protection (by enclosing) and serves as lever for muscles to act on
Bone (solid)	Skeleton	Provides support and protection (by enclosing) and levers for muscles to act on
Blood (fluid)	Within blood vessels	Transports oxygen and carbon dioxide, nutrients, hormones, and wastes; helps fight infections

- *Dense connective tissue.* Dense connective tissue, also called *fibrous tissue*, consist mainly of collagen fibers. They include:

  - *Cartilage.* **Cartilage** provides a cushion between bones and helps maintain the structure of certain body parts (ear, nose). Cartilage contains specialized cells called *chondrocytes* that reside in pockets of cells in the matrix called *lacunae*. These are suspended in a firm gel extracellular matrix that contains protein fibers for strength and ground substance for resilience. Cartilage does not contain blood vessels, so the tissue obtains nutrients and removes wastes through diffusion. There are three types of cartilage:

    - *Hyaline*—found at the end of long bones and provides support, flexibility, and reduces friction. It is the most abundant form of cartilage.

    - *Elastic*—more flexible than hyaline cartilage, elastic cartilage is found in the pinna of the ear.

    - *Fibrocartilage*—forms the outer part of the intervertebral disks that cushion the vertebral bodies. Fibrocartilage is also found between the bones of the pelvis and in selected joints. It contains fewer cells than hyaline or elastic cartilage.

  - *Bone.* Bone provides protection and support for the organism. Bone contains specialized cells called **osteocytes**, situated in lacunae. Bone, along with cartilage and joints, makes up the bulk of the skeletal system. The matrix in bones contains calcium that gives the bones strength.

  - *Ligaments.* Ligaments hold bone together and contain both elastic and collagen fibers.

  - *Tendons.* Tendons connect muscle to bone and allow for movement of the organism. Collagen fibers run the length of tendons giving them strength.

Specialized connective tissues include:

- *Blood.* Blood is a collection of cells in a liquid matrix. The proteins in blood, under normal conditions, do not form fibers. Approximately half of the cells in blood are red blood cells. The remaining cells are white blood cells and platelets.

- *Lymph.* Lymph is the fluid within the lymphatic system. The lymphatic system is a network of organs, lymph nodes, lymph ducts, and lymph vessels that produce and transport lymph from tissues to the bloodstream. The lymphatic system is a major component of the body's immune system.

Muscle Tissue

Muscle tissues are specialized for contraction. They contain muscle cells that contract when stimulated. This allows for movement of the organism and for movement of substances through the organism. There are three types of muscle tissue (Figure 12-76 and Table 12-12):

FIGURE 12-76 Diagram and chart of the three muscle tissue types.

Table 12-12 Types of Muscle Tissue

Type	Description	Example Locations	Functions
Skeletal	Long, cylindrical cells; multiple nuclei per cell; obvious striations	Muscles attached to bones	Provides voluntary movement
Cardiac	Branching, striated cells; one nucleus; specialized junctions between cells	Wall of heart	Contracts and propels blood through the circulatory system
Smooth	Cells taper at each end; single nucleus; arranged in sheets; no striations	Walls of digestive system, blood vessels, and tubules of urinary system	Propels substances or objects through internal passageways

- *Skeletal muscle.* Skeletal muscle is usually attached to bones—hence the name. When skeletal muscle contracts, bones are moved. Skeletal muscles are under voluntary control. Skeletal muscle contains striations (alternating dark and light bands) that give them a characteristic appearance under the microscope.

- *Smooth muscle.* Smooth muscle does not contain the striations seen in skeletal muscle—hence the name. Smooth muscle is under involuntary control and found in internal organs such as the digestive system, blood vessels, and bladder. Smooth muscle plays a major role in moving food through the digestive tract and removing waste. It is also important in the control of blood pressure and perfusion.

- *Cardiac muscle.* Cardiac muscle is found only in the heart and contains striations. Cardiac muscle cells are tightly connected to other cardiac muscle cells by special junctions at the plasma membranes called *intercalated discs*. These discs allow the rapid transmission of electrical impulses from one cell to another. Cardiac muscle cells are almost totally dependent on aerobic metabolism to obtain the energy needed to continue contracting. Because of this, cardiac muscle cells contain large numbers of mitochondria and abundant reserves of oxygen stores in myoglobin. Energy reserves are maintained in the form of glycogen and lipid inclusions.

Nervous Tissue

The last type of tissue is nervous tissue, is found in the brain, spinal cord, and peripheral nerves. Approximately 98 percent of nervous tissue is located in the brain and spinal cord. Nervous tissue conducts electrical impulses from one part of the body to another and controls numerous body functions.

There are two types of cells found in nervous tissue: **neurons** and **neuroglia**. Neurons are responsible for transmitting electrical impulses (Figure 12-77). The neuroglia, often simply called *glial cells*, support, insulate, and protect neurons (Figure 12-78).

Neoplasia

Neoplasia is an abnormal type of tissue growth where the cells grow and multiply in an uncontrolled fashion. In neoplasia, the factors that normally control cell and tissue growth are lost, resulting in a continuing increase in the number of dividing cells. This mass of uncontrolled cell growth is referred to as a **tumor**.

All cell lines go through the process of differentiation. That is, primitive nonspecialized cells called **stem cells** mature into specific cell types, depending on function. Some stem cells will mature to muscle cells, others will become connective tissue cells, and so on. Cells that have not differentiated are those that have either remained in an early stage or regressed to an early stage in a process called *anaplasia*. Neoplastic cells are often less differentiated than normal cells from the same tissue or are totally undifferentiated.

As discussed before, all cells go through differentiation and adaptation. The processes of hypertrophy, hyperplasia, atrophy, and metaplasia can all occur in response

Neuron

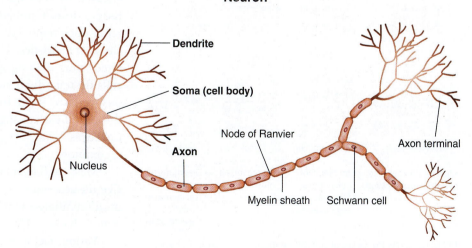

FIGURE 12-77 Neuron.

Neuroglia

Three kinds of neuroglia:
astrocyte (purple)
oligodendrocyte (blue)
microglia (green)

FIGURE 12-78 Neuroglia.

Cancer Development

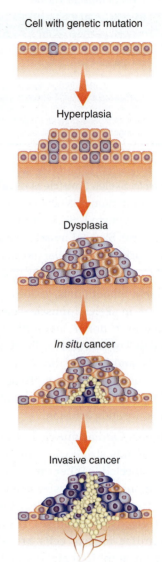

FIGURE 12-80 Abnormal cell development, progressing to invasive cancer.

to stress. However, some cells will develop abnormal growth patterns. When these cells are examined under a microscope, some of the cells may look abnormal. Such cells are called **dysplastic** or *atypical*. Most often the abnormalities are seen in the nucleus of the cell. A common example of dysplasia is abnormal cervical cells found on a Pap smear. These vary in their level of dysplasia with the highest level being considered cancerous (*carcinoma in situ*). (Figure 12-79)

Neoplasia, by definition, means "new growth." The tumors may be benign or malignant. Benign and malignant tumors have different characteristics. For example, benign neoplastic lesions are slow growing, are usually encased by cells that are adherent, do not invade local tissue, do not spread to other body areas, and do not recur once removed. Cancerous tumors have the opposite characteristics. They grow fast and are not encapsulated, thus making removal more difficult. Malignant cells do not adhere together well, thus allowing cancerous cells to shed to other areas of the body—often through the bloodstream in a process called **metastasis**. Cancer is locally invasive (Figure 12-80), and recurrence is common.

Most cancers are either of epithelial origin or connective tissue origin. Some tumors contain cells that are so undifferentiated that the cell of origin cannot be determined (Table 12-13).

Various factors have been associated with the development of cancer, termed *oncogenesis*. Among these oncogenic

Differentiation

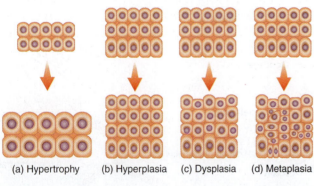

FIGURE 12-79 Processes of cell differentiation: hypertrophy, hyperplasia, dysplasia, neoplasia.

Table 12-13 Tumor Origins and Names

Origin/Prefix	Cell Type	Benign Tumor	Malignant Tumor
Epithelial			
Adeno-	Gland	Adenoma	Adenocarcinoma
Basal cell	Basal cell	Basal cell adenoma	Basal cell carcinoma
Squamous cell	Squamous cell	Keratoacanthoma	Squamous cell carcinoma
Melano-	Pigmented cell	Mole	Melanoma
Terato-	Multipotential cell	Teratoma	Teratocarcinoma
Supporting/Connective			
Chandro-	Cartilage	Chondroma	Chondrosarcoma
Fibro-	Fibroblast	Fibroma	Fibrosarcoma
Hemangio-	Blood vessel	Hemangioma	Hemangiosarcoma
Leiomyo-	Smooth muscle	Leiomyoma	Leiomyosarcoma
Lipo-	Fat	Lipoma	Liposarcoma
Meningio-	Meninges	Meningioma	Meningiosarcoma
Myo-	Muscle	Myoma	Myosarcoma
Osteo-	Bone	Osteoma	Osteosarcoma
Rhabdomyo-	Striated muscle	Rhabdomyoma	Rhabdomyosarcoma
Blood/Lymphatic			
Lympho-	Lymphocyte		Lymphoma or lymphocytic leukemia
Erythro-	Erythrocyte		Erythrocytic leukemia
Myelo-	Bone marrow		Myeloma or myelogenous leukemia

factors are carcinogens and radiation (Figure 12-81). Carcinogens are chemicals capable of causing cancer. Radiation is also capable of causing cancer—most often tumors of the skin and internal organs, and leukemia. Radiation can result from several sources and damages the genetic material in the cell, possibly resulting in a mutation. Some mutations repair themselves, others remain but do not cause adverse effects, and yet others result in the development of cancer. Whereas carcinogens and radiation have been proven to cause cancer, several other factors remain highly suspect. These include such possible causes of cancer as viruses, genetics, environmental factors, hormones, and perhaps chronic infection or irritation.

Viruses that produce cancers are called *oncogenic viruses*. That is, genetic material within the virus (either RNA or DNA), called an *oncogene*, can cause malignant transformation of host cells when they are incorporated into the host cell DNA. The link between certain viruses and cancer is fairly strong. As already noted, human papillomavirus (HPV) has been found to be a cause of cervical cancer in women. Chronic infections with hepatitis B virus

(HBV) and hepatitis C virus (HCV) have been associated with the development of hepatocellular carcinoma. Whether this results from the virus itself or the resultant infection and inflammation caused by the virus remains unclear.

Genetics is thought to be responsible for some cancers. Although the link between genetics and cancer has not been definitively made, it is clear that some families tend to develop cancers, whereas others do not. In these cases, the environment may be a confounding variable. A number of genes have been identified that play a role in the development of some cancers. Persons born with one of these genes may be more prone to cancer yet may not ultimately develop cancer.

The environment is a definite risk factor for the development of cancer. Some environmental factors have been documented to be carcinogenic. Asbestos exposure, for example, has been linked to a rare form of cancer called mesothelioma. These tumors are more common in people who have a history of significant exposures to asbestos. Bladder cancer was noted to be more common in printing press operators. The cause was later linked to a chemical

Oncogenesis

FIGURE 12-81 Oncogenesis (development of cancer).

(benzidine) in the ink. Again, in these cases there is an identified carcinogen.

Our environment is so diverse and there are so many possible carcinogens present that many have not been clearly linked to the development of cancers. Radiation is also present in the environment. For example, the incidence of thyroid cancers increased markedly in Japan after the United States dropped atomic bombs on the cities of Nagasaki and Hiroshima in 1945. When the nuclear reactor at the Chernobyl nuclear plant in Ukraine exploded in 1986, more than five million people were exposed to the resulting radiation. Subsequently, that nuclear disaster has produced the biggest group of cancers ever from a single incident, with almost 2,000 cases of thyroid cancer being documented since the reactor explosion. Consequences of the disruptions to nuclear power plants in Japan resulting from the severe earthquake and tidal wave in 2011 are yet to develop and be analyzed.

Hormones are thought to play a role in the development of certain cancers. Some tumors, especially tumors of the breast, have been found to have receptors for the female hormone estrogen. Breast cancers with estrogen receptors have increased growth while estrogen is present and decreased growth or even tumor regression when estrogen is removed. The administration of estrogen to men with prostate cancer sometimes inhibits cancer growth.

The process of developing a malignant neoplasia is called **carcinogenesis** and occurs in three stages: initiation, promotion, and progression (Figure 12-82). *Initiation* is the event that begins the transformation from normal tissue to cancer. As just discussed, the factor may be a carcinogen, radiation, or a combination of factors. Initiation does not mean that malignancy will ultimately develop, just that the process has started. For example, a carcinogen such as tar from tobacco will bind to the DNA in the susceptible cells, causing errors in replication and the subsequent formation of dysplastic daughter cells. Dysplasia can result in anaplasia.

The second phase is *promotion*. A promoter can be a carcinogen or any of the factors discussed earlier that are associated with cancer development. Promotion is necessary for the continued development of the tumor and speeds up the process. The growth rate increases because the cells divide more rapidly. During promotion, cells begin to change from dysplasia to anaplasia. However, the promotion stage is still considered precancerous.

Carcinogenesis

FIGURE 12-82 Carcinogenesis (development of a malignant neoplasia).

The last stage in carcinogenesis is *progression*. At this point, a malignancy exists and the cells are anaplastic in appearance. The more poorly differentiated and primitive the cells are in appearance, the faster will be the growth of the tumor. Progression is followed by growth and, subsequently, local tissue invasion and possible metastasis. Unfortunately, in many cases, cancer is not diagnosed until this stage of carcinogenesis.

Once cancer develops, it becomes invasive. If the affected tissue is a squamous epithelium, and the tumor has not extended past the basement membrane, it is considered carcinoma *in situ*. Cancer spreads along tissue planes and attaches to various tissues. Sometimes, individual cells or clumps of cells will be shed from the primary tumor and travel through a blood vessel or lymphatic channel to another part of the body, where they will begin to develop a secondary tumor (metastasis). The distal spread of tumor cells makes treatment difficult and often causes death.

Cancer cells are usually graded by the degree of cell differentiation present. The grade affects the prognosis (likely outcome). The grading system is as follows:

- *Grade X.* The grade cannot be assessed (undetermined grade). Prognosis: undetermined.

- *Grade 1.* The cells are well differentiated and closely resemble the cells of the tissue of origin. Few mitotic figures (cells undergoing division) are seen (low grade). Prognosis: good.

- *Grade 2.* The cells are moderately differentiated, with some structural similarity to the tissue of origin. Moderate mitotic figures are seen (intermediate grade). Prognosis: fair.

- *Grade 3.* The cells are poorly differentiated, with little resemblance to the tissue of origin. Many mitotic figures are seen (high grade). Prognosis: fair to poor.

- *Grade 4.* The cells are undifferentiated or dedifferentiated, appear bizarre and primitive, and do not resemble the tissue of origin. Many mitotic figures are seen (high grade). Prognosis: poor.

Grading is somewhat subjective. Nevertheless, the higher the grade, the more the cells are undifferentiated and the worse the prognosis.

Often, cancer is *staged* based on numerous findings, but primarily indicating the degree to which the cancer is spread. Stages 1 to 4 are usually described, with stage 1 being the least advanced state of the cancer's progression and stage 4 being the most advanced. Staging is usually based on the size of the tumor, whether lymph nodes contain cancer, and whether the cancer has spread from the original site to other parts of the body. Staging is particularly important in planning treatment strategies and in determining the prognosis.

PART 5: Disease at the Organ Level
Genetic and Other Causes of Disease

When we think of disease at the **organ** level, at the level of **organ systems**, and at the level of the total human **organism**, we are likely to think first of infections caused by pathogens, including bacteria, viruses, fungi, and parasites. In recent years, great strides have been made in the medical treatment of infectious diseases, but—as we have been discussing throughout this chapter—many diseases result from genetic causes, which have been far more difficult to identify and treat. The picture is additionally complicated by the fact that many diseases result from a combination of genetic and environmental factors (including lifestyle factors), as well as factors such as age and gender.

Even a family history of a particular disease does not necessarily mean that the disease has a purely genetic origin, because families also share environmental and lifestyle factors that may cause or contribute to the family disease. Although family history may point to the possibility of genetic causes, these cannot be confirmed, much less treated, until scientists are able to make definitive identifications of the defective genes or chromosomes that cause or contribute to particular diseases.

At present, there is increasing progress in identifying and understanding genetic and other noninfectious causes of disease. Many promising advances toward gene therapies (the replacement of defective genes with normal genes) and other therapies for diseases have been made.

Genetics, Environment, Lifestyle, Age, and Gender

As noted earlier, our inherited traits are determined by molecules of deoxyribonucleic acid, or DNA, which form structures called genes that reside on larger structures called chromosomes within the nuclei of all our cells. We inherit our genetic structure from our parents. Every one of a person's somatic cells (all the cells except the sex cells) contains 46 chromosomes. The sex cells, however, contain only 23 chromosomes each. The sex cells contribute these 23 chromosomes to the offspring. Thus, the offspring receives 23 chromosomes from the father and 23 chromosomes from the mother, resulting in a total of 46 chromosomes. Occasionally, one or more of a person's genes or chromosomes is abnormal; this may cause a congenital disease (one we are born with) or a propensity toward acquiring a disease later in life.

Some diseases are thought to be purely genetic. For example, cystic fibrosis, which affects mainly people of European origin, and sickle cell disease, which affects mainly people of African origin, are known to be caused by disorders of single genes. They affect different populations to a different degree because of the evolutionary history of those populations. A genetic disease may be caused by a single defective gene or by several defective genes or chromosomes. Single-gene causes are, obviously, easier for medical researchers to identify and potentially devise treatments for than are other, more complex genetic causes of disease.

Other diseases are caused by a combination of genetic and environmental factors and are called *multifactorial disorders.* For example, type 2 (adult-onset) diabetes has a very high correlation with family history of the disease. However, it is also affected by environmental and lifestyle factors such as a high-fat or high-carbohydrate diet and lack of exercise, which result in obesity, and with age. (There is a higher incidence of type 2 diabetes in overweight people, and the disease tends to appear in middle age or later.) Heart disease, which is highly correlated with family history and age, also has a gender/hormonal factor: Women appear to be somewhat protected from heart disease before menopause, when their bodies are still producing estrogen. Following menopause, women quickly "catch up" with men in the development of heart disease.

Clinical practitioners and epidemiologists, respectively, study disease from the point of view of their effects on individuals and from the point of view of their effects on populations as a whole.

- *Effects on individuals.* Physicians and other clinical practitioners study the effects of diseases on individuals, and find it instructive to view the development of diseases as products of the interactions among three factors: *host, agent,* and *environment.* This establishes a framework for determining how one, or a combination, of these factors may precipitate a disease state. Genetic predisposition, gender, and ethnic origin are determinants related to the host. These may interact with a specific agent, in a specific type of environment, to cause illness. The agent may be a bacterium, toxin, gunshot, or other pathophysiologic process. The environment may be defined by the local climate, socioeconomic or demographic features, culture, religion, and associated factors. Determination of how the host, agent, and environment interact may yield solutions to curing a disease process. Injury and trauma are now being viewed as "diseases," in the sense of how the interaction of host, agent, and environment may contribute to an understanding of what, heretofore, have been perceived as social problems.

- *Effects on populations.* Epidemiologists, who study the effects of diseases on populations, generally report disease data with three basic measures: *incidence, prevalence,* and *mortality. Morbidity,* a term commonly used in discussing disease statistics, can be more precisely reported as incidence and prevalence. *Incidence* is the number of new cases of the disease that are reported in a given period of time, usually 1 year. *Prevalence* is the proportion of the total population who are affected by the disease at a given point in time. (Prevalence is higher than incidence, as those who acquire the disease each year are added to those who already have the disease.) *Mortality* is the rate of death from the disease.

Epidemiologists and clinical practitioners are now collaborating to study risk factors, such as the relationship between smoking and lung cancer. Risk factor analysis is both statistical and complex. Although the correlation of smoking to lung cancer is extremely high, not everyone who smokes develops lung cancer, and not everyone who develops lung cancer has been a smoker. Risk factor analysis would compare the number of smokers to nonsmokers among lung cancer cases, the pack/year (number of packs per day × number of years) history of the smokers with lung cancer, factors that might have aggravated or mitigated the effects of smoking, and so on.

Family History and Associated Risk Factors

It is important for those who have a family history of a particular disease not to conclude that acquiring the disease is their destiny and there is nothing they can do about it. This is not always true. Most diseases with a genetic component that come on during adulthood also have associated risk factors that can be modified to prevent, delay, or reduce the impact of the disease.

Consider the variety of possible risk factors for disease: People who live in less-developed countries are often at higher risk for disease from microorganisms flourishing in their water supply and disease transmission caused by poor sanitation. Physical conditions commonly seen in larger U.S. cities as well as rural areas, such as inadequate housing, poor nutrition, and little or no medical attention, potentiate disease transmission. Chemical factors such as smoke, smog, illicit drug use, occupational chemical exposure, and additives in our food are causative agents for a variety of diseases.

Personal habit is among the most publicized—and controllable—causes of disease in our society. For example, predisposing factors for cardiovascular disease include smoking, excessive alcohol consumption, inactivity, and obesity. Unfortunately, changes in individual lifestyle often occur only after a disease has already manifested itself. As we age, the predisposing factors and causative agents take their toll. The body's ability to defend itself against disease decreases as a result of the effects of aging on our immunologic system and other compensatory mechanisms.

Following is a discussion of some of the most common diseases in which both genetics and other risk factors play a role. You will notice, as you read, that the causation of various diseases varies widely, and that although the causes are known for some diseases, the causes of other diseases are still not clearly understood.

Immunologic Disorders

A number of immunologic disorders, such as rheumatic fever, allergies, and asthma, are more prevalent among those with a family history of the disorder but also involve other risk factors.

Rheumatic fever is an inflammatory reaction to an infection but is not an infection itself. There seems to be a hereditary factor, but inadequate nutrition and crowded living conditions are contributing factors.

Allergies often have a family history factor (and some allergies can be passed from the mother to the fetus during pregnancy). However, allergic reactions are triggered by exposure to allergens and can usually be controlled by avoiding or reducing the presence of allergens, as well as with medication.

Asthma sufferers may inherit the propensity for airway-narrowing in response to various stimuli, but other triggering factors may be identified and, perhaps, controlled, including stress, overexertion, exposure to cold air, and stimuli such as pollens, dust mites, cockroach detritus, and smoke.

Cancer

A wide variety of family history and environmental factors are included among the risk factors for cancer. Some kinds of cancer, such as breast and colorectal cancer, tend to cluster in families and seem to have a combination of genetic and environmental causes. Others, such as lung cancer, are more strongly identified with environmental causes.

For *breast cancer,* the greatest risk factor is female gender. The second highest risk factor is age. Approximately two out of three women with invasive breast cancer are diagnosed after age 55. A history of breast cancer in a first-degree relative (mother, sister, or daughter) increases the risk by two or three times. Some progress has been made in identifying genes for certain breast cancers. Lifestyle factors such as lack of exercise and obesity may contribute slightly to the incidence of breast cancer, but this has not been proven.

As with breast cancer, *colorectal cancer* risk factors include age (with the incidence rising after age 40 and peaking between 60 and 75) and family history (incidence in a first-degree relative increases the risk by two or three times). There are gender factors, with rectal cancer being more common in men and colon cancer more common in women. Diet may also be a risk factor, although recent studies have failed to confirm a link between a high-fat, low-fiber diet and colorectal cancer. (However, a high-fat, low-fiber diet has been positively linked to heart disease and other health problems.)

The causes of *lung cancer* are overwhelmingly environmental. Smoking has been identified as the main cause of 90 percent of lung cancers in men and 70 percent of lung cancers in women. Lung cancer can also be caused by inhaling substances such as asbestos, arsenic, and nickel, usually in the workplace.

Endocrine Disorders

The most common endocrine disorder is *diabetes mellitus,* which is a leading cause of blindness, heart disease, kidney failure, and premature death. The causes of diabetes are complex and still not well understood.

There are two major types of diabetes: type 1 and type 2. Type 1 diabetes usually occurs before age 40, sometimes in childhood. Although it is less prevalent than type 2 diabetes (accounting for about 20 percent of diabetes cases), it is more severe. In the type 1 diabetic, the pancreas produces no or almost no insulin, which is required for the cellular utilization of glucose, the body's chief source of energy. Type 1 diabetics must take insulin daily. There is some association of type 1 diabetes with family history (siblings of type 1 diabetics have a 6 percent risk, compared with 0.3 percent in the general population), and medical researchers have pinpointed some possible genetic factors. Other causative factors may include autoimmunity disorders and viral infections that invade the pancreas and destroy the insulin-producing cells.

Type 2 diabetes accounts for about 80 percent of all diabetes cases. It usually occurs after age 40 and the incidence increases with age. It clusters much more strongly in families than does type 1 diabetes (siblings of type 2 diabetics have a 10 to 15 percent risk). In contrast to type 1 diabetes, in which there is a total lack of insulin, type 2 diabetes is associated with a decreased insulin receptor response or a decrease in insulin production. Diet and exercise may also be factors, as the majority of type 2 diabetics are obese. Type 2 diabetes can often be controlled with diet and exercise or with oral medications.

Hematologic Disorders

Hereditary coagulation disorders have been studied by geneticists and physicians in great detail. Hereditary hematologic disorders have many causes, such as gene alteration and histocompatibility (tissue interaction) dysfunctions.

Hemophilia is a bleeding disorder that is caused by a genetic clotting factor deficiency. It can be mild, but if severe, it can cause not only serious bruising but also bleeding into the joints, which can lead to crippling deformities. A slight bump on the head can cause bleeding within the skull, often resulting in brain damage and death. The heredity is sex linked (associated with the sex chromosomes), inherited through the mother, and affects male children almost exclusively. There is no cure, but administration of concentrated clotting factors can improve the condition.

Hemochromatosis is another genetic disorder, but this time it is caused by a histocompatibility complex dysfunction. It is marked by excessive absorption and accumulation of iron in the body, causing weight loss, joint pain, abdominal pain, palpitations, and testicular atrophy in males. It is treated by removing blood from the body at intervals.

Not all blood disorders are genetic. Environmental factors, for example, can cause *anemia* (reduction in circulating red blood cells). For instance, some antihypertensive medications and other drugs may cause a drug-induced hemolytic (red-blood-cell–destroying) anemia.

Cardiovascular Disorders

The cardiovascular system can be greatly affected by genetic disorders. Disorders such as *prolongation of the QT interval* (a delay between depolarization and repolarization of the ventricles as revealed in an electrocardiogram) and *mitral-valve prolapse* (an upward ballooning of the valve between the left ventricle and atrium that allows blood to regurgitate back into the atrium when the ventricle contracts) tend to cluster in families.

The American Heart Association lists heredity as a major risk factor for cardiovascular disease. Those with parents who have *coronary artery disease* (deposits on the walls of the coronary arteries that reduce blood flow to the heart muscle) have an approximately fivefold greater risk of developing the disease than those whose parents do not have it. This is why it is important to ask about family history of congenital heart disease (CHD), hypertension, and stroke when assessing patients with possible cardiovascular disease. However, environmental factors, such as a diet high in saturated fats and cholesterol (or a diet high in carbohydrates) and lack of exercise, also play a large role in cardiovascular disease.

Hypertension (high blood pressure) is a major risk factor not only for cardiac disease, but also for stroke and kidney disease. Studies of family history show that approximately 20 to 40 percent of the causation of hypertension is genetic. The remaining causative factors, then, are environmental, and may include high sodium ingestion, lack of physical activity, stress, and obesity.

Not all cardiac disorders have a genetic component. For example, *cardiomyopathy* (disease affecting the heart muscle) is thought to occur secondarily to other causes, such as infectious disease, toxin exposure, connective tissue disease, or nutritional deficiencies, which may be partially or totally environmental.

Renal Disorders

Renal (kidney) failure is caused by a variety of factors (primarily hypertension) that may eventually require a patient to receive dialysis treatment several times a week. As the location of dialysis treatment shifts from medical centers to homes and community satellite centers, EMS personnel are increasingly being called to deal with the complications of dialysis. These include problems with vascular access devices (shunts, fistulas), localized infection and sepsis, and electrolyte abnormalities (hyperkalemia), which can result in cardiac arrest.

Rheumatic Disorders

Gout is a condition that may have both genetic and environmental causes. It is characterized by severe arthritic pain caused by deposit of crystals in the joints, most commonly in the great toe. The crystals form as the result of an abnormally high level of uric acid in the blood that may be caused when the kidneys do not excrete enough uric acid or by high production of uric acid. High production of uric acid may be caused by a hereditary metabolic abnormality. Although the underlying cause may be genetic, attacks of gout can be triggered by environmental factors such as trauma, alcohol consumption, ingestion of certain foods, stress, or other illnesses. Patients with gout also have a tendency to develop *kidney stones*.

Gastrointestinal Disorders

Gastrointestinal disorders have a variety of causes, and the causes of some are not known. *Lactose intolerance*, for example, is usually identified by the inability of the patient to tolerate milk and some other dairy products. The patient lacks lactase, the enzyme that usually breaks down lactose in the digestive tract. This enzyme deficiency may be congenital (inborn) or may develop later on. It is more common in those of Asian, African, Native American, or Mediterranean ancestry than it is among northern and western Europeans.

Crohn's disease is a chronic inflammation of the wall of the digestive tract that usually affects the small intestine, the large intestine, or both. The cause is not known, but medical researchers have focused on immune system dysfunction, infection, and diet as the major probabilities. A similar disorder is ulcerative colitis, in which the large intestine becomes inflamed and develops ulcers. As with Crohn's disease, the cause is not known, but an overactive immune response is suspected, and heredity seems to play a role.

Peptic ulcers develop when the normal protective structures and mechanisms, such as mucus production, break down and areas in the lining of the stomach or duodenum are inflamed by stomach acid and digestive juices. Environmental factors, bacterial infection (by *Helicobacter pylori*), diet, stress, and alcohol consumption are thought to play roles in the development of peptic ulcers. Many medications, particularly nonsteroidal anti-inflammatory medications, are associated with ulcer formation.

Cholecystitis is an inflammation of the gallbladder that usually results from blockage by a gallstone. There may be a genetic predisposition for gallstone formation. Gallstones are more prevalent in women and in some groups such as Native Americans and Mexican Americans. Other risk factors include age, a high-fat diet, and obesity.

Obesity can be defined as being more than 20 percent over the ideal body weight. Obesity has both an environmental and a familial risk of transmission. Research has shown that children whose parents are obese have a much-increased chance of developing obesity. Environmental factors such as proper nutrition and exercise may not be modeled or taught by obese parents, but there also seems to be a genetic factor to many cases of obesity. Obesity has been linked to, or defined as a cause for, diseases such as hypertension, heart disease, and vascular diseases.

Neuromuscular Disorders

Diseases of the nervous and muscular systems also have a variety of causes. *Huntington's disease* (which results in uncontrollable jerking and writhing movements) and muscular dystrophy (which results in progressive muscle weakness) are both known to be caused by genetic defects.

Multiple sclerosis (which affects the nerves of the eye, brain, and spinal cord) seems to have some hereditary factor, with clustering among close relatives. Its exact cause is unknown, but it seems to result when the virus-triggered autoimmune response begins to attack the myelin sheath that protects the nerves.

Alzheimer's disease is thought to cause about 50 percent of dementias, or progressive mental deterioration. Its cause is unknown, but it does cluster strongly in families and appears to be either caused or influenced by specific gene abnormalities.

Psychiatric Disorders

Genetic and biological causes of psychiatric disorders are being studied and increasingly understood. An example is *schizophrenia*, which affects about 1 percent of the population worldwide and is more prevalent than Alzheimer's

disease, diabetes, or multiple sclerosis. The schizophrenic loses contact with reality and suffers from hallucinations, delusions, abnormal thinking, and disrupted social functioning. People who develop schizophrenia are now thought to be "biologically vulnerable" to the disease, but what makes them vulnerable is not fully understood. The cause may be a genetic predisposition or some problem that occurs before, during, or after birth or a viral infection of the brain.

Another common psychiatric disorder is *manic-depressive illness,* now called *bipolar disorder,* in which the person experiences alternating periods of depression and mania or excitement. It can be mild or severe enough to interfere with the patient's ability to work or function socially. Manic-depressive illness affects about twice as many people as schizophrenia. It is believed to be hereditary, but the exact gene deficit has not yet been discovered.

Hypoperfusion

Hypoperfusion (shock) is a condition that is progressive (that is, it triggers a self-worsening cycle of pathophysiologic events) and fatal if not corrected. It can occur for many reasons, such as trauma, fluid loss, myocardial infarction, infection, allergic reaction, spinal cord injury, and other causes. Although causes differ, all forms of shock have the same underlying pathophysiology at the cellular and tissue levels.

The Physiology of Perfusion

As discussed earlier, all body cells require a constant supply of oxygen and other essential nutrients (primarily glucose), whereas waste products, such as carbon dioxide, must be constantly removed. The circulatory system, in conjunction with the respiratory and gastrointestinal systems, provides the body's cells with these essential nutrients and removal of wastes. This is accomplished by the passage of blood through the capillaries, the small vessels that interface with body cells, while oxygen, carbon dioxide, nutrients, and wastes are exchanged by movement across the capillary walls and cell membranes. This constant and necessary passage of blood through the body's tissues is called **perfusion.**

Inadequate perfusion of body tissues is **hypoperfusion,** which is commonly called **shock.** Shock occurs first at a cellular level. If allowed to progress, the tissues, organs, organ systems, and, ultimately, the entire organism are affected.

Components of the Circulatory System

Perfusion is dependent on a functioning and intact circulatory system. A derangement in any component of the

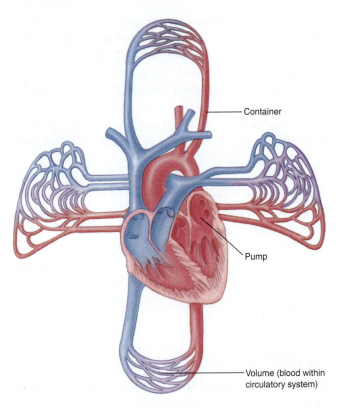

Container

Pump

Volume (blood within circulatory system)

FIGURE 12-83 Components of the circulatory system.

system can adversely affect perfusion (Figure 12-83). The three components of the circulatory system are:

- The pump (heart)
- The fluid (blood)
- The container (blood vessels)

THE PUMP The heart is the pump of the cardiovascular system. It receives blood from the venous system, pumps it to the lungs for oxygenation, and then pumps it to the peripheral tissues. The amount of blood ejected by the heart in one contraction is referred to as the **stroke volume**. Factors affecting stroke volume include:

- Preload
- Cardiac contractile force
- Afterload

Preload is the amount of blood delivered to the heart during diastole (when the heart fills with blood between contractions). Preload depends on venous return. The venous system is a capacitance, or storage, system. That is, it can be contracted or expanded, to some extent, as needed to meet the physiologic demands of the body. When additional oxygenated blood is required, the venous capacitance is reduced, thus

increasing the amount of blood delivered to the heart. The greater the preload, the greater the stroke volume.

Preload also affects **cardiac contractile force**. The greater the volume of preload, the more the ventricles are stretched. The greater the stretch, up to a certain point, the greater will be the subsequent cardiac contraction. This is referred to as the *Frank-Starling mechanism* and can be illustrated through the example of a rubber band. The more the rubber band is stretched, the greater will be its velocity when released.

In addition, cardiac contractile strength is affected by circulating hormones called **catecholamines** (epinephrine and norepinephrine) controlled by the sympathetic nervous system. Catecholamines enhance cardiac contractile strength by action on the beta-adrenergic receptors on the surface of the cells.

Finally, stroke volume is affected by **afterload**. Afterload is the resistance against which the ventricle must contract. This resistance must be overcome before ventricular contraction can result in ejection of blood. Afterload is determined by the degree of peripheral vascular resistance (defined later). This, in effect, is due to the amount of vasoconstriction present. The arterial system can be expanded and contracted to meet the metabolic demands of the body. The greater the resistance offered by the arterial system, the less the stroke volume.

The amount of blood pumped by the heart in 1 minute is referred to as the **cardiac output**. It is a function of stroke volume (milliliters per beat) and heart rate (beats per minute). Cardiac output is usually expressed in liters per minute. It can be defined by this equation:

$$\text{Stroke volume} \times \text{Heart rate} = \text{Cardiac output}$$

The preceding equation illustrates the factors that can affect cardiac output. An increase in stroke volume or an increase in heart rate can increase cardiac output. Conversely, a decrease in stroke volume or a decrease in heart rate can decrease cardiac output. The blood pressure is dependent on both cardiac output and peripheral vascular resistance.

$$\text{Cardiac output} \times \text{Peripheral vascular resistance} = \text{Blood pressure}$$

Peripheral vascular resistance is the pressure against which the heart must pump. Since the circulatory system is a closed system, increasing either cardiac output or peripheral vascular resistance will increase blood pressure. Likewise, a decrease in cardiac output or a decrease in peripheral vascular resistance will decrease blood pressure.

The body strives to keep the blood pressure relatively constant by employing *compensatory mechanisms* and **negative feedback loops**. As noted earlier, baroreceptors in the carotid sinuses and in the arch of the aorta closely monitor blood pressure. If blood pressure increases, the baroreceptors send signals to the brain that cause the blood pressure to return to its normal values. This is accomplished by decreasing the heart rate, decreasing the preload, or decreasing peripheral vascular resistance.

The baroreceptors are also stimulated if the blood pressure falls. The heart rate is increased, as is the strength of the cardiac contractions. There is also arteriolar constriction, venous constriction (which results in decreased container size), and overall increased peripheral vascular resistance. Also, the adrenal medulla (the inner portion of the adrenal gland) is stimulated. This results in the secretion of epinephrine and norepinephrine, which further enhance the response.

THE FLUID   Blood is the fluid of the cardiovascular system. It is a viscous fluid; that is, it is thicker and more adhesive than water. As a result, blood flows more slowly than water. Blood, which consists of the plasma and the formed elements (red cells, white cells, and platelets), transports oxygen, carbon dioxide, nutrients, hormones, metabolic waste products, and heat.

An adequate amount of blood is required for perfusion. Because the cardiovascular system (the heart and blood vessels) is a closed system, the volume of blood present must be adequate to fill the container, as described later.

Natriuretic Peptides   The heart has been found to have endocrine functions, especially through substances called **natriuretic peptides (NPs)**. These substances are involved in the long-term regulation of sodium and water balance, blood volume, and arterial pressure. There are two of these substances of interest: *atrial natriuretic peptide (ANP)* and *brain natriuretic peptide (BNP)*. ANP is manufactured, stored, and released by the heart's atrial muscle cells in response to such things as atrial distention and sympathetic stimulation. BNP is manufactured, stored, and released by the heart's ventricular muscle cells in response to ventricular dilation and sympathetic stimulation. BNP was first identified in the brains of rats, which is why it was named brain natriuretic peptide, although it was later found to be manufactured in both the brain and in the ventricles.

Natriuretic peptides serve as a sort of counterregulatory system to the renin–angiotensin system. They are involved in the long-term regulation of sodium and water balance, blood volume, and arterial blood pressure. These hormones decrease aldosterone release from the adrenal cortex, which increases the glomerular filtration rate (GFR) and produces natriuresis (sodium loss) and diuresis (water loss). It also decreases renin release by decreasing angiotensin II. This results in a reduction in blood volume and thus a reduction in central venous pressure (CVP), cardiac output (CO), and arterial blood pressure. Chronic elevation of natriuretic peptides appears to decrease arterial

Physiology of the Natriuretic Peptides

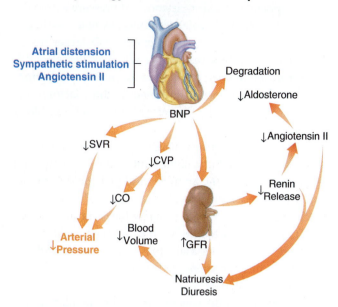

FIGURE 12-84 Physiology of the natriuretic peptides.

blood pressure primarily by decreasing peripheral vascular resistance (Figure 12-84).

BNP levels are elevated in congestive heart failure (CHF) and have become a marker for the presence of CHF. BNP (marketed as nesiritide) can be administered as a treatment for acute decompensated CHF.

THE CONTAINER   Blood vessels (arteries, arterioles, capillaries, venules, and veins) serve as the container of the cardiovascular system. The blood vessels can be thought of as a continuous, closed, and pressurized pipeline by which blood moves throughout the body. Whereas the heart functions as the pump of the circulatory system, the blood vessels—under the control of the autonomic nervous system—can regulate blood flow to different areas of the body by adjusting their size, as well as by selectively rerouting blood through the microcirculation.

Whereas the arteries and veins, like the heart, are subject to direct stimulation from sympathetic portions of the autonomic nervous system, the *microcirculation* (comprising the small vessels: the arterioles, capillaries, and venules) is primarily responsive to local tissue needs. The capability of some vessels in the capillary network to adjust their diameter permits the microcirculation to selectively supply undernourished tissue, while temporarily bypassing tissues with no immediate need. Capillaries have a sphincter at the origin of the capillary (between arteriole and capillary), called the *precapillary sphincter,* and another at the end of the capillary (between capillary and venule), called *the postcapillary sphincter.* The precapillary sphincter responds to local tissue conditions, such as acidosis and hypoxia, and opens as more arterial blood is needed. The postcapillary sphincter opens when blood is to be emptied into the venous system.

Blood flow through the vessels is regulated by two factors: peripheral vascular resistance and pressure within the system. Peripheral vascular resistance, as noted earlier, is the resistance to blood flow. Vessels with larger inside diameters offer less resistance, whereas vessels with smaller inside diameters offer greater resistance. Peripheral vascular resistance is governed by three factors—the length of the vessel, the diameter of the vessel, and blood viscosity.

There is very little resistance to blood flow through the aorta and arteries, but a significant change in peripheral resistance occurs at the arterioles and precapillary sphincters. This is because the inside diameter of the arteriole is much smaller, as compared to that of the aorta and arteries. Additionally, the arteriole has the ability to make a pronounced change in its diameter, as much as fivefold. It tends to do this in response to local tissue needs and autonomic nervous signals.

Contraction of the venous side of the vascular system results in decreased capacitance and increased cardiac preload. The arterial system, however, provides systemic vascular resistance. An increase in arterial tone increases resistance, which increases blood pressure.

Oxygen Transport

Oxygen is brought into the body via the respiratory system. During inspiration, approximately 500 to 800 mL of atmospheric air is taken in through the upper and lower airways, coming to rest in the alveoli of the lungs.

Surrounding the alveoli are capillaries that are perfused by the pulmonary circulation. The blood that comes into the pulmonary capillaries is oxygen-depleted blood that was returned from the body to the right atrium of the heart, then pumped by the right ventricle of the heart into the pulmonary arteries and thence into the pulmonary capillaries.

The air in the alveoli contains a concentration of about 13.6 percent oxygen. This is less than the 21 percent concentration of oxygen in atmospheric air because of various factors, including the fact that some air always remains in the alveoli from earlier respirations and oxygen is constantly being absorbed from this air. Nevertheless, alveolar air is far richer in oxygen than blood that enters the pulmonary capillaries.

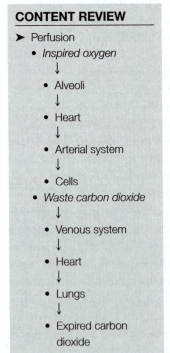

CONTENT REVIEW

➤ Perfusion
- *Inspired oxygen*
  ↓
- Alveoli
  ↓
- Heart
  ↓
- Arterial system
  ↓
- Cells
- *Waste carbon dioxide*
  ↓
- Venous system
  ↓
- Heart
  ↓
- Lungs
  ↓
- Expired carbon dioxide

Another way of stating this is that the *partial pressure of oxygen* present in air in the alveoli of the lungs is greater than the partial pressure of oxygen in the blood within the pulmonary circulation. (In a mix of gases, the portion of the total pressure exerted by each component of the mix is known as the *partial pressure* of that component.) For this reason, oxygen from the alveoli diffuses across the alveolar–capillary membrane and into the bloodstream—from the area of greater partial pressure to the area of lower partial pressure.

The red blood cells "pick up" this oxygen while passing through the pulmonary capillary bed. Oxygen binds to the hemoglobin molecules of the red blood cells, which serve as the primary carriers of oxygen within the bloodstream. Normally, between 95 and 100 percent of the hemoglobin is saturated with oxygen. Approximately 97 percent of oxygen is transported reversibly bound to hemoglobin, whereas the remaining 3 percent is transported as a gas dissolved in the plasma. The oxygen-enriched blood then circulates back to the heart through the venous side of the pulmonary circulation. Passing through the left atrium and into the left ventricle, the oxygen-enriched blood is pumped throughout the body via the systemic circulation.

On reaching capillaries throughout the body, the oxygen-rich blood interfaces with the tissues. The tissues contain cells that are oxygen deficient as a result of normal metabolic activity. Because the partial pressure of oxygen is greater in the bloodstream than in the cells, oxygen will diffuse from the red blood cells across the capillary wall–cell membrane barrier, into the cells and tissues.

Overall, the movement and utilization of oxygen in the body is dependent on the following conditions:

- Adequate concentration of inspired oxygen
- Appropriate movement of oxygen across the alveolar–capillary membrane into the arterial bloodstream
- Adequate number of red blood cells to carry the oxygen
- Proper tissue perfusion
- Efficient offloading of oxygen at the tissue level

The dependence on this set of conditions for oxygen movement and utilization is known as the **Fick principle**.

Waste Removal

The waste products of cellular metabolism are expelled from the cells and carried away by the blood. Carbon dioxide leaves the bloodstream during the oxygen–carbon dioxide exchange, which occurs through the alveolar–capillary membranes. The majority of carbon dioxide (approximately 70 percent) is transported in the form of bicarbonate ion (HCO_3^-). Only 23 percent is reversibly bound to hemoglobin (carbon dioxide binds to a different site on hemoglobin than oxygen does). Only 7 percent of carbon dioxide is transported as a gas dissolved in the plasma. Carbon dioxide is ultimately eliminated by exhalation from the lungs. Some cellular waste products are expelled into the interstitial fluid and picked up by the lymphatic system. These ultimately flow through the lymph channels into the thoracic duct. The thoracic duct empties the waste products into the venous side of the circulatory system. Other wastes are cleansed from the blood by the kidneys and excreted as urine. Finally, some cellular waste products are emptied into the gastrointestinal system and expelled in the feces.

There is some local control of both tissue perfusion and waste removal. When the amounts of metabolic waste products (such as lactic acid) increase, the tissues subsequently become acidotic. This local acidosis causes nearby precapillary sphincters to relax, thus opening the capillaries and increasing perfusion of the affected tissues. This provides increased capacity for waste elimination and response to local metabolic demands.

The Pathophysiology of Hypoperfusion

Causes of Hypoperfusion

Hypoperfusion (shock) is almost always a result of inadequate cardiac output. A number of factors can decrease effective cardiac output. These include:

- Inadequate pump
  - Inadequate preload
  - Inadequate cardiac contractile strength
  - Inadequate heart rate
  - Excessive afterload
- Inadequate fluid
  - Hypovolemia (abnormally low circulating blood volume)
- Inadequate container
  - Dilated container without change in fluid volume (inadequate systemic vascular resistance)
  - Leak in container

Occasionally, hypoperfusion can develop even when cardiac output is adequate. This can happen when cell metabolism is so excessive that the body cannot increase perfusion enough to meet the cells' metabolic requirements. It can also happen when abnormal circulatory patterns develop, so that circulating blood is bypassing critical tissues.

As mentioned earlier, the conditions that lead to hypoperfusion can result from a number of underlying causes, such as infection, trauma and hemorrhage, loss of plasma through burns, severe cardiac arrhythmia, central

nervous system dysfunction, and many others. But the outcome is always the same: inadequate delivery of oxygen and essential nutrients to, and removal of wastes from, all the tissues of the body, especially the critical tissues (brain, heart, kidneys).

> **CONTENT REVIEW**
> ➤ Causes of Hypoperfusion (Shock)
> - Inadequate pump (heart malfunction)
> - Inadequate fluid (hypovolemia)
> - Inadequate container (dilated or leaking blood vessels)

Shock at the Cellular Level

Shock is a complex phenomenon. The causes vary. The signs and symptoms vary. At the simplest level, however, shock is inadequate tissue perfusion. Additionally, all types of shock have this in common: The ultimate outcome is impairment of cellular metabolism. Two characteristics of impaired cellular metabolism in any type of shock are impaired oxygen use and impaired glucose use.

IMPAIRED USE OF OXYGEN One characteristic of any type of shock is that the cells are either not receiving enough oxygen or are unable to use it effectively. This may be caused by hypoperfusion resulting from reduced cardiac function, inadequate blood volume, or vasodilation (pump, fluid, or container problems). It may result from insufficient red cells to carry the oxygen, from fever that increases cellular oxygen demand, or from chemical disruption of cellular metabolism.

When the cells don't receive enough oxygen or cannot use it effectively, they change from **aerobic metabolism** to **anaerobic metabolism**, a far less efficient means of producing energy—as explained in the following text.

The primary energy source for the cells is glucose, taken into the cell with the aid of insulin. Glucose does not provide energy until it is broken down inside the cell. The first stage of glucose breakdown, called glycolysis, is anaerobic (does not require oxygen). Glycolysis produces pyruvic acid as an end product but yields very little energy. Thus, by itself, glycolysis is an inefficient utilization of glucose. Therefore, in a normal state of metabolism, a second stage of glucose breakdown is required. During this second stage, which is aerobic (requires oxygen), pyruvic acid is further degraded into carbon dioxide, water, and energy in a process termed the Krebs or citric acid cycle. The energy yield of this second-stage aerobic process is much higher than from the first-stage anaerobic process (Figure 12-85).

During shock, or any condition in which the cells do not receive adequate oxygen or cannot use it effectively, glucose breakdown can complete only the first-stage, anaerobic process of glycolysis and cannot enter into the second-stage, aerobic, citric acid cycle. This causes an accumulation of the end product of glycolysis, pyruvic acid. In

(a) Stage one: Anaerobic metabolism

Glucose

Small amount
of energy

Pyruvic
acid

Lactic acid

No oxygen

Anaerobic metabolism
(without oxygen)

(b) Stage two: Aerobic metabolism

Glucose

Energy

Aerobic metabolism
(with oxygen)

Oxygen

FIGURE 12-85 Glucose breakdown. (a) Stage one, glycolysis, is anaerobic (does not require oxygen). It yields pyruvic acid, with toxic byproducts such as lactic acid, and very little energy. (b) Stage two is aerobic (requires oxygen). In a process called the Krebs or citric acid cycle, pyruvic acid is degraded into carbon dioxide and water, which produces a much higher yield of energy.

these cases, pyruvic acid is quickly degraded to lactic acid. If oxygen is promptly restored to the cells, lactic acid will be reconverted to pyruvic acid. However, if time elapses and the cellular hypoxia is not corrected, lactic acid and other metabolic acids will accumulate. One outcome is that the acidic condition of the blood reduces the ability of hemoglobin in red blood cells to bind with and carry oxygen, which compounds the problem of cellular oxygen deprivation.

The energy that is produced during glucose breakdown is in the form of the chemical adenosine triphosphate (ATP), which is essential to all metabolic processes in the cells. As just noted, the amount of energy, or ATP, produced during first-stage, anaerobic glycolysis is very small. Without oxygen, when the process of glucose breakdown stops after glycolysis (during which very little energy has been produced), cellular stores of ATP are used up much faster than they can be replaced, so all the processes of cellular metabolism are gravely impaired.

Because of changes to the internal cell and because blood flow has been slowed by the decreased pumping action and vasodilation, sludging of the blood occurs. This further impedes blood flow. Thus, the normal diffusion of nutrients and wastes in and out of the cells is disrupted and the balance of the cellular electrolytes is altered. Lysosomes, the organelles that assist in digestion of nutrients, are normally enclosed by a membrane that prevents the digestive enzymes from damaging other cell components. Now the lysosomes rupture, releasing the lysosomal enzymes into the cell. The sodium–potassium pumping mechanism fails, changing the electrical charge of the cells' internal environment. There is an increase in sodium and water (because water follows sodium) inside the cells, causing cellular edema. The cell membrane then ruptures,

allowing lysosomal enzymes and other cellular contents to leak into the interstitial spaces. Cellular death soon follows.

IMPAIRED USE OF GLUCOSE The same factors that reduce delivery of oxygen to the cells also reduce delivery of glucose to the cells. In addition, uptake of glucose by the cells may be disrupted by fever, cell damage, or the presence of bacteria, toxins, histamine, or other substances produced or activated by the body's immune and inflammatory responses to disease or injury. Compensatory mechanisms activated by shock may also be responsible for substances that inhibit glucose uptake, including catecholamines and the hormones cortisol and growth hormone.

Glucose that is prevented from entering the cells remains in the blood, resulting in a condition of high serum glucose, or hyperglycemia. Because glucose is the substance from which cells produce energy, the consequences of reduced glucose delivery and uptake are critical.

In the absence of an adequate supply of glucose, certain body cells can create fuel for energy production by converting other substances to glucose. One source is glycogen, the form of glucose that cells store and hold in reserve. Cells convert glycogen to glucose in a process called *glycogenolysis.* However, there is very little stored glycogen in cells other than the liver, kidneys, and muscles. When glycogen reserves are depleted, which typically occurs in 4 to 8 hours, the cells will then derive energy from the breakdown of fats (*lipolysis*) and from the conversion of noncarbohydrate substrates, such as amino acids from proteins, to glucose (*gluconeogenesis*). The energy costs of glycogenolysis and lipolysis are high and contribute to the failure of cells—but the depletion of proteins in gluconeogenesis will ultimately cause organ failure (Figure 12-86).

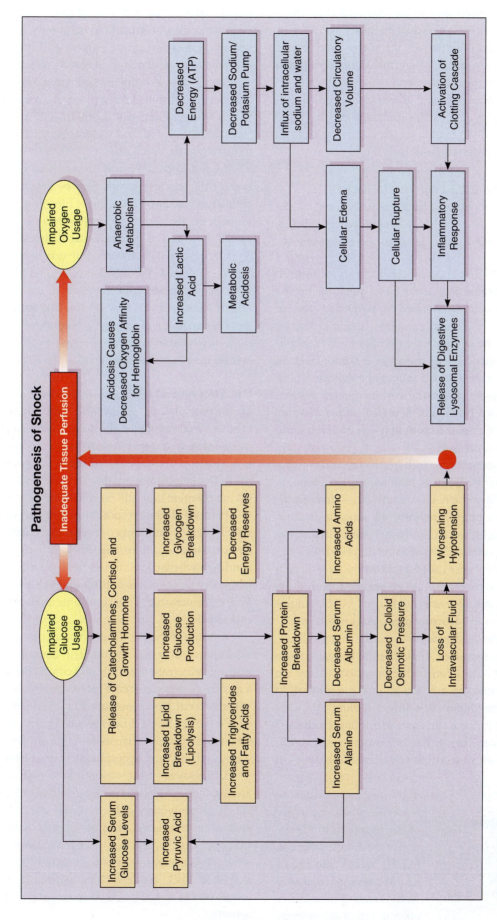

FIGURE 12-86 The pathogenesis of shock in the human.

In addition, the anaerobic breakdown of proteins produces ammonia, which is toxic to the cells, and urea, which leads to uric acid, which is also toxic to cells. Finally, when cellular metabolism is impaired, the waste products of metabolism build up in the cells, further impairing cell function and damaging cell membranes.

Impaired use of oxygen and glucose soon leads to cellular death. Cellular death will ultimately lead to tissue death, tissue death will lead to organ failure, and organ failure will lead to death of the individual.

Compensation and Decompensation

Usually, the body is able to compensate for any of the changes previously described. However, when the compensatory mechanisms fail, shock develops and may progress.

COMPENSATION In shock, the fall in cardiac output, detected as a decrease in arterial blood pressure by the baroreceptors, activates several body systems that attempt to reestablish a normal blood pressure—a process known as *compensation*. The sympathetic nervous system stimulates the adrenal gland of the endocrine system to secrete the catecholamines epinephrine and norepinephrine. These chemicals profoundly affect the cardiovascular system, causing an increased heart rate, increased cardiac contractile strength, and arteriolar constriction—all of which serve to elevate the blood pressure.

Another compensatory mechanism, the *renin–angiotensin system*, aids the body in maintaining an adequate blood pressure. When the renin–angiotensin system is activated by a fall in blood pressure, the enzyme *renin* is released from the kidneys into the systemic circulation. Renin acts on a specialized plasma protein called *angiotensin* to produce a substance called *angiotensin I*. Angiotensin I is converted to *angiotensin II* by an enzyme found in the lungs called *angiotensin-converting enzyme (ACE)*. Angiotensin II is a potent vasoconstrictor. As angiotensin II causes the diameter of the vascular container to decrease, the blood pressure increases. Angiotensin II also stimulates the production of aldosterone, a hormone secreted by the adrenal cortex (outer layer of the adrenal gland) that, in turn, stimulates the kidneys to reabsorb sodium, and, subsequently, water (as noted earlier, "water follows sodium") into peritubular capillaries. The intravascular volume is maintained, and elimination of water by the kidneys is reduced.

Another endocrine response by the pituitary gland results in the secretion of antidiuretic hormone (ADH), which also causes the kidneys to reabsorb water, creating an additive effect to that of aldosterone.

CONTENT REVIEW
➤ Bodily Responses to Shock
• Compensated shock
• Decompensated shock
• Irreversible shock

The spleen, capable of storing more than 300 mL of blood, can expel up to 200 mL of blood into the venous circulation and can contract, consequently increasing blood volume, preload, cardiac output, and blood pressure in response to a sudden drop in blood pressure.

Some passive compensatory responses also occur, with beneficial fluid shifts taking place as a result of simple diffusion. With volume loss, the hydrostatic pressure in capillary beds is reduced, and water from the interstitial spaces diffuses into the capillaries.

All the aforementioned mechanisms work to compensate for the shock state, and may be able to restore normal circulatory volume—if excessive bleeding is managed and the shock state has not progressed too far. In this case, the patient is said to be in **compensated shock**.

Once normal circulatory function and blood pressure are reestablished, the blood pressure will "feed back" on all the compensatory mechanisms so that all systems can return to normal. In this way, negative feedback loops work to maintain stability by "signaling" the systems to cease the compensatory responses. In this way, stability and homeostasis are maintained.

DECOMPENSATION If the conditions causing shock are too serious, or progress too rapidly, compensatory mechanisms may not be able to restore normal function. In those cases, *decompensation* is said to occur, and the patient is in a state of **decompensated shock**, also called *progressive shock*. During decompensated or progressive shock, medical intervention may still be able to correct the condition.

Because all the "responding" systems have a point at which they can no longer sustain their action (i.e., a limited duration of action), the shock state may progress to a condition where correction, either by the body's own compensatory mechanisms or through medical intervention, is no longer possible. This condition is known as **irreversible shock**.

A critical factor in the downward spiral of decompensation is cardiac depression. The compensatory mechanisms that increase heart rate and contractile strength create a greatly increased demand for oxygen by the myocardium. When arterial blood pressure has fallen sufficiently, however, coronary blood flow is reduced below the level necessary to adequately perfuse the myocardium. The heart is weakened and cardiac output falls even further.

Depression of the vasomotor center of the brain is another consequence of reduced blood pressure. In early shock, as previously discussed, the sympathetic nervous system is stimulated to cause release of catecholamines that support the function of the circulatory system. But when blood pressure falls to a certain point, in the late stages of shock, reduced blood supply to the vasomotor center results in a slowing, then stoppage, of sympathetic activity.

Metabolic wastes, products of anaerobic metabolism, are released into the slower-flowing blood. The blood in the capillary beds becomes acidic, causing formation of minute blood clots ("sludged" blood), which further slows the flow of blood. And a more generalized, systemic acidosis develops, causing further deterioration of cells and tissues, including the capillary walls.

Capillary cells, like other cells, suffer from lack of oxygen and other nutrients, as well as from the ravages of acidosis. This begins to cause permeability of the capillaries and leakage of fluid into the interstitial spaces. This is another self-perpetuating process, as the decreased circulating volume and anaerobic metabolism cause further cell hypoxia and increased permeability.

Cellular deterioration progresses to tissue deterioration, which progresses to organ failure. (See Multiple Organ Dysfunction Syndrome, later in the chapter.) Medical intervention may save the patient if initiated early enough, but when enough damage has been done to cells, tissues, and organs, no known treatment can help the patient to recover. Medical therapies may support function for a while, but death becomes inevitable.

Types of Shock

Shock is usually classified according to the cause. Some newer terminology classifies shock as *cardiogenic* (caused by impaired pumping power of the heart), *hypovolemic* (caused by decreased blood or water volume), *obstructive* (caused by an obstruction that interferes with return of blood to the heart, such as a pulmonary embolism, cardiac tamponade, or tension pneumothorax), and *distributive* (caused by abnormal distribution and return of blood resulting from vasodilation, vasopermeability, or both, as in neurogenic, anaphylactic, or septic shock).

Another, more familiar terminology classifies shock as *cardiogenic, hypovolemic, neurogenic, anaphylactic,* and *septic*. The following discussion of types of shock uses these classifications.

Although all types of shock ultimately have the same effects on the body's cells, tissues, and organs, it is important to try to identify the underlying cause, because correcting the cause is the most important element in reversing the condition and saving the patient's life. Many of the treatments that you, as a paramedic, will provide for the shock patient will be the same, no matter

what the cause or type of shock is, but some differ in important ways. For example, providing IV fluid boluses, which may be appropriate to support circulating volume in the hypovolemic patient, would not be indicated for the patient in cardiogenic shock with pulmonary edema.

Cardiogenic Shock

An inability of the heart to pump enough blood to supply all body parts is referred to as **cardiogenic shock**. Cardiogenic shock is usually the result of severe left ventricular failure secondary to acute myocardial infarction or congestive heart failure. The reduced blood pressure that accompanies this form of shock aggravates the situation by decreasing coronary artery perfusion. With decreased coronary perfusion, the heart muscle becomes even more damaged, thus establishing a vicious cycle that ultimately results in complete pump failure.

During cardiogenic shock, as noted earlier, the activation of compensatory mechanisms can actually worsen the situation. When the peripheral resistance increases in an attempt to maintain blood pressure, the myocardial workload increases. This, in turn, increases the myocardial oxygen demand, further aggravating myocardial ischemia and infarction. Cardiac output is further depressed and ejection fraction (the percentage of blood in the ventricle that is ejected with each beat) is decreased (Figure 12-87).

The most common cause of cardiogenic shock is severe left ventricular failure, but a number of other factors can have the same result. These include chronic progressive heart disease such as cardiomyopathy, rupture of the papillary heart muscles or intraventricular septum, and end-stage valvular disease (mitral stenosis or aortic regurgitation).

Most patients who experience cardiogenic shock will have normal blood volume. However, some patients will be hypovolemic from an excessive use of prescribed diuretics or the severe diaphoresis that accompanies some acute cardiac events. Patients may also experience relative hypovolemia (neurogenic shock) from the vasodilatory (vessel dilation) effects of drugs such as nitroglycerin.

EVALUATION AND TREATMENT A major difference between cardiogenic and other types of shock is the presence of pulmonary edema (excess fluid in the lungs), which will probably result in a complaint of difficulty breathing. There may be diminished lung sounds as fluid enters the interstitial spaces of the lungs. As fluid levels rise, wheezes, crackles, or rales may be heard. A productive cough may develop, characterized by white- or pink-tinged foamy sputum. Cyanosis (a dusky blue-gray skin color) is typical, resulting from the decreased diffusion of oxygen across the alveolar–capillary interface, decreasing oxygen delivery to cells that are already hypoxic because of decreased blood pressure and perfusion. Other signs of shock include altered mentation (resulting from reduced perfusion of the

CONTENT REVIEW
➤ Two Classifications of Shock
Classification #1
- Cardiogenic shock
- Hypovolemic shock
- Obstructive shock
- Distributive shock

Classification #2
- Cardiogenic shock
- Hypovolemic shock
- Neurogenic shock
- Anaphylactic shock
- Septic shock

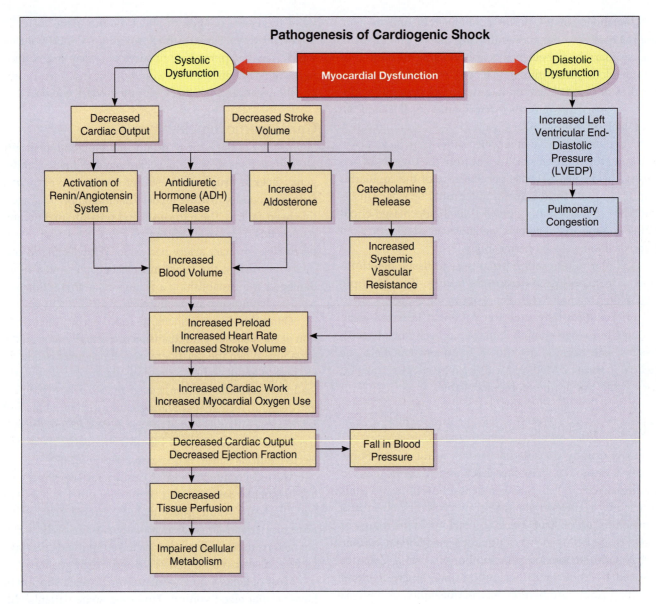

FIGURE 12-87 The pathogenesis of cardiogenic shock.

brain) and oliguria (diminished urination resulting from compensatory mechanisms that stimulate reabsorption of water by the kidneys to enhance circulating volume).

Treatment of cardiogenic shock includes the supportive measures that should be provided for shock of any origin: Ensure an open airway, administer supplemental oxygen if the patient is hypoxic and assist ventilations if necessary (to support oxygenation of myocardial and other body cells), and keep the patient warm (because impaired cellular metabolism is no longer producing enough energy to keep body temperature normal).

Hypovolemic Shock

Shock due to a loss of intravascular fluid volume is referred to as **hypovolemic shock**. Possible causes of hypovolemic shock include:

- Internal or external hemorrhage (This type of hypovolemic shock is also known as hemorrhagic shock.)

- Traumatic injury
- Long bone or open fractures
- Severe dehydration from vomiting or diarrhea
- Plasma loss from burns
- Excessive sweating
- Diabetic ketoacidosis with resultant **osmotic diuresis**

Hypovolemic shock can also be due to internal third-space loss (loss from intracellular or, more commonly, from intravascular spaces into the interstitial spaces). Such a condition can occur with bowel obstruction, peritonitis, pancreatitis, or liver failure resulting in ascites (accumulation of fluid within the abdominal cavity) (Figure 12-88).

EVALUATION AND TREATMENT The signs of hypovolemic shock are considered the "classic" signs of shock. The mental status becomes altered, progressing from anxiety to lethargy or combativeness to unresponsiveness. The

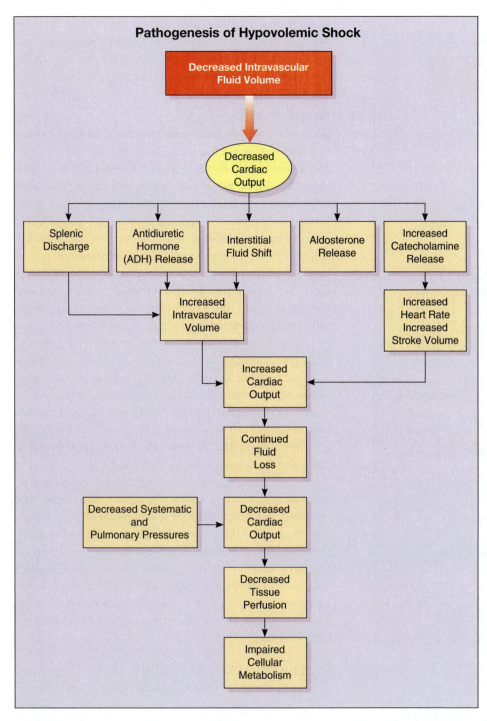

Pathogenesis of Hypovolemic Shock

Decreased Intravascular Fluid Volume

↓

Decreased Cardiac Output

Splenic Discharge | Antidiuretic Hormone (ADH) Release | Interstitial Fluid Shift | Aldosterone Release | Increased Catecholamine Release

Increased Intravascular Volume

Increased Heart Rate Increased Stroke Volume

Increased Cardiac Output

Continued Fluid Loss

Decreased Systematic and Pulmonary Pressures → Decreased Cardiac Output

Decreased Tissue Perfusion

Impaired Cellular Metabolism

FIGURE 12-88 The pathogenesis of hypovolemic shock.

skin becomes pale, cool, and clammy (sweaty). The blood pressure may be normal during compensated shock, but then begins to fall. The pulse may be normal in the beginning, then become rapid, finally slowing and disappearing. As the kidneys continue to reabsorb water, urination decreases. Cardiac arrhythmias may develop in late shock, deteriorating to asystole (absence of heartbeat).

Although it is accepted practice to administer crystalloid or colloid solutions to replace fluids lost through vomiting, diarrhea, burns, excessive sweating, or osmotic diuresis, the replacement of fluids in trauma patients is quite controversial. It has been demonstrated that the body provides a natural compensation for low-flow states when the systolic pressure is maintained between 70 and 85 mmHg. In a few studies, elevating the systolic blood pressure to greater than 85 mmHg has been associated with worsened outcomes. The worsened outcomes are attributed to the fact that aggressive fluid resuscitation, before the source of bleeding is repaired, causes progressive dilution of the blood, which decreases the oxygen-carrying capacity of the blood. Thus, many surgeons and EMS medical directors are now recommending administering only enough fluid to maintain a systolic blood pressure between 70 and 85 mmHg—a process called "permissive hypotension."

Neurogenic Shock

Neurogenic shock results from injury to either the brain or the spinal cord. Spinal cord injuries can result in an imbalance between sympathetic and parasympathetic tone depending on the level of the spinal cord injured. This can result in an interruption of nerve impulses to the arteries. The arteries lose tone and dilate, causing a relative hypovolemia. There has been no loss of fluid, but the container has been enlarged. With this inappropriate vasodilation, a disproportionate amount of blood collects in the capillary bed. This reduces venous return, cardiac output, and arterial blood pressure. Sympathetic nerve impulses to the adrenal glands are lost, which prevents the release of catecholamines and their compensatory effects. With injury high in the cervical spine, there may be interruption of impulses to the peripheral nervous system, causing paralysis and loss of sensation. The respiratory and cardiac centers of the brain may also be affected.

The usual cause of neurogenic shock is central nervous system injury. Neurogenic shock is most commonly due to

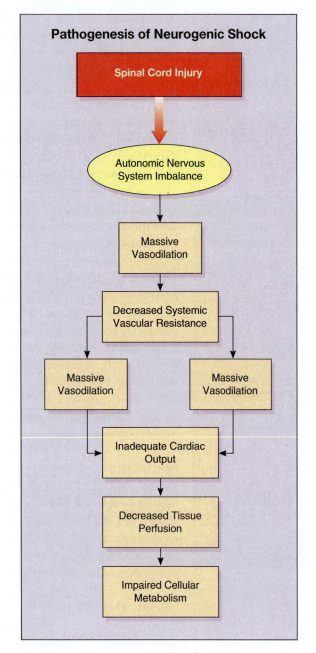

Pathogenesis of Neurogenic Shock

Spinal Cord Injury

↓

Autonomic Nervous System Imbalance

↓

Massive Vasodilation

↓

Decreased Systemic Vascular Resistance

↓   ↓

Massive Vasodilation   Massive Vasodilation

↓   ↓

Inadequate Cardiac Output

↓

Decreased Tissue Perfusion

↓

Impaired Cellular Metabolism

FIGURE 12-89 The pathogenesis of neurogenic shock.

an injury that has resulted in severe spinal cord injury or total transection of the cord (which may be called *spinal shock*) or injury or deprivation of oxygen or glucose to the medulla of the brain (Figure 12-89).

EVALUATION AND TREATMENT   The vasodilation in neurogenic shock causes warm, red skin, and sweat gland malfunction causes dry skin—in contrast to the cool, pale, sweaty skin associated with hypovolemic shock. Because of the lack of compensatory stimulation from catecholamine release, the patient will have a low blood pressure and a slow pulse even in the early stages—again, in contrast to hypovolemic shock.

Treatment for neurogenic shock or spinal shock is similar to treatment for other types of shock and includes

support of the airway, oxygenation, ventilation, maintenance of body temperature, and intravenous access. Spinal shock is characterized by hypotension, reflex bradycardia, and warm, dry skin.

Anaphylactic Shock

When a foreign substance enters the body, the immune system responds to rid the body of the invader. (See the discussion of immunity later in this chapter.) This usually happens with no noticeable effects, and the person is not even aware that an immune response is taking place. Some foreign substances (antigens) provoke an exaggerated immune response (allergic response) that will cause noticeable symptoms such as a rash (as from contact with poison ivy) or swollen, irritated airway passages (as with hay fever). In rare cases, an allergic response is very severe and life threatening. This kind of severe allergic response is called **anaphylaxis**, or *anaphylactic shock* (Figure 12-90).

An anaphylactic reaction usually occurs very rapidly. Signs and symptoms most often appear within a minute or less, but occasionally may appear an hour or more after exposure. Generally, the faster the reaction develops, the more severe it is likely to be. Death can occur before the patient can get to a hospital, so prompt intervention is critical. This is a situation in which the paramedic at the scene can make the difference between life and death.

Anaphylactic reactions can be triggered by a variety of substances, including foods (especially nuts, eggs, and shellfish), venoms, aspirin or nonsteroidal anti-inflammatory drugs (NSAIDS), hormones (animal-derived insulin), preservatives, and others. The most rapid and severe reactions are usually caused by substances injected directly into the bloodstream, which is one reason that penicillin injections and hymenoptera stings (e.g., from bees, wasps, and hornets) are the most common causes of fatal anaphylactic reactions.

EVALUATION AND TREATMENT   Because the immune responses involved in anaphylaxis can affect different body systems, the signs and symptoms can vary widely, as follows:

- Skin
  - Flushing
  - Itching
  - Hives
  - Swelling
  - Cyanosis
- Respiratory system
  - Breathing difficulty
  - Sneezing, coughing
  - Wheezing, stridor

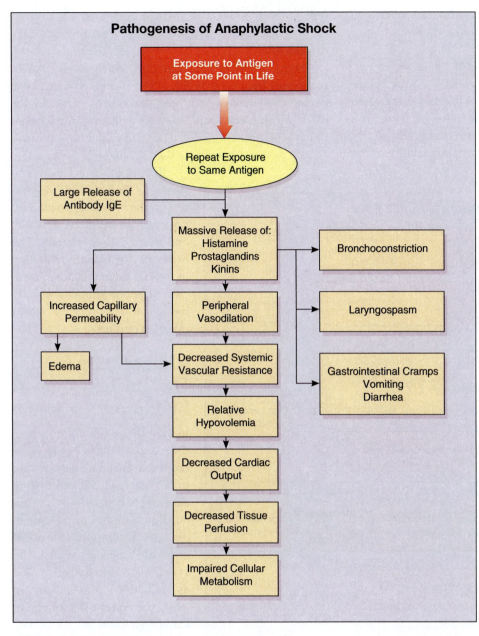

FIGURE 12-90 The pathogenesis of anaphylactic shock.

- Laryngeal edema
- Laryngospasm
- Cardiovascular system
  - Vasodilation
  - Increased heart rate
  - Decreased blood pressure
- Gastrointestinal system
  - Nausea, vomiting
  - Abdominal cramping
  - Diarrhea
- Nervous system
  - Altered mental status
  - Dizziness

- Headache
- Seizures
- Tearing

The patient may present with an altered mental status that can progress to unresponsiveness, so gather a brief history as soon as possible, including previous allergic reactions and any information about what the patient may have ingested or been exposed to that could have caused the present reaction. Be sure the patient is no longer in contact with the allergen; if a stinger is in the skin, scrape it away with a fingernail or scalpel blade.

Because laryngeal edema is often a problem, protecting the patient's airway will be your first concern. Administer oxygen by nonrebreather mask or, as necessary, by endotracheal intubation. The anaphylactic response causes depletion of circulatory volume by promoting capillary permeability and leaking of fluid into interstitial spaces, so establish an IV of crystalloid solution (normal saline or lactated Ringer's) for volume support.

The primary treatment for anaphylaxis is pharmacological. In addition to oxygen, epinephrine is usually administered (if the patient has a history of anaphylaxis, he may be carrying a prescribed spring-loaded epinephrine injector), as are antihistamines (diphenhydramine), corticosteroids (methylprednisolone, hydrocortisone, dexamethasone), and vasopressors (dopamine, norepinephrine, epinephrine). Occasionally an inhaled beta agonist (albuterol) may be required. Follow local protocols.

Septic Shock

Septic shock begins with *septicemia* (also called *sepsis*), an infection that enters the bloodstream and is carried throughout the body. The person may have septicemia for some time before septic shock develops, but eventually toxins released by the invading organism overcome the compensatory mechanisms. Unless it is corrected, septic shock will cause the dysfunction of more than one organ system, resulting in multiple organ dysfunction syndrome (discussed in the next section) (Figure 12-91).

EVALUATION AND TREATMENT The signs and symptoms of septic shock are progressive. In the beginning, cardiac output is increased, but toxins causing vasodilation may prevent an increase in blood pressure. The person may seem to be sick, but not alarmingly so. By the last stages, toxins have increased permeability of the blood vessels to the point where great amounts of fluid are lost from the vasculature and blood pressure falls drastically.

Signs and symptoms can vary widely as the patient progresses from early to late stages of septic shock. Some patients may have a high fever, but others, especially the elderly or the very young, may have no fever or may even be hypothermic. The skin can be flushed, if fever is present, or very pale and cyanotic in the late stages.

The most susceptible organ system is the lungs and respiratory system, so the patient may present with breathing difficulty and altered lung sounds. The brain may be infected, resulting in altered mental status. Suspicion of septic shock is usually based on a history of recent infection or illness.

Multiple Organ Dysfunction Syndrome

In the 1970s, a syndrome of multiple organ failure began to be noticed in hospital intensive care units. Medical advances were allowing patients to survive serious illness and trauma—only to die later of complications of the original disease or injury. The syndrome was described in 1975 as *multisystem organ failure*. In 1991, the American College of Chest Physicians and the Society of Critical Care Medicine named it **multiple organ dysfunction syndrome (MODS)**.

MODS is the progressive impairment of two or more organ systems resulting from an uncontrolled inflammatory response to a severe illness or injury. Sepsis and septic shock are the most common causes of MODS, with MODS being the end stage. (The progression from infection to sepsis to septic shock to MODS is known as *systemic inflammatory response syndrome*, or SIRS.)

Actually, MODS can result from any severe disease or injury

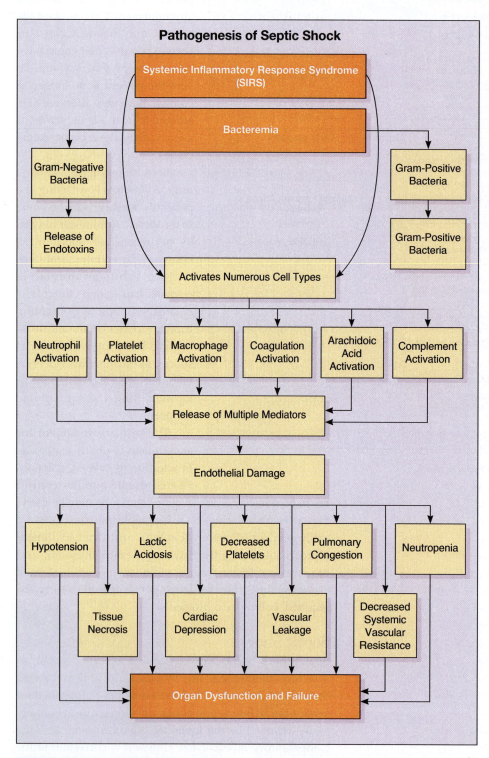

FIGURE 12-91 The pathogenesis of septic shock.

that triggers a massive systemic inflammatory response—including trauma, burns, surgery, circulatory shock, acute pancreatitis, acute renal failure, and others. Risk factors include age (>65), malnutrition, and preexisting chronic disease such as cancer or diabetes. With a mortality rate of 60 to 90 percent, MODS is the major cause of death following sepsis, trauma, and burn injuries.

Pathophysiology of MODS

MODS occurs in two stages. In primary MODS, organ damage results directly from a specific cause such as ischemia or inadequate perfusion resulting from an episode of shock, trauma, or major surgery. There are stress and inflammatory responses (discussed in detail later in this chapter) to this initial injury, but they may be mild and not readily detectable. However, during this response, neutrophils and macrophages (cells that attack and destroy bacteria, protozoa, foreign cells, and cell debris) as well as mast cells (cells that produce histamine and other components of allergic response) are thought to be "primed" by cytokines (proteins released during an inflammatory or immune response).

The next time there is an insult, such as an additional injury or ischemia or infection—even though the insult may be mild—the primed cells are activated, producing an exaggerated inflammatory response, known as secondary MODS.

Now, the inflammatory response enters a self-perpetuating cycle. As inflammatory mediators are released by the injured organ, they enter the circulation, activating inflammatory responses in organ systems throughout the body. These mediators, especially cytokines such as tumor necrosis factor (TNF) and interleukin 1 (IL-1), damage the endothelium (cells that line the blood vessels, the heart, and body cavities). Gram-negative bacteria, if present, release endotoxins that also damage endothelial cells. The injured endothelial cells release factors that aggravate the inflammation and cause vasodilation. The injured epithelium becomes permeable, allowing leakage of fluid into interstitial spaces, and loses much of its anticoagulation function, which allows formation of tiny blood clots (thrombi) in the microvasculature.

The secondary insult also triggers an exaggerated neuroendocrine response. Catecholamine release causes many of the manifestations of MODS, including tachycardia, increased metabolic rates, and increased oxygen consumption. Release of a variety of hormones contributes to the hypermetabolism, and release of endorphins contributes to vasodilation. Additionally, plasma protein systems are activated: specifically, the complement system, the coagulation system, and the kallikrein–kinin system. Plasma proteins are key mediators of the inflammatory response. When activated, each of these systems triggers a cascade of responses with the overall result of increased vasodilation,

vasopermeability, cardiovascular instability, endothelial damage, and clotting abnormalities.

As a result of the release of the inflammatory mediators and toxins and the plasma protein cascades, a massive immune/inflammatory and coagulation response develops. Vascular changes (vasodilation, increased capillary permeability, selective vasoconstriction, and microvascular thrombi) continue and worsen. Two metabolites that are released have opposing vascular effects: Prostacyclin, also called prostaglandin I_2 (PGI$_2$), is a vasodilator, whereas thromboxane A_2 (TXA$_2$) is a vasoconstrictor. They are released in differing amounts within different organ tissues, contributing to a maldistribution of blood flow to organs and organ systems.

As noted earlier, the release of catecholamines stimulates hypermetabolism within the body cells, which, in turn, creates a greatly increased oxygen demand. Because of lung damage, **hypoxemia** and hypoperfusion, a severe oxygen supply/demand imbalance, develop. As the cells switch from aerobic to anaerobic metabolism, fuel supplies within the cells (ATP and glucose) are used up faster than they can be replenished. Without adequate ATP, the cells lose their ability to operate the sodium–potassium pump, which is essential to cardiac function. The myocardium is profoundly weakened. Cellular lysosomes begin to break down, releasing lysosomal enzymes that damage the cell membrane and the surrounding cells. Large amounts of lactic acid are released, contributing to acidosis, which further damages the cells. The overall response is similar to that seen in septic and anaphylactic shock, except on a larger scale.

Clinical Presentation of MODS

The cumulative effects of MODS at the cellular and tissue levels begin to cause the breakdown of organ systems: The organs that fail first are not necessarily the organs where the initial insult occurred, and there is a lag time between the initial insult and the onset of organ failure. Dysfunction may develop in the pulmonary, gastrointestinal, hepatic, renal, cardiovascular, hematologic, and immune systems. There is decreased cardiac function and myocardial depression, caused by the factors discussed earlier, possibly abetted by release of myocardial depressant factor (MDF) and a decrease in beta-adrenergic receptors in the heart. The smooth muscle of the vascular system fails with consequent release of capillary sphincters and increased vasodilation.

MODS does not occur in one intense crisis. It will usually develop over a period of two, three, or more weeks. There is no specific therapy for MODS, and the only chance of rescuing the patient from its self-perpetuating spiral toward death is early recognition and initiation of supportive measures. For this reason, it is important to understand how MODS usually presents in the first 24 hours after initial resuscitation.

Although MODS will usually be detected in the hospital rather than the out-of-hospital setting, there may be occasions when a patient who has not been hospitalized or has returned home from the hospital is the subject of a call to EMS, or when a patient being transported by EMS from one facility to another is suffering from MODS.

The most common presentation of MODS over time is as follows:

24 hours after resuscitation

- Low-grade fever
- Tachycardia (rapid heart rate)
- Dyspnea (breathing difficulty)
- Altered mental status
- General hypermetabolic, hyperdynamic state

Within 24 to 72 hours

- Pulmonary (lung) failure begins

Within 7 to 10 days

- Hepatic (liver) failure begins
- Intestinal failure begins
- Renal (kidney) failure begins

Within 14 to 21 days

- Intensified renal and hepatic failure
- Gastrointestinal collapse
- Immune system collapse

After 21 days

- Hematologic (blood system) failure begins
- Myocardial (heart muscle) failure begins
- Altered mental status resulting from encephalopathy (brain infection)
- Death

PART 6: The Body's Defenses Against Disease and Injury

Self-Defense Mechanisms

So far in this chapter, we have discussed normal body conditions (the normal cell and its environment: fluids and electrolytes, the acid–base balance) and how the body may be attacked or injured (cellular injury, infection, genetic and other causes of disease, hypoperfusion, and multiple organ dysfunction syndrome). In the remainder of the chapter, we will discuss how the body defends itself from infection and injury.

It is important to keep in mind that the body has powerful ways of defending and healing itself (restoring homeostasis) and that medical intervention is needed only when, on occasion, these natural defense mechanisms are unequal to the task and become overwhelmed.

Infectious Agents

Bacteria

Bacteria are single-celled organisms that consist of internal cytoplasm surrounded by a rigid cell wall. Bacteria are prokaryotic cells that, unlike the eukaryotic cells of the human body, lack an organized nucleus and other intracellular organelles. Bacteria can reproduce independently, but they need a host to supply food and other support. Inside the body, they achieve this by binding to host cells.

Bacteria can be cultured and identified readily in most hospital laboratories. Many bacteria are categorized according to their appearance under the microscope after staining with several dyes referred to as *Gram stains*. Some bacteria stain blue, whereas others stain red. Bacteria that stain blue are referred to as *Gram-positive* bacteria. They are somewhat similar to one another in their structure. Bacteria that stain red are referred to as *Gram-negative* bacteria. They are also somewhat similar to one another in their structure.

Bacteria can cause many of the common infections in medicine, including middle ear infections in children, many cases of tonsillitis, and meningitis. (These kinds of infections can also be caused by viruses, which are discussed in the next section.) Most bacterial infections respond to treatment with drugs called **antibiotics**. Once administered, antibiotics kill or inhibit the growth of invading bacteria. As mentioned earlier, the bacterial cell membrane is the site of action for many antibiotics. Once the cell membrane is broken down, phagocytes (cells that ingest and destroy pathogens and other foreign and abnormal substances) can begin to destroy the bacterium. A variety of antibiotic drugs have been developed with mechanisms of action tailored to different types of bacteria. However, the broad variety of infectious bacteria, and their ability to develop resistance to drugs, makes developing antibiotics to battle them a difficult job.

Some bacteria protect themselves by forming a capsule outside the cell wall that protects the organism from digestion by phagocytes. Some bacteria, such as *Mycoplasmic* bacteria, have no protective capsule but rely on other mechanisms to survive and attack the body. *Mycobacterium tuberculosis*, which has no protective capsule, can actually survive and be transported by phagocytes. Other bacteria simply multiply faster than the body's defense systems can respond. Still others overpower the body's defenses by producing

---

CONTENT REVIEW

➤ Infectious Agents
- Bacteria
- Viruses
- Fungi
- Parasites
- Prions

enzymes and toxins that attack and injure cells and produce hypersensitivity reactions.

Simple infection is not the only consequence of a bacterial invasion. Many bacteria release poisonous chemicals, or *toxins.* There are two types of toxins produced by bacteria: exotoxins and endotoxins. **Exotoxins** are proteins secreted and released by the bacterial cell during its growth. They travel throughout the body via the blood or lymph, ultimately causing problems. For example, botulism toxin, released by the bacterium *Clostridium botulinum,* blocks the release of cholinergic neurotransmitters at neuromuscular junctions and elsewhere in the autonomic nervous system, causing systemic paralysis. Another example is tetanus, which is caused by the bacterium *Clostridium tetani.* The actual infection by the bacteria themselves is mild and may be limited, for example, to the site of a puncture wound in the foot. However, on entering the body, the bacteria release their toxin, *tetanospasmin.* This toxin then travels through the blood to the skeletal muscles, causing the spastic rigidity classically seen in tetanus.

Endotoxins are complex molecules that are contained in the cell walls of certain Gram-negative bacteria. Endotoxins can be released during the destruction of the bacterial cell by phagocytes or even when the bacterial cell is attacked by an antibiotic, so antibiotics cannot control the endotoxic effects of bacteria. When released, endotoxins trigger the inflammatory process and produce fever. In the bloodstream, they can cause widespread clotting within the blood vessels, capillary damage, and hypotension, as well as respiratory distress and fever—a condition known as *endotoxin shock.* Endotoxins can survive even when the cell that produced them is dead.

Depending on their amount and site of release, the effects of toxins can be local or systemic. When a bacterial organism enters the circulatory system, its released toxins can spread throughout the body. The systemic spread of toxins through the bloodstream is known as **septicemia,** or *sepsis,* and is a grave medical illness.

The body counters the bacterial invasion and release of enzymes and toxins through activation of the immune system. The immune system will mobilize foreign-cell–destroying macrophages (a type of white blood cell) to the site of infection in an attempt to rid the body of the foreign pathogen. As the macrophages attempt to destroy the bacteria, they release substances known as *pyrogens.* Pyrogens are responsible for causing the increase in temperature known as fever. Pyrogens act on the thermoregulation center in the hypothalamus to cause the increased body temperature, which is thought to aid in the destruction of pathogens.

Viruses

Most infections are caused by **viruses.** Viruses are much smaller than bacteria and can be seen only with an electron microscope. In addition, they cannot grow without the assistance of another organism. In fact, viruses are referred to as *intracellular parasites,* since they must invade the cells of the organism they infect.

A virus has no organized cellular structure except a protein coat (capsid) surrounding the internal genetic material, deoxyribonucleic acid (DNA) or ribonucleic acid (RNA). With no organized cellular structure or cellular organelles, viruses are incapable of metabolism. Once inside a cell, they take over, using the cellular enzymes to replicate and produce more viruses, which decreases synthesis of macromolecules vital to the host cell.

Some viruses develop a coating in addition to the capsid, called an *envelope.* The envelope and the protein capsid allow the virus to resist destruction by the phagocytes of the immune system. However, because viruses cannot reproduce outside a host cell, if the virus does not find a host cell, it will die.

The symptoms of a virus may not be readily apparent because it is hidden within the host cell. After replication is complete, the virus will sometimes destroy the host cell. In other cases, a virus will remain dormant within a cell for months or years. An example is the *varicella zoster* virus, which causes childhood chicken pox and may then remain dormant, only to cause shingles in the adult decades later. Some viruses form a long-term symbiotic (living in close association) relationship with the host cell, resulting in a persistent but unapparent infection.

Viruses do not produce toxins, but they can still cause very serious illnesses. Some viruses are capable of altering the host cell to induce a malignancy (cancer). Others, such as the *human immunodeficiency virus (HIV),* which causes AIDS, can proliferate, attacking cells of the immune system and destroying its ability to ward off infections of all types.

Unlike bacteria, viruses are very difficult to treat. Once a virus infects a cell, it can be killed only by destroying the infected cell. Drugs have not yet been developed that can selectively destroy cells infected by viruses while leaving uninfected cells unharmed. This partially explains the dilemma facing researchers trying to find a cure for AIDS. An additional problem is that some viruses mutate (change) frequently, which is why a new flu vaccine must be developed for every flu season. Fortunately, most viral illnesses are mild and fairly self-limiting. (Because viral agents must spread from cell to cell, the immune system is eventually able to "catch" them outside a host cell and destroy them.) Even so, at present, viruses usually cannot be treated with more than symptomatic care.

Other Agents of Infection

Other biological agents that cause human infection include *fungi* (the plural of *fungus*) and parasites.

Fungi, which includes yeasts and molds, are more like plants than animals. Fungi rarely cause human disease other than minor skin infections such as athlete's foot and some common vaginal infections. Fungus infections are called *mycoses*. Patients with an impaired immune system, such as HIV patients or patients with organ transplants, suffer fungal infections more commonly than healthy people. In such patients, the fungi can invade the lungs, blood, and several organs. Treatment of complicated, deep fungal infections has proven difficult, even in the hospital setting.

Parasites range in size from protozoa (single-celled animals not much larger than bacteria) to large intestinal worms. Parasites tend to be more common in developing nations than in the United States. Treatment depends on the organism and the location.

Prions are the most recently recognized classification of infectious agents. Initially thought to be slow-acting viruses, prions differ from viruses in that they are smaller, are made entirely of proteins, and do not have protective capsids.

For more about infectious diseases, see the Medical Emergencies chapter titled "Infectious Diseases."

Three Lines of Defense

There are three chief lines of self-defense against infection and injury. One involves anatomic barriers. The other two—the inflammatory response and the immune response—rely on actions of the leukocytes (white blood cells). Each line of defense can be characterized as external or internal, nonspecific or specific (Table 12-14)—characterizations you may want to keep in mind as you read the following sections and compare the ways these defenses protect the body.

Before an infectious agent can attack the body, it has to get past the body's natural anatomic barrier, the epithelium (the skin and the mucous membranes that line the respiratory, gastrointestinal, and genitourinary tracts). The epithelium is more than just a physical barrier; it also provides a chemical defense against infection. The sebaceous glands of the skin secrete fatty and lactic acids, which attack bacteria and fungi. Sweat, tears, and saliva secreted by other glands contain bacteria-attacking

CONTENT REVIEW

➤ Three Lines of Defense against Infection and Injury
  • Anatomic barriers
  • Inflammatory response
  • Immune response

Table 12-14 Three Lines of Defense against Infection and Injury

	External	Internal	Nonspecific	Specific
Anatomic barriers	External		Nonspecific	
Inflammatory response		Internal	Nonspecific	
Immune response		Internal		Specific

Table 12-15 Characteristics of the Inflammatory and Immune Responses

	Inflammatory Response	Immune Response
Speed	Fast	Slow
Specificity	Nonspecific	Specific
Duration (memory)	Transient (no memory)	Long-term (memory)
Involving which plasma systems	Multiple plasma protein (complement, coagulation, kinin systems)	One plasma protein (immunoglobulin)
Involving which cell type	Multiple cell types (granulocytes, monocytes, macrophages)	One blood cell type (lymphocytes)

enzymes. Various mechanical responses also work to get rid of invading substances. For example, the invader may be coughed or sneezed out of the respiratory tract, flushed out of the urinary tract, or eliminated from the gastrointestinal tract by vomiting or diarrhea.

The anatomic defenses are *external* and *nonspecific*. They are considered external because they prevent substances from penetrating the skin or the coverings of internal passageways. They are nonspecific because they defend against all invaders, such as foreign bodies, chemicals, or microorganisms, without targeting any specific type of invader.

If an invading foreign body, chemical, or microorganism penetrates the anatomic barriers and begins to attack internal cells and tissues, two other lines of defense are triggered: the inflammatory response and the immune response. These twin responses of the immune system have contrasting characteristics of speed, specificity, duration (memory), and of the plasma systems and cell types that are involved in the response (Table 12-15).

The *inflammatory response,* or *inflammation,* begins within seconds of injury or invasion by a pathogen. As noted earlier, it is nonspecific, attacking any invader by surrounding it with cells and fluids to isolate, destroy, and eliminate it. Inflammation is mediated by multiple plasma protein systems, especially the complement system, the coagulation system, and the kinin system (which will be explained later) and involves a variety of cell types as it attacks the invader.

The *immune response* develops more slowly (one type of response requires a second exposure after priming by the first exposure to the invader). The immune response is specific, in that it will develop a specialized response for each different invader. It is mediated by just one plasma protein system (immunoglobulin) and attacks the invader mainly with a single cell type (lymphocytes, which are one type of leukocyte, or white blood cell).

Inflammation and the immune response interact in many ways. We will discuss the immune response first, because understanding the immune response is necessary for understanding some parts of the inflammatory response.

The Immune Response

How the Immune Response Works: An Overview

Most viruses, bacteria, fungi, and parasites—as well as noninfectious substances such as pollens, foods, venoms, drugs, and others that may enter the body—have proteins on their surface called **antigens**. The immune system detects these antigens as being foreign, or "non-self," and responds to produce substances called **antibodies** that combine with antigens to control or destroy them. This is known as the **immune response**. As part of this process, *memory cells* "remember" the antigen and will trigger an even faster and more effective response to destroy the same antigen if it enters the body again. Such long-term protection against specific foreign substances is known as **immunity**.

Characteristics of the Immune Response and Immunity

The immune response and immunity can be classified in various ways: natural versus acquired immunity, primary versus secondary immune responses, and humoral versus cell-mediated immunity.

Natural versus Acquired Immunity
Natural immunity is not generated by the immune response. It is inborn, part of the genetic makeup of the individual or of the species in general. For example, the measles virus cannot reproduce in canine cells, so dogs are naturally immune to measles. Conversely, canine distemper cannot thrive within human cells, so humans are naturally immune to that disease. (Some diseases, however, such as leukemia, can affect more than one species.)

Acquired immunity develops as an outcome of the immune response. Acquired immunity can be either active or passive. *Active acquired immunity* is generated by the host's (infected person's) immune system after exposure to an antigen. *Passive acquired immunity* is transferred to a person from an outside source. For example, a mother may transfer antibodies through the placenta to the fetus. Or antibodies may be administered to a patient as an immune serum to aid the body's response to a dangerous invader such as rabies, tetanus, or snake venom. Active acquired immunity is long-lasting. Passive acquired immunity is temporary.

Primary versus Secondary Immune Responses
There are two phases to the immune response to an antigen: the primary immune response and the secondary immune response.

On exposure to an antigen, B lymphocyte cells (explained in the next section) produce antibodies to attack the antigen. These antibodies are called **immunoglobulins**, which are proteins present in the plasma portion of the blood. There are five classes of immunoglobulins—IgM, IgG, IgA, IgE, and IgD.

On first exposure to an antigen, after a lag time of five to seven days, the presence of IgM antibodies can be detected in the blood, with a lesser presence of IgG antibodies. This constitutes the **primary immune response**, also called the *initial immune response.* If there is no further exposure to the antigen, the antibodies are catabolized (broken down)—but the immune system has been "primed." If there is a second exposure to the antigen, the body responds much faster, and a far greater quantity of IgG antibodies is produced. The level of IgG antibodies, with their memory for the specific antigen, will remain elevated for many years. This constitutes the **secondary immune response**, also called the *anamnestic* (or memory-assisting) *immune response.*

The primary and secondary immune responses together create active acquired immunity to the specific antigen.

Humoral versus Cell-Mediated Immunity
A special type of leukocyte (white blood cell) is the **lymphocyte**. Lymphocytes (which constitute about 20 to 35 percent of all leukocytes) are responsible for several critical functions of the immune response, including recognizing foreign antigens, producing antibodies (the immunoglobulins such as IgM and IgG, previously mentioned), and developing memory (Figure 12-92)

As lymphocytes mature, they become one of several types, including B lymphocytes and T lymphocytes. **B lymphocytes** do not attack antigens directly. Instead, they produce the antibodies (immunoglobulins) that attack antigens. B lymphocytes also develop memory, and confer long-term immunity to specific antigens. This type of immunity is called **humoral immunity**. (*Humor* refers to

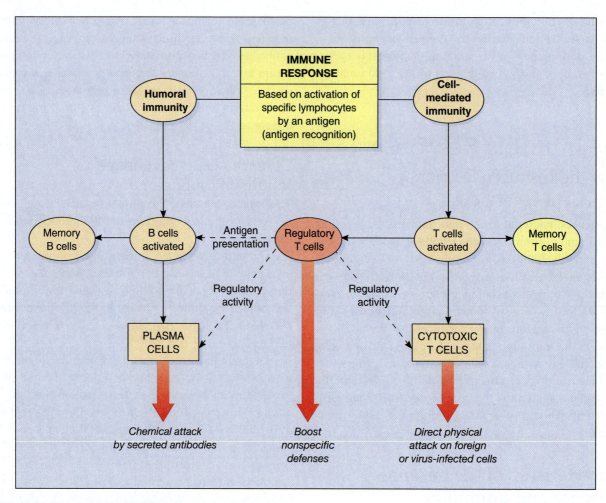

FIGURE 12-92 Humoral and cell-mediated immunity—an overview.

the blood and other fluids of the body; *humoral immunity* refers to the long-lasting antibodies and memory cells present in the blood and lymph.) (Figure 12-93)

T lymphocytes do not produce antibodies. Instead, they recognize the presence of a foreign antigen and attack it directly. This type of immunity is called **cell-mediated immunity** (Figure 12-94).

LYMPHOCYTES AND THE LYMPHATIC SYSTEM

Lymphocytes—including B lymphocytes, T lymphocytes, and secretory lymphocytes (discussed later)—are circulated through the body as part of the lymphatic system. Lymph (the fluid of the lymphatic system) consists primarily of interstitial fluid carrying proteins, bacteria, and other substances. (As discussed earlier in the chapter, most interstitial fluid reenters the bloodstream via the capillaries, but the small amount that does not reenter the capillaries is carried away by the lymphatic system.)

Lymph is carried through the lymphatic vessels, which are parallel to but separate from the blood vessels, and is filtered through *lymph nodes* in various parts of the body. Eventually, the lymph empties into one of two lymphatic ducts in the thorax. The smaller of the two is the *right lymphatic duct*, which drains lymph from the right arm, the right

side of the head, and the right side of the thorax. The larger is the *thoracic duct*, which is located in the left thorax and receives lymph from the rest of the body. These ducts drain the lymph into the right and left subclavian veins, respectively, and the lymph then travels through the bloodstream. The cycle is completed as the lymph is returned from the blood to the tissues to the lymphatic system. In this way, lymph, and the lymphocytes it carries, are circulated through the blood and lymphatic system again and again.

The B lymphocytes and T lymphocytes carried by the blood and the lymphatic system are the key elements in humoral and cell-mediated immunity, which will be discussed in more detail in the next sections.

Induction of the Immune Response

The immune response must be triggered, or induced. The following sections discuss the role of antigens and immunogens, histocompatibility, and blood groups in induction of the immune response.

Antigens and Immunogens

Antigens that can trigger the immune response are called **immunogens**. Not every antigen is an immunogen. In

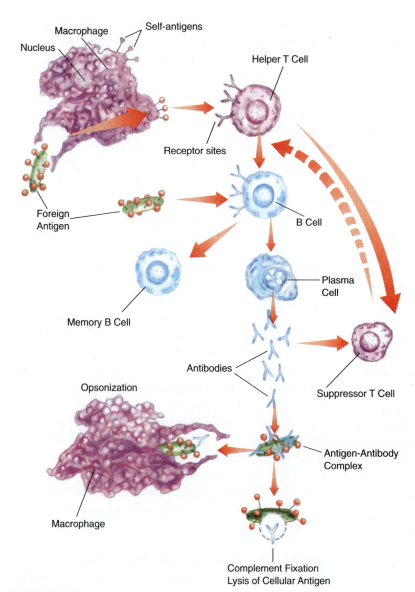

Macrophage — Self-antigens

Nucleus

Helper T Cell

Receptor sites

Foreign Antigen

B Cell

Memory B Cell

Plasma Cell

Antibodies

Opsonization

Suppressor T Cell

Macrophage

Antigen-Antibody Complex

Complement Fixation
Lysis of Cellular Antigen

FIGURE 12-93 Humoral immune response.

As mentioned earlier, the body can distinguish between self and non-self, or foreign, antigens. Normally, the immune system is not triggered by self-antigens. In fact, the immune system does not just "tolerate" self-antigens, it also actively protects them through suppression of the immune system by T lymphocytes and a special antibody called anti-idiopathic antibody.

Large molecules, such as proteins, polysaccharides, and nucleic acids, are the most likely to trigger the immune response. Smaller molecules, such as amino acids, monosaccharides, and fatty acids, are less likely to induce the immune response. Some small molecules, however, can function as **haptens**, meaning that they can become immunogenic when combined with larger molecules.

More complex molecules, and molecules that are present in sufficient numbers, are more likely to trigger an immune response. Additionally, different routes of entry can stimulate different types of cell-mediated or humoral immune response (which dictates the route by which serum antigens may be administered, such as intravenous, subcutaneously, orally, intraperitoneally, intranasally). Other substances present in the body can help to stimulate the immune response. Also, as noted earlier, the person's genetic makeup can affect the ability to respond to antigens.

other words, not every antigen is capable of triggering the immune response. As an example, antigens are present on various helpful bacteria that reside within our bodies, but the immune response is not triggered by these antigens.

What makes a molecule an antigen is a chemical structure that is capable of reacting with existing components of the immune system, such as antibodies and T lymphocytes. However, having this chemical structure, the ability to *react* once the immune system has been triggered, is not enough to *trigger* the immune system in the first place. To be immunogenic—able to trigger an immune response—an antigen must have certain additional characteristics.

Characteristics of Antigenic Immunogenicity

- Sufficient foreignness
- Sufficient size
- Sufficient complexity
- Presence in sufficient amounts

Macrophage Nucleus Self-antigens

Receptor sites Helper T Cell

Foreign Antigen

Memory T Cell Cytotoxic T Cell Suppressor T Cell

Chemically destroys foreign cells Produces cytokines to attract macrophages

FIGURE 12-94 Cell-mediated immune response.

Histocompatibility Locus Antigens

The body recognizes whether a substance is self or non-self as a result of certain antigens that are present on almost all cells of the body, except the red blood cells. These antigens are called **HLA antigens** (for *histocompatibility locus antigens*—or *human leukocyte antigens,* because these antigens were originally found on leukocytes). HLA antigens are the antigens that the body recognizes as self or foreign. The chief genetic source of HLA antigens has been identified as genes located at several sites (loci) on chromosome 6 that are known as the **major histocompatibility complex (MHC)**.

HLA antigens determine the suitability, or compatibility, of tissues and organs that will be grafted or transplanted from a donor. The more closely related the donor and recipient are, the more likely the recipient's body is to accept the graft or transplant. Why? Every person receives half his genetic inheritance from each parent.

Like all genes, the genes that produce HLA antigens occur as pairs (alleles) on corresponding loci on pairs of chromosomes. A group of alleles on one chromosome is called a *haplotype*. Every person has two HLA haplotypes, one on each of the pair of chromosomes. Of each pair of chromosomes (and the HLA haplotypes they carry), the person inherits one from his father and one from his mother.

Because each parent has two haplotypes, but only one gets passed along to each child (to pair up with one from the other parent), various combinations of inherited haplotypes are possible among the children of those parents. In general, each child will share one haplotype with half his siblings, both haplotypes with a quarter of his siblings, and no haplotypes with a quarter of his siblings.

Siblings and other close relatives are generally considered first as donors of tissues and organs because they have the highest likelihood of histocompatibility—hence the least likelihood of the immune system's rejecting the graft or transplant. (Identical twins, who come from the same egg fertilized by the same sperm, have identical genetic makeups and identical haplotypes. Therefore, they are the most reliable match for grafts and transplants.)

Other factors besides HLA makeup can affect the success of a graft or transplant, so they sometimes fail, even when from a histocompatible donor. However, histocompatibility is the most important factor in graft and transplant success.

Blood Group Antigens

HLA antigens do not exist on the surface of erythrocytes (red blood cells), but other antigens, known as the blood group antigens, do. There are more than 80 of these red cell antigens that have been grouped into a number of different blood group systems. The two groups that trigger the strongest immune response are the Rh system and the ABO system.

THE Rh SYSTEM   The **Rh blood group** is named for the rhesus monkey, in which it was first identified. One of several antigens in this group is known as Rh antigen D, or the **Rh factor**. Rh factor is present in about 85 percent of North Americans (Rh positive), but absent in about 15 percent (Rh negative).

Incompatibility between Rh positive and Rh negative blood can cause harmful immune responses. For example, if a patient with Rh negative blood receives a transplant of Rh positive blood, a primary immune response is triggered. If there is a second transfusion of Rh positive blood, a severe transfusion reaction may result.

Hemolytic disease of the newborn may result from Rh incompatibility between mother and fetus. Problems will usually not occur in a first pregnancy where the mother is Rh negative and the fetus is Rh positive, because few fetal erythrocytes cross the placental barrier to the mother. However, a significant number of fetal erythrocytes do enter the mother's bloodstream at birth when the placenta separates from the uterus. These may (depending on several factors) activate a primary immune response and development of Rh antibodies. If the fetus in her next pregnancy is also Rh positive, the mother's Rh antibodies can cross the placenta and destroy the red blood cells of the fetus. This is actually a rare occurrence. Rh incompatibility occurs in only about 10 percent of pregnancies, and because not all such incompatibilities actually produce Rh antibodies in the mother, only about 5 percent of women ever have babies with hemolytic disease, even after numerous pregnancies.

THE ABO SYSTEM   The **ABO blood groups** are formed because there are two types of antigens that may be present on the surface of red blood cells. These antigens are named A and B. Persons with blood type A carry only A antigens on their red blood cells. Those with blood type B carry only B antigens. Those with blood type AB carry both, and those with blood type O carry neither (Table 12-16).

An immune response will be activated in a person with type A blood who receives a transfusion of type B blood, which is recognized as non-self. The same will happen when a person with type B blood receives type A blood. People with type O blood are known as *universal*

Table 12-16 Blood Groups—ABO System

Blood Type	Antigen Present on Erythrocyte	Antibody Present in Serum
O	None	Anti-A, Anti-B
AB	A and B	None
B	B	Anti-A
A	A	Anti-B

Table 12-17 Compatibility among ABO Blood Groups

Cells of Donor	Reaction with Serum of Recipient			
	AB	B	A	O
AB	−	+	+	+
B	−	−	+	+
A	−	+	−	+
O	−	−	−	−

− = No Reaction
+ = Reaction

donors, because type O blood has no antigens that will trigger an immune response in any other group. Those with type AB blood are known as *universal recipients*, because they have both types of antigens and will not produce antibodies in response to any other blood groups (Table 12-17).

ABO incompatibility between mother and fetus is more common than Rh incompatibility, occurring in about 20 to 25 percent of pregnancies. However, only 10 percent of ABO incompatibilities will result in hemolytic disease of the infant.

Humoral Immune Response

Earlier, we identified the humoral immune response as the long-lasting response provided by production in the bloodstream of antibodies (immunoglobulins) and memory cells by B lymphocytes (review Figure 12-93). This is sometimes called the *internal* or *systemic immune system*. Another kind of humoral immunity is provided by secretions at the body surfaces, such as sweat and saliva, and is sometimes called the *external, mucosal,* or *secretory immune system*. These types of humoral immune responses will be discussed in the following sections.

B Lymphocytes

The blood cells that are involved in immune response, as noted earlier, are lymphocytes, which are one type of white blood cell. Lymphocytes are generated from *stem cells* in the bone marrow, from which all blood cells are generated. Lymphocytes then take one of two paths as they mature. In one path, lymphocytes that travel through the thymus gland mature into T lymphocytes, which are involved in cell-mediated immunity and will be discussed in detail later. On the other path, lymphocytes that travel through a set of lymphoid tissues, including the spleen and lymph nodes, mature into B lymphocytes, which are involved in humoral immunity.

Each mature B cell recognizes, through an antigen receptor on its surface, a single type of antigen and then produces antibodies to that antigen. But since there are many, many kinds of antigens—and since exactly which foreign antigens may ever invade the body cannot be antic-

ipated—how does a B cell develop a receptor that is specialized to a specific antigen?

It is thought that this specialization of B cells takes place through the processes of clonal diversity and clonal selection. **Clonal diversity** is generated as the precursors of mature B cells develop in the bone marrow. During this process, a B cell precursor develops receptors for every possible kind of antigen it may ever encounter. Later, after the immature B cells have migrated into the peripheral lymphoid organs, primarily the spleen and the lymph nodes, antigen that is present in the system reacts with the appropriate receptors on the surfaces of B cell clones, which is the process of **clonal selection**.

Clonal selection activates the immature B cell, prompting it to proliferate and differentiate, the end result being the mature B cell that produces plasma cells that secrete immunoglobulin antibodies into the blood and secondary lymphoid organs. The mature B cell also produces **memory cells** that will trigger a swifter and stronger immune response if they encounter the same antigen again (the secondary immune response). The process of clonal selection is probably responsible (during the primary immune response) for the lag time of five to seven days between introduction of an antigen and the first detectable appearance of antibodies in the blood.

Immunoglobulins

IMMUNOGLOBULINS AND ANTIBODIES Antibodies are proteins secreted by plasma cells that are produced by B cells in response to an antigen. All antibodies are immunoglobulins, but researchers have not yet determined whether all immunoglobulins function as antibodies.

THE STRUCTURE OF IMMUNOGLOBULINS The structure of immunoglobulin molecules consists of Y-shaped chains, arranged somewhat differently in the different immunoglobulin classes (Figure 12-95). At the two "upper" tips of the Y are the *antigen-binding sites*. The interaction of amino acids with parts of the chain determines the shape of the immunoglobulin molecule's antigen-binding site. The shape of the antigen-binding site determines which antigen the immunoglobulin molecule will bind to—because there is an area on the antigen (the antigenic determinant) that will fit the shape of the antigen-binding site like a key in a lock (Figure 12-96). In some cases, substitution of a single amino acid changes the conformation of the antigen-binding site and, therefore, the antigen it will combine with.

THE FUNCTIONS OF ANTIBODIES An antibody circulates in the blood or is suspended in body secretions until it meets and binds to its specific antigen. The antibody can then have either a direct or an indirect effect on the target antigen that results in inactivation or destruction of the antigen. Both direct and indirect effects result from the binding

FIGURE 12-95 Some immunoglobulin (antibody) structures.

FIGURE 12-96 Antigen–antibody binding. The shape of the antigen fits the shape of the antigen-binding site on the immunoglobulin (antibody) molecule like a key in a lock.

of antibodies and antigens, forming **antigen–antibody complexes**, also called *immune complexes*.

Direct Effects of Antibodies on Antigens

- *Agglutination*—A soluble antibody combines with a solid antigen, causing it to clump together.

- *Precipitation*—The antigen–antibody complex precipitates out of the blood and is carried away by body fluids.

- *Neutralization*—The antibody, in combining with the antigen, inactivates the antigen by preventing it from binding to receptors on the surface of body cells.

Indirect Effects of Antibodies on Antigens

- *Enhancement of phagocytosis—Phagocytosis* is one of the chief processes of inflammation (described later in the chapter) in which certain types of white blood cells (neutrophils and macrophages) ingest and digest foreign substances. The actions of antibodies can encourage phagocytosis.

- *Activation of plasma proteins*—Antibodies can activate plasma proteins of the complement system (described later) that, in turn, attack and destroy antigens.

Through the direct and indirect effects previously described, antibodies serve four main functions: neutralizing bacterial toxins, neutralizing viruses, opsonizing bacteria, and activating portions of the inflammatory response.

- ***Neutralization of bacterial toxins.*** As noted earlier, many bacteria produce harmful toxins that increase their pathogenic effect. However, bacterial toxins sow the seeds of their own destruction by triggering the humoral immune response. In this case the antigen–antibody complex is a *toxin–antitoxin complex*. Antibodies neutralize the bacterial toxins by occupying their antigenic determinant sites, which prevents them from binding to and harming tissue cells. Detection of specific antitoxins aids in the diagnosis of disease. Vaccines against diseases such as diphtheria and tetanus work by injecting a form of the bacterial toxin, which is altered to greatly reduce its toxic effects but to retain its immunogenicity.

- ***Neutralization of viruses.*** Antibodies can prevent some viruses from attaching to and entering body cells. The antibodies attach to the viruses, causing agglutination or fostering phagocytosis. The effectiveness of antibodies against viruses depends on whether the virus circulates in the bloodstream (as with polio and flu) or spreads by direct cell-to-cell contact (as with measles and herpes). Antibodies against the latter may help prevent the initial infection but cannot prevent the spread or recurrence of an established infection. Vaccines are effective against some viral infections such as influenza, rubella, and polio.

- *Opsonization of bacteria.* Many bacteria have an outer capsule that is resistant to phagocytosis. Opsonization coats the bacteria with opsonin, a substance that makes them vulnerable to phagocytosis. Antibodies themselves are opsonins, and they also cause opsonization by a plasma protein that is a component of the complement system.

- *Activation of inflammatory processes.* When the antigen-binding sites at the "upper" tips of the Y-shaped immunoglobulin molecule bind to an antigen, the "lower" tip activates elements of the inflammatory response, transmitting the information that a foreign invader has entered the body. The inflammatory response (which will be described later) enhances the attack by the immune system against the invader.

CLASSES OF IMMUNOGLOBULINS As noted earlier, there are five classes of immunoglobulins:

IgM—the antibody that is produced first during the primary immune response. It is the largest immunoglobulin.

IgG—the antibody that has "memory" and recognizes repeated invasions of an antigen. IgG comprises 80 to 85 percent of immunoglobulins in the blood. It is the major class of immunoglobulin in the immune response and has four subclasses. IgG is responsible for antibody functions such as agglutination, precipitation, and complement activation.

IgA—the antibody present in mucous membranes. One subclass of IgA is the predominant immunoglobulin in body secretions. The other subclass of IgA is present mostly in the blood.

IgE—the least-concentrated immunoglobulin in the circulation. It is the principal antibody that contributes to allergic and anaphylactic reactions and to the prevention of parasitic infections.

IgD—an antibody that is present in very low concentrations; little is known about its role. It is present principally on the surfaces of developing B cells.

ANTIBODIES AS ANTIGENS A molecule that functions as an antibody in the human body can function as an antigen if it enters the body of another person or a member of another species. To function in the role of antigens,

antibody molecules usually contain antigenic determinants with which the antigen-binding sites on other antibodies can combine.

The antigenic determinants on human antibody molecules are classified into three groups:

- *Isotypic antigens* are species-specific. That is, they are the same within a given species but differ from those within other species. For example, isotypic antigens in human serum would function as antigens if injected into a rabbit.

- *Allotypic antigens* can differ between members of the same species. The serum from a person with one form of allotype might function as an antigen in another person.

- *Idiotypic antigenic determinants* can differ within the same individual. For example, IgG subclass 3 molecules produced against mumps and those produced against tetanus in the same person will differ from each other.

MONOCLONAL ANTIBODIES Most antigens have multiple antigenic determinants, which stimulate a response from multiple clones of B lymphocytes. This is known as a *polyclonal response.* Each B cell clone secretes antibody that is slightly different from that of the other clones. Recently, researchers have been working with monoclonal antibodies. A **monoclonal antibody**, produced in the laboratory, is very pure and specific to a single antigen. Monoclonal antibodies are being put to a variety of cutting-edge and experimental uses, including identification of infectious organisms, blood and tissue typing, and treatment of autoimmune diseases and some cancers.

The Secretory Immune System

The **secretory immune system** (also known as the *external* or *mucosal immune system*) consists of lymphoid tissues beneath the mucosal endothelium. These tissues secrete substances such as sweat, tears, saliva, mucus, and breast milk. Some antibodies are present in these secretions (mostly IgA, with some IgM and IgG) and can help defend the body (or the nursing baby) against antigens that have not yet penetrated the skin or the mucous membranes.

The secretory immune system's primary function is to protect the body from pathogens that are inhaled or ingested. Other mechanisms must be functioning adequately to complete that task. For example, gastric acid helps destroy pathogens, and mechanisms such as blinking, sneezing, coughing, and peristalsis (the wavelike muscle contractions that move substances through the passageways of the digestive system) help move pathogens out of the system.

The lymphocytes of the secretory immune system follow a different developmental path after leaving the bone marrow than do the lymphocytes of the systemic immune system. As they mature, systemic lymphocytes migrate through the spleen and lymph nodes, whereas lymphocytes of the secretory system travel through the lacrimal (tear-producing) and salivary glands and through mucosal-associated lymphoid tissues in the bronchi, breasts, intestines, and genitourinary tract.

Secretory lymphocytes circulate through the lymphatic system and bloodstream in a pattern that is different from the circulatory pattern of the systemic lymphocytes. Secretory lymphocytes are returned from the blood through the tissues to the mucosal-associated lymphoid tissues, rather than to the lymphoid tissues of the systemic immune system.

The secretory immune system is the body's first line of defense against pathogens, whereas the systemic immune system is the body's last line of defense.

Cell-Mediated Immune Response

Some lymphocytes develop into B cells, which are responsible for *humoral immunity*, which we have discussed in the prior sections. Other lymphocytes develop into T cells, which are responsible for *cell-mediated immunity*, the subject of this section (review Figure 12-94).

A key difference between the two is that B cells do not attack pathogens directly. Instead, they produce antibodies that combine with antigens on the surfaces of pathogenic cells. The antibodies remain in the bloodstream for a long time and will attack the antigen again on any subsequent exposure. Thus, the humoral immunity created by B cells is long-lasting. T cells, however, do not produce antibodies. Rather, they attack pathogens directly, and the immunity they create, called cell-mediated immunity, is temporary.

Another key distinction is that one kind of T cell (helper T cells) is responsible for activating both T cells (in cell-mediated immune response) and B cells (in humoral immune response). (To compare humoral and cell-mediated responses, review Figures 12-92 through 12-94.

T Lymphocytes and Their Major Effects

In contrast to B lymphocytes, which travel through the spleen and lymph nodes as they mature, T cells travel through the thymus gland (hence the name *T cell*).

T cells become specialized through processes that are similar to the processes described earlier for B cells: clonal diversity and clonal selection. After generation by stem cells in the bone marrow, lymphocytes destined to become T cells travel to the thymus. There, through the process of *clonal diversity*, maturing T cells develop the capacity to recognize all the antigens they will ever encounter. Later, after the T cells have migrated into the peripheral lymphoid organs, they undergo the process of *clonal selection*. In this process, the immature T cells encounter antigens that react with appropriate receptors on the surfaces of the T cells, causing them to proliferate and differentiate into five different types of mature T cells, each with distinct functions.

Five Types of Mature T Cells

- *Memory cells* induce secondary immune responses.
- *Td cells* transfer delayed hypersensitivity (allergic responses) and secrete proteins called *lymphokines* that activate other cells, such as macrophages.
- *Tc cells* are cytotoxic cells that directly attack and destroy cells that bear foreign antigens.
- *Th cells* are *helper cells* that facilitate both cell-mediated and humoral immune processes.
- *Ts cells* are *suppressor cells* that inhibit both cell-mediated and humoral immune processes.

As a result of this specialization, T cells are capable of attacking an antigen in a variety of ways. The major effects of cell-mediated immune response result from the specialized functions of the four types of T cells: memory, delayed hypersensitivity, cytotoxicity, and control.

MEMORY Memory cells "remember" an antigen and trigger the immune response to any repeated exposure to that antigen.

DELAYED HYPERSENSITIVITY Td cells (delayed hypersensitivity cells) are involved in allergic reactions and the inflammatory response. They produce substances (lymphokines) that communicate with and influence the behavior of other cells.

CYTOTOXICITY Tc cells (cytotoxic cells) mediate the direct killing of target cells, such as cells that have been infected by a virus, tumor cells, or cells in transplanted organs (Figure 12-97).

CONTROL Th (helper) cells and Ts (suppressor) cells effect control of both humoral and cell-mediated immune responses. Th cells facilitate the response; Ts cells inhibit the response.

Cellular Interactions in Immune Response

The immune and inflammatory responses are interacting, not separate. For example:

Sequence of Events	Interaction
Macrophages released during an inflammatory response activate the helper T cells (Th cells).	Inflammatory response interacting with cell-mediated immune response
The helper T cells (Th cells) activate other T cells, and they also activate B cells.	Cell-mediated immune response interacting with humoral immune response
Delayed hypersensitivity T cells (Td cells) stimulate the production of more macrophages.	Cell-mediated immune response interacting with inflammatory response

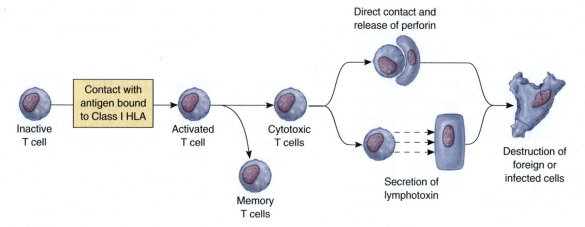

FIGURE 12-97 The physiology of cytotoxic T cells.

The three key interactions that occur during an immune response (review Figures 12-93 and 12-94) are:

1. Antigen-presenting cells (macrophages) interact with Th (helper) cells.
2. Th (helper) cells interact with B cells.
3. Th (helper) cells interact with Tc (cytotoxic) cells.

Cytokines

Cytokines, proteins produced by white blood cells, are the "messengers" of the immune response. When released by one cell, they can bind with nearby cells, affecting their function. They can also bind with the same cell that produced them and alter the function of that cell. They help to regulate cell functions during both inflammatory and immune responses. For example, a cytokine must be released by a macrophage to facilitate activation of a helper T cell.

A cytokine that is released by a macrophage is called a **monokine** ("mono" because a macrophage is a kind of monocyte, a single-nucleus white blood cell). A cytokine that is released by a lymphocyte (a T cell or B cell) is called a **lymphokine**. Types of cytokines include proteins known as *interleukins, interferon,* and *tumor necrosis factor.*

Antigen Processing, Presentation, and Recognition

A sequence of three processes is necessary before an immune response can begin:

1. Antigen processing (by macrophages)
2. Antigen presentation (by macrophages)
3. Antigen recognition (by T cells or B cells)

More will be said later in the chapter about how macrophages are released during the inflammatory response. For now, keep in mind that a *macrophage* is a large cell (a type of white blood cell) that will ingest and destroy or partially destroy an invading organism. As it does so, the invader's antigens are released into the cytosol (fluid interior) of the macrophage cell. The ingestion of an invading organism and breakdown of its antigens is the beginning of **antigen processing**.

Once the macrophage has broken down the antigens, it then expresses these antigen fragments and "presents" them on its own surface, along with its own self-antigens. When these two markers on the surface of the macrophage—the foreign antigens and the self-antigens—are recognized by helper T cells, the helper T cells are activated.

Because macrophages (and other macrophagelike cells) present portions of antigen on their surfaces, they are called **antigen-presenting cells (APCs)**.

The helper T cells recognize the presented antigen through receptors on their surfaces. There are two types of receptors. One type, called a **T cell receptor (TCR)**, is antigen-specific; that is, it will respond to only one specific antigen. The other type, CD4 or CD8 receptors, will respond no matter what antigen is presented.

As discussed earlier, the body recognizes whether an antigen is self or non-self as a result of HLA antigens. For presentation of an antigen to be effective, the antigen must be in a complex with either class I or class II HLA antigens. The HLA class determines which cells will respond. Th (helper) cells respond only to class II HLA antigens. Tc (cytotoxic) cells and Ts (suppressor) cells respond only to class I HLA antigens.

In addition to the antigen–receptor interaction, another requirement for intercellular communication between the macrophage cell and the T cell is an interaction between *self-adhesion molecules* on the surface of the macrophage and the T cell. These molecules, in connecting, strengthen the interactions between the cells.

The macrophage also produces the cytokine interleukin-1 (IL-1), which helps the T cell respond to the presented antigens.

T Cell and B Cell Differentiation

T cells and B cells are not differentiated until antigens present in the system react with the appropriate receptors on the cell surfaces. As previously described, this reaction occurs as a result of antigen processing and presentation by macrophages and antigen recognition by the T or B cell. The presence of secreted cytokines is also usually necessary to facilitate the antigen–receptor reaction.

Once a reaction between antigen and T cell receptor takes place, the immature T cells proliferate and differentiate, depending on the specific receptors and antigens involved, into Th, Tc, Td, Ts, and memory cells.

After stimulation by Th cells or direct recognition of antigen, B cells will proliferate and produce antibodies differentiated as IgM, IgG, IgA, IgE, and IgD immunoglobulins.

Control of T Cell and B Cell Development

Several parameters control immune responses, activating them when needed but stopping or inhibiting them when not needed, thus preventing them from destroying the body's own tissues. As noted earlier, Ts (suppressor) cells help suppress immune responses; so do some macrophages and other monocytes.

The exact function of suppressor cells is still not fully understood. Some suppressor cells seem to affect antigen recognition, whereas others seem to suppress the proliferation that follows antigen recognition. Tolerance of self-antigens seems to be another function of suppressor cells.

Fetal and Neonatal Immune Function

The human infant develops some immune response capabilities, even *in utero*, but the immune response system is normally not fully mature when the infant is born. For example, in the last trimester, the fetus can produce a primary immune response involving mostly IgM antibody to some infections. The ability to produce IgG and IgA antibodies is underdeveloped.

To protect the child *in utero* and during the first few months after birth, maternal antibodies cross the placenta into the fetal circulation. In the placenta, specialized cells called *trophoblasts* separate maternal from fetal blood. The trophoblastic cells actively transport the large immunoglobulin cells from maternal to fetal circulation. This transport is so effective that the level of antibodies in the umbilical cord is sometimes higher than in the mother's blood.

After birth, when antibodies can no longer be transported from the mother's blood, the levels of antibodies in the newborn's blood begin to drop as the immunoglobulins present at birth are catabolized, while the infant's ability to produce immunoglobulins on its own is still not fully developed. The levels are generally at their lowest at about 5 or 6 months of age (when many infants experience recurrent respiratory tract infections). Then, as the immune system matures, the levels of immunoglobulin begin to rise.

Aging and the Immune Response

As the human body ages, immune function begins to deteriorate. B cell antibody production is affected, but the primary assault is on T cell function. The thymus, which is the organ responsible for T cell development, reaches its maximum size at sexual maturity and then decreases in size until, in middle age, it has shrunk by 65 percent. Circulating T cells do not decrease, but T cell function may diminish. Men and women over age 60 generally have decreased hypersensitivity (allergic) responses and decreased T cell response to infections.

For a summary of the immune response, see Figure 12-98.

Inflammation
Inflammation Contrasted to the Immune Response

Inflammation, also called the *inflammatory response*, is the body's response to cellular injury. It differs from the immune response in many ways. As you read the following sections, keep in mind that:

- The immune response develops *slowly*; inflammation develops *swiftly*.

- The immune response is *specific* (targets specific antigens); inflammation is *nonspecific* (it attacks all unwanted substances in the same way). In fact, inflammation is sometimes called "the nonspecific immune response."

- The immune response is *long-lasting* (memory cells will remember an antigen and trigger a swift response on reexposure, even years later); inflammation is *temporary*, lasting only until the immediate threat is conquered—usually only a few days to two weeks.

- The immune response involves *one type of white blood cell* (lymphocytes); inflammation involves *platelets and many types of white blood cells* (the granulatory cells called neutrophils, basophils, and eosinophils; and the monocytes that mature into macrophages).

- The immune response involves *one type of plasma protein* (immunoglobulins, also called antibodies); inflammation involves *several plasma protein systems* (complement, coagulation, and kinin).

However, the immune response and inflammation are interdependent. For example, macrophages that are developed during the inflammatory response must ingest antigens before helper T cells can recognize them and trigger

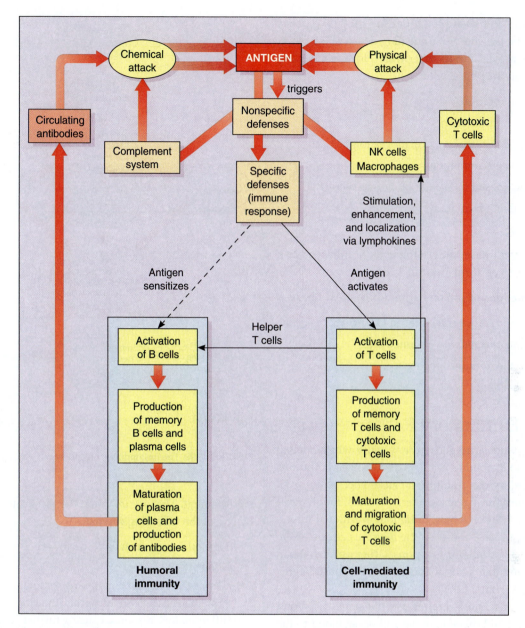

FIGURE 12-98 The immune response.

the immune response. Conversely, IgE antibody produced by B cells during an immune response can stimulate mast cells to activate inflammation.

Although inflammation differs from the immune response in many ways, inflammation and the immune response are both considered to be part of the body's immune system.

How Inflammation Works: An Overview

Inflammation is somewhat easier to understand than the immune response, because we have all observed it. The immune response is often hidden; your body's immune system may be knocking out an infectious antigen without your ever being aware of it. However, if you cut your finger, you will probably be acutely aware of the inflammatory process. You will actually see the redness and swelling and feel the pain. You may observe the formation of pus. As days go by, you will see the progress of wound healing and, perhaps, scar formation.

This is not to say that inflammation is simple; in its way, it is as complex as the immune response. There are several phases to

CONTENT REVIEW

➤ Phases of Inflammation
- *Phase 1:* Acute inflammation (if healing not accomplished, move to Phase 2)
- *Phase 2:* Chronic inflammation (if healing not accomplished, move to Phase 3)
- *Phase 3:* Granuloma formation
- *Phase 4:* Healing (may take place after any of the first three phases)

inflammation. After each phase, healing may take place, and that will be the end of it. If healing doesn't take place, inflammation moves into its next phase. However, healing is the goal of all the phases.

Phases of Inflammation

Phase 1: Acute inflammation

    (If healing doesn't take place, moves to phase 2)

Phase 2: Chronic inflammation

    (If healing doesn't take place, moves to phase 3)

Phase 3: Granuloma formation

Phase 4: Healing

During each phase, the components of inflammation work together to perform four functions.

The Four Functions of Inflammation (during All Phases)

- Destroy and remove unwanted substances
- Wall off the infected and inflamed area
- Stimulate the immune response
- Promote healing

Acute Inflammatory Response

Acute inflammation is triggered by any injury, whether lethal or nonlethal, to the body's cells. As discussed earlier in this chapter, cell injury can result from causes such as hypoxia, chemicals, infectious agents (bacteria, viruses, fungi, parasites), trauma, heat extremes, radiation, nutritional imbalances, genetic factors, and even the injurious effects of the immune and inflammatory responses themselves. When cells are injured, the acute inflammatory response begins within seconds (Figure 12-99).

The basic mechanics are always the same: (1) Blood vessels contract and dilate to move additional blood to the site. Then, (2) vascular permeability increases so that (3) white cells and plasma proteins can move through the capillary walls and into the tissues to begin the tasks of destroying the invader and healing the injury site (Figure 12-100).

Mast Cells

Mast cells, which resemble bags of granules, are the chief activators of the inflammatory response. They are not blood cells. Instead, they reside in connective tissues just outside the blood vessels.

Mast cells activate the inflammatory response through two functions: *degranulation* and *synthesis* (Figure 12-101).

CONTENT REVIEW

➤ Mast Cell Functions
- Degranulation
- Synthesis

Degranulation

Degranulation is the process by which mast cells empty granules from their interior into the extracellular

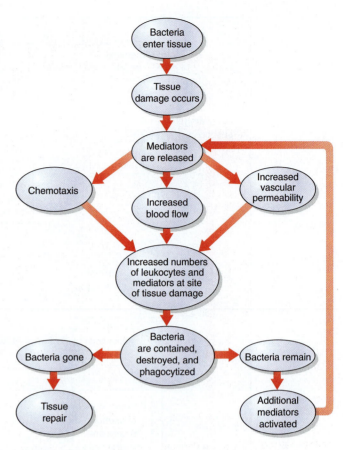

FIGURE 12-99 The inflammatory response.

environment. This occurs when the mast cell is stimulated by one of the following events:

- *Physical injury*, such as trauma, radiation, or temperature extremes
- *Chemical agents*, such as toxins, venoms, enzymes, or a protein released by neutrophils (the latter an example of inflammatory response causing further cellular injury)
- *Immunologic and direct processes*, such as hypersensitivity (allergic) reactions involving release of IgE antibody or activation of complement components (discussed later)

During degranulation, biochemical agents in the mast cell granules are released, notably vasoactive amines and chemotactic factors.

VASOACTIVE AMINES **Histamine** is a vasoactive amine (organic compound) released during degranulation of mast cells. The effect of vasoactive amines is the constriction of the smooth muscle of large vessel walls and dilation of the postcapillary sphincter, resulting in increased blood flow at the injury site.

Basophils (a type of white blood cell) also release histamine, with the same effect. Additionally, **serotonin**, released by platelets, can have effects of both vasoconstriction and vasodilation that may affect blood flow to the affected site.

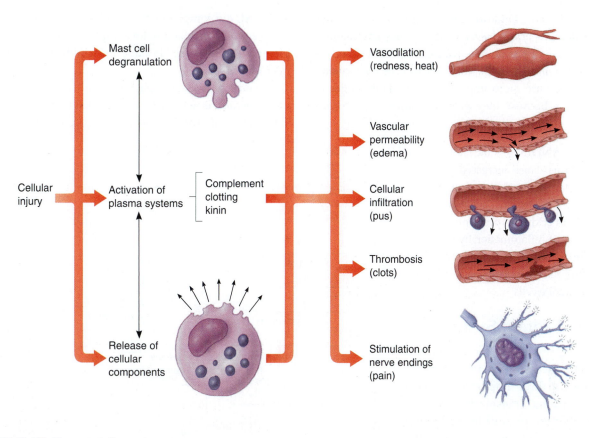

FIGURE 12-100 The acute inflammatory response.

CHEMOTACTIC FACTORS Another consequence of degranulation of mast cells is the release of **chemotactic factors**. Chemotactic factors are chemicals that attract white cells to the site of inflammation. This attraction of white cells is called **chemotaxis**.

Synthesis

When stimulated, mast cells synthesize, or construct, two substances that play important roles in inflammation: leukotrienes and prostaglandins.

Cause: Mast cell stimulated by:
- Physical injury (e.g., trauma, radiation, temperature extremes)
- Chemical agent (e.g., toxin, venom, enzyme, neutrophil-produced protein)
- Immunologic process (e.g., allergic reaction/IgE antibody, activated complement)

Plasma membrane

Granules

Result: Degranulation (release of histamine, serotonin, and chemotactic factors)

Result: Synthesis (construction of leukotrienes and prostaglandins)

Nucleus

FIGURE 12-101 Mast cell degranulation and synthesis.

LEUKOTRIENES **Leukotrienes** are also known as *slow-reacting substances of anaphylaxis (SRS-A)*. They have actions similar to those of histamines—vasoconstriction, vasodilation, and increased permeability—as well as chemotaxis. However, they are more important in the later stages of inflammation, because they promote slower and longer-lasting effects than histamines.

PROSTAGLANDINS Like leukotrienes, **prostaglandins** cause increased vasodilation, vascular permeability, and chemotaxis. They are also the substances that cause pain. In addition, prostaglandins act to control some inflammation by suppressing release of histamine from mast cells and suppressing release of lysosomal enzymes from some white cells.

Plasma Protein Systems

The actions of white blood cells and other components of inflammation are mediated by three important **plasma protein systems**. (Plasma proteins are proteins that are present in the blood.) One group of plasma proteins, the immunoglobulins, or antibodies, are key factors in the immune response, as discussed earlier. Three other plasma protein systems are critical to inflammation: the complement system, the coagulation system, and the kinin system.

Important to an understanding of these plasma protein systems is the concept of **cascade**. In a cascade, a first action is stimulated, that action causes the next action, which causes the next action, and so on until a final action has been completed.

The Complement System

The **complement system** consists of 11 proteins (numbered C-1 through C-9, plus factors B and D) and comprises about 10 percent of all the proteins that circulate in the blood. The complement proteins lie inactive in the blood until they are activated. The complement system can be activated by formation of antigen–antibody complexes, by products released by invading bacteria, or by components of other plasma protein systems.

Once the C-1 complement is activated, the *complement cascade* proceeds through the rest of the sequence of proteins. When

activated, the complement system takes part in almost all the events of the inflammatory response. The last few complements in the cascade have the ability to directly kill microorganisms.

There are two chief pathways by which the complement cascade is activated and proceeds: the classic pathway and the alternative pathway (Figure 12-102).

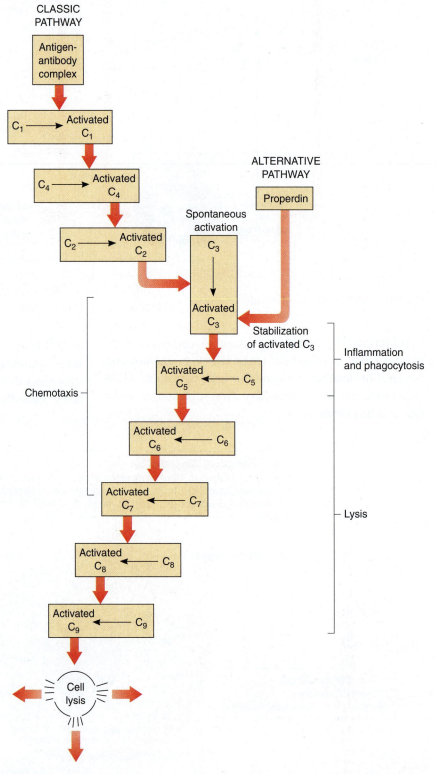

FIGURE 12-102 The complement cascade. The classic pathway is activated at C1, whereas the alternative pathway is activated at C3.

THE CLASSIC PATHWAY
In the classic pathway, the complement system is activated by formation of an antigen–antibody complex during the immune response. Complement factor C-1 is activated, and the cascade proceeds through complement factor C-9. Only a few antigen–antibody complexes are required to activate the complement cascade. The enzymes that are formed stimulate formation of increasing numbers of enzymes as the cascade proceeds, so that a very large response ensues, even from a small initial stimulus.

A number of effects that result from the complement cascade assist in destroying or limiting the damage of the invading organism. These include opsonization (coating) and phagocytosis (ingesting) of the organism, lysis (rupturing of bacterial cell membranes), agglutination (causing invading organisms to clump together), neutralization of viruses, chemotaxis of white cells, increased blood flow, and increased permeability. Complement proteins also lodge in the tissues and help to prevent spread of the infection.

THE ALTERNATIVE PATHWAY In some instances, the complement cascade can be activated without an intervening antigen–antibody complex formed by the immune response. Substances produced by some invading organisms are capable of reacting with complement factors B and D, which produce a substance that activates complement factor C-3, and the complement cascade then proceeds to its end.

Because the alternative pathway begins without waiting for the development of an antigen–antibody complex, it is much faster than the classic pathway and acts as part of the first line of inflammatory defense.

The Coagulation System

The **coagulation system**, also called the *clotting system*, forms a network at the site of inflammation. The network is composed primarily of a protein called *fibrin*, which is the end product of the coagulation cascade. The fibrinous network stops the spread of infectious agents and products of inflammation, keeps microorganisms "corralled" in the area of greatest phagocyte concentration, forms a clot that stops bleeding, and forms the foundation for repair and healing (Figure 12-103).

The *coagulation cascade* can be activated by many substances released during tissue destruction and infection. As with the complement cascade, the coagulation cascade can be activated through either of two pathways. The pathways of coagulation cascade activation are the extrinsic pathway

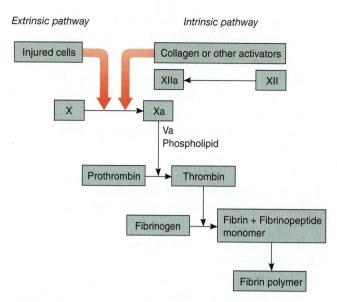

FIGURE 12-103 The coagulation cascade.

and the intrinsic pathway. The *extrinsic pathway* of coagulation begins with injury to the vascular wall or surrounding tissues. It requires exposure of the blood to a tissue factor that originates outside the blood. The *intrinsic pathway* of coagulation begins with exposure to elements in the blood itself, such as collagen from a traumatized vessel wall.

As with the complement cascade, the two pathways converge at a certain point and continue toward the same end product, fibrin. Substances produced during the complement cascade also enhance the inflammatory response, including increase of vascular permeability and chemotaxis.

The Kinin System

The **kinin system** has, as its chief product, *bradykinin*, which causes vasodilation, extravascular smooth muscle contraction, increased permeability, and possibly chemotaxis. It also works with prostaglandins to cause pain. Its effects are similar to the effects of histamine, but bradykinin works more slowly than histamine and so is probably more important during the later phases of inflammation.

The *plasma kinin cascade* is triggered by factors associated with the coagulation cascade. The sequence of the kinin cascade is conversion of prekallikrein to kallikrein, which then converts kininogen to kinin. Another source of kinin is the tissue kallikreins in saliva, sweat, tears, urine, and feces. Whatever the source, kinin is the end product, with bradykinin being the chief kinin.

Control and Interaction of Plasma Protein Systems

Control of the plasma protein systems is important for two reasons:

• The inflammatory response is essential for protection of the body from unwanted invaders. Its functioning must be guaranteed. Therefore, there are numerous means of stimulating the inflammatory response, including those of the plasma protein systems.

- Conversely, the inflammatory processes are powerful and potentially very damaging to the body. Therefore, they must be controlled and confined to the site of injury or infection. Obviously, there are a variety of mechanisms that regulate or inactivate inflammatory responses.

The inflammatory response is controlled at a number of levels and by a variety of mechanisms. For example, many components of inflammation are destroyed within seconds by enzymes from the blood plasma. Antagonists (substances or actions that counteract other substances or actions) exist for histamine, kinins, complement components, and other components of the inflammatory response.

An example of antagonistic control of inflammation is the function of histamine receptors. Histamine works by attaching itself to two types of receptors on the surface of target cells, H1 and H2 receptors. H1 receptors, when contacted by histamine, promote inflammation. H2 receptors are antagonistic to H1 receptors; when contacted by histamine, H2 receptors inhibit inflammation, mainly by suppressing leukocyte function and mast cell degranulation. In this way, the inflammatory action of histamine is triggered when needed, yet kept within bounds.

Most of the inflammatory processes interact; a substance or action that activates one element tends to activate others as well. For example, plasmin, an important factor in clot formation in the coagulation cascade, also has a role in activating the complement and kinin cascades. Conversely, controls on inflammatory processes also tend to interact. For example, a substance known as C1 esterase inhibitor inhibits plasmin activation that, in turn, tends to inhibit the coagulation, complement, and kinin cascades.

An example of what happens when interacting controls fail is the genetic deficiency of C1 esterase inhibitor. Its absence seems to permit uncontrolled activation of plasmin and triggering of the three plasma protein cascades when the patient undergoes emotional distress. This results in out-of-control effects typical of inflammation, including extreme edema of the gastrointestinal and respiratory tracts and the skin. The patient may die as a result of laryngeal swelling.

In other words, inflammatory processes have to be both reliably started and reliably stopped. Normally, this is ensured by the interacting processes of activation and control.

Cellular Components of Inflammation

An important term to remember in connection with inflammation is **exudate**, a collective term for all the helpful substances, including white cells and plasma, that move out of

the capillaries into the tissues to attack unwanted substances and promote healing. This occurs in the sequence outlined below.

> **CONTENT REVIEW**
> ➤ Inflammation Sequence
> - Vascular response
> - Increased permeability
> - Exudation of white cells

Sequence of Events in Inflammation

1. *Vascular Response.* The first response of inflammation is vascular. First, arterioles near the site constrict, followed by vasodilation of the postcapillary venules. The result is an increase in blood flow to the injury site. One result is increased pressure within the microcirculation (arterioles, capillaries, and venules), which helps to exude plasma and blood cells into the tissues.

   When plasma and blood cells move out of the microcirculation, pressure is decreased, and blood moves more sluggishly, thickening and becoming sticky. White cells migrate to the vessel walls and adhere to them—a phenomenon known as **margination** that is important in the next two events.

2. *Increased permeability.* At the same time, chemical substances cause the endothelial cells of the vessel walls to constrict, creating openings between the cells in the vessel walls.

3. *Exudation of white cells.* The white cells adhering to the vessel walls now squeeze out through the openings and into the tissues. Ordinarily, white cells are too large to move through vessel walls. The inflammation-caused constriction of vessel-wall cells that creates openings between them and allows white cells to squeeze through is known as **diapedesis**.

Earlier, we discussed lymphocytes, which are the category of white cells involved in the immune response. The inflammatory response involves two other categories of white cells: granulocytes and monocytes (Table 12-18). **Granulocytes** (like mast cells, discussed earlier) have the appearance of a bag of granules, hence their name. They are also called *polymorphonuclear cells* because they have

---

Table 12-18 Types of White Blood Cells (Leukocytes)

Lymphocytes (25–30 percent of all white blood cells)*
T cells
B cells

Granulocytes**
Neutrophils (55–70 percent of all white blood cells)
Basophils
Eosinophils

Monocytes**
Monocytes (immature) become macrophages (mature)**

*Involved in the immune response.
**Involved in inflammation.

multiple nuclei. There are three types of granulocytes: *neutrophils, eosinophils,* and *basophils.* **Monocytes**, so named because they have a single nucleus, change and mature when they become involved in inflammation. Monocytes are the largest normal blood cell. During inflammation, they grow to several times their original size, becoming *macrophages.*

All the granulocytes and monocytes are **phagocytes**, blood cells that have the ability to ingest other cells and substances such as bacteria and cell debris. (The word comes from the Greek *phagein,* meaning "to eat," and *cyte,* for "cell"—so a phagocyte is a cell that eats.) A phagocyte behaves something like Pac-Man® in the video game, destroying its "enemies" by swallowing them up. The most important phagocytes involved in inflammation are the neutrophils and the macrophages.

Neutrophils are the first phagocytes to reach the inflamed site. They ingest bacteria, dead cells, and cell debris, and then they die. Neutrophils can begin phagocytosis quickly because they are already mature cells. *Macrophages* come along later, because they first have to go through the process of maturing from their parent monocytes.

Eosinophils, basophils, and platelets also migrate to the site to join the inflammatory response. These cells function with assistance from plasma proteins of the complement, coagulation, and kinin systems, acting to kill microorganisms, remove the dead cells and debris, and prepare the site for healing.

Eosinophils are the primary defense against parasites. They contain large numbers of lysosomes. The eosinophils attach themselves to parasites and degranulate, depositing the caustic lysosomes, and killing the parasites by damaging their surfaces. Eosinophils also release chemicals that control the vascular effects of serotonin and histamine. Additionally, eosinophils help to control the inflammatory response, preventing it from spreading beyond the area where it is needed by degrading vasoactive amines, thereby limiting their effects.

Basophils are thought to function in the same way within the blood as mast cells do outside the blood, releasing histamines and other chemicals that control constriction and dilation of vessels.

Platelets, another cellular component of the inflammatory response, are fragments of cytoplasm that circulate in the blood. When cellular injury occurs, platelets act with components of the coagulation cascade to promote blood clotting. Platelets also release serotonin, a substance with effects similar to those of histamine.

Cellular Products

As mentioned earlier, *cytokines* are proteins produced by white blood cells that act as "messengers" between cells. They are important in mediating both immune and inflammatory responses. Cytokines produced by lymphocytes are called *lymphokines.* Cytokines produced by macrophages and monocytes are called *monokines.*

Actually, cytokines are produced by a wide variety of cells, including some that are not part of the immune system. They play a wide variety of roles. Cytokines can interact in a synergistic manner (so their combined effect is greater than the sum of their individual contributions) or they can interact in an antagonistic manner (so they inhibit or cancel out each other's actions). Examples of the variety of sources and activities of cytokines can be found among the interleukins, lymphokines, and interferon.

Interleukins (ILs) are an important group of cytokines. They are produced by both lymphocytes and macrophages. Interleukin-1 is a lymphocyte-stimulating factor. As noted earlier, during the immune response macrophages that ingest antigens release IL-1, which assists helper T cells to respond to the antigens. It also enhances production of IL-2 by the helper T cells, which encourages antibody production. As part of the inflammatory process, IL-1 produced by macrophages induces neutrophilia, the proliferation of neutrophils.

Lymphokines are produced by T cells as a result of antigen stimulation during the immune response. In turn, these lymphokines stimulate monocytes to develop into macrophages, a critical phase of the inflammatory response. Different kinds of lymphokines have different effects. One type, called *migration-inhibitory factor (MIF),* inhibits macrophages from migrating away from the site of inflammation. Another type, called *macrophage-activating factor (MAF),* enhances the phagocytic activities of macrophages.

Interferon is a cytokine that is critical in the body's defense against viral infection. It is a small, low-molecular-weight protein produced and released by cells that have been invaded by viruses. It doesn't kill viruses, nor does it have any effect on a cell that is already infected by a virus. However, interferon prevents viruses from migrating to and infecting healthy cells.

Systemic Responses of Acute Inflammation

The three chief manifestations of acute inflammation are fever, leukocytosis (proliferation of circulating white cells), and an increase in circulating plasma proteins.

Endogenous pyrogen is a fever-causing chemical that is identical to IL-1 and is released by neutrophils and macrophages. It is released after the cell engages in phagocytosis or is exposed to a bacterial endotoxin or to an antigen-antibody complex. Fever can have both beneficial and harmful effects. On one hand, an increase in temperature can create an environment that is inhospitable to some invading microorganisms. On the other hand, fever may increase susceptibility of the infected person to the effects of endotoxins associated with some Gram-negative bacterial infections.

In some infections, the number of circulating leukocytes, especially neutrophils, increases. Several components of the inflammatory response stimulate production of neutrophils, including a component of the complement system. Phagocytes produce a factor that induces production of granulocytes, including neutrophils, eosinophils, and basophils.

Plasma proteins called *acute phase reactants,* produced mostly in the liver, increase during inflammation. Their synthesis is stimulated by interleukins. Many of these act to inhibit and control the inflammatory response.

Chronic Inflammatory Responses

Defined simply, chronic inflammation is any inflammation that lasts longer than two weeks. It may be caused by a foreign object or substance that persists in the wound—for example, a splinter, glass, or dirt—or it may accompany a persistent bacterial infection. This can occur because some microorganisms have cell walls with a high lipid or wax content that resist phagocytosis. Other microorganisms can survive inside a macrophage. Still others produce toxins that persist even after the bacterium is dead, continuing to incite inflammatory responses. Inflammation can also be prolonged by the presence of chemicals and other irritants.

During chronic inflammation, large numbers of neutrophils—the phagocytes that were first on the scene during acute inflammation—degranulate and die. Now, the neutrophils are replaced by components that have taken longer to develop, and there is a large infiltration of lymphocytes from the immune response and of macrophages that have matured from monocytes. In addition to attacking foreign invaders, macrophages produce a factor that stimulates *fibroblasts,* cells that secrete collagen, a critical factor in wound healing.

As neutrophils, lymphocytes, and macrophages die, they infiltrate the tissues, sometimes forming a cavity that contains these dead cells, bits of dead tissue, and tissue fluid, a mixture called **pus.** Enzymes present in pus eventually cause it to self-digest, and it is removed through the epithelium or the lymphatic system.

Occasionally, when macrophages are unable to destroy the foreign invader, a **granuloma** will form to wall off the infection from the rest of the body. The granuloma is formed as large numbers of macrophages, other white cells, and fibroblasts are drawn to the site and surround it. Cells decay within the granuloma, and the released acids and lysosomes break the cellular debris down to basic components and fluid. The fluid eventually diffuses out of the granuloma, leaving a hollow, hard-walled structure buried in the tissues. Some granulomas persist for the life of the individual. Granuloma formation is common in leprosy and tuberculosis, which are caused by mycobacteria, bacteria that resist destruction by phagocytes.

Tissue repair and possible scar formation are the final stages of inflammation and will be discussed in more detail later.

Local Inflammatory Responses

All the manifestations observed at the local inflammation site result from (1) vascular changes and (2) exudation. Redness and heat result from vascular dilation and increased blood flow to the area. Swelling and pain result from the vascular permeability that permits infiltration of exudate into the tissues.

Exudate has three functions:

- To dilute toxins released by bacteria and the toxic products of dying cells
- To bring plasma proteins and leukocytes to the site to attack the invaders
- To carry away the products of inflammation (e.g., toxins, dead cells, pus)

The composition of exudate varies with the stage of inflammation and the type of injury or infection. Early exudate (serous exudate) is watery with few plasma proteins or leukocytes, as in a blister. In a severe or advanced inflammation, the exudate may be thick and clotted (fibrinous exudate), as in lobar pneumonia. In persistent bacterial infections, the exudate contains pus (purulent, or suppurative, exudate), as with cysts and abscesses. If bleeding is present, the exudate contains blood (hemorrhagic exudate).

The lesions (infected areas or wounds) that result from inflammation vary, depending on the organ affected. In myocardial infarction, cellular death results in the replacement of dead tissue by scar tissue. An infarction of brain tissue may result in liquefactive necrosis, in which the dead cells liquefy and are contained in walled cysts. In the liver, destroyed cells result in the regeneration of liver cells.

Keep in mind that inflammation can only occur in vascularized tissues (tissues to which blood can flow). When perfusion is cut off, as in a gangrenous limb or a limb distal to a tourniquet, inflammation cannot take place—and without inflammation, healing cannot take place.

Resolution and Repair

Healing begins during acute inflammation and may continue for as long as two years. The best outcome is **resolution**, the complete restoration of normal structure and function. This can happen if the damage was minor, there are no complications, and the tissues are capable of **regeneration** through the proliferation of the remaining cells. If resolution is not possible, then **repair** takes place, with scarring being the end result. This happens if the wound is large, an abscess or granuloma has formed, or fibrin remains in the damaged tissues.

Both resolution and repair begin in the same way, with **debridement** ("cleaning up") of the site of inflammation. Debridement involves the phagocytosis of dead cells and debris and the dissolution of fibrin cells (scabs). After debridement, there is a draining away of exudate, toxins, and particles from the site, and vascular dilation and permeability are reversed. At this point, either regeneration and resolution or repair and scar formation will take place.

Minor wounds with little tissue loss, like paper cuts, close and heal easily. They are said to heal by **primary intention**. More extensive wounds require more complex processes of sealing the wound, filling the wound, and contracting the wound and are said to heal by **secondary intention**.

Both resolution and repair proceed in two overlapping phases: reconstruction and maturation. Reconstruction begins three or four days after injury or infection and takes about two weeks. Maturation begins several days after injury or infection and can take up to two years.

Reconstruction
Reconstruction of a wound proceeds through four steps: initial wound response, granulation, epithelialization, and contraction.

INITIAL RESPONSE The first step of healing is the sealing off of the wound by a clot (scab) that contains a mesh of fibrin and trapped red and white blood cells. The fibrin mesh is formed as a result of activation of the coagulation cascade. The fibrin traps platelets, which enhance the seal. The fibrin seal creates a barrier to bacterial invasion and a framework for collagen to fill the wound.

Eventually the fibrin clot is dissolved by enzymes and cleared away through debridement by macrophages and any remaining neutrophils. The clot will then be replaced by normal tissue (in the case of resolution) or by scar tissue (in the case of repair).

GRANULATION Repair begins with **granulation**. Granulation tissues grow inward from the healthy connective tissues surrounding the wound. The granulation tissues are filled with capillaries. Some capillaries differentiate into venules and arterioles. Similarly, new lymph channels develop in the granulation tissues.

The granulation tissues are surrounded by macrophages. The macrophages secrete fibroblast-activating factor, which stimulates fibroblasts to enter the tissues and secrete collagen. The macrophages also secrete angiogenesis factor, which causes formation of the capillary buds,

and an unidentified factor that stimulates epithelial factors to grow over the wound.

EPITHELIALIZATION While granulation is taking place and the original clot, or scab, is being dissolved, **epithelialization** takes place. Epithelial cells move in under the scab, separating it from the wound surface, and providing a protective covering for the healing wound.

CONTRACTION Six to twelve days after the injury, **contraction** begins as the wound edges begin to move inward. Contraction is caused by myofibroblasts in the granulation tissues. These are similar to the collagen-secreting fibroblasts, but myofibroblasts contain parallel fiber bundles in their cytoplasm similar to those in smooth muscle cells. They exert a contractile force as they connect to neighboring cells, slowly bringing the wound edges together.

Maturation
At the end of the reconstructive phase, collagen deposition, tissue regeneration, and wound contraction are seldom completed. These processes may continue into the maturation phase, possibly for years. During **maturation**, scar tissue is remodeled; blood vessels disappear, leaving an avascular scar; and the scar tissue becomes stronger.

Only epithelial, hepatic (liver), and bone marrow cells are capable of the total regeneration by mitosis known as hyperplasia (discussed earlier in the chapter). In most wounds, healing produces new tissues that are not structured exactly like the original tissues. Typically, repaired tissues regain about 80 percent of their original strength.

Dysfunctional Wound Healing
Dysfunctional healing can result in an insufficient repair, an excessive repair, or a new infection. Causes of dysfunctional healing vary; they include disease states such as diabetes, hypoxemia, nutritional deficiencies, and the use of certain drugs. Dysfunctional healing can occur during the inflammatory response or during reconstruction.

DYSFUNCTIONAL HEALING DURING INFLAMMATION During inflammation, several factors can disrupt healing. If bleeding hasn't stopped, healing can be delayed by clotting that takes up space and inhibits granulation and by blood-cell debridement from the site. Blood is also a hospitable medium for infection, which in turn exacerbates inflammation and delays healing.

If there is excess fibrin in the wound, this, too, must be cleared away so as not to delay healing. Sometimes excess fibrin causes *adhesions,* fibrous bands that bind organs together and pose a significant problem if they occur in the abdominal, pleural, or pericardial cavities.

Other problems that can arise during inflammation include hypovolemia, which inhibits inflammation (remember that perfusion is necessary to inflammation), and anti-inflammatory steroid drugs that inhibit macrophage and fibroblast migration.

DYSFUNCTIONAL HEALING DURING RECONSTRUCTION A number of factors can disrupt the phases of reconstruction. For example, various nutritional deficiencies can inhibit collagen synthesis. Collagen synthesis can also become excessive, causing the formation of raised scars. Steroid drugs can suppress epithelialization.

Wounds can also be disrupted by pulling apart. Surgical wounds are sometimes disrupted as a result of strain or obesity. In some cases—frequently with burns—wound contraction is excessive, resulting in a deformity called *contracture.* Internal contractures may occur in cirrhosis of the liver, duodenal strictures caused by improper healing of an ulcer, or esophageal strictures from lye burns.

Positioning, exercises, surgery, and administration of drugs can sometimes help to prevent or correct the results of dysfunctional wound healing.

Age and the Mechanisms of Self-Defense

Newborns and the elderly are particularly susceptible to problems of insufficient immune and inflammatory responses.

As noted earlier in the chapter, neonates generally go through a phase at about 5 or 6 months of age when immune system protection received from their mother is depleted and their own immune system is still immature, making them particularly susceptible to respiratory tract infections. Inflammatory responses are similarly immature in the neonate. For example, neutrophils and monocytes may not be capable of chemotaxis, the release of chemical factors that attract other white cells to the site of infection. This makes newborns prone to infections such as cutaneous abscesses and cutaneous candidiasis. As another example, the deficiency of a component of the complement cascade in infants can cause a severe, overwhelming sepsis or meningitis when infants are infected by bacteria for which they do not have transferred maternal antibody.

The elderly also have difficulties with both the immune and the inflammatory responses. As discussed earlier in the chapter, B cell and especially T cell functions of the immune system decrease markedly after age 60. The elderly are also prone to impaired wound healing. This is thought not to be due to the normal processes of aging but rather to the higher incidence of chronic diseases such as diabetes and cardiovascular disease in the elderly. Also, many elderly persons take prescribed anti-inflammatory steroids for conditions such as arthritis, and these inhibit inflammation. Decreased perfusion contributes to hypoxia

in the wound bed, inhibiting inflammation and healing. Unfortunately, the elderly are also more prone to wounding as the protective fat layer diminishes and skin loses its elasticity and becomes more vulnerable to tearing. Diminished sensitivity, mobility, and balance also lead to falls and wounds.

Variances in Immunity and Inflammation

Sometimes the immune and inflammatory systems work "too well" and sometimes not well enough. Hypersensitivity reactions are an example of the former, and immune deficiency diseases are an example of the latter.

Hypersensitivity: Allergy, Autoimmunity, and Isoimmunity

Immune responses are normally protective and helpful. **Hypersensitivity**, however, is an exaggerated and harmful immune response. The word *hypersensitivity* is often used as a synonym for *allergy.* However, *hypersensitivity* is also used as an umbrella term for allergy and two other categories of harmful immune response, which are defined as follows:

Three Types of Hypersensitivity

- **Allergy**—an exaggerated immune response to an environmental antigen, such as pollen or bee venom.
- **Autoimmunity**—a disturbance in the body's normal tolerance for self-antigens, as in hyperthyroidism or rheumatic fever.
- **Isoimmunity** (also called *alloimmunity*)—an immune reaction between members of the same species, commonly of one person against the antigens of another person, as in the reaction of a mother to her infant's Rh negative factor or in transplant rejections.

The exact cause of such pathological immune responses is not known, but at least three factors seem to be involved: (1) the original insult (exposure to the antigen); (2) the person's genetic makeup, which determines susceptibility to the insult; and (3) an immunologic process that boosts the response beyond normal bounds.

Hypersensitivity reactions are classified as **immediate hypersensitivity reactions** or **delayed hypersensitivity reactions**, depending on how long it takes the secondary reaction to appear after reexposure to an antigen. The swiftest immediate hypersensitivity reaction is *anaphylaxis,* a severe allergic response that usually develops within minutes of reexposure. (Review the section on anaphylactic shock earlier in this chapter. Also see the Medical Emergencies chapter titled "Immunology.")

Mechanisms of Hypersensitivity

Usually, when a hypersensitivity reaction takes place, inflammation is triggered that results in destruction of healthy tissues. Four mechanisms, or types, of hypersensitivity that cause this destructive reaction have been identified.

Mechanisms of Hypersensitivity Reaction

• Type I—IgE-mediated allergen reactions
• Type II—tissue-specific reactions
• Type III—immune-complex-mediated reactions
• Type IV—cell-mediated reactions

In reality, hypersensitivity reactions are not so easy to categorize. Most involve more than one type of mechanism.

TYPE I—IgE REACTIONS As noted earlier in the chapter, IgE is the type of immunoglobulin (antibody) that contributes most to allergic and anaphylactic reactions. The first exposure to the allergen (antigen that causes allergic reaction) stimulates B lymphocytes to produce IgE antibodies. These bind to receptors on mast cells in the tissues near blood vessels. On reexposure (or after several reexposures), the allergen binds to the IgE on the mast cell, which causes degranulation of the mast cell, release of histamine, and triggering of the inflammatory process.

The potency of the inflammatory response is controlled in two ways. As discussed earlier, H1 receptors on target cells promote inflammation when contacted by histamine, whereas H2 receptors inhibit inflammation when contacted by histamine. Another control mechanism is the autonomic nervous system, which stimulates production of chemical mediators (epinephrine, acetylcholine) that govern release of inflammatory mediators from the mast cells and the degree to which target cells will respond to inflammatory processes.

The clinical indications of type I IgE-mediated responses are the familiar signs and symptoms of allergic and anaphylactic response.

Clinical Indications of IgE-Mediated Responses

• *Skin*—flushing, itching, urticaria (hives), edema
• *Respiratory system*—breathing difficulty, laryngeal edema, laryngospasm, bronchospasm
• *Cardiovascular system*—vasodilation and permeability, increased heart rate, increased blood pressure
• *Gastrointestinal system*—nausea, vomiting, cramping, diarrhea
• *Nervous system*—dizziness, headache, convulsions, tearing

There is a genetic component to Type I, IgE-mediated responses. Some individuals suffer from *atopia*, in which higher amounts of IgE are produced, and there are more receptors for IgE on the mast cells. In families in which one parent has an allergy, approximately 40 percent of the offspring will also have allergies. If both parents are atopic, approximately 80 percent of their offspring will also be atopic.

Anaphylactic reactions are life threatening. Therefore, people who have reason to believe they are susceptible need to find out what specific allergens they are sensitized to so they can avoid them. A number of tests have been developed that are successful in making these identifications. Additionally, there has been some success in desensitizing some individuals by injecting small but increasing doses of the offending allergen over a long period of time. Research in desensitization techniques is ongoing.

TYPE II—TISSUE-SPECIFIC REACTIONS Most cells of the body present HLA antigens, the antigens that the body recognizes as self or non-self. In addition to HLA antigens, most tissues have other antigens, but these are not the same in all tissues. They are called *tissue-specific antigens* because they exist on the cells of only some body tissues. An immune response against one of these antigens will affect only the organs or tissues that present that particular antigen; this is called a *tissue-specific reaction*.

There are four mechanisms by which Type II tissue-specific reactions attack cells. The first involves the complement system. Antibody bound to the antigen of the target cell initiates the complement cascade, which causes lysis (dissolving) of the cell's plasma membrane. The second mechanism is clearance of the target cells by macrophages. In the third mechanism, antibody bound to the antigen on the target cell also binds to cytotoxic cells, which release toxins that destroy the target cell. In the fourth mechanism, the antibody disables the target cell by occupying receptor sites on the cell, preventing them from binding to molecules that are needed for normal cell functioning.

TYPE III—IMMUNE-COMPLEX-MEDIATED REACTIONS Type III immune-complex-mediated reactions result from antigen-antibody complexes (also called *immune complexes*) that, as discussed earlier, are formed when antibody circulating in the blood or suspended in body secretions meets and binds to a specific antigen. The immune complexes generally circulate for a time before finally being deposited in vessel walls or other tissues. For this reason, which organs are affected may have very little connection with where or how the antigen or the immune complex originated.

The harmful effects of the immune complex result from the activation of the complement system. Some complement fragments are chemotactic for (attract) neutrophils. The neutrophils attempt to ingest the immune complexes but frequently fail because the complexes are bound to the tissues. During this attempt, the neutrophils release large quantities of damaging lysosomal enzymes into the tissues.

The nature and course of immune complex diseases vary tremendously. This results from the fact that immune complex formation is dynamic and constantly changing. There can be variations in the quantity and quality of circulating antigen and the antigen-antibody ratio. Also, many immune complexes bind complement components effectively, which causes complement levels in the blood to fluctuate. In some cases, the interaction between complement and the immune complexes results in dissolving the complex and mitigating its effects. As a result of these factors, immune complex diseases are characterized by tremendous variability in symptoms and periods of alternating remission and exacerbation.

Some immune complex diseases are systemic and some are localized. Systemic immune complex diseases are called *serum sickness*. They typically present with fever, enlarged lymph nodes, rash, and pain, commonly affecting the blood vessels, joints, and kidneys. *Raynaud's phenomenon* is a form of serum sickness in which temperature governs deposition of immune complexes in the peripheral circulation. Typical presentations include numbness in the fingers and toes, followed by cyanosis and gangrene or redness and pain.

Arthus reaction is an example of a localized immune complex disease. It results from the interaction of an environmental antigen with preformed antibody lodged in the walls of blood vessels. A typical inflammatory response follows, resulting in edema, hemorrhage, clotting, and tissue damage. The antigen can enter the body through injection, ingestion, or inhalation. Examples of arthus reactions are skin reactions following inoculations, gastrointestinal reactions to ingestion of wheat products, or hemorrhagic inflammation of the alveoli following inhalation of fungus from a source such as moldy hay.

TYPE IV—CELL-MEDIATED TISSUE REACTIONS
Types I, II, and III hypersensitivity reactions are mediated by antibody. Type IV reactions are activated directly by T cells and do not involve antibody. There are two cell-mediated mechanisms. One involves lymphokine-producing T cells (Td cells). The other involves cytotoxic T cells (Tc cells). The lymphokine produced by Td cells activates other cells such as macrophages. The Tc cells attack antigen-bearing cells directly and destroy them with the toxins they produce.

Graft rejection and contact allergic reactions such as poison ivy are examples of Type IV reactions. There may also be Type IV components to autoimmune diseases such as rheumatoid arthritis, in which the self-antigen is a protein present in joint tissues, and insulin-dependent diabetes, in which the self-antigen is a protein on the cell of the pancreas that produces insulin.

CONTENT REVIEW
➤ Three Hypersensitivity Targets
• Environmental antigens (targeted by *allergic responses*)
• Self-antigens (targeted by *autoimmune responses*)
• Other person's antigens (targeted by *isoimmune responses*)

Targets of Hypersensitivity

Antigens, the proteins or "markers" on the surface of cells, are the targets of the immune response and of the exaggerated immune response called hypersensitivity. As noted earlier, cells bearing these antigens can come from one of three sources: the environment, the person's own body, or another person. The source of the target antigen is what defines the type of hypersensitivity, as follows:

Type of Hypersensitivity	Targeted Antigen
Allergy	Environmental antigens
Autoimmunity	Self-antigens
Isoimmunity	Other person's antigens

IN ALLERGY The antigens that are the targets of allergic reaction are called *allergens*. Allergens typically occur on cells from such environmental sources as ragweed, molds, certain foods such as shellfish or peanuts, animal sources such as cat dander, cigarette smoke, and components of house dust. Often, an allergen is contained in a capsule that is too large to be phagocytosed or is surrounded by a nonallergenic coating. The actual allergen is not released until the capsule or coating is broken down by enzymes. Most allergens are low-molecular-weight immunogens or haptens (which are too small to cause an immune response unless they bind with larger molecules).

In some situations, an allergen combines with components of the host tissue (tissues of the person's body) to form a new substance, called a *neoantigen*, which, in turn, induces an allergic response. For example, a drug such as penicillin, which causes an allergic reaction in some people, is a hapten. It does not cause an allergic reaction until it binds to proteins on the plasma membranes of host cells. The immune system attacks the neoantigen and destroys the cell it is bound to as well. In the case of penicillin, which attaches to red blood cells, the immune response kills the red cells and causes anemia.

IN AUTOIMMUNITY The immune system normally recognizes the person's own tissues as self and tolerates the self-antigens presented by the body's own cells. If the body generated an immune response to its own tissues, it would destroy itself. Autoimmunity is a form of exactly this undesirable situation: There is a breakdown in the body's tolerance for self-antigens, and the immune system begins to attack the body's own cells.

Tolerance for self-antigens begins in the embryo when any lymphocytes that react to self-antigens are eliminated or suppressed. Several causes of a later breakdown in tolerance have been identified.

For example, some cells are *sequestered* (hidden) from the immune system by existing in areas of the body that are not drained by lymph (for example, the cornea and the testicles). If these cells become exposed to the immune system (e.g., during trauma), the body may recognize them as foreign and initiate an autoimmune response.

A neoantigen can trigger an immune response to the cells it is bound to. Infectious diseases can also trigger autoimmune responses in one of two ways. A foreign infectious antigen, in binding with an antibody, can form an immune complex that lodges in host tissues and causes an autoimmune response to the cells of those tissues. Additionally, a foreign antigen may resemble a self-antigen to such a degree that the antibody to the foreign antigen also attacks the self-antigen.

Suppressor T cell dysfunction is another cause of autoimmune disorders. In normal immune function, some T cells develop clones that attack self-antigens. Suppressor T cells are thought to have the function of suppressing these autoimmune responses. However, if the suppressor T cells dysfunction, the autoimmune response caused by T cell clones is able to develop.

The original insult that causes the autoimmune response is usually easy to identify—for instance, an administered drug causing autoimmune anemia or a recent infection such as rubella causing autoimmune encephalitis. In other cases, the causative insult cannot be identified. In these cases, the autoimmune disease is thought to have resulted from a prior infection that is no longer traceable.

Genetic causes are actually easier to identify than pathological causes. Most autoimmune diseases are familial. All affected family members may not have the same disorder, but each may have a different autoimmune disorder or a disorder characterized by hypersensitivity responses.

IN ISOIMMUNITY In isoimmunity, one member of a species has an immune reaction to cells from another member of the same species. In humans, two types of isoimmune disorders are most common, as discussed earlier in this chapter. One type consists of transient neonatal diseases, in which the mother becomes sensitized to fetal antigens, as in Rh negative sensitivity. The other type is encountered in the rejection of grafts or transplants from one person to another.

Autoimmune and Isoimmune Diseases

A number of diseases are recognized or suspected to have an autoimmune or isoimmune basis. The following are some examples:

- *Graves' disease* is thought to be caused by an antibody that stimulates overproduction of thyroid hormone. People with Graves' disease have the symptoms of hyperthyroidism (e.g., elevated heart rate and blood pressure, increased appetite, increased activity level) plus a visibly enlarged thyroid gland (goiter), bulging eyes, and sometimes raised areas of skin over the shins. A pregnant woman with Graves' disease can pass the antibody and the disease along to the newborn.

- *Rheumatoid arthritis* is a disease that causes inflammation of the joints and eventual destruction of the interior of the joint. Its exact cause is not known, but it is recognized as an autoimmune disorder, probably involving antibody reactions to self-antigen in the collagen of the joints.

- *Myasthenia gravis* is a disease caused by antibody response to self-antigens on acetylcholine receptors and the striations of skeletal and cardiac muscle. It is characterized by abnormal function of the neuromuscular junction, resulting in episodes of muscular weakness. Like Graves' disease, the mother's antibody can bind with receptors on the infant's muscle cells, causing neonatal muscle weakness.

- *Immune thrombocytopenic purpura (ITP)* presents with pinhead-sized red spots on the skin, unexplained bruises, and bleeding from the gums and nose and into the stool. It is characterized by a low platelet count. The exact cause is not known, but an autoimmune disorder in which antibodies destroy the person's own platelets appears to be involved. Maternal antibodies can also destroy platelets in the neonate.

- *Isoimmune neutropenia* occurs when a mother has developed antibodies that attack and severely reduce the level of neutrophils in her blood. The antibody in the maternal blood can also attack and destroy neutrophils in the blood of the neonate.

- *Systemic lupus erythematosus (SLE)*, also called simply *lupus,* is an autoimmune disease in which a variety of antibodies to self-antigens are developed that then attack nucleic acids, red blood cells, coagulation proteins, lymphocytes, platelets, and many other targets within the person's own body. The disease causes episodal inflammations of joints, tendons, and other connective tissues and organs. The diversity of antibodies in maternal blood can cause a variety of problems, such as congenital heart defects, in the infant.

- *Rh and ABO isoimmunization,* or hemolytic disease of the newborn, was discussed earlier in the chapter. It is an isoimmune disease that causes severe anemia in the neonate. Immune problems occur if antigens on fetal red blood cells are different from antigens on maternal red blood cells.

Deficiencies in Immunity and Inflammation

Immune deficiency disorders result from impaired function of some component of the immune system, including phagocytes, complement, and lymphocytes (T cells and B cells), with lymphocyte dysfunction being the primary cause. Immune deficiency can be congenital (inborn) or acquired (after birth). The most common manifestations of immune deficiency are recurrent infections, because the body's ability to ward off invaders has been damaged.

Congenital Immune Deficiencies

Congenital, or primary, immune deficiency develops if the development of lymphocytes in the fetus or embryo is impaired or halted. Different immune-deficiency diseases may develop, depending on whether the T cells, the B cells, or both have been affected.

In the *DiGeorge syndrome,* there is a lack or partial lack of thymus development, resulting in a severe decrease in T cell production and function. *Bruton agammaglobulinemia* is caused by impaired development of B cell precursors, resulting in B cells that cannot produce IgM or IgD antibodies. In *bare lymphocyte syndrome,* lymphocytes and macrophages are unable to produce Class I or Class II HLA antigens, which disrupts the ability of cells to recognize self or non-self substances, resulting in severe infections that are usually fatal before age 5.

Sometimes there is a defect that depresses the function of just a small portion of the immune system. For example, in *Wiskott-Aldrich syndrome,* IgM antibody production is reduced. *Selective IgA deficiency* is the most common immune deficiency. IgA is the antibody present in mucous membranes. People with IgA deficiency frequently suffer from sinus, lung, and gastrointestinal infections.

Some immune system deficiencies cause a decreased ability to respond to one particular antigen. For example, in *chronic mucocutaneous candidiasis,* the T lymphocytes are unable to respond against candida infections.

Acquired Immune Deficiencies

Acquired, or secondary, immune deficiencies develop after birth and do not result from genetic factors. They can be caused by or associated with pregnancy, infections, and diseases such as diabetes or cirrhosis. The elderly are more prone to acquired immune deficiencies than the young. Among the factors that can severely affect immune function are nutritional deficiencies, medical treatment, trauma, and stress. Of special interest is the fatal acquired immune disorder AIDS.

CONTENT REVIEW
➤ Two Types of Immune Deficiency
- Congenital (inborn)
- Acquired (after birth)

NUTRITIONAL DEFICIENCIES Critical deficits in calorie or protein ingestion can lead to depression of T cell production and function. Complement activity, neutrophil chemotaxis, and the ability of neutrophils to kill bacteria are also seriously affected by starvation. Zinc deficiencies and vitamin deficiencies can affect both B cell and T cell function.

IATROGENIC DEFICIENCIES Iatrogenic deficiencies are those that are caused by medical treatment. Some drugs depress blood cell formation in the bone marrow. Others trigger immune responses that destroy granulocytes. Immunosuppressive drugs administered in the treatment for transplants, cancer, or autoimmune diseases suppress B and T cell function and antibody production. Radiation treatment for cancer exacerbates this effect. Surgery and anesthesia also can suppress B and T cell function, with severely depressed white cell levels persisting for several weeks after surgery. Surgical removal of the spleen depresses humor response against encapsulated bacteria, depresses IgM levels, and decreases the levels of opsonins.

DEFICIENCIES CAUSED BY TRAUMA Burn victims are especially susceptible to bacterial infection. Not only has the normal barrier presented by the skin been disrupted, but thermal burns also appear to decrease neutrophil function, complement levels, and other immune functions while increasing immunosuppressive functions, which further depress immune function.

DEFICIENCIES CAUSED BY STRESS It has long been suggested that persons undergoing emotional stress (major stresses such as divorce, but also minor stresses such as studying for final exams) are more prone to illness. The speculation was that stress has deleterious effects on immune function. Research into the possible mechanisms of stress-induced immune deficiency are just getting under way. (Stress and susceptibility to disease will be discussed later in the chapter.)

AIDS AIDS is an acronym for *acquired immunodeficiency syndrome,* which has become the best known acquired immune deficiency disorder. AIDS is a syndrome of disorders that develop from infection with **HIV,** the *human immunodeficiency virus.*

HIV is a retrovirus; that is, it carries its genetic information in RNA rather than DNA molecules. As a retrovirus, HIV infects target cells by binding to receptors on their surfaces, then inserting the HIV RNA into the cell. There, the RNA is converted into DNA and becomes part of the infected cell's genetic material. HIV can remain dormant inside the host cell for years; however, once the cell is activated (and the mechanism by which this occurs is not fully understood), HIV proliferates, kills the host cell, and can then infect other cells. The result is a pervasive breakdown of the immune defenses, making the body vulnerable to a wide variety of infections and disorders.

HIV can infect anyone, male or female, homosexual or heterosexual, mostly through the exchange of body fluids during sexual intercourse or through injection. In the United States, most cases to date have involved homosexual men and intravenous drug users. However, preventive measures (safe sex practices—including use of condoms—and clean-needle programs) have reduced the incidence of HIV/AIDS among homosexual populations and drug users. An increasing proportion of new patients are women who have acquired the infection during heterosexual intercourse. In other parts of the world, HIV/AIDS occurs equally among men and women.

The possibility of acquiring HIV/AIDS by contact with patients or accidental needle sticks fostered something of a panic among health care workers when AIDS first spread so alarmingly in the United States in the 1970s. Following recommendations by OSHA, universal precautions (Standard Precautions) have been widely adopted—including the use of disposable gloves, protective eyewear, masks, and gowns, as appropriate, to avoid contact with any body fluids, along with improved techniques for handling needles and other sharps. These measures have proved effective in reducing the fear of HIV/AIDS infection and in making such infections very rare among health care workers.

Until recently, more than 90 percent of those with AIDS have died within five years of the development of severe symptoms. This picture has improved somewhat in developed nations with the initiation of treatments involving multiple chemotherapies (treatment "cocktails") that have shown success in prolonging life, greatly improving feelings of health and well-being, and suppressing measurable blood levels of HIV.

It is not yet known if such treatments can eradicate HIV and cure AIDS. One fear is that the treatments suppress, but do not totally destroy, the HIV virus, which "hides" somewhere in the body, waiting to proliferate at some later date. Another fear is that HIV will develop strains that are resistant to the treatments that appear to be successful in the short term. Nevertheless, the success of these treatments has caused the first feelings of optimism since AIDS was identified. Preventive measures have also

helped to greatly reduce the number of new cases reported in the United States. In some parts of the world, however, including Africa and Asia, HIV/AIDS is still spreading at an extremely alarming rate, with seriously inadequate reporting, prevention, and treatment.

Replacement Therapies for Immune Deficiencies

Advances have been made in the treatment of immune deficiencies through the use of replacement therapies, such as those listed below.

Replacement Therapies

Gamma globulin therapy. Gamma globulin is administered to individuals with B cell deficiencies that cause immunoglobulin (antibody) deficiencies.

Transplantation and transfusion. HLA-matched bone marrow is transplanted into patients suffering *severe combined immune deficiencies (SCID)*, which is caused by a lack of the stem cells from which T cells and B cells develop. In patients who lack a thymus or have a defective thymus, fetal thymus tissue may be transplanted. Enzyme deficiencies that cause SCID have been treated with transfusions of red blood cells that contain the needed enzyme. Other substances have been transfused into individuals to help restore T cell function and reactivity against certain antigens.

Gene therapy. Therapies involving identification of defective genes that are responsible for immune disorders, and replacement of these defective genes with cloned normal genes, are in the early stages of development and use.

Stress and Disease

Stress is a word that is used a lot in modern life. You might have a stressful job, or feel stressed out by too many demands on your job, or be going through a lot of emotional stress in connection with a personal relationship. In some situations, you may be acutely aware of some of the physiologic components of stress—for example, sweaty palms and a pounding heart just before you have to get up and give a speech. If so, you already have a basic understanding of stress that can help you grasp the physiologic and medical concepts of stress and how stress is related to disease.

Concepts of Stress

Today, it is commonly understood that mind and body interact. It was not always so. In fact, the concept that psychological states influence physiologic states—and,

CONTENT REVIEW
➤ General Adaptation
  Syndrome (GAS)
  • *Stage I*—Alarm
  • *Stage II*—Resistance,
    or adaptation
  • *Stage III*—Exhaustion

particularly, that there is a cause–effect relationship between stress and disease—date primarily from the work of Hans Selye, an Austrian-born Canadian physician and educator, in the 1940s.

General Adaptation Syndrome

Dr. Selye was not studying stress when he made his discovery. Instead, he was trying to identify a new sex hormone. He was injecting ovarian extracts into laboratory rats when he discovered the following triad of physiologic effects:

Triad of Stress Effects

• Enlargement of the cortex (outer portion) of the adrenal gland

• Atrophy of the thymus gland and other lymphatic structures

• Development of bleeding ulcers of the stomach and duodenum

Dr. Selye soon discovered that this triad of effects was not a response only to the ovarian extracts. The same effects occurred when he subjected the rats to other stimuli, such as cold, surgical injury, and restraint. He concluded that the triad of effects was not specific to any particular stimulus but comprised a nonspecific response to any noxious stimulus, or stressor. (**Stress** is generally defined as a state of physical and/or psychological arousal to a stimulus. Dr. Selye originally intended to use the word *stress* for the stimulus, or cause, but through a mistranslation of his work, *stress* came to mean the arousal, or effect. Dr. Selye then coined the word **stressor** for the stimulus/cause.)

Because the same responses occurred to a wide array of stimuli, Dr. Selye named it the **general adaptation syndrome (GAS)**. Later, he identified three stages in the development of GAS:

Stages of GAS

• *Stage I, alarm.* The sympathetic nervous system is aroused and mobilized in the "fight-or-flight" response syndrome. Pupils dilate, heart rate increases, and bronchial passages dilate. In addition, blood glucose levels rise, digestion slows, blood pressure rises, and the flow of blood to the skeletal muscles increases. At the same time, the endocrine system is aroused, resulting in secretion of hormones by the pituitary and adrenal glands that enhance the body's readiness to meet the challenge.

• *Stage II, resistance, or adaptation.* The person begins to cope with the situation. Sympathetic nervous system

responses and circulating hormones return to normal. In most situations, this is the last stage; the stress is resolved. If the stress is very severe or prolonged, however, stress is not resolved and stage III occurs.

• *Stage III, exhaustion.* This is the stage sometimes known as "burnout." During this stage, the triad of physiologic effects described by Dr. Selye occurs. The person can no longer cope with or resolve the stress, and physical illness may ensue.

The stages of GAS begin with **physiologic stress**, defined by Dr. Selye as a chemical or physical disturbance in the cells or tissue fluid produced by a change, either in the external environment or within the body itself, that requires a response to counteract the disturbance. Selye identified three components of physiologic stress: (1) the stressor that initiates the disturbance, (2) the chemical or physical disturbance the stressor produces, and (3) the body's counteracting (adaptational) response.

Psychological Mediators and Specificity

Since Dr. Selye defined GAS, others who have studied adaptation to stress have refined the concept. For example, more attention has been paid to the psychological mediators of stress. Experiments have shown that there isn't a direct correlation between stressor and response. People react differently to the same stressor. One person may take in stride the same situation that greatly upsets another person, and the degree of physiologic response may be governed more by the psychological, emotional, or social response to the stressor than to the stressor itself. In particular, research has demonstrated pituitary gland and adrenal cortex sensitivity to emotional/psychological/social influences.

Another way in which recent research has diverged from Dr. Selye's original hypotheses regards specificity. Dr. Selye postulated that the triad of physiologic responses he identified were nonspecific, or the same for any stressor. It is now thought that, although the triad of responses he identified may occur in response to a wide variety of stressors, the total body response to different stressors must be specific—that is, targeted toward correction of the specific disturbance. For example, the body reacts to cold by shivering, and to heat through vasodilation and sweating.

Homeostasis as a Dynamic Steady State

An older definition of homeostasis states that the body maintains itself at a "constant" composition. More recently, homeostasis has been described as a **dynamic steady state**. This takes into account the concept of **turnover**, the continual synthesis and breakdown of all body substances (e.g., fats, proteins). Thus, the internal environment of the body is always changing, not constant, but the net effect of all the changes is the dynamic (always changing), yet steady (tending always toward normal balance) state.

Stressors cause a series of reactions that alter the dynamic steady state. Usually, there is a return to normal, which may be rapid or slow. If a disturbance in the dynamic steady state—for example, a high blood glucose level—is prolonged and a causative stressor is no longer present, it is considered a sign of disease.

Stress Responses

Alteration of the immune system is the ultimate outcome of a stress response that resists quick and successful adaptation. The interactions of psychological, neurologic/endocrine, and immunologic factors that lead to this outcome are known as **psychoneuroimmunologic regulation**.

The **stress response** is initiated by a stressor. The input of the stressor into the central nervous system, as mediated by the person's psychological response, leads to production of corticotropin-releasing factor (CRF) from the hypothalamus, which, in turn, stimulates responses by the sympathetic nervous system and the endocrine system (neuroendocrine regulation), which then affect the immune

system. This chain of events is outlined in Figure 12-104 and described in the next sections.

Neuroendocrine Regulation

As previously mentioned, when a person encounters a stressor and has a psychological response to the stressor, the sympathetic nervous system is stimulated by *corticotropin-releasing factor (CRF)*. In turn, this stimulates release of catecholamines, cortisol, and other hormones.

CATECHOLAMINES Sympathetic nervous system stimulation results in the release of norepinephrine (noradrenalin) and epinephrine (adrenalin), which constitute the category of hormones called *catecholamines*. The nerves of the sympathetic nervous system exit the spine at the thoracic and lumbar levels, and norepinephrine is released into the synaptic spaces (the spaces between the presynaptic ganglia and the postsynaptic nerves).

> **CONTENT REVIEW**
>
> ➤ Hormones Released in Response to Stress
> - Catecholamines (norepinephrine and epinephrine)
> - Cortisol
> - Beta endorphins
> - Growth hormone
> - Prolactin

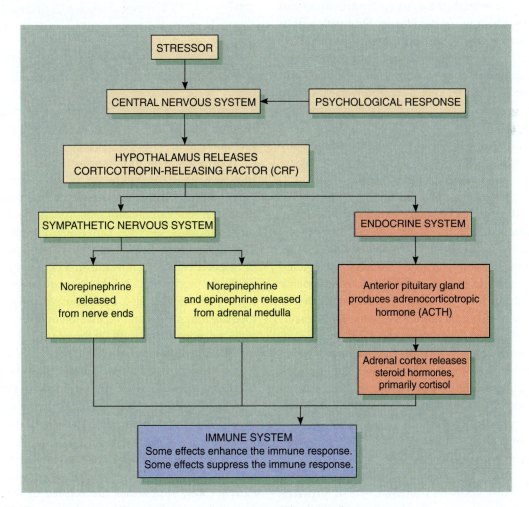

FIGURE 12-104 The stress response: effects on the sympathetic nervous, endocrine, and immune systems.

Additionally, sympathetic nervous system stimulation results in direct stimulation of the adrenal medulla, the inner portion of the adrenal gland. The adrenal medulla, in turn, releases the norepinephrine and epinephrine into the circulatory system. Approximately 80 percent of the hormones released by the adrenal medulla are epinephrine, and norepinephrine accounts for the remaining 20 percent. Once released, these hormones are carried throughout the body, where their effects (preparing the body to deal with stressful situations) act on hormone receptors.

Both epinephrine and norepinephrine interact with specialized adrenergic receptors on the membranes of target organs. These receptors are located throughout the body. Once stimulated by the appropriate hormone, they cause a response in the organ or organs they control.

The adrenergic receptors are generally divided into five types, designated alpha 1 (α_1), alpha 2 (α_2), beta 1 (β_1), beta 2 (β_2), and beta 3 (β_3). The α_1 receptors cause peripheral vasoconstriction, mild bronchoconstriction, and stimulation of metabolism. The α_2 receptors are found on the presynaptic surfaces of sympathetic neuroeffector junctions. Stimulation of α_2 receptors is inhibitory. These receptors serve to prevent over-release of norepinephrine in the synapse. When the level of norepinephrine in the synapse gets high enough, the α_2 receptors are stimulated and norepinephrine release is inhibited. Stimulation of β_1 receptors causes increases in heart rate, cardiac contractile force, and cardiac automaticity and conduction. Stimulation of β_2 receptors causes vasodilation and bronchodilation. Stimulation of β_3 receptors causes fat to be broken down in adipose tissues and heat production in muscle tissue.

All the effects of the catecholamines prepare the body to "fight-or-flight" in response to a stressor. Their physiologic effects are summarized in Table 12-19.

CORTISOL **Cortisol** is another hormone produced in response to stress. The corticotropin-releasing factor (CRF) that stimulates the sympathetic nervous system, as previously discussed, simultaneously stimulates the anterior pituitary gland to produce *adrenocorticotropic hormone (ACTH)*, which, in turn, stimulates the adrenal cortex to produce a variety of steroid hormones, primarily cortisol.

One of the primary functions of cortisol is the stimulation of gluconeogenesis. It enhances the elevation of blood glucose by other hormones and also inhibits peripheral uptake and oxidation of glucose by the cells. Because of these functions, it has the overall effect of elevating blood glucose.

Cortisol also affects protein metabolism—increasing synthesis of proteins in the liver but increasing breakdown of proteins in the muscle, lymphoid tissue, fatty tissues, skin, and bone. The breakdown of proteins results in increased blood levels of amino acids. Cortisol

Table 12-19 Physiologic Effects of Catecholamines

Organ	Effects
Brain	Increased blood flow Increased glucose metabolism
Cardiovascular system	Increased contractile force and rate Peripheral vasoconstriction
Pulmonary system	Increased ventilation Bronchodilation Increased oxygen supply
Liver	Increased glucose production Increased gluconeogenesis Increased glycogenolysis Decreased glycogen synthesis
Gastrointestinal and genitourinary tracts	Decreased protein synthesis
Muscle	Increased glycogenolysis Increased contraction Increased dilation of skeletal muscle vasculature
Skeleton	Decreased glucose uptake and utilization (insulin release decreased)
Adipose (fatty) tissue	Increased lipolysis Increased fatty acids and glycerol
Skin	Decreased blood flow
Lymphoid tissue	Increased protein breakdown (shrinkage of lymphoid tissue)

also promotes lipolysis (fat breakdown) in the extremities and lipogenesis (fat synthesis and deposition) in the face and trunk.

Cortisol acts as an immunosuppressant by inhibiting protein synthesis, including synthesis of immunoglobulins (antibodies). Additionally, it reduces the numbers of lymphocytes, eosinophils, and macrophages in the blood. In large amounts, cortisol can cause lymphoid atrophy. Through a series of actions, cortisol diminishes the actions of helper T cells, which results in a decrease in B cells and antibody production. It inhibits production of interleukin-1 and interleukin-2 and, consequently, blocks cell-mediated immunity and generation of fever. It inhibits the accumulation of leukocytes at the site of inflammation and inhibits release of substances that are critical in the inflammatory response, including kinins, prostaglandins, and histamine. Cortisol also inhibits fibroblast proliferation during inflammatory response, which, in turn, causes poor wound healing and increased susceptibility to wound infection.

In the gastrointestinal tract, cortisol increases gastric secretions, occasionally enough to cause ulcer formation. Cortisol also suppresses the release of sex hormones, including testosterone and estradiol.

The immunosuppressive actions of cortisol seem clearly harmful, yet its production in response to stress indicates that it is beneficial in protecting against stress. Its beneficial effects in stress, however, are not well understood. It has been suggested that its promotion of gluconeogenesis helps ensure an adequate source of glucose as energy for body tissues, especially nerve tissues. Pooled amino acids from protein breakdown may promote protein synthesis in some cells. Its depressive influence on inflammatory responses may play a role in decreasing peripheral blood flow and redirecting blood to critical organs or sites of injury. Suppression of immune function may also help prevent tissue damage that results from prolonged immune responses. The physiologic effects of cortisol are summarized in Table 12-20.

OTHER HORMONES In addition to the catecholamines and cortisol, other hormones are associated with stress response. For example, *beta-endorphins* (endogenous opiates) are released into the blood from the pituitary gland, or possibly the central nervous system, in response to CRF stimulation. They may play a part in regulating ACTH secretion and inhibiting CRF secretion, which means that beta-endorphins may exercise a control over the stress response. The beta-endorphins also are associated with decreased pain sensitivity and increased feelings of well-being, which may help to moderate the psychological response to a stressor.

Growth hormone (GH) is released by the anterior pituitary gland. GH affects protein, lipid, and carbohydrate metabolism and immune function. Its levels have been noted to increase after stressful experiences such as electroshock, cardiac catheterization, and surgery. However, the levels of GH become depressed with prolonged stress. *Prolactin* is released by the anterior pituitary gland and is necessary for breast development and lactation. Levels of prolactin have been noted to rise after a variety of stressful stimuli. *Testosterone* is a hormone produced in the testicles and also by the adrenal cortex in both males and females. It is necessary for development of male sexual characteristics and also affects many metabolic activities. Many stressful activities lead to a decrease in testosterone, which is thought to be a result of increased cortisol levels. Some competitive sports activities, however, appear to increase testosterone levels.

Role of the Immune System in Stress

During a stress response, as noted earlier, there is a complex interaction among the nervous and endocrine systems and the immune system. As a consequence, a variety of immune-related disorders are associated with stress.

The specific mechanisms by which stress leads to immune-related disorders is the subject of ongoing research but is not yet well understood. However, research points to the substances that serve as communicators between the cells of the nervous system, the endocrine system, and the immune system—including hormones, neurotransmitters, neuropeptides, and cytokines—as the pathways of cause and effect.

The pathway is not a straight line. The directional arrows of cause and effect move forward, backward, and

Table 12-20 Physiologic Effects of Cortisol

Function	Effects
Carbohydrate metabolism	Diminished peripheral uptake/use of glucose; promotes gluconeogenesis; elevates blood glucose levels
Protein metabolism	Increases protein synthesis in liver; depresses protein synthesis in other tissues; depresses immunoglobulin production
Inflammatory effects	Decreases blood levels of lymphocytes, macrophages, eosinophils; decreases leukocytes at inflammation site; delays healing/promotes wound infection
Lipid metabolism	Increases lipolysis in extremities, lipogenesis in face and trunk
Immune reserves	Decreases lymphoid tissue mass; decreases circulation white cells; inhibits production of interleukin-1 and interleukin-2; blocks cell-mediated immunity and generation of fever
Digestive function	Promotes gastric secretions; at high levels, causes ulceration
Urinary function	Enhances production of urine
Connective tissue function	Decreases proliferation of fibroblasts (delays healing)
Muscle function	Maintains normal contractility and work output for skeletal and cardiac muscle
Bone function	Decreases bone formation
Cardiovascular function	Maintains normal blood pressure; assists arteriole constriction; supports myocardial function
Central nervous system function	Modulates perceptual/emotional functioning and daytime arousal

in circles. Many components of the immune system can be affected by the factors produced by the neuroendocrine system. Conversely, immune system products can affect components of the neuroendocrine system. Here are two examples (Figure 12-105):

- *Pathway 1: Central nervous system to immune system.* The central nervous system *stimulates* the hypothalamus to produce CRF, which *stimulates* the pituitary gland to produce ACTH, which *stimulates* the

adrenal gland to secrete cortisol, which *suppresses* the development of macrophages, T cells, B cells, and natural killer (NK) cells, a lymphocyte specially adapted to recognize and kill virally infected cells and malignant cells.

- *Pathway 2: Immune system to central nervous system.* During immune system response, macrophages secrete cytokines which stimulate the hypothalamus to secrete CRF (which begins Pathway 1 again).

These are only two examples of the many pathways and interactions that take place among the nervous, endocrine, and immune systems.

The suppression of immune system function that is caused by stress-related products of the sympathetic nervous and endocrine systems—especially catecholamines and cortisol—has been linked to a number of immune-mediated diseases, as listed in Table 12-21.

Stress, Coping, and Illness Interrelationships

Research has shown that the ability to cope with stress has significant effects on associated illnesses. Those who cope positively with stress have a reduced chance of becoming ill in the first place and a better chance of getting better or getting better faster if they do become ill. Conversely, those who don't cope as well with stress have a greater chance of becoming ill or of prolonging the course of illness or of not surviving an illness.

Physiologic stress is caused by events that directly affect the body, such as a burn, extreme cold, or starvation. *Psychological stress* consists of the unpleasant emotions caused by life events, such as taking exams or a divorce. The effects that these stresses will have on the body depend on the individual's ability to cope with them. Some people are "thrown" by events others would perceive as relatively minor, such as a traffic jam or a sprained ankle. Others can take in stride events that others would find very difficult, such as loss of a job or a long-term disability.

The effects of stress, including the degree to which stress causes or affects illness, are moderated by the type, duration, and severity of the stressor in combination

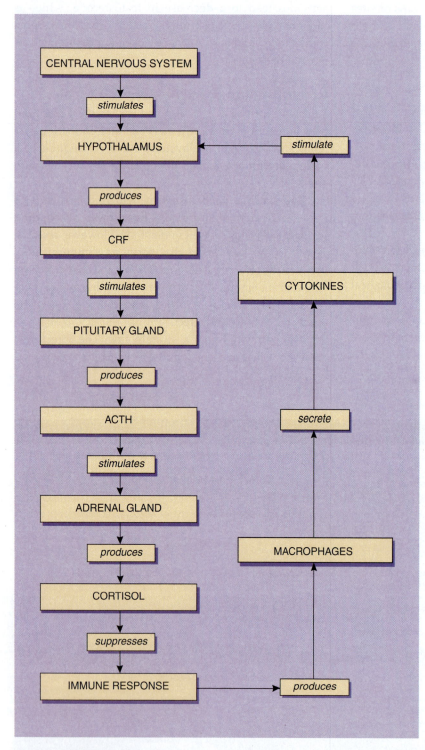

FIGURE 12-105 Interactions among the nervous, endocrine, and immune systems.

Table 12-21 Stress- and Immune-Related Diseases and Conditions

Target Organ	Diseases and Conditions
Cardiovascular system	Coronary artery disease Hypertension Stroke Arrhythmias
Muscles	Tension headaches Muscle-related backaches
Connective tissues	Rheumatoid arthritis
Pulmonary system	Asthma Hay fever
Immune system	Immunosuppression or immune deficiency
Gastrointestinal system	Ulcer Irritable bowel syndrome Ulcerative colitis
Genitourinary system	Diuresis Impotence
Skin	Eczema Acne
Endocrine system	Diabetes mellitus
Central nervous system	Fatigue Depression Insomnia

with the individual's perception and ability to cope with it. Stressors that are the most likely to have a negative effect on immunity and disease have been characterized as those that are not only undesirable but also are uncontrollable and that overtax the person's ability to cope.

Effective and ineffective coping has been seen to have potentially different effects in healthy persons, symptomatic persons (those who already have some manifestations of disease), and persons who are undergoing medical treatment.

Potential Effects of Stress Based on Effectiveness of Coping

- *In a healthy person:*

  Effective coping → Transient effects, return to normal function

  Ineffective coping → Significant stress effects, illness

- *In a symptomatic person:*

  Effective coping → Little or no effect on symptoms

  Ineffective coping → Exacerbation of symptoms, illness

- *In a person undergoing medical treatment:*

  Effective coping → Person does not perceive the treatment itself as stressful → Treatment is more likely to have a positive effect on symptoms and the course of illness

  Ineffective coping → Person perceives the treatment itself as stressful → Treatment is more likely to have a negative effect on symptoms and the course of illness

Because of the importance of coping ability in the interplay between stress and illness, attention is increasingly being paid to providing counseling and support systems—including family members, friends, and other support networks—to assist persons who are ill or in stressful life situations. There is recognition that supporting the patient's ability to cope is a critical adjunct to medical treatment itself.

Summary

The cell is the basic unit of life. It contains all the components needed to turn nutrients into energy, remove waste products, reproduce, and carry on other essential life functions. The body's cells interact via electrochemical substances including hormones, neurotransmitters, neuropeptides, and cytokines. The cells exist in an environment of fluids and electrolytes. When something interferes with normal cell function, the normal cell environment, or normal cell intercommunication, disease can begin or advance.

Groups of cells that perform similar functions form tissues. A group of tissues functioning together is an organ. A group of organs that work together is an organ system.

Perfusion of the tissues is necessary to provide essential nutrients to the cells (especially oxygen and glucose) and to remove wastes. Inadequate perfusion, called hypoperfusion or shock, can be caused by a problem in any of the three parts of the cardiovascular system (the heart, the blood vessels, or the blood), sometimes abetted by problems with the respiratory or gastrointestinal system in which the normal intake and transfer of oxygen and glucose may be interrupted. If not corrected, positive feedback mechanisms can enhance the process of shock, creating a downward spiral toward irreversible shock, possible multiple organ dysfunction syndrome (MODS), and death.

Cells can be injured in a variety of ways, including hypoxia, chemicals, infectious agents, immunologic/inflammatory injuries, and others. Diseases can be caused by genetic factors, environmental factors, or a combination of factors (multifactorial diseases).

The body responds to cellular injury in a variety of ways to restore homeostasis, the body's normal dynamic steady state. Cells can adapt through atrophy, hypertrophy, hyperplasia, metaplasia, and dysplasia. Negative feedback mechanisms work to correct, or compensate for, shock—if shock has not progressed too far.

The body's chief means of self defense is the immune system and the immune and inflammatory responses, which work to attack and destroy infectious agents and other unwanted invaders. Occasionally, the immune response system works "too well," as in hypersensitivity reactions, or not well enough, as in immune deficiency disorders. Stress can also contribute to disease through the interactions of the nervous, endocrine, and immune systems.

Keep in mind that an understanding of the cell is essential to an understanding of all of these physiologic and pathophysiologic systems and processes. The more you understand what is happening at the cellular level, the better you will be able to understand the disease/injury process. This will help you make better decisions for treatment and transport of your patient.

You Make the Call

You have volunteered to work at a high school rodeo for your fire department. You and another paramedic take the backup EMS unit to the arena. This event brings in participants from several states. More than 300 people are expected to attend. On arrival at the arena, you park the unit at the designated spot and move your equipment to the "first-aid room."

Shortly after the rodeo is under way, an elderly gentleman stumbles into the first-aid room and slumps onto the treatment table. He states that he feels very weak and wants to be "checked out." You perform a quick assessment. The patient is pale but dry. His pulse rate is 110 beats per minute, blood pressure is 110/60, and his respirations are 36 per minute. You notice the characteristic odor of ketones on his breath. You ask the patient if he is diabetic. He says he is, but has not had his insulin in two days, as he ran out of syringes. A finger-stick glucose reads "HIGH." On further exam, you note that the patient's mucous membranes are very dry.

1. Explain the physiologic basis for the patient's apparent dehydration.

2. Describe the role of insulin in glucose transport into the cell.

3. Prepare a prehospital treatment plan given the information provided.

See Suggested Responses to "You Make the Call" at the end of this book.

Review Questions

1. The clear liquid portion of the cytoplasm in a cell is called _____

   a. cytosol.

   b. plasma.

   c. synovial fluid.

   d. aqueous humor.

2. The _____ are the energy factories, sometimes called the "powerhouses," of the cells.

   a. lysosomes

   b. mitochondria

   c. Golgi apparatuses

   d. endoplasmic reticula

3. Which property of nerve cells results in the ability to transmit an electrical impulse in response to a stimulus>
   a. Excitability
   b. Automaticity
   c. Conductivity
   d. Contractility

4. _____ tissue has the capability of contraction when stimulated.
   a. Nerve
   b. Muscle
   c. Connective
   d. Epithelial

5. What is the term for the body's natural tendency to keep the internal environment and metabolism steady and normal?
   a. Positive responsiveness
   b. Positive feedback system
   c. Metabolism
   d. Homeostasis

6. _____ is the study of disease and its causes.
   a. Pathology
   b. Physiologic disruption
   c. Physiology
   d. Pathophysiology

7. _____ is an increase in the number of cells through cell division, resulting from an increased workload.
   a. Multiplasia
   b. Metaplasia
   c. Hypertrophy
   d. Hyperplasia

8. What is the "force" or pressure that helps to push plasma out from a capillary bed>
   a. Osmotic
   b. Hydrostatic
   c. Oncotic
   d. Filtration

9. Water accounts for approximately _____ percent of the total body weight.
   a. 40
   b. 50
   c. 60
   d. 70

10. The fluid found outside cells and within the circulatory system is the _____ fluid.
    a. synovial
    b. interstitial
    c. intravascular
    d. extracellular

11. The most frequently occurring anions include all of the following except _____
    a. chloride.
    b. calcium.
    c. phosphate.
    d. bicarbonate.

12. The mechanism(s) that most commonly result in accumulation of water in the interstitial space include is/are _____
    a. lymphatic obstruction.
    b. an increase in hydrostatic pressure.
    c. increased permeability of the capillary membrane.
    d. all of the above.

13. _____ are proteins secreted by plasma cells in response to an antigen.
    a. Clonal antigens
    b. Antibodies
    c. Antibiotics
    d. Haptens

14. Progressive impairment of two or more organ systems resulting from an uncontrolled inflammatory response to a severe illness or injury is called _____
    a. ALS.
    b. MODS.
    c. ARDS.
    d. AODS.

15. An advanced stage of shock in which the body's compensatory mechanisms are no longer able to maintain normal perfusion is called _____
    a. reversible shock.
    b. compensated shock.
    c. homeostatic shock.
    d. decompensated shock.

16. Which of the following is *not* a commonly used prehospital IV fluid?
    a. D_5W
    b. Normal saline
    c. Lactated Ringer's
    d. Chloride solution.

17. The human somatic cell nucleus contains _____ chromosomes.
    a. 48
    b. 46
    c. 24
    d. 23

18. The amount of blood ejected by the heart in one contraction is referred to as the_____
    a. preload.
    b. afterload.
    c. stroke volume.
    d. cardiac force.

19. The energy that is produced during glucose breakdown is in the form of the chemical _____
    a. ATP.
    b. APT.
    c. TAP.
    d. PTA.

20. Obstructive shock is caused by an obstruction of blood through the heart, and can be caused by

    _____

    a. cardiac tamponade.

    b. pulmonary embolism.

    c. tension pneumothorax.

    d. all of the above.

21. What is the best description of shock?

    a. Inadequate blood flow

    b. Inadequate blood flow and inadequate oxygenation

    c. Inadequate blood flow, inadequate oxygenation, and inadequate waste removal to organs

    d. Inadequate blood flow, inadequate oxygenation, and inadequate wate removal to organs and cells

22. With a mortality rate of _____ percent, MODS is the major cause of death in patients with significant injuries or illnesses.

    a. 40–50   c. 60–90

    b. 50–60   d. 80–90

23. People with type_____ blood are known as universal donors, because this type of blood has no antigens that will trigger an immune response in any other group.

    a. A   c. O

    b. B   d. AB

24. _____ cells are the chief activators of the inflammatory response.

    a. T   c. Immune

    b. Mast   d. Histamine

25. _____ occurs when a mother has developed antibodies that attack and severely reduce the level of neutrophils in her blood.

    a. Myasthenia gravis

    b. Rheumatoid arthritis

    c. Isoimmune neutropenia

    d. Systemic lupus erythematosus

See Answers to Review Questions at the end of this book.

References

1. Behar, D. M., E. Metspala, T. Kivisild, et al. "The Matrilineal Ancestry of Ashkenazi Jewry: Portrait of a Recent Founder Event." *Am J Hum Genet* 78 (2006): 487–497.

2. Lotti, M., L. Bergamo, and B. Murer. "Occupational Toxicology of Asbestos-Related Malignancies." *Clin Toxicol (Phla)* 48 (2010): 485–496.

3. Hendricks, K. A., J. S. Simpson, and R. D. Larsen. "Neural Tube Defects along the Texas-Mexico Border, 1993–1995." *Am J Epidemiol* 15 (1999): 1119–1127.

4. Williams, D. "Radiation Carcinogenesis: Lessons from Chernobyl." *Oncogene* 27 (Suppl 2) (2008): S9–S18.

5. Harman, D. "Aging: A Theory Based upon Free Radical and Radiation Chemistry." *J Gerontol* 11 (1956): 298–300.

Further Reading

Bledsoe, B. E. and R.W. Benner. *Critical Care Paramedic.* Upper Saddle River, NJ: Brady/Pearson/Prentice-Hall, 2006.

Bledsoe, B. E. "EMS Needs a Few More Cowboys." *Journal of Emergency Medical Services (JEMS)* 28(12) (2003): 112–113.

Bledsoe, B. E. "Where Are the Wise Men?" *Emergency Medical Services (EMS)* 31(10) (2002): 172.

Grayson, S. *En Route: A Paramedic's Stories of Life, Death, and Everything in Between.* New York: Kaplan Publishing, 2009.

Page, J. O. *Simple Advice.* Carlsbad, CA: JEMS Publishing, 2002.

Page, J. O. *The Magic of 3 A.M.: Essays on the Art and Science of Emergency medical Services.* Carlsbad, CA: JEMS Publishing, 2002.

Page, J. O. *The Paramedics.* Morristown, NJ: Backdraft Publications, 1979.

Perry, M. *Population 485: Meeting Your Neighbors One Siren at a Time.* New York, NY: Harper-Collins, 2002.

Chapter 13
Emergency Pharmacology

Bryan Bledsoe, DO, FACEP, FAAEM

STANDARD
Pharmacology (Principles of Pharmacology; Emergency Medications)

COMPETENCY
Integrates comprehensive knowledge of pharmacology to formulate a treatment plan intended to mitigate emergencies and improve the overall health of the patient.

 ## Learning Objectives

Terminal Performance Objective: After reading this chapter, you should be able to apply concepts of pharmacology to the assessment and management of patients.

Enabling Objectives: To accomplish the terminal performance objective, you should be able to:

1. Define key terms introduced in this chapter.

2. Explain the chemical, generic, brand, and official names of drugs, and the four main sources of material from which drugs are created.

3. Identify reliable reference materials for drug information.

4. Describe each of the components of a drug profile.

5. Explain how key drug legislation applies to the paramedic's role in administering drugs.

6. Discuss the processes of drug research and development for marketing, and the FDA classification of newly approved drugs.

7. Explain the responsibilities with respect to administering medications, including medication delivery to special patient populations.

8. Explain key principles of pharmacokinetics.

9. Describe each of the routes of drug administration.

10. Describe the various forms of drugs and any storage considerations they may have.

11. Explain key principles of pharmacodynamics.

12. Describe unintended adverse effects of drug administration and how various factors, such as age, body mass, concurrent medications, and others, can alter drug responses.

13. Describe the characteristics of drugs used to affect the central nervous system.

14. Describe the characteristics of drugs used to affect the autonomic nervous system.

15. Describe the characteristics of drugs used to affect the cardiovascular system.

16. Describe the characteristics of drugs used to affect the respiratory system.

17. Describe the characteristics of drugs used to affect the gastrointestinal system.

18. Describe the characteristics of drugs used to affect the eyes and ears.

19. Describe the characteristics of drugs used to affect the endocrine system.

20. Describe the characteristics of drugs used to affect the male and female reproductive system and those that affect sexual behavior.

21. Describe the characteristics of drugs used to treat cancer, infection and inflammation, the skin.

22. Describe the characteristics of drugs used to supplement the diet, and those used for poisoning and overdoses.

KEY TERMS

active transport, p. 362

adjunct medication, p. 373

adrenergic, p. 388

affinity, p. 368

agonist, p. 368

agonist–antagonist, p. 368

analgesia, p. 373

analgesic, p. 373

anesthesia, p. 373

anesthetic, p. 375

antacid, p. 420

antagonist, p. 368

antiarrhythmic, p. 403

antibiotic, p. 430

anticoagulant, p. 414

antiemetic, p. 421

antifibrinolytic, p. 415

antihistamine, p. 418

antihyperlipidemic, p. 415

antihypertensive, p. 408

antineoplastic agent, p. 428

antiplatelet, p. 414

antitussive, p. 419

assay, p. 357

autonomic ganglia, p. 387

autonomic nervous system, p. 387

bioassay, p. 357

bioavailability, p. 364

bioequivalence, p. 357

biologic half-life, p. 370

biotransformation, p. 365

blood–brain barrier, p. 365

carrier-mediated diffusion, p. 362

cholinergic, p. 388

competitive antagonism, p. 369

diffusion, p. 363

diuretic, p. 408

dose packaging, p. 360

down-regulation, p. 368

drug-response relationship, p. 370

drugs, p. 354

duration of action, p. 370

efficacy, p. 368

enteral route, p. 366

expectorant, p. 419

extrapyramidal symptoms, p. 382

facilitated diffusion, p. 362

fibrinolytic, p. 415

filtration, p. 363

first-pass effect, p. 365

free drug availability, p. 361

glucagon, p. 425

hemostasis, p. 414

histamine, p. 418

hydrolyze, p. 365

hypnosis, p. 378

immunity, p. 431

insulin, p. 425

ionize, p. 364

irreversible antagonism, p. 369

laxative, p. 420

leukotrienes, p. 417

medications, p. 354

metabolism, p. 365

minimum effective concentration, p. 370

mucolytic, p. 419

neuroeffector junction, p. 387

neuroleptanesthesia, p. 375

neuroleptic, p. 382

neuron, p. 388

neurotransmitter, p. 387

noncompetitive antagonism, p. 369

onset of action, p. 370

organic nitrates, p. 413

osmosis, p. 363

oxidation, p. 365

parasympatholytic, p. 390

parasympathomimetic, p. 390

parenteral route, p. 366

partial agonist, p. 368

passive transport, p. 363

pathogen, p. 431

pharmacodynamics, p. 362

Case Study

Paramedics Jo Henderson and her partner, Scott Parker, are dispatched to a rural residence just outside of town on a "chest pain" call. The response time is approximately 8 minutes. Emergency Medical Responders from the Alamo Fire Department are already on the scene. As they pull up to the well-kept brick home, a woman waves to them from the front porch. She tells them that she is the patient's wife and shows them through the house to the den, where her husband is seated in an overstuffed recliner. The patient is Reverend Charles Allen, a 54-year-old Methodist minister, who is well known to the paramedics. He is conscious and alert, but in obvious distress. He is breathing at a rate of 24 breaths per minute with some difficulty. His skin is pale and diaphoretic. While Jo gets a brief history from him, she checks his radial pulse and finds that it is strong and regular at a rate of 84 beats per minute. Scott is busy attaching ECG electrodes and a pulse oximeter. The Emergency Medical Responders have already started oxygen administration with a nonrebreather mask. They inform Jo and Scott that the patient's blood pressure is 150/90 mmHg.

Reverend Allen tells Jo he is experiencing a "heaviness" in his chest, which is making it difficult for him to breathe. He says it feels as though "an elephant is sitting on it." He rates the discomfort as an 8 out of 10 and says it began about 15 minutes earlier, while he was watching television. He denies any other complaints and has no relevant medical history, takes no medications, and has no allergies. Per system standing orders, Jo administers 325 milligrams of chewable aspirin to her patient while she listens to his lungs. He has clear breath sounds in all fields. Jo asks Scott to place a saline lock while she administers 0.4 milligram (1/150 grain) of nitroglycerin (NitroStat) sublingually. The patient's pain has decreased somewhat, but he is still very uncomfortable and is now complaining of nausea. Jo has him place another nitroglycerin under his tongue while she administers 4 milligrams of ondansetron (Zofran) intravenously. She asks

him to hold still while she runs a 12-lead ECG, and then she moves him to the ambulance for transport to the nearest cardiac center.

Jo anticipates an approximately 75-minute transport time to Our Lady of the Sea Hospital. The local community hospital closed several years ago due to financial reasons, forcing patients to drive 60 miles to a neighboring town for their health care needs. Because of this, EMS has become even more important to the small community. Jo reassesses her patient and finds that he is still having chest discomfort, but he now rates it as a 6 out of 10. She administers another 2 milligrams of morphine sulfate intravenously. She notices that the ECG shows ST elevation in leads V_2 through V_6, indicating an anterolateral injury. Jo confirms the key findings of the history to determine whether her patient is a candidate for prehospital fibrinolytic therapy. Finding no contraindications for fibrinolytic therapy, she contacts the hospital to notify the staff. The medical direction physician reviews the patient's risk factors and confirms that there are no contraindications to fibrinolytic therapy. Jo faxes him a copy of the 12-lead. He agrees with the paramedics' assessment of anterolateral myocardial ischemia and authorizes Jo to administer recombinant tissue plasminogen activator (rtPA) via a standardized protocol. The protocol includes an initial 15-mg bolus over 1 to 2 minutes followed by a timed infusion over the next 90 minutes. Following the bolus, Jo prepares and starts the infusion using a programmed IV pump. Jo carefully documents the time at which the rtPA bolus was administered. In addition, they are to continue titrating the morphine sulfate, with the goal of eliminating all discomfort.

Jo continues to administer morphine incrementally until Reverend Allen reports that he is free of discomfort. She carefully monitors his blood pressure and pulse rate throughout transport. On arrival at the hospital, the patient is moved to the chest pain unit of the emergency department. Initial laboratory studies and a chest X-ray are obtained. The patient is placed on a 12-lead ECG monitor. The paramedics note marked improvement in the ST segment elevation seen earlier in leads V$_2$ through V$_6$. The patient remains pain free. Shortly thereafter, he is taken to the intensive care unit and has an uneventful night.

The next morning, he undergoes cardiac catheterization and coronary angiography. Unfortunately, Reverend Allen has rather severe coronary artery disease, with several high-grade blockages. The cardiologists determine that he has too much disease for percutaneous

coronary intervention (PCI). The patient is referred to cardiovascular surgery. The next day, he undergoes four-vessel coronary artery bypass grafting (CABG). He does well in surgery and afterward. Thanks to the efforts of the paramedics, he has no permanent myocardial injury from the heart attack.

Reverend Allen is discharged from the hospital four days later and begins an aggressive cardiac rehabilitation program. Six weeks later, he is able to resume his usual activities and returns to the pulpit, much to the satisfaction of his parishioners.

Introduction

The use of herbs and minerals to treat the sick and injured has been documented as long ago as 2000 B.C.E. Ancient Egyptians, Arabs, and Greeks probably passed formulations down through generations by word of mouth for centuries until they were finally recorded in pharmacopoeias. By the end of the Renaissance, pharmacology was a distinct and growing discipline, separate from medicine. During the seventeenth and eighteenth centuries, tinctures of opium, coca, and digitalis were available. The related concept of vaccination with biological extracts began in 1796 with Edward Jenner's smallpox inoculations. By the nineteenth century, atropine, chloroform, codeine, ether, and morphine were in use. The discoveries of animal insulin and penicillin in the early twentieth century dramatically changed the treatment of endocrine/metabolic and infectious diseases. Now, in the twenty-first century, recombinant DNA technology has produced human insulin and recombinant tissue plasminogen activator (rtPA). These drugs have markedly changed the treatment of diabetes and cardiovascular disease.

Currently in the United States, the Food and Drug Administration (FDA) is allowing many previously prescription-only drugs to become available over the counter. This is due in part to growing consumer awareness in health care and also in part to consumer marketing by the pharmaceutical industry. The industry is actively seeking drugs that appeal widely to the consumer for treatments and cures. Pharmaceutical research to limit aging or increase the life span is growing rapidly. The federal government also offers incentives to pharmaceutical companies to research drugs for rare diseases. These so-called orphan drugs are often expensive to investigate and have a limited sales potential, making them less profitable to develop and manufacture than others.

General principles of pharmacology are presented in this chapter, which is divided into two parts:

Part 1: Basic Pharmacology

Part 2: Drug Classifications

PART 1: Basic Pharmacology
General Aspects
Names

Drugs may be broadly defined as foreign substances placed into the body. The term *drugs* is also used as a synonym for **medications**, chemicals used to diagnose, treat, or prevent disease. **Pharmacology** is the study of drugs and their actions on the body. To study and converse about pharmacology, health care professionals must have a systematic method for naming drugs. The most detailed name for any drug is its chemical description, which states its chemical composition and molecular structure. Ethyl-1-methyl-4-phenylisonipecotate hydrochloride, for example, is a chemical name. A generic name is usually suggested by the manufacturer and confirmed by the United States Adopted Name Council. It becomes the Federal Drug Administration's (FDA's) official name when listed in the *United States Pharmacopeia* (USP), the official standard for information about pharmaceuticals in the United States. In the case of N-Phenyl-N-(1-(2-phenylethyl)-4-piperidinyl) propanamide, the generic name is fentanyl citrate, USP. To foster brand loyalty among its customers, the manufacturer gives the drug a brand name (sometimes called a trade name or proprietary name)—in our example, Sublimaze or Duragesic. The brand name is a proper name and should be capitalized. Most manufacturers also register the name as a trademark, so the stylized ® or ™ may follow the name, as in Duragesic®. Another example is the widely prescribed sedative Valium:

Chemical Name: 7-chloro-1,3-dihydro-1-methyl-5-phenyl-2H-1,4-benzodiazepin-2-one

Generic Name: diazepam

Official Name: diazepam, USP

Brand Name: Valium®

Sources

The four main sources of drugs are plants, animals, minerals, and the laboratory (synthetic). Plants may be the oldest source of medications; primitive people probably used them directly as "herbal" medicines. Indirectly, plant extracts such as gums and oils have long been a source of medications. Examples include the purple foxglove, a source of digitalis (a glycoside), and deadly nightshade, a source of atropine (an alkaloid). Animal extracts are another important source of drugs. For many years, the primary sources of insulin for treating diabetes mellitus were the extracts of bovine (cow) and porcine (pig) pancreas. Minerals are inorganic sources of drugs such as calcium chloride and magnesium sulfate. Synthetic drugs are created in the laboratory. They may provide alternative sources of medications for those found in nature, or they may be entirely new medications not found in nature.

Reference Materials

Obtaining information on drugs can be difficult. Using multiple sources of information about drugs is usually a good idea. Every book about drugs, including this one, has a disclaimer regarding doses and current uses, referring the reader to local medical direction for the final word. Using multiple sources and comparing the authors' statements about a drug may lead you to the best available information. The USP is a nongovernmental, official public standards-setting authority for prescription and over-the-counter medicines and other health care products manufactured or sold in the United States. EMS providers, however, generally like small, short guides that they can carry in a shirt pocket. These usually include important details about drugs that out-of-hospital providers administer, along with a long list of commonly prescribed drugs and their classes. These EMS guides will be useful if you clearly understand the drugs used in your system and have a working knowledge of commonly prescribed drug classes.

Drug inserts, the printed fact sheets that drug manufacturers supply with most medications, contain information prescribed by the FDA. The *Physician's Desk Reference*, a compilation of these drug inserts, also includes three indices and a section containing photographs of drugs. It is among the most popular references, but it contains only factual information and must be interpreted by informed readers. The American Hospital Formulary Service publishes *Drug Information* annually as a service to the American Society of Health-System

Pharmacists. It contains an authoritative listing of monographs on virtually every drug used in the United States. A less bulky reference to keep in an ambulance might be one of the many drug guides for nurses. They contain information on hundreds of drugs in a format much like the EMS drug guides, but they also offer information on commonly prescribed drugs rather than only on emergency drugs. The American Medical Association also publishes a useful reference, the *AMA Drug Evaluation.* The Internet provides an enormous amount of information, but you must be especially cautious when using it as a source, because it allows anyone with a computer to be a publisher, with no requirement for accuracy. Examples of reputable Internet-based reference sites include the following:

- Drugs.com
- Rxlist.com
- WebMD
- *eMedicine*
- *Micromedix*

There are several widely available pharmacology reference programs for smartphones. Among these are:

- *Epocrates*
- *Skyscape/DrDrugs*
- *MediMath*
- *Lexi-comp*

Components of a Drug Profile

A drug's profile describes its various properties. As a paramedic student, you will become familiar with drug profiles as you study specific medications. A typical drug profile will contain the following information:

- *Names.* These most frequently include the generic and trade names, although the occasional reference will include chemical names.
- *Classification.* This is the broad group to which the drug belongs. Knowing classifications is essential to understanding the properties of drugs.
- *Mechanism of action.* The way in which a drug causes its effects; its pharmacodynamics.

Cultural Considerations

Folk Remedies. Many cultures place great trust in herbal and folk remedies. Some have been proven beneficial by modern research. It is important to ask about them when you obtain your patient's history. Some folk medications can contain potentially toxic compounds, such as those containing lead or arsenic.

- *Indications.* Conditions that make administration of the drug appropriate (as approved by the FDA).

- *Pharmacokinetics.* How the drug is absorbed, distributed, and eliminated; typically includes onset and duration of action.

- *Side effects/adverse reactions.* The drug's untoward or undesired effects.

- *Routes of administration.* How the drug is given.

- *Contraindications.* Conditions that make it inappropriate to give the drug. Unlike conditions when the drug is simply not indicated, a contraindication means that a predictable harmful event will occur if the drug is given in this situation.

- *Dosage.* The amount of the drug that should be given.

- *How supplied.* This typically includes the common concentrations of the available preparations; many drugs come in different concentrations.

- *Special considerations.* How the drug may affect pediatric, geriatric, or pregnant patients.

Drug profiles may also include other components, such as its interactions with other drugs or with foods, when appropriate.

Legal Aspects

Knowing and obeying the laws and regulations governing medications and their administration will be an important part of your career. These laws and regulations come from three distinct authorities: federal law, state laws and regulations, and individual agency regulations.

Federal

Drug legislation in the United States has been aimed primarily at protecting the public from adulterated or mislabeled drugs. The *Pure Food and Drug Act of 1906*, enacted to improve the quality and labeling of drugs, named the *United States Pharmacopeia* as this country's official source for drug information. The *Harrison Narcotic Act of 1914* limited the indiscriminate use of addicting drugs by regulating the importation, manufacture, sale, and use of opium, cocaine, and their compounds or derivatives. *The Federal Food, Drug and Cosmetic Act of 1938* empowered the FDA to enforce and set premarket safety standards for drugs. In 1951, the *Durham-Humphrey Amendments* to the 1938 act (also known as the prescription

CONTENT REVIEW

➤ Drug Laws and Regulations
- Federal law
- State laws and regulations
- Individual agency regulations

Legal Considerations

Follow Orders of the Medical Director. The administration of medications by a paramedic is allowed only by express physician order. This can be either verbal or through approved written standing orders. Always follow your medical director's orders in regard to medication administration.

---

drug amendments) required pharmacists to have either a written or verbal prescription from a physician to dispense certain drugs. It also created the category of over-the-counter medications. The *Kefauver-Harris Amendment* was an amendment to the Federal Food, Drug and Cosmetic Act, added in 1962, that required pharmaceutical manufacturers to provide proof of the safety and effectiveness of their drugs before being granted approval to produce and market the products. This also stopped the process of remarketing inexpensive generic drugs under new "trade names." The *Comprehensive Drug Abuse Prevention and Control Act* (also known as the Controlled Substances Act) of 1970 is the most recent major federal legislation affecting drug sales and use. It repealed and replaced the Harrison Narcotic Act.

The federal government strictly regulates controlled substances because of their high potential for abuse. Because not all drugs cause the same level of physical or psychological dependence, they do not all need to be regulated in the same way. To accommodate their differences, the *Controlled Substance Act of 1970* created five schedules of controlled substances, each with its own level of control and record keeping requirements (Table 13-1). Most emergency medical services administer only a few controlled substances—usually a narcotic analgesic, such as morphine sulfate or fentanyl, and a benzodiazepine anticonvulsant, such as diazepam or lorazepam.

The majority of the remaining drugs provided by an EMS are prescription drugs—those whose use the FDA has designated sufficiently dangerous to require the supervision of a health care practitioner (physician, dentist, and, in some states, nurse practitioner or certified physician assistant). For emergency medical services, this means that the physician medical director is, in effect, prescribing the drugs in advance, based on the assessments and judgments of EMS providers in the field.

Over-the-counter (OTC) medications are generally available in small doses and, when taken as recommended, present a low risk to patients. Of the few OTC drugs that EMS providers administer, acetaminophen and aspirin are probably the most commonly used. Although laws vary from state to state, they still require most EMS providers to obtain a physician's order (either written, verbal, or standing) to administer OTC drugs.

Table 13-1 Schedules of Drugs According to the Controlled Substances Act of 1970

Schedule	Description	Examples
Schedule I	High abuse potential; may lead to severe dependence; no accepted medical indications; used for research, analysis, or instruction only	Heroin, LSD, mescaline
Schedule II	High abuse potential; may lead to severe dependence; accepted medical indications	Opium, cocaine, morphine, codeine, oxycodone, hydrocodone, methadone, secobarbital
Schedule III	Less abuse potential than Schedule I and II; may lead to moderate or low physical dependence or high psychological dependence; accepted medical indications	Limited opioid amounts or combined with noncontrolled substances; acetaminophen with codeine, buprenorphine
Schedule IV	Low abuse potential compared to Schedule III; limited psychological and/or physical dependence; accepted medical indications	Diazepam, lorazepam, phenobarbital
Schedule V	Lower abuse potential compared to Schedule IV; may lead to limited physical or psychological dependence; accepted medical indications	Limited amounts of opioids; often for cough or diarrhea

Federal drug laws require that certain substances be appropriately secured, distributed, and accounted for. Because of the complexity of this issue and the large variability of drugs used in EMS systems across the country, specific answers to these concerns are not practical here. Consult your local protocols, laws, and most importantly, your medical director for guidance in this area.

State

State laws vary widely. Some states have legislated which medications are appropriate for paramedics to give, whereas others have left those decisions to local control. Local control varies as well. In some areas, regional EMS authorities set the local standards; in others, the individual medical directors and department directors do. In all cases, however, the physician medical director can delegate to paramedics the authority to administer medications, either by written, verbal, or standing order. You must know the laws of the state where you practice.

Local

In each community, local leaders are responsible for ensuring public safety. Local EMS agencies have the responsibility to create local policies and procedures to ensure the public well-being. An excellent example of a local procedure protecting the patient (and thereby the individual EMS provider and agency) would be a requirement to use a pulse oximeter whenever a patient is sedated or paralyzed. Even though this requirement would not have the force of law, it would locally help to ensure that local EMS providers do not overlook hypoxia in these patients.

Standards

Because some generic drugs affect patients differently than their brand name counterparts do, standardization

of drugs is a necessity. Despite FDA standards, drugs sold or distributed by various manufacturers may have biological or therapeutic differences. An **assay** determines the amount and purity of a given chemical in a preparation in the laboratory (in vitro). Although two generically equivalent preparations may contain the same amount of a given chemical (drug), they may have different therapeutic effects. This relative therapeutic effectiveness of chemically equivalent drugs is their **bioequivalence**. Bioequivalence is determined by a **bioassay**, which attempts to ascertain the drug's availability in a biological model (in vivo). Again, the USP is the official standard for the United States.

Drug Research and Bringing a Drug to Market

The pharmaceutical industry is highly motivated to bring profitable new drugs to market. Proving the safety and reliability of these new drugs, however, requires extensive research. Even though better understanding of biology is shortening the time needed to bring a new drug to market, the process still takes many years. To ensure the safety of new medications, the FDA has developed a process for evaluating their safety and efficacy. This process, illustrated in Figure 13-1, adds even more time to the development cycle. Initial drug testing begins with the study of both male and female mammals. After testing a drug's toxicity, researchers evaluate its pharmacokinetics—how it is absorbed, distributed, metabolized (biotransformed), and excreted—in animals. These animal studies also help determine the drug's therapeutic index (the ratio of its lethal dose to its effective dose). If the results of animal testing are satisfactory, the FDA designates the drug as an investigational new drug (IND), and researchers can then test it in humans.

New Drug Development Timeline

FIGURE 13-1 New drug development timeline.

(United States Food and Drug Administration website, http://www.fda.gov/fdac/special/newdrug/testing.html)

Phases of Human Studies

Human studies take place in four phases.

PHASE 1 The primary purposes of phase 1 testing are to determine the drug's pharmacokinetics, toxicity, and safe dose in humans. These studies are usually carried out on limited populations of healthy human volunteers; some drugs with a high risk of untoward effects will not be tested on healthy individuals.

PHASE 2 When phase 1 studies prove that the drug is safe, it is tested on a limited population of patients who have the disease it is intended to treat. The primary purposes of phase 2 studies are to find the therapeutic drug level and watch carefully for toxic and side effects.

PHASE 3 The main purposes of phase 3 testing are to refine the usual therapeutic dose and to collect relevant data on side effects. Gathering the significant amounts of

data needed for these goals requires a large patient population. Phase 3 studies are usually *double-blind*. That is, neither the patient nor the researcher knows whether the patient is receiving a placebo or the drug until after the study has been completed. This keeps personal biases from affecting the reporting of results. Some phase 3 studies are controlled studies, which are like placebo studies except that, instead of a placebo, the patient receives a treatment that is known to be effective. Occasionally, a double-blind study will be ended sooner than planned if the early results are convincing.

Once phase 3 studies are completed, the manufacturer files a new drug application (NDA) with the Food and Drug Administration, which then evaluates the data collected in the investigation's first three phases. At this point, the FDA decides whether to conditionally approve manufacturing and marketing the drug in the United States. The FDA's abbreviated new drug application (ANDA) process may significantly shorten this process for generic equivalents of currently approved drugs.

PHASE 4   Phase 4 testing involves postmarketing analysis during conditional approval. Once a drug is being used in the general population, the FDA requires the drug's maker to monitor its performance. Many drugs have been discontinued after marketing when previously unknown effects became apparent. One example would be the antiemetic thalidomide. Because children and pregnant women are generally excluded from the first three phases of testing, the premarket testing did not reveal that thalidomide caused birth defects in the children of pregnant women who took it.

FDA Classification of Newly Approved Drugs

The FDA has developed a method for immediately classifying new drugs. This method of drug classification uses a number and a letter for each new drug in the IND phase or on NDA review by the FDA. The manufacturer has a right to contest this classification and have it changed before the final classification is established.

Numerical Classification (Chemical)

1. A new molecular drug
2. A new salt of a marketed drug
3. A new formulation or dosage form not previously marketed
4. A new combination not previously marketed
5. A drug that is already on the market, a generic duplication
6. A product already marketed by the same company (This designation is used for new indications for a marketed drug.)
7. A drug product on the market without an approved NDA (drug was marketed prior to 1938)

Letter Classification (Treatment or Therapeutic Potential)

A. Drug offers an important therapeutic gain (P-priority)
B. Drug that is similar to drugs already on the market (S-similar)

Other Classifications

A. Drugs indicated for AIDS and HIV-related disease
B. Drugs developed to treat life-threatening or severely debilitating illness
C. An orphan drug

Patient Care Using Medications

Paramedics are responsible for the standard of care for patients in their charge. They are, therefore, personally responsible—legally, morally, and ethically—for the safe and effective administration of medications. The following guidelines will help you to meet that responsibility:

- Know the precautions and contraindications for all medications you administer.
- Practice proper techniques.
- Know how to observe and document drug effects.
- Maintain a current knowledge of pharmacology.
- Establish and maintain professional relationships with other health care providers.
- Understand the pharmacokinetics and pharmacodynamics.
- Have current medication references available.
- Take careful drug histories, including:
  - Name, strength, and daily dose of prescribed drugs
  - Over-the-counter drugs
  - Vitamins
  - Herbal medications
  - Folk medicine or folk remedies
  - Allergies
- Evaluate the compliance, dosage, and adverse reactions.
- Consult with medical direction when appropriate.

Six Rights of Medication Administration

No pharmacology chapter would be complete without discussing the six rights of medication administration. They include the right medication, the right dose, the right time, the right route, the right patient, and the right documentation.

RIGHT MEDICATION   When following a physician's verbal medication order, repeat the order back to him to confirm that you both intend the same thing for the patient. Inspect the label on the drug at least three times before giving the medication to the patient: first, as you remove the medication from the drug box or cabinet; second, as you draw the medication into the syringe or dole the tablet into a cup; and third, immediately before you administer the medication. Failure to confirm the medication name is one of the most common medication administration errors. If you have any question about a drug, do not administer it without confirmation. Showing the medication container to your partner and asking for confirmation is an easy way to further ensure that you are giving the right drug.

CONTENT REVIEW

➤ Six Rights of Medication Administration
  - Right medication
  - Right dose
  - Right time
  - Right route
  - Right patient
  - Right documentation

RIGHT DOSE To reduce medication errors, many drugs come in unit **dose packaging**. That is, the package contains a single dose for a single patient. Dosages of many emergency drugs, however, are based on patient weight, so a prefilled syringe may not contain the exact amount a patient needs. You will have to calculate the correct dose. One good practice for identifying potential medication errors is to consider the number of unit dose packages needed for a single dose. If your calculations tell you to open 10 vials for one dose of medication, for example, prudence requires you to check the calculation and dose carefully. The package may contain a unit dose of the wrong medication, or you may have miscalculated.

RIGHT TIME Even though paramedics usually give medications in urgent and emergent situations rather than on a schedule, timing can still be very important. Giving nitroglycerin tablets too soon may precipitate hypotension; if epinephrine is not repeated on time during cardiac arrest, it may not help to lower the threshold for defibrillation. Take care to give medications punctually and to document their administration promptly.

RIGHT ROUTE Often, you will have to choose among several treatments for a particular problem. In these cases, knowing the principles of pharmacokinetics can help greatly in giving your patient the medication via the right route. For example, your knowledge that you should administer epinephrine intravenously rather than subcutaneously to the patient in anaphylactic shock because knowing that his blood is being shunted away from the skin will guide you to the proper administration route.

RIGHT PATIENT As the paramedic's role in health care expands, you will find yourself caring for more people than just "the patient in the back of the truck." You will deal with multiple patients, and the potential for giving medication to the wrong patient will be real. You will have to identify patients by name before administering medications.

RIGHT DOCUMENTATION The drugs you administer in the field do not stop affecting your patients when they enter the hospital. As a result, you must completely document all your care, especially any drugs you have administered, so that long after you have gone on to your next call, other providers will know what drugs your patient has taken.

Special Considerations

PREGNANT PATIENTS Whenever you administer drugs to a woman of childbearing years, you must consider the possibility that she is pregnant. Treating pregnant patients clearly means treating two patients. Although emphasis appropriately seems to center on the mother during care,

you must understand that many drugs that affect the mother also affect the fetus. A drug's possible benefits to the mother must clearly outweigh its potential risks to the fetus. For example, some situations such as cardiac arrest justify giving the mother medications that may harm the fetus because the drug's possible harm to the fetus is clearly outweighed by the fetus's certain death if the mother dies.

> **CONTENT REVIEW**
> ➤ Special Considerations
>   • Pregnant patients
>   • Pediatric patients
>   • Geriatric patients

Patho Pearls

Medications That Cross the Placenta. Some medications cross the placenta and affect the fetus. Because of this, it is prudent to ask whether a female patient might be pregnant before administering a medication. In addition, some medications cross into the breast milk and can potentially affect a breast-feeding baby.

Pregnancy presents two particular pharmacological problems: changes in the mother's anatomy and physiology, and the potential for drugs to harm the fetus. Because the mother is supporting the fetus entirely, her heart rate, cardiac output, and blood volume will increase. This altered maternal physiology can affect the onset and duration of action of many medications. During the first trimester of pregnancy, the ingestion of some drugs (**teratogenic drugs**) may potentially deform, injure, or kill the fetus. During the last trimester, drugs administered to the mother may pass through the placenta to the fetus. Some of these drugs will have unwanted effects on the fetus. Others may not be metabolized and/or excreted, possibly resulting in toxic accumulations. Additionally, a breast-feeding mother's milk may pass some drugs to her infant.

Under some conditions, of course, the health and safety of mother and fetus demand the use of drugs during the pregnancy. Examples include pregnancy-induced diabetes, hypertension, and seizure disorders. To help health care providers determine when drugs are needed during pregnancy, the FDA has developed the classification system shown in Table 13-2. Always consult medical direction for any questions about drug safety in pregnancy.

PEDIATRIC PATIENTS Several physiologic factors affect pharmacokinetics in newborns and young children. These patients' absorption of oral medications is less than an adult's because of various differences in gastric pH, gastric emptying time, and low enzyme levels. A newborn's skin is thinner than an older patient's and is therefore more permeable to topically administered drugs. This can result in unexpected toxicity. Older children still have less gastric acid than adults do, but their gastric emptying times reach an adult's around the sixth to eighth month of life. Because

Table 13-2 FDA Pregnancy Categories

Category	Description
A	Adequate studies in pregnant women have not demonstrated a risk to the fetus in the first trimester or later trimesters.
B	Animal studies have not demonstrated a risk to the fetus, *but* there are no adequate studies in pregnant women. OR Adequate studies in pregnant women have not demonstrated a risk to the fetus in the first trimester and there is no risk in the last trimester, *but* animal studies have demonstrated adverse effects.
C	Animal studies have demonstrated adverse effects, *but* there are no adequate studies in pregnant women; however, benefits may be acceptable despite the potential risks. OR No adequate animal studies or adequate studies of pregnant women have been done.
D	Fetal risk has been demonstrated. In certain circumstances, benefits could outweigh the risks.
X	Fetal risk has been demonstrated. This risk outweighs any possible benefit to the mother. Avoid using in pregnant or potentially pregnant patients.

FIGURE 13-2 A Broselow tape is useful for calculating drug dosages for pediatric patients.

children up to a year old have diminished plasma protein concentrations, drugs that bind to proteins have higher **free drug availability**. That is, a greater proportion of the drug will be available in the body to cause either desired or undesired effects. Water distribution is different in the neonate as well. Neonates have a much higher proportion of extracellular fluid (nearly 80 percent) than adults (50 to 55 percent). This higher amount of water means a greater volume and, with less than expected protein binding, may require higher drug doses. The premature infant is especially susceptible to drugs penetrating the *blood–brain barrier* because his immature connective tissues form a weaker obstacle.

The newborn's metabolic rates may be much lower than an adult's, but they rise rapidly and by a few years of age may triple those of an adult. These metabolic rates then decline steadily until early adolescence, when they reach adult levels. A newborn's low metabolic rate and incompletely developed hepatic system put him at higher risk for toxic interactions. Neonates' metabolic pathways also are different from an adult's, meaning that some drugs will not have the expected effect or may have other, unexpected effects. Finally, the neonatal renal and hepatic systems' immaturity delays elimination of many drugs and their metabolites. Dosing schedules may have to be adjusted to accommodate longer half-lives until these systems mature at about 6 months to 1 year of age.

With all these factors, a pediatric patient's drug function can differ radically from an adult's. Pediatric drug dosages must be individualized to minimize the risks of toxicity. Body surface area and weight are the two most common factors in calculating dosages. The Broselow tape gives a good approximation of average height/weight ratio for children. It bases its calculations on the child's height (length), and assumes the child's weight is at the fiftieth percentile for his height (Figure 13-2). The Broselow tape addresses primarily drugs administered in the critical care setting.

GERIATRIC PATIENTS Significant changes in pharmacokinetics may also occur in patients older than about 60 years. They may absorb oral medications more slowly due to decreased gastrointestinal motility. Decreased plasma protein concentration may alter distribution of drugs in their systems, leaving drugs free that would otherwise have been protein bound. Body fat increases and muscle mass decreases with age; therefore, lipid-soluble drugs may have greater deposition, thereby lowering the amount of available drug. Absorption and distribution of intramuscular injections may change if volumes are inappropriate for the remaining muscle mass. Because the liver primarily handles biotransformation, depressed liver function in an aging patient may delay or prolong drug action. The aging process may also slow elimination by the renal system.

Older patients are also more likely to be on multiple medications or to have multiple underlying disease processes. Various medication interactions can have a severe impact on patients. For example, sildenafil (Viagra) and nitroglycerin taken together may cause severe hypotension. Underlying diseases may affect therapeutics in unexpected ways. Congestive heart failure, for instance, may cause congestion of the gastrointestinal tract's vasculature, delaying the absorption of oral medications. The congestive heart failure patient may also have compromised renal function, delaying his elimination of drugs.

Pharmacology

Pharmacology is the study of drugs and their interactions with the body. Drugs do not confer any new properties on cells or tissues; they only modify or exploit existing functions. They may be given for their local action (in which case systemic absorption of the drug is discouraged) or for systemic action. Although generally given for a specific effect, drugs tend to have multiple actions at multiple sites, so they must be thought of in terms of their systemic effects rather than in terms of an isolated single effect. Pharmacology's two major divisions are pharmacokinetics and pharmacodynamics. We have already indicated that **pharmacokinetics** addresses how drugs are transported into and out of the body and that **pharmacodynamics** deals with their effects once they reach the target tissues.

Pharmacokinetics

Strictly defined, pharmacokinetics is the study of the basic processes that determine the duration and intensity of a drug's effect. These four processes are absorption, distribution, biotransformation, and elimination.

Review of Physiology of Transport

Pharmacokinetics is dependent on the body's various physiologic mechanisms that move substances across the body's compartments. These mechanisms can be broken down into two broad categories based on their energy requirements and then further classified. A mechanism is referred to as **active transport** if it requires the use of energy to move a substance. This energy is achieved by the breakdown of high-energy chemical bonds found in chemicals such as ATP (adenosine triphosphate). ATP is broken down into ADP (adenosine diphosphate), liberating a considerable amount of biochemical energy. A common example of an active transport mechanism is the sodium–potassium (Na^+–K^+) pump. This is a protein pump that actively moves potassium ions into the cell and sodium ions out of the cell. Because this movement goes *against* the ions' concentration gradients, it must use energy (Figure 13-3).

Sodium/Potassium Pump

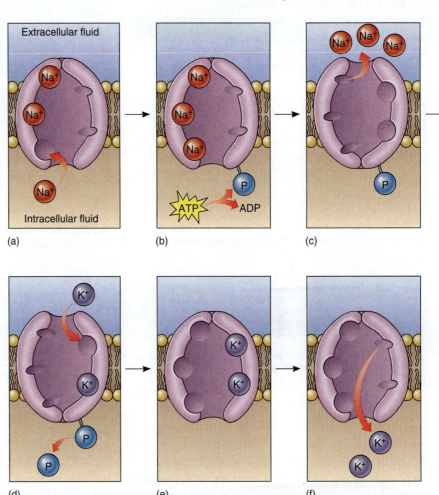

FIGURE 13-3 Primary active transport by the Na^+/K^+ pump. The pump possesses three sodium-binding sites and two potassium-binding sites. ATP is used to power the pump, which transports sodium ions outside the cell and potassium ions into the cell against their electrochemical gradients. (a) Intracellular Na^+ ions bind to the pump protein. (b) The binding of three Na^+ ions triggers phosphorylation of the pump by ATP. (c) Phosphorylation induces a conformational change in the protein that allows the release of Na^+ in the extracellular fluid. (d) Extracellular K^+ ions bind to the pump protein and trigger release of the phosphate group. (e) Loss of the phosphate group allows the protein to return to its original conformation. (f) K^+ ions are released to the inside of the cell, and the Na^+ sites become again available for binding.

Large molecules, such as glucose and most of the amino acids, do not readily pass through the cell membrane because of their size. These molecules are moved across the cell membrane with the help of special "carrier" proteins found on the surface of the target cells. These large molecules are "carried" across the cell membrane in a special transport process called **carrier-mediated diffusion** or **facilitated diffusion**. These mechanisms typically do not require the expenditure of energy. Once the molecule to be transported binds with the carrier protein, the configuration of the cell membrane changes, allowing the large molecule to enter the target cell. Insulin, an important hormone secreted by the endocrine pancreas, can increase the rate of carrier-mediated glucose transport from 10- to 20-fold.

FIGURE 13-4 Transport of a glucose molecule across a cell membrane by a carrier protein. (a) A carrier protein with an empty binding site. (b) Binding of a glucose molecule to the protein's binding site, which faces the extracellular surface of the cell. (c) Conformational change in the carrier protein, such that the binding site now faces the interior of the cell. (d) Release of the glucose molecule. The binding site is once again empty. (e) Return of the carrier to its original conformation. The carrier is now ready to bind another glucose molecule.

Facilitated Diffusion

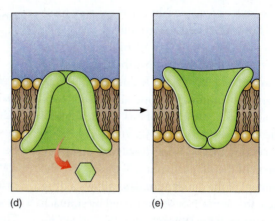

This is the principal mechanism by which insulin controls glucose use in the body (Figure 13-4).

Most drugs travel through the body by means of **passive transport**, the movement of a substance without the use of energy. This requires the presence of concentration gradients in a solution. Diffusion and osmosis are forms of passive transport. **Diffusion** involves the movement of solute in the solution, whereas **osmosis** involves the movement of the solvent (usually water). In diffusion, the solute's molecules or ions move *down* their concentration gradients from an area of higher concentration to an area of lower concentration. Conversely, in osmosis the solvent's molecules move *up* the concentration gradient from an area of low solute concentration to an area of higher solute concentration. Another way of looking at this is to think of osmosis as simply the diffusion of solvent from an area of high *solvent* concentration to an area of low *solvent* concentration (Figure 13-5). A final type of passive transport is **filtration**. This is simply the movement of molecules across a membrane down a *pressure* gradient, from an area of high pressure to an area of lower pressure. This pressure typically results from the hydrostatic force of blood pressure.

Absorption

When a drug is administered to a patient it must find its way to the site of action. If a drug is given orally or injected into any place except the bloodstream,

Diffusion

When solutes are differently concentrated on two sides of membranes, molecules cross in both directions until equilibrium is reached.

Osmosis

When there is more of a solute such as salt on one side of the membrane, water is drawn across the membrane to dilute the greater concentration until the concentration is equal on both sides.

FIGURE 13-5 Diffusion is the movement of solute from an area of higher concentration to an area of lower concentration. Osmosis is the movement of water from an area of lower solute concentration to an area of higher solute concentration.

its absorption into the bloodstream is the first step in this process. (Because drugs given intravenously or intraarterially enter directly into the bloodstream, no absorption needs to occur.) Several factors affect a drug's absorption. The body absorbs most drugs faster when they are given intramuscularly than when they are given subcutaneously. This is because muscles are more vascular than subcutaneous tissue. Of course, anything that slows blood flow will delay absorption. Shock and hypothermia are just two examples. Conversely, processes such as fever and hyperthermia increase peripheral blood flow and speed absorption.

Drugs given orally (enterally) must first survive the digestive processes before being absorbed across the mucosa of the gastrointestinal system. If a drug is not soluble in water, it will have difficulty being absorbed. Time-released medications take advantage of this with an enteric coating that releases the medication slowly. Some drugs have an enteric coating that will not dissolve in the more acidic environment of the stomach, but will dissolve in the alkaline environment of the duodenum. This allows a drug that would irritate the stomach or be destroyed by stomach acid to be passed through the stomach into the duodenum and absorbed there. Besides being able to survive stomach acid, a drug must also be somewhat lipid (fat) soluble to cross the cells' lipid two-layered (bilayered) membranes. Many drugs **ionize**, or become electrically charged or polar, following administration. Generally, ionized drugs do not absorb across the membranes of cells (lipid bilayers), but fortunately, most drugs do not fully ionize. In addition, ions can be transported across the cell membrane through the use of carrier proteins (Figure 13-6). In other instances, they reach an equilibrium between their ionized and nonionized forms, and the nonionized form can be absorbed. A drug's pH also affects the extent to which it ionizes. A drug that is a weak acid will ionize much more substantially in an alkaline environment than in an acidic environment; conversely, an alkaline drug will ionize more readily in an acidic environment than in an alkaline environment. For example, aspirin (an acidic drug) does not dissociate well in the stomach (an acidic environment) and is therefore readily absorbed there.

The nature of the absorbing surface and the blood flow to the administration site also affect drug absorption. The rate of absorption is directly related to the amount of surface area available for absorption. The greater the area, the faster the absorption. Much of the gastrointestinal system has multiple invaginations, or folds, that increase its surface area. Also, the greater blood flow is to an area, the faster will be the rate of absorption. Again, the GI tract has

Ion Transport

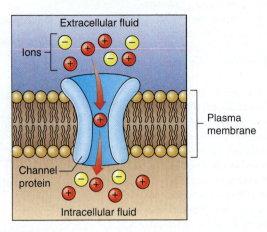

FIGURE 13-6 Transport of ions across a cell membrane through a channel protein.

a rich vascular system with many capillaries that perfuse its absorbing surfaces, allowing nutrients (and drugs) to diffuse into the bloodstream.

Finally, the drug's concentration affects its absorption. Because drugs diffuse in the body, the higher their concentration, the more rapidly the body will absorb them. This principle is frequently used when giving a "loading dose" of a drug and following it with a "maintenance infusion." The loading dose is typically a larger dose of the same concentration of the drug. On occasion, a more concentrated solution of the drug is used as the loading dose. Regardless, the desired effect is to rapidly raise the amount of the drug in the system to a therapeutic level. This is typically followed by a continuous infusion of the drug at a lower concentration, or slower administration rate, to keep it at the therapeutic level.

Bioavailability is the measure of the amount of a drug that is still active after it reaches its target tissue. This is the bottom line as far as absorption is concerned. The goal of administering a drug is to ensure sufficient bioavailability of the drug at the target tissue in order to produce the desired effect, after considering all the absorption factors.

Distribution

Once a drug has entered the bloodstream, it must be distributed throughout the body. Most drugs will pass easily from the bloodstream, through the interstitial spaces, into the target cells. Some drugs, however, will bind to proteins found in the blood—most commonly, albumin—and remain in the body for a prolonged time. They thus have a sustained release from the bloodstream and a prolonged period of action. The therapeutic effects of a drug are primarily due to the unbound portion of the drug in the blood. A drug that is bound to plasma proteins cannot cross membranes and reach the target cells. Thus, only the unbound drug is in equilibrium with the target cells and can cross the cell membranes.

Changing the bloodstream's pH can affect the protein-binding action of a drug. Tricyclic antidepressants (TCAs), for instance, are strongly bound to plasma proteins. Making the blood more alkaline increases protein binding of the TCA molecules. Therefore, in addition to supportive therapy, serious overdoses of TCAs are treated by administering sodium bicarbonate. Sodium bicarbonate makes the blood more alkaline (raises the pH), causing increased binding of the TCA to serum proteins. Cumulatively, this decreases the amount of free drug in the blood, thus decreasing the adverse effects. Sodium bicarbonate administration also facilitates elimination of the drug through the urine.

The presence of other serum protein-binding drugs can also affect drug–protein binding. For example, the drug warfarin (Coumadin) is highly protein bound (99 percent). Its therapeutic effects are due to the 1 percent of the drug that is unbound and circulating in the bloodstream. Aspirin molecules bind to the same binding site on the serum proteins as do warfarin molecules. Thus, when aspirin is administered to a patient on warfarin, it displaces some of the protein-bound warfarin, increasing the amount of free (unbound) warfarin in the blood. Even if it displaces only 1 percent of the total warfarin, it effectively doubles the available warfarin. This can lead to unwanted side effects, such as hemorrhage.

Albumin is one of the chief proteins in the blood that is available for binding with drugs. When albumin levels are low (hypoalbuminemia), as occurs in malnutrition, drugs that are normally protein bound rise to much greater blood levels than anticipated. For example, consider a patient who has been taking warfarin without difficulty. If he develops hypoalbuminemia, his normal dose of warfarin will result in much more of the drug being available in the body, possibly leading to dangerous bleeding.

Certain organs exclude some drugs from distribution. For example, the tight junctions of the capillary endothelial cells in the central nervous system (CNS) vasculature form a **blood–brain barrier**. These cells are packed together so tightly that only non–protein-bound, highly lipid-soluble drugs can cross into the CNS. The so-called **placental barrier** can likewise prevent drugs from reaching a fetus, although it is not the solid barrier that its name implies. The fetus is exposed to almost every drug that the mother takes. However, because any drug must traverse the maternal blood supply and cross the capillary membranes into the placental (fetal) circulation, delivering drugs to a fetus requires them to be lipid soluble, nonionized, and non–protein-bound. This may slow some drugs or reduce their placental transfer to benign levels.

Other drugs are deposited in specific tissues. Fatty tissue, for example, can serve as a drug depot, or reservoir.

Because blood flow is lower in fatty areas than in muscular areas, fatty tissue is a relatively stable depot; it can neither absorb nor release a large amount of drug in a short time. Similarly, bones and teeth can accumulate high amounts of drugs that bind to calcium, especially tetracycline antibiotics.

Biotransformation

Like other chemicals that enter the body, drugs are metabolized, or broken down into different chemicals (metabolites). The special name given to the **metabolism** of drugs is **biotransformation**. Biotransformation has one of two effects on most drugs: (1) It can transform the drug into a more or less active metabolite, or (2) it can make the drug more water soluble (or less lipid soluble) to facilitate elimination. Some drugs, such as lidocaine, are totally metabolized before elimination, others only partially, and still others not at all. The body will transform some molecules of most drugs and eliminate others without transformation. Protein-bound drugs are not available for biotransformation. Some so-called **prodrugs** (or parent drugs) are not active when administered, but biotransformation converts them into active metabolites.

Many biotransformation processes occur in the liver. The endoplasmic reticula of hepatocytes (liver cells) contain microsomal enzymes that perform much of the metabolizing. (Smaller quantities of these enzymes are also found in the kidney, lung, and GI tract.) Because the blood supply from the GI tract passes through the liver via the portal vein, all drugs absorbed in the GI tract pass through the liver before moving on through the systemic circulation. The first pass through the liver may partially or completely inactivate many drugs. This **first-pass effect** is why some drugs cannot be given orally but instead must be given intravenously to bypass the GI tract and prevent first-pass hepatic metabolism. It is also why drugs that can be given either orally or intravenously may require a much higher oral dose than IV dose. Because we can observe the extent of first-pass metabolism, we can predict how much to increase a dose of an oral medication to deliver an effective amount of the drug into the general circulation.

The liver's microsomal enzymes react with drugs in two ways: phase I, or nonsynthetic reactions; and phase II, or synthetic reactions. *Phase I reactions* most often **oxidize** the parent drug, although they may reduce it or **hydrolyze** it. These nonsynthetic reactions make the drug more water soluble to ease excretion. A number of drugs and chemicals increase the activity of, or induce, the microsomal enzyme that causes phase I reactions. This means that more enzyme is produced, and drugs will be metabolized more rapidly. Because the microsomal enzymes are nonspecific, they can be induced by one drug or chemical and then biotransform other drugs or chemicals. *Phase II reactions*, which are also called conjugation reactions, combine the prodrug or its metabolites with an endogenous (naturally occurring) chemical, usually making the drug more polar and easier to excrete.

Elimination

Whether they are unchanged or metabolized before elimination, most drugs (toxins and metabolites) are excreted in the urine. Some are excreted in the feces or in expired air.

Renal excretion occurs through two major processes: glomerular filtration and tubular secretion. Glomerular filtration is a function of glomerular filtration pressure, which in turn results from blood pressure and blood flow through the kidneys. Conditions that affect blood pressure and blood flow can affect renal elimination. Specialized transport systems in the walls of the proximal kidney tubules secrete drugs into the urine. These "pumps" are active transport systems and require energy in the form of adenosine triphosphate (ATP) to function. Some are specialized and transport only specific chemicals, whereas others can transport a range of similar chemicals. When drugs compete for the same pump, toxicity or other unwanted effects can result; however, combinations of some drugs can take advantage of this specialization to prolong their circulation. For example, probenecid blocks renal tubular pumps and competes for them with many antibiotics, among them penicillin, ampicillin, and oxacillin. Thus, probenecid is sometimes given with those antibiotics to increase and prolong their blood levels.

The same factors that affect absorption at any other site also affect reabsorption in the renal tubules. Of particular concern is the urine pH. Lipid-soluble and nonionized molecules are readily reabsorbed. Changing the urine pH (usually by administering sodium bicarbonate to make it more alkaline) can affect the reabsorption in the renal tubules. For example, if a drug becomes ionized in a more alkaline environment, then making the urine more alkaline will interfere with reabsorption and cause more of the drug to be excreted.

Some drugs and their metabolites can be eliminated in the expired air. This is the basis of the breath test that police use to determine a driver's blood alcohol level. Ethanol is released in the expired air in proportion to its concentration in the bloodstream. Although the liver degrades most ingested ethanol, exhalation releases a measurable quantity. Drugs also can be excreted in the feces. In enterohepatic circulation, if a drug (or its metabolites) is excreted into the intestines from bile, the body may reabsorb the drug and experience a sustained effect. Additionally, drugs may be excreted through sweat, saliva, and breast milk. Excretion through sweat glands is rarely a significant mechanism for elimination. Excretion through mammary glands becomes a concern when nursing mothers take medications.

Drug Routes

The route of a drug's administration clearly has an impact on the drug's absorption and distribution. The route's impact on biotransformation and elimination may not be so clear. The bloodstream will more quickly absorb and distribute water-soluble drugs if given in more vascular compartments than if given in less vascular compartments. Oral or nasogastric administration of alkaline drugs may allow the gastric acids to neutralize the drug and prevent its absorption. The liver's first-pass effect may biotransform some orally administered drugs and degrade them almost immediately.

> **CONTENT REVIEW**
> ➤ Drug Routes
> • Enteral
> • Parenteral

ENTERAL ROUTES   Enteral routes deliver medications by absorption through the gastrointestinal tract, which goes from the mouth to the stomach and on through the intestines to the rectum. They may be oral, orogastric/nasogastric, sublingual, buccal, or rectal.

- *Oral (PO).* The oral route is good for self-administered drugs. Most home medications are administered by this route. The drug must be able to tolerate the acidic gastric environment and be absorbed. Few emergency drugs are administered through this route.

- *Orogastric/nasogastric tube (OG/NG).* This route is generally used for oral medications when the patient already has the tube in place for other reasons.

- *Sublingual (SL).* This is a good route for self-administration and excellent absorption from the sublingual capillary bed without the problems of gastric acidity or absorption.

- *Buccal.* Absorption through this route between the cheek and gum is similar to sublingual absorption.

- *Rectal (PR).* This route is usually reserved for unconscious or vomiting patients or patients who cannot cooperate with oral or IV administration (small children).

PARENTERAL ROUTES   **Broadly defined, parenteral denotes any area outside the gastrointestinal tract; however, additional, specific criteria apply to parenteral drug administration. **Parenteral routes typically use needles to inject medications into the circulatory system or tissues. Consequently, some forms of parenteral drug delivery afford the most rapid drug delivery and absorption.

- *Intravenous (IV).* With its rapid onset, this is the preferred route in most emergencies.[1]

- *Endotracheal (ET).* This is an alternative route for *selected* medications in an emergency.[2]

- *Intraosseous (IO).* The intraosseous route delivers drugs to the medullary space of bones. Most often used as an alternative to IV administration in pediatric emergencies, it also sees limited use in adults.

- *Umbilical.* Both the umbilical vein and umbilical artery can provide an alternative to IV administration in newborns.[3]

- *Intramuscular (IM).* The intramuscular route allows a slower absorption than IV administration, as the drug passes into the capillaries.

- *Subcutaneous (SC, SQ, SubQ).* This route is slower than the IM route, because the subcutaneous tissue is less vascular than the muscular tissue.

- *Inhaled/nebulized.* This route, which offers very rapid absorption, is especially useful for delivering drugs whose target tissues are in the lungs.

- *Topical.* Topical administration delivers drugs directly to the skin.

- *Transdermal.* For drugs that can be absorbed through the skin, the transdermal route allows slow, continuous release.

- *Nasal.* Useful for delivering drugs directly to the nasal mucosa, the nasal route has an expanding role in delivering systemically acting drugs.

- *Instillation.* Instillation is similar to topical administration, but places the drug directly into a wound or an eye.

- *Intradermal.* For allergy testing, intradermal administration delivers a drug or biological agent between the dermal layers.

Drug Forms

Drugs come in many forms. Solid forms, generally given orally, include the following:

- *Powders.* Although they are not as popular as they once were, some powdered drugs are still in use.

- *Tablets.* Powders compressed into a disklike form.

- *Suppositories.* Drugs mixed with a waxlike base that melts at body temperature, allowing absorption by rectal or vaginal tissue.

- *Capsules.* Gelatin containers filled with powders or tiny pills; the gelatin dissolves, releasing the drug into the gastrointestinal tract.

Liquid drugs are usually solutions of a solid drug dissolved in a solvent. Some can be given parenterally, whereas others must be given enterally.

- *Solutions.* The most common liquid preparations. Generally water based; some may be oil based.

- *Tinctures.* Prepared using an alcohol extraction process; some alcohol usually remains in the final drug preparation.

- *Suspensions.* Preparations in which the solid does not dissolve in the solvent; if left alone, the solid portion will precipitate out.

- *Emulsions.* Suspensions with an oily substance in the solvent; even when well mixed, globules of oil separate out of the solution.

- *Spirits.* Solution of a volatile drug in alcohol.

- *Elixirs.* Alcohol and water solvent, often with flavorings added to improve the taste.

- *Syrups.* Sugar, water, and drug solutions.

Some drugs come in a gaseous form. The most common drug supplied this way is oxygen. Paramedics may also find nitrous oxide (N_2O) used as an inhaled analgesic in ambulances and emergency departments.

Drug Storage

Certain guidelines should dictate the manner in which drugs are stored; their properties may be altered by the environment in which they are stored. Some EMS units are parked in heated stations, but others are kept outdoors and exposed to the elements. EMS systems must consider the storage requirements of all drugs and diluents when deciding operational issues such as vehicle design and posting policies (as occur in system status management). This rapidly becomes a clinical issue because the actual potency of most medications is altered if they are not stored in proper conditions. Examples of variables to consider when determining the proper method of drug storage include temperature, light, moisture, and shelf life.

Pharmacodynamics

When we consider a drug's pharmacodynamics, or effects on the body, we are specifically interested in its mechanisms of action and the relationship between its concentration and its effect.

Actions of Drugs

Drugs can act in four different ways. They may bind to a receptor site, change the physical properties of cells, chemically combine with other chemicals, or alter a normal metabolic pathway. Each of these actions involves a physiochemical interaction between the drug and a functionally important molecule in the body.

DRUGS THAT ACT BY BINDING TO A RECEPTOR SITE Most drugs operate by binding to a **receptor**. Almost all drug receptors are protein molecules on the surfaces of cells. They are part of the body's normal regulatory stimulation/inhibition function, and can be stimulated or inhibited by chemicals. . Each different receptor's name generally corresponds to the drug that stimulates it. For example, if an opiate stimulates the receptor, then the receptor is an opioid receptor. When multiple drugs stimulate the same receptor, standard practice is to use the generic name.

The force of attraction between a drug and a receptor is their **affinity**. The greater the affinity, the stronger the bond. Different drugs may bind to the same type of receptor site, but the strength of their bond may vary. The binding site's shape determines its receptivity to other chemicals, whether they are drugs or endogenous substances. These binding sites are relatively specific—a nonopiate drug generally will not affect an opiate binding site, although occasionally a drug with a similar receptor binding site will unexpectedly cross react. Receptors can also have subtypes. At least five subtypes of adrenergic receptors, for example, are important to paramedic practice.

A drug's pharmacodynamics also involves its ability to cause the expected response, or **efficacy**. Just as different drugs may have different affinities for a site, they may also have different efficacies; that is, drug A may cause a stronger response than drug B. Affinity and efficacy are not directly related. Drug A may cause a stronger response than drug B, even though drug B binds to the receptor site more strongly than drug A.

When a drug binds with its specific type of receptor, a chemical change occurs that ultimately leads to the drug's effect. In most cases, drugs will either stimulate or inhibit the cell's normal biochemical actions. In fact, a drug cannot impart a new function to a cell. Some drugs may interact with a receptor and directly result in the desired effect. Other drugs, however, may interact with a receptor and cause the release or production of a second compound. This secondary compound, or **second messenger**, includes such compounds as calcium or cyclic adenosine monophosphate (cAMP). Cyclic AMP is the most common second messenger. It has a multitude of effects inside the cell. These secondary messengers are particularly important in the endocrine system, as they occur principally in endocrine glands. Once cAMP is formed inside the cell, it activates still other enzymes, usually in a cascading action. That is, the first enzyme activates another enzyme, which activates a third enzyme, and so forth. This is important in that it amplifies the action so that even a small amount of a drug (or hormone) acting on the cell surface can initiate a powerful, cascading, activating force for the entire cell.

The number of receptors on a target cell usually does not remain constant on a daily basis, or even from minute to minute. This is because the receptor proteins are often destroyed during the course of their function. At other times, they are either reactivated or remanufactured by the protein-manufacturing mechanism of the cell. Binding of a drug (or hormone) to a target cell receptor causes the number of available receptors to decrease. This process is known as **down-regulation** of the receptors. It results in a decreased responsiveness of the target cell to the drug or hormone as the number of available active receptors decreases. In other cases, but less commonly, a drug (or hormone) can cause the formation of more receptors than normal. This process, **up-regulation**, increases the target tissue's sensitivity to the particular drug or hormone.

Chemicals that stimulate a receptor site generally fall into two broad categories—agonists and antagonists. **Agonists** bind to the receptor and cause it to initiate the expected response. **Antagonists** bind to a site but do not cause the receptor to initiate the expected response. Some drugs, **agonist–antagonists** (also called **partial agonists**), may do both. Nalbuphine (Nubain), for instance, stimulates some of the opioid agonists' analgesic properties but partially blocks others such as respiratory depression (Figure 13-7).

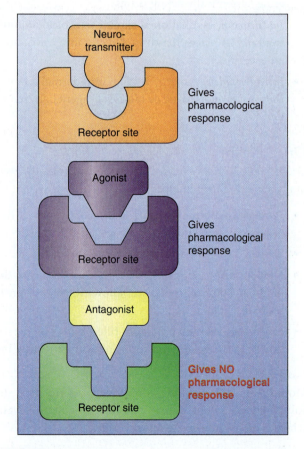

FIGURE 13-7 Receptor site interactions. (top) Naturally occurring neurotransmitter binds to receptor site and creates a physiologic response. (middle) Administered drug (agonist) binds to the receptor site and creates a physiologic response. (bottom) A drug (antagonist) binds to the receptor site but does not cause a physiologic response and prevents agonists from binding to the receptor site.

Receptor-mediated drug actions work like a lock (the receptor) and key (the agonist). If you put the key in the lock and turn it, the lock will open. An antagonist is like a key that fits into the lock but will not turn and cannot open the lock. Target tissues generally have many receptors, so to take the analogy another step, imagine that to get maximal effect a single key (agonist) must move around and open many doors (trigger many biochemical responses). An agonist–antagonist would be a key that unlocks and opens a door but gets stuck in the lock. That is, the drug will cause the expected effect, but that drug will also block another drug from triggering the same receptor. This **competitive antagonism** is considered *surmountable* because a sufficiently large dose of the agonist can overcome the antagonism.

Noncompetitive antagonism can also occur. Continuing the lock, key, and door analogy, imagine that the door is barred. This antagonism would be *insurmountable*; no amount of agonist could overcome it. Noncompetitive antagonism occurs because the binding of the antagonist at a different site causes a deformity of the binding site that actually prevents the agonist from fitting and binding. **Irreversible antagonism** may also occur when a competitive antagonist permanently binds with a receptor site. When this occurs, no amount of agonist will stimulate the receptor. For the effects of such an antagonist to wear off, the body must create new receptors.

Two drugs may appear to be antagonists while actually acting independently. This physiologic antagonism can occur when one drug's effects counteract another's. Although neither agent chemically affects the other, their net effect is antagonistic. An example of a receptor, agonist, antagonist, and agonist–antagonist can be described using an opiate receptor. These receptors occur naturally in the brain and respond to natural endorphins. Morphine sulfate acts as an agonist. It binds to the opiate receptor and causes the expected response of pain relief. Naloxone (Narcan) acts as an antagonist. It will bind to the opiate receptor, but will not initiate the pain relief. It will prevent morphine sulfate from binding to the site and thus effectively blocks the morphine and its response. If the patient is given nalbuphine (Nubain), an agonist–antagonist, it will bind to the opiate receptor and relieve pain, but it is less efficacious than morphine. The nalbuphine blocks morphine from the receptor like an antagonist but stimulates the receptor on its own like an agonist, although to a lesser extent.

DRUGS THAT ACT BY CHANGING PHYSICAL PROPERTIES Some drugs change the physical properties of a part of the body. Drugs that change the osmotic balance across membranes are good examples of this type of drug action. The osmotic diuretic mannitol (Osmotrol), for instance, increases urine output by increasing the blood's osmolarity, or osmotic "pull." This increased osmolarity triggers the normal regulatory systems to decrease water reabsorption in the renal tubules, thereby reducing the total amount of water in the body.

DRUGS THAT ACT BY CHEMICALLY COMBINING WITH OTHER SUBSTANCES Drugs that participate in chemical reactions that change the chemical nature of their substrates (the chemical or substance on which a drug acts) play a large role in paramedic practice. For example, isopropyl alcohol, which is often used to disinfect skin before percutaneous needle insertion for phlebotomy or IV cannulation, denatures the proteins on the surface of bacterial cells. This ruptures the cells, destroying the bacteria. The antacids are another example. They act by chemically neutralizing the hydrochloric acid in the stomach. Sodium bicarbonate given intravenously chemically neutralizes some of the acids in the bloodstream, effectively making the blood more alkalotic.

DRUGS THAT ACT BY ALTERING A NORMAL METABOLIC PATHWAY Some anticancer and antiviral drugs are chemical analogs of normal metabolic substrates. In a process that has been dubbed a counterfeit incorporation mechanism, these drugs can be incorporated into the products of metabolism of cancer cells. Because these drugs are not really the expected substrate, the anticipated product either will not form or, if formed, will be substantially or completely inactive.

Responses to Drug Administration

When a drug is administered, a response is obviously anticipated. The actual response may be the one desired, or it may be an unintended **side effect**. Most, if not all, drugs have at least some minor side effects. Because our knowledge of pharmacology and physiology has not yet arrived at the point at which we can engineer the perfect drug, we must weigh the need for the desired response against the dangers of side effects. In essence, every time we give a medication, we must carefully weigh the risks against the benefits. Although undesirable, side effects are predictable. Iatrogenic responses, however, are not predicted. In general, the term *iatrogenic* refers to a disease or response induced by the actions of a care provider. Derived from the Greek *iatros* (physician) and *gennan* (to produce), it literally means *physician produced*. Negligence is not the only cause of iatrogenic responses. Some common unintended adverse responses to drugs include:

- *Allergic reaction.* Also known as hypersensitivity; this effect occurs as the drug is antigenic and activates the immune system, causing effects that are normally more profound than seen in the general population.

- *Idiosyncrasy.* A drug effect that is unique to the individual; different than seen or expected in the population in general.

- *Tolerance.* Decreased response to the same amount of drug after repeated administrations.

- *Cross tolerance.* Tolerance for a drug that develops after administration of a different drug. Morphine and other opioid agents are common examples. Tolerance for one agent implies tolerance for others as well.

- *Tachyphylaxis.* Rapidly occurring tolerance to a drug. May occur after a single dose. This typically occurs with sympathetic agonists, specifically decongestant and bronchodilation agents.

- *Cumulative effect.* Increased effectiveness when a drug is given in several doses.

- *Drug dependence.* The patient becomes accustomed to the drug's presence in his body and will suffer from withdrawal symptoms on its absence. The dependence may be physical or psychological.

- *Drug Interaction.* The effects of one drug alter the response to another drug.

- *Drug antagonism.* The effects of one drug block the response to another drug.

- *Summation.* Also known as an additive effect. Two drugs that both have the same effect are given together, analogous to $1 + 1 = 2$.

- *Synergism.* Two drugs that both have the same effect are given together and produce a response greater than the sum of their individual responses, analogous to $1 + 1 = 3$.

- *Potentiation.* One drug enhances the effect of another. A common example is promethazine (Phenergan) enhancing the effects of morphine.

- *Interference.* The direct biochemical interaction between two drugs; one drug affects the pharmacology of another drug.

Drug-Response Relationship

To have its optimal desired or therapeutic effects, a drug must reach appropriate concentrations at its site of action. The magnitude of the response therefore depends on the dosage and the drug's course through the body over time. Factors that can affect the drug's concentration may be pharmaceutical (the dosage form's disintegration and the drug's dissolution), pharmacokinetic (the drug's absorption, distribution, metabolism, and excretion), or pharmacodynamic (drug-receptor interaction). To predict how the drug will affect different people, a **drug-response relationship** thus correlates different amounts of drug to the resultant clinical response.

Most of the information needed to describe drug-response relationships comes from **plasma-level profiles**, which describe the lengths of onset, duration, and

Legal Considerations

Safety First. Administration of medications is one area where a paramedic or advanced EMT differs from the EMT. Most EMT skills, even if performed incorrectly, rarely have the potential to harm the patient. However, many advanced skills, if performed improperly, can severely harm or even kill the patient. Prehospital administration of emergency medications has saved countless lives. However, there have been instances in which patients have been given the wrong medication or an incorrect dose of the correct medication, resulting in harm to the patient. Because of this, you must be extremely vigilant regarding medication administration. Be certain always to confirm orders and write them down. Follow the six "rights" of medication administration. Double check your drugs and expiration dates, the doses, the timing of administration, and the intended route of administration. Make sure the medication is being given to the right patient. Following administration, constantly monitor your patient for the desired effects as well as any possible side effects. Accurately document your findings, including any untoward effects. It is essential that you make prehospital medication administration as safe as possible for both the patient and you.

termination of action, as well as the drug's minimum effective concentration and toxic levels. The **onset of action** is the time from administration until a medication reaches its **minimum effective concentration** (the minimum level of drug necessary to cause a given effect). The length of time the amount of drug remains above this level is its **duration of action**. **Termination of action** is measured from when the drug's level drops below the minimum effective concentration until it is eliminated from the body.

The ratio of a drug's lethal dose for 50 percent of the population (LD_{50}) to its effective dose for 50 percent of the population (ED_{50}) is its **therapeutic index** (TI) or LD_{50}/ED_{50}. The therapeutic index represents the drug's margin of safety. As the range between effective dose and lethal dose decreases, the value of TI decreases; that is, it becomes closer to 1. TI values of close to 1 indicate a very small margin of safety. In other words, the effective dose and lethal dose of a drug whose TI value is close to 1 are nearly the same. This drug would be very difficult to effectively dose without causing toxicity.

The last component of the drug-response relationship, the **biologic half-life**, is the time the body takes to clear one-half of the drug. Although the rates of metabolism and excretion both affect it, a drug's half-life ($t_{1/2}$) is independent of its concentration. For example, if the concentration of a drug were 500 mcg/dL after administration and 250 mcg/dL in 10 minutes, then its half-life would be 10 minutes. After another 10 minutes, 125 mcg/dL would remain.

Factors Altering Drug Response

Different individuals may have different responses to the same drug given. Factors that alter the standard drug-response relationship include the following:

- *Age.* The liver and kidney functions of infants are not yet fully developed, so the response to drugs may be altered. Likewise, as we age, the functions of these organs begin to deteriorate. As a result, infants and the elderly are most susceptible to having an altered response to a drug.

- *Body mass.* The more body mass a person has, the more fluid is potentially available to dilute a drug. A given amount of drug will cause a higher concentration in a person with little body mass than in a much larger person. Thus, most drug dosages are stated in terms of body mass. For example, the standard dose of fentanyl for a patient in pain is 1.0 mcg/kg. A 100-kg patient will receive 100 mcg of fentanyl, whereas a 50-kg patient will receive only 50 mcg.

- *Sex.* Most differences in drug response due to sex result from the relative body masses of men and women. The different distribution and amounts of body fat also affect the amounts of drug available at any given time.

- *Environmental milieu.* Various stimuli in a patient's environment affect his response to a given drug. This is most clearly seen with drugs affecting mood or behavior. The same dose of an antianxiety medication such as diazepam (Valium) will have different effects, depending on the patient's mood or surroundings. For example, if the patient were afraid of heights, his usual dose of diazepam would not be likely to help him remain calm while rappelling from the top of a tall building. Surrounding conditions may also affect the distribution or elimination of a drug. Heat, for example, causes vasodilation and increases perspiration, both of which may alter the rate at which the body distributes and eliminates a drug.

- *Time of administration.* If a patient takes a drug immediately after eating, its absorption will be different than if he took the same drug before breakfast in the morning. Some drugs may cause nausea if taken on an empty stomach and must therefore be taken only after eating.

- *Pathological state.* Several disease states alter the drug-response relationship. Most notable are renal and hepatic dysfunctions, both of which may lead to excess accumulation of a drug in the body. Renal failure is likely to decrease elimination of drugs, whereas hepatic failure may decrease or inhibit their metabolism, prolonging their duration of action. Acid–base disturbances may alter a drug's solubility or the extent to which it ionizes, thus changing its absorption rate.

- *Genetic factors.* Genetic traits such as the lack of specific enzymes or lowered basal metabolic rate alter drug absorption or biotransformation and thus modify the patient's response.

- *Psychological factors.* A patient's mental state can also affect his response to a drug. The best-known example of this is the placebo effect. Essentially, if a patient believes that a drug will have a given effect, then he is much more likely to perceive that the effect has occurred.

Drug–Drug Interactions

Drug–drug interactions occur whenever two or more drugs are available in the same patient. The interaction can increase, decrease, or have no effect on their combined actions. Any number of variables may cause these drug–drug interactions, including the following:

- One drug could alter the rate of intestinal absorption.

- The two drugs could compete for plasma protein binding, resulting in one's accumulation at the other's expense.

- One drug could alter the other's metabolism, thus increasing or decreasing either's bioavailability.

- One drug's action at a receptor site may be antagonistic or synergistic to another's.

- One drug could alter the other's rate of excretion through the kidneys.

- One drug could alter the balance of electrolytes necessary for the other drug's expected result.

In addition to drug-drug interactions, other types of interactions are possible. They include a drug's effects on the rate of absorption of food and nutrients, alteration of enzymes, and food-initiated alteration of drug excretion. Alcohol consumption and smoking may also cause interactions with drugs. Finally, some drugs are incompatible with each other. As an example, catecholamines such as epinephrine will precipitate in an alkaline solution such as sodium bicarbonate.

CONTENT REVIEW

➤ Factors Affecting Drug-Response Relationship
- Age
- Body mass
- Sex
- Environment
- Time of administration
- Pathology
- Genetics
- Psychology

PART 2: Drug Classifications

Classifying Drugs

The enormous amount of material that you must learn about pharmacology can easily become overwhelming. The best way to surmount this challenge is to break the information into manageable groups. Drugs can be classified in many ways. You will often find them listed by the body system they affect, by their mechanism of action, or by their indications. Drugs also can be classified by source or by chemical class. Understanding the properties of drug classes (or the model drug of a class) can increase your understanding of drugs and quicken your learning of new drugs.

Grouping medications according to their uses is a very practical way of classifying them. For example, one class of drugs is used to treat heart arrhythmias, whereas another treats hypertension. Although the specific dosing regimens and contraindications vary among medications within any class, their general properties are consistent. If you understand those general principles, learning the specific information about individual medications becomes much easier. Thinking in terms of prototypical medications usually helps to describe each classification. A **prototype** is a drug that best demonstrates the class's common properties and illustrates its particular characteristics.

In the rest of this chapter, we will look at specific classifications of medications that, as a paramedic, you will commonly either administer or encounter. Even though you may not frequently administer medications from every classification, knowing how they work remains important. It will help you to understand the implications of medications your patients may be taking themselves or getting from another caregiver. An example often cited to demonstrate the importance of understanding the classes of medications, even those that you will rarely administer, is the patient who has taken an overdose of tricyclic antidepressants. Based on your knowledge of this classification, you will know to increase your index of suspicion for hypotension and abnormal cardiac rhythms.

Drugs Used to Affect the Nervous System

The two major divisions of the nervous system are the central nervous system and the peripheral nervous system (Figure 13-8). The *central nervous system* includes the brain and spinal cord; all nerves that originate and terminate within either the brain or the spinal cord are considered central. The *peripheral nervous system* comprises everything else. If a neuron originates within the brain and terminates outside the spinal cord, it is part of the peripheral nervous system, which, in turn, consists of the somatic nervous system and the autonomic nervous system. The *somatic nervous system* controls voluntary, or motor, functions. The *autonomic nervous system,* which controls involuntary, or automatic, functions, is further divided into the sympathetic and parasympathetic nervous systems. The two major groupings of medications used to affect the nervous system are those that affect the central nervous system and those that affect the autonomic nervous system.

Central Nervous System Medications

Many pathological conditions involve the central nervous system (CNS). As a result, a great number of drugs have been developed to affect the CNS, including analgesics, anesthetics, drugs to treat anxiety and insomnia, anticonvulsants, stimulants, psychotherapeutic agents (antidepressants and antimanic agents), and drugs used to treat specific nervous system disorders such as Parkinson's disease. Obviously, this is a very broad classification with many different types of agents. Having a firm grasp on the basic physiology involved will help you to understand the various drugs you encounter.

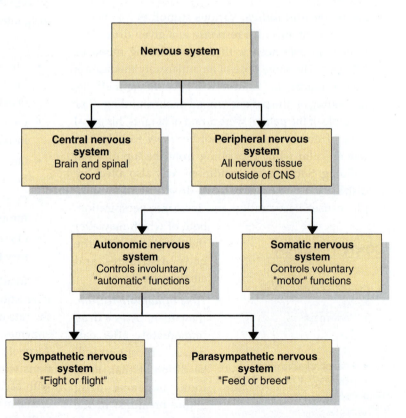

FIGURE 13-8 Functional organization of the autonomic nervous system within the overall nervous system.

Analgesics and Antagonists

Analgesics are medications that relieve the sensation of pain. The distinction between **analgesia**, the absence of the sensation of *pain,* and **anesthesia**, the absence of *all* sensation, is important. Whereas an analgesic decreases the specific sensation of pain, an anesthetic prevents all sensation, often impairing consciousness in the process. A frequently used class of medications, analgesics are available by prescription or over the counter. The two basic subclasses of analgesics are opioid agonists and their derivatives and nonopioid derivatives. Opioid antagonists, which we also discuss in this section, reverse the effects of opioid analgesics; **adjunct medications** enhance the effects of other analgesics.

OPIOID AGONISTS   An opioid is chemically similar to opium, which is extracted from the poppy plant and has been used for centuries for its analgesic and hallucinatory effects. Opium and all its derivatives effectively treat pain because of their similarity to natural pain-reducing peptides called *endorphins.* Endorphins and, by extension, opioid drugs work through opiate receptors and decrease by decreasing the sensory neurons' ability to propagate pain impulses to the spinal cord and brain. At least five types of opiate receptors have been identified (Table 13-3).

The prototype opioid drug is morphine. Several of morphine's effects make it useful for clinical practice. At therapeutic doses, morphine causes analgesia, euphoria,

Table 13-3 Opiate Receptor Types

Receptor Name	Abbreviation	Effects
mu₁	μ_1	Analgesia, euphoria
mu₂	μ_2	Respiratory and physical depression, miosis, and reduced GI motility
delta	δ	Analgesia, dysphoria, psychotomimetic effects (i.e., hallucinations), and respiratory and vasomotor stimulation
kappa	κ	Analgesia, sedation, and miosis, respiratory depression, and dysphoria
sigma	σ	Psychotomimetic (i.e., hallucinations), dysphoria, and possibly dilation of the pupils
epsilon	ε	Effects uncertain

sedation, and miosis (pupil constriction). It also decreases cardiac preload and afterload, which makes it useful in treating myocardial infarction and pulmonary edema. At higher doses, it may cause respiratory depression and hypotension (Figure 13-9). Table 13-4 details common opioids used in EMS.[4–10]

NONOPIOID ANALGESICS   Three broad types of nonopioid medications also have analgesic properties, several of which also share antipyretic (fever-fighting) properties.

Opiate Receptors

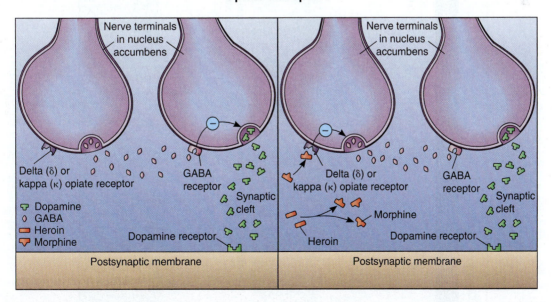

FIGURE 13-9 The effects of opiates on opiate receptors. Opiates modify the action of dopamine in selected areas of the brain, which form part of the brain's "reward pathway." After crossing the blood–brain barrier, opiates act on the various opioid receptors. This binding inhibits the release of GABA from the nerve terminal, reducing the inhibitory effect of GABA on dopaminergic neurons. The increased activation of dopaminergic neurons and the release of dopamine into the synaptic cleft results in activation of the postsynaptic membrane. Continued activation of the dopaminergic reward pathway leads to the feelings of euphoria and the "high" associated with opiate use. Morphine is a powerful agonist at the opioid mu receptor subtype, and activation of these receptors has a strong activating effect on the dopaminergic reward pathway.

Table 13-4 Common Opioids

Name	Classification	Action	Indications	Contraindications	Doses	Routes	Adverse Effects	Other
Morphine *Duramorph*	Narcotic (opioid) Ⅱ	Analgesia and sedation through binding to opiate receptors	• Moderate–severe pain	• Hypotension • Hypersensitivity to the drug	2–10 mg	IV, IO, IM, SQ, PO	• Hypotension • Syncope • Tachycardia • Bradycardia • Apnea • Nausea • Vomiting • Respiratory depression	• Use appropriate monitors • Naloxone is an antagonist
Hydromorphone *Dilaudid*	Narcotic (opioid) Ⅱ	Analgesia and sedation through binding to opiate receptors	• Moderate–severe pain	• Hypersensitivity to the drug	0.5–2.0 mg	IV, IO, IM, SQ, PO	• Nausea • Vomiting • Cramps • Respiratory depression	• Use appropriate monitors • Naloxone is an antagonist
Fentanyl *Sublimaze*	Narcotic (opioid) Ⅱ	Analgesia through binding to opiate receptors	• Moderate–severe pain • Anesthetic	• Hypersensitivity to the drug	50–100 mcg	IV, IO, IM, SQ, IN	• Nausea • Vomiting • Cramps • Chest wall rigidity • Respiratory depression	• Use appropriate monitors • Naloxone is an antagonist
Meperidine *Demerol*	Narcotic (opioid) Ⅱ	Analgesia through binding to opiate receptors	• Moderate–severe pain	• Hypersensitivity to the drug • Patients receiving monamine oxidase inhibitors (MAOIs)	25–100 mg	IV, IO, IM, SQ, PO	• Nausea • Vomiting • Euphoria • Dysphoria • Respiratory depression	• Use appropriate monitors • Naloxone is an antagonist

These are *salicylates*, such as aspirin; *nonsteroidal anti-inflammatory drugs (NSAIDs)*, such as ibuprofen and ketorolac; and *para-aminophenol* derivatives, such as acetaminophen. The drugs in each of these classes affect the production of prostaglandins and cyclooxygenase, important neurotransmitters involved in the pain response. Table 13-5 details common nonopioid analgesics.

OPIOID ANTAGONISTS Opioid antagonists are useful in reversing the effects of opioid drugs. Typically, this is necessary to treat respiratory depression. Naloxone (Narcan) is the prototype opioid antagonist. It competitively binds with opioid receptors but without causing the effects of opioid bonding. It is commonly used to treat overdoses of heroin and other opioid derivatives; however, it has a shorter half-life than most opioid drugs, so repeated doses may be necessary to prevent its unwanted side effects. Table 13-6 details common opiate antagonists.[11–13]

ADJUNCT MEDICATIONS Adjunct medications are given concurrently with other drugs to enhance their effects. Although they may have only limited or no analgesic properties by themselves, combined with a true analgesic they either prolong or intensify its effect. Examples of adjunct medications are benzodiazepines (diazepam [Valium], lorazepam [Ativan], midazolam [Versed]), antihistamines (promethazine [Phenergan]), and caffeine. We will discuss many of these agents in separate sections.

OPIOID AGONIST–ANTAGONISTS An opioid agonist–antagonist displays both agonistic and antagonistic properties. Pentazocine (Talwin) is the prototype for this class. Nalbuphine (Nubain) was commonly used in field care. It is an agonist because, like opioids, it decreases pain response, and it is an antagonist because it has fewer respiratory depressant and addictive side effects. Butorphanol (Stadol) is another common opioid agonist–antagonist. Although rarely used in modern EMS, these drugs are detailed in Table 13-7.

Anesthetics

Unlike analgesics, an **anesthetic** induces a state of anesthesia, or loss of sensation to touch or pain. Anesthetics are useful during unpleasant procedures such as surgery or electrical cardioversion. At low levels of anesthesia, patients may have a decreased sensation of pain but remain conscious. **Neuroleptanesthesia**, a type of anesthesia that combines this effect with amnesia, is useful in procedures that require the patient to remain alert and responsive.

Anesthetics as a group tend to cause respiratory, central nervous system (CNS), and cardiovascular depression. Different agents affect these systems to different degrees and are typically chosen for their ability to produce the desired effect with minimal side effects. Anesthetic agents are rarely used singly; rather, several different agents are typically given together to achieve a balanced anesthetic result. For example, intubating a conscious patient requires his natural gag reflex to be inhibited. Neuromuscular blocking agents such as succinylcholine are used to induce paralysis. Because this would be a terribly frightening and potentially painful procedure, antianxiety, amnesic, and analgesic agents are also given to produce the desired anesthetic effect.

Anesthetics are given either by inhalation or injection. The gaseous anesthetics given by inhalation include halothane, enflurane, and nitrous oxide. The first clinically useful anesthetic was ether, a gas. Its discovery marked a new generation in surgical care, but it is very flammable. The modern gaseous anesthetics are much less volatile, but still decrease consciousness and sensation as required. These drugs, by some as-yet-unidentified mechanism, hyperpolarize neural membranes, making depolarization more difficult. This decreases the firing rates of neural impulses and, therefore, the propagation of action potentials through the nervous system, thus reducing sensation. These effects appear to depend on the gases' solubility. The rate of onset of anesthesia further depends on several additional factors, including cardiac output, inhaled concentration of gas, pulmonary minute volume, and end organ perfusion. Because these gases clear mostly through the lungs, respiratory rate and depth affect the duration of their effect. Although halothane is the prototype of inhaled anesthetics, nitrous oxide is the only medication in this class with which you are likely to have much involvement.

Most anesthetics used outside the operating room are given intravenously. This gives them a considerably faster onset and shorter duration, making them much more useful in emergency care. Paramedics use these agents primarily to assist with intubation in rapid-sequence intubation. They include several pharmacological classes, such as ultra-short-acting barbiturates (thiopental [Pentothal] and methohexital [Brevital]), benzodiazepines (diazepam [Valium] and midazolam [Versed]), and opioids (fentanyl [Sublimaze] and remifentanil [Ultiva]). We discuss barbiturates' and benzodiazepines' mechanisms of action in the section on antianxiety and sedative–hypnotics.[14–15]

Anesthetics are also given locally to block sensation for procedures such as suturing and most dentistry. These agents are injected into the skin around the nerves that innervate the area of the procedure. They decrease the nerve's ability to depolarize and propagate the impulse from this area to the brain. Cocaine's first clinical use was as a topical anesthetic of the eye in 1884. The current prototype of this class is lidocaine (Xylocaine). It is frequently mixed with epinephrine. The epinephrine causes local vasoconstriction, decreasing bleeding and systemic absorption of the drug.

Table 13-5 Common Nonopioid Analgesics

Name	Classification	Action	Indications	Contraindications	Doses	Routes	Adverse Effects	Other
Acetaminophen *Tylenol, OFIRMEV (injectable)*	Nonnarcotic analgesic, antipyretic (para-aminophenol derivative)	Exact mechanism uncertain, but felt to inhibit cyclooxygenase	• Mild–moderate pain • Fever	• Hypersensitivity to the drug • Alcoholism • Chronic liver disease	325–650 mg	PO, IV	• Rare	• Can be liver toxic—use minimal dose necessary
Ibuprofen *Motrin* *Advil*	NSAID	Anti-inflammatory and antipyretic through inhibition of prostaglandins	• Mild–moderate pain • Fever • Inflammation	• Hypersensitivity to the drug • Bronchospasm • Angioedema	200–800 mg	PO	• Nausea • Vomiting • GI bleeding • Allergic reactions	• Commonly causes gastric upset
Ketorolac *Toradol*	NSAID	Anti-inflammatory and antipyretic through inhibition of prostaglandins	• Mild–moderate pain • Fever • Inflammation • Renal colic	• Hypersensitivity to the drug • Bronchospasm • Angioedema	30 mg (IV and elderly) 60 mg IM	IV, IM	• Nausea • Vomiting • GI bleeding • Allergic reactions	• Can cause dizziness and headache
Aspirin	NSAID	Anti-inflammatory and antipyretic through inhibition of thromboxane A_2	• Mild–moderate pain • Fever • Platelet aggregation inhibitor	• Hypersensitivity to the drug • Bronchospasm • Angioedema • Patients receiving monamine oxidase inhibitors (MAOIs)	350–650 mg	PO	• Nausea • Vomiting • GI bleeding • Allergic reactions	• Commonly causes gastric upset • Avoid enteric-coated aspirin in chest pain

Table 13-6 Common Opioid Antagonists

Name	Classification	Action	Indications	Contraindications	Doses	Routes	Adverse Effects	Other
Naloxone *Narcan*	Opiate antagonist	Opioid antagonist without opiate agonist properties (it has no activity when given in the absence of an opiate agonist)	• Partial reversal of opiate drug effects • Opiate overdose	• Hypersensitivity to the drug	0.4–2.0 mg	IV, IO, SQ, IN, nebulizer	• Fever • Chills • Nausea • Vomiting • Diarrhea • Opiate withdrawal	• Administer enough to reverse respiratory depression and avoid full narcotic withdrawal syndrome
Nalmefene *Revex*	Opiate antagonist	Opioid antagonist without opiate agonist properties (it has no activity when given in the absence of an opiate agonist)	• Partial reversal of opiate drug effects • Opiate overdose	• Hypersensitivity to the drug	0.5–1.0 mg	IV, IM, SQ, IO	• Fever • Chills • Nausea • Vomiting • Diarrhea • Opiate withdrawal	• Duration of effect much longer than naloxone

Table 13-7 Opioid Agonists–Antagonists

Name	Classification	Action	Indications	Contraindications	Doses	Routes	Adverse Effects	Other
Nalbuphine *Nubain*	Opiate agonist–antagonist	Analgesia and sedation through binding to opiate receptors. It also has some opiate receptor antagonistic properties.	• Moderate–severe pain	• Hypersensitivity to the drug • Opiate dependence • Respiratory depression	10–20 mg	IV, IO, SQ	• Sedation • Dizziness • Nausea • Vomiting • Opiate withdrawal	• Use with caution in patients with liver and renal disease
Butorphanol *Stadol* Ⓝ	Opiate agonist–antagonist	Analgesia and sedation through binding to opiate receptors. It also has some opiate receptor antagonistic properties.	• Moderate–severe pain	• Hypersensitivity to the drug • Opiate dependence • Respiratory depression	1–4 mg	IV, IM, SQ, IO, IN	• Sedation • Dizziness • Nausea • Vomiting • Opiate withdrawal	• Use with caution in patients with liver and renal disease

Antianxiety and Sedative–Hypnotic Drugs

Antianxiety and sedative–hypnotic drugs are generally used to decrease anxiety, induce amnesia, and assist sleeping and as part of a balanced approach to anesthesia. **Sedation** refers to a state of decreased anxiety and inhibitions. Sedation is often quantified and classified by the level of sedation. The American Society of Anesthesiologists (ASA) uses the following system:

- *Minimal sedation*, also called anxiolysis, is characterized by a normal response to verbal stimuli.

- *Moderate sedation*, also called conscious sedation, is characterized by purposeful response to verbal and/or tactile stimulation.

- *Deep sedation* is characterized by purposeful response to repeated or painful stimulation.

- *General anesthesia* is characterized by unarousable unresponsiveness, even with painful stimulation.

Hypnosis in this context refers to the instigation of sleep. Sleep may be categorized as either rapid-eye-movement (REM) or non-rapid-eye-movement (non-REM). REM sleep is characterized by rapid eye movements and lack of motor control. Most dreaming is thought to occur during REM sleep. Insomnia, or difficulty sleeping, typically presents with increased latency (the period of time between lying down and going to sleep) or awakening during sleep.

The two main pharmacological classes within this functional class are benzodiazepines and barbiturates. Alcohol is also in this functional class. Benzodiazepines and barbiturates work in similar ways. Benzodiazepines are frequently prescribed for oral use and are relatively safe and effective for treating general anxiety and insomnia. Barbiturates, which have broader general depressant activities and a higher potential for abuse, are used much less frequently than benzodiazepines. Before the release of benzodiazepines in the 1960s, however, barbiturates were the drug of choice for treating anxiety and insomnia.

Benzodiazepine Receptors

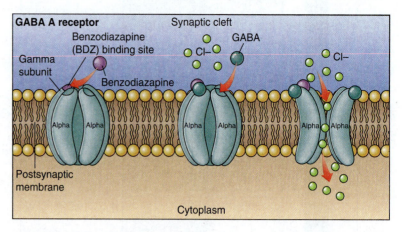

FIGURE 13-10 The effects of benzodiazepines on GABA A receptors. Their binding causes a conformational change in the receptor that results in an increase in GABA A receptor activity. BDZs do not substitute for GABA, which bind at the alpha subunit, but increase the frequency of channel-opening events, which leads to an increase in chloride ion conductance and inhibition of the action potential.

Both benzodiazepines and barbiturates hyperpolarize the membrane of central nervous system neurons, which decreases their response to stimuli. Gamma-aminobutyric acid (GABA) is the chief inhibitory neurotransmitter in the central nervous system. GABA receptors are dispersed widely throughout the CNS on proteins that make up chloride ion channels in the cell membrane. When GABA combines with these receptors, the channel "opens" and chloride, which is more prevalent outside the cell, diffuses through the channel. As chloride is an anion, or negative ion, it makes the inside of the cell more negative than the outside. This hyperpolarizes the membrane and makes it more difficult to depolarize. Depolarization therefore requires a larger stimulus to cause the cell to fire. Both benzodiazepines and barbiturates increase the GABA receptor–chloride ion channel complexes' potential for binding with GABA, and both are dose dependent (Figure 13-10). At low doses, they decrease anxiety and cause sedation (See Tables 13-8 and 13-9.) As the dose increases, they induce sleep (hypnosis) and, at higher doses, anesthesia. Because benzodiazepines only increase the effectiveness

Table 13-8 Levels of Sedation

	Minimal Sedation (Anxiolysis)	**Moderate Sedation/Analgesia (Conscious Sedation)**	**Deep Sedation/Analgesia**	**General Anesthesia**
Responsiveness	Normal response to verbal stimulation	Purposeful response to verbal or tactile stimulation	Purposeful response after repeated or painful stimulation	Unarousable, even with painful stimulation
Airway	Unaffected	No intervention required	Intervention may be required	Intervention often required
Spontaneous Ventilations	Unaffected	Adequate	May be inadequate	Frequently inadequate
Cardiovascular Function	Unaffected	Usually maintained	Usually maintained	May be impaired

Table 13-9 Ramsey Sedation Score

Score	Responsiveness
1	Patient is anxious and agitated or restless, or both.
2	Patient is cooperative, oriented, and tranquil.
3	Patient responds to commands only.
4	Patient exhibits brisk response to light glabellar (between eyebrows—just above the nose) tap or loud auditory stimulus.
5	Patient exhibits a sluggish response to light glabellar (between eyebrows—just above the nose) tap or loud auditory stimulus.
6	Patient exhibits no response.

of GABA, the amount of GABA present limits their effects. This actually makes benzodiazepines much safer than barbiturates, which at high doses can actually mimic GABA's effects and thus can have unlimited effects. Benzodiazepines and barbiturates are also useful in treating convulsions. Common sedatives and hypnotics are detailed in Table 13-10.

Just as opiates have an antagonist in naloxone (Narcan), benzodiazepines have an antagonist in flumazenil (Romazicon). Flumazenil competitively binds with the benzodiazepine receptors in the GABA receptor–chloride ion channel complex without causing the effects of benzodiazepines. This reverses the sedation from benzodiazepines, but it can occasionally have untoward consequences, specifically if a patient depends on benzodiazepines for seizure control, is withdrawing from alcohol, or is taking tricyclic antidepressants. In these cases, the patient may develop seizures following the administration of flumazenil.

Antiseizure or Antiepileptic Drugs

Seizures are a state of hyperactivity of either a section of the brain (partial seizure) or all of the brain (generalized seizure). They may or may not be accompanied by convulsions. Therefore, although the medications in this functional class may be called anticonvulsants, they are more appropriately referred to as antiseizure or antiepileptic drugs. The goal of seizure management is to balance eliminating the seizures against the side effects of the medications used to treat them. Controlling seizures is a lifelong process for most patients and requires diligent compliance with medication dosing regimens.

Partial (or focal) seizures erupt from a specific focus and are described in terms of alterations in consciousness or behavior. These may be further divided into simple or complex partial seizures based on the specific area of the brain in which the focus is located. Complex partial seizures are also known as psychomotor seizures and are characterized by repetitive motions.

Generalized seizures involve both hemispheres of the brain and are described in terms of visible motor activity. Generalized tonic–clonic seizures involve periods of muscle rigidity (tonic stage) followed by spasmodic twitching (clonic stage) and then flaccidity and a gradual return to consciousness (postictal stage). Absence seizures are also generalized but do not have obvious convulsions. They involve brief losses of consciousness that may occur hundreds of times a day. Absence seizures are treated differently from other types of seizures. Finally, status epilepticus is a life-threatening condition characterized by uninterrupted tonic–clonic seizures lasting more than 30 minutes or by two or more tonic–clonic seizures without an intervening lucid interval. The preferred therapy for each type of seizure differs.

Seizures are treated through several general mechanisms. The most common is direct action on the sodium and calcium ion channels in the neural membranes. Phenytoin (Dilantin) and carbamazepine (Tegretol) both inhibit the influx of sodium into the cell, thus decreasing the cell's ability to depolarize and propagate seizures. Valproic acid and ethosuximide act similarly, but they interact with calcium channels in the hypothalamus, where absence seizures typically begin. These two drugs are particularly useful because they are specific to hyperactive neurons and therefore have few side effects. Other medications such as benzodiazepines and barbiturates interact with the GABA receptor–chloride ion channel complex, as explained in the section on antianxiety and sedative–hypnotic drugs.

Antiseizure medications comprise several pharmacological classes, including benzodiazepines (diazepam [Valium] and lorazepam [Ativan]), barbiturates (phenobarbital [Luminal]), hydantoins (phenytoin [Dilantin] and fosphenytoin [Cerebyx]), succinimides (ethosuximide [Zarontin]), and miscellaneous medications such as valproic acid (Depakote), felbamate (Felbatol), lacosamide (VIMBAT), lamotrigene (Lamictal), levetiracetam (Keppra), and gabapentin (Neurontin). Table 13-11 lists the preferred medication for treating each type of seizure.

Central Nervous System Stimulants

Stimulating the central nervous system is desirable in certain circumstances such as fatigue, drowsiness, narcolepsy, obesity, and attention deficit hyperactivity disorder. Broadly, two techniques may accomplish this:

- Increasing the release or effectiveness of excitatory neurotransmitters
- Decreasing the release or effectiveness of inhibitory neurotransmitters

Within the functional class of CNS stimulants are three pharmacological classes: amphetamines, methylphenidates, and methylxanthines.

Table 13-10 Common Sedatives/Hypnotics

Name	Classification	Action	Indications	Contraindications	Doses	Routes	Adverse Effects	Other
Benzodiazepines								
Diazepam *Valium*	Benzodiazepine Ⓒ	Binds to Type A GABA receptors, causing sedation	• Anxiety • Seizures • Sedation • Muscle relaxation	• History of hypersensitivity to the drug	2–10 mg	IV, IM, IO, PO, rectal	• Hypotension • Sedation • Amnesia • Respiratory depression • Nausea • Vomiting	• Incompatible with other medications because it is not water soluble. • Can cause irritation with injection. • Flumazenil is an antagonist.
Midazolam *Versed*	Benzodiazepine Ⓒ	Binds to Type A GABA receptors, causing sedation	• Anxiety • Sedation • Seizures	• History of hypersensitivity to the drug	1–5 mg	IV, IM, IO,	• Hypotension • Sedation • Amnesia • Respiratory depression • Nausea • Vomiting	• Flumazenil is an antagonist.
Lorazepam *Ativan*	Benzodiazepine Ⓒ	Binds to Type A GABA receptors, causing sedation	• Anxiety • Sedation • Seizures	• History of hypersensitivity to the drug	1–4 mg	IV, IM, IO, PO, rectal	• Hypotension • Sedation • Amnesia • Respiratory depression • Nausea • Vomiting	• Flumazenil is an antagonist.
Dissociative Agents								
Ketamine *Ketalar*	Dissociative anesthetic Ⓒ	Causes dissociation between the cortical and limbic system	• Sedation • Analgesia	• History of hypersensitivity to the drug • Hypertension	0.5–1.0 mg/kg (IV); 2–4 mg/kg (IM)	IV, IM	• Hallucinations	• All monitors should be in place. • Resuscitative equipment should be immediately available.
Miscellaneous Agents								
Nitrous Oxide	Sedative/anesthetic gas	CNS depressant	• Pain • Sedation	• COPD • Pneumothorax • Bowel obstruction	Self-administered	Inhalation	• Dizziness • Hallucinations • Nausea • Vomiting • Altered mental status	• Should not be used in any patient who cannot comprehend verbal instructions or who is intoxicated with alcohol or other medications.
Propofol *Diprivan*	Nonbarbiturate, nonbenzodiazepine sedative	Uncertain, but appears to potentiate GABA receptors	• Sedation	• History of hypersensitivity to the drug • Hypersensitivity of soy or egg products	25–75 mcg/kg/min	IV	• Pain on induction • Nausea • Vomiting • Respiratory depression	• All monitors should be in place. • Resuscitative equipment should be immediately available.
Etomidate *Amidate*	Nonbarbiturate, nonbenzodiazepine sedative	Appears to modulate GABA receptors	• Sedation	• History of hypersensitivity to the drug	0.1–0.3 mg/kg	IV	• Myoclonic jerks • Respiratory depression • Laryngospasm	• Does not have analgesic properties. • Calcium–channel blockers can prolong respiratory depression. • Can cause increased cortisol levels. • All monitors should be in place. • Resuscitative equipment should be immediately available.

Table 13-11 Antiseizure Medications

Type of Seizure	Drug of Choice
Partial seizures	Phenytoin
	Carbamazepine
	Oxacarbazepine
	Felbamate
	Lacosamide
	Lamotrigene
	Levetiracetam
Generalized seizures	Carbamazepine
	Phenytoin
	Phenobarbital
	Lamotrigene
	Levetiracetam
	Gabapentin
Absence seizures	Valproic acid
	Ethosuximide

The amphetamines also include methamphetamine and dextroamphetamine. These drugs all increase the release of excitatory neurotransmitters including norepinephrine and dopamine. Norepinephrine is the primary cause of these drugs' effects, which include an increased wakefulness and awareness as well as a decreased appetite (Figure 13-11). Amphetamines' most common uses, therefore, are treating drowsiness and fatigue and suppressing the appetite. Most of amphetamines' side effects result from overstimulation; they include tachycardia and other arrhythmias, hypertension, convulsions, insomnia, and occasionally psychoses with hallucinations and agitation. Examples of this class include amphetamine sulfate (the prototype) and dextroamphetamine (Dexedrine).

Methylphenidate, marketed as Ritalin, is the most commonly prescribed drug for attention deficit hyperactivity disorder (ADHD). Although it is chemically different from the amphetamines, its pharmacological mechanism of action is similar. Also, like the amphetamines, it has a high abuse potential and is therefore listed as a Class II controlled substance. Although treating hyperactivity with a stimulant may seem odd, it is quite effective. Frequently, the cause of inappropriate behavior in a child with ADHD is his inability to concentrate or focus. Ritalin's stimulant effects increase this ability, and the unwanted behavior often diminishes.

The methylxanthines include caffeine, aminophylline, and theophylline. Although caffeine, the prototype drug in this class, has few clinical uses, it is frequently ingested in coffee, colas, and

chocolates. Theophylline's relaxing effects on bronchial smooth muscle make it helpful in treating asthma. The methylxanthines' mechanism of action is unclear, but it seems to block adenosine receptors. Adenosine is an endogenous neurotransmitter that is used clinically for certain types of tachycardias. Because methylxanthines block the adenosine receptors, larger-than-normal doses may be needed to achieve the desired result. This class's side effects are similar to those of the amphetamines, but they have a much lower potential for abuse and are not controlled drugs.

Psychotherapeutic Medications

Psychotherapeutic medications treat mental dysfunction. Unlike other disease states, we do not thoroughly understand the pathophysiology of mental dysfunction; therefore, we base much of our pharmacological treatment of these conditions on our limited knowledge and on clinical correlation (scientific observation that these medications are indeed effective, even if we do not fully understand their mechanism). Medications are typically only one tactic in a balanced strategy for treating mental illness. Depending on the specific disorder, physicians

Amphetamine Actions

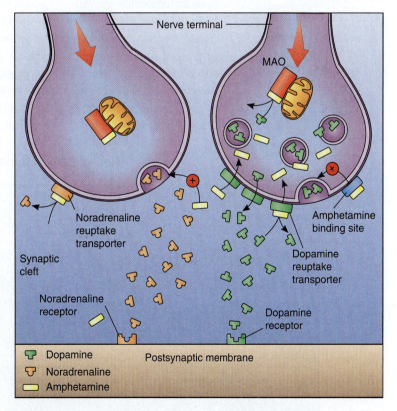

FIGURE 13-11 The mechanism of action of amphetamines. High-dose amphetamines can modify the action of dopamine and norepinephrine in the brain. At high doses, amphetamine increases the concentration of dopamine in the synaptic cleft. High-dose amphetamine has a similar effect on norepinephrine neurons; it can induce the release of norepinephrine into the synaptic cleft and inhibit the norepinephrine reuptake transporter.

will use other treatments such as psychotherapy and electroconvulsive therapy in conjunction with pharmaceutical interventions.

Although we do not completely understand these diseases' specific pathologies, they seem to involve the monoamine neurotransmitters in the central nervous system. These neurotransmitters (norepinephrine, dopamine, serotonin) have been implicated in the control and regulation of emotions. Imbalances in these neurotransmitters, especially dopamine, appear to be at least involved with, if not responsible for, most mental disease. Regulating these and other excitatory and inhibitory neurotransmitters forms the basis for psychopharmaceutical therapy. Schizophrenia appears to be related to an increased release of dopamine, so treatment is aimed at blocking dopamine receptors. Depression seems to be related to inadequate amounts of these neurotransmitters, so treatment is aimed at increasing their release or duration.

The major diseases treated with psychotherapeutic medications are schizophrenia, depression, and bipolar disorder. *The Diagnostic and Statistical Manual of Mental Disorders*, fifth edition (DSM-5), published by the American Psychiatric Association, gives schizophrenia's chief characteristics as a lack of contact with reality and disorganized thinking. Its many different manifestations include delusions, hallucinations (auditory more frequently than visual), disorganized and incoherent speech, and grossly disorganized or catatonic behavior. Schizophrenia is typically treated with antipsychotic

medications, frequently in conjunction with medications from other classes such as antianxiety drugs or antidepressants. **Extrapyramidal symptoms** (EPS), a common side effect of antipsychotic medications, include muscle tremors and parkinsonism-like effects. As a result, antipsychotic medications are also known as **neuroleptic** (literally, *affecting the nerves*) drugs.

The two chief pharmaceutical classes of antipsychotics and neuroleptics are phenothiazines and butyrophenones. Both have been mainstays of psychiatry since the mid-1950s and are considered traditional antipsychotic drugs. Medications in this group block dopamine, muscarinic acetylcholine, histamine, and alpha$_1$ adrenergic receptors in the central nervous system. These medications' therapeutic effects appear to come from blocking the dopamine receptors; their side effects are fairly well understood to originate in blocking the other receptors. The phenothiazines' and butyrophenones' mechanisms of action are the same; they differ only in potency and pharmacokinetics. The distinction between potency and strength is important. Strength refers to the drug's concentration, whereas potency is the amount of drug necessary to produce the desired effect. Although the phenothiazines are considered low-potency and the butyrophenones are considered high-potency, they both produce the same effect. The differences in potency and pharmacokinetics determine which class of medication will be prescribed. Chlorpromazine (Thorazine) is the prototype phenothiazine; haloperidol (Haldol) is the prototype of the butyrophenones (Figure 13-12).

CONTENT REVIEW
➤ Major Diseases Treated with Psychotherapeutic Medications
• Schizophrenia
• Depression
• Bipolar disorder

CONTENT REVIEW
➤ Major Classes of Antipsychotic Medications
• Phenothiazines
• Butyrophenones
• Atypicals

Neuroleptic Actions

FIGURE 13-12 The mechanism of action of haloperidol. Haloperidol is an older "typical," or "first-generation" drug. It is nonselective and binds to a broad range of receptors. It can bind to dopamine, histamine, and α$_2$ adrenergic receptors in the brain.

Because the phenothiazines' and the butyrophenones' mechanisms of action are identical, their common side effects are also similar: extrapyramidal symptoms from cholinergic blockade in the basal ganglia of the cerebral hemispheres; orthostatic hypotension from blockage of alpha$_1$ adrenergic receptors; sedation; and sexual dysfunction. Treatment for these side effects typically involves modifying the drug dose. Diphenhydramine (Benadryl), an antihistamine with anticholinergic properties, is indicated for treating acute dystonic reactions (manifestations of EPS), which often present with tongue and neck spasm. Patients with a newly prescribed antipsychotic may experience these effects and contact EMS. Fortunately, treatment with diphenhydramine is effective and rapid. Orthostatic hypotension is treated in the usual fashion, described in the chapter "Hemorrhage and Shock."

Other medications used to treat psychotic conditions are considered atypical antipsychotics. Although their mechanisms of action are similar to those of the traditional antipsychotics, the atypical antipsychotics block more specific receptors. This specificity allows them to function much like traditional antipsychotics but without causing the prominent extrapyramidal symptoms. These drugs include clozapine (Clozaril), risperidone (Risperdal), ziprasidone (Geodon), and olanzapine (Zyprexa). See Table 13-12.

Another functional class of psychotherapeutic medications includes the antidepressants. The DSM-5 characterizes major depressive episodes as causing significantly depressed mood, loss of interest in things that normally give the patient pleasure, weight loss or gain, sleeping disturbances, suicide attempts, feelings of hopelessness and helplessness, loss of energy, agitation or withdrawal, and an inability to concentrate. Although the specific pathology of this disease is not yet known, it appears to be related to an insufficiency of monoamine neurotransmitters (norepinephrine and serotonin). Thus, the pharmaceutical interventions for this disease appear to increase the number of neurotransmitters released in the brain. The several ways of doing this include increasing the amount of neurotransmitter produced in the presynaptic terminal, increasing the amount of neurotransmitter released from the presynaptic terminal, and blocking the neurotransmitter's reuptake (reabsorption by the presynaptic terminal). This results in a net increase in the neurotransmitter. The antidepressants comprise three pharmacological classes: tricyclic antidepressants, selective serotonin reuptake inhibitors, and monoamine oxidase inhibitors.

Tricyclic antidepressants (TCAs) are frequently used in treating depression because they are effective, relatively safe, and have few significant side effects when taken in therapeutic dosages. TCAs act by blocking the reuptake of norepinephrine and serotonin, thus extending the duration of their action (Figure 13-13). Unfortunately, they also have anticholinergic properties that cause many side effects, including blurred vision, dry mouth, urinary retention, and tachycardia. Another frequent side effect, orthostatic hypotension, is likely due to the alpha$_1$ adrenergic blockade. This is commonly seen when patients try to stand up too quickly and become dizzy. Additionally, because TCAs can lower the seizure threshold, patients with existing seizure disorders are at risk for convulsions. Unfortunately, when taken in overdose, TCAs can have very significant cardiotoxic effects—including myocardial infarction and arrhythmias—that make them a favored means of attempting suicide among depressed patients. Partly because of this potential for overdose, TCAs have fallen behind the newer selective serotonin reuptake inhibitors as the drug of choice for depression. Overdoses of these medications also frequently cause marked hypotension. Treatment of TCA

CONTENT REVIEW

➤ Major Classes of Antidepressant Medications
- TCAs
- SSRIs
- MAOIs

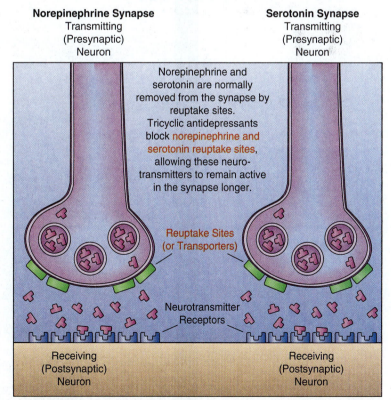

Tricyclic Antidepressants

FIGURE 13-13 The mechanism of action of tricyclic antidepressants (TCAs), blocking the reuptake of serotonin and norepinephrine.

Table 13-12 Antipsychotics

Name	Classification	Action	Indications	Contraindications	Doses	Routes	Adverse Effects	Other
Haloperidol *Haldol*	Butyrophenone	Blocks dopamine receptors associated with mood and behavior	• Psychosis	• Hypotension • Hypersensitivity to the drug	2–10 mg	IM, PO	• Extrapyramidal reactions • Insomnia • Restlessness • Dry mouth • Hypotension • Tachycardia	• Hypotension more common in patients taking antihypertensives.
Chlorpromazine *Thorazine*	Phenothiazine	Blocks dopamine receptors associated with mood and behavior	• Psychosis • Intractable hiccups	• Hypotension • Hypersensitivity to the drug	25–50 mg	IM, PO	• Extrapyramidal reactions • Insomnia • Restlessness • Dry mouth • Hypotension • Tachycardia	• Hypotension more common in patients taking antihypertensives.
Ziprasidone *Geodon*	Unclassified antipsychotic	Inhibits uptake of serotonin and dopamine	• Psychosis • Tourette's syndrome	• Hypersensitivity to the drug	50–100 mcg	IM, PO	• Extrapyramidal reactions • Insomnia • Restlessness • Dry mouth • Hypotension • Tachycardia	• Carbamazepine (Tegretol) can decrease ziprasidone levels.

overdoses is primarily supportive, with sodium bicarbonate given to increase the excretion of TCAs by alkalinizing the urine. The prototype tricyclic antidepressant, imipramine (Tofranil), was also the first one on the market. Other common examples include amitriptyline (Elavil), desipramine (Norpramin), and nortriptyline (Pamelor).

Selective serotonin reuptake inhibitors (SSRIs) are a recent addition to the antidepressants. The prototype, fluoxetine (Prozac), is the most widely prescribed antidepressant in the United States. These drugs' antidepressant effects are comparable to those of the TCAs, but because the SSRIs selectively block the reuptake of serotonin, they do not affect dopamine or norepinephrine. Nor do they block histaminic or cholinergic receptors, thus avoiding many of the TCAs' side effects (Figure 13-14). The primary adverse reactions to SSRIs are sexual dysfunction, headache, and nausea. Other selective serotonin reuptake inhibitors include sertraline (Zoloft), citalopram (Celexa), escitalopram (Lexapro), and paroxetine (Paxil).

A third pharmacological class of psychotherapeutic medications includes the monoamine oxidase inhibitors (MAOIs). The monoamine neurotransmitters are thought to be insufficient in depression. Monoamine oxidase, an enzyme, metabolizes monoamines into inactive metabolites. MAOIs inhibit monoamine oxidase and block the monoamines' breakdown, thus increasing their availability (Figure 13-15). Monoamine oxidase is also present in the liver and has a significant role in metabolizing foods that contain tyramine, a substance that increases the

MAO Inhibitors

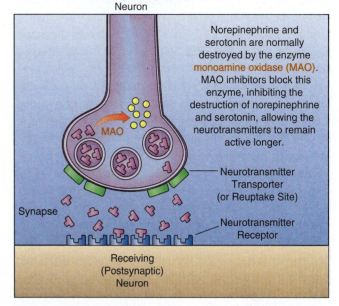

FIGURE 13-15 The mechanism of action of monamine oxidase inhibitors (MAOIs).

release of norepinephrine. The MAOIs' major side effect is hypertensive crisis brought on by the consumption of foods rich in tyramine, such as cheese and red wine. By inhibiting monoamine oxidase, these drugs also decrease the body's ability to inactivate tyramine; they therefore promote the release of norepinephrine, a potent vasopressor. Because of this and other unwanted side effects, MAOIs are not commonly used anymore; rather, they are reserved for treating depression that is refractory to TCAs and SSRIs. The prototype of this class is phenelzine (Nardil).

Patients with bipolar disorder (manic depression) exhibit cyclic swings from mania to depression, with periods of normalcy in between. According to the DSM-5, the manic phases of this disease are characterized by hyperactivity, thoughts of grandeur or inflated self-esteem, decreased need for sleep, increased goal-oriented behavior, increased productivity, flight of ideas (moving from thought to thought with little connection between them), distractibility, and increased risk taking. Lithium is the drug of choice for the management of bipolar disorder. It is frequently given in conjunction with benzodiazepines or antipsychotics. Lithium's mechanism of action is unknown, but it effectively decreases the signs of mania without causing sedation. Adverse reactions include headache, dizziness, fatigue, nausea, and vomiting. Recently, two antiseizure medications—carbamazepine (Tegretol) and valproic acid (Depakote)—have proven successful in treating bipolar disorder.

SSRI Antidepressants

FIGURE 13-14 The mechanism of action of selective serotonin reuptake inhibitors (SSRIs).

Drugs Used to Treat Parkinson's Disease

Parkinson's disease is a nervous disorder caused by the destruction of dopamine-releasing neurons in the *substantia nigra,* a part of the basal ganglia, which is a specialized area of the brain involved in controlling fine movements. Dysfunction of parts of the basal ganglia causes the extrapyramidal symptoms (EPS) often seen as a side effect of antipsychotic medications.

Parkinson's disease is characterized by dyskinesia (dysfunctional movements) such as involuntary tremors, unsteady gait, and postural instability. Severe cases also involve bradykinesia (slow movements) and akinesia (the absence of movement). In the later stages, patients frequently present with psychological impairment, including dementia, depression, and impaired memory. Parkinson's is a progressive disease that usually begins in middle age with subtle signs and progresses to a state of incapacitation. Although no treatments can cure Parkinson's or even slow its progression, treating the symptoms can return some function to the patient. The goal in treating these patients is to restore their ability to function without causing unacceptable side effects. Some remarkably effective drugs are available. Unfortunately, they usually are effective for only several years. After that, signs and symptoms return and often are more severe than before treatment began.

The medications that are effective in treating Parkinson's disease are also effective in treating the EPS of antipsychotics. This is because fine motor control is based in part on a balance between inhibitory and excitatory neurotransmitters. In the basal ganglia, dopamine, an inhibitory transmitter, opposes acetylcholine, an excitatory neurotransmitter. Parkinson's disease and the medications that cause EPS both decrease the number of presynaptic terminals that release dopamine in the basal ganglia. This allows the excitatory stimulus of acetylcholine to dominate, ultimately impeding fine motor control.

Pharmacological therapy for Parkinson's disease seeks to restore the balance of dopamine and acetylcholine. This may be done either by increasing the stimulation of dopamine receptors or by decreasing the stimulation of acetylcholine receptors. Drugs can do this either through dopaminergic effects or through anticholinergic effects. Dopaminergic effects increase the release of dopamine from the neuron, directly stimulate the dopamine receptors, or decrease the breakdown of however much dopamine is being released. Anticholinergic effects prevent acetylcholine's effects either by reducing the amount of the neurotransmitter released or by directly blocking the acetylcholine receptors.

Dopamine cannot be given directly to Parkinson's disease patients because it cannot cross the blood–brain barrier and consequently would be ineffective in treating the disease, while still causing many side effects. The drug of choice in treating Parkinson's disease, therefore, is levodopa, an inactive drug that readily crosses the blood–brain barrier. Levodopa is absorbed by the dopamine-releasing neuron terminals, where the enzyme decarboxylase metabolizes it into dopamine, thus increasing the amount of dopamine available for release. Levodopa is very effective and reduces symptoms in the vast majority of patients. As previously mentioned, however, symptoms will return within a period of years as the disease progresses. Levodopa's side effects include nausea, vomiting, and ironically, for unknown reasons, dyskinesias. Because it is converted to dopamine, levodopa may also have cardiovascular effects, including tachycardias and hypertension.

When given alone, levodopa is metabolized primarily outside the brain, where it is ineffective. To prevent this, Sinemet, the most popular anti-Parkinson preparation available, combines levodopa with an inactive ingredient, carbidopa. Although carbidopa by itself produces no effects, it prevents levodopa's conversion into dopamine in the periphery. Because carbidopa does not cross the blood–brain barrier, however, levodopa can still be metabolized in the CNS. This decreases the incidence of cardiovascular side effects and enables lower doses of levodopa to be effective. Sinemet's side effects are essentially those of levodopa by itself. Nausea and vomiting, stimulated from within the CNS, remain problematic.

Another dopaminergic medication, amantadine (Symmetrel), promotes the release of dopamine from the dopamine-releasing neurons that remain unaffected by the disease. It has a rapid onset but generally becomes ineffective in less than a year. Although it can be effective alone, it is usually given in conjunction with Sinemet or levodopa. Several other medications, such as bromocriptine, directly stimulate the dopamine receptors instead of attempting to increase the amount of dopamine released.

One additional dopaminergic approach is to decrease the breakdown of dopamine after it has been released. The enzyme responsible for breaking down monoamines such as norepinephrine, dopamine, and serotonin is monoamine oxidase. (We have previously described monoamine oxidase inhibitors in our discussion of their role in depression.) One monoamine oxidase inhibitor, selegiline (Carbex), is specific for monoamine oxidase type B. This MAO-B enzyme is involved only in the breakdown of dopamine. (MAO-A is responsible for breaking down norepinephrine and serotonin.) By selectively inhibiting the breakdown of dopamine, selegiline increases the amount available for binding with dopamine receptors, thus promoting the dopamine–acetylcholine balance. This selective blockage avoids increased norepinephrine levels that can lead to undesired tachycardia and hypertension.

As opposed to dopaminergic medications, which act on the dopamine side of the dopamine–acetylcholine balance, anticholinergic medications act on the acetylcholine side to block the acetylcholine receptors. The prototype anticholinergic, atropine, was initially used in this context with success, but it also had the typical peripheral anticholinergic side effects of blurred vision, dry mouth, and urinary hesitancy. More recently developed medications affect the CNS more than they do the peripheral nervous system. The prototype centrally acting anticholinergic medication is benztropine (Cogentin). Another example is diphenhydramine (Benadryl), which is more frequently administered for its antihistaminic properties.

Autonomic Nervous System Medications

The **autonomic nervous system** is the part of the nervous system that controls involuntary (automatic) actions. Many medications used in out-of-hospital care directly affect the autonomic nervous system. It is essential that you have a good understanding of this aspect of the nervous system and the ways in which emergency medications affect it.

The two functional divisions of the autonomic nervous system are the sympathetic nervous system and the parasympathetic nervous system. The sympathetic nervous system allows the body to function under stress. It is often referred to as the fight-or-flight aspect of the nervous system. The parasympathetic nervous system, however, primarily controls vegetative functions such as digestion of food. It is often referred to as the feed-or-breed or the rest-and-repose aspect of the nervous system. The parasympathetic nervous system and the sympathetic nervous system work in constant opposition to control organ responses. For example, the sympathetic nervous system stimulates specific receptors in the heart that increase the heart rate. At the same time, the parasympathetic nervous system stimulates specific receptors that decrease the heart rate. The net result is the resting heart rate. When the body's physiologic needs dictate an increased heart rate, the sympathetic stimuli dominate the parasympathetic effects. Conversely, when the body needs to rest (with a decreased heart rate), the parasympathetic stimuli predominate.

Basic Anatomy and Physiology of the Autonomic Nervous System

The autonomic nervous system arises from the central nervous system. The nerves of the autonomic nervous system exit the central nervous system and subsequently enter specialized structures called **autonomic ganglia**. In the autonomic ganglia, the nerve fibers from the central nervous system interact with nerve fibers that extend from the ganglia to the various target organs. Autonomic nerve fibers that exit the central nervous system and terminate in the autonomic ganglia are called **preganglionic nerves**. Autonomic nerve fibers that exit the ganglia and terminate in the various target tissues are called **postganglionic nerves**. The ganglia of the sympathetic nervous system are located close to the spinal cord, whereas the ganglia of the

parasympathetic nervous system are located close to the target organs (Figure 13-16).

No actual physical connection exists between two nerve cells or between a nerve cell and the organ it innervates. Instead, there is a space, or **synapse**, between nerve cells. The space between a nerve cell and the target organ is a **neuroeffector junction**. Specialized chemicals called **neurotransmitters** conduct the nervous impulse between nerve cells or between a nerve cell and its target organ.

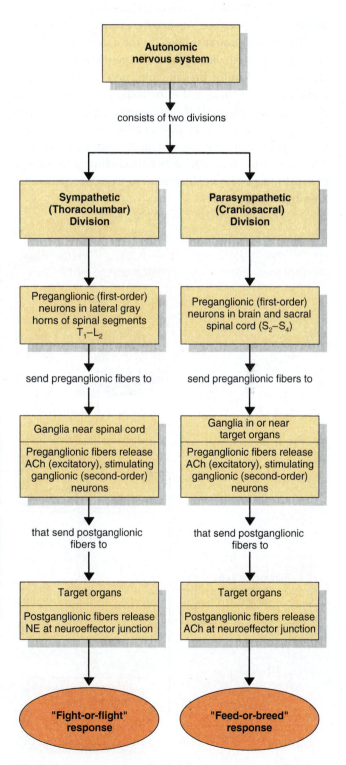

FIGURE 13-16 Components of the autonomic nervous system.

Neurotransmitters are released from presynaptic **neurons** and subsequently act on postsynaptic neurons or on the designated target organ. When released by the nerve ending, the neurotransmitter travels across the synapse and activates membrane receptors on the adjoining nerve or target tissue. The neurotransmitter is then either deactivated or taken back up into the presynaptic neuron.

The two neurotransmitters of the autonomic nervous system are acetylcholine (ACh) and norepinephrine. Acetylcholine is used in the preganglionic nerves of the sympathetic nervous system and in both the preganglionic and postganglionic nerves of the parasympathetic nervous system. Norepinephrine is the postganglionic neurotransmitter of the sympathetic nervous system. Synapses that use acetylcholine as the neurotransmitter are **cholinergic** synapses. Synapses that use norepinephrine as the neurotransmitter are **adrenergic** synapses.

Drugs Used to Affect the Parasympathetic Nervous System

The parasympathetic nervous system arises from the brainstem and the sacral segments of the spinal cord. The preganglionic neurons of the parasympathetic nervous system are typically much longer than those of the sympathetic nervous system, because the ganglia are located close to the target tissues. Parasympathetic nerve fibers that leave the brainstem travel within four of the cranial nerves: the oculomotor nerve (III), the facial nerve (VII), the glossopharyngeal nerve (IX), and the vagus nerve (X). These fibers synapse in the parasympathetic ganglia with short postganglionic fibers that then continue to their target tissues. Postsynaptic fibers innervate much of the body, including the intrinsic eye muscles, the salivary glands, the heart, the lungs, and most of the organs of the abdominal cavity. The sacral segment of the parasympathetic nervous system forms distinct pelvic nerves that innervate ganglia in the kidneys, bladder, sex organs, and the terminal portions of the large intestine (Figure 13-17).

FIGURE 13-17 Organization of the parasympathetic division of the autonomic nervous system.

Stimulation of the parasympathetic nervous system results in the following conditions:

- Pupillary constriction
- Secretion by digestive glands
- Reduction in heart rate and cardiac contractile force
- Bronchoconstriction
- Increased smooth muscle activity along the digestive tract

These and other functions facilitate the processing of food, energy absorption, relaxation, and reproduction (Figure 13-18).

All preganglionic and postganglionic parasympathetic nerve fibers use acetylcholine as a neurotransmitter. ACh, when released by presynaptic neurons, crosses the synaptic cleft and activates receptors on the postsynaptic neurons or on the neuroeffector junction. ACh is also the neurotransmitter for the somatic nervous system and is present in the neuromuscular junction. ACh is very short-lived. Within a fraction of a second after its release, it is deactivated by another chemical, acetylcholinesterase. Acetic acid and choline, which are produced when ACh is deactivated, are taken back up by the presynaptic neuron (Figure 13-19).

The parasympathetic system has two main types of ACh receptors, nicotinic and muscarinic. Knowing these receptors' locations and functions will greatly simplify learning the functions of drugs in this class (Table 13-13). Nicotinic$_N$ (neuron) receptors are found in all autonomic ganglia, where acetylcholine serves as the presynaptic neurotransmitter of both the parasympathetic and sympathetic nervous systems. Nicotinic$_M$ (muscle) receptors are found at the neuromuscular junction and initiate muscular contraction as part of the somatic nervous system. Muscarinic receptors are found in many organs throughout the body and are primarily responsible for promoting the parasympathetic response. Table 13-14

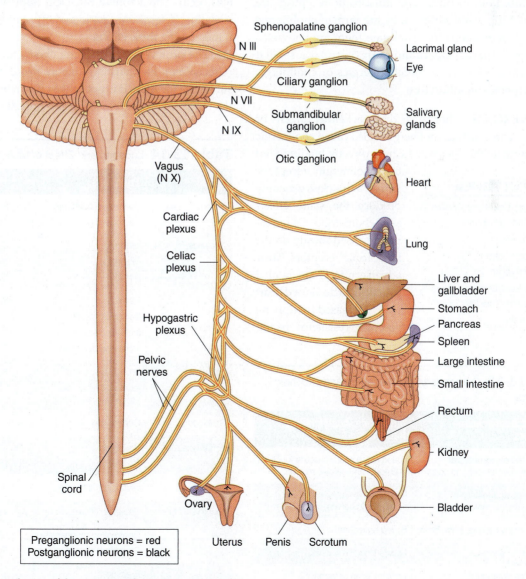

FIGURE 13-18 Distribution of the parasympathetic postganglionic fibers.

FIGURE 13-19 Physiology of a cholinergic synapse. Acetylcholine is released from the presynaptic nerve and stimulates receptors on the postsynaptic nerve. Subsequently, acetylcholinesterase breaks down the acetylcholine and the presynaptic nerve fiber takes up the products.

summarizes the locations and actions of the muscarinic receptors.

Because both nicotinic and muscarinic receptors are specialized for acetylcholine, they are termed cholinergic receptors. Medications that stimulate them are known as cholinergics (**parasympathomimetics**), and those that block them are known as anticholinergics or cholinergic blockers (**parasympatholytics**).

CHOLINERGICS Cholinergic drugs act either directly or indirectly. Direct-acting cholinergics (also called cholinergic esters) simulate the effects of ACh by directly binding with the cholinergic receptors. Drugs in this class generally produce the same effects as cholinergic stimulation, focused mostly on the muscarinic receptors. Their adverse effects are related primarily to decreased heart rate, decreased peripheral vascular resistance result-ing in hypotension, and excessive salivation, urination, defecation, and sweating. Vomiting and abdominal cramps may also occur. The acronym SLUDGE (*s*alivation, *l*acrimation, *u*rination, *d*efecation, *g*astric motility, *e*mesis) is helpful for remembering these effects.

The prototype direct-acting cholinergic is bethanechol (Urecholine). Its pharmacokinetics make it a good clinical substitute for ACh. It is not broken down by cholinesterase, the enzyme responsible for destroying ACh, and therefore

---

CONTENT REVIEW

➤ Sludge Effects of Cholinergic Medications
- *S*alivation
- *L*acrimation
- *U*rination
- *D*efecation
- *G*astric motility
- *E*mesis

Table 13-13 Comparison of Muscarinic and Nicotinic Receptors

Nicotinic Acetylcholine Receptors	Muscarinic Acetylcholine Receptors
Found at the neuromuscular junction of skeletal (only) muscles.	Found at the neuromuscular junction of smooth and cardiac muscle.
Found on postganglionic parasympathetic nerves.	Found on postganglionic sympathetic nerves.
Found on many neurons in the brain.	Found on glands.
Nicotine is an agonist.	Muscarine is an agonist.
Curare is an antagonist.	Atropine is an antagonist.

Table 13-14 Location and Effect of Muscarinic Receptors

Organ	Functions	Location
Heart	Decreased heart rate	Sinoatrial node
	Decreased conduction rate	Atrioventricular node
Arterioles	Dilation	Coronary
	Dilation	Skin and mucosa
	Dilation	Cerebral
GI tract	Relaxed	Sphincters
	Increased motility	
	Increased salivation	Salivary glands
	Increased secretion	Exocrine glands
Lungs	Bronchoconstriction	Bronchiole smooth muscle
	Increased mucus production	Bronchial glands
Gallbladder	Contraction	
Urinary bladder	Relaxation	Urinary sphincter
	Contraction	Detrusor muscle
Liver	Glycogen synthesis	
Lacrimal glands	Secretion (increased tearing)	Eye
Eye	Contraction for near vision	Ciliary muscle
	Constriction	Pupil
Penis	Erection	

it has a longer duration of action. Most of its effects are on muscarinic receptors in the urinary bladder and gastrointestinal tract. It may be given orally or subcutaneously. Thus, it is used primarily to increase micturition (urination) and peristalsis. Adverse effects are rare but related to its parasympathomimetic effects. Another direct-acting cholinergic medication, pilocarpine, is used as a topical treatment for glaucoma.

Indirect-acting cholinergic drugs affect acetylcholinesterase. By inhibiting its actions in degrading acetylcholine, they prolong the cholinergic response. These drugs affect both muscarinic and nicotinic receptors and therefore have little specificity. Their uses are limited primarily to treating myasthenia gravis, some types of poisoning, and glaucoma, as well as for reversing nondepolarizing neuromuscular blockade.

The two basic types of indirect-acting cholinergic drugs are reversible inhibitors and irreversible inhibitors. Both types bind with cholinesterase (ChE), acting as a substitute for ACh. In doing so, they prevent ChE from destroying ACh. The difference between the reversible and irreversible inhibitors is how long they remain bound with cholinesterase. The reversible inhibitors remain bound with cholinesterase much longer than ACh but eventually release it. The irreversible inhibitors, too, will eventually release cholinesterase, but they remain bound for so long that, from a practical standpoint, they can be considered irreversible.

Neostigmine (Prostigmin) is the prototype reversible cholinesterase inhibitor. It is used to treat myasthenia gravis, an illness characterized by muscle weakness and progressive fatigue. This illness is an autoimmune disease that destroys the nicotinic$_M$ receptors at the neuromuscular junction. With fewer of these receptors, muscles cannot be stimulated as well and weakness occurs. Neostigmine treats the symptoms of myasthenia gravis by blocking the degradation of ACh, thereby prolonging its effects and increasing motor strength. Its primary side effects are due to the stimulation of muscarinic receptors and include the SLUDGE responses. Fortunately, these responses may be treated effectively with a cholinergic blocker. Neostigmine can also reverse a nondepolarizing neuromuscular blockade. This use is fairly uncommon, however, because such blockades typically are administered only intentionally as part of anesthesia or before intubation.

Physostigmine (Antilirium) is another reversible cholinesterase inhibitor. Its mechanism is similar to neostigmine's, with their primary difference being in their pharmacokinetics. Whereas neostigmine is poorly absorbed across the cell membrane, physostigmine crosses rapidly and therefore has a shorter onset and may be given in lower doses. Physostigmine's chief use is for reversing overdoses of atropine, an anticholinergic drug that blocks muscarinic receptors.

Irreversible cholinesterase inhibitors have only one clinical function—the treatment of glaucoma—and only one drug, echothiophate (Phospholine Iodide), has been approved for that purpose. Cholinesterase inhibitors, however, are very useful as insecticides (organophosphates), and, unfortunately, their mechanism of action is also very attractive for makers of chemical weapons. They are the chief component in nerve gases such as VX and sarin. They cause extensive stimulation of cholinergic receptors, ultimately resulting in the SLUDGE response. Toxic levels may also affect nicotinic$_M$ receptors, leading to paralysis. Treatment for such toxic exposures involves drugs such as high doses of atropine or pralidoxime (Protopam, 2-PAM) to block the effects of the accumulating ACh. Pralidoxime can encourage irreversible cholinesterase inhibitors to release cholinesterase.

ANTICHOLINERGICS Anticholinergic agents oppose the parasympathetic (cholinergic) nervous system. Just as there are multiple types of cholinergic receptors, there are multiple classes of cholinergic receptor antagonists. We will discuss agents that selectively block muscarinic and nicotinic receptors, as well as nonselective blockers (ganglionic blockers). A special subclass of nicotinic receptor blocking agents is neuromuscular blocking drugs.

Muscarinic Cholinergic Antagonists Cholinergic antagonists block the effects of acetylcholine almost exclusively at the muscarinic receptors. They are often called anticholinergics or parasympatholytics. They work by competitively binding with muscarinic receptors without stimulating them. As a result, these receptors cannot bind with ACh.

The prototype anticholinergic drug is atropine, which is widely used to block muscarinic receptors and is commonly administered in the field. Found in the plant *Atropa belladonna*, atropine is one of several drugs classified as belladonna alkaloids (scopolamine is also in this classification). Readily absorbed through both enteral and parenteral routes, it has therapeutic effects at dose-dependent levels at most sites with muscarinic receptors. At low doses, atropine decreases secretion from salivary and bronchial glands as well as from the sympathetically innervated sweat glands. At moderate doses, it increases heart rate and causes mydriasis (dilated pupils) and blurry vision. At higher doses, it decreases gastric motility and stomach acid secretion. Atropine is also useful in reversing overdoses of muscarinic agonists (cholinergics or cholinesterase inhibitors). Its side effects, which are predictable, include dry mouth, blurred vision and photophobia, urinary retention, increased intraocular pressure, tachycardia, constipation, and

CONTENT REVIEW

➤ Types of Parasympathetic Acetylcholine Receptors
- Muscarinic
- Nicotinic
  - Nicotinic$_N$ (neuron)
  - Nicotinic$_M$ (muscle)

anhidrosis (decreased sweating), which may cause hyperthermia. A helpful mnemonic for remembering the effects of atropine overdose is "hot as hell, blind as a bat, dry as a bone, red as a beet, mad as a hatter."

Scopolamine is another belladonna anticholinergic. Its actions are similar to atropine's, but unlike atropine, scopolamine causes sedation and antiemesis. Thus, its primary purpose is to prevent motion sickness. It is available as a transdermal patch.

Several synthetic medications mimic the effects of the belladonna alkaloids while minimizing their side effects. Ipratropium bromide (Atrovent), an inhaled anticholinergic, is effective in treating asthma because it relaxes the bronchial smooth muscle and causes bronchodilation. It is frequently administered along with an inhaled beta-adrenergic agonist. Because it is inhaled and has little systemic effect, ipratropium bromide avoids many of atropine's side effects (Table 13-15).

Other anticholinergic drugs include dicyclomine (Bentyl) and benztropine (Cogentin).

Nicotinic Cholinergic Antagonists Nicotinic cholinergic antagonists block acetylcholine only at nicotinic sites. They include ganglionic blocking agents that block the nicotinic$_N$ receptors in the autonomic ganglia and neuromuscular blocking agents that block nicotinic$_M$ receptors at the neuromuscular junction.

GANGLIONIC BLOCKING AGENTS Ganglionic blockade is produced by competitive antagonism with acetylcholine at the nicotinic$_N$ receptors in the autonomic ganglia. This can, in effect, turn off the entire autonomic nervous system. The two drugs in this class are trimethaphan (Arfonad) and mecamylamine (Inversine). Both are used to treat hypertension. The adverse effects of ganglionic blockade include signs associated with antimuscarinic drugs like atropine—dry mouth, blurred vision, urinary retention, and tachycardia. Other adverse effects arising from the vasodilation and decreased preload caused by sympathetic blockage include profound hypotension, with orthostatic hypotension even more evident. Trimethaphan is administered primarily for hypertensive crisis when other treatments are ineffective. These agents are almost never used anymore because they are not selective and many superior agents are available.

NEUROMUSCULAR BLOCKING AGENTS Neuromuscular blockade produces a state of paralysis without affecting consciousness. Imagine how terrifying it would be to be fully conscious and aware but completely paralyzed, unable to move or breathe. Neuromuscular blockade is caused by competitive antagonism of nicotinic$_M$ receptors at the neuromuscular junction. This is useful during surgery as part of anesthesia and during electroconvulsive therapy for depression. These agents are most often used in the field to facilitate intubation.

Neuromuscular blocking agents are either depolarizing or nondepolarizing, depending on their mechanism of action. Most are nondepolarizing; only one depolarizing drug, succinylcholine (Anectine), is commonly used in the clinical setting. Tubocurarine, though not frequently used clinically, is the oldest neuromuscular blocker and the prototype nondepolarizing agent. It produces neuromuscular blockade by binding with the nicotinic$_M$ receptor sites without causing muscle depolarization. Succinylcholine acts in the same manner, but like acetylcholine, it does cause muscle depolarization when it binds with the nicotinic$_M$ receptor. It is useful as a neuromuscular blocker because, in contrast to ACh, which rapidly separates from the receptor, it remains bound, preventing the muscle's repolarization. Several nondepolarizing agents are available; the specific agent chosen depends on its rate of onset and duration of action. Succinylcholine has the shortest onset and duration of action because it has a naturally occurring enzyme, pseudocholinesterase, which degrades it.[16,17] See Table 13-16.

GANGLIONIC STIMULATING AGENTS Nicotinic$_N$ receptors reside at the ganglia of both the parasympathetic and sympathetic nervous systems. The alkaloid nicotine stimulates these receptors. Nicotine is found in tobacco and, although it has no therapeutic uses, is of interest for two reasons. Historically, nicotine, along with muscarine, led to a much better understanding of the autonomic nervous system's specific receptors. Also, it is one of the most abused drugs in the world.

Nicotine may cause a variety of responses, most of which are dose related. At low doses, like those from smoking, nicotine causes excitation at the autonomic ganglia. This affects both the parasympathetic and sympathetic nervous systems. The parasympathetic response causes increased salivation, peristalsis, and secretion of gastric acid. The sympathetic response causes the release of norepinephrine and epinephrine. These lead to increases in heart rate, myocardial contractility, vasoconstriction, and blood pressure, all of which increase the heart's workload. Sympathetic stimulation also increases awareness and suppresses fatigue and appetite.

Nicotine administration devices such as gum and transdermal patches are available for use in smoking cessation. Their actions are similar to the actions of nicotine inhaled in smoke.

Table 13-15 Parasympatholytic Medications

Name	Classification	Action	Indications	Contraindications	Doses	Routes	Adverse Effects	Other
Atropine	Muscarinic anticholinergic (parasympatholytic)	Selectively blocks muscarinic receptors inhibiting parasympathetic stimulation	• Bradycardia • Antidote for organophosphate poisoning • Premedication for RSI	• Hypersensitivity to the drug	0.5–2.0 mg	IV, IO	• Blurred vision • Dry Mouth • Dilated pupils • Confusion	• Organophosphate poisonings may require a significantly higher dose
Ipratropium *Atrovent*	Muscarinic anticholinergic (parasympatholytic)	Selectively blocks muscarinic receptors inhibiting parasympathetic stimulation	• Bronchospasm associated with obstructive lung disease (asthma, COPD)	• Hypersensitivity to the drug	500 mcg	Inhaled	• Blurred vision • Dry Mouth • Dilated pupils • Cough • Confusion	• Typically administered with a beta agonist (although not as frequently)

Table 13-16 Neuromuscular Blocking Agents

Name	Classification	Action	Indications	Contraindications	Doses	Routes	Adverse Effects	Other
Succinylcholine *Anectine*	Depolarizing neuromuscular blocker	Binds to ACh receptors at the neuromuscular junction, causing depolarization and subsequent paralysis	• Rapid sequence intubation (RSI)	• Hyperkalemia • Neuromuscular disease • Crush injury • Burns • Increased intracranial pressure • Severe trauma	1–2 mg/kg	IV, IO	• Hyperkalemia • Bradycardia • Prolonged paralysis • Malignant hyperthermia • Increased intracranial pressure • Muscle fasciculations • Trismus	• These agents should be used only by persons skilled in their use, competent at complicated airway management, and with all necessary resuscitative equipment available.
Vecuronium *Norcuron*	Nondepolarizing neuromuscular blocker	Binds to ACh receptors at the neuromuscular junction, causing paralysis	• Rapid sequence intubation (RSI)	• Hypersensitivity to the drug	0.1–0.15 mg/kg	IV, IO	• Skeletal muscle weakness • Malignant hyperthermia • Apnea	• These agents should be used only by persons skilled in their use, competent at complicated airway management, and with all necessary resuscitative equipment available.
Rocuronium *Zemuron*	Nondepolarizing neuromuscular blocker	Binds to ACh receptors at the neuromuscular junction, causing paralysis	• Rapid sequence intubation (RSI)	• Hypersensitivity to the drug	1 mg/kg	IV, IO	• Hypertension • Hypotension • Skeletal muscle weakness • Malignant hyperthermia • Apnea	• These agents should be used only by persons skilled in their use, competent at complicated airway management, and with all necessary resuscitative equipment available.

Drugs Used to Affect the Sympathetic Nervous System

The sympathetic nervous system arises from the thoracic and lumbar regions of the spinal cord. Preganglionic nerves leave the spinal cord through the spinal nerves and end in the sympathetic ganglia. There are two types of sympathetic ganglia: sympathetic chain ganglia and collateral ganglia (Figure 13-20). In addition, special preganglionic sympathetic nerve fibers innervate the adrenal medulla. Postganglionic nerves that exit the sympathetic chain ganglia extend to several peripheral target tissues of the sympathetic nervous system. When stimulated, these fibers have several effects. They include:

- Stimulation of secretion by sweat glands
- Constriction of blood vessels in the skin
- Increase in blood flow to skeletal muscles
- Increase in the heart rate and force of cardiac contractions
- Bronchodilation
- Stimulation of energy production

The collateral ganglia are located in the abdominal cavity. Nerves leaving the collateral ganglia innervate many of the organs of the abdomen. Stimulation of these fibers causes several conditions. They include:

- Reduction of blood flow to abdominal organs
- Decreased digestive activity
- Relaxation of smooth muscle in the wall of the urinary bladder
- Release of glucose stores from the liver

Sympathetic nervous system stimulation also results in direct stimulation of the adrenal medulla, the inner portion of the adrenal gland (Figure 13-21). The adrenal medulla, in turn, releases the hormones norepinephrine (noradrenalin) and epinephrine (adrenalin) into the circulatory system.

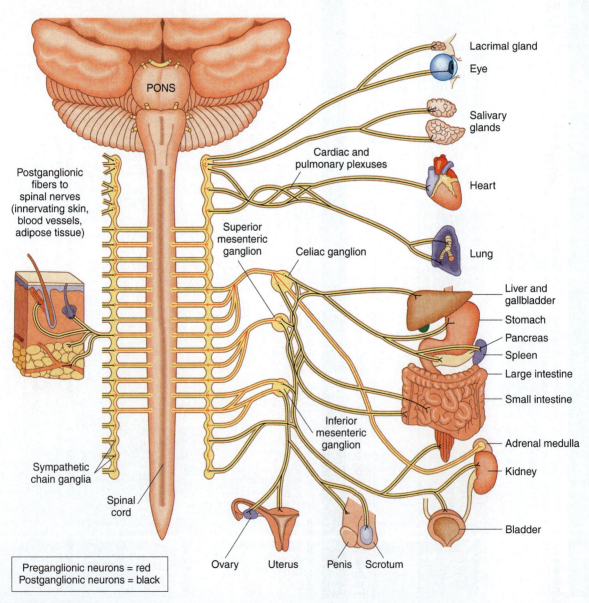

FIGURE 13-20 Distribution of sympathetic postganglionic fibers.

FIGURE 13-21 Organization of the sympathetic division of the autonomic nervous system.

Approximately 80 percent of the hormones released by the adrenal medulla are epinephrine, and norepinephrine constitutes the remaining 20 percent. Once released, these hormones are carried throughout the body, where they cause their intended effects by acting on hormone receptors. The release of norepinephrine and epinephrine by the adrenal medulla stimulates tissues that are not innervated by sympathetic nerves. In addition, it prolongs the effects of direct sympathetic stimulation. All these effects serve to prepare the body to deal with stressful and potentially dangerous situations.

ADRENERGIC RECEPTORS Sympathetic stimulation ultimately results in the release of the hormone norepinephrine from postganglionic nerves. The norepinephrine subsequently crosses the synaptic cleft and interacts with adrenergic receptors on the postsynaptic nerves. Shortly thereafter, the norepinephrine is either taken up by the presynaptic neuron for reuse or broken down by enzymes present within the synapse (Figure 13-22). Sympathetic stimulation also results in the release of the hormones epinephrine and norepinephrine from the adrenal medulla.

In addition, both epinephrine and norepinephrine interact with specialized adrenergic receptors on the membranes of the target organs. These receptors are located throughout the body. Once stimulated by the appropriate hormone, they cause a response in the organ or organs they control.

The two known types of sympathetic receptors are the adrenergic receptors and the dopaminergic receptors. The adrenergic receptors are generally divided into four types. These five receptors are designated alpha 1 (α_1), alpha 2 (α_2), beta 1 (β_1), beta 2 (β_2), and beta 3 (β_3). The α_1 receptors cause peripheral vasoconstriction, mild bronchoconstriction, and stimulation of metabolism. The α_2 receptors are found on the presynaptic surfaces of sympathetic neuroeffector junctions. Stimulation of α_2 receptors is inhibitory. These receptors serve to prevent overrelease of norepinephrine in the synapse. When the level of norepinephrine in the synapse gets high

FIGURE 13-22 Physiology of an adrenergic synapse. Norepinephrine is released from the presynaptic nerve and stimulates receptors on the postsynaptic nerve. Subsequently, the norepinephrine is either taken up by the presynaptic nerve or deactivated by enzymes in the synapse.

enough, the α_2 receptors are stimulated, and norepinephrine release is inhibited. Stimulation of β_1 receptors causes increases in heart rate, cardiac contractile force, and cardiac automaticity and conduction. Stimulation of β_2 receptors causes vasodilation and bronchodilation. Stimulation of β_3 receptors promotes the breakdown of lipids for energy production. It has long been thought that dopaminergic receptors cause some degree of dilation of the renal, coronary, and cerebral arteries. However, recent studies have questioned whether such an effect exists. Several studies have demonstrated that low-dose dopamine infusions actually worsen renal function instead of improving it. Other studies have not been able to demonstrate improved bowel perfusion with dopamine administration.

Medications that stimulate the sympathetic nervous system are **sympathomimetics**. Medications that inhibit the sympathetic nervous system are called **sympatholytics**. Some medications are pure alpha agonists, whereas others are pure alpha antagonists. Some medications are pure beta agonists, whereas others are pure beta antagonists. Medications such as epinephrine stimulate both alpha and beta receptors. Other medications, such as the bronchodilators, are termed beta selective, as they act more on β_2 receptors than on β_1 receptors.

The sympathetic nervous system releases norepinephrine from postganglionic end terminals and epinephrine from the adrenal medulla. These neurotransmitters bind with adrenergic receptors. (Epinephrine is also called adrenalin because of its release from the adrenal medulla; hence the term *adren*-ergic.) There are two main types of adrenergic receptors, each with two subtypes. These receptors' effects depend primarily on their locations. Table 13-17 describes the chief locations and primary actions of each receptor.

The primary clinical purpose for medications that stimulate α_1 receptors is peripheral vasoconstriction. Constriction of the arterioles increases afterload, whereas constriction of venules increases preload (decreasing venous capacitance or "pooling"). Both these effects

increase systolic and diastolic blood pressure and represent the chief therapeutic indication for alpha$_1$ agonists. Stimulation of α_1 receptors locally may be useful in combination with local anesthetics. The main reason to add the α_1 agonist in this context is to cause local vasoconstriction so the systemic absorption of the anesthetic will decrease, and its duration will increase. Alpha$_1$ agonists are also useful topically to decrease nasal congestion caused by dilation and engorgement of nasal blood vessels. The primary adverse responses to α_1 agonist agents are hypertension and local tissue necrosis. If a medication with significant α_1 properties infiltrates the surrounding tissue or distal body parts

Table 13-17 Location of Adrenergic Receptors and Effects of Stimulation

Receptor	Response to Stimulation	Location
Alpha 1 (α_1)	Constriction	Arterioles
	Constriction	Veins
	Mydriasis	Eye
	Ejaculation	Penis
Alpha 2 (α_2)	Presynaptic terminal inhibition*	
Beta 1 (β_1)	Increased heart rate	Heart
	Increased conductivity	
	Increased automaticity	
	Increased contractility	
	Renin release	Kidney
Beta 2 (β_2)	Bronchodilation	Lungs
	Dilation	Arterioles
	Inhibition of contractions	Uterus
	Tremors	Skeletal muscle
Beta 3 (β_3)	Lipolysis	Adipose tissue
Dopaminergic	Vasodilation (increased blood flow)	Kidney

*Stimulation of α_2 adrenergic receptors inhibits the continued release of norepinephrine from the presynaptic terminal. It is a feedback mechanism that limits the adrenergic response at that synapse. These receptors have no other identified peripheral effects.

such as fingers, toes, earlobes, or nose, inadequate local blood flow due to profound vasoconstriction will likely kill the tissue. In addition, α_1 stimulation may cause reflex bradycardia due to the feedback mechanism that regulates blood pressure. As baroreceptors detect a rise in blood pressure, heart rate decreases to compensate.

Alpha$_1$ antagonism is indicated almost exclusively for controlling hypertension. By preventing the peripheral vasoconstriction of α_1 stimulation, these agents decrease blood pressure. They are also useful in treating local tissue necrosis caused by infiltration of α_1 agonists. Injecting α_1 antagonists into the area surrounding the infiltration prevents tissue death from excessive vasoconstriction. The effects of pheochromocytoma, a tumor of the adrenal medulla that causes the release of large amounts of catecholamine, may be treated with an α_1 blocker. The most common adverse effects of α_1 antagonism are orthostatic hypotension and reflex tachycardia. Just as α_1 stimulation may increase blood pressure and cause a baroreceptor-mediated bradycardia, the hypotension from α_1 blockage may lead to reflex tachycardia from the same mechanism. Other side effects include nasal congestion and inhibition of ejaculation. These agents may also increase blood volume. This is ironic, as their primary indication is hypertension. As another feedback mechanism detects hypotension, the kidneys begin to reabsorb sodium and water to increase blood volume. This is typically addressed by use of a diuretic concomitant with the α_1 antagonist.

Beta$_1$ stimulation increases heart rate, contractility, and conduction. Its primary indications are cardiac arrest and hypotension resulting from inadequate pumping. During cardiac arrest, β_1 activation may stimulate contractions or increase the force of any existing contractions. Even if the heart is only fibrillating, these agents may increase the effectiveness of electrical defibrillation. In cardiogenic shock, when the heart is not pumping with enough force to overcome the afterload created by peripheral vascular resistance, β_1 agonists can adequately increase the contractions' force. The chief adverse effects of β_1 agonists include tachycardia, arrhythmias, and chest pain from increasing workload.

Beta$_1$ antagonists are among the most frequently prescribed medications in the United States. Their most common use is to control blood pressure. By blocking the effects of β_1 stimulation, they decrease heart rate (chronotropy) and contractility (inotropy). These agents are also effective in treating supraventricular tachycardias because they decrease the rate of impulse generation at the SA node (negative chronotropic effects) while also slowing conductivity through the AV node (negative dromotropic effects). Blocking β_1 stimulation also helps treat angina pectoris and reduces the recurrence of myocardial infarction. Its main adverse effects are symptomatic bradycardia, hypotension, and AV block.

Beta$_2$ agonists are used to treat asthma and other conditions with excessive narrowing of the bronchioles. By stimulating β_2 receptors in the lungs, these agents relax the bronchial smooth muscle and cause bronchodilation. Beta$_2$ agonists can also cause uterine smooth muscle relaxation, which may help to suppress preterm labor. Their primary adverse effects are muscle tremors and "bleed over" effects on unintended β_1 stimulation such as tachycardias.

Although β_2 blockade serves no clinically useful purpose, nonselective beta-blockers have side effects of β_2 blockade. Chief among these is bronchoconstriction and inhibition of glycogenolysis, the release of stored glycogen by the liver and skeletal muscles. Beta$_2$ stimulation causes glycogenesis. Antagonizing the β_2 receptors can inhibit this release. Although this is not typically a problem for most people, it can be very problematic for diabetics. It not only makes hypoglycemia more likely, but also masks one of its common early warning signs, tachycardia.

ADRENERGIC AGONISTS Drugs that stimulate the effects of adrenergic receptors work either directly, indirectly, or through a combination of the two. The direct-acting agents bind with the receptor and cause the same response as the normal neurotransmitter. In fact, most of the drugs in this category are either synthetically produced versions of the naturally occurring neurotransmitter or derivatives of those synthetically produced versions. The indirect-acting agents stimulate the release of epinephrine from the adrenal medulla and of norepinephrine from the presynaptic terminals. In turn, the epinephrine and norepinephrine stimulate the adrenergic receptors. The mixed actions of direct–indirect-acting medications combine these mechanisms.

The most frequently used adrenergic agents are chemically and functionally similar to the endogenous neurotransmitters. These drugs, which are called catecholamines, include norepinephrine, epinephrine, and dopamine.[18,19] Synthetic catecholamines are also available. They include dobutamine and isoproterenol. Noncatecholamine adrenergic agents, including ephedrine, phenylephrine, and terbutaline, also affect the adrenergic receptors and have useful clinical applications.

> **CONTENT REVIEW**
> ➤ Common Catecholamines
> - Natural
>   - Epinephrine
>   - Norepinephrine
>   - Dopamine
> - Synthetic
>   - Isoproterenol
>   - Dobutamine

Patho Pearls

Adrenergic Agonists: Effects of Repeated Doses. Many adrenergic agonists (Table 13-18), particularly decongestants and respiratory drugs, can result in tachyphylaxis. That is, repeated doses of the same drug have decreasing effects. In these cases, it may be prudent to change to a similar drug in the same family. The effects of a different drug can often be significantly better.

Table 13-18 Adrenergic Agonists

Name	Classification	Action	Indications	Contraindications	Doses	Routes	Adverse Effects	Other
Vasopressors								
Epinephrine	Sympathetic agonist	α and β adrenergic agonist (β effects more pronounced although dose-related)	• Cardiac arrest • Symptomatic bradycardia • Normovolemic hypotension • Allergies/anaphylaxis • Severe bronchospasm	• Few in the emergency setting	0.3–1.0 mg	IV, IO, IM, SQ, ET, inhaled	• Palpitations • Anxiety • Tremulousness • Headache • Dizziness • Hypertension • Can worsen cardiac ischemia	• Two preparations are commonly available: • 1:1,000 (1 mg/mL) • 1:10,000 (1 mg/10 mL)
Norepinephrine *Levophed*	Sympathetic agonist	α and β adrenergic agonist (α effects more pronounced)	• Normovolemic hypotension • Septic shock • Cardiogenic shock	• Should not be used in hypovolemia until volume replacement has occurred	0.1–0.5 mcg/kg/min (titrate to effect)	IV	• Palpitations • Anxiety • Tremulousness • Headache • Dizziness • Hypertension • Can worsen cardiac ischemia • Reflex bradycardia	• Extravasation can cause localized tissue damage. • Best administered through a central line.
Dopamine *Intropin*	Sympathetic agonist	α and β adrenergic agonist	• Normovolemic hypotension • Symptomatic bradycardia • Septic shock • Cardiogenic shock	• Should not be used in hypovolemia until volume replacement has occurred	2–20 mcg/kg/min (titrated to effect)	IV	• Palpitations • Anxiety • Tremulousness • Headache • Dizziness • Hypertension • Can worsen cardiac ischemia • Reflex bradycardia	• Extravasation can cause localized tissue damage. • Best administered through a central line. • Proposed renal benefit has been disproven.
Dobutamine *Dobutrex*	Synthetic sympathetic agonist	α and β adrenergic agonist (inotropic properties more pronounced than chronotropic properties)	• Congestive heart failure	• Should not be used in hypovolemia until volume replacement has occurred	2–20 mcg/kg/min (titrate to effect)	IV	• Palpitations • Anxiety • Tremulousness • Headache • Dizziness • Hypertension • Can worsen cardiac ischemia • Reflex bradycardia	• Extravasation can cause localized tissue damage. • Best administered through a central line. • Other agents preferred in cardiogenic shock.

Medication	Class	Description	Contraindications	Dosage	Route	Side Effects	Special Considerations
Phenylephrine *Neo-Synephrine*	Sympathetic agonist	Almost a pure α agonist causing vasoconstriction	• Avoid in cardiogenic shock	100–180 mcg/min (0.5–2.0 mcg/kg/min and titrate to effect)	IV	• Palpitations • Anxiety • Tremulousness • Headache • Dizziness • Can worsen cardiac ischemia • Reflex bradycardia	• Can be applied topically to nasal mucosa to shrink tissues prior to nasal procedures.
Bronchodilators			• Normovolemic hypotension • Septic shock • Spinal shock				
Albuterol *Ventolin, Proventil*	β agonist	β agonist with preference for β_2 adrenergic receptors	• Known hypersensitivity to the medication	2.5 mg (SVN); 90 mcg (MDI)	Inhalation	• Palpitations • Anxiety • Tremulousness • Headache • Dizziness • Tachycardia	• The patient's heart rate and SpO_2 should be monitored during treatment.
Levalbuterol *Xopenex*	β agonist	β agonist with preference for β_2 adrenergic receptors. It is a racemic isomer of albuterol.	• Known hypersensitivity to the medication	0.63 mc (SVN)	Inhalation	• Palpitations • Anxiety • Tremulousness • Headache • Dizziness • Tachycardia	• The patient's heart rate and SpO_2 should be monitored during treatment.
Metaproterenol *Alupent*	β agonist	β agonist with preference for β_2 adrenergic receptors	• Known hypersensitivity to the medication	0.2–0.3 mL of solution containing 15 mg/mL (SVN); 0.65 mg (MDI)	Inhalation	• Palpitations • Anxiety • Tremulousness • Headache • Dizziness • Tachycardia	• The patient's heart rate and SpO_2 should be monitored during treatment.
Terbutaline *Brethine*	β agonist	Relatively nonselective β agonist	• Known hypersensitivity to the medication	0.25 mg	Inhalation SQ	• Palpitations • Anxiety • Tremulousness • Headache • Dizziness • Tachycardia	• The patient's heart rate and SpO_2 should be monitored during treatment.
Racemic Epinephrine S_2	Sympathetic agonist	Relatively nonselective β agonist. It is a mix of both racemic isomers of epinephrine.	• Known hypersensitivity to the medication	0.25–0.75 mL of a 2.5% solution	Inhalation	• Palpitations • Anxiety • Tremulousness • Headache • Dizziness • Tachycardia	• The patient's heart rate and SpO_2 should be monitored during treatment.

Indications (from uses column):
- Phenylephrine: Normovolemic hypotension; Septic shock; Spinal shock
- Albuterol: Bronchospasm; Allergies/anaphylaxis; Hyperkalemia
- Levalbuterol: Bronchospasm; Allergies/anaphylaxis; Hyperkalemia
- Metaproterenol: Bronchospasm; Allergies/anaphylaxis; Hyperkalemia
- Terbutaline: Bronchospasm; Allergies/anaphylaxis; Hyperkalemia; Preterm labor
- Racemic Epinephrine: Croup

Table 13-19 Adrenergic Receptor Specificity

Medication	Receptor				
	Alpha₁	Alpha₂	Beta₁	Beta₂	Dopaminergic
Phenylephrine	✓				
Norepinephrine	✓	✓	✓		
Ephedrine	✓	✓	✓	✓	
Epinephrine	✓	✓	✓	✓	
Dobutamine			✓		
Dopamine*			✓		✓
Isoproterenol			✓	✓	
Terbutaline				✓	

*Receptor specificity is dose dependent. The higher the dose, the fewer dopaminergic effects are seen.

Almost all the drugs in this section act on more than one type of receptor. Their specificity varies and is important in determining their uses. Table 13-19 lists their actions on various receptors.[20–21]

ADRENERGIC ANTAGONISTS   Unlike most adrenergic agonists, the majority of available adrenergic antagonists are remarkably selective in which receptor they affect. This selectivity, however, occurs only at therapeutic doses. At higher doses, most agents lose their selectivity and begin affecting other receptors as well.

The two basic subcategories of alpha adrenergic antagonists are "noncompetitive, long-acting" and "competitive, short-acting." They differ chiefly in the stability of their bond with the receptor. The prototype noncompetitive, long-acting alpha antagonist is phenoxybenzamine (Dibenzyline). The prototype competitive, short-acting antagonist is prazosin (Minipress). Prazosin also is the prototype for all alpha adrenergic antagonists. Phentolamine (Regitine) is an important nonselective alpha antagonist because of its effects in reversing tissue necrosis caused by catecholamine infiltration.

Beta adrenergic antagonists are more commonly referred to as beta-blockers. Propranolol (Inderal) is the prototype beta-blocker. It is a nonselective antagonist, which means that it blocks both β₁ and β₂ receptors. It is used to treat tachycardia, hypertension, and angina, all results of β₁ blockade. Because it is nonselective, it also has the side effects of β₂ blockade—bronchoconstriction and inhibited glycogenolysis. Propranolol was the first clinically employed beta-blocker, but its use has declined since the development of more selective β₁ antagonists. The prototype of these cardioselective beta-blockers is metoprolol (Lopressor). At normal doses, metoprolol is selective for only β₁ receptors; therefore, it does not cause propranolol's problematic side effects for asthmatics and diabetics. Atenolol (Tenormin) is another commonly used cardioselective beta-blocker.

SKELETAL MUSCLE RELAXANTS   Skeletal muscle relaxants are used to treat muscle spasm from injury and muscle spasticity from CNS injuries or diseases such as multiple sclerosis. Treatment can involve centrally acting agents or direct-acting agents.

The centrally acting muscle relaxants' mechanism is not clear, but it appears to be associated with general sedation. The prototype centrally acting skeletal muscle relaxant is baclofen (Lioresal), which is indicated in the treatment of spasticity. Although baclofen is effective in the treatment of muscle spasticity, it is generally ineffective in muscle spasm. Several drugs are effective in treating muscle spasm, including cyclobenzaprine (Flexeril) and carisoprodol (Soma).

The prototype of the direct-acting muscle relaxants is dantrolene (Dantrium). Unlike the centrally acting agents, dantrolene's mechanism is well understood. It decreases the release of calcium from the sarcoplasmic reticulum in response to action potentials propagated from the neuromuscular junction. This calcium is required for the cross-bridge binding of the actin and myosin filaments in the muscle fibers responsible for contraction. Dantrolene is indicated for treating the spasticity associated with multiple sclerosis and cerebral palsy. It is also indicated for treating malignant hyperthermia, which is seen, on rare occasion, with some anesthetics and succinylcholine. This hyperthermia results from muscular contractions. Because dantrolene decreases these contractions, the heat that they generate also decreases. Dantrolene is not effective in treating muscle spasm.

Drugs Used to Affect the Cardiovascular System

Cardiovascular drugs have traditionally comprised one of the largest parts of the paramedic's pharmacological "toolbox." Although this is changing with the expansion of paramedic practice, cardiovascular care (and agents used in that care) remains an important and integral part of a paramedic's knowledge base.

Cardiovascular Physiology Review

To understand cardiovascular pharmacology, you must first understand how electrical conduction and mechanical contraction work together to produce an organized and effective pumping action. In this section, we briefly review the anatomy and physiology of the heart and then discuss the generation of electrical impulses and the creation of arrhythmias. Then we discuss how each classification acts on arrhythmias.

The heart is essentially a two-sided pump. The right side is a low-pressure pump responsible for pulmonary circulation, and the left side is a high-pressure pump responsible for systemic circulation. The human heart has four chambers: two atria and two ventricles. The atria receive blood from the pulmonary and systemic circulation and pass it on to the ventricles, where most of the pumping pressure originates (Figure 13-23). Because the left side of the heart must generate substantially higher pressures than the right, the left ventricle's muscular wall is much larger than those of the other chambers. The atria accept blood and allow it to pour passively into the ventricles. Just before the ventricles contract, the atria contract to "top off" the volume of blood in the ventricles. After this atrial "kick" fills the ventricles, they contract, forcing blood out of the heart. The myocardial muscle contraction depends on three factors: (1) electrical stimulation from the conduction system, (2) adequate amounts of ATP (energy), and (3) adequate amounts of the calcium ion. ATP and calcium are both needed for the thin and thick filaments to combine and shorten the muscle. To pump blood effectively, the entire heart must contract in a precise sequence. Both atria contract at the same time from the top down (toward the AV valves). A slight delay allows the ventricles to fill completely with blood, and then both ventricles contract simultaneously from the bottom up (toward the semilunar valves). This entire cycle must repeat itself continually.

Impulse Generation and Conduction

The key to the precise cardiac cycle is the electrical conduction system (Figure 13-24). This system is composed of specialized cardiac tissue that generates electrical impulses and conducts them rapidly throughout the heart to

ensure that the chambers contract in proper sequence. The sinoatrial (SA) node is the heart's dominant pacemaker. It spontaneously generates electrical impulses (action potentials) that are propagated through intraatrial pathways to the atrioventricular (AV) node, where conduction is

Superior vena cava

Pulmonary trunk

Left pulmonary arteries

Left pulmonary veins

Right atrium

Left ventricle

Right ventricle

Inferior vena cava

FIGURE 13-23 Blood flow through the heart.

SA node

atrial pathways

AV node

AV junction

Bundle of His

Interventricular septum

Right bundle branch

Left bundle branch

Purkinje fibers

Purkinje network

FIGURE 13-24 Cardiac conductive system.

delayed momentarily. This delay gives the ventricles time to fill completely. The impulse then travels from the AV node throughout the ventricles via the bundle of His and the Purkinje network.

All myocardial tissue, both contractile and conductive, has the ability to self-generate electrical impulses (automaticity) and to propagate those impulses to surrounding tissue. It does this through the movement of ions across the cell membrane. At rest (when not stimulated), the cell membrane is polarized with a slight electrical charge. This charge is present because there are more positive ions out-

side the cell than inside, resulting in a slight negative charge on the inside. The primary ions involved are sodium (Na^+) on the outside of the cell and potassium (K^+) on the inside. Calcium (Ca^{++}), which is responsible for muscle contraction, is present in storage vesicles surrounding the cell. These vesicles are called the *sarcoplasmic reticulum*. The cell membrane is said to depolarize when this charge is eliminated or reversed. When an impulse is generated and conducted to the muscle cells, the process of depolarization and repolarization begins. Figure 13-25 depicts the sequence of ion movements in the depolarization and repolarization of

Action potential of cardiac contractile (muscle) tissue depends upon activation of fast sodium channels (opening the gates) via stimulus from pacing cells.

Action potential of cardiac pacing cells slows influx of Ca^{++} (leaking) and, to a lesser extent, Na^+ is responsible for automaticity or spontaneous depolarization. Class IV antiarrhythmics inhibit these calcium channels and decrease heart rate.

FIGURE 13-25 Ion movements in the depolarization and repolarization of slow and fast potentials.

both slow and fast potentials. Fast potentials occur in cardiac muscle tissue, as well as in the ventricular conduction system; slow potentials occur in the pacemaker cells of the SA and AV nodes.

Cyclic activity in the fast potentials has five phases. Phase 0, which represents depolarization, results from a rapid influx of Na^+ ions into the cell. This makes the inside of the cell more positive than the outside and is normally caused by the arrival of an impulse generated elsewhere in the heart, such as the SA node. Sodium stops entering the cell once the inside has become positive. Phases 1 through 3 represent repolarization. In phase 1, K^+ begins to leave the cell, slowly returning the cell to its normal negative charge. Phase 2 interrupts with an influx of Ca^{++} into the cell. Remember, the muscles are using calcium inside the cell for contraction. This plateau phase delays repolarization and is important for medications that affect the strength of contraction. Phase 3 is marked by a cessation of calcium influx and the rapid efflux of potassium. Phase 4 is normally a flat stage representing the resting membrane potential. However, in pathological states, phase 4 may include a slow influx of sodium that will gradually make the inside of the cell more positive. When the interior of the cell reaches a point called its *threshold potential*, the cell will depolarize without waiting for an impulse. Many antiarrhythmics have their mechanism of action during this phase 4 depolarization.

The slow potentials, though similar to the fast ones, have several important distinctions. First, they are located in the dominant pacemakers of the heart. Second, they depolarize differently. Notice in Figure 13-25 how phase 4 normally exhibits a gradually increasing slope toward the threshold potential. Whereas sodium causes depolarization (phase 0) of the fast potentials, a gradual influx of calcium causes it in the slow potentials. The slow potentials normally undergo a gradual, phase 4 depolarization. Although we do not know the exact mechanism, this gradual depolarization clearly is responsible for the spontaneous generation of impulses in the SA and AV nodes. Although the AV node also has these slow potentials, the SA node's rate of depolarization is faster, making it the heart's dominant pacemaker.

Arrhythmia Generation

Arrhythmias are generated at various places in the heart through either abnormal impulse formation (automaticity) or abnormal conductivity. The most prevalent types of arrhythmias are tachycardia (too fast) and bradycardia (too slow). An imbalance between the sympathetic and parasympathetic nervous systems most often causes these arrhythmias. Typically, excessive parasympathetic stimulation through muscarinic receptors causes bradycardias, which are treated with anticholinergic medications. Tachycardias, however, have a variety of causes and are treated with the antiarrhythmics we discuss in this section.

As mentioned earlier, fast-potential means of depolarization dominate most of the heart, including the muscle cells and the ventricular conduction system. This process normally does not include a phase 4 depolarization; rather, depolarization most often happens in response to an impulse generated in the SA node and propagated to the cell. In pathological conditions such as ischemia, myocardial infarction, and excessive sympathetic stimulation, these tissues will develop phase 4 depolarization and generate an impulse abnormally. This abnormal impulse will then be propagated throughout the heart. These are considered ectopic foci, meaning the focus for the electrical impulse generation originated somewhere other than where it normally should.

Another cause of both abnormal beats and abnormal rhythms is abnormal conduction. Figure 13-26 shows how an irregularity in the conduction system can generate arrhythmias. The inverted Y in that diagram represents the Purkinje network attaching to a single muscle fiber (represented by the horizontal bar under the Y). Impulses normally travel down both legs of the Y and begin depolarizing the muscle tissue. The muscle tissue depolarizes in both directions and meets in the middle of the Y, where it ends because the tissue is now refractory in both directions. In pathological conditions, a section of one of the Purkinje fibers has what amounts to a one-way valve that allows impulses to travel in only one direction. The impulse travels down the good leg and depolarizes the muscle fiber, which then propagates the impulse in both directions, unhindered by a refractory period in the opposing direction. Then the impulse will travel up the other leg of the Y, through the one-way valve. If the tissue of the other leg is no longer in the absolute refractory phase, the impulse will continue back down the first leg. This can create either an early beat or, if circumstances are just right, a very rapid reentrant rhythm (a so-called circus rhythm).

Classes of Cardiovascular Drugs

The drugs used to treat cardiovascular disease generally fall into the two broad functional classifications of antiarrhythmics, also called antidysrhythmics, and antihypertensives.

Antiarrhythmics

Antiarrhythmic drugs are used to treat and prevent abnormal cardiac rhythms. Table 13-20 describes the pharmacological classes of antiarrhythmics. Although

CONTENT REVIEW
➤ Antiarrhythmics
Antiarrhythmics are routinely classified in the Vaughn-Williams and Singh Classification System.
- I: Na^+ channel blockers
  - 1A
  - 1B
  - 1C
- II: Beta-blockers
- III: K^+ channel blockers
- IV: Miscellaneous Ca^{++} channel blockers
- V: Miscellaneous

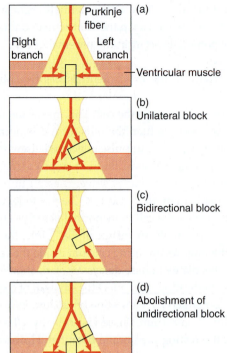

FIGURE 13-26 Reentrant pathways.

these medications are useful in treating arrhythmias, they can also cause them or deterioration in existing rhythms when used inappropriately (Table 13-21).

SODIUM CHANNEL BLOCKERS (CLASS I) All the medications in this general class affect the sodium influx in phases 0 and 4 of fast potentials. This slows the propagation of impulses down the specialized conduction system of the atria and ventricles, although it does not affect the SA or AV node.

Class IA drugs include quinidine (Quinidex), procainamide (Pronestyl), and disopyramide (Norpace). In addition to slowing conduction, these drugs also decrease the repolarization rate. This widens the QRS complex and prolongs the QT interval. Although quinidine is usually

considered the prototype for this class, we will use procainamide here because it is administered more frequently in emergency medicine. Procainamide is indicated in the treatment of atrial fibrillation with rapid ventricular response and ventricular arrhythmias. Quinidine has a similar mechanism of action, but it also has anticholinergic properties that may induce unintended tachycardias.

Class IB drugs include lidocaine (Xylocaine), phenytoin (Dilantin), tocainide (Tonocard), and mexiletine (Mexitil). Unlike Class IA drugs, Class IB drugs increase the rate of repolarization. They also reduce automaticity in ventricular cells, which makes them effective in treating rhythms originating from ectopic ventricular foci. Several of the drugs in this class are also used for other purposes. Lidocaine, the prototype, is frequently used with epinephrine

Table 13-20 Antiarrhythmic Classifications and Examples

General Action	Class	Prototype	ECG Effects
Sodium channel blockers	IA	Quinidine, procainamide*, disopyramide	Widened QRS, prolonged QT
	IB	Lidocaine*, phenytoin, tocainide, mexiletine	Widened QRS, prolonged QT
	IC	Flecainide*, propafenone	Prolonged PR, widened QRS
	I (Miscellaneous)	Moricizine*	Prolonged PR, widened QRS
Beta-blockers	II	Propranolol*, acebutolol, esmolol	Prolonged PR, bradycardias
Potassium channel blockers	III	Bretylium*, amiodarone	Prolonged QT
Calcium channel blockers	IV	Verapamil*, diltiazem	Prolonged PR, bradycardias
Miscellaneous		Adenosine, digoxin	Prolonged PR, bradycardias

* Prototype.

Table 13-21 Antiarrhythmics

Name	Classification	Action	Indications	Contraindications	Doses	Routes	Adverse Effects	Other
Amiodarone *Cordarone*	Class III antiarrhythmic	Prolongs action potential and duration in cardiac tissues through sodium, potassium, and calcium channels; blocks α and β adrenergic receptors.	May be considered for: • Ventricular tachycardia • Ventricular fibrillation that is unresponsive to CPR, defibrillation, and vasopressor therapy	• Breastfeeding • Bradycardia • High-grade heart block • Hypersensitivity to the drug	150–300 mg	IV	• Hypotension • Bradycardia • Prolonged PR, QRS, and QT	• Constant ECG monitoring • Now first-line agent in ventricular fibrillation and tachycardia
Lidocaine *Xylocaine*	Class Ib antiarrhythmic; local anesthetic	Amide-type local anesthetic; slows depolarization and automaticity	May be considered for: • Ventricular tachycardia • Ventricular fibrillation that is unresponsive to CPR, defibrillation, and vasopressor therapy • Local anesthetic	• Should not be administered to patients receiving IV calcium channel blockers	1.0–1.5 mg/kg	IV	• Drowsiness • Slurred speech • Confusion • Seizures • Hypotension	• Use with caution when administered with other antiarrhythmics
Procainamide *Pronestyl*	Class Ia antiarrhythmic; local anesthetic	Ester-type local anesthetic; reduces automaticity and AV conduction	• Ventricular tachycardia with pulse • Pre-excited atrial fibrillation	• Should not be administered to patients receiving IV calcium channel blockers	20–50 mg/min	IV	• Drowsiness • Slurred speech • Confusion • Seizures • Hypotension	• Carefully monitor ECG (QRS duration) during administration
Phenytoin *Dilantin*	Class Ib antiarrhythmic; anticonvulsant	Depresses automaticity and AV conduction; reduces voltage and spread of electrical discharges in motor cortex	• Life-threatening arrhythmias from digitalis toxicity • Seizures	• Bradycardia • High-grade heart block • Hypersensitivity to the drug	15–18 mg/kg	IV	• Drowsiness • Dizziness • Headache • Hypotension • Arrhythmias • Nausea • Vomiting	• Fosphenytoin is preferred for seizure management
Adenosine *Adenocard*	Nucleoside	Slows AV conduction; short half-life	• Supraventricular tachyarrhythmias	• Atrial fibrillation • *Torsades des pointes* • Atrial fibrillation	6 mg	IV	• Facial flushing • Headache • Chest pain • Nausea	• Should be given by rapid IV push followed by saline bolus • Arrhythmias common following administration

(Continued)

Table 13-21 Antiarrhythmics *(Continued)*

Name	Classification	Action	Indications	Contraindications	Doses	Routes	Adverse Effects	Other
Esmolol *Brevibloc*	Class II antiarrhythmic; beta blocker	Slows heart rate through selective blockade of β_1 receptors; short half-life	• Tachycardia	• Asthma • Heart block • Bradycardia • Cardiogenic shock	50–100 mcg/kg/min	IV	• Bradycardia • Hypotension • Congestive heart failure • Lethargy	• Hypotension is common but dose related • Should not be administered to patients receiving IV calcium channel blockers
Labetalol *Trandate, Normodyne*	Class II antiarrhythmic; beta blocker	Lowers blood pressure through nonselective blockade of β receptors (and limited blockade of α_2 receptors)	• Hypertensive emergency	• Asthma • Heart block • Bradycardia • Cardiogenic shock	10–20 mg	IV, PO	• Bradycardia • Hypotension • Congestive heart failure • Lethargy	• Should not be administered to patients receiving IV calcium channel blockers
Dittiazem *Cardizem*	Class IV antiarrhythmic; calcium channel blocker	Lowers blood pressure by relaxing vascular smooth muscle; slows AV conduction	• Rapid ventricular rate associated with atrial fibrillation • Stable narrow-complex tachyarrhythmias	• Hypotension • Congestive heart failure • Cardiogenic shock • Wide-complex ventricular tachycardia	15–20 mg	IV	• Nausea • Vomiting • Dizziness • Headache • Hypotension	• Can be given as IV bolus or IV infusion • Calcium chloride can reverse some of the untoward effects
Magnesium Sulfate	Mineral/electrolyte	Physiologic calcium-channel blocker; bronchodilator	• *Torsades des pointes* • Asthma • Hypertensive disorders of pregnancy	• High-degree heart blocks • Shock • Dialysis • Hypocalcemia • Ventricular fibrillation/pulseless ventricular tachycardia in adult patients	1–2 g	IV	• Flushing • Sweating • Bradycardia • Respiratory depression • Hypothermia	• Can cause cardiac conduction problems in conjunction with digitalis

as a local anesthetic, and phenytoin (Dilantin) is most commonly used as an antiseizure medication. Lidocaine was once the drug of choice for treating ventricular tachycardia and ventricular fibrillation. Prophylactic administration of lidocaine was once thought to benefit patients with myocardial infarction. Recent studies, however, have shown it to be relatively ineffective. When given in overdose, lidocaine has significant CNS side effects, including tinnitus, confusion, and convulsions.

Class IC drugs include flecainide (Tambocor) and propafenone (Rythmol). They decrease conduction velocity through the atria and ventricles, as well as through the bundle of His and the Purkinje network. Like the Class IA drugs, they delay ventricular repolarization. Both these medications, which are administered orally, are given to prevent recurrence of ventricular arrhythmias, but both also have proarrhythmic properties; that is, they are likely to cause arrhythmias as well as treat them. They also depress myocardial contractility and are therefore reserved for potentially lethal ventricular arrhythmias that do not respond to any other conventional therapy.

Moricizine (Ethmozine) is similar to the other Class I drugs but has additional properties that exclude it from the other subclasses. Like the other drugs in this class, it blocks sodium influx during fast potential depolarization, thereby decreasing conduction velocity, but it can also depress myocardial contractility. Like the Class IC drugs, it is reserved for the treatment of ventricular arrhythmias refractory to other conventional therapy.

BETA-BLOCKERS (CLASS II)   The drugs in this class, propranolol (Inderal), acebutolol (Sectral), and esmolol (Brevibloc), are all beta adrenergic antagonists. Propranolol is nonselective, whereas acebutolol and esmolol are both selective for the β_1 receptors in the heart. (The mechanism of action at the β_1 receptor is described in the section on adrenergic antagonists.) Of the many beta-blockers, these are the only ones approved for the treatment of arrhythmias. They are indicated in the treatment of tachycardias resulting from excessive sympathetic stimulation. The β_1 receptor in the heart is attached to the calcium channels. Blocking the β_1 receptors thus blocks the calcium channel and prevents the gradual influx of calcium in phase 0 of the slow potential. As a result, the effects of beta-blocker therapy on arrhythmias are almost identical to those of calcium channel blockers. Propranolol is the prototype Class II drug. Because it is nonselective, it also blocks the effect of β_2 receptors, which leads to many of its side effects. Other side effects are consistent with those discussed in the section on drugs that affect the sympathetic nervous system.

POTASSIUM CHANNEL BLOCKERS (CLASS III)   Potassium channel-blocking drugs are also known as antiadrenergic medications because of their complex actions on

sympathetic terminals. They include bretylium (Bretylol) and amiodarone (Cordarone); bretylium is the prototype. Their mechanism of action is on the potassium channels in the fast potentials. By blocking the efflux of potassium, bretylium prolongs repolarization and the effective refractory period. It was indicated in the treatment of ventricular fibrillation and refractory ventricular tachycardia. It causes an initial release of norepinephrine at the sympathetic end terminals, followed by an inhibition of that neurotransmitter's release. This delayed repolarization prolongs the QT interval; consequently, bretylium's primary and frequent side effect is hypotension. It is now rarely used.[22]

CALCIUM CHANNEL BLOCKERS (CLASS IV)   Calcium channel blockers' effect on the heart is almost identical to that of beta-blockers. They decrease SA and AV node automaticity, but most of their usefulness arises from decreasing conductivity through the AV node. They effectively slow the ventricular conduction of atrial fibrillation and flutter, and they can terminate supraventricular tachycardias originating from a reentrant circuit. Verapamil (Calan) and diltiazem (Cardizem) are the only two calcium channel blockers that affect the heart. Verapamil is the prototype. Their chief side effect is hypotension and bradycardia. The section on antihypertensives discusses calcium channel blockers in more detail.

MISCELLANEOUS ANTIARRHYTHMICS   Adenosine (Adenocard) and digoxin (Lanoxin) are both effective antiarrhythmics. Magnesium is the drug of choice in *torsades de pointes,* a type of polymorphic ventricular tachycardia. We briefly discuss each here.

Adenosine does not fit any of the previous categories. It is an endogenous nucleoside with a very short half-life (about 10 seconds). It acts on both potassium and calcium channels, increasing potassium efflux and inhibiting calcium influx. This results in a hyperpolarization that effectively slows the conduction of slow potentials, such as those found in the SA and AV nodes. It has little effect on the fast potentials in the ventricles and is not particularly effective on ventricular tachycardias or atrial fibrillation or flutter. Because of its short half-life, its side effects are short lived, but they can be alarming. They include facial flushing, shortness of breath, chest pain, and marked bradycardias. Adenosine must be given as a rapid IV push, as the drug is metabolized rapidly. Doses should be increased in patients taking adenosine blockers such as aminophylline or caffeine. They should be decreased in patients taking adenosine uptake inhibitors such as dipyridamole (Persantine) and carbamazepine (Tegretol).

Digoxin (Lanoxin) is a paradoxical drug. Its many effects on the heart make it both an effective antiarrhythmic and a potent proarrhythmic (generator of arrhythmias). Although we do not clearly understand its specific actions on the heart's electrical activity, we do understand its effects. Digoxin decreases the intrinsic firing rate in the SA node, whereas it decreases conduction velocity in the AV node. Both these effects are due to its increasing the strength of the parasympathetic effects on the heart. In the Purkinje fibers and ventricular myocardial cells, it decreases the effective refractory period and increases automaticity, both of which may explain its ability to increase ventricular arrhythmias. To compound this, by depressing SA node activity, digoxin makes ectopic ventricular beats more likely to assume the pacing activity of the heart. Its side effects include bradycardias, AV blocks, postventricular contractions (PVCs), ventricular tachycardia, ventricular fibrillation, and atrial fibrillation. Actually, there are few arrhythmias that digoxin does not produce. In addition, digoxin has a very narrow therapeutic index, meaning that it is difficult to find a patient's effective dose without producing side effects. Digoxin also increases cardiac contractility. It is indicated for atrial fibrillation with rapid ventricular conduction and chronic treatment of congestive heart failure.

Magnesium is the drug of choice in *torsades de pointes,* a polymorphic ventricular tachycardia, and in other ventricular arrhythmias refractory to other therapy. Its mechanism of action is not known, but it may act on the sodium or potassium channels or on $Na^+K^+ATPase$.

Antihypertensives

Hypertension affects more than 50 million people in the United States alone and is a major contributor to coronary artery disease, stroke, and blindness. Fortunately, available drugs can effectively manage blood pressure with limited side effects in the vast majority of patients. Multiple studies have shown conclusively that controlling blood pressure decreases both morbidity and mortality.

Blood pressure is the force of blood against the arteries' walls as the heart contracts and relaxes. It is equal to cardiac output times the peripheral vascular resistance:

Blood pressure = Cardiac output × Peripheral vascular resistance

Cardiac output is equal to the heart rate times the stroke volume:

Cardiac output = Heart rate × Stroke volume

Antihypertensive agents can manipulate each of these factors. The primary determinant of peripheral vascular resistance is the diameter of peripheral arterioles, which are affected by α_1 receptors. Heart rate is affected by both muscarinic receptors of the parasympathetic nervous system and β_1 receptors of the sympathetic nervous system; however, hypertension control typically manipulates only β_1 receptors. Stroke volume is affected by contractility and volume. Recall that Starling's law says that preload and stroke volume are proportionate; that is, as preload

increases, stroke volume increases (up to a point), and as preload decreases, stroke volume decreases. Drugs that affect blood volume control hypertension by manipulating preload.

Several pharmacological classes of medications are used to control blood pressure. The major approaches to dealing with hypertension are diuretics, beta-blockers and other antiadrenergic drugs, angiotensin-converting enzyme (ACE) inhibitors, calcium channel blockers, and direct vasodilators. Of these, diuretics and beta-blockers are the most frequently prescribed, and they are effective in many patients. The remaining agents are used when diuretics or beta-blockers are contraindicated or when those approaches are not effective, although ACE inhibitors are gaining increasing popularity. Often, physicians must prescribe multiple drugs to manage hypertension effectively. In these cases, they will pick one drug from two or more classes that complement each other. For example, a physician might prescribe a diuretic with a beta-blocker. [23]

> **CONTENT REVIEW**
>
> ➤ Pharmacological Classes of Antihypertensives
> - Diuretics
> - Beta-blockers and antiadrenergic drugs
> - ACE inhibitors
> - Calcium channel blockers
> - Direct vasodilators

DIURETICS **Diuretics** reduce circulating blood volume by increasing the amount of urine. This reduces preload to the heart, which, in turn, reduces cardiac output. The main categories of diuretics include loop diuretics (high-ceiling diuretics), thiazides, and potassium-sparing diuretics. They all affect the reabsorption of sodium and chloride and create an osmotic gradient that decreases the reabsorption of water. These classes differ according to which area of the nephron they affect. In general, the earlier in the nephron the drug works, the more sodium and water will be affected. Almost all electrolytes and other small particles in the blood are filtered through the glomerulus. Most sodium and water (approximately 65 percent) are reabsorbed in the proximal convoluted tubule. Another 20 percent are reabsorbed in the thick portion of the ascending loop of Henle, whereas only about 1 to 5 percent are recaptured in the distal convoluted tubule and collecting duct. Therefore, a drug that decreases sodium reabsorption in the proximal convoluted tubule will cause the kidneys to excrete more water than will a drug that works on the distal convoluted tubule.

Loop diuretics profoundly affect circulating blood volume. In fact, they decrease blood volume so well that they are typically considered excessive for treating moderate hypertension. They are, however, one of the primary tools in treating left ventricular heart failure (congestive heart failure). They are used for hypertension typically because other diuretics have failed. Furosemide (Lasix) is the prototype of this class. Furosemide blocks sodium reabsorption in the thick portion of the ascending loop of Henle (hence, the name *loop diuretic*). In doing so, it decreases the pull of water from the tubule and into the capillary bed, thus decreasing fluid volume. Furosemide's main side effects are hyponatremia, hypovolemia, hypokalemia, and dehydration. Because the decrease in volume is most noticeable as decreased preload, orthostatic hypotension is a problem. Reflex tachycardia may also occur as the baroreceptors detect a decreased blood pressure and attempt to compensate by increasing heart rate. This happens in individuals with hypertension because the homeostatic "thermostat" has been set too high. In other words, the body believes that what is actually hypertension is normal and tries to maintain a higher blood pressure than is healthy. This reflex tachycardia is frequently treated with concurrent administration of a loop diuretic with a β_1 blocker. Hypokalemia is frequently treated by increasing dietary potassium intake (bananas are rich in potassium) or by prescribing potassium supplements. An unexplained side effect of loop diuretics is ototoxicity (tinnitus and deafness). Administering loop diuretics slowly can decrease ototoxicity.

Thiazides have a mechanism similar to loop diuretics. The main difference is that the thiazides' mechanism affects the early part of the distal convoluted tubules and therefore cannot block as much sodium from reabsorption. Thiazides are often the drugs of choice in hypertension treatment because they can decrease fluid volume sufficiently to prevent hypertension but not so much that they promote hypotension. The prototype thiazide is hydrochlorothiazide (HydroDIURIL). This class has essentially the same side effects as loop diuretics. One important distinction is that thiazides depend on the glomerular filtration rate, whereas loop diuretics do not. Thus, loop diuretics may be preferred for patients with renal disease.

Potassium-sparing diuretics have a slightly different mechanism from other diuretics. Although they still affect sodium absorption, they do so by inhibiting either the effects of aldosterone on the distal tubules (as does spironolactone) or the specific sodium–potassium exchange mechanism (as does triamterene). Acting so late in the nephritic loop, these agents are not very potent diuretics. In fact, they are rarely used alone but instead are typically administered in conjunction with either a loop diuretic or a thiazide diuretic. They are useful as adjuncts to other diuretics because they not only decrease sodium reabsorption (although in small volumes) but also increase potassium reabsorption. This helps to limit the other diuretics' hypokalemic effects. Spironolactone (Aldactone) is the prototype potassium-sparing diuretic.

Though not used in the treatment of hypertension, osmotic diuretics are important because they alter the reabsorption of water in the proximal convoluted tubule. To do this, they use an osmotically large sugar molecule that is freely filtered through the glomerulus and pulls water after it. Mannitol (Osmitrol), the prototype osmotic diuretic, is used to treat increased intracranial and intraocular pressure.

ADRENERGIC INHIBITING AGENTS Inhibiting the effects of adrenergic stimulation can also control hypertension. Several broad mechanisms accomplish this: beta adrenergic antagonism, centrally acting alpha adrenergic antagonism, adrenergic neuron blockade, α_1 blockade, and alpha/beta blockade.

Beta Adrenergic Antagonists From Table 13-17 in our earlier discussion of β_1 blockers, you will recall that most β_1 receptors are in the heart but some also exist in the juxtaglomerular cells of the kidney. Selective β_1 blockade is useful in treating hypertension for several reasons. It decreases contractility, thereby directly decreasing cardiac output. It also reduces reflex tachycardia by inhibiting sympathetically induced compensatory increases in heart rate. Finally, it represses renin release from the kidneys, which, in turn, inhibits the vasoconstriction activated by the renin–angiotensin–aldosterone system. The prototype selective β_1 blocker is metoprolol (Lopressor); the prototype nonselective beta-blocker is propranolol (Inderal). The section on β_1 blockers discussed these agents' side effects.

Centrally Acting Adrenergic Inhibitors Centrally acting adrenergic inhibitors reduce hypertension by inhibiting CNS stimulation of adrenergic receptors. In effect, they are CNS α_2 agonists. Recall that α_2 receptors are located on the presynaptic end terminals in the sympathetic nervous system. When stimulated, they inhibit the release of norepinephrine to counterbalance sympathetic stimulation. By increasing the stimulation of α_2 receptors in the section of the CNS responsible for cardiovascular regulation, centrally acting adrenergic inhibitors decrease the sympathetic stimulation of both α_1 and β_2 receptors. The net effect is to decrease heart rate and contractility by decreasing release of norepinephrine at β_1 receptors and to promote vasodilation by decreasing norepinephrine release at α_1 receptors at vascular smooth muscle. The prototype drug in this category is clonidine (Catapres). Although it does have some side effects—notably, drowsiness and dry mouth—clonidine is a relatively safe and frequently prescribed antihypertensive agent. Methyldopa (Aldomet) is another centrally acting antihypertensive with a mechanism similar to clonidine.

Peripheral Adrenergic Neuron Blocking Agents Like the centrally acting adrenergic inhibitors, peripheral adrenergic neuron blocking agents work indirectly to decrease stimulation of adrenergic receptors. They do this by decreasing the amount of norepinephrine released from sympathetic presynaptic terminals. These agents are no longer commonly used.

The prototype of this class is reserpine (Serpalan). Reserpine has two actions that decrease the amount of norepinephrine released. First, it decreases the synthesis of norepinephrine. Second, it exposes norepinephrine in the terminal vesicles to monoamine oxidase, an enzyme that destroys it. This decreases stimulation of α_1 receptors, resulting in peripheral vasodilation, and of β_1 receptors, resulting in decreased heart rate and contractility. The decreased peripheral vascular resistance and cardiac output in turn lower blood pressure.

Reserpine also decreases synthesis of several CNS neurotransmitters (serotonin and other catecholamines). This causes reserpine's primary adverse effect, depression. Reserpine, therefore, is not frequently used as an antihypertensive. Additional side effects include gastrointestinal cramps and increased stomach acid production. Other drugs with similar actions include guanethidine (Ismeline) and guanadrel (Hylorel).

Alpha$_1$ Antagonists This chapter's section on drugs affecting the sympathetic nervous system discusses the α_1 receptor antagonists in detail. Only their specific action will be repeated here. The prototype selective α_1 antagonist is prazosin (Minipress). It decreases blood pressure by competitively blocking the alpha$_1$ receptors, thereby inhibiting the sympathetically mediated increases in peripheral vascular resistance. By causing the arterioles to dilate, prazosin directly decreases afterload. By causing the venules to dilate, it promotes venous pooling, which decreases preload. The decreased afterload and preload help to lower blood pressure. Terazosin (Hytrin) is another drug with similar properties.

Combined Alpha/Beta Antagonists Labetalol (Normodyne) and carvedilol (Coreg) competitively bind with both α_1 and β_1 receptors, increasing their antihypertensive actions. Hypertension is treated by decreasing β_1-mediated vasoconstriction, which, again, decreases both preload and afterload. Beta$_1$ blockade decreases heart rate, contractility, and renin release from kidneys. By blocking the release of renin, which promotes vasoconstriction, these agents decrease peripheral vascular resistance even further. Labetalol is commonly used to treat hypertensive crisis and is rapidly replacing the use of sublingual nifedipine (Procardia) for this purpose.

ANGIOTENSIN-CONVERTING ENZYME (ACE) INHIBITORS Agents in this class interrupt the renin–angiotensin–aldosterone system (RAAS) by preventing the conversion of angiotensin I to angiotensin II. Angiotensin II is one of the most potent vasoconstrictors yet discovered. By decreasing the amount of circulating angiotensin II, peripheral vascular resistance can be decreased, which leads to a decrease in blood pressure.

The juxtaglomerular apparatus in the kidneys releases renin in response to decreases in blood volume, sodium concentration, and blood pressure. Renin acts as an enzyme to convert the inactive protein angiotensinogen into angiotensin I. Neither angiotensinogen nor angiotensin I has much pharmaceutical effect, but angiotensin-converting enzyme (ACE) almost immediately converts angiotensin I in the blood into angiotensin II. (ACE is found in the lumen of almost all vessels and is found in the lungs in very high concentrations.) Angiotensin II causes both systemic and local vasoconstriction, with more pronounced effects on arterioles than on venules. It also lessens water loss by decreasing renal filtration secondary to renal vasoconstriction. Finally, angiotensin II also increases the release of aldosterone, a corticosteroid produced in the adrenal cortex. Aldosterone, in turn, increases sodium and water reabsorption in the distal convoluted tubule of the nephrons (Figure 13-27).

ACE inhibitors are very effective in treating hypertension and have also seen success in managing heart failure and renal failure. ACE inhibitors block the conversion of angiotensin I to angiotensin II, thereby providing a host of beneficial effects for patients with hypertension. These include a rapid decrease in arteriolar constriction, which lowers peripheral vascular resistance and afterload. Although it does cause some dilation of the venules, this effect is limited. Because of the limited decrease in preload, orthostatic hypotension, common in other antihypertensives, is not a significant concern with ACE inhibitors. These agents also appear to be effective in preventing some of the untoward structural changes in the heart and blood vessels that angiotensin II causes over time.

The prototype ACE inhibitor is captopril (Capoten). Captopril acts like all ACE inhibitors to prevent hypertension. Its main advantage is the absence of side effects common to other antihypertensives. It does not interfere with beta receptors, so it does not decrease the ability to exercise or respond to hemorrhage. It does not cause potassium loss like many diuretics, and it does not cause depression or drowsiness. Because it has no effect on sexual desire or performance, it is much more attractive to many patients who might not comply with other medications. Other common ACE inhibitors include enalapril (Vasotec), benazepril (Lotensin), and lisinopril (Zestril). These medications are all taken orally. For intravenous use in hypertensive crisis, enalaprilat (Vasotec I.V.) is available.

The most dangerous side effect of ACE inhibitors is pronounced hypotension after the first dose. This can be minimized by reducing initial doses, and it does not reoccur. The main adverse effects of continual use are a persistent cough and angioedema.

Renin-Angiotensin-Aldosterone System

FIGURE 13-27 The renin–angiotensin–aldosterone system.

ANGIOTENSIN II RECEPTOR ANTAGONISTS This recently developed classification of antihypertensive drugs also acts on the renin–angiotensin–aldosterone system. Angiotensin II receptor antagonists achieve the same effects as the ACE inhibitors without the side effects of cough or angioedema. The prototype of this new class is losartan (Cozaar).

CALCIUM CHANNEL BLOCKING AGENTS We have already discussed two calcium channel blockers, verapamil and diltiazem, in the section on antiarrhythmics. Another structural subclass of calcium channel blockers is the dihydropyridines. The prototype dihydropyridine is nifedipine (Procardia, Adalat). Nifedipine, as well as the other members of the dihydropyridines, differs from verapamil and diltiazem in that it does not affect the calcium channels of the heart at therapeutic doses. Rather, it acts only on the vascular smooth muscle of the arterioles. These agents act by blocking the calcium channels in the arterioles. Calcium, which is required for muscle contraction, is released from the sarcoplasmic reticulum on activation by an action potential. When it enters the muscle cell through calcium channels, muscle contraction ensues. Blocking the calcium channels prevents the arterioles' smooth muscle from contracting and therefore dilates these vessels. When this occurs, peripheral vascular resistance decreases, and blood pressure falls as a result of lower afterload. Because nifedipine has little effect on veins, it does not cause a corresponding drop in preload and consequently avoids orthostatic hypotension. Although nifedipine does not affect the cardiac electrical conduction system, it is effective in dilating the coronary arteries and arterioles and thereby helps to increase coronary perfusion. The primary indications for nifedipine are angina pectoris and chronic treatment of hypertension. Its primary side effects include reflex tachycardia (responding to baroreceptor response to decreased blood pressure), facial flushing, dizziness, headache, and peripheral edema. It has been used commonly for the emergent reduction of blood pressure in the field; however, labetalol and nicardipine are replacing it.

DIRECT VASODILATORS We have already discussed several drugs that cause vasodilation. Two specific classes of vasodilators are those that dilate arterioles and those that dilate both arterioles and veins. All these drugs are used to decrease blood pressure.

Selective dilation of arterioles causes a decrease in peripheral vascular resistance or afterload. This is the resistance that the heart must overcome to eject blood. Decreasing peripheral vascular resistance lowers blood pressure, increases cardiac output, and reduces cardiac workload. However, dilating the veins increases capacitance and decreases preload, the amount of blood in the heart prior to contraction. Starling's law tells us that as preload increases, so do stroke volume and cardiac output (up to a point). By decreasing preload, venodilators decrease both blood pressure and cardiac output.

Hydralazine (Apresoline) is the prototype for the selective arteriole dilators. It is effective in decreasing peripheral vascular resistance and afterload and thus lowering blood pressure. Its primary side effects are reflex tachycardia and increased blood volume. Both occur as a compensatory mechanism to lowered blood pressure, and both have the effect of increasing cardiac workload. As a result, hydralazine is almost always prescribed in conjunction with a beta-blocker and a diuretic. It is frequently used in the treatment of pregnancy-induced hypertension.

Minoxidil (Loniten) is another selective arteriole dilator with properties similar to those of hydralazine. One side effect deserves comment. It produces hypertrichosis (excessive hair growth) in about 80 percent of those taking it. Although this is particularly irritating when it occurs all over a patient's body, it can become a therapeutic effect when the drug is applied as a topical ointment. Minoxidil is marketed in this form as Rogaine for promoting hair growth in men.

Unlike hydralazine, sodium nitroprusside (Nipride) acts on both arterioles and veins. It is the fastest acting antihypertensive available and is the drug of choice in hypertensive emergencies. It is very potent and is given via controlled IV infusion. Its effects are almost immediate and end within minutes of drug cessation; therefore, blood pressure must be carefully and continuously monitored during infusion, preferably in the ICU. Sodium nitroprusside has several significant side effects. Obviously, hypotension can be a problem when this medication is not administered carefully. Because cyanide and thiocyanate are byproducts of nitroprusside metabolism, other adverse effects include cyanide poisoning and thiocyanate toxicity.

Ganglionic Blocking Agents Ganglionic blocking agents are nicotinic$_N$ antagonists. The prototype is trimethaphan (Arfonad). Because nicotinic$_N$ receptors exist at the ganglia of both the sympathetic and the parasympathetic nervous systems, competitive antagonism of these receptors turns off the entire autonomic nervous system, which is obviously not a very selective approach. When this happens, the effects on each organ system are determined by the predominant autonomic tone (the division of the ANS that normally has the greater influence on that organ). Because the arteries and veins have predominant sympathetic control, they dilate in response to trimethaphan administration. This reduces both preload and afterload, and blood pressure drops. Trimethaphan also directly affects vascular smooth muscle, causing dilation and the release of histamine, which is also a vasodilator. Mecamylamine (Inversine) is the other ganglionic blocking drug available in the United States, although it is not commonly used anymore.

Cardiac Glycosides The cardiac glycosides occur naturally in the foxglove plant. The two drugs in the class, digoxin (Lanoxin) and digitoxin (Crystodigin), are chemically related. These drugs are also known as digitalis glycosides. Digoxin is the prototype. One of the ten most frequently prescribed medications in the country, it is indicated for heart failure and some types of arrhythmias. Digoxin's mechanism of action is complex. It blocks the effects of Na$^+$K$^+$ATPase, an enzyme responsible for returning ion flow to normal levels after muscle depolarization. By interfering with this sodium–potassium pump, digoxin increases the intracellular levels of sodium. Because sodium is also involved in a reciprocal exchange with calcium, a buildup of intracellular sodium leads to a similar buildup of intracellular calcium. These elevated levels of intracellular calcium increase the strength of muscle contraction and are the basis for digoxin's primary indication. Digoxin reduces the symptoms of congestive heart failure by increasing myocardial contractility and cardiac output. This diminishes the dilation of the heart's chambers frequently seen in left heart failure because it enables the heart to effectively pump blood out of its ventricles, thus decreasing the engorgement typical of this condition. Increasing cardiac output decreases the sympathetic discharge mediated by baroreceptor reflexes, resulting in reduced afterload. Furthermore, digoxin indirectly lessens preload by increasing renal blood flow, which results in higher glomerular filtration and decreased blood volume. Digoxin also has antiarrhythmic effects, which we discuss more thoroughly in the section on antiarrhythmic medications.

Although digoxin effectively treats the symptoms of heart failure, it also is potentially dangerous. Its therapeutic index is very small, and the individual variability is large. This leads to toxicity in some individuals even though they have normal digoxin levels. Digoxin's chief adverse effects are arrhythmias. In fact, digoxin frequently induces some of the same arrhythmias it is used to treat. Other side effects include fatigue, anorexia, nausea and vomiting, and blurred vision with a yellowish haze and halos around dark objects.

Other Vasodilators and Antianginals The drugs discussed in this section have vasodilatory properties that are useful in reducing blood pressure, but they are most commonly used to treat angina. The three basic types of angina pectoris (chest pain) are stable (exertional) angina; unstable angina; and variant, or Prinzmetal's, angina. Stable and unstable angina have the same pathophysiology and differ only by causation: Stable angina occurs after exercise as a result of increased myocardial oxygen demand; unstable angina occurs without exertion. Both result from an imbalance between myocardial supply and demand. A buildup of plaque (atherosclerosis) along the walls of coronary arteries decreases these vessels' diameter and, as a result, the amount of blood flow to the heart. The same imbalance causes Prinzmetal's angina but it results from vasospasm instead of plaque buildup. The medications discussed in this section all either increase oxygen supply or decrease oxygen demand.

In addition to their previously discussed use as antihypertensives and antiarrhythmics, calcium channel blockers have a role in the treatment of angina. The three calcium channel blockers most frequently used for this purpose are verapamil (Calan, Isoptin), diltiazem (Cardizem), and nifedipine (Procardia). Recall that calcium is an integral part of both depolarization and muscle contraction. The effects of blocking its entry into the cells are twofold. All these agents directly affect vascular smooth muscle, leading to dilation of the arterioles and, to a lesser degree, of the venules. This arterial dilation decreases peripheral vascular resistance and, as a result, afterload, which in turn directly decreases the workload of the heart and myocardial oxygen demand.

Verapamil and diltiazem also reduce SA and AV node conductivity, which can decrease reflex tachycardia and arrhythmias. Nifedipine has relatively few effects on the heart and, thus, has limited antiarrhythmic properties. The calcium channel blockers are effective in all forms of angina. A primary side effect of these agents is hypotension.

Organic nitrates are potent vasodilators used to treat all forms of angina. First used clinically in 1879, nitroglycerin (Nitrostat) is the oldest of these drugs and is the category's prototype. Other agents include isosorbide (Isordil, Sorbitrate) and amyl nitrite. Nitroglycerin acts on vascular smooth muscle via a complex series of events to decrease intracellular calcium, thus causing vasodilation. Nitroglycerin primarily dilates veins rather than arterioles. This decreases preload and thus decreases myocardial workload, which is its primary antianginal effect. In Prinzmetal's angina, nitroglycerin reverses coronary artery spasm and increases oxygen supply.

Nitroglycerin is very lipid soluble, which allows it to cross membranes easily. Because of this, it is readily absorbed and can be administered via sublingual, buccal, and transdermal routes. The primary concern with nitroglycerin is orthostatic hypotension, a side effect more common in the presence of right ventricular failure. Other common side effects include headache and reflex tachycardia. Headache is frequently used as an indicator of the effectiveness of nitroglycerin, which rapidly loses its potency when exposed to light. Although orthostatic hypotension is a serious concern with the administration of nitroglycerin, this condition typically responds well to fluid infusions.[24] Table 13-22 details common nitrates.

Table 13-22 Nitrates

Name	Classification	Action	Indications	Contraindications	Doses	Routes	Adverse Effects	Other
Nitroglycerin *Nitrostat*	Nitrate	Relaxes vascular smooth muscle causing vasodilation, decreased cardiac work, and improved coronary blood flow.	• Chest pain • Congestive heart failure	• Hypotension • Increased intracranial pressure	0.4 mg	SL (tablet or spray)	• Headache • Dizziness • Weakness • Tachycardia • Hypotension	• Tablets will lose effectiveness after exposure to air. • Monitor BP closely.
Nitroglycerin paste	Nitrate	Relaxes vascular smooth muscle causing vasodilation, decreased cardiac work, and improved coronary blood flow.	• Chest pain • Congestive heart failure	• Hypotension • Increased intracranial pressure	0.5–1.0 inch	Transdermal	• Headache • Dizziness • Weakness • Tachycardia • Hypotension	• Do not get paste on your finger, as this may cause a headache. • Monitor BP closely.

Hemostatic Agents

Hemostasis is the stoppage of bleeding. It is a series of events in response to a tear in a blood vessel. Damage to the vessel's intima (innermost layer) exposes the underlying collagen and triggers a release of two naturally occurring substances, adenosine diphosphate (ADP) and thromboxane A_2 (TXA_2). Both ADP and TXA_2 stimulate the aggregation of platelets and vasoconstriction. The vasoconstriction decreases the flow of blood past the tear, thus allowing the newly "sticky" platelets to form a plug that temporarily occludes the bleeding.

Although this plug effectively halts bleeding for the short term, it must be reinforced to continue the stoppage until the tear can be permanently repaired. Stabilizing the plug requires a complex cascade of events involving the activation of naturally occurring factors and ending with the conversion of prothrombin into thrombin. The thrombin then converts fibrinogen into fibrin, a strandlike substance that attaches to the vessel's surface and contracts in a mesh web over the platelet plug to form a blood clot. Several of the factors involved need vitamin K to carry out their functions. A vitamin K deficiency inhibits clotting and makes uncontrolled bleeding more likely. Conversely, limiting the clotting cascade to the immediate area of the vessel injury is important for obvious reasons. The protein antithrombin III is key in this process. Antithrombin III binds with several of the factors needed for clotting, thus inhibiting their ability to coagulate.

Once the vessel has been permanently repaired, the fibrin mesh must be broken down. This process, called *fibrinolysis*, involves another cascading system that ends with the activation of plasminogen into plasmin, which in turn breaks up the clot. Tissue plasminogen activator, a substance in the tissue, activates this last conversion.

Thrombi (blood clots that obstruct vessels or heart cavities) are the primary pathology in several clinical conditions, including myocardial infarction, stroke, and pulmonary embolism. Drugs can effectively treat the causes of these conditions by decreasing platelet aggregation (**antiplatelet** drugs), by interfering with the clotting cascade (anticoagulants), or by directly breaking up the thrombus (fibrinolytics).

PLATELET AGGREGATION INHIBITORS **Platelet aggregation inhibitors** decrease the formation of platelet plugs. The prototype antiplatelet drug is aspirin. Aspirin inhibits cyclooxygenase, an enzyme needed for the synthesis of thromboxane A_2 (TXA_2). Remember that TXA_2 causes platelets to aggregate and promotes local vasoconstriction. By inhibiting TXA_2, aspirin decreases the formation of

> **CONTENT REVIEW**
>
> ➤ Drugs Used to Treat Thrombi
> - Antiplatelets
> - Anticoagulants
> - Fibrinolytics

platelet plugs and potential thrombi. Aspirin, as well as other antiplatelet and anticoagulant drugs, has no effect on existing thrombi; it only curbs the formation of new thrombi. Aspirin is indicated in the acute treatment of developing myocardial infarction. It is also useful in preventing the reoccurrence of MI and of ischemic stroke following transient ischemic attacks (TIAs).

One of aspirin's primary side effects is bleeding. Aspirin also may lead to an increase in gastric ulcers, which are a frequent source of gastrointestinal hemorrhage. By both stimulating the development of a potential source of bleeding as well as blocking an important mechanism for stopping that bleeding, aspirin can cause dangerous blood loss. Other antiplatelet drugs include dipyridamole (Persantine). A major class of drugs in this family includes the adenosine diphosphate (ADP) and glycoprotein IIB/IIIA inhibitors such as ticlopidine (Ticlid), abciximab (ReoPro), clopidogrel (Plavix), eptifibatide (Integrilin), tirofiban (Aggrastat), and ticlopidine (Ticlid).[25]

ANTICOAGULANTS **Anticoagulants** interrupt the clotting cascade. The two main types of anticoagulants are parenteral and oral. The prototype parenteral anticoagulant is heparin, a substance derived from the lungs of cattle or the intestines of pigs. Its primary mechanism of action is to enhance antithrombin III's ability to inhibit the clotting cascade. Because heparin is very polar, it is very poorly absorbed and must be given parenterally. Heparin injections and infusions are indicated in treating and preventing deep vein thrombosis, pulmonary embolism, and some forms of stroke. Heparin also is used frequently in conjunction with fibrinolytics to treat myocardial infarction. Finally, it is used to keep rubber-capped IV catheters (Hep-Locks) free from clots. As you would expect, bleeding is heparin's primary side effect. Other untoward effects include thrombocytopenia (decreased platelet counts) and allergic reactions. Heparin is measured in units rather than milligrams. A unit is that amount of heparin necessary to keep 1 mL of sheep plasma from clotting for 1 hour. Using this measurement is necessary because heparin's potency varies greatly when measured in milligrams.

Low-molecular-weight heparin (enoxaparin [Lovenox]) has become increasingly popular in emergency medicine. Normal heparin has a molecular weight of 5,000 to 30 000 Da, whereas low-molecular-weight heparin has a molecular weight of 1,000 to 10 000 Da. Because of this, low-molecular-weight heparin has greater bioavailability, is easier to dose, and has fewer effects on platelet function.

Protamine sulfate is available as a heparin antagonist. Protamine can reverse the effects of heparin in the presence of dangerous and unintended bleeding by binding with heparin. This prevents heparin from binding with antithrombin III and enhancing its anticlotting abilities.

The prototype oral anticoagulant is warfarin (Coumadin). Warfarin's history serves as a useful reminder of its primary side effect. Warfarin was first developed as a rat poison that killed through uncontrolled bleeding. After noticing that a patient who attempted suicide by ingesting warfarin did not, in fact, die, its clinical use was investigated. Needless to say, this drug's primary side effect is bleeding.

Warfarin prevents coagulation by antagonizing the effects of vitamin K, which is needed for the synthesis of multiple factors involved in the clotting cascade. It is prescribed for chronic use to prevent thrombi in high-risk patients such as those who have hip replacements or artificial heart valves or those who are in atrial fibrillation. Because warfarin easily crosses the placental barrier and has dangerous *teratogenic* (capable of causing malformations) properties, it is contraindicated in pregnant patients. It also interacts adversely with many other medications. Like heparin, warfarin may lead to bleeding. In cases of overdose, you may give vitamin K as an antidote.

FIBRINOLYTICS Fibrinolytics (also called *thrombolytics*) act directly on thrombi to break them up. The several available fibrinolytics share a similar mechanism of action. Through a chemical conversion, these drugs activate enzymes that dissolve thrombi or clots. The prototype drug of this class is streptokinase (Streptase). Other fibrinolytics include alteplase (rtPA), tenecteplase (TNKase), and anistreplase (Eminase). These medications all dissolve clots effectively; they differ primarily in their administration and risk of bleeding side effects.

Streptokinase, which is derived from the streptococci bacterium, is the oldest available fibrinolytic. Its mechanism of action is to promote plasminogen's conversion to plasmin. Because plasmin dissolves the fibrin mesh of clots, it can directly treat the cause of most myocardial infarctions and some strokes, as opposed to antiplatelet agents and anticoagulants, which can only prevent potential future thrombi. Streptokinase also breaks down fibrinogen, the precursor to fibrin. Although this action does not serve a clinical purpose (the problematic clot has already been formed), it does play an important role in streptokinase's chief side effect, bleeding. Other side effects include allergic reaction, hypotension, and fever.

Alteplase (Activase) is produced by recombinant DNA technology that is identical to the naturally occurring tissue plasminogen activator (hence its common name, rtPA). The window of opportunity for fibrinolytic therapy is limited. Because of this, some EMS systems administer fibrinolytics in the prehospital setting.[26]

ANTIFIBRINOLYTICS Antifibrinolytics inhibit the activation of plasminogen to plasmin, prevent the breakup of fibrin (fibrinolysis) and maintain clot stability. They are used to prevent excessive bleeding and have an evolving role in the management of trauma.

The most commonly used antifibrinolytic is tranexamic acid (TXA). It has been shown to limit bleeding and decrease the need for transfusion in trauma patients. TXA is relatively inexpensive and easy to administer. It has a good safety profile and is being used in several EMS systems—especially those with long transport times.[27]

Antihyperlipidemic Agents

Elevated levels of low-density lipoproteins (LDLs) have been clearly indicated as a causative factor in coronary artery disease. Lipoproteins are essentially transport mechanisms for lipids (triglycerides and cholesterol). Because lipids are insoluble in plasma, the body coats them in a plasma-soluble shell in order to transport them to their target destinations. Lipoproteins are categorized as very-low-density (VLDL), low-density (LDL), intermediate-density (IDL), and high-density (HDL). Low-density lipoproteins contain most of the cholesterol in the blood and are required for transporting cholesterol from the liver to the peripheral tissues. Conversely, high-density lipoproteins (HDLs) carry cholesterol from the peripheral tissues to the liver, where it is broken down.

HDLs have been described as "good" cholesterol because they lower blood cholesterol levels and decrease the risk of coronary artery disease (CAD). LDLs are known as "bad" cholesterol because they increase blood cholesterol levels and the risk of CAD. As blood cholesterol levels increase, fatty plaque is deposited under the arteries' endothelial tissues. Atherosclerosis then develops, and coronary arteries decrease in diameter. Coronary vasoconstriction, in turn, reduces blood flow to the heart and, in times of increased myocardial oxygen demand, may lead to angina. Also, newly deposited plaque is often unstable. Typically, the plaque is under the endothelial tissues, which cap the plaque deposits. As the deposits age, the cap usually becomes fairly stable. In some cases, however, the cap breaks open and exposes the plaque to the blood. When this happens, platelet aggregation and coagulation begin. If the developing clot breaks free of the vessel, it becomes a thrombus and may completely occlude a coronary artery, leading to myocardial infarction.

The goal in lowering LDL levels is to prevent atherosclerosis and subsequent CAD. While raising HDL levels would help accomplish this, no pharmaceutical means of doing so currently exists. By far, the best way to lower LDL levels remains dietary modification. If this is not sufficient, several classifications of **antihyperlipidemic** medications may be used. The most common are drugs that inhibit hydroxymethylglutaryl coenzyme A (HMG CoA) reductase. The liver must have HMG CoA to synthesize cholesterol. By inhibiting this enzyme, HMG CoA agents lower LDL levels; however, they also increase the number of LDL receptors in the liver, causing a further uptake of LDL.

Five HMG CoA reductase inhibitors are available. Because the names of all five end in *statin,* these agents are also known as statins. They include lovastatin (Mevacor) and simvastatin (Zocor). Lovastatin is the HMG CoA reductase inhibitors' prototype. Overall, these drugs are well tolerated. Their chief side effects are headache, rash, and flushing. In rare cases, they may cause hepatotoxicity and lead to liver failure.

Bile acid-binding resins can also reduce LDL levels. Inert substances that have no direct biological activity, these agents pass straight through the GI system without being absorbed and are excreted in feces. They are useful, however, in that they indirectly increase the number of LDL receptors in the liver by binding with bile acids, thus decreasing their availability. Because the liver needs cholesterol to synthesize bile acids, it must have more cholesterol to compensate for the decrease in bile acids. The body therefore increases the LDL receptors on the liver. As more LDLs remain in the liver, their levels in the blood drop. Because the body does not absorb bile acid-binding agents, they have no systemic effects. Their chief untoward effect is constipation. Cholestyramine (Questran) is the prototype.

Drugs Used to Affect the Respiratory System

Drugs that affect the respiratory system are useful for several purposes. The most obvious is the treatment of asthma, but this class also includes cough suppressants, nasal decongestants, and antihistamines.

Antiasthmatic Medications

Asthma is a common disease that decreases pulmonary function and may limit daily activities. It typically presents with shortness of breath, wheezing, and coughing. Its basic pathophysiology has two components: bronchoconstriction and inflammation. Typically, a response to some sort of allergen sets both of these processes in motion. Common culprits include pet dander, mold, and dust. Cold air, tobacco smoke, or other pollutants may bring on acute episodes of shortness of breath in patients with existing asthma.

The response to asthma typically begins with an allergen's binding to an antibody on mast cells. This causes the mast cell membrane to rupture and release its contents, including histamine, leukotrienes, and prostaglandins. These cause immediate bronchoconstriction, followed by a slower inflammatory response that can lead to mucus plugs and a further decrease in airway size. The inflammation may, in turn, cause a hyperreactivity to stimuli, and

allergens that might not normally produce dyspnea may lead to an acute attack.

Drug treatment of asthma aims to relieve bronchospasm and decrease inflammation. Specific approaches are categorized as beta$_2$ selective sympathomimetics, nonselective sympathomimetics, methylxanthines, anticholinergics, glucocorticoids, and leukotriene antagonists. Cromolyn (Intal), a frequently used anti-inflammatory agent, does not fit neatly into any of those categories. Table 13-23 summarizes these agents.

BETA$_2$ SPECIFIC AGENTS   Drugs that are selective for β_2 receptors are the mainstay in treating asthma-induced shortness of breath. Albuterol (Proventil, Ventolin) is the prototype of this class. In general, these agents relax bronchial smooth muscle, which results in bronchodilation and relief from bronchospasm. Agents from this class are first-line therapy for acute shortness of breath and may also be used daily for prophylaxis. Most are administered via metered dose inhaler or nebulizer. Albuterol and terbutaline may both be taken orally, and terbutaline may be given by injection. These medications' β_2 specificity is not absolute; some patients may experience β_1 effects such as tachycardia or arrhythmias. Patients may also experience

Table 13-23 Drugs Used in the Treatment of Asthma

Mechanism of Action	Medication
Bronchodilators	
Nonspecific agonists	Epinephrine
	Ephedrine
Beta$_2$ specific agonists	
Inhaled (short-acting)	Albuterol (Ventolin, Proventil), Metaproterenol (Alupent), Terbutaline (Brethine), Bitolterol (Tornalate)
Inhaled (long-acting)	Salmeterol (Serevent)
Methylxanthines	Theophylline (Theo-Dur, Slo-Bid), Aminophylline
Anticholinergics	Atropine
	Ipratropium (Atrovent)
Anti-inflammatory agents	
Glucocorticoids	
Inhaled	Beclomethasone (Beclovent), Flucticasone (Flovent), Triamcinolone (Azmacort)
Oral	Prednisone (Deltasone)
Injected	Methylprednisolone (Solu-Medrol)
	Dexamethasone (Decadron)
Leukotriene antagonists	Zafirlukast (Accolate)
	Zileuton (Zyflo)
	Montelukast (Singulair)
Mast-cell membrane stabilizer	Cromolyn (Intal)

tremors resulting from the stimulation of β_2 receptors in smooth muscles. Overall, these agents are very safe.

NONSELECTIVE SYMPATHOMIMETICS Medications that stimulate both β_1 and β_2 receptors, as well as α receptors, are rarely used to treat asthma because they have the undesired effects of increased peripheral vascular resistance and increased risks for tachycardias and other arrhythmias. Nonselective drugs include epinephrine, ephedrine, and isoproterenol. Epinephrine is the only nonselective sympathomimetic in common use today, because of the availability of selective agents. It may be given subcutaneously for patients who have severe bronchospasm that does not respond to other treatments.

METHYLXANTHINES The methylxanthines are CNS stimulants that have additional bronchodilatory properties. They were once first-line therapy for asthma, but now they are used only when other drugs such as β_2 specific agents are ineffective. We do not know the methylxanthines' specific action, but they may block adenosine receptors. The prototype methylxanthine, theophylline, is taken orally. Aminophylline, an IV medication, is rapidly metabolized into theophylline and, therefore, has identical effects. These agents' chief side effects are nausea, vomiting, insomnia, restlessness, and arrhythmias. Aminophylline is still used occasionally in the emergency treatment of acute asthma attacks.

ANTICHOLINERGICS Ipratropium (Atrovent) is an atropine derivative given by nebulizer. Because stimulating the muscarinic receptors in the lungs results in constriction of bronchial smooth muscle, ipratropium, a muscarinic antagonist, causes bronchodilation. Ipratropium is inhaled and, therefore, has no systemic effects. Ipratropium and β_2 agonists like albuterol act along different pathways, so their concurrent administration has an additive effect. Ipratropium's most common side effect is dry mouth. This results from the local effects of the drug that remains in the oropharynx after administration.

GLUCOCORTICOIDS Glucocorticoids have anti-inflammatory properties. They lower the production and release of inflammatory substances such as histamine, prostaglandins, and leukotrienes, and they reduce mucus and edema secondary to decreasing vascular permeability. These drugs may be inhaled or taken orally, or they may be given intravenously in emergencies. The prototype inhaled glucocorticoid is beclomethasone; the prototype oral glucocorticoid is prednisone. Primarily preventive, they are taken on a regular schedule, as opposed to the as-needed administration of the β_2 agonists. An injectable glucocorticoid (methylprednisolone) is available for use secondary to β_2 agonists in emergencies. When inhaled, glucocorticoids cause few side effects. Those are due mostly to direct exposure on the oropharynx, and gargling after taking the drug can decrease them. Likewise, side effects from the intravenous administrations of methylprednisolone in emergencies are not likely. When given orally or intravenously over long periods, however, glucocorticoids may have profound side effects, including adrenal suppression and hyperglycemia.

Another anti-inflammatory agent used to prevent asthma attacks is cromolyn (Intal), an inhaled powder. Although it is not a glucocorticoid, its actions are similar. The inhaled glucocorticoids are relatively safe, but cromolyn is even safer. In fact, it is the safest of all antiasthma agents. Its only side effects are coughing or wheezing due to local irritation caused by the powder. Cromolyn is often used for preventing asthma in adults and children. It is also a useful prophylaxis before activities known to cause shortness of breath, such as exercise or mowing grass.

LEUKOTRIENE ANTAGONISTS Leukotrienes are mediators released from mast cells on contact with allergens. They contribute powerfully to both inflammation and bronchoconstriction. Consequently, agents that block their effects are useful in treating asthma. Leukotriene antagonists can either block the synthesis of leukotrienes or block their receptors. Zileuton (Zyflo) is the prototype of those that block the synthesis of leukotrienes. Zafirlukast (Accolate) is the prototype of those that block their receptors.

Drugs Used for Rhinitis and Cough

Rhinitis (inflammation of the nasal lining) comprises a group of symptoms including nasal congestion, itching, redness, sneezing, and rhinorrhea (runny nose). Either allergic reactions or viral infections such as the common cold may cause it. Drugs that treat the symptoms of rhinitis and cold are commonly found in over-the-counter remedies. In addition, nasal decongestants, antihistamines, and cough suppressants are available in prescription medications. Although manufacturers of cold medications often combine several drugs in one product intended to treat multiple symptoms, we discuss each class separately.

NASAL DECONGESTANTS Nasal congestion is caused by dilated and engorged nasal capillaries. Drugs that constrict these capillaries are effective nasal decongestants. The main pharmacological classification in this functional category is α_1 agonists. Alpha$_1$ agonists may be given either topically or orally. The chief examples of these agents—phenylephrine, pseudoephedrine, and phenylpropanolamine—can be administered either as a mist or in drops. Topical administration reduces systemic effects but has the undesired local effect of rebound congestion, a form of tolerance. Rebound congestion occurs after long-term use (longer than 7 consecutive days). As the drug wears off, congestion becomes progressively worse. This effect ends when the patient stops taking the drug; however, the longer the patient has been using the drug, the more unpleasant stopping becomes. While pseudoephedrine is an over-the-counter (OTC) medication, it is often placed behind the pharmacy counter because pseudoephedrine is one of the ingredients used in the clandestine manufacturing of methamphetamine.

ANTIHISTAMINES **Antihistamines** arrest the effects of histamine by blocking its receptors. **Histamine** is an endogenous substance that affects a wide variety of organ systems. It is noted for its role in allergic reaction. In the vasculature, histamine binds with H_1 receptors to cause vasodilation and increased capillary permeability. In the lungs, H_1 receptors cause bronchoconstriction. In the gut, H_2 receptors cause an increase in gastric acid release. Histamine also acts as a neurotransmitter in the central nervous system. Histamine is synthesized and stored in two types of granulocytes: tissue-bound mast cells and plasma-bound basophils. Both types are full of secretory granules, which are vesicles containing inflammatory mediators such as histamine, leukotrienes, and prostaglandins, among others. When these cells are exposed to allergens, they develop antibodies on their surfaces. On subsequent exposures, the antibodies bind with their specific allergen. The secretory granules then migrate toward the cell's exterior and fuse with the cell membrane. This causes them to release their contents. Although some available medications stabilize this membrane to prevent the release of these substances, the traditional antihistamines work by antagonizing the histamine receptors.

Although they are commonly thought of as a nuisance, histamines are useful in our immune systems. Only when our immune systems overreact do allergies such as hay fever or cedar fever send us running for the antihistamines. The typical symptoms of allergic reaction include most of those associated with rhinitis. Severe allergic reactions (anaphylaxis) may cause hypotension. Although histamines play a major role in mild and moderate allergic reactions, their part in anaphylaxis is minimal; therefore,

antihistamines are at best only a secondary drug for treating anaphylaxis. (Epinephrine is the drug of choice.)

Just as there are H_1 and H_2 histamine receptors, there are H_1 and H_2 histamine receptor antagonists. When most people refer to antihistamines, they are thinking of H_1 receptor antagonists. These agents were in popular use long before the discovery of the H_2 receptors. (We discuss H_2 receptor antagonists in the section on drugs used to treat peptic ulcer disease.) The chief side effect of antihistamines is sedation, which the early antihistamines all caused to some degree. Now a second generation of antihistamines that do not cause sedation is available.

The first-generation antihistamines comprise several chemical subclasses. Examples include alkylamines (chlorpheniramine [Chlor-Trimeton]), ethanolamines (diphenhydramine [Benadryl] and clemastine [Tavist]), and phenothiazines (promethazine [Phenergan]). The different classes of agents have the same actions, but they differ in the degree of sedation they cause and in their ability to block other, nonhistamine receptors. Several antihistamines also have significant anticholinergic properties. In fact, some are used specifically for their anticholinergic effects, notably promethazine and dimenhydrinate (Dramamine), which are used to reduce motion sickness. Other than the sedation that first-generation antihistamines cause, these agents' primary side effects are constipation and the effects of muscarinic blockade, such as dry mouth. Because they can thicken bronchial secretions, antihistamines should not be used in patients with asthma.

The second-generation antihistamines include loratadine (Claritin), cetirizine (Zyrtec), and fexofenadine (Allegra). These agents' actions are similar to the first generation's, with the notable exception that they do not cross the blood–brain barrier and therefore do not cause sedation. In addition, their H_1 receptor antagonism is more pronounced, and their anticholinergic actions are greatly diminished. See Table 13-24 for common antihistamines.

Table 13-24 Antihistamines

Name	Classification	Action	Indications	Contraindications	Doses	Routes	Adverse Effects	Other
Diphenhydramine *Benadryl*	Antihistamine	Nonselectively blocks H_1 and H_2 histamine receptors	• Allergies • Extrapyramidal reactions • Parkinson's disease • Sedation • Anaphylaxis	• Hypersensitivity to the drug • Glaucoma • Pregnancy	25–50 mg	IV, IM, IO, PO	• Drowsiness • Dizziness • Sedation • Dry mouth	• If given IM, give deep in muscle
Cimetidine *Tagamet*	Antihistamine	Selectively blocks H_2 histamine receptors	• Duodenal/peptic ulcer • Anaphylaxis	• Hypersensitivity to the drug	300 mg	IV, IM, PO	• Diarrhea • Drowsiness • Dizziness	• Can be used as an adjunct for severe allergic reactions and anaphylaxis

COUGH SUPPRESSANTS Coughing is a complex reflex that depends on functions in the CNS, the PNS, and the respiratory muscles. It is a defense mechanism that aids the removal of foreign particles such as smoke and dust. A productive cough is one in which these particles are actually being coughed up. In general, treating a productive cough is not appropriate, as it is performing a useful function. An unproductive cough, however, usually results from an irritated oropharynx and can be troublesome. The three classifications of cough suppressants include one that is supported by evidence and two that are not. **Antitussive** medications suppress the stimulus to cough in the central nervous system. This functional class includes two specific pharmacological types, opioids and nonopioids. The two most common opioid antitussives are codeine and hydrocodone. Both inhibit the stimulus for coughing in the brain but also produce varying degrees of euphoria. The doses required for cough suppression are not high enough to cause euphoria, but these drugs still have the potential for abuse. The nonopioid antitussives, in contrast, do not have the potential for abuse. Dextromethorphan is the leading drug in this class. Although it is almost never given alone, it is the most common antitussive used in over-the-counter combination products for treating cold and flu symptoms. Diphenhydramine (Benadryl) is also used as a nonopioid antitussive, although its mechanism of action is not clear. Finally, the locally acting anesthetic benzonatate (Tessalon) depresses the cough stimulus by directly reducing oropharyngeal irritation. **Expectorants** are intended to increase the productivity of cough, and **mucolytics** make mucus more watery and, therefore, easier to cough up; however, little data support the effectiveness of either of these approaches to cough suppression.

Drugs Used to Affect the Gastrointestinal System

The main purposes of drug therapy in the gastrointestinal system are to treat peptic ulcers, constipation, diarrhea, and emesis, and to aid digestion.

Drugs Used to Treat Peptic Ulcer Disease

Peptic ulcer disease (PUD) is characterized by an imbalance between factors in the gastrointestinal system that increase acidity and those that protect against acidity. PUD may manifest as indigestion, heartburn, or, more seriously, as perforated ulcers. If the imbalance becomes too severe, parts of the lining of the GI system may be eaten away, exposing the tissue and vasculature underneath to the highly acidic environment of the stomach or duodenum.

The GI system's structure fits its function. Many mucus-lined folds surround the GI lumen. The cells of these folds secrete acids needed to help break down foods; they secrete protective mucus that prevents the acid from injuring the underlying tissue; and finally, they secrete bicarbonates, which buffer the effects of acids on the GI system's absorbing surfaces. To absorb the digested nutrients and supply the mucus-producing cells of the lumen wall with oxygen, the entire GI system is very vascular. If the protective lining covering these vessels is removed, hemorrhage may occur.

Several pathological factors oppose the GI system's defenses. Contrary to popular belief, the most common cause of peptic ulcer disease is not stress or alcohol, but the *Helicobacter pylori* bacterium. *H. pylori* infests the space between the endothelial cells and the mucus lining of the stomach and duodenum. It can remain there for decades, protected against the acid environment by the mucus layer. Although we are still uncertain how this bacteria promotes ulcers, it apparently decreases the body's ability to produce the protective mucus lining. *H. pylori* by itself, however, does not cause ulcers. Many people remain infected for years and years without signs of PUD. Evidently, predisposing and contributing factors combine with *H. pylori* to cause ulceration. Some of these factors include smoking and long-term use of nonsteroidal anti-inflammatory drugs (NSAIDs) such as aspirin and acetaminophen.

The approaches to treating PUD include antibiotics and drugs that block or decrease the secretion of gastric acid. Most often they are used in conjunction with each other. First, and most effective, are antibiotics. When the *H. pylori* infection is eliminated, the signs of PUD resolve, and recurrence is low. Typically, three antibiotics will be used to ensure elimination of the bacteria and prevent resistance. Common medications for this purpose include bismuth (Pepto-Bismol), metronidazole (Flagyl), amoxicillin (Amoxil), and tetracycline (Achromycin V).

Drugs that block or decrease the secretion of gastric acid include H_2 receptor antagonists (H2RAs), proton pump inhibitors, and anticholinergic agents. Mucosal protectants and antacids are also used.

H_2 receptors occur throughout the gut on the membranes of the parietal cells lining the GI lumen. When stimulated with histamine, they increase the action of $H^+K^+ATPase$, an enzyme that exchanges potassium for hydrogen, leading to increased gastric acid secretion. Acetylcholine and prostaglandin receptors appear along with H_2 receptors. Stimulating the ACh receptors (muscarinic receptors) increases gastric acid secretion; stimulating the prostaglandin receptors inhibits it.

H₂ RECEPTOR ANTAGONISTS   H₂RA agents block the H₂ receptors in the gut. This inhibits gastric acid secretion and helps return the balance between protective and aggressive factors. Four approved H₂RAs are in use: cimetidine (Tagamet), ranitidine (Zantac), famotidine (Pepcid), and nizatidine (Axid Pulvules). Cimetidine is the oldest of these and serves as the prototype. These agents' primary therapeutic use is for ulcers, gastroesophageal reflux, heartburn or acid indigestion, and preventing aspiration pneumonia during anesthesia. Most of these agents have few significant side effects, with the exception of cimetidine, which may lead to decreased libido, impotence, and CNS effects in some patients. Although these agents could technically be called antihistamines, that name by tradition is reserved for the H₁ antagonists. The H₂RAs have no effect on the H₁ receptors and are of no value in allergic reactions.

PROTON PUMP INHIBITORS   Proton pump inhibitors act directly on the $K^+H^+ATPase$ enzyme that secretes gastric acid. Omeprazole (Prilosec) and lansoprazole (Prevacid) are examples. Omeprazole is the prototype. These agents irreversibly block this enzyme, which means that the body must produce new enzyme in order to begin secreting acid again. This gives proton pump inhibitors a long duration of effect. Side effects are minor and rare, occurring in less than 1 percent of patients. They include diarrhea and headache.

ANTACIDS   **Antacids** are alkalotic compounds used to increase the gastric environment's pH. Most available products are either aluminum, magnesium, calcium, or sodium compounds. They are used in conjunction with other approaches to PUD and are available over the counter for relief of acid indigestion and heartburn.

ANTICHOLINERGICS   Although it might seem that all muscarinic blocking agents would be effective in decreasing gastric acid secretion, most atropine-like drugs produce too many unwanted effects and, therefore, are not used. The one exception is pirenzepine (Gastrozepine), because of its ability to selectively block the ACh receptors in the gut.

Drugs Used to Treat Constipation

Laxatives decrease the firmness of stool and increase the water content. Although an uninformed public frequently uses these agents unnecessarily, they are effective in some situations, specifically with patients for whom excessive strain is inappropriate. These patients include those with recent episiotomy, hemorrhoids, colostomies, or cardiovascular disease (for whom excessive straining may decrease heart rate).

Laxatives are traditionally grouped into four categories based on their mechanism of action: bulk-forming, surfactant, stimulant, and osmotic. The bulk-forming agents, such as methylcellulose (Citrucel) and psyllium (Metamucil), produce a response almost identical to normal dietary fiber intake. Fiber is undigestible and unabsorbable; therefore, it remains in the lumen of the GI system and is passed more or less intact in stool. Most water absorption takes place in the colon. Fiber (or bulk-forming laxatives) in the colon absorbs water, leading to a softer, more bulky stool. Fiber can also provide nutrients for bacteria living in the colon. These bacteria feed and provide even more bulk. The enlarged stool stimulates stretch receptors in the colonic wall, which increases peristalsis. Softening the stool also lessens strain on defecation.

The **surfactant** laxatives include docusate sodium (Colace). They decrease surface tension, which increases water absorption into the feces. They also increase water secretion and limit its reabsorption by the intestinal wall.

Stimulant laxatives increase motility. Like the surfactant laxatives, they also increase water secretion and decrease its absorption. The prototype stimulant laxative is phenolphthalein (Ex-Lax, Correctol). Bisacodyl (Bisacolax) is another example.

The osmotic laxatives are poorly absorbed salts that increase the feces' osmotic pull, thereby increasing their water content. Magnesium hydroxide, the active ingredient in milk of magnesia, is the prototype of this class.

CONTENT REVIEW

➤ Categories of Laxatives
  - Bulk-forming
  - Stimulant
  - Osmotic
  - Surfactant

Drugs Used to Treat Diarrhea

Diarrhea is the abnormally frequent passage of soft, liquid stool. It is a symptom of an underlying disease, usually a bacterial infection. It may be caused by an increased gastric motility (the stool does not stay in the colon long enough to have much water absorbed), increased water secretion, or decreased water absorption. Even though it is a nuisance, diarrhea is often a helpful process because it increases the expulsion of the offending agent. It is usually self-correcting and does not need to be treated. When treatment is necessary, either specific or nonspecific agents may be used. A specific agent directly treats the cause, usually bacteria. As you would expect, antibiotics are a common specific antidiarrheal medication.

Drugs Used to Treat Emesis

Emesis is a complex process that involves different parts of the brain, as well as receptors and muscles in the stomach and inner ear. The two involved parts of the brain include the vomiting center in the medulla and the chemoreceptor trigger zone (CTZ). The vomiting center stimulates vomiting directly, whereas the CTZ does so indirectly.

The vomiting center is stimulated by H_1 and ACh receptors in the pathway between itself and the inner ear, by sensory input from the eyes and nose (unpleasant or disturbing sights and smells), and by other parts of the brain in response to anxiety or fear. The CTZ stimulates the vomiting center in response to stimuli from serotonin receptors in the stomach and bloodborne substances such as opioids and ipecac.

Stimulating emesis is rarely desired, but it can be useful in treating certain types of overdoses or poisonings. Ipecac is the drug of choice when stimulating emesis is indicated. It stimulates the CTZ which, in turn, stimulates the vomiting center.

ANTIEMETICS Unlike causing emesis, preventing emesis is frequently desirable. **Antiemetics** are indicated in conjunction with chemotherapy, which may cause violent nausea and vomiting. Antiemetics are also indicated in the prophylactic treatment of motion sickness.

Multiple transmitters are involved in the vomiting reflex. They include serotonin, dopamine, acetylcholine, and histamine. Drugs that interfere with any of these transmitters can decrease or prevent nausea and vomiting. This functional class includes several pharmacological subclasses: serotonin antagonists, dopamine antagonists, anticholinergics, and cannabinoids.

SEROTONIN ANTAGONISTS The prototype serotonin antagonist is ondansetron (Zofran). It blocks the serotonin receptors in the CTZ, the stomach, and the small intestine. It is very effective in the treatment of nausea and vomiting associated with chemotherapy, and, unlike the dopamine antagonists, it does not cause extrapyramidal effects such as dystonia and ataxia. Its most common side effects are headache and diarrhea.

DOPAMINE ANTAGONISTS Both phenothiazines and butyrophenones effectively block dopamine receptors in the CTZ. (This chapter's section on psychotherapeutic medications discusses both of these medications at length.) The phenothiazines include prochlorperazine (Compazine) and promethazine (Phenergan), whereas the butyrophenones include haloperidol (Haldol) and droperidol (Inapsine). Agents from both classes cause side effects of extrapyramidal effects and sedation. Another dopamine antagonist, metoclopramide (Reglan), is neither a phenothiazine nor a butyrophenone. It is unique in that it blocks both serotonin and dopamine receptors in the CTZ. Table 13-25 details common antiemetics.

CANNABINOIDS The cannabinoids are derivatives of tetrahydrocannabinol (THC) and are effective antiemetics used to treat chemotherapy-induced nausea and vomiting. The two available agents are dronabinol (Marinol) and nabilone (Cesamet). Because both agents are essentially the same as THC (the active ingredient in marijuana), their side effects include euphoria similar to that of marijuana. While those effects may be desirable for some, they may be intensely unpleasant for others.

Drugs Used to Aid Digestion

Several drugs are available to aid the digestion of carbohydrates and fats. These agents are similar to endogenous digestive enzymes released into the duodenum in response to vagal stimulation. Occasionally, supplemental enzymes are necessary for patients whose vagal stimulus has been surgically severed or whose duodenum has been bypassed. Two of these drugs are pancreatin (Entozyme) and pancrelipase (Viokase). Their chief side effects are nausea, vomiting, and abdominal cramping.

Drugs Used to Affect the Eyes

Ophthalmic drugs are used to treat conditions involving the eyes, primarily glaucoma and trauma. In addition, some ophthalmic agents are used in diagnosing and examining the eyes.

Glaucoma is a degenerative disease that affects the optic nerve. Its causative factors are not clear; however, correlations are known between it and several risk factors, including intraocular pressure, race (its rate is three times higher among African Americans than among whites), and age. The medications used to treat glaucoma are all aimed at reducing intraocular pressure (IOP). Beta-blockers and cholinergics are the most common. Beta-blockade decreases IOP by an unknown mechanism. Timolol (Timoptic) and betaxolol (Betoptic) are examples of this class. Pilocarpine (Isopto Carpine) is the prototype cholinergic drug for treating glaucoma. It stimulates muscarinic receptors in the eye to cause miosis (pupil constriction) and ciliary muscle contraction, which indirectly lowers IOP. Drugs from these classes are given topically. Beta-blockers have few side effects, whereas pilocarpine causes blurred vision and local irritation.

Some diagnostic procedures call for causing mydriasis (pupil dilation) and cycloplegia (paralysis of the ciliary muscles used to focus vision). The two pharmacological approaches to doing this involve anticholinergics or adrenergic agonists. In this functional class, atropine solutions (such as Atropisol) and scopolamine solutions (such as Isopto Hyoscine) are typical anticholinergics; phenylephrine solution (AK-Dilate) is the class's principal adrenergic

Table 13-25 Antiemetics

Name	Classification	Action	Indications	Contraindications	Doses	Routes	Adverse Effects	Other
Prochlorperazine *Compazine*	Phenothiazine	Suppresses the CTZ; has antihistaminic effects	• Nausea • Vomiting • Anxiety • Psychosis	• Hypersensitivity to the drug or the phenothiazine class • Small children • Pregnancy	5–10 mg	IV, IM, IO, PO	• Drowsiness • Dizziness • Sedation • Dry mouth • Extrapyramidal symptoms	• Can potentiate CNS depressants (e.g., alcohol).
Promethazine *Phenergan*	Phenothiazine	Suppresses the CTZ; has antihistaminic effects	• Nausea • Vomiting	• Hypersensitivity to the drug	12.5–25 mg	IV, IM, PO	• Drowsiness • Dizziness • Sedation • Dry mouth • Extrapyramidal symptoms	• Can potentiate CNS depressants (e.g., alcohol). • Extravasation can cause local tissue injury. • Rarely used.
Droperidol *Inapsine*	Antidopaminergic	Blocks dopamine receptors (D₂)	• Nausea • Vomiting • Psychosis	• Hypersensitivity to the drug • Prolonged QTc on ECG	1.25–2.50 mg	IV, IM,	• QTc prolongation • Hypotension • Tachycardia	• Has "black box warning" due to possible QT prolongation.
Ondansetron *Zofran*	Serotonin antagonist	Selectively blocks 5-HT₃ serotonin receptors, including those in the CTZ and vagus nerve terminals	• Nausea • Vomiting	• Hypersensitivity to the drug	4–8 mg	IV, IM, PO, SL	• Dizziness • Lightheaded	• Commonly used in emergency medicine because of good safety profile.

agonist. This chapter's sections on anticholinergics and adrenergic agonists discuss these pharmacological classes in more detail.

Tetracaine (Pontocaine) is a local anesthetic of the ester class. (It is related to cocaine, another ester, but not to lidocaine, an amide.) It is used to decrease pain and sensation in the eye from trauma or during ophthalmic procedures.

Drugs Used to Affect the Ears

Most drugs used to treat conditions involving the ear are aimed at eliminating underlying bacterial or fungal infections or at breaking up impacted earwax. Chloramphenicol (Chloromycetin Otic) and gentamicin sulfate otic solution (Garamycin) are common antibiotics; carbamide peroxide (Auro Ear Drops) and carbamide peroxide and glycerin (Ear Wax Removal System) are both used to treat earwax. Finally, several drugs are available to treat swimmer's ear, an inflammation/irritation of the external ear. They include isopropyl alcohol (Auro-Dri Ear Drops) and boric acid and isopropyl alcohol (Aurocaine 2).

Some drugs used for other purposes have ototoxic (harmful to the organs or nerves that produce hearing or balance) properties if taken in overdose or administered too quickly. The most common ototoxic symptom is tinnitus, or ringing in the ears. Drugs with ototoxic properties include aspirin and other NSAIDs, some antibiotics (including erythromycin and vancomycin), and the diuretic furosemide (Lasix).

Drugs Used to Affect the Endocrine System

The endocrine system and nervous system together are chiefly responsible for the regulatory activities that maintain homeostasis. The nervous system, with its direct connections between nerves and organs, may be thought of as a "wired" system, whereas the endocrine system, which releases hormones directly into the bloodstream, may be thought of as "wireless." The endocrine system comprises the following glands: pituitary (anterior and posterior lobes), pineal, thyroid, parathyroid, thymus, adrenal, pancreas, ovaries, and testes. (Table 13-26 lists the specific hormones that each gland releases.) Of these, the pituitary is commonly referred to as the master gland because of its role in controlling the other endocrine glands. (The hypothalamus, in turn, controls many of the pituitary's functions.) Once in the bloodstream, the hormones from these glands circulate widely throughout the body. To be effective, however, they must bind with very specific receptors. This discussion focuses on the pharmacological actions of drugs that affect the various endocrine glands.

Drugs Affecting the Pituitary Gland

The pituitary gland is made up of a posterior lobe and an anterior lobe. It sits in the *sella turcica*, a depression of the sphenoid bone, and is physically connected to the hypothalamus. The posterior pituitary hormones are actually synthesized in the hypothalamus and then migrate into the posterior pituitary, where they are released on hypothalamic stimulation. In contrast, the hormones of the anterior

Table 13-26 Summary of Hormone Actions

Gland	Hormone	Action
Posterior pituitary	Oxytocin	Uterine contraction, milk ejection
	Vasopressin (ADH)	Retains salt and water, increases ECF volume
Anterior pituitary	Thyroid-stimulating hormone (TSH)	Increases metabolic rate
	Growth hormone (GH)	Increases use of stored fats, decreases glucose use
	Adrenocorticotropic hormone (ACTH)	Stimulates adrenal cortex to release hormones
	Follicle-stimulating hormone (FSH)	Males: sperm production
		Females: stimulates growth and development of ovarian follicles
	Luteinizing hormone (LH)	Males: responsible for secretion of testosterone by testes
		Females: ovulation, secretion of estrogen and progesterone
	Prolactin (PRL)	Enhances breast development and milk production
Thyroid	Thyroid hormone	Increases metabolic rate
Parathyroid	Parathyroid hormone	Increases calcium in ECF
Pancreas	Insulin	Decreases blood glucose
	Glucagon	Increases blood glucose
Adrenal	Glucocorticoids	Increases blood glucose, prevents inflammation

pituitary are synthesized in that lobe. The hypothalamus secretes releasing hormones into a portal system that carries them into the anterior pituitary, where they stimulate the release of the anterior pituitary hormones. There are six main anterior pituitary hormones.

ANTERIOR PITUITARY DRUGS The only conditions treated with anterior pituitary-like drugs are those associated with abnormal growth, specifically dwarfism, acromegaly, and gigantism. Dwarfism is caused by a deficiency of growth hormone, and therapy is aimed at hormone replacement. Somatrem (Protropin) and somatropin (Humatrope) are both essentially the same as the endogenous growth hormone, acting indirectly to increase skeletal growth as well as cell numbers by stimulating another hormone, insulinlike growth factor 1 (IGF-1), to cause its effects. These drugs' primary side effects are pain and redness at the injection site. Some cases of inadvertent gigantism have been reported, but this can be avoided with careful observation.

Acromegaly and gigantism are caused by excesses of growth hormone, usually resulting from a tumor. The treatment of choice is surgical removal of the tumor, but octreotide (Sandostatin) is available for pharmacological intervention. Octreotide is a synthetic drug with actions similar to somatostatin, the endogenous growth hormone inhibiting hormone. Its main action inhibits the release of growth hormone. Octreotide's many side effects include bradycardia, diarrhea, and stomach distress.

POSTERIOR PITUITARY DRUGS The two posterior pituitary hormones are oxytocin and antidiuretic hormone. Oxytocin is discussed in the section on drugs affecting labor and delivery. Antidiuretic hormone (ADH) increases water reabsorption in the renal collecting tubules, thus promoting the retention of water and a more concentrated urine. Physiologically, ADH is a key component in regulating blood volume, blood pressure, and electrolyte balance. Clinically, ADH analogs are used to treat diabetes insipidus and nocturnal enuresis (bedwetting). Diabetes insipidus, unlike diabetes mellitus, is caused by inadequate amounts of centrally acting ADH. This causes a profound polyuria and polydipsia. At higher doses, ADH can cause vasoconstriction and increased blood pressure—hence its other name, vasopressin. Vasopressin (Pitressin), desmopressin (Stimate), and lypressin (Diapid) are all available to reverse this ADH deficiency. Desmopressin is also available for administration via intranasal spray for nocturnal enuresis.[29]

Drugs Affecting the Parathyroid and Thyroid Glands

The parathyroid glands are primarily responsible for regulating calcium levels. Hypoparathyroidism leads to decreased levels of calcium and vitamin D. Treatment,

therefore, is through calcium and vitamin D supplements. Hyperparathyroidism leads to high levels of calcium. Because it usually results from tumors, the treatment of choice is surgical removal of all or part of the parathyroid glands.

The thyroid gland produces thyroid hormones, which play a vital role in regulating growth, maturation, and metabolism. Hypothyroidism can occur in children or adults. When it develops in children, it is known as cretinism and manifests itself as dwarfism and mental retardation with characteristic features. Because most growth and maturation in adults is complete, adult onset of hypothyroidism appears as decreased metabolic rate, weight gain, fatigue, and bradycardia. In some cases, myxedema (facial puffiness) may be present. Treatment is aimed at thyroid hormone replacement. The prototype drug, levothyroxine (Synthroid), is also the most commonly used. A synthetic analog of T_4 (thyroxine), one of the thyroid hormones, levothyroxine generally has no significant side effects when taken in therapeutic doses. Overdose may lead to thyrotoxicosis or thyroid storm. Thyrotoxicosis is a condition in which hyperthyroidism causes an increase in thyroid hormones. Thyroid storm is a severe form of thyrotoxicosis in which the manifestations of the disease increase to life-threatening proportions. Thyroid storm is characterized by tachycardic arrhythmias, angina, hypertension, and hyperthermia.

Goiters are enlargements of the thyroid gland. They are typically caused by insufficient dietary iodine. In developed countries, goiter is much rarer than in undeveloped countries and is most commonly caused by Hashimoto's disease, a chronic autoimmune disease. Treatment of goiters is aimed at supplementing the inadequate iodine.

Hyperthyroidism is caused by excessive release of thyroid hormones, typically as a result of tumors. The most common cause of hyperthyroidism in the United States is Graves' disease. It presents with tachycardia, hypertension, hyperthermia, nervousness, insomnia, increased metabolic rate, and weight loss. In severe cases, exophthalmos (protrusion of the eyeballs) may occur. Treatment is typically surgical removal of all or part of the thyroid gland. Radioactive iodine (^{131}I) may also be given for radiation therapy. Propylthiouracil (PTU) may be given alone or as adjunct therapy to surgery or radiation in treating hyperthyroidism.

Drugs Affecting the Adrenal Cortex

The adrenal cortex synthesizes and secretes three classes of hormones: glucocorticoids, mineralocorticoids, and androgens. The glucocorticoids and mineralocorticoids are referred to collectively as corticosteroids, adrenocorticoids, or corticoids. As their name implies, glucocorticoids increase the production of glucose by enhancing carbohydrate metabolism, promoting gluconeogenesis, and reducing peripheral glucose utilization. The most important glucocorticoid is cortisol. The mineralocorticoids regulate salt and water balance. The primary mineralocorticoid is aldosterone. The androgens are important hormones in regulating sexual maturation and development.

Two diseases typify the disorders associated with the adrenal cortex: Cushing's disease and Addison's disease. Cushing's disease is characterized by hypersecretion of adrenocorticotropic hormone, an anterior pituitary tropic hormone that increases the synthesis of corticoids, leading to excessive glucocorticoid secretion. Common signs and symptoms include hyperglycemia, obesity, hypertension, and electrolyte imbalances. Addison's disease is characterized by hyposecretion of corticoids as a result of damage to the adrenal gland. Common signs and symptoms include hypoglycemia, emaciation, hypotension, hyperkalemia, and hyponatremia.

Treatment of Cushing's disease is typically surgical. Symptomatic pharmacological intervention with an antihypertensive (potassium-sparing diuretics such as spironolactone [Aldactone] or ACE inhibitors such as captopril [Capoten]) may be necessary. Drugs that may inhibit the synthesis of corticosteroids (antiadrenals) may also be used as an adjunct to surgery or radiation. In high doses, the antifungal agent ketoconazole (Nizoral) is an effective temporary antiadrenal drug. At such doses, however, it may cause liver dysfunction.

Treatment of Addison's disease is aimed at replacement therapy. Cortisone (Cortistan) and hydrocortisone (Solu-Cortef) are the drugs of choice. Occasionally, a specific mineralocorticoid is necessary. Fludrocortisone (Florinef Acetate) is the only mineralocorticoid available.[28]

Drugs Affecting the Pancreas

Diabetes mellitus is the most important disease involving the pancreas. Diabetes mellitus (as opposed to diabetes insipidus, which involves inadequate ADH secretion) involves inappropriate carbohydrate metabolism. Traditionally, the term *diabetes* used alone refers to diabetes mellitus, of which the two main types are, logically, type 1 and type 2. Type 1 diabetes is also known as insulin-dependent diabetes mellitus, or IDDM. It results from an inadequate release of insulin from the beta cells of the pancreatic islets. Patients with type 1 diabetes rely on insulin replacement therapy to survive. Because IDDM typically manifests itself at an early age (usually before 30 years), it is also commonly called juvenile onset diabetes. Most diabetics have type 2 diabetes, which is also referred to as non–insulin-dependent diabetes mellitus (NIDDM) or adult onset diabetes. It results from a decreased responsiveness to insulin and a lack of synchronization between insulin release and blood glucose levels. Type 2 diabetes typically

begins later in life (after age 40) and almost always occurs in patients with obesity. Because they have functioning beta cells that release insulin, type 2 diabetics usually do not depend on insulin replacement. Gestational diabetes, a third type, occurs transitionally during pregnancy. Gestational diabetes is a form of stress-induced diabetes in which the mother cannot effectively manage her blood glucose levels during pregnancy without medical intervention. Gestational diabetes resolves itself within hours to days after delivery.

The two main substances involved with regulating blood glucose are insulin and glucagon. Both are secreted from the pancreas and both are used to manage diabetes. Secreted from the beta cells of the pancreatic islets of Langerhans in response to increased blood glucose levels, **insulin** increases cellular transport of glucose, potassium, and amino acids. It also converts glucose into glycogen for storage in the liver and in skeletal muscle. Finally, insulin promotes cell growth and division.

Glucagon, too, is secreted from the pancreatic islets, but by alpha cells rather than by the insulin-producing beta cells. Glucagon's actions are the direct opposite of insulin's; it increases both glycogenolysis (glycogen breakdown into glucose) and gluconeogenesis (the synthesis of glucose from glycerol and amino acids). Thus, while insulin decreases blood glucose levels, glucagon increases them.

Patients with either type 1 or type 2 diabetes may experience both hyperglycemia and hypoglycemia. Hyperglycemia more often results from the disease, but hypoglycemia is a common side effect of treatment. The main intervention for patients with type 1 diabetes is insulin replacement therapy. Several insulin preparations are available. The most effective therapy for patients with type 2 diabetes is usually weight loss through diet modification and exercise. When this is not effective, oral hypoglycemic agents (e.g., metformin [Glucophage]) and, occasionally, insulin are used. Finally, glucagon and diazoxide (both can be considered hyperglycemic agents) are occasionally used for treating emergency hypoglycemia.

INSULIN PREPARATIONS Insulin comes from one of three sources. Initially, it came from either beef or pork intestines. Now, recombinant DNA technology has made human insulin available (that is, insulin synthesized with a human RNA template, not harvested directly from humans). Insulin preparations differ primarily in their onset and duration of action and in their incidence of allergic reaction. Insulin preparations may be short acting, intermediate acting, or long acting, depending on their onset and duration of action. (Table 13-27 lists insulin preparations.)

Insulin is also classified as natural (regular) or modified. As their name suggests, the natural insulins are used as they occur in nature. The other insulin preparations have been modified to increase their duration of action and

Table 13-27 Insulin Preparations

Classification	Trade Name	Source	Onset (Hrs)	Peak (Hrs)	Duration (Hrs)
Rapid-acting			0.25+	<0.75–2.5	3.5–5.0
Lispro Insulin	Humalog	Human			
Aspart Insulin	NovoRapid	Human			
Short-acting or regular	Humulin R	Human	0.5–10	2.0–5.0	5.0–8.0
	Novolin R	Human			
	Iletin II R	Pork			
Intermediate-acting or NPH	Humulin N	Human	1–2	4–12	14–18
	Novolin N	Human			
	Iletin II NPH	Pork			
Premixed	Humulin 70/30	Human	0.5–1.0	2–12	14–18
	Humulin 50/50	Human			
	Novolin 70/30	Human			
	Novolin 50/50	Human			
Intermediate-acting	Humulin L	Human	2–4	7–15	12–24
	Iletin II Lente	Pork			
Long-acting	Humulin U	Human	3–4	8–24	24–28
	Ultralente				
Insulin Glargine	Lantus	Human	>1.5	No peak	>20

thus decrease the frequency of their administration. All insulin preparations are given subcutaneously, with the exception of regular insulin, which may also be given intravenously. Insulin is not available as an oral medication because the digestive enzymes would rapidly render it inactive; therefore, IDDM patients must take multiple injections every day of their lives. This may discourage compliance in some patients.

The modified insulin preparations include NPH (neutral protamine Hagedorn) insulin, which is regular insulin attached to a large protein designed to delay absorption, and the Lente series, which is attached to zinc. Two preparations of Lente insulin are available by themselves, Lente and Ultralente. A third, Semilente insulin, is available only in a combination product with other insulins.

Insulin preparations are used for lifelong replacement therapy in IDDM and for emergency treatment of hyperglycemia and hyperkalemia in nondiabetics. (Recall that insulin also increases potassium uptake by cells and is therefore useful in lowering potassium levels.) These preparations' primary side effect is unintended hypoglycemia. Because β_2 adrenergic blockers can hide the effects of hypoglycemia, patients may not recognize this condition's signs until they cannot care for themselves. Also, beta-blockers decrease the release of glucagon, so these patients' hypoglycemia may be even worse. Insulin preparations derived from beef or pork, as well as the Lentes, may lead to allergic reactions. The natural human insulin preparations do not have this effect.

ORAL HYPOGLYCEMIC AGENTS   Oral hypoglycemic agents are used to stimulate insulin secretion from the pancreas in patients with NIDDM. These agents are ineffective in people with type 1 diabetes because those patients cannot secrete insulin. This functional class comprises four pharmacological classes: sulfonylureas, biguanides, alpha-glucosidase inhibitors, and thiazolidinediones. The sulfonylureas were the first class of oral hypoglycemics available and as such are also known as first-generation or second-generation oral hypoglycemics, depending on when they were released. Drugs in this class include tolbutamide (Orinase), chlorpropamide (Diabinese), glipizide (Glucotrol), and glyburide (Micronase). They work by increasing insulin secretion from the pancreas and may also increase tissue response to insulin. Their major side effect is hypoglycemia.

The only agent in the biguanide class is metformin (Glucophage). It decreases glucose synthesis and increases glucose uptake. It does not stimulate the release of insulin from the pancreas and therefore does not cause hypoglycemia. Its primary side effects are nausea, vomiting, and decreased appetite.

Alpha-glucosidase inhibitors include acarbose (Precose) and miglitol (Glyset). They work by delaying carbohydrate metabolism, which moderates the increase in blood glucose that occurs after meals. These agents' primary side effects are flatulence, cramps, diarrhea, and abdominal distention resulting from colonic bacteria feeding on the increased number of carbohydrates remaining in fecal matter.

Thiazolidinediones are a new class of oral hypoglycemic agents unrelated to the others. The only drug in this class is troglitazone (Rezulin). It works by promoting tissue response to insulin and thus making the available insulin more effective. Troglitazone has no major side effects.

HYPERGLYCEMIC AGENTS   Two hyperglycemic agents, glucagon and diazoxide (Proglycem), act to increase blood glucose levels. Glucagon is indicated for the emergency treatment of patients with hypoglycemia. It will frequently be given intramuscularly to hypoglycemic patients in whom an IV line is unobtainable. Occasional side effects are nausea and vomiting and, rarely, allergic reactions. Diazoxide (Proglycem) inhibits insulin release and is typically used only for patients with hyperinsulin secretion resulting from pancreatic tumors; it is more commonly used for hypertension. It is not indicated for treating diabetes-induced hypoglycemia.

$D_{50}W$ (50 percent dextrose in water) is a sugar solution given intravenously for acute hypoglycemia. Its primary side effect is local tissue necrosis if infiltration occurs. Many EMS systems have transitioned from $D_{50}W$ to $D_{10}W$ (10 percent dextrose in water). $D_{10}W$ is less expensive and equally effective. Furthermore, it causes less persistent hyperglycemia following administration. It is less hypertonic than $D_{50}W$ and that decreases the likelihood of tissue damage if the solution extravasates.

Drugs Affecting the Female Reproductive System

The main groups of drugs affecting the female reproductive system are estrogens, progestins, oral contraceptives, drugs affecting uterine contraction, and those used to treat infertility.

ESTROGENS AND PROGESTINS   Estrogens are produced in females by the ovaries and the ovarian follicles, and in pregnancy, the placenta. Outside of pregnancy, the ovaries are the principal source of estrogens. The principal ovarian estrogen is estradiol, of which there are many commercial preparations. The principal indication for estrogen is replacement therapy in postmenopausal women. After menopause, estrogen levels drop significantly and have been indicated as the cause of menopausal symptoms such as hot flashes and vaginal dryness and as an increased risk factor for osteoporosis. Hormone replacement therapy (HRT) with estrogen has been shown to alleviate menopausal symptoms and reverse the increased risk for osteoporosis; however, it is not without its own risks. Recent studies have shown increased chances of breast cancer and stroke associated with hormone replacement therapy. Side effects include nausea, fluid retention, and breast tenderness. The nausea usually diminishes after several months of therapy. Estrogen is also administered in cases of delayed puberty in girls as a result of hypogonadism.

The progestins' principal noncontraceptive use is to counteract the untoward effects of estrogen on the endometrium in hormone replacement therapy for postmenopausal women. They are also used to treat amenorrhea, endometriosis, and dysfunctional uterine bleeding.

ORAL CONTRACEPTIVES   Oral contraception is an effective means of preventing pregnancy. All oral contraceptives' primary mechanism of action is the prevention of ovulation, which makes the endometrium less favorable for implantation and promotes the development of a thick mucus plug that blocks access to sperm through the cervix. These contraceptives are either a combination of estrogen and progestin or, in the case of "mini-pills," progestin only. They may also be classified based on their administration cycle as monophasic, biphasic, or triphasic. These classes differ in how they alter the dose of estrogen or progestin throughout the menstrual cycle. Many different preparations are available, although they all work in similar fashion. In general, these drugs are well tolerated and have few side effects. The oral contraceptives' chief side effects are unintended pregnancy (in less than 3 percent of users), thromboembolism (this risk is much lower with the newer low-estrogen dose preparations), hypertension, and abnormal uterine bleeding. They are in wide use and are one of the most widely prescribed drug classes. They are the second most popular means of birth control after surgical sterilization (male and female combined).

UTERINE STIMULANTS AND RELAXANTS   Drugs that increase uterine contraction (uterine stimulants) are oxytocics (oxytocin means rapid birth). Drugs that relax the uterus or inhibit uterine contraction are tocolytics.

The primary indications for administration of an oxytocic are to induce labor and to treat severe postpartum hemorrhage. Oxytocin is available commercially as Pitocin and Syntocinon. The uterus becomes increasingly sensitive to oxytocin throughout gestation, progressing from relatively insensitive before pregnancy to very sensitive around the time of labor. Oxytocin's chief side effect, water retention, is rarely significant and only so if large volumes of fluid have been administered without careful ongoing assessment. Ergonovine (Ergotrate), a derivative of a rye fungus, is a powerful uterine stimulant. It increases both the force and duration of contraction. Because of this increased duration, ergonovine is only used in the treatment of postpartum hemorrhage.

The tocolytics relax uterine smooth muscle by stimulating the β_2 receptors in the uterus. The two β_2 agonists commonly used for this purpose are terbutaline (Brethine) and ritodrine (Yutopar). Terbutaline's primary use is to treat asthma, but it is commonly used to delay labor even though the FDA does not currently approve it for that purpose. Both agents decrease both the force and frequency of contraction. Their chief side effects are the same as those of the other beta$_2$ agonists used to treat asthma: tremors and tachycardia. Occasionally, hyperglycemia may result from glycogenolysis in the liver.

INFERTILITY AGENTS A number of conditions may cause infertility, which is the inability to become pregnant, and medications can treat only some of them. Most infertility drugs are developed for women and promote maturation of ovarian follicles. Clomiphene (Clomid), urofollitropin (Metrodin), and menotropins (Pergonal) are all within this class, although each of them acts by a different mechanism. These agents' side effects include ovarian enlargement or cysts, abdominal pain, and menstrual irregularities.

Drugs Affecting the Male Reproductive System

Drugs that affect the male reproductive system include those that treat testosterone deficiency and benign prostatic hyperplasia. Testosterone replacement therapy may be indicated in testosterone deficiency caused by cryptorchidism (failure of one or both of the testes to descend during puberty), orchitis (testicular inflammation), or orchidectomy (testicular removal). It is also used in delayed puberty. Preparations include testosterone enanthate, methyltestosterone (Metandren), and fluoxymesterone (Halotestin).

Benign prostatic hyperplasia is an enlarged prostate. This is a common but problematic age-related disease. By the age of 70, close to 75 percent of men will have symptoms severe enough to seek therapy. These symptoms may include urinary hesitancy and retention. Treatment has traditionally been surgery, but several drugs are available, including finasteride (Proscar), which interferes with the production of an enzyme involved with prostate growth. Side effects may include rash, breast tenderness, headache, impotence, and decreased libido.

Drugs Affecting Sexual Behavior

For centuries, cultures have searched for drugs that would increase libido and sexual potency. Ironically, the reverse has most commonly been found. The largest category of drugs affecting sexual behavior do so as a side effect of their intended purpose. Many drug classifications decrease libido in both sexes and inhibit erection and ejaculation. Examples include antihypertensives (beta-blockers, centrally acting alpha antagonists, and diuretics) and antianxiety/antipsychotic medications (benzodiazepines, phenothiazines, MAO inhibitors, and tricyclic antidepressants).

Many drugs are purported to increase libido. The most notable of these is cantharis (Spanish fly). Despite common belief, no evidence indicates that cantharis actually increases sexual appetite. Indeed, it can produce some very dangerous side effects. Hallucinogens such as LSD and marijuana, as well as alcohol, are also commonly believed to heighten sexuality. Any such effect from these agents is likely an indirect result of decreased inhibitions or anxiety. These drugs all have very different effects, depending on each individual's unique physiology, expectations before use, and surrounding circumstances. They have no proven direct physiologic effect on sexual gratification.

Levodopa (L-dopa), an anti-Parkinson's drug, has demonstrated increased libido and improved erectile ability as a side effect of treatment. Whether this results directly from increased autonomic stimulation or indirectly from improved self-esteem achieved in therapy, any improvement seems to be only temporary. Several drugs have been developed that aid in erectile dysfunction. Erectile dysfunction becomes more frequent with age or with certain diseases such as diabetes or cardiovascular disease. Drugs that aid in erectile dysfunction increase blood supply to the penis. These include sildenafil (Viagra), vardenafil (Levitra), and tadalafil (Cialis). These drugs act by relaxing vascular smooth muscle, which increases blood flow to the corpus cavernosum, the spongelike tissue on the sides of the penis responsible for erection. These drugs are unique in that they have no effect in the absence of sexual stimulation. Other drugs used to treat impotence have caused prolonged and painful erections (priapism). The chief side effect of sildenafil is seen when it is used in combination with nitrates. The combined effect of relaxing vascular smooth muscle may lead to a dangerously decreased preload, which may lower blood pressure and lead to myocardial infarction. Prehospital personnel should be aware of this important interaction.

If you are called on to treat a patient with chest pain who has taken sildenafil, vardenafil, or tadalafil recently, do not give him nitroglycerin or any other nitrate. Table 13-28 details hormones and related agents.

Drugs Used to Treat Cancer

Drugs used to treat cancer are called **antineoplastic agents**. A detailed discussion of the many different antineoplastic agents is beyond the scope of this text; however, this section briefly overviews their main classes and prototype drugs.

Cancer involves the modification of cellular DNA leading to an abnormal growth of tissues. Of the many known types of cancer, only a few are successfully treated with chemotherapy. In fact, most cancers are best treated by surgical removal of the tumor. Unfortunately, many of the more lethal cancers do not involve a compact growth; rather, they affect the formed elements of the blood, especially leukocytes. Treating these widely dispersed cancers

Table 13-28 Hormones and Related Agents

Name	Classification	Action	Indications	Contraindications	Doses	Routes	Adverse Effects	Other
Vasopressin *Pitressin*	Hormone (analog of antidiuretic hormone)	Non-adrenergic vasoconstrictor; promotes fluid retention in the kidney	• Normovolemic hypotension	• Few in the emergency setting	40 units	IV	• Blanching of the skin • Abdominal cramping • Nausea • Hypertension	• Benefits in cardiac arrest are questionable.
Oxytocin *Pitocin*	Hormone (oxytocin)	Oxytocic; causes uterine contractions and lactations	• Postpartum vaginal bleeding • Induction/augmentation of labor	• Anything other than postpartum bleeding (in the prehospital setting)	10–20 units in 500 mL IV; 3–10 units (IM)	IV, IM	• Anaphylaxis • Arrhythmias	• Ensure placenta (and possible additional baby) has delivered before administering.
Glucagon	Hormone (glucagon)	Elevates blood glucose levels through conversion of glycogen to glucose and other factors	• Hypoglycemia • Beta-blocker overdose	• Hypersensitivity to the drug	0.25–0.5 units (IV); 1.0 mg IM	IV, IM, IO	• Few in the emergency setting	• Less effective in patients with decreased glycogen stores (e.g., alcoholics).
Insulin *Humulin, NovoLog, Novolin*	Hormone (insulin)	Causes glucose uptake by the cells thus lowering blood glucose levels	• Diabetes • Hyperglycemia • Diabetic ketoacidosis	• Hypoglycemia • Normoglycemia	Varies	IV, SQ	• Few in the emergency setting	• Dosages of the various insulin types vary significantly.
Dextrose, 50%	Carbohydrate	Substrate for carbohydrate metabolism	• Hypoglycemia	• None in the emergency setting	12.5–25.0 g	IV, PO	• Local venous irritation common • Tissue injury	• Less concentrated solutions (e.g., 10%) equally effective with fewer side effects.
Dextrose, 10%	Carbohydrate	Substrate for carbohydrate metabolism	• Hypoglycemia	• None in the emergency setting	100 mL	IV, IO	• Local venous irritation common • Tissue injury	• Preferred over D$_{50}$W due to improved safety profile and cost.
Methylprednisolone	Hormone (analog of corticosteroid)	Anti-inflammatory; suppresses immune response	• Asthma • COPD • Anaphylaxis	• Hypersensitivity to the drug	125–250 mg	IV, IO	• GI bleeding • Increases blood glucose levels	• Effects are delayed and not typically seen in the prehospital setting.

with surgery is not possible, as there is nothing for the surgeon to remove.

Chemotherapy is not nearly as safe or devoid of side effects as antibiotic therapy; however, scientists have yet to identify any unique characteristics of cancer cells that would allow them to develop drugs specific to those cells. Because cancer is the abnormal growth of normal cells, drugs that kill cancerous cells therefore also kill noncancerous cells. Chemotherapy is thus largely a balancing act aimed at maximizing the kill rate of cancer cells while minimizing the death of normal tissue. The one characteristic that most cancer cells share is rapid cell division and replication. Consequently, most antineoplastic agents have their greatest effect on cancer cells during mitosis and on young, small cancers that are undergoing rapid growth.

The agents used to kill cancer cells are grouped according to their mechanism of action. Antimetabolite drugs mimic some of the enzymes and proteins needed for DNA replication but do not have the same effects; therefore, they prevent cells from reproducing. Their prototype is fluorouracil (Adrucil). Alkylating agents that interfere with DNA splitting include cyclophosphamide (Cytoxan) and mechlorethamine (Mustargen). Mitotic inhibitors also interfere with cell division; they include vinblastine (Velban) and vincristine (Oncovin).

Chemotherapy's primary side effects include nausea, vomiting, and other gastrointestinal disturbances, as well as hair loss and weakness. Almost all antineoplastic agents cause severe side effects and are given in conjunction with antiemetics.

Drugs Used to Treat Infectious Diseases and Inflammation

Infectious diseases are typically caused by bacteria, viruses, or funguses and may be treated with antimicrobial drugs developed to fight those particular invaders. We discuss each broad class here.

ANTIBIOTICS   An **antibiotic** agent may either kill the offending bacteria (bactericidal agents) or so decrease the bacteria's growth that the patient's immune system can effectively fight the infection (bacteriostatic agents). In general, all these agents share one of several mechanisms. Drugs in the penicillin and cephalosporin classes, as well as vancomycin (Vancocin), are bactericidal and act by inhibiting cell wall synthesis. Unlike animal cells, bacteria have hypertonic cell cytoplasm and depend on the rigid and relatively impermeable cell wall to maintain integrity. When cell wall synthesis is inhibited, osmotic pressure pulls water into the cell, and the cell ruptures, killing the bacteria. The

macrolide, aminoglycoside, and tetracycline antibiotics inhibit protein synthesis, preventing the bacterial cell from replicating and thus spreading infection. These agents are usually bacteriostatic but can be bactericidal at high doses. Typical side effects from antibiotics include gastrointestinal dysfunction, which commonly results from a decrease in the natural gastrointestinal bacteria that inhabit the colon.

Patho Pearls

Antibiotic Resistance. The misuse and overuse of antibiotics have contributed to a phenomenon known as *antibiotic resistance*. This resistance develops when potentially harmful bacteria change in a way that reduces or eliminates the effectiveness of antibiotics. Stated another way, the bacteria are "resistant" and continue to multiply in the presence of therapeutic levels of an antibiotic. It is estimated that each year at least two million people in the United States become infected with bacteria that are resistant to antibiotics and at least 23,000 people die each year as a direct result of these infections. Antibiotics are effective only in the treatment of bacterial infections. Most common infections are viral and antibiotics are of no benefit. Patients and health care professionals alike can play an important role in combating antibiotic resistance. Patients should not demand antibiotics when a health care professional says the drugs are not needed. Health care professionals should prescribe antibiotics only for infections they believe to be caused by bacteria.

ANTIFUNGAL AND ANTIVIRAL AGENTS   Fungi are parasitic microorganisms that cannot synthesize their own food. Fungal infections (mycoses) may be treated with several drugs. The azole antifungals inhibit fungal growth. Their prototype is ketoconazole (Nizoral). Drugs used to treat viruses work by a variety of mechanisms and include acyclovir (Zovirax) and zidovudine (Retrovir), which is commonly known as AZT. Protease inhibitors are one of the more promising classes of drugs for treating viruses such as HIV. Indinavir (Crixivan) is the prototype of this class.

OTHER ANTIMICROBIAL AND ANTIPARASITIC AGENTS   Although most diseases treated with the medications discussed in this section are uncommon in developed countries, they are leading causes of death in third-world countries. They include malaria, tuberculosis, leprosy, amebiasis, and helminthiasis. Tuberculosis is increasingly appearing in the United States in patients with compromised immune systems.

Malaria is a parasitic infection common in the tropics. It is transmitted by certain types of mosquitoes or, less commonly, by blood transfusion. Drugs used to treat malaria are called schizonticides. They include chloroquine (Aralen), mefloquine (Lariam), and quinine. Treatment is aimed at either preventing infestation (prophylactic treatment for individuals traveling to high-risk areas) or killing the parasites in infected patients.

Tuberculosis is caused by bacteria that are transmitted through airborne droplets from the coughing and sneezing of infected patients. The bacteria can grow only in well-oxygenated areas. Because of the route of infection and the need for oxygen, most patients with tuberculosis have infestations in the lungs. Once in the lungs, the bacteria are typically "walled off," or enclosed in tubercules, and become dormant and noninfective. If the patient's immune system is compromised, the bacteria may become active again and begin to cause symptoms. Drugs commonly used to treat tuberculosis include isoniazid (Nydrazid, INH) and rifampin (Rifadin).

Amebiasis is a parasitic infection of the intestines common in tropical areas. Transmission most frequently occurs via the oral–fecal route from eating poorly cooked food contaminated by cooks who wash their hands inadequately. Drugs used to treat amebiasis include paromomycin (Humatin) and metronidazole (Flagyl).

Helminthiasis is caused by parasitic worms (helminths), including flatworms and roundworms. These worms usually invade the host's intestinal tract and attach themselves to the lumen wall with hooks or suckers. They cause symptoms by depriving the host of nutrients (especially in children); by obstructing the intestinal lumen, which leads to bowel obstruction; and by producing toxins. Treatment is aimed at either killing the organism outright or destroying its ability to latch onto the intestinal wall so it passes with the patient's feces. These drugs include mebendazole (Vermox) and niclosamide (Niclocide).

Leprosy, also known as Hansen's disease, is caused by bacteria. It leads to characteristic lesions, foot drop (plantar flexion), and plantar ulceration. Drugs used to treat it include dapsone (DDS, Avlosulfon) and clofazimine (Lamprene).

NONSTEROIDAL ANTI-INFLAMMATORY DRUGS
NSAIDs (nonsteroidal anti-inflammatory drugs) are commonly used as analgesics and antipyretics (fever reducers). Many, including acetaminophen and ibuprofen, are available over the counter. As a group, these agents interfere with the production of prostaglandins, thereby interrupting the inflammatory process. NSAIDs are indicated for the relief of pain, fever, and inflammation associated with common headache, arthritis, dysmenorrhea, and orthopedic injuries. They are also commonly prescribed to relieve pain following trauma and surgery. Other NSAIDs include ketorolac (Toradol), piroxicam (Feldene), and naproxen (Naprosyn).

URICOSURIC DRUGS
Uricosuric drugs are used to treat and prevent acute episodes of gout. Gout is an inflammatory disease caused by an altered metabolism of uric acid and marked by hyperuricemia (high levels of uric acid in the blood). It may present with acute episodes characterized by pain and swelling of joints. Left untreated, gout may lead to crystal deposits in various parts of the body that can cause kidney stones, nephritis, and atherosclerosis. Drugs used to treat gout include colchicine and allopurinol (Zyloprim).

SERUMS, VACCINES, AND OTHER IMMUNIZING AGENTS
The human body has a complex series of systems that help prevent disease. The most important of these are the anatomic barriers such as the skin and mucous membranes that block the entrance of **pathogens** (disease-causing organisms, including viruses and bacteria). If pathogens get past these protective barriers, our immune system comes into play. This system consists of the spleen, lymph nodes, thymus, leukocytes, and proteins called antibodies in plasma. The ability to respond to pathogens is called **immunity**.

Immunity may be acquired passively or actively. It is passively acquired when antibodies pass directly into a person, either through artificial routes such as injection or through natural routes such as the placenta or breast milk. Immunity may also be actively acquired in response to the presence of a pathogen.

Actively acquired immunity occurs when T lymphocytes (a type of leukocyte that becomes specialized in the thymus gland) comes in contact with a new pathogen. The body produces an infinite variety of T cell configurations. When the pathogen comes into contact with a T cell that is specific to it, that T cell begins to reproduce rapidly. Some of these cells become involved in the immune response to the pathogen, whereas others act as "memory" cells. The cells involved in the immune response either directly attack the pathogen (cell-mediated immunity) or activate the complement system, a complex cascade of events that leads to the immune response. The memory cells remain in the body in higher numbers so the next time this specific pathogen enters the body, a much faster response is possible. At the same time, B cells (lymphocytes that differentiate or become more specialized in the body, as opposed to the thymus) that are specific for the invading pathogen begin to produce antibodies for that antigen. This process is called humoral immunity or antibody immunity. When an antibody contacts its specific antigen, it forms a complex that triggers the complement system, leading to the immune response.

Serums and vaccines may augment the immune system. A **serum** is a solution containing whole antibodies for a specific pathogen. The antibodies give the recipient temporary, passive immunity. A **vaccine** contains a modified pathogen that does not actually cause disease but still stimulates the development of antibodies specific to it. These pathogens may be either dead or attenuated (having a decreased disease-causing ability).

The best age for vaccination against disease is within the first two years of life, as the immune system is fairly immature. Table 13-29 summarize the recommended schedule for immunization.

Table 13-29   Recommended Childhood (0–18 Years) Immunization Schedule United States, 2015

Figure 1. Recommended immunization schedule for persons aged 0 through 18 years – United States, 2015.

(FOR THOSE WHO FALL BEHIND OR START LATE, SEE THE CATCH-UP SCHEDULE (FIGURE 2)).

These recommendations must be read with the footnotes that follow. For those who fall behind or start late, provide catch-up vaccination at the earliest opportunity as indicated by the green bars in Figure 1. To determine minimum intervals between doses, see the catch-up schedule (Figure 2). School entry and adolescent vaccine age groups are shaded.

Vaccine	Birth	1 mo	2 mos	4 mos	6 mos	9 mos	12 mos	15 mos	18 mos	19–23 mos	2–3 yrs	4–6 yrs	7–10 yrs	11–12 yrs	13–15 yrs	16–18 yrs
Hepatitis B[1] (HepB)	1st dose	←2nd dose→			←——— 3rd dose ———→											
Rotavirus[2] (RV) RV1 (2-dose series); RV5 (3-dose series)			1st dose	2nd dose	See footnote 2											
Diphtheria, tetanus, & acellular pertussis[3] (DTaP: <7 yrs)			1st dose	2nd dose	3rd dose			←— 4th dose —→				5th dose				
Tetanus, diphtheria, & acellular pertussis[4] (Tdap: ≥7 yrs)														(Tdap)		
Haemophilus influenzae type b[5] (Hib)			1st dose	2nd dose	See footnote 5		3rd or 4th dose, See footnote 5									
Pneumococcal conjugate[6] (PCV13)			1st dose	2nd dose	3rd dose		←— 4th dose —→									
Pneumococcal polysaccharide[6] (PPSV23)																
Inactivated poliovirus[7] (IPV: <18 yrs)			1st dose	2nd dose	←——— 3rd dose ———→							4th dose				
Influenza[8] (IIV; LAIV) 2 doses for some: See footnote 8					Annual vaccination (IIV only) 1 or 2 doses						Annual vaccination (LAIV or IIV) 1 or 2 doses		Annual vaccination (LAIV or IIV) 1 dose only			
Measles, mumps, rubella[9] (MMR)					See footnote 9		←— 1st dose —→					2nd dose				
Varicella[10] (VAR)							←— 1st dose —→					2nd dose				
Hepatitis A[11] (HepA)							←— 2-dose series, See footnote 11 —→									
Human papillomavirus[12] (HPV2: females only; HPV4: males and females)														(3-dose series)		
Meningococcal[13] (Hib-MenCY ≥6 weeks; MenACWY-D ≥9 mos; MenACWY-CRM ≥2 mos)							See footnote 13							1st dose		Booster

Legend:
- Range of recommended ages for all children
- Range of recommended ages for catch-up immunization
- Range of recommended ages during which catch-up is encouraged and for certain high-risk groups
- Range of recommended ages for certain high-risk groups
- Not routinely recommended

This schedule includes recommendations in effect as of January 1, 2015. Any dose not administered at the recommended age should be administered at a subsequent visit, when indicated and feasible. The use of a combination vaccine generally is preferred over separate injections of its equivalent component vaccines. Vaccination providers should consult the relevant Advisory Committee on Immunization Practices (ACIP) statement for detailed recommendations, available online at http://www.cdc.gov/vaccines/hcp/acip-recs/index.html. Clinically significant adverse events that follow vaccination should be reported to the Vaccine Adverse Event Reporting System (VAERS) online (http://www.vaers.hhs.gov) or by telephone (800-822-7967). Suspected cases of vaccine-preventable diseases should be reported to the state or local health department. Additional information, including precautions and contraindications for vaccination, is available from CDC online (http://www.cdc.gov/vaccines/recs/vac-admin/contraindications.htm) or by telephone (800-CDC-INFO [800-232-4636]).

This schedule is approved by the Advisory Committee on Immunization Practices (http://www.cdc.gov/vaccines/acip), the American Academy of Pediatrics (http://www.aap.org), the American Academy of Family Physicians (http://www.aafp.org), and the American College of Obstetricians and Gynecologists (http://www.acog.org).

NOTE: The above recommendations must be read along with the footnotes of this schedule.

Note: This schedule plus the catch-up schedule for those who fall behind or start late and the accompanying footnotes can be found at http://www.cdc.gov/vaccines/schedules/downloads/child/0-18yrs-child-combined-schedule.pdf

IMMUNE SUPPRESSING AND ENHANCING AGENTS
Available drugs can either suppress the immune system (immunosuppressants) or enhance it (immunomodulators). Suppressing the immune system is indicated to prevent the rejection of transplanted organs and grafted skin. Azathioprine (Imuran) is a commonly used immunosuppressant that acts by decreasing cell-mediated reactions and suppressing antibody production.

Immunomodulating agents enhance the natural immune reaction in immunosuppressed patients such as those with HIV. Zidovudine (Retrovir), commonly known as AZT, and several protease inhibitors such as ritonavir (Norvir) and saquinavir (Invirase) are examples of these agents.

Drugs Used to Affect the Skin

Dermatologic drugs are used to treat skin irritations. They are common over-the-counter medications. The many different general preparations include baths, soaps, solutions, cleansers, emollients (Lubriderm, Vaseline), skin protectants (Benzoin), wet dressings or soaks (Domeboro Powder), and rubs and liniments (Ben-Gay, Icy Hot). Prophylactic agents such as sunscreens are also available to help prevent skin disease and irritation.

Drugs Used to Supplement the Diet

Many disease processes affect the production, distribution, and utilization of essential dietary nutrients. Additionally, the body's intricate balance of fluid (including specific amounts of electrolytes) is a vital component of maintaining homeostasis. Dietary supplements can help to maintain needed levels of these essential nutrients and fluids.

Vitamins and Minerals

Vitamins are organic compounds necessary for many different physiologic processes, including metabolism, growth, development, and tissue repair. The body absorbs most vitamins through the gastrointestinal tract following dietary ingestion. Vitamins must be obtained from the diet, as the body cannot manufacture them. In developed countries, healthy adults usually receive adequate amounts of vitamins and do not need supplements. Vitamin supplements may, however, be indicated for special populations, including pregnant and nursing women, patients with absorption disorders, the chronically ill, surgery patients,

alcoholics, and the malnourished. Additionally, people on a strict vegetarian or vegan diet may need supplemental vitamins. Vitamins are either fat soluble or water soluble. The liver stores the fat-soluble vitamins (A, D, E, and K), so the patient will become deficient only after long periods of inadequate vitamin intake. Vitamin D is unique in that the skin produces it with exposure to sunlight. The water-soluble vitamins (C and those in the B complex) must be routinely ingested, as the body does not store them. After short periods of deprivation, patients may begin to experience vitamin deficiency. The B complex vitamins are grouped only because they occur together in foods; otherwise, they share no significant characteristics. The individual B vitamins are named for the order in which they were discovered (B_1, B_2, B_3, and so forth). These vitamins also have specific names. For example, B_1 is also known as thiamine, a vitamin that plays a key role in carbohydrate metabolism. It was once commonly administered in the prehospital setting for presumed Wernicke's encephalopathy (a disease commonly seen in chronic alcoholics that results from a deficiency in thiamine).[30] However, it has been determined that delaying administration to the hospital setting saves money and is just as effective. Table 13-30 details selected vitamins.

Iron is an essential mineral necessary for oxygen transport and several metabolic processes. Iron supplements are the most common mineral supplement. They are indicated for iron deficiency.

Fluids and Electrolytes

Water comprises approximately 60 percent of a person's total body weight. The specific composition and amounts of this fluid are vital to a patient's well-being. The specific amounts of electrolytes such as calcium, potassium, sodium, and chlorine are similarly important. The chapter "Pathophysiology" reviews the physiology of fluids and electrolytes and discusses acid–base balance. The indications and contraindications for administering fluids and electrolytes, as well as these medications' interactions, are covered in the chapters titled "Intravenous Access and Medication Administration" and "Hemorrhage and Shock."

Drugs Used to Treat Poisoning and Overdoses

The treatment for poisoning and overdose depends greatly on the substance involved. In general, therapy aims at eliminating the substance by emptying the gastric contents, by increasing gastric motility to decrease the time available for absorption, by alkalinizing the urine with sodium bicarbonate (for tricyclic antidepressant and salicylate overdose), or by filtering the substance from the

Table 13-30   Vitamin Sources and Deficiencies

Vitamin	Problems Resulting from Deficiency	Source
Fat Soluble		
A	Night blindness, skin lesions	Butter, yellow fruit, green leafy vegetables, milk
D	Bone and muscle pain, weakness, softening of bones	Fish, fortified milk, exposure to sunlight
E	Hyporeflexia, ataxia, anemia	Nuts, green leafy vegetables, wheat
K	Increased bleeding	Liver, green leafy vegetables
Water Soluble		
B_1 (thiamine)	Peripheral neuritis, depression, anorexia, poor memory	Whole grain, beef, pork, peas, beans, nuts
B_2 (riboflavin)	Sore throat, stomatitis, painful or swollen tongue, anemia	Milk, eggs, cheese, green leafy vegetables
B_3 (niacin)	Skin eruptions, diarrhea, enteritis, headache, dizziness, insomnia	Meat, eggs, milk
B_6 (pyridoxine)	Skin lesions, seizures, peripheral neuritis	Liver, meats, eggs, vegetables
B_9 (folic acid)	Megaloblastic anemia	Liver, fresh green vegetables, yeast
B_{12} (cyanocobalamin)	Irreversible nervous system damage, pernicious anemia	Fish, egg yolk, milk
C	Scurvy	Citrus fruits, tomatoes, strawberries

blood with dialysis. Activated charcoal may be used as a gastric absorbent.[31]

Actual antidotes are few; however, some medications are effective in treating certain overdoses or poisonings. General mechanisms for antidote action include receptor site antagonism, blocking enzyme actions involved with metabolism of the substance, and chelation (binding the substance with a stable compound such as iron so it becomes inactive). Specific antidotes include acetylcysteine (Mucomyst) for acetaminophen overdose and deferoxamine for iron chelation. Organophosphates are a common ingredient in insecticides and herbicides as well as chemical weapons. They are aggressive acetylcholinesterase (AChE) inhibitors that prevent the breakdown of acetylcholine, leading to overstimulation of the parasympathetic nervous system as well as neuromuscular junctions. Signs and symptoms of this overstimulation may be remembered by the acronym SLUDGE (salivation, lacrimation, urination, defecation, gastric motility, and emesis). Other signs include bradycardia, hypotension, bronchospasm, muscle fasciculations, miosis (pupil constriction), and respiratory arrest. The antidotes for organophosphate poisoning are atropine and pralidoxime (2-PAM, Protopam). Atropine antagonizes ACh, whereas pralidoxime breaks the organophosphate–acetylcholinesterase bond, freeing AChE to break down the excess ACh. Hydroxocobalamin is now available as an antidote for cyanide poisoning. Hydroxocobalamin is a precursor to cyanocobalamin (vitamin B_{12}). When administered, it chelates the cyanide molecule from cytochrome oxidase, thus restoring normal energy production. It has largely replaced the old cyanide antidote kit.[32] See Table 13-31 for common antidotes.

Table 13-31 Common Antidotes

Name	Classification	Action	Indications	Contraindications	Doses	Routes	Adverse Effects	Other
Naloxone *Narcan*	Opiate antagonist	Opioid antagonist without opiate agonist properties (it has no activity when given in the absence of an opiate agonist)	• Partial reversal of opiate drug effects • Opiate overdose	• Hypersensitivity to the drug	0.4–2.0 mg	IV, IO, SQ, IN, nebulizer	• Fever • Chills • Nausea • Vomiting • Diarrhea • Opiate withdrawal	• Administer enough to reverse respiratory depression and avoid full narcotic withdrawal syndrome.
Flumazenil *Romazicon*	Benzodiazepine antagonist	Competitively blocks benzodiazepines at the GABA/benzodiazepine receptor complex	• Benzodiazepine overdose	• Hypersensitivity to the drug	0.2 mg	IV	• Fatigue • Headache • Nervousness • Dizziness	• Administer with caution in patients dependent on benzodiazepines, as life-threatening withdrawal (including seizures) can occur.
Hydroxocobalamin *Cyanokit*	Cyanide antidote	Chelates cyanide from cytochrome oxidase forming cyanocobalamin (vitamin B_{12})	• Cyanide or suspected cyanide poisoning	• None in the emergency setting	5–10 g	IV	• Chromaturia • Red skin • Rash • Hypertension • Nausea • Headache	• Be prepared to continue full resuscitative measures following administration.
Amyl nitrite	Cyanide antidote	Vasodilator; oxidizes hemoglobin to methemoglobin which reacts with cyanide ion to form cyanomethemoglobin, that is enzymatically degraded	• Cyanide poisoning	• None in the emergency setting	1–2 inhalants	Inhaled	• Headache • Weakness • Dizziness • Flushing • Tachycardia • Orthostatic hypotension	• Headache and hypotension common. • Can worsen hypoxia in the setting of carbon monoxide poisoning.
Sodium nitrite	Cyanide antidote	Vasodilator; oxidizes hemoglobin to methemoglobin which reacts with cyanide ion to form cyanomethemoglobin, which is enzymatically degraded	• Cyanide poisoning	• Should not be administered to asymptomatic patients	150–300 mg	IV	• Headache • Weakness • Dizziness • Flushing • Tachycardia • Orthostatic hypotension	• Headache and hypotension common. • Can worsen hypoxia in the setting of carbon monoxide poisoning.
Sodium thiosulfate	Cyanide antidote	Converts cyanide to thiocyanate, which is removed by the kidneys	• Cyanide poisoning	• None in the emergency setting	12.5 g	IV	• Nausea • Vomiting • Joint pain • Psychosis	• Should be administered as part of the standard (Pasadena) cyanide kit.
Pralidoxime *2-PAM, Protpam*	Organophosphate antidote	Reactivates cholinesterase; deactivates certain organophosphates	• Organophosphate poisoning	• Poisonings other than organophosphates	1–2 g over 30 minutes	IV	• Excitement • Manic behavior • Laryngospasm • Tachycardia	• Always protect rescue personnel from the poison. • 2-PAM administration should always follow atropinization.

Summary

Pharmacology is a cornerstone of paramedic practice. Paramedics must have a solid understanding of its foundations (legal issues, terminology, drug forms, and routes), pharmacokinetics, and pharmacodynamics if they are to practice their profession safely. Additionally, paramedics must understand not only the medications they personally administer, but also the medications that their patients are taking on an ongoing basis. You are personally, ethically, and legally responsible for every medication you administer. If medical direction orders you to give a medication or a dosage that is potentially dangerous, it is your responsibility to question and even refuse to administer a harmful medication or dosage.

Even though you are not likely to remember everything in this chapter after your first reading, with diligent study and practice you can master this information. This chapter has barely broken the surface of pharmacology. To continue your education, you should take the time to understand the mechanisms and interactions of the medications your patients are taking. If you do not already know them (you will not, in the majority of cases, as you begin your career), look them up. Many very useful drug references are available today. Most are small and can be easily carried with you on a smart phone, on your unit, or in your station.

Pharmacology is a dynamic field with new discoveries being made every day. Emergency treatments are constantly changing, based on the latest results of pharmacological studies. If you take your responsibilities as a paramedic seriously and practice lifelong learning, remaining current on the latest changes in this field, you can be confident in your ability to give your patients the care they deserve.

You Make the Call

You and your partner are caring for a 62-year-old man with acute pulmonary edema and cardiogenic shock. He is responsive only to painful stimuli, has ashen skin, and is very diaphoretic. He is in obvious respiratory distress, with a rate of 36 per minute. You note bilateral crackles in all fields. His blood pressure is 82/50, and his heart rate is 108. The SpO_2 is 84 percent. The ECG shows atrial fibrillation. You immediately have your partner begin assisting the patient's ventilations with a bag-valve mask and 100 percent high-concentration oxygen. You place a continuous positive airway pressure (CPAP) device set at 5 cm/H_2O. You establish a saline lock and begin to administer a dopamine infusion through one of them at 6 mcg/kg/min and move the patient to your unit for transport to the hospital.

The dopamine appears to be helping, as your patient's blood pressure rises to 110/60; however, your partner is having an increasingly difficult time bagging the patient, whose oxygen saturation has not risen above 86 percent. You decide to perform a facilitated intubation and administer the following medications: 0.5 mg of atropine and 5.0 mg of midazolam (Versed). Your partner administers 1.5 mg/kg of succinylcholine. After placing a size 8.0 ET tube, you confirm placement and secure the tube. Now that the patient is being successfully ventilated, you turn your attention back to the pulmonary edema. As you are delivering your patient to the ED staff, you note that his color and breath sounds have improved remarkably and the pulse oximeter now reads 96 percent.

1. What is dopamine and what is its mechanism of action?

2. What was the purpose of the dopamine infusion?

3. What is atropine's mechanism of action?

4. Why was midazolam administered before succinylcholine?

5. What are succinylcholine's classification and mechanism of action?

See Suggested Responses to "You Make the Call" at the end of this book.

Review Questions

1. The study of drugs and their interactions with the body is called _____
   a. physiology.
   b. toxicology.
   c. pharmacology.
   d. pharmacopeia.

2. A drug or other substance that blocks the actions of the sympathetic nervous system is called

   _____
   a. adrenergic.
   b. sympatholytic.
   c. sympathomimetic.
   d. anticholinergic.

3. Which drug is frequently used in the treatment of pregnancy-induced hypertension?
   a. Coreg
   c. Captopril
   b. Apresoline
   d. Nifedipine

4. Because they can thicken bronchial secretions, you should not use _____ in patients with asthma.
   a. mucolytics
   b. antitussives
   c. antihistamines
   d. antiarrrhythmics

5. The following describes a Schedule _____ drug: High abuse potential; may lead to severe dependence; accepted medical indications.
   a. I
   c. III
   b. II
   d. IV

6. _____is an example of an anticholinergic drug used in the treatment of asthma
   a. Prednisone
   c. Proventil
   b. Atrovent
   d. Beclovent

7. The drug name found in the *United States Pharmacopeia* (USP) is its _____
   a. official name.
   b. chemical name.
   c. generic name.
   d. trade name.

8. The drug name that is derived from a drug's basic molecular structure is referred to as its

   _____
   a. official name.
   b. chemical name.
   c. generic name.
   d. trade name.

9. The proprietary name of a drug, such as Valium, is the same as the _____
   a. official name.
   b. chemical name.
   c. generic name.
   d. trade name.

10. Drug legislation was instituted in 1906 by the

    _____
    a. Narcotics Act.
    b. Cosmetics Act.
    c. Pure Food and Drug Act.
    d. Pharmacology Act.

11. _____ drugs may be similar to those existing in nature, or they may be entirely new medications not found in nature.
    a. Plant
    c. Synthetic
    b. Animal
    d. Mineral

12. The six rights of medication administration include the right _____
    a. dose.
    b. time.
    c. route.
    d. all of the above.

13. In which type of medication route is the drug subject to the "first-pass effect"?
    a. Oral
    c. Subcutaneous
    b. Intramuscular
    d. Intravenous

14. Drugs manufactured in gelatin containers are called

    _____
    a. pills.
    c. capsules.
    b. tablets.
    d. extracts.

15. A drug's pharmacodynamics involves its ability to cause the expected response, or _____
    a. affinity.
    b. efficacy.
    c. side effect.
    d. contraindication.

16. A type of anesthesia that combines decreased sensation of pain with amnesia, while the patient remains conscious, is a(n) _____
    a. opioid.
    b. nonopioid.
    c. anesthetic.
    d. neuroleptanesthesia.

17. _____ agents block the parasympathetic nervous system.

    a. Cholinergic

    b. Adrenergic

    c. Antiadrenergic

    d. Anticholinergic

18. In antiarrhythmic classifications, Class IA drugs include all of the following except

    _____

    a. quinidine.

    b. lidocaine.

    c. procainamide.

    d. disopyramide.

19. One of aspirin's primary side effects is _____

    a. stasis.

    b. bleeding.

    c. headache.

    d. seizures.

20. _____ are mediators released from mast cells on contact with allergens, and contribute to the inflammation response of the immune system.

    a. BNP modulators

    b. Leukotrienes

    c. Glucocorticoids

    d. Methylxanthines

See Answers to Review Questions at the end of this book.

References

1. Olasveengen, T. M., K. Sunde, C. Brunborg, J. Thowsen, P. A. Steen, and L. Wik. "Intravenous Drug Administration during Out-of-Hospital Cardiac Arrest: A Randomized Trial." *JAMA* 302 (2009): 2222–2229.

2. Niemann, J. T., S. J. Stratton, B. Cruz, and R. J. Lewis. "Endotracheal Drug Administration during Out-of-Hospital Resuscitation: Where Are the Survivors?" *Resuscitation* 53 (2002): 153–157.

3. Fowler, R., J. V. Gallagher, S. M. Isaacs, E. Ossman, P. Pepe, and M. Wayne. "The Role of Intraosseous Vascular Access in the Out-of-Hospital Environment (Resource Document to NAEMSP Position Statement)." *Prehosp Emerg Care* 11 (2007): 63–66.

4. Thomas, S. H., O. Rago, T. Harrison, P. D. Biddinger, and S. K. Wedel. "Fentanyl Trauma Analgesia Use in Air Medical Scene Transports." *J Emerg Med* 29 (2005): 179–187.

5. Galinski, M., F. Dolveck, S. W. Borron et al. "A Randomized, Double-Blind Study Comparing Morphine with Fentanyl in Prehospital Analgesia." *American Journal of Emergency Medicine* 23 (2005): 114–119.

6. Green, R., B. Bulloch, A. Kabani, B. J. Hancock, and M. Tenenbein. "Early Analgesia for Children with Acute Abdominal Pain." *Pediatrics* 116 (2005): 978–983.

7. Kanowitz, A., T. M. Dunn, E. M. Kanowitz, W. W. Dunn, and K. Vanbuskirk. "Safety and Effectiveness of Fentanyl Administration for Prehospital Pain Management." *Prehosp Emerg Care* 10 (2006): 1–7.

8. Meine, T. J., M. T. Roe, A. Y. Chen et al. "Association of Intravenous Morphine Use and Outcomes in Acute Coronary Syndromes: Results from the CRUSADE Quality Improvement Initiative." *Am Heart J* 149 (2005): 1043–1049.

9. Rickard, C., P. O'Meara, M. McGrail, D. Garner, A. McLean, and P. Le Lievre. "A Randomized Controlled Trial of Intranasal Fentanyl vs. Intravenous Morphine for Analgesia in the Prehospital Setting." *Am J Emerg Med* 25 (2007): 911–917.

10. Pace, S. and T. F. Burke. "Intravenous Morphine for Early Pain Relief in Patients with Acute Abdominal Pain." *Acad Emerg Med* 3 (1996): 1086–1092.

11. Barton, E. D., C. B. Colwell, T. Wolfe et al. "Efficacy of Intranasal Naloxone as a Needleless Alternative for Treatment of Opioid Overdose in the Prehospital Setting." *J Emerg Med* 29 (2005): 265–271.

12. Kelly, A. M., D. Kerr, P. Dietze, I. Patrick, T. Walker, and Z. Koutsogiannis. "Randomised Trial of Intranasal versus Intramuscular Naloxone in Prehospital Treatment for Suspected Opioid Overdose." *Med J Aust* 182 (2005): 24–27.

13. Robertson, T. M., G. W. Hendey, G. Stroh, and M. Shalit. "Intranasal Naloxone Is a Viable Alternative to Intravenous Naloxone for Prehospital Narcotic Overdose." *Prehosp Emerg Care* 13 (2009): 512–515.

14. Holsti, M., B. L. Sill, S. D. Firth, F. M. Filloux, S. M. Joyce, and R. A. Furnival. "Prehospital Intranasal Midazolam for the Treatment of Pediatric Seizures." *Pediatr Emerg Care* 23 (2007): 148–153.

15. Kress, J. P. and Hall J. B. "Sedation in the Mechanically Ventilated Patient." *Crit Care Med* 34 (2006): 2541–2546.

16. Bulger, E. M., M. K. Copass, D. R. Sabath, R. V. Maier, and G. J. Jurkovich. "The Use of Neuromuscular Blocking Agents to Facilitate Prehospital Intubation Does Not Impair Outcome after Traumatic Brain Injury." *J Trauma* 58 (2005): 718–723; discussion 723–724.

17. Wyer, P. C., P. Perera, Z. Jin et al. "Vasopressin or Epinephrine for Out-of-Hospital Cardiac Arrest." *Ann Emerg Med* 48 (2006): 86–97.

18. Ong, M. E., E. H. Tan, F. S. Ng et al. "Survival Outcomes with the Introduction of Intravenous Epinephrine in the Management of Out-of-Hospital Cardiac Arrest." *Ann Emerg Med* 50 (2007): 635–642.

19. De Backer, D., P. Biston, J. Devriendt et al. "Comparison of Dopamine and Norepinephrine in the Treatment of Shock." *N Engl J Med* 362 (2010): 779–789.

20. Delbridge, T., R. Domeier, and C. B. Key. "Prehospital Asthma Management." *Prehosp Emerg Care* 7 (2003): 42–47.

21. Christianson, G., A. Woolf, and K. R. Olson. "β-Blocker Ingestion: An Evidence-Based Consensus Guideline for Out-of-Hospital Management." *Clinical Toxicology* 43 (2005): 131–146.

22. Marill, K. A., I. S. deSouza, D. K. Nishijima, T. O. Stair, G. S. Setnik, and J. N. Ruskin. "Amiodarone Is Poorly Effective for the Acute Termination of Ventricular Tachycardia." *Ann Emerg Med* 47 (2006): 217–224.

23. Kessler, C. S. and Y. Joudeh. "Evaluation and Treatment of Severe Asymptomatic Hypertension." *Am Fam Physician* 81 (2010): 470–476.

24. Tang, W. H. "Pharmacological Therapy for Acute Heart Failure." *Cardiol Clin* 25 (2007): 539–551; vi.

25. Anderson, J. L., C. D. Adams, E. M. Antman et al. "ACC/AHA 2007 Guidelines for the Management of Patients with Unstable Angina/Non ST-Elevation Myocardial Infarction: A Report of the American College of Cardiology/American Heart Association Task Force on Practice Guidelines (Writing Committee to Revise the 2002 Guidelines for the Management of Patients with

Unstable Angina/Non ST-Elevation Myocardial Infarction): Developed in Collaboration with the American College of Emergency Physicians, the Society for Cardiovascular Angiography and Interventions, and the Society of Thoracic Surgeons: Endorsed by the American Association of Cardiovascular and Pulmonary Rehabilitation and the Society for Academic Emergency Medicine." *Circulation* 116 (2007): e148–e304.

26. Pedley, D. K., K. Bissett, E. M. Connolly et al. "Prospective Observational Cohort Study of Time Saved by Prehospital Thrombolysis for ST Elevation Myocardial Infarction Delivered by Paramedics." *BMJ* 327 (2003): 22–26.

27. Ausset, S, Glassberg E, Nadler R, et al. "Tranexamic Acid as Part of Remote Damage-Control Resuscitation in the Prehospital Setting: A Critical Appraisal of the Medical Literature and Available Alternatives." *J Trauma Acute Care Surg* 2015;78:S70–S75.

28. Gueugniaud, P. Y., J. S. David, E. Chanzy et al. "Vasopressin and Epinephrine vs. Epinephrine Alone in Cardiopulmonary Resuscitation." *N Engl J Med* 359 (2008): 21–30.

29. Knapp, B. and C. Wood. "The Prehospital Administration of Intravenous Methylprednisolone Lowers Hospital Admission Rates for Moderate to Severe Asthma." *Prehosp Emerg Care* 7 (2003): 423–426.

30. Donnino, M. W., J. Vega, J. Miller, and M. Walsh. "Myths and Misconceptions of Wernicke's Encephalopathy: What Every Emergency Physician Should Know." *Ann Emerg Med* 50 (2007): 715–721.

31. Manoguerra, A. S. and D. J. Cobaugh. "Guidelines for the Management of Poisoning Consensus Panel. Guideline on the Use of Ipecac Syrup in the Out-of-Hospital Management of Ingested Poisons." *Clin Toxicol (Phila)* 43 (2005): 1–10.

32. Borron, S. W., F. J. Baud, P. Barriot, M. Imbert, and C. Bismuth. "Prospective Study of Hydroxocobalamin for Acute Cyanide Poisoning in Smoke Inhalation." *Ann Emerg Med* 49 (2007): 794–801, 801.e1–e2.

Further Reading

Bledsoe, Bryan E. and Dwayne E. Clayden. *Prehospital Emergency Pharmacology.* 7th ed. Upper Saddle River, NJ: Pearson/Prentice Hall, 2011.

Katzung, Bertram G. *Basic and Clinical Pharmacology.* 11th ed. Philadelphia: McGraw-Hill Medical, 2009.

Shannon, Margaret T., Billie Ann Wilson, and Carolyn L. Stang. *Prentice Hall's Health Professionals Drug Guide 2009–2010.* Upper Saddle River, NJ: Pearson/Prentice Hall, 2010.

Chapter 14
Intravenous Access and Medication Administration

Bryan Bledsoe, DO, FACEP, FAAEM

STANDARD
Pharmacology (Medication Administration)

COMPETENCY
Integrates comprehensive knowledge of pharmacology to formulate a treatment plan intended to mitigate emergencies and improve the overall health of the patient.

 ## Learning Objectives

Terminal Performance Objective: After reading this chapter, you should be able to apply concepts of pharmacology to the assessment and management of patients.

Enabling Objectives: To accomplish the terminal performance objective, you should be able to:

1. Define key terms introduced in this chapter.

2. Apply the six rights of medication administration when administering patient medications.

3. Recognize situations involving medication administration in which you should communicate directly with a medical direction physician.

4. Select the appropriate standard precautions for all medication administration situations.

5. Demonstrate principles of medical asepsis in the administration of medications.

6. Describe the procedures, precautions, risks, equipment, advantages, and disadvantages of each of the routes of percutaneous,

pulmonary, enteral, and parenteral medication administration.

7. Prepare medications for administration from a variety of types of packaging, including vials, nonconstituted vials, ampules, prefilled syringes, and packaging for intravenous solutions.

8. Describe the indications, contraindications, procedure, equipment, and risks associated with peripheral intravenous access.

9. Discuss the purposes of central venous access and the various types of catheters used.

10. Describe the characteristics of various intravenous fluids, including colloids, crystalloids, and blood.

11. Discuss individual components of an IV administration set along with the different types of administration sets and their appropriate indications for use.

12. Identify the common intravenous cannulas used in the out-of-hospital environment and individual indications for use.

13. List common location for intravenous cannulation by the paramedic, and describe the basic steps necessary to initiate a patent IV line in each location.

14. Name the common factors affecting the IV flow rates, and list the complications of IV access.

15. Describe the steps needed to access the IV line for bolus and infusion of medications, and how to change the intravenous bag when empty.

16. Discuss the alternatives to intravenous line initiation for medication therapy, such as saline locks, heparin locks, and venous access devices.

17. Explain the advantages, disadvantages, and use of electromechanical infusion devices in the out-of-hospital environment.

18. Discuss the emerging role of ultrasound-guided intravenous access.

19. Identify the indications, equipment, procedure, and complications of obtaining a blood sample from a patient.

20. Identify the indications, contraindications, equipment, procedure, and complications of intraosseous infusion initiation.

21. Given the variety of medication dosages, drug packaging, and patient factors, precisely calculate intravenous infusion rates and drug dosages.

KEY TERMS

administration tubing, p. 472

air embolism, p. 483

ampule, p. 458

anticoagulant, p. 483

antiseptic, p. 446

asepsis, p. 445

aural medication, p. 450

blood tube, p. 492

blood tubing, p. 474

bolus, p. 457

buccal, p. 448

burette chamber, p. 473

cannula, p. 472

cannulation, p. 469

catheter inserted through the needle/intracatheter, p. 476

central venous access, p. 470

circulatory overload, p. 483

colloidal solution, p. 470

concentration, p. 503

crystalloid, p. 471

desired dose, p. 503

disinfectant, p. 446

dosage on hand, p. 503

drip chamber, p. 472

drip rate, p. 472

drop former, p. 472

drops, p. 472

drugs, p. 443

embolus, p. 482

enema, p. 457

enteral route, p. 452

extension tubing, p. 473

extravasation, p. 481

extravascular, p. 490

gauge, p. 458

hemoconcentration, p. 494

hemolysis, p. 494

heparin lock, p. 487

hepatic alteration, p. 456

hollow-needle catheter, p. 475

Huber needle, p. 489

hypertonic, p. 471

hypodermic needle, p. 458

hypotonic, p. 471

induced therapeutic hypothermia (ITH), p. 471

infusion, p. 463

infusion controller, p. 490

infusion pump, p. 490

infusion rate, p. 507

inhalation, p. 450

injection, p. 450

intracatheter, p. 476

intradermal, p. 463

intramuscular, p. 465

intraosseous, p. 494

intravenous (IV) access, p. 469

intravenous fluid, p. 470

isotonic, p. 471

IV catheter, p. 475

local, p. 445

Luer sampling needle, p. 494

Case Study

It is early in February, and clouds heavy with snow loom not far in the distance. Paramedic Susan Adams watches the sky and hopes she will get off work on time, before the storm hits. Suddenly the tones drop, alerting her and her partner, Advanced EMT Todd Michaels, of a 28-year-old female patient with shortness of breath. After acknowledging the call and confirming the location with their GPS device, Susan and Todd get under way. In preparation, Susan dons gloves and eye protection. Additionally, she reviews the likely causes of shortness of breath in a 28-year-old patient.

As Susan and Todd pull up to the residence, they observe a well-kept house. A woman frantically waves them inside, shouting that her daughter cannot breathe. Quickly, they grab the airway kit, cardiac monitor, and medication bag, then cautiously enter the residence.

Once inside, Susan and Todd begin to size up the scene. Immediately to their left, they find the female patient seated on a chair in the tripod position. Quick observation reveals her to be in considerable respiratory distress and exhibiting cyanosis around the lips and in the extremities. Even without a stethoscope, Susan detects expiratory wheezing.

Susan promptly introduces herself and Todd to the patient and asks what is wrong. Because the patient can barely talk, Susan cannot obtain a specific chief complaint. Recognizing a life-threatening situation, she gains consent for treatment and turns her attention to the primary assessment.

The patient is responsive but exhibits lethargy and fatigue from the increased work of breathing and hypoxia. Inspection of her oral cavity reveals no foreign bodies or other obstructions. Susan deems the patient able to maintain her airway and forgoes a nasopharyngeal airway adjunct.

The patient is tachypneic at 36 breaths per minute. Tidal and minute volumes are shallow. Todd obtains a pulse oximetry reading (SpO_2) of 86 percent on room air. Exhaled carbon dioxide ($EtCO_2$) is 55 mmHg. A quick two-point auscultation reveals expiratory wheezing in the upper lobes of both the right and left lungs. Because the patient will not tolerate the assistance of ventilations with a bag-valve mask, Susan applies 100 percent oxygen.

Without missing a beat, Susan proceeds to evaluate the circulatory system. The patient's radial pulse is weak and rapid, with accompanying cool, diaphoretic skin. Again, Susan notes cyanosis.

Realizing that the situation is critical, Susan turns to the patient's mother while Todd applies the cardiac monitor and obtains vital signs. When Susan asks about a history of asthma, the mother confirms it and adds that this particular episode has been occurring over the past day and a half. Her daughter's metered-dose inhaler of albuterol has not provided any relief as it has in the past. Aside from the asthma, the patient has no other medical history. She has no allergies and has not eaten or drunk anything today.

Confident that she is dealing with an asthmatic patient, Susan performs a detailed secondary assessment. She accordingly notes bilateral distention of the jugular veins and retractions at the suprasternal notch and intercostal spaces, along with nasal flaring and pursed lips. Quickly she auscultates breath sounds from the posterior thorax in a six-point pattern. She observes bilateral expiratory wheezing in the apices of the lungs with no net air movement in the bases.

Todd informs Susan of the patient's vital signs: pulse, 116 beats per minute; respirations, 56 per minute; and blood pressure, 152/94 mmHg. With the primary assessment and history obtained, Susan begins emergency interventions. The cardiac monitor displays sinus tachycardia with no ectopy.

As Todd obtains a venous blood sample and establishes an IV line, Susan assembles a nebulizer and adds a solution of 2.5 mg of albuterol and 500 mcg of ipratropium (diluted in 3 mL of normal saline) to the chamber. She gives the nebulizer, complete with medication, to the patient for self-administration. Susan proceeds to administer 125 mg of methylprednisolone (Solu-Medrol) intravenously. Todd prepares the cot and loads the patient for transport. The patient is exhibiting minimal improvement with the nebulizer treatment. Susan places a continuous positive airway pressure (CPAP) mask and begins CPAP with 100 percent oxygen. The patient quickly starts to pink up. The albuterol is placed in an in-line delivery system so the patient receives the medication through the CPAP device.

En route to the hospital, Susan performs reassessment by evaluating the components of the primary assessment and the effects of all interventions. The patient now is more alert and breathes easier. Her pulse oximetry reads 92 percent, and her expiratory wheezing has subsided significantly. Her $EtCO_2$ has dropped to 50 mmHg. Susan now notes air movement in the bases of the lungs. Additionally, the cyanosis and diaphoresis have almost subsided, and vital signs have returned to normal limits. Because the pulse oximeter reading is still low and some residual wheezing persists, Susan gives another nebulized treatment of 2.5 mg of albuterol (without ipratropium). She alerts the receiving hospital.

Once at the hospital, Susan and Todd turn over care to the emergency department staff. Later they find out that the woman was admitted for overnight observation with the diagnosis of acute exacerbation of asthma. She is doing fine and is expected to be released in the morning.

Introduction

Drugs are foreign substances placed into the human body. **Medications** are drugs used for medical purposes. They serve a variety of purposes, such as controlling specific diseases like hypertension or helping the body cure diseases such as cancer and infection.

Medication administration will be an important part of the medical care you provide as a paramedic. You may have to use medications to correct or prevent many life-threatening situations. You may also use them to stabilize or comfort a patient in distress. In addition to your knowledge of particular medications and their properties from the "Emergency Pharmacology" chapter, you must also be thoroughly skilled in medication administration. Specific medications require specific routes and administration techniques. Their effectiveness depends directly on their correct route of delivery. Incorrect or sloppy medication administration can have tremendous legal implications for the paramedic. More important, it equates to poor care that can harm or even kill the patient.

This chapter discusses the routes and techniques you will use to correctly deliver your patient's medications. It is divided into three parts:

Part 1: Principles and Routes of Medication Administration

Part 2: Intravenous Access, Blood Sampling, and Intraosseous Infusion

Part 3: Medical Mathematics

PART 1: Principles and Routes of Medication Administration

General Principles

As a paramedic, you are responsible for ensuring that all emergency medications are in place and ready for immediate use. Therefore, you must know your local medication distribution system. You will have to know where to obtain and replace each medication as it expires or is used, as another patient may require it at any time. You also will have to thoroughly document the administration and restocking of narcotics, as many local, state, and federal agencies mandate such record keeping.

Always be certain that you correctly give all medications in the right dose. Medication errors may prove disastrous in terms of patient care and legal responsibility. Your knowledge of medication indications, contraindications,

➤ Six Rights of Drug
  Administration
  • Right person
  • Right drug
  • Right dose
  • Right time
  • Right route
  • Right documentation

side effects, dosages, and routes of administration is crucial to effective patient care. (See the "Emergency Pharmacology" chapter.)

You can attain effective pharmacological therapy and eliminate medication errors by following the "six rights" of medication administration:

Right person. Ensure that the patient receiving the medication is the right person. Generally, you will provide one-on-one attention. In a clinical setting, however, keeping track of multiple patients proves more challenging.

Right medication. Ensure that you administer the proper medication. Many medications are contained in similar appearing packages. To avoid inadvertently delivering the incorrect medication, read the label! Administering the incorrect medication can have disastrous consequences.

Right dose. Be certain that you administer the exact dosage of any medication. The correct dose may be standardized or require calculation. Never underdose or overdose a patient.

Right time. Timing their administration is important for many medications. Typically, in the emergent setting, you will quickly administer the necessary emergency medications. During transfers and critical care transports, you may have to administer other medications at preestablished intervals.

Right route. Specific medications require specific delivery routes. You must be familiar not only with the properties of individual medications, but also with their different routes of administration.

Right documentation. Documenting medication administration is of paramount importance. You must record all appropriate information about every medication you administer. Pertinent information includes, but is not limited to, medication name(s), dose, route of delivery, person administering, time administered, and patient response to the medication—both good and bad.

In the field, you will be responsible for the safe and appropriate delivery of medications. If you ever doubt the use or dosage of a medication, contact medical direction immediately. You must repeat back, or echo, all medication orders issued by on-line medical direction. For example, if medical direction ordered you to administer 25 mg of diphenhydramine (Benadryl), you would echo, "Medic 101 copies the medication order for 25 mg of diphenhydramine

to be administered slow IV push." By echoing, you confirm your reception and understanding of the order. If medical direction has issued an inappropriate medication or dosage, echoing may bring it to light and elicit an immediate correction. If you still find the order questionable after echoing, diplomatically request clarification or ask about the intent.

Pharmacological therapy permits you to function as an extension of the physician. No room exists for medication errors, as once a medication is given it is difficult, if not impossible, to retrieve. In addition, withholding a needed medication can have catastrophic consequences. Concentration and knowledge are the keys to this component of paramedic care.

Medical Direction

Paramedics do not practice autonomously. You will operate under the license of a medical director who is responsible for all of your actions. This responsibility extends to the administration of medications.

The medical director (or the EMS system) determines which medications you will use and the routes by which you will deliver them. Some states have a "state medication list" whereby the medications a service carries are dictated by law or a legislative or regulatory agency. Although some medications can be administered via off-line medical direction (written standing orders), you may need specific authorization for others after consulting on-line or direct medical direction. You must strictly abide by all of your medical director's guidelines.

Knowing all medication administration protocols is essential, especially which medications to administer under standing orders and which to deliver only after getting authorization from medical direction. You can ill afford to waste valuable time looking up procedures and directives for the critical patient who requires immediate medication therapy. Furthermore, because inappropriate medication delivery can have serious consequences, you may face severe legal ramifications even if your patient suffers no harm.[1, 2]

Standard Precautions

Establishing routes for medication delivery presents the constant potential for exposure to blood and other body fluids. Formerly called *body substance isolation (BSI)*, the strategy is now called **Standard Precautions**. In 1996 (and updated in 2011), the Centers for Disease Control and Prevention (CDC) established a single set of guidelines called Standard Precautions. These guidelines are measures to decrease your risk of exposure. The purpose of Standard Precautions is to ensure that you take the same precautions for every patient (Table 14-1).

Table 14-1 Summary of Standard Precautions

Component	Recommendations
Hand hygiene	After touching blood, body fluids, secretions, excretions, and contaminated items; immediately after removing gloves; between patient contacts.
Personal protective equipment (PPE)	*Gloves* For touching blood, body fluids, secretions, excretions, contaminated items; for touching mucous membranes and nonintact skin.
	Gown During procedures and patient-care activities when contact of clothing/exposed skin with blood/body fluids, secretions, and excretions is anticipated.
	Mask, eye protection (goggles), face shield* During procedures and patient-care activities likely to generate splashes or sprays of blood, body fluids, or secretions, especially suctioning or endotracheal intubation
Soiled patient-care equipment	Handle in a manner that prevents transfer of microorganisms to others and to the environment; wear gloves if visibly contaminated; perform hand hygiene.
Environmental control	Develop procedures for routine care, cleaning, and disinfection of environmental surfaces, especially frequently touched surfaces in patient-care areas.
Textiles and laundry	Handle in a manner that prevents transfer of microorganisms to others and to the environment.
Needles and other sharps	Do not recap, bend, break, or hand-manipulate used needles; if recapping is required, use a one-handed scoop technique only; use safety features when available; place used sharps in puncture-resistant container.
Patient resuscitation	Use mouthpiece, resuscitation bag, other ventilation devices to prevent contact with mouth and oral secretions.
Patient placement	Prioritize for single-patient room if patient is at increased risk of transmission, is likely to contaminate the environment, does not maintain appropriate hygiene, or is at increased risk of acquiring infection or developing adverse outcome following infection.
Respiratory hygiene/cough etiquette	Instruct symptomatic persons to cover mouth/nose when sneezing/coughing; use tissues and dispose in no-touch receptacle; observe hand hygiene after soiling of hands with respiratory secretions; wear surgical mask if tolerated or maintain spatial separation, >3 feet if possible.

During aerosol-generating procedures on patients with suspected or proven infections transmitted by respiratory aerosols (e.g., SARS), wear a fit-tested N95 or higher respirator in addition to gloves, gown, and face/eye protection.

During most patient care, you will wear gloves and eye protection (Figure 14-1). A mask is often required for procedures and patient care conditions when there is an increased likelihood that splashes or sprays of blood, body fluids, or secretions may occur. This is especially important during suctioning, endotracheal intubation, and other airway procedures. Remarkably, the simplest standard precaution is often the most neglected: handwashing. Washing your hands before and after patient contact is one of the most effective ways to decrease your exposure to infectious material. The chapter "Workforce Wellness and Safety" includes a thorough discussion of Standard Precautions.

Medical Asepsis

Medical **asepsis** (*a-*, without; *sepsis*, infection) describes a medical environment free of pathogens. Many paramedic procedures, especially those related to medication administration, place the patient at increased risk for infection. The external environment is full of microorganisms, many of them pathogenic. Techniques such as intravenous access or endotracheal intubation can allow pathogens to enter the patient's body, where they may cause **local** or **systemic** complications. Medical asepsis practices, including the use of sterilization, disinfectants, and antiseptics, guard against this hazard.

Sterilization

A truly aseptic environment is a sterile one. A **sterile** environment is free of all forms of life. Generally, environments are sterilized with extensive heat or chemicals. A sterile environment is difficult to attain in the out-of-hospital setting. Consequently, you must practice medically clean

FIGURE 14-1 Standard Precautions should be followed on each possible patient encounter.

techniques to minimize your patient's risk of infection. **Medically clean** techniques involve the careful handling of sterile equipment to prevent contamination. For example, much of the equipment used for medication administration is packaged sterilely. Once you open the package, you must use a medically clean technique to keep the equipment clean and uncontaminated until you use it. If you drop a piece of equipment on a dirty surface, you should discard it and obtain a new piece. Other medically clean techniques, including hand washing, glove changing, and discarding equipment that is in opened packages, help to prevent equipment and patient contamination. Remember, too, that many patients have lowered immunity levels or carry infectious diseases. Thus, keeping the ambulance and equipment clean is another essential medically clean procedure.

Disinfectants and Antiseptics

When administering medications, you must use disinfectants and antiseptics to ensure local cleanliness. Do not confuse disinfectants and antiseptics; the distinction between them is important. **Disinfectants** are toxic to living tissue. You will therefore use them only on nonliving surfaces or objects such as the inside of an ambulance or laryngoscope blades after use. Never use disinfectants on living tissue. **Antiseptics** are not toxic to living tissue. They destroy or inhibit pathogenic microorganisms that already exist on living surfaces and are generally used to cleanse the local area before a needle puncture. Common antiseptics include alcohol and iodine preparations, used either alone or together. Frequently, antiseptics are diluted disinfectants.

Disposal of Contaminated Equipment and Sharps

Blood and body fluid can harbor infectious material that endangers the health care provider, family, bystanders, or the patient himself. Many times, the patient is infected with pathogenic organisms long before signs and symptoms appear. Therefore, you must treat all blood and body fluids as potentially infectious.

Medication administration commonly involves needles in direct contact with the patient's blood and body fluid. Once used, a needle presents a significant risk. Inadvertent needle sticks, the most common accident in health care, can transmit diseases between the patient and paramedic. Properly handling needles and other sharps before and after patient use can prevent many of these accidental needle sticks. To

---

CONTENT REVIEW

➤ Needle Handling Precautions
- Minimize tasks in a moving ambulance.
- Properly dispose of all sharps.
- Recap needles only as a last resort.

---

minimize or eliminate the risk of an accidental needle stick, take these precautions:

- *Minimize the tasks you perform in a moving ambulance.* Use needles as sparingly as possible in the back of a moving ambulance. When appropriate, perform all interventions involving needles on scene. If en route, it may occasionally be necessary to have the driver pull the ambulance to the side of the road and stop briefly. Most paramedics become quite proficient at completing these procedures in a moving ambulance.

- *Immediately dispose of used sharps in a sharps container.* A **sharps container** is a rigid, puncture-resistant container clearly marked as biohazardous. You can deposit whole needles and prefilled syringes in it, thus eliminating the need for bending or cutting. Some sharps containers have adapters that permit the easy removal of needles from blood draw equipment and syringes. You should also dispose of items such as used ampules in the sharps container. Avoid dropping sharps onto the floor for later disposal. In the heat of the moment, you may forget the sharp or mentally misplace it.

- *Recap needles only as a last resort.* If you absolutely must recap a needle, never use two hands to do so. Instead, use the "one-handed scoop" method. First, place the cap on the bench top and hold the syringe in one hand. Keep the other hand by your side. Next, slip the needle into the cap. Finally, lift it up and snap it on securely using only one hand and dispose of it properly (Figure 14-2).

By law, every medical organization must have a biological hazard exposure plan. Be familiar with yours. If you are exposed to blood or other body substances, follow the plan and immediately notify the appropriate resources. Remember that prevention is the best medicine.[3]

Medication Administration and Documentation

When administering medications, proper and thorough documentation is extremely important. You must record all information concerning the patient and the medication, including:

- Indication for medication administration
- Dosage and route delivered
- Patient response to the medication—both positive and negative

You must also document the patient's condition and vital signs before medication administration, as well as after. In addition to communicating all information to those to whom you transfer care, you must record it on a copy of the patient care report.

FIGURE 14-2 The "one-hand scoop" is the safest way to recap a needle when it must be recapped.

In emergent and nonemergent situations alike, you will administer a variety of medications through a variety of delivery routes. The routes of medication administration fall into four basic categories: percutaneous, pulmonary, enteral, and parenteral. Technically, medications delivered through the rectum and pulmonary system are **topical medications**; however, accepted practice classifies these routes separately. Which route you use will depend on the medication you are administering and your patient's status.

Percutaneous Medication Administration

Percutaneous medications are those that are applied to and absorbed through the skin or the mucous membranes. They are easy to administer, and they bypass the digestive tract, making their absorption more predictable.

Transdermal Administration

Medications given by the **transdermal** (*trans-*, across; *dermal*, skin) route promote slow, steady absorption. Nitroglycerin, hormones, and analgesics are commonly administered transdermally. Transdermal delivery can also produce localized effects, as with anti-inflammatories and other bacteriostatic and softening agents. Applying medication locally avoids passing larger quantities of the medication through the entire body, where it is not needed. Transdermal medications include lotions, ointments, creams, foams, wet dressings, adhesive-backed applications, and suppositories.

To administer a transdermal medication, use the following technique:

1. Use Standard Precautions and avoid contaminating the medication and inadvertently getting it on your skin.

2. Clean and dry your patient's skin at the administration site.

3. Apply medication to the site as specified by

the manufacturer. Avoid overdosing or underdosing when using lotion, ointment, cream, or foam.

4. Leave the medication in place for the required time. Monitor the patient for desirable or adverse effects.

You may need to place a dressing over the medication to protect the site and quantity of medication. Carefully follow all recommendations. Administration may vary subtly, depending on the form of medication and the specific manufacturer's instructions.

Several factors can affect how quickly the skin absorbs transdermal medications. Thin skin, overdose, or penetrating solvents can increase the absorption rate. Conversely, thick skin, scar tissue, or peripheral vascular disease can decrease the rate. If these factors are present, consider alternative sites or dosage adjustments.

Mucous Membranes

The mucous membranes absorb medications at a moderate to rapid rate. Similar to transdermal administration, medication delivery through the mucous membranes avoids the digestive tract and complications associated with that route. You can deliver medications through the mucous membranes at several sites (sublingual, buccal, ocular, nasal, and aural). However, specific medications are made for specific sites and generally are not interchangeable.

Sublingual

Sublingual medications are absorbed through the mucous membranes beneath the tongue (*sub-*, below; *lingual*, tongue). The sublingual region is extremely vascular and permits rapid absorption with systemic delivery. These medications are generally dissolvable tablets or sprays. One commonly administered sublingual medication is nitroglycerin.

To administer a medication via the sublingual route, follow these steps (Figure 14-3):

1. Use Standard Precautions.

2. Confirm the indication, medication, dose, sublingual route, and expiration date.

3. Have your patient lift his tongue toward the top and back of his oral cavity.

4. Place the pill or direct spray between the underside of the tongue and the floor of the oral cavity. Have your patient relax his tongue and mouth. If administering a tablet, instruct the patient to let the tablet dissolve and not to swallow it.

5. Monitor the patient for desirable or adverse effects.

> **CONTENT REVIEW**
>
> ➤ Mucous Membrane Medication Sites
> - Tongue
> - Cheek
> - Eye
> - Nose
> - Ear

FIGURE 14-3 Sublingual medication administration. Place the pill or direct spray between the underside of the tongue and the floor of the oral cavity.

Buccal

The **buccal** region lies in the oral cavity between the cheek and gums. Buccal medications are generally tablets. Hormonal and enzyme preparations are typically given buccally.

To administer a medication buccally, follow these steps (Figure 14-4):

1. Use Standard Precautions.

2. Confirm the indication, medication, dose, buccal route, and expiration date.

FIGURE 14-4 Buccal medication administration. Place the medication between the patient's cheek and gum.

3. Place the medication between the patient's cheek and gum. Instruct the patient to allow the pill or other preparation to dissolve. Ensure that the patient does not swallow the medication.

4. Monitor the patient for desirable or adverse effects.

Ocular

Ocular medications are topical medications that are administered through the mucous membranes of the eye. These are typically local medications for alleviating eye pain, treating infection, decreasing intraocular pressure, or lubricating the eyelid. Medications delivered by way of the eye are labeled for ophthalmic use and packaged as drops or ointments.

If medication is to be administered only to one eye, be sure to medicate the correct eye. The following abbreviations were formerly used to designate right, left, or both eyes:

o.d.   right eye (*oculus dexter*)

o.s.   left eye (*oculus sinister*)

o.u.   both right and left eyes (*oculus uterque*)

However, to avoid confusion, it is preferred to simply write "left eye," "right eye" or "both eyes."

To administer a medication via eye drops, use the following technique (Figure 14-5):

1. Use Standard Precautions.

2. Have your patient lie supine or lay his head back and look toward the ceiling.

3. Pull the lower eyelid downward to expose the conjunctival sac. Never touch the eye.

4. Use a medicine dropper to place the prescribed dosage on the conjunctival sac. Never administer medications directly on the eye unless specifically instructed.

5. Instruct the patient to hold his eye(s) shut for 1 to 2 minutes.

Ocular medications may also be packaged as ointments. To apply an ointment, follow the same procedure as above, but carefully squeeze the ointment onto the conjunctival sac. If you administer too much medication, carefully blot away the excess drops or ointment with sterile gauze. The ointment will melt as it warms to body temperature and will spread smoothly across the surface of the eye.

Nasal

The mucous membranes of the nose are another port for topical medication delivery. Given through the nares (nostrils), these **nasal medications** are usually drops or sprays intended for local effect. A commercial device called the mucosal atomization device (MAD) is commonly used. Often, these medications are aerosolized to provide better distribution to the nasal mucosa. The intranasal route can be used for analgesia (particularly in children), sedation, epistaxis, and to reduce nasal congestion from nasotracheal intubation.[4,5,6,7]

To administer a medication via the nose, use the following technique (Figure 14-6):

1. Use Standard Precautions, including face mask.

2. Have the patient blow his nose and tilt his head backward.

3. Use a medicine dropper or squeezable nebulizer to administer the medication into the appropriate nare(s) according to the manufacturer's instructions (Figure 14-7).

4. Hold the naris or nares shut and/or tilt the head forward to distribute the medication.

5. Monitor the patient for desirable and undesirable effects.

Aural

Some medications are delivered to the mucous membranes of the ear and ear canal through drops or medicated gauze.

FIGURE 14-5 Eyedrop administration. Use a medicine dropper to place the prescribed dosage on the conjunctival sac.

FIGURE 14-6 Nasal medication administration.

FIGURE 14-7 Mucosal atomization device (MAD) for intranasal administration of emergency medications.

These **aural medications** primarily treat local infections and ear pain. Use the following technique to administer medicated drops (Figure 14-8):

1. Use Standard Precautions.
2. Confirm the indication, medication, dose, and expiration date.
3. Determine the correct ear for administration.
4. Have the patient lie in the lateral recumbent position with the affected ear upward.
5. Manually open the ear canal: For adult patients, pull the ear up and back; for pediatric patients, pull it down and back.
6. Administer the appropriate dose of medication with a medicine dropper.
7. Have the patient continue to lie with his ear up for 10 minutes.
8. Monitor the patient for desirable and undesirable effects.

Using medicated gauze or cotton is generally reserved for the hospital setting. If your local protocols permit you to administer these medications, follow the procedure

previously outlined, gently inserting the gauze into the ear instead of instilling medicated drops. Avoid tightly packing the ear canal.

CONTENT REVIEW

➤ Pulmonary Medication Mechanisms
  • Nebulizer
  • Metered dose inhaler
  • Endotracheal tube

Pulmonary Medication Administration

Special medications can be administered into the pulmonary system via **inhalation** or **injection**. Generally in the form of gases, powders, fine mists, or liquids, these medications include those that promote bronchodilation for respiratory emergencies. Other inhaled medications are mucolytics, antibiotics, and topical steroids. Inhalation can also be used for humidification and pulmonary decongestion.

Nebulizer

Typically, medications administered by inhalation are delivered with the aid of a small volume nebulizer (SVN) or handheld nebulizer (HHN). A **nebulizer** uses pressurized oxygen or air to disperse a liquid into a fine aerosol spray or mist. Inhalation carries the aerosol into the lungs. Figure 14-9 illustrates a typical nebulizer. The specific design depends on the manufacturer, but they all work on the same principle and typically have the same parts:

- Mouthpiece
- Medication reservoir
- Oxygen port
- Relief valve
- Oxygen tubing
- Oxygen source

FIGURE 14-8 Aural medication administration. Manually open the ear canal and administer the appropriate dose.

FIGURE 14-9 Typical small-volume nebulizer (SVN) setup.

To administer a medication with a nebulizer, follow these steps:

1. Use Standard Precautions including a mask.

2. Put the medication in the medication reservoir. If the medication is not diluted, combine it with 3 to 5 mL sterile saline solution. This will allow adequate aerosolization. Screw the reservoir in place.

3. Assemble the nebulizer.

4. Attach oxygen tubing to the oxygen port and oxygen source.

5. Set the oxygen source regulator for 5 to 8 liters per minute.

   Note: Never set the oxygen pressure outside this range. Less than 5 liters per minute will not create enough pressure to aerosolize the medication. More than 8 liters per minute will create too much pressure and destroy the oxygen tubing or nebulizer at its weakest point. Furthermore, because of pressure restrictions, do not attach the nebulizer to an oxygen humidifier.

6. Place the nebulizer in the patient's mouth. Instruct him to exhale and then seal his lips around the mouthpiece. Then have him hold the nebulizer and slowly inhale as deeply as possible. On maximum inhalation, instruct the patient to hold in the medication for 1 to 2 seconds before exhaling. This permits maximum deposition and absorption. Continue this process until the medication is completely gone. Typically, this takes 3 to 5 minutes.

Nebulizers also come preattached to an oxygen face mask in both pediatric and adult sizes (Figure 14-10). Use nebulization face masks for pediatric or adult patients who cannot hold the nebulizer. Nebulizers can also be used with CPAP devices when indicated (Figure 14-11).[8] They can also be used in patients who are intubated and receiving mechanical ventilation (Figure 14-12).

FIGURE 14-11 Nebulized medications can be administered through most CPAP masks.

FIGURE 14-12 In-line administration of nebulized medication in an intubated patient.

For a nebulizer to be effective, the patient must have an adequate tidal volume and respiratory rate. If the tidal volume is shallow or respiratory rate low, the medication will not move from the nebulizer into the lungs. For patients with a poor tidal and/or respiratory rate who cannot pull the medication into their lungs, you can connect the nebulizer to a bag-valve mask, a CPAP device, and/or an endotracheal tube.

Metered Dose Inhaler

Inhaled medications may also be delivered through a **metered dose inhaler** (MDI). These small, handheld devices produce a medicated spray for inhalation. Patients with conditions such as asthma or COPD use metered dose inhalers to deliver a specific, or metered, dose of medication. A metered dose inhaler consists of two parts, a medication canister and a plastic shell and mouthpiece (Figure 14-13). Some MDIs come equipped with a spacer. The spacer is a cylindrical canister between the inhaler

FIGURE 14-10 SVN medication administration through mask.

FIGURE 14-13 Metered dose inhaler.

and the mouthpiece. Prior to self-administration, the patient will depress the inhaler, sending a measured dose of medication into the spacer. The patient will then breathe in and out of the spacer through the mouthpiece, thus inhaling the medication into the lungs. The spacer system is particularly useful for patients who have a hard time operating and inhaling directly from the MDI, which is common in the elderly and in young children. The spacer, when used in conjunction with an MDI, is very effective.

MDIs are usually self-administered. However, if your patient is incapacitated, you may have to physically assist with the administration or educate the patient or his caregivers in its use. To assist a patient in the use of an MDI, follow this technique:

1. Insert the medication canister into the plastic shell.
2. Remove the cap from the mouthpiece. Make sure the cap is clean.
3. Gently shake the MDI for 2 to 5 seconds.
4. Instruct the patient to maximally exhale.
5. Place the mouthpiece in the patient's mouth and have him form a seal with his lips.
6. As the patient inhales, press the canister's top downward to release the medication.
7. Have the patient hold his breath for several seconds.
8. Remove the inhaler from the patient's mouth and instruct him to breathe slowly.
9. If a second dose is necessary, wait according to the manufacturer's instructions. Then repeat.

In an acute respiratory emergency involving a patient with an MDI, always use a nebulizer instead of the MDI. The MDI delivers a small amount of medication, but the nebulizer delivers larger quantities of medication mixed with water and oxygen.

Nebulizers and MDIs offer several advantages. In respiratory emergencies, less medication is needed because

it reaches its exact site of action. The lower dosage is less likely to promote side effects, and if the patient has an adverse reaction, implementing or discontinuing medication delivery is easy. Furthermore, because the patient can hold the nebulizer, he will benefit from feeling more in control of his overall therapy. Most important, if your patient is hypoxic you can administer inhaled medications with supplemental oxygen.

The nebulizer and MDI also have disadvantages. Moving the aerosolized medication into the lungs depends on adequate ventilation. For the patient with a poor tidal and minute volume, nebulized medications are ineffective, as the medication cannot reach its site of action. In these cases, you should use the nebulizer in conjunction with a bag-valve mask and/or endotracheal tube. In addition, the patient must exhibit an adequate level of consciousness and manual dexterity to hold the nebulizer and follow instructions correctly.

Endotracheal Tube

Although they are infrequently used, you can administer certain medications such as lidocaine (Xylocaine), vasopressin, epinephrine, atropine, and naloxone (Narcan) through an endotracheal tube if an intravenous line or intraosseous line is unavailable. Delivering liquid medications into the lungs theoretically permits rapid absorption through the pulmonary capillaries. However, recent research has shown that the administration of medications via an endotracheal tube is not as effective as once thought.

When using an endotracheal tube, you must increase conventional IV dosages from two to two and one-half times. You also should dilute the medication in normal saline to create 10 mL of solution and then quickly inject it down the endotracheal tube. Several ventilations must follow to aerosolize the medication and enhance its absorption. Ideally, you can pass a commercially manufactured catheter through the endotracheal tube and inject the medication through it.[9]

Enteral Medication Administration

The **enteral route** is the delivery of medication to be absorbed through the gastrointestinal tract. The gastrointestinal tract, or alimentary canal, travels from

CONTENT REVIEW
➤ Endotracheal Medications
  • Lidocaine
  • Vasopressin
  • Epinephrine
  • Atropine
  • Naloxone

CONTENT REVIEW
➤ Enteral Routes
  • Oral
  • Gastric tube
  • Rectal

Mouth

Esophagus

Stomach

Large intestine

Small intestine

Rectum

Anus

FIGURE 14-14 Gastrointestinal tract.

the mouth to the stomach and on through the intestines to the rectum (Figure 14-14). You can administer enteral medications orally, through a gastric tube, or rectally.

Several advantages make the gastrointestinal tract the most common route for medication delivery. Aside from sheer convenience, it is the least expensive route, and its use requires little equipment and minimal training. In some instances, after you have delivered a medication you may be able to retrieve it by inducing vomiting, by removing it from the rectum, or simply by having the patient spit it out.

Conversely, enteral medication administration poses several disadvantages. Physical activity, emotions, or food can significantly alter the gastrointestinal tract's chemical and physical environment, making absorption unreliable. In addition, as all blood from the stomach and small intestine must pass through the hepatic circulatory system (portal circulation), the liver's condition can reduce the medication's effectiveness. A dysfunctional liver can significantly alter medication distribution and, in extreme cases, metabolize therapeutic medications into inert or harmful substances. Furthermore, a patient resistant to or

noncompliant in taking medications makes administration via the enteral route very difficult.

Oral Administration

Oral medication administration denotes any medication taken by mouth (oral) and swallowed into the gastrointestinal (GI) tract. From the GI tract, the medication is absorbed and distributed throughout the body. When administering a medication by the oral route, you must be sure that the patient has an adequate level of consciousness to support his airway. Administering an oral medication to a patient who cannot support his airway may result in an airway occlusion or aspiration into the lungs. If aspiration into the lungs occurs, aspiration pneumonia and its deadly consequences may occur.

Medications for oral delivery come in a variety of forms, either solid or liquid.

- *Capsules.* Capsules contain liquid, dry, or beaded medication in a soluble casing. For maximum effectiveness, the patient must swallow them whole.
- *Tablets.* Tablets comprise medicated powder compressed into a small, solid disk. Typically, tablets may be scored to permit breaking in half or quarters when lower dosages are required.
- *Enteric coated/time-release capsules and tablets.* These forms of medication release the medication gradually as layers of the capsule or tablet slowly erode. Time-release capsules or tablets must be swallowed whole.
- *Elixirs.* Elixirs are liquid medications combined with alcohol or placed in a sweetened fluid.
- *Emulsions.* Emulsions are medications combined with a fat or oil emulsifier.
- *Lozenges.* Lozenges are solid forms of medication that slowly dissolve in the mouth, thus permitting gradual swallowing.
- *Suspensions.* A suspension is a liquid that contains small particles of solid medication.
- *Syrups.* A syrup is a concentrated solution of sugar in water or another liquid to which a medication is added.

Equipment for Oral Administration

Administering oral medications is simple and easy. The basic equipment that you may need depends on the medication and the patient's status:

- *Soufflé cup.* A soufflé cup is a paper or plastic cup. Placing a solid medication in a soufflé cup makes it easy to see and minimizes contact with the provider's hands.

- *Medicine cup.* A medicine cup is a plastic or glass cup with volumetric measurements on the side. It facilitates giving specific amounts of liquid medication. When you pour medication into the cup, the liquid does not form a flat surface but clings to the sides at a higher level, forming a *meniscus.* To compensate for the meniscus, measure the medication toward the center, at its lowest level.

- *Medicine dropper.* A medicine dropper has markings for measuring liquid volumes. You will use it for special medications and to administer medications to children or patients who cannot tolerate other forms of oral medication.

- *Teaspoon.* You will use these accurately sized measuring spoons to administer liquid medications. A teaspoon normally holds 5 mL of fluid; however, the volume of household teaspoons varies significantly. To ensure accurate medication administration, use a measured teaspoon or syringe.

- *Oral syringe.* Oral syringes are calibrated plastic syringes without a hypodermic needle. They are considered the most accurate oral means of administering liquid-based medications. When administering a medication with the oral syringe, place the end of the syringe in the patient's mouth and deliver only as much medication as the patient can safely swallow. Several administrations may be necessary to deliver a complete dose.

- *Nipple.* For the neonate or infant, liquid medication can be delivered with a plastic nipple.

General Principles of Oral Administration

To administer medications orally, use the following technique:

1. Use Standard Precautions.

2. Note whether to administer the medication with food or on an empty stomach.

3. Gather any necessary equipment such as a soufflé cup or teaspoon; mix liquids or suspensions, or otherwise prepare medications as needed.

4. Have your patient sit upright (when not contraindicated).

5. Place the medication into your patient's mouth. Allow self-administration when possible; assist when needed.

6. Follow administration with 4 to 8 ounces of water or other liquid. Swallowing a liquid pushes the medication into the stomach.

7. Ensure that the patient has swallowed the medication and it is not hidden in his mouth. For some pediatric and psychiatric patients, you may have to visually confirm that the patient has swallowed the medication by inspecting the oral cavity.

Gastric Tube Administration

For patients who have difficulty swallowing or whose nutritional status is poor, you may place a gastric tube to support or completely supplement nutritional requirements. Gastric tubes are also used in instances of medication overdose, trauma, and upper gastrointestinal bleeding. They may be surgically inserted directly into the stomach through the abdomen or indirectly through the nose (nasogastric tube) or mouth (orogastric tube). Placing a gastric tube through the abdominal wall is reserved for the hospital setting. *Before administering any medication through a gastric tube or other enteral tube, ensure that it is indeed an enteral tube and not a similar-looking device such as a chronic ambulatory peritoneal dialysis (CAPD) catheter.* In some EMS systems, paramedics insert orogastric or nasogastric tubes in the field for emergencies. A properly placed gastric tube allows enteral medication delivery. Few emergency medications are administered via a nasogastric or orogastric tube. Other medications, many used in the nonacute setting, also are administered via the gastric tube. With modification, most oral medications can be administered this way. However, you should avoid administering time-release capsules and enteric-coated tablets through a gastric tube, as crushing them for delivery destroys their slow-release mechanism. Also, ensure that the medication has been sufficiently crushed so as not to become trapped and occlude the gastric tube.

To administer a medication via a gastric tube, use the following technique (Procedure 14-1):

1. Use Standard Precautions.

2. Confirm proper tube placement. Disconnect the tube from the drainage or suction unit or clamping device. Clamp the tube from the drainage or suction unit to prevent gastric contents spilling from either device. Attach a cone-tipped syringe to the proximal end of the gastric tube. Gently inject air while auscultating over the stomach. Following this, withdraw the plunger while observing for the presence of gastric fluid or contents, which indicates appropriate placement. Leave the tube disconnected from the drainage or suction unit.

3. Irrigate the gastric tube. To irrigate the gastric tube, draw up 50 to 100 mL of normal saline into a cone-tipped syringe. Insert the syringe into the open end of the gastric tube. With the syringe tip pointed at the floor, gently inject the saline into the tube. If the saline encounters resistance, look for problems such as tube kinking. Have the patient lie on his left side and

Procedure 14–1   Medication Administration through a Nasogastric Tube

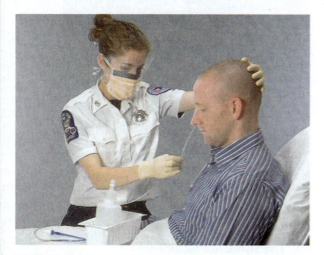

14-1A Confirm proper tube placement.

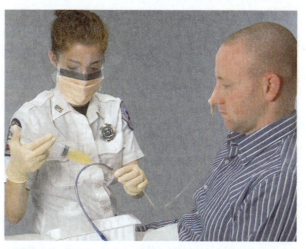

14-1B Withdraw the plunger while observing for the presence of gastric fluid or contents.

14-1C Instill medication into the gastric tube.

14-1D Gently inject the saline.

14-1E Clamp off the distal tube.

reattempt injection. If the saline still meets resistance, reattach the tube to the drainage or suction unit and contact medical direction for further directives.

4. Prepare the medication(s) for delivery. Crush tablets or empty capsules into 30 mL of warm water. Ensure that all particles are small so they will not occlude the tube. You may administer liquid medications without further preparation.

5. Draw the medication into a 30 to 50 mL cone-tipped syringe and place the tip into the open gastric tube. Gently administer the medication into the gastric tube; forceful application may create considerable distention and patient discomfort.

6. Draw 50 to 100 mL of warm normal saline into a cone-tipped syringe and attach it to the open end of the gastric tube. Gently inject the saline. This facilitates the medication's passage into the stomach and rinses the tube, ensuring that the patient receives the entire dose. Repeated administrations may be necessary.

7. Clamp off the distal tube. Use a commercially manufactured device or hemostat to clamp shut the distal portion of the gastric tube for approximately 30 minutes after you administer the medication. Do not reattach to the drainage or suction unit. This will prevent the medication's inadvertent removal from the stomach.

If you must refill the syringe in order to administer the full dosage of medication, do not allow the syringe to empty completely before you detach it from the gastric tube. This prevents drawing air into the syringe and then introducing it into the stomach, which causes discomfort.

Rectal Administration

The rectum's extreme vascularity promotes rapid medication absorption. Additionally, because medications given rectally do not pass through the liver, they are not subject to **hepatic alteration**; thus, their absorption is more predictable.

In the emergency setting, you may give certain medications rectally if you cannot establish an intravenous line or use the oral route. These include diazepam (Valium) or lorazepam (Ativan) for protracted seizures or aspirin for cardiac or neurologic emergencies. In the nonacute setting, you may administer sedatives, antiemetics, or other specially prepared medications rectally.

Rectal administration may prove advantageous with the unconscious or pediatric patient, or when administering medications with an objectionable taste or odor. Unfortunately, medication absorption may be erratic if gross fecal matter exists. In addition, some medications may cause considerable anal or rectal irritation.

Rectal medications come in a variety of forms. In the emergency setting, they are typically liquid, thus permitting

FIGURE 14-15 Catheter placement on needleless syringe.

easy administration and rapid absorption. To administer a rectal medication in the emergent setting, follow this technique:

1. Use Standard Precautions.

2. Confirm the indication for administration and dose, and draw the correct quantity of medication into a syringe.

3. Place the hub of a 14-gauge Teflon catheter (removed from the IV catheter) on the end of a needleless syringe (Figure 14-15).

4. Insert the Teflon catheter into the patient's rectum and inject the medication. Try to keep the medication in the lower part of the rectum. Administration higher in the rectum may result in the medication's being absorbed by veins that deliver the medication to the portal circulation.

5. Withdraw the catheter and hold the patient's buttocks together, thus permitting retention and absorption.

An alternative technique utilizes a small endotracheal tube instead of the Teflon IV catheter. Remove the 15/22-mm BVM adapter and connect a syringe to the proximal end of the tube (Figure 14-16). Lubricate the tube and insert it into the rectum. Inject the medication, remove the tube, and hold the buttocks together.

In the nonemergent setting, suppositories or enemas are common methods for rectal administration. Because your responsibilities as a paramedic may include nonemergent clinical settings, you should master these techniques.

FIGURE 14-16 Syringe attached to endotracheal tube for rectal administration.

FIGURE 14-17 Prepackaged enema container.

Additionally, the rectal route may prove beneficial for a pediatric patient who resists oral administration or for whom IV access proves impractical.

Suppositories are medications packaged in a soft, pliable form. Generally refrigerated until they are used, they begin to melt at body temperature in the rectum. Some are lubricated to ease insertion. Suppositories can be lubricated by running a small amount of lukewarm tap water over the suppository prior to insertion. To administer a suppository, manually insert it into the rectum. Hold the buttocks shut for 5 to 10 minutes to allow for retention and absorption.

An **enema** is typically a liquid **bolus** of medication that is injected into the rectum. Medications given via this route are typically referred to as small-volume enemas. They are typically prepackaged in a squeezable container with a rectal tip (Figure 14-17).

To administer a medicated small-volume enema, use the following technique:

1. Use Standard Precautions and confirm the need for administration via a small volume enema.

2. Place the patient on his left side. Flex his right leg to expose the anus.

3. Insert the prelubricated rectal tip into the anus and advance 3 to 4 inches.

4. Gently squeeze the medicated solution of the bottle into the rectum and colon.

5. Hold the buttocks together to enhance absorption into the rectal and intestinal tissue.

Only medications with specific guidelines for rectal administration should be delivered through this route. Do not administer rectal medications in the presence of diarrhea, rectal bleeding, hemorrhoids, or any other situation involving severe anal irritation.

Parenteral Medication Administration

Parenteral route denotes the administration of medication outside the gastrointestinal tract. Broadly, this encompasses pulmonary and some topical forms of medication

delivery; however, additional, specific criteria apply to parenteral administration. Typically, the parenteral route involves the use of needles as medications are injected into the circulatory system or tissues. Consequently, some forms of parenteral medication delivery afford the most rapid medication delivery and absorption.

Syringes and Needles

Frequently, giving medications via the parenteral route requires a syringe and hypodermic needle.

Syringe

A **syringe** is a plastic tube with which liquid medications can be drawn up, stored, and injected. Syringes range in size from 1 to 100 mL and greater. Remember that although medication dosages are generally given by weight (g/mg/mcg), syringes represent volume. Therefore, you must be prepared to mathematically convert these measurements.

A syringe's two major components are a barrel and a plunger (Figure 14-18). The tube-like barrel, or body, functions as a reservoir for medication. Markings on its side calibrate its overall volume. Smaller syringes are calibrated in 0.10-mL intervals, larger syringes in 1.0-mL intervals.

The plunger is a device that fits into the barrel. At one end it has a handle for pulling or pushing. At the opposite end, a rubber stopper fits snugly into the barrel. Pulling on the plunger draws material into the barrel; pushing on it expels material from the barrel. The rubber

FIGURE 14-18 Syringe.

end forms a tight seal from which the fluid medication cannot escape.

The junction of the fluid and rubber stopper measures the total volume of liquid in the syringe. The barrel's maximum volume should correspond closely to the volume of medication needed. For example, to administer 2 mL of medication, a 3-mL syringe would prove most appropriate.

An adapter at the syringe's distal end is compatible with the hub of an IV catheter or, as many cases will require, a hypodermic needle.

Hypodermic Needle

The **hypodermic needle** is a hollow metal tube used with the syringe to administer medications. It is sharp enough to easily puncture tissues, blood vessels, or IV medication ports.

The hypodermic needle's primary components include a hilt and shaft. The hilt is a threaded plastic tube that screws securely onto the syringe's distal adapter. The shaft is a thin metal tube through which medications can flow from the syringe into the delivery site. A bevel at the shaft's distal end accounts for its sharpness (Figure 14-19).

Hypodermic needles come in a variety of gauges and lengths. A needle's **gauge** describes its diameter. Generally, hypodermic needle gauges range from 18 to 27. The gauge and actual diameter are inversely related: the higher the gauge, the smaller the diameter. Thus, a 25-gauge needle's diameter is smaller than an 18-gauge needle's. Conversely, a 20-gauge needle's diameter is larger than a 22-gauge needle's. Hypodermic needle lengths generally range from ⅜ to 1½ inches. The package label lists the size of the syringe and the gauge and length of the hypodermic needle.

Because syringes and hypodermic needles frequently involve invasive procedures, they are packaged sterile. Never use either a syringe or a hypodermic needle from a package that has been opened or tampered with. Used hypodermic needles are sharp and present a biohazard. Dispose of them immediately after you complete any task involving their use. Many modern needles are designed for safe needle disposal without recapping the needle (Figure 14-20). These decrease the possibility of accidental needle stick injuries and are preferred in the emergency setting.

FIGURE 14-19 Hypodermic needle.

FIGURE 14-20 Safety needles help to minimize the possibility of needle stick injuries.

Medication Packaging

All medications delivered by the parenteral route are liquids. They are packaged in a variety of containers with which you must be familiar, as obtaining medication from each type requires a different procedure. The kinds of parenteral medication containers include the following:

- Glass ampules
- Single and multidose vials
- Nonconstituted medication vials
- Nebulizer vials
- Prefilled syringes
- Intravenous medication fluids

You must also be thoroughly familiar with the information included on the labels of all medication containers:

- *Name of medication.* The label lists both the generic and trade name of the medication. Always ensure that you have selected the right medication.
- *Expiration date.* All medications have an expiration date after which they cannot be used. Never use an expired medication.
- *Total dose and concentration.* The total dose of medication is the total weight (g/mg/mcg) of medication in the container. The concentration represents the weight of the medication per volume of fluid. For example, if 10 mg of a medication were packaged in 10 mL of fluid, the total dose would be 10 mg, and the concentration would be 10 mg/10 mL or 1 mg/mL. Beware—identical medications can be packaged in different dosages and concentrations.

These labels are printed directly on the vial, ampule, prefilled syringe, or IV medication bag. Always use them to confirm the correct medication.

Glass Ampules

An **ampule**, or amp, is a breakable glass vessel containing liquid medication. It has a cone-shaped top, thin neck, and circular tubular base for storing the medication (Figure 14-21). The thin neck is a vulnerable point at which you intentionally break the ampule to retrieve its contents. Ampules usually range in volume from 1 to 5 mL. The least-expensive form of medication packaging, they contain single doses of medication. It is essential to use a filter needle when drawing medication up from a glass ampule. This will help to filter any small glass shards that may be present.

To obtain medication from a glass ampule you will need a syringe and needle. Use the following technique (Procedure 14-2):

1. Confirm medication indications and patient allergies.
2. Confirm the ampule label (medication name, dose, and expiration).

FIGURE 14-21 Ampules.

Procedure 14–2   Obtaining Medication from a Glass Ampule

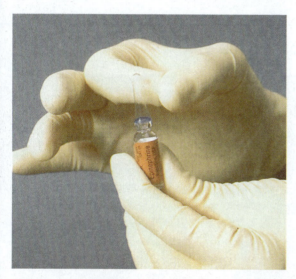

14-2A Hold the ampule upright and tap its top to dislodge any trapped solution.

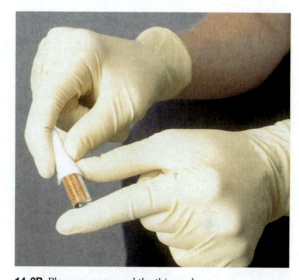

14-2B Place gauze around the thin neck . . .

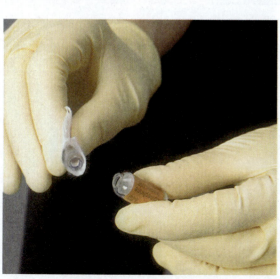

14-2C . . . and snap it off with your thumb.

14-2D Draw up the medication.

3. Hold the ampule upright and tap its top to dislodge any trapped solution.

4. Place gauze around the thin neck and snap it off with your thumb.

5. Place the tip of the hypodermic needle inside the ampule and withdraw the medication into the syringe.

6. Reconfirm the indication, medication, dose, and route of administration.

7. Administer the medication appropriately via the indicated route.

8. Properly dispose of the needle, syringe, and broken glass ampule.

Single and Multidose Vials

Vials are plastic or glass containers with a self-sealing rubber top (Figure 14-22). Vials may contain single or multiple doses of medication; the self-sealing rubber top prevents

FIGURE 14-22 Vials.

leakage from punctures and permits multiple accesses with a syringe and hypodermic needle. The medication inside the vial is packaged in a vacuum.

To obtain medication from a vial, follow these steps (Procedure 14-3):

1. Confirm medication indications and patient allergies.

2. Confirm the vial label (name, dose, and expiration).

Procedure 14–3   Obtaining Medication from a Vial

14-3A Confirm the vial label.

14-3B Prepare the syringe and hypodermic needle.

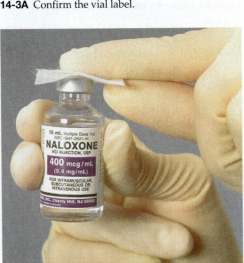

14-3C Cleanse the vial's rubber top.

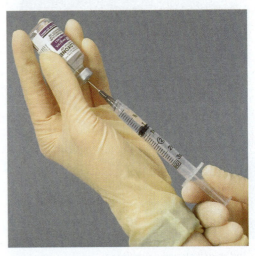

14-3D Insert the hypodermic needle into the rubber top and inject the air from the syringe into the vial.

3. Determine the volume of medication to be administered.

4. Prepare the syringe and hypodermic needle. Because the vial is vacuum packed, you will have to replace the volume of medication removed with air to maintain equilibrium in the vial. Withdraw the plunger to draw a volume of air into the syringe equal to the volume of medication to be administered. This technique permits easy medication retrieval from the vial.

5. Cleanse the vial's rubber top with an antiseptic alcohol preparation.

6. Insert the hypodermic needle into the rubber top and inject the air from the syringe into the vial. Then withdraw the appropriate volume of medication.

7. Reconfirm the indication, medication, dose, and route of administration.

8. Administer appropriately via the indicated route.

9. Properly dispose of the needle, syringe, and vial.

Nonconstituted Medication Vial

The **nonconstituted medication vial** extends the viability and storage time of medications that have a short shelf life or are unstable in liquid form. The nonconstituted medication vial actually consists of two vials, one containing a powdered medication and one containing a liquid mixing solution (Figure 14-23). To prepare the medication you must mix it, or reconstitute it, by withdrawing the liquid solution from its vial and placing it in the powdered medication's vial. In a **Mix-o-Vial** system, the two vials are joined and you must squeeze them together to break the seal and mix.

To prepare a medication from a nonconstituted medication vial, use the following technique (Procedure 14-4):

1. Confirm medication indications and patient allergies.

2. Confirm the vial's label (name, dose, expiration date).

3. Remove all solution from the vial containing the mixing solution, using the same procedure as you would to withdraw medication from a single or multidose vial.

4. With an alcohol preparation, cleanse the top of the vial containing the powdered medication and inject the mixing solution.

5. Gently agitate or shake the vial to ensure complete mixture.

6. Determine the volume of newly constituted medication to be administered.

7. Prepare the syringe and hypodermic needle. Because the vial is vacuum packed, you will have to replace the volume of medication removed with air to retain equilibrium in the vial. By withdrawing the plunger, place into the syringe a volume of air equal to the volume of medication that will be removed. This technique permits easy medication retrieval from the vial.

8. Cleanse the medication vial's rubber top with an antiseptic alcohol preparation.

9. Insert the hypodermic needle into the rubber top and withdraw the appropriate volume of medication.

10. Reconfirm the indication, medication, dose, and route of administration.

11. Administer appropriately via the indicated route.

12. Monitor the patient for the desired effects.

13. Properly dispose of the needle and syringe.

Prefilled or Preloaded Syringes

Prefilled or **preloaded syringes** are packaged in tamper-proof containers with the medication already in the syringe. Because the syringe is prefilled, you do not need to draw the medication from another source. Generally, prefilled syringes contain standard dosages, thus decreasing the chance of dosage error.

The prefilled syringe consists of two parts, a syringe and a glass tube prefilled with liquid medication. The plastic syringe is similar to those described earlier; however, it does not have a plunger. Rather, you screw the prefilled glass tube into the syringe barrel and secure it (Figure 14-24). Pushing the glass container into the syringe barrel expels the medication through the attached hypodermic needle.

Follow these steps to administer a medication from a prefilled syringe:

1. Confirm medication indications and patient allergies.

2. Confirm the prefilled syringe label (name, dose, and expiration date).

FIGURE 14-23 The nonconstituted drug vial actually consists of two vials, one containing a powdered medication and one containing a liquid mixing solution.

FIGURE 14-24 Prefilled syringes.

Procedure 14–4   Preparing Medication from a Nonconstituted Drug Vial

14-4A Inspect the medication. Check the label and the expiration date.

14-4B Compress the plunger to mix the solution and the solvent.

14-4C Shake the vial to adequately mix the solution.

14-4D Remove the protective covering to expose the diaphragm.

14-4E Uncap the syringe and prepare to withdraw the medication.

14-4F Insert the needle through the diaphragm.

14-4G Withdraw the medication from the vial.

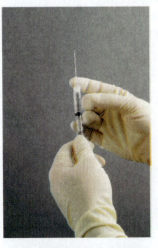

14-4H Expel any air from the syringe.

14-4I Administer the medication and properly dispose of the needle.

3. Assemble the prefilled syringe. Remove the pop-off caps and screw together.

4. Reconfirm the indication, medication, dose, and route of administration.

5. Administer appropriately via the indicated route.

6. Properly dispose of the needle and syringe.

Intravenous Medication Solutions

Medicated solutions are another form of parenteral medication. They are packaged in an IV bag and administered as an IV **infusion**. IV medication solutions may be pre-mixed, or you may have to mix them. The section on intravenous medication infusions later in this chapter discusses their actual preparation and administration.

Parenteral Routes

Parenterally administered medications can be absorbed locally or systemically. In addition, depending on the route of administration, their absorption rate may be slow, sustained, or rapid. Parenteral delivery bypasses the digestive tract, thus making the medication's absorption, action, and onset more predictable. Because parenteral routes use hypodermic needles that contact body fluids, the risk of disease transmission is ever present.

Parenteral medication delivery employs the following routes:

- Intradermal injection
- Subcutaneous injection
- Intramuscular injection
- Intravenous access
- Intraosseous infusion

Specific medications require specific routes of parenteral delivery; therefore, you must be competent with every route. In this section, we will discuss the specialized equipment, medications, and routes for intradermal, subcutaneous, and intramuscular injections. Because of their complexity, we will discuss intravenous access and intraosseous infusions separately in the following sections.

Whether you are administering a parenteral injection or an IV bolus or infusion, you should explain the entire procedure to the patient to help alleviate his anxiety. Finally, remember that hypoperfusion (hypovolemia or peripheral vascular disease, for instance) may significantly reduce parenteral absorption.

Intradermal Injection

Using a syringe and hypodermic needle, **intradermal** injections deposit medication into the dermal

FIGURE 14-25 Intradermal injection.

layer of the skin (*intra-*, within; *derma*, skin). The amount of medication placed in the dermal layer is quite small, typically less than 1 mL (Figure 14-25).

Capillaries in the dermis afford a very slow rate of absorption, with little or no systemic distribution. Rather, the bulk of medication remains localized in the area of administration. Intradermal delivery proves useful for allergy testing and tuberculin skin testing (PPD or Mantoux) and for administering local anesthetics during suturing, wound debridement, and IV establishment.

The forearm and upper back are preferred sites for intradermal injections. They have little hair and are highly visible. Additionally, you should look for sites free of superficial blood vessels, which increase the chance for systemic absorption.

To administer an intradermal injection, you will need the following equipment:

- Personal protective equipment
- Antiseptic preparations
- Packaged medication
- Tuberculin syringe (1 mL)
- 25- to 27-gauge needle, ⅜ to 1 inch long
- Sterile gauze and adhesive bandage

To administer an intradermal injection, follow these steps (Procedure 14-5):

1. Assemble and prepare the needed equipment.

2. Use Standard Precautions and confirm the medication, indication, dosage, and need for intradermal injection.

3. Draw up medication as appropriate.

4. Prepare the site with antiseptic solution. The intended site must be cleansed of pathogens, therein decreasing the likelihood of infection. Generally, you will use alcohol or similar antiseptics. To appropriately cleanse the site, start at the site itself and work outward with an expanding circular motion. This motion will push pathogens away from the intended site of puncture.

5. Pull the patient's skin taut with your nondominant hand.

Procedure 14–5   Intradermal Administration

14-5A Assemble and prepare the needed equipment.

14-5B Check the medication.

14-5C Draw up the medication.

14-5D Prepare the administration site.

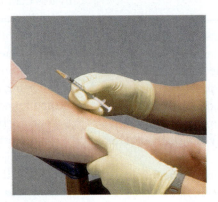

14-5E Pull the patient's skin taut.

14-5F Insert the needle, bevel up, at a 10° to 15° angle.

14-5G Remove the needle and cover the puncture site with an adhesive bandage.

14-5H Monitor the patient.

6. Insert the needle, bevel up, just under the skin, at a 10° to 15° angle.

7. Slowly inject the medication; look for a small bump or wheal to form as medication is deposited and collects in the intradermal tissue.

8. Remove the needle and dispose of it in the sharps container.

9. Place the adhesive bandage over the site; use the gauze for hemorrhage control if needed.

Do not rub or massage the injection site. This promotes systemic absorption and nullifies the advantage of localized effect.

Subcutaneous Injection

Subcutaneous injections place medication into the subcutaneous tissue (*sub-*, below; *cutaneous*, skin). The subcutaneous layer consists of loose connective tissue between the skin and muscle (Figure 14-26). The subcutaneous tissue

FIGURE 14-26 Subcutaneous injection.

FIGURE 14-27 Subcutaneous injection sites (injection sites shown in red).

has few blood vessels and thus promotes slow, sustained absorption, which prolongs a medication's effect on the body. Like intradermal injections, no more than 1.0 mL of medication is administered subcutaneously. Administering more than 1.0 mL of medication can cause irritation and, possibly, an abscess.

Administer subcutaneous injections where you can easily pinch the skin on the upper arms, thighs, or occasionally, the abdomen (Figure 14-27). Easily pinched skin contains more subcutaneous tissue and readily separates from the muscle. All sites should be free of superficial blood vessels, nerves, and tendons. Additionally, avoid areas with tattoos or bruising.

To perform a subcutaneous injection, you will need the following equipment:

- Personal protective equipment
- Antiseptic preparations
- Packaged medication
- Syringe (1 to 3 mL)
- 24- to 26-gauge hypodermic needle, ⅜ to 1 inch long
- Sterile gauze and adhesive bandage

To administer a subcutaneous injection, use the following technique (Procedure 14-6):

1. Assemble and prepare equipment.
2. Use Standard Precautions and confirm the medication, indication, dosage, and need for subcutaneous injection.
3. Draw up the medication as appropriate.
4. Prepare the site with antiseptic solution.
5. Gently pinch a 1-inch fold of skin.
6. Insert the needle just into the skin at a 45° angle with the bevel up.
7. Pull the plunger back to aspirate tissue fluid.
8. If blood appears, the hypodermic needle is in a blood vessel and absorption will be too rapid. Start the procedure over with a new syringe.

9. If no blood appears, proceed with step 10.
10. Slowly inject the medication.
11. Remove the needle and dispose of it in a sharps container.
12. Place an adhesive bandage over the site; use the gauze for hemorrhage control if needed.
13. Monitor the patient.

After you give the injection, gently rubbing or massaging the site will help initiate systemic absorption.

Some authorities recommend using an air plug in the syringe. This is approximately 0.1 mL of air that follows the injection and pushes the medication further into the subcutaneous tissue, thus preventing leakage or medication loss. To place an air plug in the syringe, aspirate approximately 0.1 mL of air into the barrel after you have drawn up the medication. Pointing the needle downward and perpendicular to the ground, tap the syringe with your finger to dislodge the air pocket. It will float to the top of the plunger, and from there it will follow the medication into the subcutaneous tissue.

You can also deliver a subcutaneous injection into the sublingual region, or fleshy tissue below the tongue. To administer a subcutaneous injection, place the hypodermic needle of a small, medication-filled syringe into the sublingual tissue and then inject the medication as appropriate. Epinephrine, in severe cases of asthma or anaphylaxis, can be administered in this manner.

Intramuscular Injection

Intramuscular injections deposit medication into muscle (*intra-*, within; *muscular*, muscle). Muscle is extremely vascular and permits systemic delivery at a moderate

Procedure 14–6 Subcutaneous Administration

14-6A Prepare the equipment.

14-6B Check the medication.

14-6C Draw up the medication.

14-6D Prep the site.

14-6E Insert the needle at a 45° angle.

14-6F Remove the needle and cover the puncture site.

14-6G Monitor the patient.

14-6H Apply an adhesive bandage to the injection site.

CONTENT REVIEW

➤ Intramuscular Injection Sites
- Deltoid
- Dorsal gluteal
- Vastus lateralis
- Rectus femoris

absorption rate. Medication absorption through muscle is also relatively predictable. To reach the muscle, a needle must penetrate the dermal and subcutaneous tissue (Figure 14-28).

Several sites are used for intramuscular injections (Figure 14-29). Depending on the site, varying quantities of medication can be delivered. These sites and their correlating volumes of medication include the following:

- **Deltoid.** The deltoid muscle is 3 to 4 fingerbreadths below the acromial process (the bony bump on the shoulder). It is highly vascular and permits easy access. You can deliver up to 2.0 mL into this muscle.

FIGURE 14-28 Intramuscular injection.

- **Dorsal gluteal.** The dorsal gluteal muscle, or buttock, is a common administration point for intramuscular injections. Injections here can deliver 5.0 mL of medication or more. They cause little discomfort, but you must avoid the large sciatic nerve, which is the leg's major motor nerve. Damage to the sciatic nerve can decrease mobility or totally paralyze the leg. To help prevent neurologic complications, envision an imaginary quadrant over the buttock; administer all injections in the upper and outer quadrant.

- **Vastus lateralis.** The *vastus lateralis* muscle of the thigh is another common site for intramuscular injection, especially for pediatric patients. As at the dorsal gluteal muscle, injections here can deliver 5 mL of medication or more. To deliver medication at this site, imagine a grid of nine boxes. Administer injections in the middle, outer box, or anterolateral part of the muscle.

- **Rectus femoris.** The *rectus femoris* lies over the femur and is closely associated with the *vastus lateralis* muscle. When utilizing the *rectus femoris* for intramuscular injection, place the medication into the center of the muscle at approximately midshaft of the femur. Up to 5 mL of medication volume can be administered into the *rectus femoris*.

When choosing a site, avoid bruised or scarred areas. Areas free of superficial blood vessels are most desirable.

To perform an intramuscular injection, you will need the following equipment:

- Personal protective equipment
- Antiseptic preparation
- Packaged medication

FIGURE 14-29 Intramuscular injection sites.

- Syringe (1 to 5 mL, depending on dosage)
- 21- to 23-gauge hypodermic needle, ⅜ to 1 inch long
- Sterile gauze and adhesive bandage

Follow these steps to administer an intramuscular injection (Procedure 14-7):

1. Assemble and prepare the needed equipment.
2. Use Standard Precautions and confirm the medication, indication, dosage, and need for intramuscular injection.
3. Draw up medication as appropriate.
4. Prepare the site with antiseptic solution.
5. Stretch the skin taut over the injection site with your nondominant hand.

6. Insert the needle just into the skin at a 90° angle with the bevel up.
7. Pull back the plunger to aspirate tissue fluid.
   - If blood appears, the hypodermic needle is in a blood vessel, and absorption of the medication will be too rapid. Start the procedure over with a new syringe.
   - If no blood appears proceed with step 8.
8. Slowly inject the medication.
9. Remove the needle and dispose of it in the sharps container.
10. Place an adhesive bandage over the site; use gauze for hemorrhage control if needed.
11. Monitor the patient.

Procedure 14–7   Intramuscular Administration

14-7A Prepare the equipment.

14-7B Check the medication.

14-7C Draw up the medication.

14-7D Prepare the site.

14-7E Insert the needle at a 90° angle.

14-7F Remove the needle and cover the puncture site.

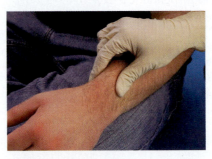

14-7G Monitor the patient.

After administration, gently rubbing or massaging the site helps to initiate systemic absorption. Do not massage the site, however, if you have administered heparin or another anticoagulant. Again, some authorities recommend a 0.1-mL air plug as described under subcutaneous injection.

Intravenous and Intraosseous Routes

Two important parenteral medication administration routes—intravenous access and intraosseous infusion—are discussed in detail in Part 2.

PART 2: Intravenous Access, Blood Sampling, and Intraosseous Infusion

Intravenous Access

Intravenous (IV) access (*intra-*, within; *venous*, vein), or **cannulation**, is a routine paramedic procedure. Circulating blood transports chemicals, proteins, and fluids throughout the body. Venous circulation can likewise deliver medications and fluids into the body and provides an invaluable tool for treating the sick and injured.

The following situations indicate intravenous access:

- Fluid and blood replacement
- Medication administration

- Obtaining venous blood specimens for laboratory analysis

Because veins are easier to locate and penetrate, venous access is preferable to arterial access. Additionally, venous circulation pressure is lower than arterial pressure and presents fewer hemorrhage control complications.

Types of Intravenous Access

Medical care providers use two types of intravenous access, peripheral and central. As a paramedic, you will most often perform peripheral intravenous access. Central venous access is rarely, if ever, performed in the out-of-hospital setting.

Peripheral Venous Access

Although challenging, **peripheral venous access** is relatively easy to master. As its name implies, it uses peripheral veins. Common sites include the arms and legs and, when necessary, the neck. Figure 14-30 illustrates the specific veins commonly accessed on the hand, forearm, and leg.

Because some patients' veins may not be readily visible, you must know venous topography. In these cases, you will have to locate veins based on anatomic layout and palpation. Exhaust all possibilities on the arms before trying to locate the veins of the legs. Leg veins are more difficult to access and present complications more frequently. For neonates and infants, you may access veins in the scalp. The "Pediatrics" chapter explains that technique.

Basilic vein

Cephalic vein

Dorsal venous network

External jugular vein

Dorsal venous arch

FIGURE 14-30 Peripheral IV access sites: veins of the arm, hand, neck, and foot.

When establishing a peripheral IV, start at the distal end of the extremity and work proximally. Once you have attempted cannulation, the disruption in blood flow hinders using veins distal to that site. However, the purpose of access also determines site selection. For example, rapid fluid administration requires larger veins like the antecubital fossa, as opposed to the smaller veins of the hand. The external jugular vein is considered a peripheral vein and can be accessed when other peripheral sites are not available.

The major advantage of peripheral venous access is that it is relatively simple to perform because visualizing and accessing the veins is usually easy. In addition, you can access peripheral veins while simultaneously doing other life-sustaining procedures such as CPR or endotracheal intubation. Conversely, peripheral veins collapse in hypovolemia or circulatory failure, thus becoming difficult to locate and access. Furthermore, the peripheral veins of geriatric patients, pediatric patients, or those with peripheral vascular disease may be fragile and difficult to cannulate. Finally, peripheral veins may roll and elude IV placement.

Central Venous Access

Central venous access uses veins located deep within the body. These include the internal jugular, subclavian, and femoral veins. They are larger than peripheral veins and will not collapse in shock. Central IV lines are placed near the heart for long-term use. Typically, they are used when medical conditions require repeated access for medication and/or fluid delivery. They also are used for transvenous pacing or for monitoring central venous pressure.

A special type of central line is the **peripherally inserted central catheter,** or **PICC,** line. PICC lines are smaller than those routinely used for central access and are threaded into the central circulation via a peripheral site (Figure 14-31). PICC lines are most often used in infants and children requiring long-term care.

Central venous access is typically restricted to the hospital setting because of its invasive nature and high risk of complications such as arterial puncture, pneumothorax, and air embolism. Central veins cannot be accessed during procedures such as CPR, and they often require a chest X-ray for placement confirmation. You may nonetheless encounter a central line during interfacility transports or in a chronically ill homebound patient. Protocols in some EMS systems allow paramedics to access existing central lines during emergency care. Still other systems allow their paramedics to place certain central lines. Always follow local protocols regarding central line access and insertion. For more information about central venous access, consult a text on advanced venipuncture techniques.

FIGURE 14-31 A peripherally inserted central catheter (PICC) is often used in patients with chronic illnesses who require repeated vascular access.

Equipment and Supplies for Venous Access

To establish intravenous access, you will need the following specialized equipment and supplies.

Intravenous Fluids

Intravenous fluids are chemically prepared solutions tailored to the body's specific needs. They replace the body's lost fluids and/or aid the delivery of IV medications. They also can keep a vein patent when no fluid or medication therapy is required.

Intravenous fluids come in three forms: colloids, crystalloids, and blood.

COLLOIDS   Colloidal solutions contain large proteins that cannot pass through the capillary membrane. Consequently, they remain in the circulatory system for a long time. In addition, colloids have osmotic properties that attract water into the circulatory system. A small quantity of colloid can significantly increase intravascular volume (volume of blood and fluid contained within the blood vessels). Common colloids include the following:

- *Plasma protein fraction (Plasmanate).* Plasmanate is a protein-containing colloid. Its principal protein, albumin, is suspended with other proteins in a saline solvent.

- *Albumin.* Albumin contains only human albumin. Each gram of albumin will retain approximately 18 mL of water in the bloodstream.

- *Dextran.* Dextran is not a protein but a large sugar molecule with osmotic properties similar to those of albumin. It comes in two molecular weights: 40,000 and 70,000 Daltons. Dextran 40 has from two to two

- *Tubing.* Intravenous administration tubing is clear and very flexible. Thus, you can watch the solution flow through the administration set, and you can manipulate the tubing in tight situations. Some medications such as intravenous nitroglycerin are chemically incompatible with regular tubing and require special tubing.

- *Clamp.* IV administration tubing has a simple plastic clamp. When slid over the tubing, the clamp completely stops the flow of solution from the IV bag to the patient. It prevents both the entrainment of air into the tubing when changing IV bags and the backflow of medication when administering medications. You can also use it to stop infusion without disturbing the flow regulator setting.

- *Flow regulator.* The flow regulator is a dial enclosed in a triangular plastic casing. It allows infinite control of flow rates ranging from a continuous stream to completely stopped. Rolling the dial toward the IV solution bag increases the drip frequency; rolling the dial towards the patient decreases the drip frequency.

- *Medication injection ports.* The **medication injection ports** have a self-sealing membrane into which you can insert a hypodermic needle for medication administration. Many sets now contain "needleless" medication ports that decrease the possibility of needlestick injuries. Their design varies, depending on the manufacturer. When possible, use the medication port nearest the patient.

- *Needle adapter.* The **needle adapter** is a rigid plastic device at the administration tubing's distal end. It is specifically constructed to fit into the hub of an intravenous cannula. Similar to the spike, the needle adapter is sterile and covered by a protective cap. If it becomes contaminated at any time, start over with a new administration set.

IV EXTENSION TUBING   **Extension tubing** is IV tubing used to extend the original macrodrip or microdrip setup (Figure 14-34). Its packaging clearly marks it as such. Like administration sets, extension tubing is sterile and must be handled accordingly.

Extension tubing also permits the paramedic to change the original administration tubing or the IV solution bag with little difficulty. For example, if you have to switch from a macrodrip set to a microdrip set, you can close the clamp on the extension and detach the primary tubing. Once you have flushed the new tubing with fluid, you place the needle adapter into the receiving port on the extension tubing and release the clamp. You can now resume fluid therapy without risking complications or having to painfully reinitiate a second IV line.

FIGURE 14-34 Extension tubing.

ELECTROMECHANICAL PUMP TUBING   Mechanical infusion devices may require specially manufactured pump tubing (Figure 14-35). Typically, pump tubing has special components that attach directly to the pump. Additionally, bladders and relief points permit you to void possible air bubbles. Many specific models of electromechanical infusion pumps require specific pump tubing. When using a mechanical infusion pump, be sure to have the appropriate tubing on hand. Consult the section on electromechanical infusion pumps for more information.

MEASURED VOLUME ADMINISTRATION SET   The **measured volume administration set** can deliver specific volumes of fluid with or without medication. It works well for patients who need specific or limited volumes of fluid, and it is especially advantageous for pediatrics, renal failure, or other patients who cannot tolerate fluid overload.

The measured volume administration set consists of either micro- or macrodrip tubing, with the addition of a large **burette chamber** marked in 1.0-mL increments

FIGURE 14-35 IV pump tubing.

FIGURE 14-36 Measured volume administration set.

(Figure 14-36). The burette chamber holds between 120 and 150 mL of fluid. The components of the measured volume administration set include the following:

- Flanged spike
- Clamp
- Airway handle
- Medication injection port
- Burette chamber
- Float valve
- Drip chamber
- Flow regulator
- Medication injection port
- Needle adapter

When opened, the airway handle on top of the burette chamber permits air to be displaced or replaced as fluid enters or exits the chamber. If a medication must be mixed in a specific amount of IV solution, you can add it through the medication administration port after correctly filling the chamber.

BLOOD TUBING Administering whole blood or blood components requires **blood tubing**, which contains a filter that prevents clots and other debris from entering the patient. Without exception, all blood must be filtered. Blood that is stored or delivered over an extended period is prone to form fibrin clots or to accumulate other debris. If these clots or debris enter the circulatory system, they can travel in the form of an embolus. Remember, once an embolus encounters a blood vessel too small for its passage,

FIGURE 14-37 Blood administration tubing.

it will lodge and effectively block all blood flow distal to the point of occlusion.

Many aeromedical and facility-based paramedics administer blood and must be familiar with blood tubing. Although most ambulances do not carry blood, paramedics may initiate normal saline with blood tubing in anticipation that whole blood or blood products will be required immediately in the emergency department (Figure 14-37).

Blood tubing comes in two configurations, straight and Y. Y tubing has two administration ports: one for blood and one for IV normal saline solution. Typically, blood is administered with normal saline. Fluids like lactated Ringer's increase the potential for blood coagulation. The two-port design permits immediate access to normal saline if the blood supply is exhausted or must be shut down, as for a transfusion reaction. When you use Y blood tubing, establish a traditional IV by connecting a bag of normal saline to the tubing. Attach the blood to the second port when needed, while maintaining strict medical asepsis. Using the flow regulator, discontinue the normal saline while opening the clamp regulating the flow of blood. Straight blood tubing has only one reservoir. Therefore, only blood is attached to the tubing. A medication administration port close to the needle adapter allows you to piggyback a secondary line of normal saline into the tubing.

MISCELLANEOUS ADMINISTRATION SETS Some tubing now has a manual dial that can set drops per minute or specific flow rates. Some manufacturers have created a single drip chamber that can create either microdrips or macrodrips, depending on the patient's need.

In-Line Intravenous Fluid Heaters

Technology now makes it possible to heat IV fluids to near body temperature in the field. Most EMS units store their IV fluids in the unit. These fluids, when opened, are at the same temperature as the ambient air. Thus, the temperature of IV fluids can vary significantly depending on where

FIGURE 14-38 Over-the-needle catheter.

in the country (or world) you work. Many patients are very prone to the development of hypothermia following fluid administration. These include the elderly, children, the frail, and those suffering from fever or similar conditions. When indicated, it is prudent to use an in-line IV fluid heater to warm the IV fluid to body temperature. These devices are designed to shut down if the IV fluid temperature exceeds body temperature. Likewise, different devices are available to meet the various flow requirements of, for example, trauma patients, pediatrics, or geriatrics.

Always use Standard Precautions. Open the unit and test the battery. Attach the in-line intravenous fluid heater between the end of the IV tubing and the extension tubing supplied with the unit. Turn the device on and monitor the indicator lights. The unit should remain with the patient on arrival at the hospital and throughout his hospital stay. It is switched to a direct current (DC) adapter on the patient's arrival at the floor.

Intravenous Cannulas

The intravenous cannula permits actual puncture and access into a patient's vein. The distal portion of the administration tubing connects to the IV cannula, thus completing the bridge between the solution bag and patient. The three basic types of IV cannulas are:

- Over-the-needle catheter
- Hollow-needle catheter
- Plastic catheter inserted through a hollow needle

OVER-THE-NEEDLE CATHETER Often called an **IV catheter** or **cannula**, an **over-the-needle catheter** comprises a semiflexible catheter enclosing a sharp metal stylet (needle) that is hollow and beveled at the distal end (Figure 14-38).

- *Metal stylet (needle).* The metal stylet permits easy puncturing of the skin and blood vessel. Blood from the vein flows through the hollow stylet to the flashback chamber.

- *Flashback chamber.* The clear plastic flashback chamber allows you to see the blood after the metal stylet has punctured the vein. Blood in the flashback chamber confirms placement of the stylet in the vein.

- *Teflon catheter.* The Teflon catheter slides over the metal stylet into a successfully punctured vein.

- *Hub.* Located on the back of the Teflon catheter, the hub receives the needle adapter of the administration tubing once removed from the metal stylet.

For peripheral venous access, the over-the-needle catheter is preferred because it is easy to place and anchor and permits freer movement of the patient. Most of these needles now have a needlestick protection mechanism that covers the exposed needle (Figure 14-39).

HOLLOW-NEEDLE CATHETER For pediatric patients or other patients with tiny, delicate veins, use **hollow-needle catheters** (Figure 14-40). These catheters do not have a Teflon tube; rather, the metal stylet itself is inserted into the vein and secured there. Because the sharp metal stylet can easily damage the vein, you must insert it very carefully. Some hollow-needle catheters have wings for guidance and securing into a vein. These hollow-needle catheters are referred to as *winged catheters* or *butterfly catheters.*

FIGURE 14-39 Safety IV catheters.

FIGURE 14-40 Hollow-needle (butterfly) catheter.

FIGURE 14-41 Catheter inserted through the needle.

CATHETER INSERTED THROUGH THE NEEDLE The **catheter inserted through the needle** is also called an **intra-catheter**. It consists of a Teflon catheter inserted through a large metal stylet (Figure 14-41). Used in the hospital setting to implement central lines, its proper placement requires great skill, as discussed previously.

The size of an intravenous cannula is expressed as its gauge. The *larger* the gauge, the *smaller* the diameter of the stylet and catheter. For example, a 22-gauge cannula is smaller than a 14-gauge cannula. The larger-diameter, 14-gauge catheter allows greater flow rates than the smaller-diameter, 22-gauge cannula. When establishing venous access, choose the cannula size most appropriate for the patient's condition. Typical uses for the various sizes of cannulas are:

- **22-gauge.** Small gauges are used for *fragile* veins such as those of the elderly or children.
- **20-gauge.** Moderate gauges are used for the average adult who does not need fluid replacement.
- **18-gauge, 16-gauge, or 14-gauge.** Larger-gauge cannulas are used to increase volume or to administer viscous medications such as dextrose. Blood can be administered only through a cannula that is 16-gauge or larger.

The largest gauge cannula that will fit into a vein is not always appropriate. A cardiac patient with large veins should not receive a 14-gauge cannula for medication administration, just as a multisystem trauma patient with good veins should not receive a 22-gauge cannula for fluid administration. Remember that intravenous access is painful and causes discomfort not only to those receiving it, but also to family members watching a loved one in distress.

Miscellaneous Equipment

The **venous constricting band** is a flat rubber band applied proximal to the intended puncture site. It impedes venous return, thereby engorging veins and making them easier to see. This helps you to select the best site and makes venipuncture easier. Never restrict arterial blood flow with the constricting band, and never leave it in place longer than 2 minutes.

Intravenous access is an invasive procedure; therefore, you must use medically clean techniques, including antiseptic preparations, to prevent infection. Applying a sterile,

impermeable dressing after venipuncture decreases the chance of infection.

Once you have established an IV, you must secure it to avoid losing the access. Medical tape and an adhesive bandage are inexpensive and easy to apply. You can also apply clear membranes over the site. Commercial devices manufactured specifically for this task are also available. Have gauze on hand for hemorrhage control if IV cannulation is unsuccessful or if blood leaks from around the site.

Obtaining a venous blood specimen at the time of venipuncture will save the patient from being stuck with a needle again later. This chapter's section on venous blood sampling discusses this technique in detail.

Intravenous Access in the Hand, Arm, and Leg

As a paramedic, you will most often establish peripheral IVs in the hand, arm, or leg. The veins in these places are relatively easy to locate and accessing them causes the patient less pain. In addition, the likelihood of complications is less with these veins than with the external jugular vein (discussed later) or central IV initiation. Therefore, the veins of the hand, arm, and leg are the primary sites for IV initiation.

To establish a peripheral IV in the hand, arm, or leg, use the following technique (Procedure 14-8):

1. Confirm indication and type of IV setup needed. Gather and arrange all supplies and equipment beforehand to make the process easy and accessible.
   - IV fluid
   - Administration set
   - Intravenous cannula
   - Tape or commercial securing device
   - Venous blood drawing equipment
   - Venous constricting band
   - Antiseptic solution

   When appropriate, explain the entire process to the patient. Apply the proper Standard Precautions—gloves, mask, and protective eyewear goggles—as IV access is invasive and presents the potential for blood exposure.

2. Prepare all needed equipment. Examine the IV fluid for clarity and expiration date. Insert the administration tubing spike in the IV solution bag's administration set port. Squeeze fluid from the IV fluid container into the drip chamber until it reaches the fill line. Open the clamp and/or flow regulator to flush the solution through the administration tubing and expel trapped air bubbles. Shut down the flow regulator and replace the cap over the needle adapter. Remember that the IV administration set is sterile; if any contamination occurs, you must replace the set with a new one.

Procedure 14–8   Peripheral Intravenous Access

14-8A Place the constricting band.

14-8B Cleanse the venipuncture site.

14-8C Insert the intravenous cannula into the vein.

14-8D Withdraw any blood samples needed.

14-8E Connect the IV tubing.

14-8F Turn on the IV and check the flow.

14-8G Secure the site.

14-8H Label the intravenous solution bag.

3. Select the venipuncture site. Acceptable sites have clearly visible veins and are free of bruising or scarring. Straight veins are easier to cannulate than crooked ones.

4. Place the constricting band proximal to the intended site of puncture. Tighten it enough to impede venous blood flow without restricting arterial blood passage. Never leave the constricting band in place for more than 2 minutes, as intrinsic changes will occur in the slowed venous blood.

5. Cleanse the venipuncture site. You must cleanse the intended site of pathogens to decrease the likelihood of infection. Alcohol and similar antiseptic solutions are the most commonly used. Start at the site itself and work outward in an expanding circle. This pushes pathogens away from the puncture site.

6. Insert the intravenous cannula into the vein. With your nondominant hand, pull all local skin taut to stabilize the vein and prevent it from rolling. With the

distal bevel of the metal stylet up, insert the cannula into the vein at a 10° to 30° angle. Continue until you feel the cannula "pop" into the vein or see blood in the flashback chamber. The metal stylet is now in the vein; however, the Teflon catheter is not. To place the catheter into the vein, carefully advance the cannula approximately 0.5 cm further. (If you are using a butterfly cannula, it has no Teflon catheter, and you must carefully advance the needle itself.)

7. Holding the metal stylet stationary, slide the Teflon catheter over the needle into the vein. Place a finger over the vein at the catheter tip and tamponade (press gently downward to occlude the vein), thus preventing blood from flowing from the catheter and/or air from entraining into the circulatory system. Carefully remove the metal stylet, retract the needle, and promptly dispose of it in the sharps container. Remove the venous constricting band.

8. Obtain venous blood samples, as discussed in the section on venous blood sampling.

9. Attach the administration tubing to the cannula. Remove the protective cap from the needle adapter and tightly secure the needle adapter into the cannula hub. Open the flow regulator and allow the fluid to run freely for several seconds. Adjust the flow rate. Do not let go of the cannula and administration tubing until you have secured them, as explained in step 10.

10. Cover the catheter and puncture site with an adhesive bandage or other commercial device. Loop the distal tubing and secure with tape. This makes the medication administration port more accessible and attaches the device to the patient more securely. Continue by taping the administration tubing to the patient, proximal to the venipuncture site.

11. Label the intravenous solution bag with the following information:

    • Date and time initiated

    • Person initiating the intravenous access

12. Continually monitor the patient and flow rate.

Intravenous Access in the External Jugular Vein

The external jugular vein is a large peripheral blood vessel in the neck, between the angle of the jaw and the middle third of the clavicle. It connects into the central circulation's subclavian vein. Because it lies so close to the central circulation, cannulation here offers many of the same benefits afforded by central venous access. Fluids and medications rapidly reach the core of the body from this site.

Consider accessing the external jugular only after you have exhausted other means of peripheral access or when a patient requires immediate fluid administration. This is an extremely painful site to access, so you typically will reserve its use for patients with a decreased or total loss of consciousness.

Cannulating the external jugular vein requires essentially the same equipment as other forms of peripheral IV access, plus a 10-mL syringe. You will not need a constricting band. To access the external jugular, use the following technique (Procedure 14-9):

1. Prepare all equipment as for peripheral IV access in an arm, hand, or leg. In addition, fill the 10-mL syringe with 3 to 5 mL of sterile saline. Attach the distal part of the syringe to the flashback chamber of a large bore, over-the-needle catheter. Use Standard Precautions.

2. Place the patient supine and/or in the Trendelenburg position. This position will increase blood flow to the chest and neck, thus distending the vein and making it easier to see. In addition, the supine-Trendelenburg position decreases the chance of air entering the circulatory system during cannulation.

3. Turn the patient's head to the side opposite of access. This maneuver makes the site easier to see and reach; do not perform it if the patient has traumatic head and/or neck injuries.

4. Cleanse the site with antiseptic solution. Start at the site of intended puncture and work outward 1 to 2 inches (2.4–5.0 cm) in ever-increasing circles.

5. Occlude venous return by placing a finger on the external jugular just above the clavicle. This should distend the vein, again allowing greater visualization and ease of puncture. Never apply a venous constricting band around the patient's neck.

6. Position the intravenous cannula parallel with the vein, midway between the angle of the jaw and the clavicle. Point the catheter at the medial third of the clavicle and insert it, bevel up, at a 10° to 30° angle.

7. Enter the external jugular while withdrawing on the plunger of the attached syringe. You will see blood in the syringe or feel a pop as the cannula enters the vein. Once inside the vein, advance the entire catheter another 0.5 cm so the tip of the Teflon catheter lies within the lumen of the vein. Then slide the Teflon catheter into the vein and remove the metal stylet, as previously described, and retract the needle. Immediately dispose of the metal stylet.

8. Obtain venous blood samples, as discussed in the section on venous blood sampling.

9. Attach the administration tubing to the IV catheter. Allow the intravenous solution to run freely for several seconds. Set the flow rate and secure as appropriate.

10. Monitor the patient for complications.

Procedure 14–9   Peripheral Intravenous Access in an External Jugular Vein

14-9A Place the patient supine or in the Trendelenburg position.

14-9B Turn the patient's head to the side opposite of access and cleanse the site.

14-9C Occlude venous return by placing a finger on the external jugular just above the clavicle.

14-9D Point the catheter at the medial third of the clavicle and insert it, bevel up, at a 10° to 30° angle.

14-9E Enter the external jugular while withdrawing on the plunger of the attached syringe.

Although using the external jugular vein has advantages, it also has distinct drawbacks. You may inadvertently puncture the airway or damage the nearby arterial vessels. Additionally, this is a painful entry site for the conscious patient. To minimize risks, perform the procedure very carefully.

Intravenous Access with a Measured Volume Administration Set

When using a measured volume administration set, follow this procedure (Procedure 14-10):

1. Prepare the tubing by closing all clamps, and insert the flanged spike into the IV solution bag's spike port.

2. Open the airway handle. Open the uppermost clamp and fill the burette chamber with approximately 20 mL of fluid. Squeeze the drip chamber until the fluid reaches the fill line. Open the bottom flow regulator to purge air through the tubing. When all air is purged, close the bottom flow regulator.

3. Continue to fill the burette chamber with the designated amount of solution.

4. Close the uppermost clamp and open the flow regulator until you reach the desired drip rate. Leave the airway handle open, so that air replaces the displaced fluid.

To refill the burette chamber, open the uppermost clamp until you have delivered the desired volume; then repeat step 4.

You can also use measured volume administration sets for continuous fluid administration. Fill the burette chamber with at least 30 mL of solution and close the airway handle. Leave the uppermost clamp open and adjust the rate with the lower flow regulator.

Intravenous Access with Blood Tubing

To establish an IV with blood tubing, use the following procedure (Procedure 14-11):

1. Prepare the tubing by closing all clamps, and insert the flanged spike into the spike port of the blood and/or normal saline solution (Y-configured tubing).

2. Squeeze the drip chamber until it is one-third full and blood covers the filter. Repeat for the normal saline if you are using Y tubing.

3. If you are using straight tubing, piggyback a secondary line of normal saline into the blood tubing, unless you plan to piggyback the straight blood tubing into a large-bore primary line.

4. Flush all tubing with normal saline and blood as appropriate.

5. Attach blood tubing to the intravenous cannula or into a previously established IV line.

Procedure 14–10   Intravenous Access with a Measured Volume Administration Set

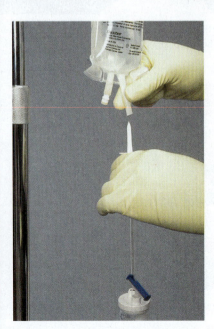

14-10A Spike the solution bag.

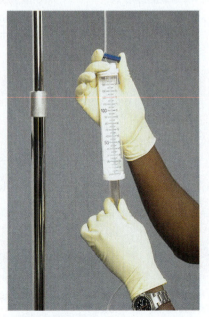

14-10B Open the uppermost clamp and fill the burette chamber with the desired volume of fluid.

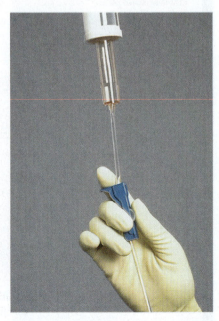

14-10C Close the uppermost clamp and open the flow regulator.

Procedure 14–11   Intravenous Access with Blood Tubing

14-11A Insert the flanged spike into the spike port of the blood and/or normal saline solution.

14-11B Squeeze the drip chamber until it is one-third full and blood covers the filter.

14-11C Attach blood tubing to the intravenous cannula or into a previously established IV line.

14-11D Open the clamp(s) and/or flow regulator(s) and adjust the flow rate.

6. Ensure patency by infusing a small amount of normal saline. Shut down when you have confirmed patency.

7. Open the clamp(s) and/or flow regulator(s) that allows blood to move from the bag to the patient. Adjust the flow rate accordingly.

8. When blood therapy is complete or must be discontinued, shut down the flow regulator from the blood supply and open the regulator(s) for the normal saline solution.

Factors Affecting Intravenous Flow Rates

If an IV does not flow properly, check for the following problems and correct them as appropriate.

- *Constricting band.* Has the venous constricting band been removed? This is probably the most common mistake both in and out of the hospital. Additionally, ensure that the patient is not wearing restrictive clothing that interferes with venous blood flow.

- *Edema at the puncture site.* Swelling at the IV site indicates fluid collection caused by infiltration. This **extravasation** occurs if you accidentally puncture the vein more than once, thus allowing IV solution and blood to escape from the second puncture and accumulate in the surrounding tissue. An infiltrated IV site is not usable.

- *Cannula abutting the vein wall or valve.* If the distal tip of the cannula butts against a wall or valve, carefully reposition it. You may have to untape and retape the cannula once you have achieved an adequate flow rate. Additionally, you may need to use an arm board to keep the patient's extremity straight, as flexion may kink the vein at the site and impede the solution's flow.

- *Administration set control valves.* Ensure that the flow regulator is open. Be sure to check the flow regulator and clamps of both the primary and any secondary or extension tubing.

- *IV bag height.* When you move the patient, you may raise the cannulation site above the IV solution bag. This interrupts the solution's gravitational flow from the bag into the patient.

- *Completely filled drip chamber.* Is the drip chamber completely filled? You can easily correct this by inverting the bag and squeezing the fluid from the drip chamber back into the bag.

- *Catheter patency.* A blood clot at the end of the Teflon catheter or needle may obstruct the flow of solution from the IV solution bag into the body. If the flow slows, increase the IV drip rate to keep the catheter or needle clear. If the flow stops completely, cleanse the medication administration port closest to the IV entry site with alcohol preparations and insert a syringe and hypodermic needle. Gently aspirate back on the syringe until the blood clot is pulled into the syringe. Never flush an IV that has stopped running because of a clot. Flushing will force the clot into the circulatory system and can cause occlusions in the heart or lungs.

If flow remains inadequate after you have eliminated all these possible causes, lower the IV bag below the insertion site. If blood flows into the IV administration tubing, the site is patent and the problem lies elsewhere. If the problem persists, remove the IV and reestablish it on another extremity, using all new equipment. If you do not observe blood return, the site is inoperable.

Complications of Peripheral Intravenous Access

Even though it is a routine procedure, intravenous access is not trouble free. It can cause a number of complications.

PAIN   Pain at the puncture site occurs during needle penetration or with extravasation. To minimize pain, use a smaller-gauge catheter or use a 1 percent lidocaine solution (without epinephrine) to anesthetize the overlying skin before insertion.

LOCAL INFECTION   Local infection occurs if you do not properly cleanse the site and thus introduce pathogens through the puncture. This complication does not become apparent until after the IV has been established for several hours.

PYROGENIC REACTION   **Pyrogens** (foreign proteins capable of producing fever) in the administration tubing or IV solution can cause a pyrogenic reaction. The abrupt onset of fever (100°F to 106°F), chills, backache, headache, nausea, and vomiting characterize these reactions. Cardiovascular collapse may also result.

Typically, a pyrogenic reaction will occur within one-half to one hour after you initiate an IV. If you suspect a pyrogenic reaction, immediately terminate the IV and reestablish access in the opposite side with new equipment and fluid.

Typically, pyrogenic reactions occur secondary to the use of intravenous solutions that have been contaminated with a microorganism or other foreign matter. Pyrogenic reactions underscore the need to discard any fluid that is cloudy or any equipment that has been opened.

> **CONTENT REVIEW**
>
> ➤ IV Troubleshooting
>   - Constricting band still in place?
>   - Edema at puncture site?
>   - Cannula abutting vein wall or valve?
>   - Administration set control valves closed?
>   - IV bag too low?
>   - Completely filled drip chamber?
>   - Catheter patent?
> ➤ IV Access Complications
>   - Pain
>   - Local infection
>   - Pyrogenic reaction
>   - Allergic reaction
>   - Catheter shear
>   - Inadvertent arterial puncture
>   - Circulatory overload
>   - Thrombophlebitis
>   - Thrombus formation
>   - Air embolism
>   - Necrosis
>   - Anticoagulants

ALLERGIC REACTION   A patient receiving IV therapy may develop an allergic reaction. Most often, allergic reactions accompany the administration of blood or colloidal (protein-containing) solutions. In addition, some patients may react to the latex in some types of IV administration tubing.

The sudden onset of hives (urticaria), itching (pruritus), localized or systemic edema, or shortness of breath may signify an allergic reaction. If you suspect an allergic reaction, stop the IV infusion and remove the IV catheter. Treat the patient as discussed in the "Immunology" chapter.

CATHETER SHEAR   A catheter shear can occur if you pull the Teflon catheter through or over the needle after you have advanced it into the vein. The soft plastic catheter will easily snag on the metal stylet's sharp point and shear off, thus forming a plastic **embolus**. Therefore, never draw the Teflon catheter over the metal stylet after you have advanced it.

INADVERTENT ARTERIAL PUNCTURE   Because arteries may lie close to veins, accidental arterial puncture may occur. Arterial blood is bright red and characteristically spurts with each contraction of the heart. When an arterial puncture occurs, immediately remove the catheter and apply direct pressure to the site for at least 5 minutes. Do not release the pressure until the hemorrhage has stopped.

CIRCULATORY OVERLOAD Circulatory overload occurs if you administer too much fluid for the patient's condition. You must monitor flow rates carefully, especially for patients with medical conditions such as kidney failure or heart failure who are intolerant of excessive fluid. Continually examine the patient for signs of circulatory overload (crackles, tachypnea, dyspnea, and jugular venous distention, as discussed in the chapter "Secondary Assessment"). If you encounter circulatory overload, adjust the flow rate.

THROMBOPHLEBITIS Thrombophlebitis, or inflammation of the vein, is particularly common in long-term intravenous therapy. Redness and edema at the puncture site are typical signs of thrombophlebitis. This complication may also present as pain along the course of the vein, sometimes accompanied by inflammation and tenderness. Typically, thrombophlebitis does not occur until several hours after IV initiation. When you suspect thrombophlebitis, terminate the IV and apply a warm compress to the site.

THROMBUS FORMATION A **thrombus**, or blood clot, can form if IV access injures the vessel wall. A thrombus may form around the catheter and occlude the movement of fluid between the IV and the blood vessel. If you suspect a thrombus, restart the IV using new equipment. Do not attempt to dislodge the clot with a fluid bolus, as this may create an embolus that causes neurologic or pulmonary complications.

AIR EMBOLISM Air embolism occurs when air enters the vein. Air embolism is most likely to occur during central venous access or when administration tubing has not been properly flushed. Failure to tamponade larger veins during cannulation may allow air into the vein.

NECROSIS Necrosis, or the sloughing off of dead tissue, occurs later in IV therapy as medication (e.g., norepinephrine, epinephrine, dopamine, dobutamine) has extravasated into the interstitial space.

ANTICOAGULANTS Anticoagulant medications such as aspirin, platelet aggregate inhibitors, warfarin (Coumadin), or heparin increase the chance of bleeding and impede hemorrhage control during IV establishment. They drastically increase the complications of hematoma or infiltration.

Changing an IV Bag or Bottle

You may sometimes have to change an IV bag or bottle. This generally occurs when only 50 mL of solution remain and you must continue therapy after those 50 mL are depleted. Changing the solution bag or bottle is a sterile process. If the equipment becomes contaminated you should dispose of it.

To change the IV solution bag or bottle, use the following technique:

1. Prepare the new IV solution bag or bottle by removing the protective cover from the IV tubing port.

2. Occlude the flow of solution from the depleted bag or bottle by moving the roller clamp on the IV administration tubing.

3. Remove the spike from the depleted IV bag or bottle. Be careful not to drop or contaminate the spike in any way.

4. Insert the spike into the new IV bag or bottle. Ensure that the drip chamber is filled appropriately.

5. Open the roller clamp to the appropriate flow rate.

If air becomes entrained within the administration tubing during this process, cleanse the medication administration port below the trapped air and insert a hypodermic needle and syringe. Pull the plunger back to aspirate the trapped air into the syringe. After you have removed the air, adjust the IV flow rate as needed.

Intravenous Medication Administration

Medications can be delivered through an existing IV line. As the IV line is seated directly into a vein, the blood rapidly absorbs these medications and distributes them throughout the body. Intravenous administration avoids many of the barriers to medication absorption in other routes. For example, medications given via the gastrointestinal tract face enzymes and other chemicals that may deactivate, exacerbate, or in some other way alter the medication being administered. Likewise, local tissues can absorb medications administered via the subcutaneous or intramuscular routes, thus preventing the total dosage from reaching the bloodstream for delivery. The two methods for administering medications through an IV line are intravenous bolus and intravenous infusion.

Intravenous Bolus

An intravenous bolus involves injecting the circulatory system with a concentrated dose of medication through the medication administration port of an established IV. This procedure requires the following equipment:

- Personal protective equipment
- Antiseptic solution
- Packaged medication
- Syringe (size depends on the volume of medication you will administer)
- 18- to 20-gauge hypodermic needle, 1 to 1.5 inches long
- Existing intravenous line with medication port

To administer an intravenous medication bolus, use the following technique (Procedure 14-12):

1. Ensure that the primary IV line is patent.
2. Confirm the medication, indication, dosage, and need for an IV bolus. Confirm that the medication is compatible with the solution being infused.

Procedure 14–12   Intravenous Bolus Administration

14-12A Prepare the equipment.

14-12B Prepare the medication.

14-12C Check the label.

14-12D Select and clean an administration port.

14-12E Pinch the line.

14-12F Administer the medication.

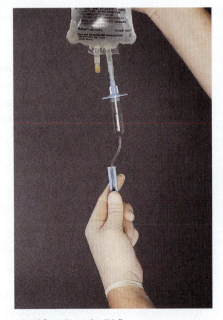

14-12G Adjust the IV flow rate.

14-12H Monitor the patient.

3. Draw up the medication or prepare a prefilled syringe as appropriate.

4. Cleanse the medication port nearest the IV site with an antiseptic preparation.

5. Insert a hypodermic needle through the port membrane.

6. Pinch the IV line above the medication port. This prevents the medication from traveling toward the fluids bag, forcing it instead toward the patient.

7. Inject the medication, as appropriate.

8. Remove the hypodermic needle and syringe and release the tubing.

9. Open the flow regulator to allow a 20-mL fluid flush. The fluid will push the medication into the patient's circulatory system.

10. Dispose of the hypodermic needle and syringe as appropriate. Monitor the patient for desired or undesired effects.

Intravenous Medication Infusion

Many cardiac medications and antibiotics are given as intravenous infusions (IV piggybacks). Intravenous medication infusions deliver a steady, continual dose of medication through an existing IV line. You may give them either as an initial dosage or to maintain medication levels after delivering an initial bolus.

Piggybacking IV infusions through an existing intravenous line gives you greater control over medication delivery and allows you to easily discontinue the infusion when therapy is complete or must be stopped. Never administer intravenous infusions as a primary IV line.

IV infusions are contained in bags or bottles of intravenous solution. If the IV infusion is premixed, read the label on the bag for the following information:

- Name of medication
- Total dosage in weight mixed in bag
- Concentration (weight per single mL)
- Expiration date

If the infusion is not premixed, make a label listing this information and attach it to the bag (Figure 14-42). Additionally, note the date and time you mixed the infusion, and initial it.

Use the following technique to administer a medication as an IV infusion (Procedure 14-13):

1. Establish a primary IV line and ensure patency.

2. Confirm administration indications and patient allergies.

3. Prepare the infusion bag or bottle. (If the infusion is premixed, continue to step 4.)

   a. Draw up the appropriate quantity of medication from its source with a syringe.

   b. Cleanse the IV bag or bottle's medication port with an antiseptic wipe.

   c. Insert the hypodermic needle into the medication port and inject the medication.

   d. Gently agitate the bag or bottle to mix its contents.

   e. Label the bag or bottle.

4. Connect administration tubing to the medication bag or bottle and fill the drip chamber to the fluid line. Most infusions require microdrip tubing. If you use a mechanical infusion pump, you may need to use special tubing.

5. Place the hypodermic needle on the administration tubing's needle adapter and flush the tubing with solution. (The needle adapter typically accepts a 20-gauge needle.)

6. Cleanse the medication administration port on the primary line with alcohol and insert the secondary line's hypodermic needle. Secure the hypodermic needle and the secondary administration line with tape or another securing device.

7. Reconfirm the indication, medication, dose, and route of administration.

8. Shut down the primary line so no fluid will flow from the primary solution bag.

9. Adjust the secondary line to the desired drip rate. If you are using a mechanical infusion pump, set it accordingly.

10. Properly dispose of the needle and syringe.

FIGURE 14-42 If an IV solution is not premixed, you will have to mix and label it yourself.

Procedure 14–13 Intravenous Infusion Administration

14-13A Select the drug.

14-13B Draw up the drug.

14-13C Select IV fluid for dilution.

14-13D Clean the medication addition port.

14-13E Inject the drug into the fluid.

14-13F Mix the solution.

14-13G Insert an administration set and connect it to the main IV line with a needle.

When the infusion is complete, shut down the secondary line with the flow regulator or a clamp. Open the primary line and adjust it to the indicated drip rate. Remove the hypodermic needle from the medication administration port and properly dispose of all contents. If required by your local protocols, retain the medication bag to verify administration and for quality assurance.

You can also use measured volume administration tubing to administer medicated infusions. First, fill the burette chamber of a measured volume administration device with a specific volume of fluid. Then you can inject the medication through the medication injection site on top of the burette chamber. You must adjust the flow rate to deliver the precise amount of medication required. In addition, you can mix the medication within the IV bag or bottles as previously described and use the measured volume administration tubing solely for administering the infusion rather than for mixing it.

Heparin Lock and Saline Lock

When a patient requires occasional IV medication drips or boluses but does not need continuous fluid, heparin locks are used. A **heparin lock** is a peripheral IV port that does not use a bag of fluid. Like a typical IV start, it places an IV cannula into a peripheral vein; however, instead of IV administration tubing, it has attached short tubing with a clamp and a distal medication port (Figure 14-43). A heparin lock decreases the risk of accidental fluid overload and electrolyte derangement. You also may withdraw blood samples from the lock if it is in a suitable vein. For short-term

FIGURE 14-43 A saline or heparin lock can be used when a patient requires occasional medications or IV drips but does not need a continuous infusion.

use, a **saline lock** may be used. Sterile saline is injected following the medication. Saline remains in the lock to keep it open. For long-term use, a heparin lock is preferred. Although it functions the same as a saline lock, a heparin lock is filled with a low-concentration solution of heparin, which aids in keeping any blood that gets into the device from clotting. Typically, a medication will be administered through the heparin lock. This is followed by a saline flush to ensure that no medication remains in the lock or hub. Then, the lock and hub are filled with a heparin solution. This aids in keeping the IV site open for a long period of time.

Initiating a heparin or saline lock requires the following equipment:

- IV cannula
- Heparin or saline lock
- Syringe with 3 to 5 mL sterile saline or commercial saline injection device
- Tape or commercial securing device
- Venous blood drawing equipment
- Venous constricting band
- Antiseptic solution
- Heparin for flush solution (if using heparin lock)—typically 10 or 100 units/mL

To place a heparin lock, follow these steps:

1. Select the venipuncture site.
2. Place the constricting band proximal to the puncture site.
3. Cleanse the venipuncture site with antiseptic solution.
4. Insert the intravenous cannula into the vein.
5. Slide the Teflon catheter into the vein.
6. Carefully remove the metal stylet, retract or protect the stylet, and promptly dispose of it into the sharps container. Remove the venous constricting band.
7. Obtain venous blood samples, as explained under "Venous Blood Sampling."
8. Attach the heparin lock tubing to the catheter hub.
9. Cleanse the medication port and inject 3 to 5 mL of sterile saline into the lock. Easy flow of the saline without edema at the puncture site indicates patency. If you encounter resistance or if edema forms, restart the procedure with new equipment. If a heparin lock is desired, fill the port with the designated heparin flush solution.
10. Apply an adhesive bandage or other commercial device. Secure the tubing to the patient.

To administer an IV medication bolus through a heparin lock, assemble the following equipment and supplies:

- Personal protective equipment
- Antiseptic solution

- Packaged medication
- Syringe (the size depends on the volume being administered)
- 18- to 20-gauge hypodermic needle 1 to 1½ inches long

After you have gathered all equipment and supplies, use the following technique to administer an IV medication bolus with a heparin or saline lock:

1. Confirm the medication, indication, dosage, and need for an IV bolus.
2. Draw up the medication or prepare a prefilled syringe as appropriate.
3. Cleanse the medication port nearest the IV site with an antiseptic solution.
4. Ensure that the plastic clamp is open.
5. Insert the hypodermic needle through the port membrane.
6. Inject the medication as appropriate.
7. Remove the hypodermic needle and dispose of it in the sharps container.
8. Follow the medication administration with a 10- to 20-mL saline flush from another syringe.
9. Properly dispose of the hypodermic needle and syringe. Monitor the patient for desired or undesired effects.

If fluid administration becomes necessary, you can unscrew the medication port and insert IV administration tubing. Periodically flush with sterile saline or heparin to prevent clot formation and occlusion at the Teflon catheter's distal end.

Venous Access Devices

A **venous access device** is an intravenous catheter that is placed into a large vein, allowing medicaion to be delivered directly into the vein. These devices are less likely to clot than peripheral intravenous lines, which are inserted into smaller veins. Venous access devices can remain in place for long periods of time; for this reason, they are used in long-term care situations. They are typically used for:

- Administration of medications (antibiotics, chemotherapy agents, and other intravenous drugs)
- Administration of fluids and nutritional compounds (hyperalimentation)
- Transfusion of blood products
- Multiple blood draws for diagnostic testing

There are three common types of venous access devices.

- *Tunnel.* Catheters can be inserted by tunneling under the skin either into the subclavian vein or into the

FIGURE 14-44 Example of a tunneled venous access device.

(© Edward T. Dickinson, MD)

internal jugular vein. The portion of the catheter where medications are administered or blood is withdrawn remains outside the skin. Common examples include the Broviac® and Hickman® catheters (Figure 14-44).

- *Medication Port.* Catheters with medication ports are placed completely below the skin. The port is a raised disk about the size of a quarter or half dollar and can be felt underneath the skin. Blood can be withdrawn or medication administered by placing a specialized tiny needle through the overlying skin into the port or reservoir. Common examples include the Portacath® and Mediport® catheters (Figure 14-45).
- *Peripherally inserted central catheter (PICC).* PICC lines are not inserted directly into the central vein. Instead, a PICC line is inserted into a large vein in the arm and then advanced into the larger subclavian vein (Figure 14-46).

FIGURE 14-45 Example of a medication port venous access device.

(Source: St Bartholomew's Hospital/Science Source)

FIGURE 14-46 Example of a PICC venous access device.

Most EMS systems have policies and procedures regarding accessing a venous access device. Use of an indwelling central venous access medication port device requires special training. Delivering a medication through the venous access device requires a special needle specific to the venous access device being used. A commonly used needle, the **Huber needle**, has an opening on the side of its shaft instead of at the tip. When the needle is placed into the injection port, this configuration allows easy administration of medication into the venous access device. Never access a venous access device unless you have the specific needle uniquely intended for that particular device. Always ask the patient, family, or nursing staff about the type of venous access device. Often, they will have a supply of needles for the device.

To administer fluids, medication, or blood through a venous access device, you must first prepare the site using the following technique:

1. Use Standard Precautions.
2. Fill a 10-mL syringe with approximately 7 mL of normal saline.
3. Place a 21- or 22-gauge Huber needle (or other specialized needle) on the end of the syringe.
4. Cleanse the skin over the injection port with an antiseptic solution.
5. Stabilize the site with one hand while inserting the Huber needle at a 90° angle. Gently advance it until it meets resistance. This signals that the needle has contacted the floor of the injection port.
6. Pull back on the plunger and observe for blood return. The presence of blood confirms placement.
7. Slowly inject the normal saline to ensure patency.

To administer the medication by intravenous bolus, use the following technique:

1. Prepare the medication, fluid, or blood for administration.
2. Attach a 21- or 22-gauge Huber needle (or other specialized needle) to the end of the syringe.
3. Cleanse the skin over the injection port with antiseptic solutions.
4. Insert the needle into the injection port at a 90° angle until the needle cannot be further advanced. Pull back on the plunger of the syringe and observe for the return of blood. The presence of blood confirms proper placement.
5. Inject the medication as appropriate.
6. Remove and dispose of the syringe appropriately.
7. With another syringe and attached specialized needle, administer a bolus of heparinized saline to clear the catheter of any blood clots or other obstruction.

If the venous access device is not patent or access proves difficult, contact medical direction for further directives.

To administer IV fluids, use the following technique:

1. Prepare a primary IV line. Be sure to prime or flush the air from the administration tubing.
2. Attach a 21- or 22-gauge Huber needle (or other specialized needle) to the primary IV administration tubing. Insert a 10-mL syringe and hypodermic needle filled with 7 mL of normal saline solution into the tubing medication delivery port nearest the venous access device.
3. Cleanse the skin over the injection port with an antiseptic solution.
4. Insert the needle into the injection port at a 90° angle until it encounters resistance.
5. Pinch the administration tubing above the medication administration port and pull back on the syringe plunger. Observe for the return of blood. The presence of blood confirms proper placement.
6. Gently inject the 7 mL of normal saline solution.
7. Set the primary line to the appropriate flow rate.

If administering a secondary medicated infusion, continue as follows:

1. Prepare a secondary line containing the fluid, blood, or medicated solution for infusion.
2. Attach a hypodermic needle to the needle adapter of the secondary line. Insert the secondary line into a medication administration port on the primary tubing.
3. Shut down the primary line and infuse the medicated solution as appropriate. Look for ease of administration as a sign of patency.

4. When infusion is complete, administer a bolus of heparinized saline to clear the catheter of any blood clots or other obstruction.

Using a venous access device is a very sterile procedure. You must take care to clean the site before delivering medications. Other complications of using a venous access device include infection, thrombus formation, and dislodgment of the catheter tip from the vein.

Electromechanical Infusion Devices

Electromechanical infusion devices permit the precise delivery of fluid and/or medications through electronic regulation. Whenever intravenous infusion occurs, electromechanical infusion pumps provide optimal delivery. Infusion devices are classified as either infusion controllers or infusion pumps.

INFUSION CONTROLLERS Infusion controllers are gravity-flow devices that regulate the fluid's passage through the pump. Because infusion controllers do not use positive pressure, they will not force fluids into the **extravascular** space if you infiltrate the vein.

INFUSION PUMPS Infusion pumps deliver fluids and medications under positive pressure (Figure 14-47). This pressure can cause complications such as hematoma or extravasation if you infiltrate the vein. Some infusion pumps contain a pressure monitor and will warn you if they encounter the increased resistance that occurs with infiltration.

Syringe-type infusion pumps are gaining popularity for medical transport. Syringe pumps deliver their medications from a medical syringe without a hypodermic needle instead of from IV solution bags, fluids, or liquid medications (Figure 14-48). You place the syringe containing the medications in the pump, which uses computerized mechanics to gradually depress the plunger at the correct rate. These compact pumps prove advantageous during transport.

FIGURE 14-48 (a) Syringe-type infusion pump in use. (b) Dual-rate syringe-type pump.

(Photo a: © Edward T. Dickinson, MD; Photo b: Courtesy of © Numia Medical Technology, LLC)

FIGURE 14-47 Modern infusion pump.

(© Edward T. Dickinson, MD)

Legal Considerations

Drawing Blood for Law Enforcement. In some regions, paramedics may be asked to draw blood for law enforcement. If this is the case in your system, make sure that you have established protocols and medical director permission before performing the task. Be advised that you may well be called to court to testify about what you saw or what you did.[10]

Manufacturers make many different electromechanical infusion pumps. Depending on the maker, pump compatibility may require specialized administration tubing. With some computerized pumps, you can enter the basic information and then the pump will perform all medical calculations internally and automatically set the drip rate. Most infusion pumps contain internal monitoring devices that sound an alarm for problems such as infiltration, occlusion, or fluid source depletion. Electronic devices are prone to malfunction, however, so you must be prepared to perform all calculations and set the drip rate manually.

Ultrasound-Guided Intravenous Access

The use of portable **ultrasound** to aid in placement of peripheral intravenous lines is now common in hospital emergency departments. With the advent of newer portable ultrasound machines it is also being used in the out-of-hospital setting.[11]

Medical ultrasound is a diagnostic imaging technique based on the application of ultrasound. Ultrasound uses sound or other vibrations having an ultrasonic frequency to image specific body structures. An ultrasound transducer probe emits and receives ultrasound waves. These waves are converted into an electrical signal (image) that can be displayed on a computer or similar screen. This gives a real-time image of the structures being observed. Blood vessels are filled with fluid (blood) and are usually easy to identify using ultrasound imaging. This technique is beneficial in patients with veins that are deep or difficult to palpate. It is also useful in shock and hypotension, when the veins are less distended.

Generally, the medium footprint linear array probe is the preferred ultrasound probe for peripheral IV insertions. A tourniquet is not required but can be used as desired. Place conductive gel on the probe and place the probe over the planned IV site. Start by placing the transducer over the antecubital fossa in a transverse orientation (Figure 14-49). The probe indicator should point to the patient's right side (operator's left side). Survey the venous anatomy. Apply pressure to compress the vessels seen. Veins will compress readily, whereas arteries will not. Arteries can be distinguished from veins as follows:

- Veins collapse easily and completely when gentle pressure is applied with the transducer.
- Arteries will not collapse completely, although slight compression of artery walls can be seen. Also, arteries will often be pulsating and the arterial walls may be thicker than venous walls.
- Color-flow Doppler and pulsed-wave spectral Doppler can help identify veins and differentiate them from arteries, if needed.

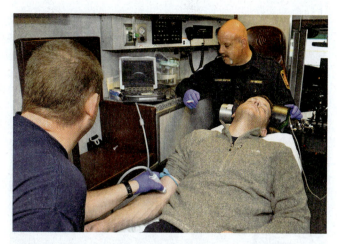

FIGURE 14-49 The use of medical ultrasound can help in placement of peripheral venous catheters.

(© Edward T. Dickinson, MD)

Once a vein is identified, hold the probe in your nondominant hand or have an assistant hold the probe in position (Figure 14-50).

Prep the skin and choose a catheter of adequate length to enter the vein. Insert the needle through the skin. Once through the skin, the needle should be visible as a shadow on the ultrasound image. Direct the needle toward the target vein. As you approach the wall of the vein, the needle will compress or tent the vein. Advance the needle into the lumen of the vein. You will often feel a subtle "pop" when this occurs (Figure 14-51).

You should notice a flash in the catheter indicating entry into the vein. Advance the catheter into the vein while withdrawing the needle. Verify placement by observing the needle within the lumen of the vein on ultrasound and by the ability to withdraw a small amount of blood. Secure the catheter in a common fashion and begin fluid or medication administration as indicated. Remove, clean, and secure the ultrasound probe.

FIGURE 14-50 Vascular anatomy of the forearm seen with ultrasound technology.

(© Edward T. Dickinson, MD)

FIGURE 14-51 Ultrasound identification of needle within the lumen of the vein.

(© Edward T. Dickinson, MD)

Venous Blood Sampling

The laboratory analysis of blood can provide valuable information about the sick and/or injured patient. The concentrations of electrolytes, gases, hormones, or other chemicals in blood can often shed light on the underlying causes of vague complaints such as dizziness or generalized weakness. Additionally, blood evaluation can confirm suspected conditions. For example, elevated cardiac enzymes in a patient's blood can confirm a suspected myocardial infarction.

In the field, you often will be the first to assess and treat an ill or injured patient. Many of your interventions can alter the blood's composition and erase important information. If you obtain venous blood samples before performing those interventions, they will enable the physician to evaluate the patient's original status.

Venous blood is commonly obtained via venipuncture. Thus, paramedics, who routinely initiate intravenous access, can simultaneously obtain blood samples. Doing so saves considerable hospital time and avoids multiple needle sticks.

You should obtain venous blood in the following situations:

- During peripheral access
- Before medication administration
- When medication administration may be needed

Never stop to draw blood if it will delay critical measures such as medication administration in cardiac arrest or transport in a multisystem trauma.

Equipment for Drawing Blood

You will need the following equipment to obtain venous blood.

BLOOD TUBES **Blood tubes** are made of glass and have color-coded, self-sealing rubber tops. Blood tube sizes for adults generally range from 5 to 7 mL—for pediatrics, from 2 to 3 mL (Figure 14-52). They are vacuum packed, and some contain a chemical anticoagulant. The different-colored tops correspond to specific anticoagulants. A label on every blood tube identifies the type of additive and its expiration date. Do not use a blood tube after its expiration date, as both the anticoagulant and the vacuum lose their effectiveness.

Using blood tubes in their correct order is essential. If you do not follow the proper sequence, the various anticoagulants will cause cross-contamination, skewing the results and rendering the blood useless. Your local EMS system and receiving hospitals can provide information about the appropriate order of tubes.

MISCELLANEOUS EQUIPMENT Depending on the technique you use to obtain venous blood, you will also need syringes, hypodermic needles, and commercially manufactured plastic sleeves called vacutainers.

Obtaining Venous Blood

Obtaining venous blood is a simple process; however, if the blood is to remain usable, you must pay strict attention to detail. You can obtain blood either from an IV catheter or directly from the vein. Which technique you use will depend on the situation. In either case, venous blood samples are best obtained from sturdy veins such as the cephalic, basilic, or median. Smaller veins such as those on the back of the hand are more likely to collapse during retrieval, making the procedure difficult to complete.

OBTAINING VENOUS BLOOD FROM AN IV CATHETER The most convenient way to obtain venous blood is through an IV catheter at the time of peripheral vascular

FIGURE 14-52 Blood tubes.

FIGURE 14-53 Vacutainer with multi-sampling needle.

access. In addition to blood tubes, you will need a tube holder (Figure 14-53). The tube holder is commonly referred to as a **vacutainer**. A special adapter needle called a *multi-draw needle* fits into the tube holder. The multidraw needle has a rubber-covered needle used to puncture the self-sealing top of the blood tube. The remaining portion of the multidraw needle protrudes from the tube holder and fits snugly into the hub of the IV catheter.

To obtain blood directly from the IV catheter, use the following procedure:

1. Assemble and prepare all equipment. Inspect the blood tubes for expiration or damage and insert the multidraw needle into the vacutainer.

    Note: Never place blood tubes into the assembled vacutainer and multidraw needle until you are ready to draw blood. This will destroy the vacuum and render the blood tube useless.

2. Establish IV access with the IV catheter. Do not connect IV administration tubing.

3. Attach the end of the multidraw needle adapter to the hub of the cannula.

4. In correct order, insert the blood tubes so that the rubber-covered needle punctures the self-sealing rubber top. Blood should be pulled into the blood tube.

5. Fill all blood tubes completely, as the amount of anticoagulant is proportional to the tube's volume. Gently agitate the tubes to mix the anticoagulant evenly with the blood.

6. Tamponade the vein and remove the vacutainer and multidraw needle. Attach the IV and ensure patency.

7. Properly dispose of all sharps.

8. Label all blood tubes with the following information:
    *   Patient's first and last name
    *   Patient's age and gender
    *   Date and time drawn
    *   Name of the person drawing the blood

If commercial equipment is not available, use a 20-mL syringe (Figure 14-54). Attach the syringe's needle adapter to the IV catheter hub and gently pull back the plunger. Blood will fill the syringe. When the syringe is full, remove it from the IV catheter and place the IV line into the IV catheter. Carefully attach a hypodermic needle to the syringe to puncture the tops of the blood tubes. In the appropriate order, place the collected blood into the blood tubes and agitate gently. When finished, properly dispose of all sharps and label the blood tubes.

OBTAINING BLOOD DIRECTLY FROM A VEIN When IV access is difficult or unobtainable, you may draw blood directly from the vein with a hypodermic needle. This technique is useful for routine sampling that will not require

FIGURE 14-54 Obtaining a blood sample with a 20-mL syringe.

FIGURE 14-55 Luer sampling needle.

further IV access. To draw blood directly from a vein, you will need the same equipment as for obtaining blood from an IV catheter, but instead of a standard needle and syringe you can use a **Luer sampling needle** (Figure 14-55). A Luer sampling needle is similar to a multidraw needle, but instead of an IV catheter adapter it has a long, exposed needle. The Luer sampling needle screws into the vacutainer, and you insert the exposed needle directly into the vein. You will also need a constricting band and antiseptic wipes.

To obtain blood directly from a vein, use the following procedure:

1. Assemble and prepare all equipment. Inspect the blood tubes for expiration or damage, and insert the multidraw needle into the vacutainer.

2. Apply the constricting band and select an appropriate puncture site.

3. Cleanse the site with antiseptic solution.

4. Insert the end of the multi-sampling needle or the Luer sampling needle into the vein and remove the constricting band.

5. In the correct order, insert each blood tube so that the rubber-covered needle punctures the self-sealing rubber top. Blood should be pulled into the tube.

6. Gently agitate the tube to evenly mix the anticoagulant with the blood. Completely fill all blood tubes, as the anticoagulant is proportional to the volume of the tube.

7. Place sterile gauze over the site and remove the sampling needle. Properly dispose of all sharps.

8. Cover the puncture site with gauze and tape or an adhesive bandage.

9. Label all blood tubes with the following information:

   - Patient's first and last name
   - Patient's age and gender
   - Date and time drawn
   - Person drawing the blood

Again, if commercial equipment is not available, you may use a 20-mL syringe. When using a syringe, attach an 18-gauge hypodermic needle to the end of the syringe and insert it into the vein. Gently pull back the plunger to fill the syringe with blood. When the syringe is full, remove the syringe and dress the puncture site. In the appropriate order, inject the collected blood into the blood tubes and gently agitate. When you have finished, properly dispose of all sharps and label the blood tubes.

Complications from drawing blood include damage to the vein wall, inadvertent removal of the IV catheter, and hemoconcentration and hemolysis of the blood sample. **Hemoconcentration** occurs when the constricting band is left in place too long, elevating the numbers of red and white blood cells in the sample. **Hemolysis** is the destruction of red blood cells. When red blood cells are destroyed, they release hemoglobin and potassium, thus rendering the blood unusable. Causes of hemolysis include vigorously shaking the blood tubes after they are filled, using too small a needle for retrieval, or too forcefully aspirating blood into or out of a syringe.

Removing a Peripheral IV

You should remove any IV that will not flow or has fulfilled its need. To do so, completely occlude the tubing with the flow regulator and/or clamp. Remove all tape or other securing devices from the tubing and the patient. Place a sterile gauze pad over the puncture site. Apply pressure to the gauze with the fingers or thumb of your nondominant hand. With your dominant hand, grasp the cannula at its hub and swiftly remove it, pulling straight back. The site may bleed, so apply direct pressure with the gauze for 5 minutes. Immediately dispose of all materials in the appropriate biohazard container. Apply an adhesive bandage or tape clean gauze over the site to protect against infection. Document that the catheter was removed intact.

Intraosseous Infusion

Intraosseous (IO) infusions involve inserting a rigid needle into the cavity of a long bone or into the sternum (*intra-*, within; *os*, bone). The bone marrow contains a network of venous sinusoids that drain into the nutrient and emissary veins. These sinusoids accept fluids and medications during intraosseous infusion and transport them to the venous system. Any solution or medication that can be administered intravenously, either bolus or infusion, can be administered by the intraosseous route.

The National Association of EMS Physicians (NAEMSP) has recommended that every EMS system should have at least one method of obtaining pediatric IO access and one method for obtaining adult IO access. Although intravenous lines remain the preferred route of vascular access, IOs provide a rapid and reliable method for administering medications and fluids when an IV cannot be established. The most frequent need for IO access will be for patients in shock and cardiac arrest. IO access may be needed in pediatric hypovolemia. Victims of multiple trauma may benefit from IO therapy, although the prevailing evidence shows that out-of-hospital fluids in trauma are of questionable benefit.[11,12]

Access Site

The bone most commonly used for pediatric and adult intraosseous access is the proximal tibia (medial and inferior to the anterior tibial tuberosity). Other insertion sites for the adult include the medial malleolus of the distal tibia, the humeral head, and the sternum (Figure 14-56). Overall, the insertion site depends on the device being used as well as the age and condition of the patient. To properly locate appropriate sites and avoid complications, you must understand the anatomy and physiology of the tibia (Figure 14-57), the other possible (device-specific) insertion sites, and the sternum. The three main sections of the tibia are the diaphysis, which comprises the middle, and the two epiphyses,

one at either end. Epiphyseal disks, or growth plates, between the diaphysis and the epiphyses allow the tibia to grow and develop and are present in children. Damage to these disks during intraosseous access can cause long-term growth complications or abnormalities in children.

Within the diaphysis, the medullary canal contains the bone marrow. When placed correctly, the distal part of the intraosseous needle will lie in the medullary canal. On either side of the proximal tibia are the medial and lateral condyles. You can identify the proximal epiphysis by palpating the condyles.

Between the condyles, on the top of the anterior tibial crest, is a palpable bump called the tibial tuberosity. The tibial

(a)

(b)

(c)

(d)

FIGURE 14-56 Intraosseous needle placement sites depend on the device being used and include (a) the proximal tibia, (b) the medial malleolus of the distal tibia, (c) the humeral head, and (d) the sternum.

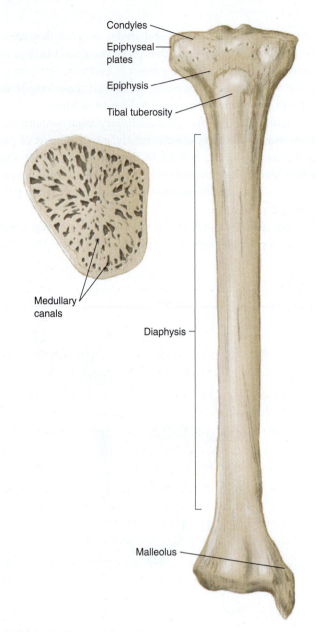

FIGURE 14-57 Anatomy of the tibia.

FIGURE 14-58 Intraosseous needle.

trocar gives strength for puncture and prevents occlusion during insertion. Upon placement, the trocar is removed. The intraosseous needle has a plastic handle for insertion and an adjustable plastic disk to stabilize the needle once it is in place. You will attach a 10-mL syringe containing 3 to 5 mL of sterile saline to the intraosseous needle. The syringe and saline are used similarly to IV access of the external jugular vein. A large-bore spinal needle with a trocar in place is an acceptable substitute for an intraosseous needle.

Other equipment for intraosseous placement is similar to that for a peripheral intravenous access line (fluid, administration tubing, tape, antiseptics, and gauze). However, you will not use a constricting band or traditional cannula. A pressure infuser is often needed for IO fluid administration. Some IO devices require a specialized adapter for flushing or using a pressure infuser. Depending on the specific intraosseous needle, you may need an adapter to connect the administration tubing and the needle.

Several commercial devices are available for both pediatric and adult intraosseous access. Although these devices differ in their mechanism and location, they still must be placed through the cortex of a bone and into the marrow cavity where fluids and medications can be administered. Examples of commercial IO access devices include the following:

- *Bone Injection Gun (B.I.G.).* The Bone Injection Gun (B.I.G.) was developed in Israel and is available in an adult and a pediatric model (Figures 14-59a and 14-59b).
- *FAST1®.* The FAST1 allows adult intraosseous placement into the sternum. This site is easy to access, and the device is easy to insert. A special needle introducer guides insertion, and a dome protects the site after placement (Figure 14-60).
- *EZ-IO™.* The EZ-IO uses a small drill to place the needle into the bone. The drill is reusable. The technique is based on the procedure routinely used by orthopedic surgeons. The manufacturer recommends placement in the proximal or distal tibia or the proximal humerus. The device is approved for both adults and children. Successful first-time placement of an intraosseous device with the EZ-IO is high (Figure 14-61).

tuberosity lies at the level of the epiphyseal growth plate. Consequently, the tibial tuberosity is extremely important in locating the appropriate pediatric intraosseous access site.

For the pediatric patient, you will establish intraosseous access on the medial aspect of the proximal tibia. This site is from two to three fingerbreadths below the tibial tuberosity. At this level, place the needle on the flat area medial to the anterior tibial crest. For adult or geriatric patients, place the needle at the distal part of the tibia, one to two fingerbreadths above the medial malleolus.

Equipment for Intraosseous Access

Intraosseous placement requires a specially designed needle and a 10-mL syringe. Manufactured specifically for IO access, an intraosseous needle is a 14- to 18-gauge hollow cannula with a sharp metal **trocar** inside (Figure 14-58). The

(a)

(b)

FIGURE 14-59 The Bone Injection Gun (B.I.G.): (a) adult model (b) pediatric model.

(Both photos: A.C.T.N.T. Healthcare Services www.bone-gun.com)

Placing an Intraosseous Infusion

To place an intraosseous line, use the following technique (Procedure 14-14):

1. Determine the indication for intraosseous access.
2. Assemble and check all equipment.

FIGURE 14-60 The FAST1® allows intraosseous placement in the sternum of an adult or adolescent (12 years of age and older).

(Pyng Medical Corp.)

FIGURE 14-61 The EZ-IO™, which uses a small drill to place the needle into the bone, is approved for both adults and children.

(Vidacare.com)

3. Position the patient. Rotate the leg toward the outside to expose the medial, proximal aspect of the tibia.
4. Locate the access site. Palpate the tibia and use all landmarks.
   - *Pediatric.* Locate the tibial tuberosity. Move from one to two fingerbreadths below the tibial tuberosity and find the flat expanse medial to the anterior tibial crest.
   - *Adult or geriatric.* Find the medial locations (based on the device you are using). These can include the tibial tuberosity, sternum, or humeral head. Be familiar with the accepted access sites, as well as the operation of the particular IO device you are using.
5. Cleanse the site with an antiseptic solution. Start at the puncture site and work outward in an expanding circular motion.
6. Perform the puncture. Holding the needle perpendicular to the puncture site, insert it with a twisting motion until you feel a decrease in resistance or a "pop." When this occurs, the needle is in the medullary canal. Do not advance it any further. Generally, you will need to insert the needle only 2 to 4 mm for entry.
7. Remove the trocar and attach the syringe. Slowly pull back the plunger to attempt aspiration into the syringe. Easy aspiration of bone marrow and blood confirms correct medullary placement.
8. Once you have confirmed placement, rotate the plastic disk toward the skin to secure the needle.
9. Remove the syringe and attach the prepared administration tubing and solution. Set the appropriate flow rate.
10. Secure the intraosseous needle as if securing an impaled object by surrounding it with bulky dressings and taping them securely in place. Commercial devices for securing an intraosseous needle are available.

Procedure 14–14   Intraosseous Medication Administration

14-14A Select the medication and prepare equipment.

14-14B Palpate the puncture site and prep with an antiseptic solution.

14-14C Make the puncture.

14-14D Aspirate to confirm proper placement.

After establishing intraosseous access, you must periodically flush the intraosseous needle to keep it patent. Failure to do so may allow the needle to become occluded, hindering medication administration.

Because the intraosseous needle is connected to the primary IV administration set and fluid, the intraosseous route can also deliver any solution or medication that can be administered by IV bolus or continuous infusion. To administer medications or solutions through the intraosseous route, use the medicinal administration port on the primary

administration tubing with the techniques as described under "Intravenous Medication Administration" ("Intravenous Medication Bolus and Intravenous Medication Infusion").

If an intraosseous infusion is complete or must be discontinued because of an adverse reaction, shut down the secondary line with the flow regulator or a clamp. Open the primary line and adjust it to the indicated drip rate. Remove the hypodermic needle from the medication administration port and properly dispose of all contents if the infusion has been exhausted.

14-14E Connect the IV fluid tubing.

14-14F Secure the needle appropriately.

14-14G Administer the medication. Monitor the patient for effects.

Intraosseous Access Complications and Precautions

Intraosseous access poses serious potential complications:

- *Fracture.* Too large a needle or too forceful an insertion can fracture the tibia, particularly in very young children.

- *Infiltration.* Infiltration occurs when IV solution collects in the local tissues instead of in the intramedullary canal. Infiltration may occur if you run fluids through an incorrectly placed needle or if a fracture has occurred. An infusion that does not run freely, or the formation of an edema at the puncture site, indicates infiltration. If infiltration occurs, immediately discontinue infusion and restart on the other leg.

- *Growth plate damage.* An improperly located puncture may damage the growth plate and result in long-term growth complications. Locating the site with proper technique is the most effective way to prevent this complication.

CONTENT REVIEW

➤ Intraosseous Access
   Complications
   • Fracture
   • Infiltration
   • Growth plate damage
   • Complete insertion
   • Pulmonary embolism
   • Infection

- *Complete insertion.* Complete insertion occurs when the needle passes through both sides of the tibia, rendering the site useless. To avoid complete puncture, stop advancing the needle once you feel the pop. If complete puncture occurs, remove the intraosseous needle with a reverse twisting motion and start again on the other leg. Apply direct pressure and a sterile dressing over the site(s) for at least 5 minutes.

- *Pulmonary embolism.* If bone, fat, or marrow particles make their way into the circulatory system, pulmonary embolism may result. Proper technique and vigilance for signs associated with pulmonary embolism (sudden onset of chest pain or shortness of breath) are important to establishing and maintaining intraosseous access.

Other complications of intraosseous access are similar to those of peripheral intravenous access. They include local infection, thrombophlebitis, air embolism, circulatory overload, and allergic reaction.

Contraindications to Intraosseous Placement

Do not attempt intraosseous placement in the following situations:

- Fracture to the tibia or femur on the side of access
- *Osteogenesis imperfecta*—a congenital bone disease that results in fragile bones
- Osteoporosis
- Establishment of a peripheral IV line

Intraosseous placement is a relatively safe intervention that can be used for the critically ill patient. Its location allows access while you perform other interventions such as CPR or endotracheal intubation. Because you probably will use intraosseous access only infrequently, you must continually refresh this skill so that you can perform it properly when needed.

PART 3: Medical Mathematics

Proper medication administration requires basic mathematical proficiency. Because medication dosages are not always standardized, you may have to calculate amounts according to your patient's age, weight, or other medically related criteria. To properly prepare and administer medications, you must understand roman numerals and be proficient in the following mathematical skills:

- Multiplication
- Division
- Fractions
- Decimal fractions
- Proportions
- Percentages

If you are deficient in one or more of these areas, refer to any text on basic and intermediate math.[13]

CONTENT REVIEW

➤ Fundamental Metric Units
   • Grams—mass
   • Meters—distance
   • Liters—volume

Metric System

Medication doses are most often expressed and measured in metric units. Accepted worldwide, the metric system is pharmacology's principal system of measurement. Once you become familiar with it, the metric system is easy to use.

The metric system's three fundamental units are grams (mass), meters (distance), and liters (volume). In pharmacology, you will frequently encounter dosages greater or less than these fundamental units. To avoid long numbers with repetitive zeros when measurements are substantially less than or greater than the fundamental unit, the metric

Cultural Considerations

The Metric System. Although the United States has been slow to adopt the metric system, it is widely used in science and medicine. As a paramedic, you must be familiar with the metric system and be able to make calculations using it.

system adds prefixes to the fundamental units. Table 14-2 lists metric prefixes.

The most commonly used prefixes in pharmacology are *kilo-, centi-, milli-,* and *micro-*. Prefixes above the fundamental units denote quantities larger than the standard gram, liter, or meter, whereas those below are smaller. The prefix *milli-* is smaller than the fundamental unit and *m* refers to 1/1,000. Thus, a *milliliter* (mL) equals 1/1,000 (one one-thousandth) of a liter. If you divided a liter into one thousand equal parts, a milliliter would equal one of those parts. Similarly, a milligram (mg) is 1/1,000 of a gram. If you divided a gram into one thousand equal parts, a milligram would equal one of those parts. The prefix *micro-* expresses 1/1,000,000. A *microgram* (mcg) is 1/1,000,000 (one one-millionth) of a gram.

Table 14-2 Metric Prefixes

Prefix	Multiplier	Abbreviation
Kilo	1,000	k
Hecto	100	h
Deka	10	D
Deci	1/10 or 0.1	d
Centi	1/100 or 0.01	C
Milli	1/1,000 or 0.001	m
Micro	1/1,000,000 or 0.000001	(mcg or μg)

Conversion between Prefixes

If you know the prefixes and their numeric equivalents, you can easily convert measurements to smaller or larger units. To convert a measurement to a smaller unit, multiply the original measurement by the numerical equivalent of the smaller measurement's prefix.

EXAMPLE 1. Convert 3 grams to milligrams.
Milligrams (1/1,000) are smaller than grams; therefore, multiply 3 by 1,000:

$$3 \, (\text{grams}) \times 1,000 \, (\text{milli}) = 3,000$$

$$3 \, \text{grams} = 3,000 \, \text{milligrams}$$

EXAMPLE 2. Convert 2.67 liters to milliliters.
Milliliters (1/1,000) are smaller than a liter; therefore, multiply 2.67 by 1,000:

$$2.67 \, \text{liters} \times 1,000 \, (\text{milli}) = 2,670$$

$$2.67 \, \text{liters} = 2,670 \, \text{milliliters}$$

To convert a measurement to a larger unit, divide the original measurement by the numerical equivalent of the smaller measurement's prefix.

EXAMPLE 3. Convert 1,600 micrograms to grams.
A microgram is 1/1,000,000 the size of a gram; therefore, divide 1,600 by 1,000,000:

$$1,600/1,000,000 = 0.0016 \, \text{grams}$$

$$1,600 \, \text{micrograms} = 0.0016 \, \text{grams}$$

When converting a measurement to or from a prefix that is not the fundamental unit, first convert the *existing* measurement to the *fundamental* measurement. Then convert the fundamental measurement to the desired unit.

EXAMPLE 4. Convert 5.6 milligrams to micrograms.
First, convert the 5.6 milligrams to grams:

$$5.6 \, \text{milligrams}/1,000 = 0.0056 \, \text{grams (g)}$$

$$5.6 \, \text{milligrams} = 0.0056 \, \text{grams}$$

Now, convert 0.0056 grams to micrograms as previously described:

$$0.0056 \, (\text{grams}) \times 1,000,000 = 5,600 \, \text{micrograms}$$

$$5.6 \, \text{milligrams} = 5,600 \, \text{micrograms}$$

For the beginner, this technique prevents confusion. The more experienced provider will be able to make a direct conversion from milligrams to micrograms.

Table 14-3 Metric Equivalents

Household	Apothecary	Metric
1 gallon	4 quarts	3.785 liters
1 quart	1 quart	0.946 liters
16 ounces	approximately 1 pint	473 milliliters
1 cup	approximately 1/2 pint	approximately 250 milliliters
1 tablespoon		approximately 16 milliliters
1 teaspoon		approximately 4 to 5 milliliters

Household and Apothecary Systems of Measure

In the past, pharmacology traditionally used the household and apothecary systems to measure medication dosages. Gradually, the metric system has replaced those systems, but you may occasionally encounter their remnants. Table 14-3 gives the metric equivalents of the household and apothecary units you will most likely confront.

Weight Conversion

Some medications' dosages are calculated according to kilograms of body weight. To convert pounds to kilograms, use the following formula:

$$\text{kilograms} = \text{pounds}/2.2$$

EXAMPLE 5. How many kilograms does a 182-lb person weigh?

$$\text{kilograms} = 182 \text{ lb}/2.2$$
$$\text{kilograms} = 82.7$$

Temperature

The international thermometric scale measures temperature in degrees Celsius. Although degrees Celsius is often cited interchangeably with degrees centigrade, the two scales are slightly different. For practical purposes, however, you can think of them both as dividing the interval between the freezing and boiling points of water into 100 equal parts, with 0° being the freezing point and 100° being the boiling point. The household measurement system, in contrast, divides the interval between the freezing and boiling points of water into 180 equal parts, with 32° being the freezing point and 212° being the boiling point. When taking a body temperature, use the following formulas to convert between degrees Fahrenheit and degrees Celsius:

$$°F = 9/5 \, °C + 32$$
$$°C = 5/9 \, (°F - 32)$$

EXAMPLE 6. Convert 98.2°F to °C.

$$°C = 5/9 \, (98.2 - 32)$$
$$°C = 5/9 \, (66.2)$$
$$°C = 36.8$$
$$98.2°F = 36.8 \, °C$$

EXAMPLE 7. Convert 28.4°C to °F.

$$°F = 9/5 \, (28.4) + 32$$
$$°F = 51.12 + 32$$
$$°F = 83.1$$
$$28.4 \, °C = 83.1 \, °F$$

Converting between the different prefixes and between different systems of measurement is crucial in calculating medication dosages. You should continually practice all conversions, not only during your formal education but also throughout your career in the emergency medical services.

Units

Some medications are measured in **units**. Penicillin, heparin, and insulin are administered in units. Units, in pharmacology, are a measure of biological activity, not of weight, mass, or volume. Thus, units do not convert among the metric, household, and apothecary systems.

Medical Calculations

Frequently, you will have to apply basic mathematical principles to calculate specific quantities before administering medications and fluids. In out-of-hospital care, the following forms of medications often require calculation:

- Oral medications
- Liquid parenteral medications
- Intravenous fluid administration
- Intravenous medication infusions

Most medications are provided in **stock solution**. Therefore, you must calculate the exact amount of medication to remove from the stock for administration. To calculate basic medication dosage, you will need three facts:

- Desired dose
- Dosage on hand
- Volume on hand

DESIRED DOSE The **desired dose** is the specific quantity of medication needed. Most dosages are expressed as a weight (grams, milligrams, or micrograms). Dosages may be standard or calculated according to body weight or age.

DOSAGE AND VOLUME ON HAND All liquid medications are packaged as concentrations. **Concentration** refers to weight per volume. A liquid medication's concentration is the medication's weight (grams, milligrams, or micrograms) per volume of liquid (mL) in which it is dissolved. For example, 50 percent dextrose (D_{50}) is packaged as a concentration of 25 grams (weight) dextrose in 50 mL (volume) of water. From the concentration, you can determine the **dosage on hand** (weight) and the **volume on hand**. For 50 percent dextrose, the dosage on hand is 25 grams and the volume on hand is 50 mL. Concentrations are identified on all medication packaging and labels.

Because you cannot see the desired dose dissolved in liquid, you must convert its weight to volume, a readily visible measurement, using the following formula:

$$\text{volume to be administered} = \frac{\text{volume on hand (desired dose)}}{\text{dosage on hand}}$$

To use this formula, you must express all weight and volume measurements with the same metric prefix. For example, if the desired dose is expressed in *milli*grams, the dosage on hand must also be expressed in *milli*grams, volume on hand in *milli*liters.

Calculating Dosages for Oral Medications

The following example illustrates how to calculate the volume of a specific medication dosage:

EXAMPLE 1. A physician orders you to administer 90 mg of acetaminophen to a pediatric patient. The liquid acetaminophen is packaged as a concentration of 500 mg in 8 mL of solution. How much of the medication will you administer?

> **MATH SUMMARY 1**
>
> $x = 8\,\text{mL} \times 90\,\text{mg}$
>
> $x = 8\,\text{mL} \times 90\,\cancel{\text{mg}}$
>
> $x = \dfrac{720\,\text{mL}\,\cancel{\text{mg}}}{500\,\cancel{\text{mg}}}$
>
> $x = 1.44\,\text{mL}$

Because you cannot see the 90 mg of acetaminophen, you must convert this weight to a volume. To do so you need these facts:

$$\text{desired dose} = 90\,\text{mg}$$
$$\text{dosage on hand} = 500\,\text{mg}$$
$$\text{volume on hand} = 8\,\text{mL}$$

Use the formula to calculate the dosage's volume:

$$\text{volume to be administered} = \frac{\text{volume on hand (8 mL)} \times \text{desired dose (90 mg)}}{\text{dosage on hand (500 mg)}}$$

$$\text{volume to be administered} = (8\,\text{mL} \times 90)/500\,\text{mg}$$

$$\text{volume to be administered} = 720\,\text{mL}/500$$

$$\text{volume to be administered} = 1.44\,\text{mL}$$

Administer 1.44 mL of solution to deliver 90 mg of acetaminophen.

Another way to calculate medication dosages is the ratio (fraction) and proportion method. A ratio (fraction) illustrates a relationship between two numbers. A proportion is the comparison of two numerically equivalent ratios. Using the variable x, the previous problem can be stated:

> **MATH SUMMARY 2**
>
> $\dfrac{8\,\text{mL}}{500\,\text{mg}} \times \dfrac{x}{90\,\text{mg}}$
>
> $x = \dfrac{720\,\text{mL}\,\cancel{\text{mg}}}{500\,\cancel{\text{mg}}}$
>
> $x = 1.44\,\text{mL}$

$$8\,\text{mL}/500\,\text{mg} = x\,\text{mL}/90\,\text{mg}$$

To solve the problem, cross-multiply the numerals:

$$\frac{8\,\text{mL}}{500\,\text{mg}} \times \frac{x}{90\,\text{mg}}$$

$$x = \frac{720\,\text{mL}\,\cancel{\text{mg}}}{500\,\cancel{\text{mg}}}$$

$$x = 1.44\,\text{mL}$$

Converting Prefixes

The following example shows how to calculate the volume to be administered when the desired dose, the dosage on hand, and the volume on hand are not all expressed in metric units with the same prefix.

EXAMPLE 2. A physician orders you to give 250 mg of a medication via IV bolus. The multidose vial contains 2 grams of the medication in 10 mL of solution. How much of the medication should you administer?

Because the desired dose is expressed as *milli*grams, the dosage on hand must be converted from grams to milligrams. In the metric system, 2 grams equal 2,000 milligrams. You now know:

$$\text{desired dose} = 250\,\text{mg}$$
$$\text{dosage on hand} = 2,000\,\text{mg}$$
$$\text{volume on hand} = 10\,\text{mL}$$

Now you can use the formula to calculate the volume to be administered:

> **MATH SUMMARY 3**
>
> $x = \dfrac{10\,\text{mL} \times 250\,\text{mg}}{2,000\,\text{mg}}$
>
> $x = \dfrac{2,500\,\text{mL}\,\cancel{\text{mg}}}{2,000\,\cancel{\text{mg}}}$
>
> $x = 1.25\,\text{mL}$

$$\text{volume to be administered} = \frac{\text{volume on hand (10 mL)} \times \text{desired dose (250 mg)}}{\text{dosage on hand (2,000 mg)}}$$

$$\text{volume to be administered} = (10\,\text{mL} \times 250\,\cancel{\text{mg}})/2,000\,\cancel{\text{mg}}$$

$$\text{volume to be administered} = 2,500\,\text{mL}\,\cancel{\text{mg}})/2,000\,\cancel{\text{mg}}$$

$$\text{volume to be administered} = 1.25\,\text{mL}$$

Administer 1.25 mL of solution to deliver 250 mg of medication.

You can also solve this problem using the ratio proportion, as follows:

$$10 \text{ mL}/2{,}000 \text{ mg} = x/250 \text{ mg}$$

$$2{,}500 \text{ mL mg} = 2{,}000 \text{ mg } x$$

$$2{,}500 \text{ mL mg}/2{,}000 \text{ mg} = x$$

$$1.25 \text{ mL} = x$$

Tablets also come in stock doses. If the dosage of one tablet or pill is more than needed, divide the tablet or pill to make the correct dose. Do not divide enteric or time-release capsules.

Calculating Dosages for Parenteral Medications

You can use the same formula to calculate specific doses and volume for parenteral medication delivery.

EXAMPLE 3. A physician wants you to administer 5 milligrams of medication subcutaneously. The ampule contains 10 mg of the medication in 2 mL of solvent. How much medication should you use?

$$\text{desired dose} = 5 \text{ mg}$$

$$\text{dosage on hand} = 10 \text{ mg}$$

$$\text{volume on hand} = 2 \text{ mL}$$

$$\text{volume to be administered} = \frac{\text{volume on hand (2 mL)} \times \text{desired dose(5 mg)}}{\text{dosage on hand (10 mg)}}$$

$$\text{volume to be administered} = (2 \text{ mL} \times 5 \text{ mg})/10 \text{ mg}$$

$$\text{volume to be administered} = 10 \text{ mL mg}/10 \text{ mg}$$

$$\text{volume to be administered} = 1.0 \text{ mL}$$

Using the ratio and proportion method, the problem is solved as follows:

$$2 \text{ mL}/10 \text{ mg} = x/5 \text{ mg}$$

$$10 \text{ mL mg}/10 \text{ mg} = x$$

$$1.0 \text{ mL} = x$$

Calculating Weight-Dependent Dosages

Occasionally, you will have to calculate the desired dose according to the patient's weight.

EXAMPLE 4. You must administer 1.5 mg/kg of lidocaine via IV bolus to a patient in stable ventricular tachycardia. The concentration of lidocaine is 100 mg in a prefilled syringe containing 10 mL of solution. The patient weighs 158 lb.

Start by converting the patient's weight to kilograms:

$$\text{kilograms} = \text{pounds}/2.2$$

$$\text{kilograms} = 158 \text{ lb}/2.2$$

$$\text{kilograms} = 71.82$$

The patient weighs approximately 72 kg.

Calculate the desired dose:

$$1.5 \text{ mg/kg} \times 72 \text{ kg} = 108 \text{ mg}$$

You now know these three facts:

$$\text{desired dose} = 108 \text{ mg}$$

$$\text{dosage on hand} = 100 \text{ mg}$$

$$\text{volume on hand} = 10 \text{ mL}$$

MATH SUMMARY 4

$$\frac{10 \text{ mL}}{2{,}000 \text{ mg}} = \frac{x}{250 \text{ mg}}$$

$$x = \frac{2{,}500 \text{ mL mg}}{2{,}000 \text{ mg}}$$

$$x = 1.25 \text{ mL}$$

MATH SUMMARY 5

$$\frac{2 \text{ mL}}{10 \text{ mg}} = \frac{x}{5 \text{ mg}}$$

$$x = \frac{10 \text{ mL mg}}{10 \text{ mg}}$$

$$x = 1.0 \text{ mL}$$

MATH SUMMARY 6

$$x = \frac{10 \text{ mL} \times 108 \text{ mg}}{100 \text{ mg}}$$

$$x = \frac{1{,}080 \text{ mL mg}}{100 \text{ mg}}$$

$$x = 10.8 \text{ mL}$$

MATH SUMMARY 7
$\dfrac{10 \text{ mL}}{100 \text{ mg}} = \dfrac{x}{108 \text{ mg}}$
$x = \dfrac{1{,}080 \text{ mL mg}}{100 \text{ mg}}$
$x = 10.8 \text{ mL}$

Use the same formula as before to calculate the volume to be administered:

$$\text{volume to be administered} = \frac{\text{volume on hand (10 mL)} \times \text{desired dose (108 mg)}}{\text{dosage on hand (100 mg)}}$$

$$\text{volume to be administered} = (10 \text{ mL} \times 100 \text{ mg})/100 \text{ mg}$$

$$\text{volume to be administered} = 1{,}080 \text{ mL mg})/100 \text{ mg}$$

$$\text{volume to be administered} = 10.8 \text{ mL}$$

Administer 10.8 mL of solution to deliver 108 mg of lidocaine.

After you have calculated the desired dose, you can solve this problem using the ratio and proportion method as previously illustrated.

Calculating Infusion Rates

To deliver fluid or medication through an IV infusion, you must calculate the correct infusion rate in drops per minute. To do so you must know the administration tubing's drip factor, as well as the volume on hand, desired dose, and dosage on hand.

Medicated Infusions

To calculate the correct IV infusion rate, use the following formula:

$$\text{drops/minute} = \frac{\text{volume on hand} \times \text{drip factor} \times \text{desired dose}}{\text{dosage on hand}}$$

EXAMPLE 5. A physician wants you to administer 2 mg per minute of lidocaine to a patient. To prepare the infusion, you mix 2 grams of lidocaine in an IV bag containing 500 milliliters of 5 percent dextrose in water (D_5W). You will use a microdrip administration set (60 drops/mL). Calculate the infusion rate.

MATH SUMMARY 8
$x = \dfrac{500 \text{ mL} \times 60 \text{ drops/mL} \times 2 \text{ mg/min}}{2{,}000 \text{ mg}}$
$x = \dfrac{60{,}000 \text{ mL drop mL mg min}}{2{,}000 \text{ mg}}$
$x = 30 \text{ drops/min}$

$$\text{desired dose} = 2 \text{ mg/minute}$$
$$\text{dosage on hand} = 2{,}000 \text{ mg (2 grams)}$$
$$\text{volume on hand} = 500 \text{ mL}$$
$$\text{drip factor} = 60 \text{ drops/mL}$$

$$\text{drops/minute} = \frac{\text{volume on hand (500 mL)} \times \text{drip factor (60 drops/mL)} \times \text{desired dose (2 mg)}}{\text{dosage on hand (2{,}000 mg)}}$$

$$\text{drops/minute} = (500 \times 60 \times 2)/2{,}000$$

$$\text{drops/minute} = (60{,}000)/2{,}000$$

$$\text{drops/minute} = 30$$

Run the infusion at 30 drops/minute to infuse 2 mg of lidocaine per minute.

Fluid Volume over Time

Fluids with or without medications may require administration over a specific period of time. To deliver the fluid correctly, you must calculate volume/time. This calculation requires the following information:

- Volume to be administered
- Drip factor of the administration set (drops/mL)
- Total time of infusion (minutes)

To calculate the **infusion rate**, use this formula:

$$\text{drops/minute} = \frac{\text{volume to be administered (drip factor)}}{\text{time in minutes}}$$

EXAMPLE 6. A physician tells you to administer 500 milliliters of normal saline solution to a patient over 1 hour (60 minutes). The administration tubing is a macrodrip set with a drip factor of 10 drops/mL. At what drip rate would you run this infusion?

$$\text{volume to be administered} = 500 \text{ mL}$$
$$\text{administration set drip factor} = 10 \text{ drops/mL}$$
$$\text{total time of infusion} = 60 \text{ minutes}$$

Calculate the infusion rate:

$$\text{drops/minute} = (500 \times 10)/60$$
$$\text{drops/minute} = 5,000/60$$
$$\text{drops/minute} = 83.3$$

MATH SUMMARY 9
$x = \dfrac{500 \text{ mL} \times 10 \text{ drops/mL}}{60 \text{ minutes}}$
$x = \dfrac{5,000 \text{ mL } 10 \text{ drops mL}}{60 \text{ min}}$
$x = 83.3 \text{ drops/min}$

Set the flow rate at approximately 83 drops per minute to infuse 500 milliliters of normal saline in almost exactly 60 minutes.

You can use the same formula to determine how long it will take to use all the fluid in a container.

EXAMPLE 7. You are transporting a patient with an IV antibiotic. The infusion rate is 45 drops/minute and the administration tubing is a microdrip set (60 drops/mL). In the 500 milliliter bag of D_5W, 150 milliliters remain. How long will it take the antibiotic to complete infusion?

Use the same formula as in example 6; however, in this instance you will find time in minutes.

$$45 \text{ drops/minute} = \frac{(150 \text{ mL})(60 \text{ drops/mL})}{x}$$
$$45 \text{ drops/minute} = \frac{9,000 \text{ mL drops mL}}{x}$$
$$x = \frac{9,000 \text{ mL drops mL}}{45 \text{ drops/minutes}}$$
$$x = 200 \text{ minutes}$$

MATH SUMMARY 10
$x = 9,000 \text{ mL}$
$\dfrac{\text{drops/mL}}{45 \text{ drops/min}}$
$x = 200 \text{ min}$

The antibiotic will complete infusion in 200 minutes, or 3 hours and 20 minutes.

Calculating Dosages and Infusion Rates for Infants and Children

Infants and children cannot tolerate under- or overdoses of medication and fluids. When you administer infusions to pediatric patients, you must calculate exact flow rates. Because infants and children differ drastically from adults in size and internal development, their dosages often depend on weight. Most weight-dependent dosages express the patient's weight in kilograms, so you must make the appropriate conversion from pounds as discussed earlier. Occasionally, you may encounter a medication that is based on body surface area (BSA). Chemotherapeutic agents for children are often based on body surface area. Although you will not initiate such medications, you may encounter them on critical care transports either by ground or air. Many aids for calculating pediatric medication doses and infusion rates are available, including charts, forms, and length-based resuscitation tapes. Even though these devices are helpful, you should not rely on them exclusively. They are no substitute for knowledge.[14]

Summary

Medication administration is a fundamental skill used in the treatment of the sick and injured. For medications to be effective, they must be *safely* delivered into the body by the *appropriate* route. Many different routes for medication delivery are available to the paramedic; however, specific medications require specific routes for administration. In addition, you must accurately calculate many medication dosages. Dosage errors and inappropriate medication administration can result in serious side effects or even death for the patient, not to mention casting serious doubt on your ability or causing loss of your certification.

Keep in mind that medication calculations can be completed by a variety of methods. What is important is to find a method that works for you and gets you the right answer every time you work a problem. Once you identify this method, stick with it and practice it, because you never know when you will need to do a calculation in less than favorable conditions.

Always remember that it is your responsibility to be familiar with all routes of medication delivery and the techniques for establishing and using them. You will use some routes of medication administration infrequently, and they will quickly fade from memory, whereas you will use other routes almost daily. Nonetheless, someone's well-being may depend on your ability to use any one of the routes of administration in an emergency. Therefore, periodic review of all routes used in medication administration is highly recommended.

You Make the Call

You have been called for a 53-year-old male patient experiencing chest pain and shortness of breath. After assessing the patient, you find him to be alert and oriented, with a clear airway, and breathing adequately at a rate of 16 breaths per minute. His distal pulses are strong, and his skin is cool and slightly diaphoretic. Your partner obtains the following vital signs: blood pressure 142/88 mmHg, pulse 92 beats per minute, and respirations 16 and easy. The patient exhibits no jugular venous distention or peripheral edema, and breath sounds are clear bilaterally. The 12-lead cardiac monitor shows a sinus rhythm with ST segment elevation in leads V_1 through V_3. The patient has no medical allergies and is on no medications. He denies any previous medical history.

In addition to high-flow, high-concentration oxygen, you elect to administer nitroglycerin, morphine sulfate, and aspirin, based on your suspicion of an acute myocardial infarction. Accordingly, you quickly establish an IV line.

1. Before administering aspirin or any other medication orally (p.o.), what major consideration must you be sure of?

2. Of the following medications and routes of delivery, which will provide the fastest and most predictable rate of absorption?
   - Aspirin—enteral tract
   - Nitroglycerin—sublingual
   - Morphine sulfate—IV bolus

3. When administered sublingually, how is the nitroglycerin absorbed into the body?

4. You elect to administer 3 mg of morphine sulfate to the patient. The medication is packaged as 10 mg in 5 mL of solution in a multidose vial. How many milliliters must you administer to give the 3 mg of morphine?

See Suggested Responses at the back of this book.

Review Questions

1. The simplest and often the most neglected form of Standard Precautions is _____
   a. handwashing.
   b. donning a gown.
   c. wearing gloves.
   d. wearing eye goggles.

2. A cleansing agent that is toxic to living tissue is_____
   a. sterile.
   b. antiseptic.
   c. disinfectant.
   d. medically clean.

3. A drug administered through the mucous membranes of the ear and ear canal is a(n) _____
   a. buccal medication.
   b. nasal medication.
   c. aural medication.
   d. ocular medication.

4. "Within the dermal layer of the skin" defines_____
   a. buccal.
   b. intradermal.
   c. subcutaneous.
   d. intramuscular.

5. The state in which solutions on opposite sides of a semipermeable membrane are in equal concentration describes a(n) _____ state.
   a. colloid
   b. isotonic
   c. hypertonic
   d. hypotonic

6. When starting an IV, never leave the constricting band in place for more than _____ minutes.
   a. 1.5
   b. 2
   c. 3
   d. 4

7. Medically clean techniques include_____
   a. handwashing.
   b. glove changing.
   c. discarding equipment in opened packages.
   d. all of the above.

8. To minimize or eliminate the risk of an accidental needle stick, the paramedic must_____
   a. recap needles using two hands.
   b. start IVs in the ambulance rather than in the patient's home.
   c. immediately dispose of used sharps in a sharps container.
   d. wash his hands before and after needle use.

9. The abbreviation _____ designates the right eye.
   a. o.u.
   b. o.p.
   c. o.d.
   d. o.s.

10. In an acute respiratory emergency involving a patient with a prescribed metered dose inhaler (MDI), always use a(n) _____ instead of the MDI.
    a. LMA
    b. ET tube
    c. nebulizer
    d. nasal airway

11. When using an endotracheal tube, you must increase conventional IV dosages from _____ to _____ times.
    a. 1, 2
    b. 2, 3
    c. 2, 2½
    d. 3½, 4

12. A _____ is a liquid that contains small particles of solid medication.
    a. syrup
    b. elixir
    c. emulsion
    d. suspension

13. _____ denotes any drug administration outside the gastrointestinal tract.
    a. Enema
    b. Enteral
    c. Parenteral
    d. Suppository

14. Which of the following is not a parenteral drug delivery route?
    a. Rectal route
    b. Intravenous access
    c. Intraosseous infusion
    d. Intramuscular injection

15. All of the following are examples of colloidal solutions except_____
    a. dextran.
    b. lactated Ringer's.
    c. hetastarch.
    d. albumin.

16. What term is used to describe inflammation of the vein, which is particularly common in long-term intravenous therapy?
    a. Necrosis
    b. Air embolism
    c. Thrombus formation
    d. Thrombophlebitis

17. Which of the following is not an enteral route of drug administration?
    a. Inhalational
    b. Oral
    c. Rectal
    d. Buccal

18. Advantages of saline and heparin locks include all of the following except_____
    a. provides a peripheral IV port.
    b. does not need continuous fluid infusion.
    c. blood samples cannot be withdrawn from the lock.
    d. decreases the risk of accidental electrolyte derangement.

19. Causes of hemolysis include_____
    a. using too small a needle for retrieval.
    b. vigorously shaking the blood tubes after they are filled.
    c. too forcefully aspirating blood into or out of a syringe.
    d. all of the above.

20. Which of the following is *not* considered a complication of intraosseous access?
    a. Local infection
    b. Air embolism
    c. Fat embolism
    d. Thrombophlebitis

21. The bone most commonly used for intraosseous access is the_____
    a. tibia.   c. fibula.
    b. femur.   d. humerus.

22. The three fundamental units of the metric system are:
    a. meters, liters, grains.
    b. grams, meters, liters.
    c. inches, pints, pounds.
    d. grams, liters, ounces.

23. 1,000 milligrams equals_____
    a. 1 kilogram.   c. 0.001 gram.
    b. 1 gram.   d. 10 grams.

24. A patient weighs 90 kg. What is his weight in pounds?
    a. 180   c. 75
    b. 41   d. 198

25. The metric prefix *hecto-* means_____
    a. 1.   c. 100.
    b. 10.   d. 1,000.

26. What is the metric unit for volume measurement?
    a. Liter   c. Gram
    b. Meter   d. Milli

27. Medical control orders you to administer Valium, 2.0 mg. The medication is in a prefilled syringe labeled 10 mg in 2 mL. You draw up the correct dose, which is_____
    a. 0.20 mL.   d. 4.0 mL.
    b. 2.0 mL.   e. none of the above.
    c. 0.4 mL.

28. To administer 35 mg of Benadryl from a syringe labeled 50 mg/mL, you would give:
    a. 1.5 mL.   d. 0.7 mg.
    b. 0.8 mL.   e. none of the above.
    c. 0.7 mL.

29. 0.75 liters converted to milliliters is_____
    a. 1,075 mL.   d. 750 mL.
    b. 1.075 mL.   e. none of the above.
    c. 75 mL.

30. Two grams is equal to_____
    a. 1,000 mg.   c. 3,000 mg.
    b. 2,000 mg.   d. 2,000 mcg.

31. 2.5 grams is equal to_____
    a. 150 mg.   d. 2,000 mcg.
    b. 1,500 mg.   e. none of the above.
    c. 2,500 mcg.

32. 1 kilogram is equal to_____
    a. 2.0 pounds.
    b. 2.2 pounds.
    c. 0.2 pounds.
    d. 2.2 kilograms.
    e. none of the above.

See Answers to Review Questions at the back of this book.

References

1. Hobgood, C., J. B. Bowen, J. H. Brice, B. Overby, and J. H. Tamayo-Sarver. "Do EMS Personnel Identify, Report, and Disclose Medical Errors?" *Prehosp Emerg Care* 10 (2006): 21–27.

2. Vilke, G. M., S. V. Tornabene, B. Stepanski, et al. "Paramedic Self-Reported Medication Errors." *Prehosp Emerg Care* 11 (2007): 80–84.

3. Harris, S. A. and L. A. Nicolai. "Occupational Exposures in Emergency Medical Service Providers and Knowledge of and Compliance with Universal Precautions." *Am J Infect Control* 38 (2010): 86–94.

4. Rickard, C., P. O'Meara, M. McGrail, D. Garner, A. McLean, and P. Le Lievre. "A Randomized Controlled Trial of Intranasal Fentanyl vs. Intravenous Morphine for Analgesia in the Prehospital Setting." *Am J Emerg Med* 25 (2007): 911–917.

5. Barton, E. D., C. B. Colwell, T. Wolfe et al. "Efficacy of Intranasal Naloxone as a Needleless Alternative for Treatment of Opioid

Overdose in the Prehospital Setting." *J Emerg Med* 29 (2005): 265–271.

6. Holsti, M., B. L. Sill, S. D. Firth, F. M. Filloux, S. M. Joyce, and R. A. Furnival. "Prehospital Intranasal Midazolam for the Treatment of Pediatric Seizures." *Pediatr Emerg Care* 23 (2007): 148–153.

7. Kelly, A. M., D. Kerr, P. Dietze, I. Patrick, T. Walker, and Z. Koutsogiannis. "Randomised Trial of Intranasal versus Intramuscular Naloxone in Prehospital Treatment for Suspected Opioid Overdose." *Med J Aust* 182 (2005): 24–27.

8. Warner, G. S. "Evaluation of the Effect of Prehospital Application of Continuous Positive Airway Pressure Therapy in Acute Respiratory Distress." *Prehosp Disaster Med* 25 (2010): 87–91.

9. Niemann, J. T., S. J. Stratton, B. Cruz, and R. J. Lewis. "Endotracheal Drug Administration during Out-of-Hospital Resuscitation: Where Are the Survivors?" *Resuscitation* 53 (2002): 153–157.

10. Harrison, G., K. G. Speroni, L. Dugan, and M. G. Daniel. "A Comparison of the Quality of Blood Specimens Drawn in the Field by EMS versus Specimens Obtained in the Emergency Department." *J Emerg Nurs* 36 (2010): 16–20.

11. Schoenfield, E., Boniface, K., Shokoohi, H. "ED Technicians Can Successfully Place Ultrasound-Guided Intravenous Catheters in Patients with Poor Vascular Access." *Am J Emerg Med* 29 (2011):496–501.

12. Fowler, R., J. V. Gallagher, S. M. Isaacs, E. Ossman, P. Pepe, and M. Wayne. "The Role of Intraosseous Vascular Access in the Out-of-Hospital Environment (resource document to NAEMSP position statement)." *Prehosp Emerg Care* 11 (2007): 63–66.

13. Leidel, B. A., C. Kirchhoff, V. Braunstein, V. Bogner, P. Biberthaler, and K. G. Kanz. "Comparison of Two Intraosseous Access Devices in Adult Patients under Resuscitation in the Emergency Department: A Prospective, Randomized Study." *Resuscitation* 81 (2010): 994–999.

14. Eastwood, K. J., M. J. Boyle, and B. Williams. "Paramedics' Ability to Perform Drug Calculations." *West J Emerg Med* 10 (2009): 240–243.

15. Bernius, M., B. Thibodeau, A. Jones, B. Clothier, and M. Witting. "Prevention of Pediatric Drug Calculation Errors by Prehospital Care Providers." *Prehosp Emerg Care* 12 (2008): 486–494.

Further Reading

Bledsoe, Bryan E. and Dwayne Clayden. *Prehospital Emergency Pharmacology.* 7th ed. Upper Saddle River, NJ: Pearson/Prentice Hall, 2012.

Campbell, John Emory and the Alabama Chapter of the American College of Emergency Physicians. *International Trauma Life Support for Prehospital Providers.* 6th ed. Upper Saddle River, NJ: Pearson/Prentice Hall, 2012.

Kee, Joyce L. and Evelyn R. Hayes. *Pharmacology: A Nursing Process Approach.* 6th ed. Philadelphia: W. B. Saunders Company, 2009.

Lesmeister, Michele B. *Math Basics for the Health Professional.* 3rd ed. Upper Saddle River, NJ: Pearson/Prentice Hall, 2009.

Martini, Frederic. *Fundamentals of Anatomy and Physiology.* 8th ed. San Francisco: Benjamin Cummings, 2008.

McKenry, Leda M., et al. *Pharmacology in Nursing.* 21st ed. St. Louis: Mosby, 2003.

McSwain, Norman E. and Scott Frame. *Prehospital Trauma Life Support.* 7th ed. St. Louis: Mosby, 2010.

Mikolaj, Alan A. *Drug Dosage Calculations for the Emergency Care Provider.* 2nd ed. Upper Saddle River, NJ: Pearson/Prentice Hall, 2003.

Chapter 15
Airway Management and Ventilation

Bryan Bledsoe, DO, FACEP, FAAEM, EMT-P
W. E. Gandy, JD, NREMTP
Darren Braude, MD, MPH, FACEP

STANDARD
Airway Management, Respiration, and Artificial Ventilation

COMPETENCY
Integrates comprehensive knowledge of anatomy, physiology, and pathophysiology into the assessment to develop and implement a treatment plan with the goal of ensuring a patent airway, adequate mechanical ventilation, and respiration for patients of all ages.

 ## Learning Objectives

Terminal Performance Objective: After reading this chapter, you should be able to apply principles of airway management and ventilation to the assessment and management of patients.

Enabling Objectives: To accomplish the terminal performance objective, you should be able to:

1. Define key terms introduced in this chapter.

2. Review the basic anatomy and physiology of the upper and lower airway, the respiratory cycle, oxygen and carbon dioxide transport, and clinical differences in the pediatric airway.

3. Describe findings consistent with upper airway obstruction and abnormal upper airway sounds.

4. Discuss the steps of the primary survey as it relates to the assessment of airway patency and ventilatory adequacy.

5. Describe the function, procedure for use, and benefits of noninvasive respiratory gas monitoring in identifying oxygenation and ventilation sufficiency.

6. Demonstrate techniques of basic airway management, including positioning, administering supplemental oxygen by a variety of devices, manual airway maneuvers, and inserting basic airway adjuncts.

7. Discuss the "Rule of Threes" as it pertains to optimal bag-valve mask ventilations.

8. Explain the importance of nonlinear thinking and action in assessment and management of problems with the airway and ventilation.

9. Identify the types, indications, contraindications, procedure for use, and limitations of the various extraglottic airway devices.

10. Describe the indications, contraindications, advantages, disadvantages, complications, equipment, and techniques for endotracheal intubation.

11. Discuss the role and use of optical and video laryngoscopy devices during patient intubation.

12. Identify multiple ways to confirm that the patient is being adequately ventilated regardless of what type of airway and ventilation device(s) are being used.

13. Identify alternative approaches to traditional endotracheal intubation to include nasal intubation, retrograde intubation, digital intubation, and lighted stylet intubation.

14. Discuss special considerations of anatomy, equipment, and procedure when intubating and ventilating pediatric patients.

15. Discuss management of post-intubation agitation and field extubation.

16. Describe the indications, contraindications, advantages, disadvantages, complications, and equipment for performing cricothyrotomy techniques.

17. Describe the pharmacology of medications commonly used in medication-assisted intubation, and the process (or order) by which rapid sequence intubation is performed.

18. Recognize predictors of a difficult airway and ventilation, and discuss techniques that can increase first-attempt intubation success rates.

19. Discuss the assessment and management of the airway and ventilation in a patient with a stoma.

20. Identify and discuss the equipment needed for effective suctioning of the nasopharynx, oropharynx, and the trachea in the intubated patient.

21. Describe the benefits of gastric decompression in the ventilated patient, to include the equipment needed and procedure for proper placement.

22. Identify the role and basic function of transport ventilators in the prehospital environment.

23. Given scenarios of patients requiring airway or ventilatory management, including patients with a difficult airway, discuss how to employ techniques to achieve adequate oxygenation.

KEY TERMS

ABCs, p. 528

alveoli, p. 519

anoxia, p. 530

apnea, p. 526

apneic oxygenation, p. 563

arterial oxygen concentration (CaO_2), p. 523

aspiration, p. 518

atelectasis, p. 520

bag-valve mask (BVM), p. 548

barotrauma, p. 582

bilevel positive airway pressure (BiPAP), p. 544

bronchi, p. 519

CaO_2, p. 523

capnography, p. 534

carbon dioxide, p. 516

compliance, p. 531

continuous positive airway pressure (CPAP), p. 544

Cormack and LeHane grading system, p. 594

cricothyroid membrane, p. 518

cyanosis, p. 530

demand-valve device, p. 550

diffusion, p. 523

dyspnea, p. 530

ear-to-sternal-notch position, p. 540

endotracheal tube (ETT), p. 559

endotracheal tube introducer, p. 560

eustachian tube, p. 517

extraglottic airway (EGA) devices, p. 550

extubation, p. 527

FiO_2, p. 524

flail chest, p. 528

free radicals, p. 533

French, p. 545

gag reflex, p. 517

glottis, p. 517

hemoglobin (Hgb), p. 523

hemoglobin oxygen saturation (SaO_2), p. 523

hemothorax, p. 524

Case Study

Ellis County Unit 947, along with a fire engine, is dispatched to a motor vehicle collision on rural County Road 664, approximately eight miles from town. This particular stretch of road is well known to paramedics because of a number of serious crashes over the last several months. The road contains numerous sharp curves and is under construction in several locations. Today, Unit 947 is staffed by paramedic Kathy Mulligan and AEMT William Benson. In addition, paramedic student Sharon Rodriguez is assigned to the unit for her paramedic field internship. There are three volunteer firefighter/EMTs on the engine.

On arrival at the scene, they find one vehicle that has apparently run off the road and struck a telephone pole. Witnesses to the crash estimate that the vehicle was traveling at approximately 45 miles per hour before striking the pole. The lone 24-year-old male occupant was ejected from the vehicle and lies face down in a ditch approximately 50 feet from the car. After ensuring scene safety and donning the appropriate

personal protective equipment, Kathy assesses the patient. She finds him to be unresponsive. William, Sharon, and the firefighters help her logroll the patient to a supine position while keeping the cervical spine in a neutral position. Sharon maintains the neck in a neutral position while Kathy opens the airway with the modified jaw-thrust technique.

The patient exhibits agonal respirations. In addition, gurgling noises are heard with each breath. After suctioning bloody secretions from his mouth, Kathy attempts to insert an oropharyngeal airway. However, the patient's teeth are tightly clenched, and the airway will not pass. Sharon places a nasal airway, and then the entire team provides three-person ventilatory support with a bag-valve-mask (BVM) unit and 100 percent oxygen. The Glasgow Coma Score is 5.

They load the patient into Unit 947 and initiate Code 3 transport to the closest Level 1 trauma center, 31 minutes away. En route, they obtain a full set of vital signs, keep the patient warm, and start a large-bore IV.

The patient's blood pressure is 167/92 mmHg, heart rate is 110, and oxygen saturation is only 88 percent, despite optimal BVM ventilation. Kathy radios to have another paramedic meet them en route so they can perform rapid sequence intubation (RSI), as their protocols require that two medics be present for this procedure.

When they meet up with the second paramedic 23 minutes from the hospital, they are still having trouble maintaining adequate oxygenation, and there is no indication of tension pneumothorax or other treatable etiology. The two medics agree that RSI is indicated. One of the firefighters maintains cervical stabilization. They give the 100-kg patient 30 mg of etomidate and 200 mg of succinylcholine. Forty-five seconds after succinylcholine was administered, the fasciculations (muscle twitches) have passed from head to toe, and the patient is flaccid.

Kathy attempts bimanual laryngoscopy, but is unable to visualize the glottis or posterior cartilages. She makes one attempt with an endotracheal tube introducer under the epiglottis, which is unsuccessful, and the patient's oxygen saturations are noted to be falling. The two medics then elect to place an LMA Supreme™ airway. They inflate the cuff and begin ventilations with high-concentration supplemental oxygen, using a self-inflating bag. The patient's oxygen saturation quickly rebounds, and they decompress the stomach with a gastric tube inserted through the dedicated channel on the device. They connect the LMA Supreme™ to the transport ventilator, and monitor capnography and other vitals. They adjust the ventilator to maintain a normal exhaled CO_2 and administer fentanyl and midazolam to keep the patient comfortable. They arrive at the trauma center 16 minutes later. The patient's blood pressure is 147/84 mmHg, heart rate is 98, oxygen saturation is 93 percent, and exhaled CO_2 is 35.

The trauma team leaves the LMA Supreme™ in place to obtain initial radiographs and CT scans, which reveal a pulmonary contusion and a large subdural hematoma that requires emergent surgical drainage. In the operating room, the patient is intubated through the LMA Supreme™, using fiber-optic guidance. Following surgery, the patient begins to regain consciousness but requires continued intubation for 72 hours because of oxygenation and ventilation issues. On day four, he is successfully extubated and moved to a regular hospital room.

Kathy and her Unit 947 team stop at the hospital to visit after the patient is extubated. He has no recall of the crash at all. The last thing he remembers is looking on the floor of his car for a CD that he dropped. One week after the crash, he is discharged to rehabilitation with minimal neurologic deficits.

Introduction

Airway management and ventilation are the first and most critical steps in the primary assessment of every patient you will encounter (unless the patient is in cardiac arrest, when chest compressions will come first). Airway management and ventilation go hand in hand. You must immediately establish and maintain an open airway while providing adequate oxygen delivery and carbon dioxide elimination for all patients. Without adequate airway maintenance and ventilation, the patient will succumb to brain injury, or even death, in as little as 4 minutes. Early detection and intervention of airway and breathing problems, including dispatcher-guided interventions by bystanders, are vital to patient survival.

Airway management and ventilation have always been taught to occur in a stepwise (linear) process. Recommended sequences include the standard ABC (airway, breathing, circulation) sequence, as well as the CAB (compressions, airway, breathing) sequence recommended by the American Heart Association for a patient who appears to be in cardiac arrest, when chest compression must come first. These established sequences (ABC and CAB) can help rescuers remember what to do in emergency situations.

With regard to airway and/or ventilation problems, paramedics should approach the patient more globally and consider the whole picture, rather than blindly following predetermined steps. You cannot assess an airway if the patient is not breathing. You cannot assess breathing if there is no airway. Therefore, airway and ventilation need to be considered and managed together. Ultimately, circulation also will depend on an intact airway and adequate ventilation and respiration. The respiratory, cardiovascular, and neurologic systems all play an important role in airway management and ventilation. Stated another way, airway and ventilation problems must be approached in a nonlinear fashion with a number of factors considered simultaneously.

Your deliberate and precise use of simple, basic airway skills is the key to successful airway management and good patient outcome. Once you have applied the basic airway techniques to properly provide oxygenation and ventilation for your patient, you can then use more sophisticated airway maneuvers and skills, if necessary, to further stabilize his airway. You must continually monitor and reassess the airway, being careful to watch for displacement of any placed airway devices, mucous plugging, equipment failure, or the development of a pneumothorax.

This chapter provides the information and skills you will need to manage even the most difficult airway. It begins with a review of the respiratory system's anatomy and physiology and then explores the primary assessment and management of the airway and ventilation. Finally, it details enhanced airway management options for the more experienced paramedic.

The chapter is divided into four parts:

Part 1: Respiratory Anatomy, Physiology, and Assessment

Part 2: Basic Airway Management and Ventilation

Part 3: Advanced Airway Management and Ventilation

Part 4: Additional Airway and Ventilation Issues

PART 1: Respiratory Anatomy, Physiology, and Assessment

Anatomy of the Respiratory System

The respiratory system provides a passage for **oxygen**, a gas necessary for energy production, to enter the body and for **carbon dioxide**, a waste product of the body's metabolism, to exit. This gas exchange, called *respiration*, requires a patent, open airway as well as adequate respiratory function. Many pathological processes can inhibit respiration. To understand the interventions that you will use to maintain adequate airway and ventilatory function, you must thoroughly understand the anatomy of the upper and lower airway.

Upper Airway Anatomy

The *upper airway* extends from the mouth and nose to the larynx (Figure 15-1). It includes the nasal cavity, oral cavity, and pharynx. The larynx joins the upper and lower airways.

The Nasal Cavity

The nasal cavity is the most superior part of the airway. The maxillary, frontal, nasal, ethmoid, and sphenoid bones comprise

the lateral and superior walls of the nasal cavity. The hard palate forms the floor of the nasal cavity. The cartilaginous and highly vascular nasal **septum** separates the right and left nasal cavities.

Several structures connect with the nasal cavity. These include the sinuses, the eustachian tubes, and the lacrimal ducts. The **sinuses** are air-filled cavities that are lined with a mucous membrane. There are four pairs of sinuses: the ethmoid sinuses, the frontal sinuses, the maxillary sinuses, and the sphenoid sinuses. The sinuses, named for the bone where they are contained, help reduce the overall weight of the head and are thought to assist in heating, purifying, and moistening inhaled air. The sinuses help trap bacteria and other substances entering the nasal cavity. Because of this, they can become infected. Fractures of the upper sinuses (sphenoids) can occasionally cause cerebrospinal fluid (CSF) to leak from the cranial cavity into the nasal cavity. Clinically, this presents with clear fluid draining from the nose (rhinorrhea) and can provide a direct route for the transmission of pathogens to the brain and associated structures.

NASAL CAVITY
- Superior, middle, and inferior turbinates
- Hard and soft palates

NASOPHARYNX
- Tonsils/adenoids
- Uvula

OROPHARYNX
- Tongue

LARYNGOPHARYNX (HYPOPHARYNX)
- Vallecula
- Epiglottis

LARYNX
- Esophagus
- Trachea

Glottic opening
Vocal cords
Thyroid cartilage
Cricothyroid membrane
Cricoid cartilage
Thyroid gland

FIGURE 15-1 Anatomy of the upper airway.

The **eustachian tubes**, or auditory tubes, connect the ear with the nasal cavity and allow for equalization of pressure on each side of the tympanic membrane. Swallowing can assist in equalizing this pressure. The **nasolacrimal ducts** drain tears and debris from the eyes into the nasal cavity. This can cause the nose to run when someone cries.

Air enters the nasal cavity through the external **nares** (nostrils). Nasal hairs just inside the external nares initially filter the incoming air. The air then proceeds into the nasal cavity, where it strikes three bony projections: the superior, middle, and inferior turbinates, or conchae. These shelflike structures, which are parallel to the nasal floor, serve as conduits into the sinuses, increase the surface area of the nasal cavity, and cause turbulent airflow. This turbulence helps to filter the air by depositing airborne particles on the **mucous membrane** lining the nasal cavity. Hairlike fibers called *cilia* propel those trapped particles to the back of the pharynx, where they are swallowed. Because the mucous membrane is covered with **mucus** and has a rich blood supply, it also immediately warms and humidifies the air entering the nose. By the time the air reaches the lower airway, it is at body temperature (37°C), 100 percent humidified, and virtually free of airborne particles. Air proceeds from the nasal cavity through internal nares into the nasopharynx.

The tissue of the nasal cavity is extremely delicate and vascular. Because of this, it is susceptible to trauma. Always remember that improper or overly aggressive placement of tubes or mechanical airways can cause significant bleeding that direct pressure might not control.

The Oral Cavity

The cheeks, the hard and soft palates, and the tongue form the mouth, or oral cavity. The lips that surround the mouth's opening are fleshy folds of skin. Behind the lips lie the gums and teeth, normally numbering 32 in the adult. Significant force is required to avulse (dislodge) or fracture the teeth. Broken or dislodged teeth can potentially obstruct the airway. The hard palate anteriorly and the soft palate posteriorly form the top of the oral cavity and separate it from the nasal cavity. The tongue, a large muscle on the bottom of the oral cavity, is the most common airway obstruction. It attaches to the mandible and the hyoid bone through a series of muscles and ligaments. The U-shaped hyoid bone is located just beneath the chin. The hyoid bone is unique: It is the only bone in the axial skeleton that does not articulate with any other bone. Instead, it is suspended by ligaments from the styloid process of the temporal bone and serves to anchor the tongue and larynx, as well as to support the trachea.

The Pharynx

The **pharynx** is a muscular tube that extends vertically from the back of the soft palate to the superior aspect of the esophagus. It allows the air to flow into and out of the respiratory tract and food and liquids to pass into the digestive system. It contains several openings, including the internal nares, the mouth, the larynx, and the esophagus.

The pharynx is divided into three regions: the nasopharynx, the oropharynx, and the laryngopharynx (hypopharynx). The nasopharynx is the uppermost region, extending from the back of the nasal opening to the plane of the soft palate. The oropharynx extends from the plane of the soft palate to the hyoid bone. The adenoids, lymphatic tissue in the mouth and nose, filter bacteria. Either hypertrophy or swelling of the adenoids from infection may make them large enough to obscure your view of the posterior pharynx. The laryngopharynx extends posteriorly from the hyoid bone to the esophagus and anteriorly to the larynx. The laryngopharynx is especially important in airway management.

Because the mouth and pharynx serve dual purposes for respiration and digestion, a number of mechanisms help prevent accidental blockage. To prevent foreign material from entering the trachea and lungs, sensitive nerves activate the body's cough and swallowing mechanisms as well as the **gag reflex**.

Located anteriorly in the hypopharynx is the epiglottis, a leaf-shaped cartilage that prevents food from entering the respiratory tract during swallowing. Just anterior and superior to the epiglottis is the **vallecula**, a fold formed by the base of the tongue and the epiglottis. It is an important landmark for endotracheal **intubation**. A series of ligaments and muscles connect the epiglottis to the hyoid bone and mandible. Immediately behind the hypopharynx are the fourth and fifth cervical vertebral bodies.

The Larynx

The **larynx** is the complex structure that joins the pharynx with the trachea (Figure 15-2). Lying midline in the neck, it is attached to and lies just inferior to the hyoid bone and anterior to the esophagus. It consists of the thyroid and cricoid cartilage (both considered tracheal cartilage), glottic opening, vocal cords, arytenoid cartilage, pyriform fossae, and cricothyroid membrane.

The main laryngeal cartilage is the shield-shaped thyroid cartilage. Larger in males than in females, the thyroid cartilage forms the anterior prominence called the Adam's apple. The arytenoid cartilage, which forms a pyramid-shaped attachment for the vocal cords posteriorly, is an important landmark for endotracheal intubation. Posteriorly, smooth muscle closes a gap in the thyroid cartilage. Directly behind the Adam's apple, the thyroid cartilage houses the glottic opening, the narrowest part of the adult trachea, which is bordered by the vocal cords. The patency of the glottic opening, or **glottis**, depends heavily on muscle tone. On either side of the glottic opening are the pyriform fossae, recesses that form the lateral borders of the larynx. The thyrohyoid membrane attaches the upper end of the thyroid cartilage to the hyoid bone.

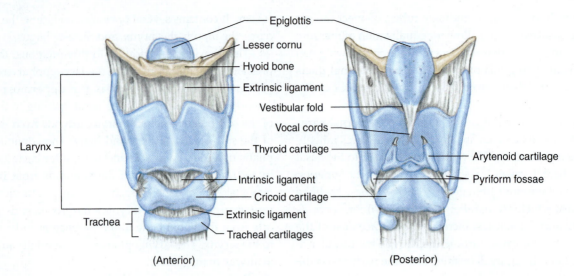

FIGURE 15-2 Internal anatomy of the upper airway.

Within the laryngeal cavity lie the true vocal cords, white bands of cartilage that regulate the passage of air through the larynx and produce voice by contraction of the laryngeal muscles. The vocal cords can also close together to prevent foreign bodies from entering the airway. The passage of an endotracheal tube between the vocal cords interferes not only with the creation of sound, but also with the protective function of coughing. Beneath the thyroid cartilage is the cricoid cartilage, which forms the inferior border of the larynx. Often it is considered the first tracheal ring. Unlike the thyroid and other tracheal cartilages, whose posterior surfaces are open and not fused, the cricoid cartilage forms a complete ring. In children, the cricoid cartilage is the narrowest part of the laryngeal airway. The fibrous **cricothyroid membrane** connects the inferior border of the thyroid cartilage with the superior aspect of the cricoid cartilage. It is the site for surgical airway techniques.

A mucous membrane lines most of the larynx. Rich with nerve endings from the vagus nerve, it is so sensitive that any irritation sparks a cough, or forceful exhalation of a large volume of air. First, air is drawn into the respiratory passageways. Next, the glottic opening shuts tightly, trapping the air within the lungs. Then the abdominal and thoracic muscles contract, pushing against the diaphragm and increasing intrathoracic pressure. The vocal cords suddenly open, and a burst of air forces foreign particles out of the lungs. The laryngeal mucous membrane is so sensitive that its stimulation by a laryngoscope or endotracheal tube can cause bradycardia (slow pulse rate), hypotension (low blood pressure), and decreased respiratory rate.

Other structures proximate to the larynx and of particular interest when you perform surgical airway procedures are the thyroid gland, carotid arteries, and jugular veins. The thyroid gland is a "bow-tie" shaped endocrine gland located in the neck. It is highly vascular and lies inferior to the cricoid cartilage. It contains two lobes, one on each side of the trachea. These lobes are joined in the middle by the isthmus that extends across the trachea. The carotid arteries run closely along the trachea. Several branches of the carotid arteries cross the trachea. Likewise, the jugular veins lie very close to the trachea. Several branches of the jugular veins, such as the superior thyroid vein, cross the trachea.

Lower Airway Anatomy

The *lower airway* extends from below the larynx to the alveoli (Figure 15-3). This is where the respiratory exchange of oxygen and carbon dioxide occurs. Helpful landmarks are the fourth cervical vertebra at the posterior superior border, and the xiphoid process anterior inferiorly, although the posterior lung extends beyond this inferiorly.

The Trachea

As air enters the lower airway from the upper airway, it first enters and then passes through the **trachea**. The trachea is a 10- to 12-centimeter-long tube that connects the larynx to the two mainstem bronchi. It contains cartilaginous, C-shaped, open rings that form a frame to keep it open. The trachea is lined with respiratory epithelium containing cilia and mucus-producing cells. The mucus traps particles that the upper airway did

CONTENT REVIEW

➤ Lower Airway Components
- Trachea
- Bronchi
- Alveoli
- Lung parenchyma
- Pleura

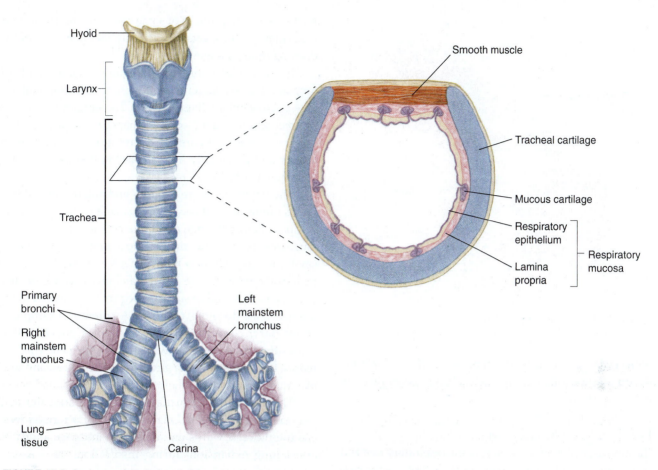

FIGURE 15-3 Anatomy of the lower airway.

not filter. The cilia then move the trapped particulate matter up into the mouth, where it is swallowed or expelled.

The Bronchi

At the carina, the trachea divides, or bifurcates, into the right and left mainstem **bronchi**. The right mainstem bronchus is almost straight, whereas the left mainstem bronchus angles more acutely to the left. Because of this, the right mainstem is often the site of aspirated foreign bodies. In addition, when an endotracheal tube is inserted too far, it tends to enter the right mainstem bronchus, thus ventilating only the right lung. Mainstem bronchi enter the lung tissue at the hilum and then divide into the secondary and tertiary bronchi. The secondary and tertiary bronchi ultimately branch into the bronchioles, or small airways.

The bronchioles are encircled with smooth muscle that contains beta-2 (β_2) adrenergic receptors. When stimulated, these β_2 receptors relax the bronchial smooth muscle, thus increasing the airway's diameter. This bronchodilation can increase the amount of air transported through the bronchiole. Conversely, parasympathetic receptors, when stimulated, cause the bronchial smooth muscles to contract, thus reducing the diameter of the bronchiole. This

bronchoconstriction can inhibit the movement of air through the bronchiole.

After approximately 22 divisions, the bronchioles turn into the respiratory bronchioles. These structures contain only muscular connective tissue and have a limited capacity for gas exchange. The respiratory bronchioles terminate at the alveoli.

The Alveoli

The respiratory bronchioles divide into the alveolar ducts, which terminate in balloonlike clusters of **alveoli** called alveolar sacs (Figure 15-4). The alveoli contain an alveolar membrane that is only one or two cell layers thick. Because of this, the alveoli comprise the key functional unit of the respiratory system. Most oxygen and carbon dioxide gas exchanges take place here, although limited gas exchange may occur in the alveolar ducts and respiratory bronchioles. The alveoli become thinner as they expand. This facilitates diffusion of oxygen and carbon dioxide. The alveoli's surface area is massive, totaling more than 40 square meters—enough to cover half a tennis court. These hollow structures resist collapse largely because of the presence of surfactant, a chemical that decreases their surface tension and makes it easier for them to expand. Alveolar collapse

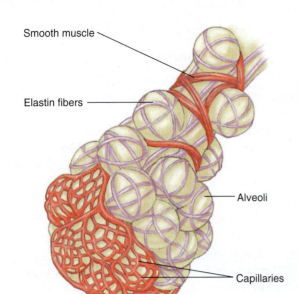

Smooth muscle

Elastin fibers

Alveoli

Capillaries

FIGURE 15-4 Anatomy of the alveoli.

(**atelectasis**) can occur if surfactant is insufficient or if the alveoli are not inflated. No gas exchange takes place in atelectatic alveoli.

The Lung Parenchyma

The alveoli are the terminal ends of the respiratory tree and the functional units of the lungs. As such, they are the core of the lung **parenchyma**. The lung parenchyma is arranged in two pulmonary lobules that form the anatomic division of the lungs. These lobules are further organized into lobes. The right lung has three lobes: the upper lobe, the middle lobe, and the lower lobe. The left lung, which shares thoracic space with the heart, has only two lobes: the upper lobe and the lower lobe.

The Pleura

Membranous connective tissue, called **pleura**, covers the lungs. The pleura consists of two layers: visceral and parietal. The visceral pleura envelops the lungs and does not contain nerve fibers. In contrast, the parietal pleura lines the thoracic cavity and does contain nerve fibers. The potential space between these two layers, called the *pleural space*, usually holds a small amount of fluid that reduces friction between the pleural layers during respiration. Occasionally, the pleura can become inflamed, causing significant pain with respiration. This condition, called *pleurisy*, is a common cause of chest pain, particularly in cigarette smokers.

The Pediatric Airway

The pediatric airway is fundamentally the same as an adult's, but you will need to know the differences in relative size and position of some components. The airway is smaller in all aspects, particularly the diameters of the openings and passageways.

In the pediatric pharynx, the jaw is smaller and the tongue relatively larger, resulting in greater potential airway encroachment (Figure 15-5). The epiglottis is much floppier and rounder ("omega" shaped). The dental (alveolar) ridge and teeth are softer and more fragile than an adult's and potentially more subject to damage from airway maneuvers.

The larynx lies more superior and anterior in children and is funnel-shaped because the cricoid cartilage is undeveloped. Before the age of 10, the cricoid cartilage is the narrowest part of the airway. Most significantly, even a small foreign body or a limited degree of swelling in the pediatric airway can be life threatening. Because of this, young children tend to suffer more problems related to the trachea than do older children. A common example is croup (laryngotracheobronchitis), a viral infection that causes the soft tissues below the glottis to swell. This can reduce the diameter of the airway, potentially causing serious problems.

The ribs and the cartilage of the pediatric thoracic cage are softer and more pliable. This lack of rigidity lessens the thoracic wall's and accessory muscles' ability to assist lung expansion during inspiration. As a result,

Relatively greater proportion of soft tissue

Larynx more superior and anterior

Epiglottis rounder and floppier

Loosely attached mucous membranes

Smaller jaw

Cricoid cartilage – narrowest part of the pediatric airway

FIGURE 15-5 Anatomy of the pediatric airway.

infants and children tend to rely more on their diaphragms for breathing. Always pay close attention to these differences when treating pediatric patients, especially those with respiratory complaints.

Physiology of the Respiratory System

Just as successful airway management requires a firm understanding of airway anatomy, a good outcome for these patients requires a working knowledge of the mechanics of oxygenation and ventilation. Your knowledge of normal respiratory physiology will lay the groundwork for your comprehension of important pathophysiology and will help you to determine which actions will ensure optimal patient care.

Respiration and Ventilation

Respiration, as noted earlier, is the exchange of gases between a living organism and its environment. Pulmonary, or external, respiration occurs in the lungs when the respiratory gases are exchanged between the alveoli and the red blood cells in the pulmonary capillaries through the capillary membranes (Figure 15-6). Cellular, or internal, respiration, however, occurs in the peripheral capillaries. It is the exchange of the respiratory gases between the red blood cells and the various body tissues. Cellular respiration in the peripheral tissue produces carbon dioxide (CO_2). The blood picks up this waste product in the capillaries and transports it as bicarbonate ions through the venous system to the lungs. Whereas respiration describes the process of gas exchange in the lungs and peripheral tissues, **ventilation** is the mechanical process that moves air into and out of the lungs. Ventilation is necessary for respiration to occur.

The Respiratory Cycle

Nothing within the lung parenchyma makes it contract or expand. Pulmonary ventilation, therefore, depends on changes in pressure within the thoracic cavity. These changes occur in a respiratory cycle involving coordinated interaction among the respiratory

system, the central nervous system, and the musculoskeletal system.

The thoracic cavity is a closed space, opening to the external environment only through the trachea. The diaphragm separates the thoracic cavity from the abdomen. When the diaphragm contracts, it draws downward, away from the thoracic cavity, thus enlarging it. Likewise, when the muscles between the ribs, or *intercostal muscles*, contract, they draw the rib cage upward and outward, away from the thoracic cavity, further increasing its volume.

The respiratory cycle begins when the lungs have achieved a normal expiration and the pressure inside the thoracic cavity equals the atmospheric pressure. At this point, respiratory centers in the brain communicate with the diaphragm by way of the phrenic nerve, signaling it to contract and thus initiate the respiratory cycle. As the size of the thorax increases in relation to the volume of air it holds, pressure within the thorax decreases, becoming lower than atmospheric pressure. This negative intrathoracic pressure invites air into the thorax through the airway. Because the visceral and parietal pleura remain in

In quiet breathing

500 mL
of inspired air

Contains: 20.94% Oxygen
79.01% Nitrogen
0.04% Carbon dioxide

150 mL
occupies the
conducting pathways
"dead space"

350 mL (together
with 150 mL of air
previously contained
in conducting pathways)
reach the alveoli

Expired air

Contains: 16.4% Oxygen
79.6% Nitrogen
4.0% Carbon dioxide

O_2

CO_2

Oxygenated blood
circulated
back to the heart

Deoxygenated
blood from the heart

FIGURE 15-6 Diffusion of gases across an alveolar membrane.

contact with each other under normal circumstances, the highly elastic lungs immediately assume the thoracic cavity's internal contour. These combined factors move air into the lungs (inspiration). At the same time, the alveoli inflate with the lungs. They become thinner as they expand, allowing oxygen and carbon dioxide to diffuse across their membranes.

When the pressure in the thoracic cavity again reaches that of the atmosphere, the alveoli are maximally inflated. Pulmonary expansion stimulates microscopic stretch receptors in the bronchi and bronchioles. These receptors signal the respiratory center by way of the vagus nerve to inhibit inspiration, and the air influx stops. This process is primarily protective, as it prevents overinflation of the lungs.

At the end of inspiration, the respiratory muscles now relax, thus decreasing the size of the chest cavity, and in turn increasing the intrathoracic pressure. The naturally elastic lungs recoil, forcing air out through the airway (expiration) until intrathoracic and atmospheric pressure are equal once again. Normal expiration is a passive process, whereas inspiration is an active process, using energy. In respiratory inadequacy, when this process fails to provide satisfactory gas exchange, the patient may use accessory respiratory muscles, such as the strap muscles of his neck and his abdominal muscles, to augment his efforts to expand the thoracic cavity.

Pulmonary Circulation

Respiration also requires an intact circulatory system. In fact, during each cardiac cycle, the heart pumps as much blood to the lungs as it pumps to the peripheral tissues. In the capillaries, these cells take oxygen from red blood cells coming from the arterial system and give up carbon dioxide to blood returning to the venous system. The venous system carries this deoxygenated blood to the right side of the heart, and the right ventricle pumps it into the pulmonary artery (Figure 15-7). The pulmonary artery immediately branches into the right and the left pulmonary arteries, each supplying its respective lung. In turn, both branches quickly fan into smaller arteries that end in the pulmonary capillaries. These capillaries are spread over the surfaces of the alveoli, where the red blood cells

exchange carbon dioxide for oxygen. The pulmonary capillaries recombine into larger veins, eventually terminating in the pulmonary vein. The pulmonary vein empties the oxygenated blood into the left atrium of the heart. Finally, the heart transports the oxygenated blood through the left ventricle and into the systemic arterial system via the aorta and its tributaries.

The lungs themselves receive little of their blood supply from the pulmonary arteries or veins. Instead, bronchial arteries that branch from the aorta supply most of their blood. Bronchial veins return this blood from the lungs to the superior vena cava.

Measuring Oxygen and Carbon Dioxide Levels

You can determine the amount of oxygen and carbon dioxide in the blood by measuring their partial pressures. **Partial pressure** is the pressure exerted by each component of a gas mixture. In other words, the partial pressure of a gas is its percentage of the mixture's total pressure. The partial pressure of oxygen at normal atmospheric pressure, for example, is the percentage of oxygen in atmospheric air (21 percent) multiplied by the atmospheric pressure at sea level (760 torr, or 14.7 pounds per square inch):

$$0.21 \times 760 \text{ torr} = 159.6 \text{ torr}$$

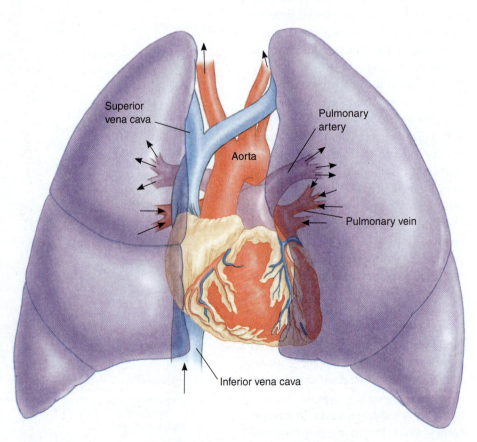

FIGURE 15-7 Pulmonary circulation.

Table 15-1 Partial Pressures and Concentrations of Gases

	Partial Pressure		Concentration	
	Atmospheric	Alveolar	Atmospheric	Alveolar
Nitrogen	597.0 torr	569.0 torr	78.62%	74.9%
Oxygen	159.0 torr	104.0 torr	20.84%	13.7%
Carbon dioxide	0.3 torr	40.0 torr	0.04%	5.2%
Water	3.7 torr	47.0 torr	0.50%	6.2%
TOTAL	760.0 torr	760.0 torr	100.00%	100.0%

(Note that torr and mmHg are the same measures of pressure.) Earth's atmosphere consists of four major respiratory gases: nitrogen (N_2), oxygen (O_2), carbon dioxide (CO_2), and water (H_2O). Although nitrogen is metabolically inert, it is needed to inflate gas-filled body cavities such as the chest. Table 15-1 lists these four respiratory gases' partial pressures and concentrations in the environment and in the alveoli.

Because alveolar partial pressure and arterial partial pressure are essentially the same in the normal lung, normal arterial partial pressures for oxygen and carbon dioxide may be expressed:

$$\text{Oxygen (PaO}_2) = 100 \text{ torr (average} = 80 - 100)$$
$$\text{Carbon dioxide (PaCO}_2) = 40 \text{ torr (average} = 35 - 45)$$

Alveolar partial pressures are abbreviated **PA** (PAO_2 and $PACO_2$), whereas arterial partial pressures are abbreviated **Pa** (PaO_2 and $PaCO_2$). Because these values are usually the same, however, they typically appear as the shortened notations PO_2 and PCO_2.

Diffusion

Diffusion is the movement of a gas from an area of higher concentration (partial pressure) to an area of lower concentration, attempting to reach equilibrium. Diffusion transfers gases between the lungs and the blood and between the blood and the peripheral tissues. The rate of diffusion of a gas across the pulmonary membranes depends on the gas's solubility in water. For example, carbon dioxide is 21 times more soluble in water than oxygen and readily crosses the pulmonary capillary membranes. In the peripheral tissues, the gradient (direction of diffusion) for CO_2 is from the tissue, where its concentration is high, to the capillary blood, where its concentration is low.

In the lungs, oxygen dissolves in water at the alveolar membrane and leaves the area of higher PO_2, the alveoli, and enters the area of lower PO_2, the venous blood in the pulmonary capillaries. Concurrently, carbon dioxide leaves the area of higher PCO_2, the arterial blood, and enters the area of lower PCO_2, the alveoli. The blood

returns from the pulmonary vein to the heart and then moves into the systemic circulation.

Oxygen Concentration in the Blood

Oxygen diffuses into the blood plasma, where most of it combines with hemoglobin and is measured as oxygen saturation (SaO_2). The remainder is dissolved in the blood and is measured as the PaO_2. Hemoglobin approaches 100 percent saturation when the PaO_2 of dissolved oxygen reaches 90 to 100 torr. Each gram of saturated hemoglobin carries 1.34 milliliters of oxygen. Oxygen saturation is the ratio of the blood's actual oxygen content to its total oxygen-carrying capacity:

$$\text{Oxygen saturation} = O_2 \text{ content}/O_2 \text{ capacity} \times 100(\%)$$

The hemoglobin molecule carries the vast majority of oxygen in the blood (approximately 97 percent). Very little oxygen dissolves in the plasma. Because partial pressure measurements detect only the amount of oxygen dissolved in the plasma and do not always reflect the total oxygen saturation of hemoglobin, they can be misleading. For example, a patient who has suffered carbon monoxide poisoning cannot transport enough oxygen to the essential tissues, because carbon monoxide displaces oxygen from the hemoglobin molecule, but an arterial blood gas sample might reveal a normal or high PaO_2. This would indicate that adequate oxygen was reaching the blood. In fact, however, an inadequate amount of hemoglobin would be available to transport the oxygen to the peripheral tissues, thus resulting in peripheral hypoxia.

The oxygen content of the arterial blood can be calculated using the following standardized equation:

$$CaO_2 = (SaO_2 \times Hgb \times 1.34) + (0.003 \times PaO_2)$$

where **CaO$_2$** is the **arterial oxygen concentration** (mL/dL), **SaO$_2$** is **hemoglobin-oxygen saturation** (%), **Hgb** indicates the amount of **hemoglobin** present (g/dL), 1.34 is a constant and represents the amount of oxygen bound to one gram of hemoglobin at one atmosphere pressure, 0.003 is the amount of oxygen dissolved in plasma (mL/g Hgb), and PaO_2 is the partial pressure of oxygen dissolved in the plasma (mmHg). Normal CaO_2 is 17 to 24 mL/dL.

Several factors can affect oxygen concentrations in the blood:

- Decreased hemoglobin concentration (anemia, hemorrhage)

- Inadequate alveolar ventilation due to low inspired-oxygen concentration, respiratory muscle paralysis, and pulmonary conditions such as emphysema, asthma, or pneumothorax

- Decreased diffusion across the pulmonary membrane when diffusion distance increases or the pulmonary membrane changes—for example, when fluid enters the space between the alveolar membrane and the pulmonary capillary membrane, as in pneumonia, chronic obstructive pulmonary disease (COPD), or pulmonary edema (swelling)

- Ventilation/perfusion mismatch occurs when a portion of the alveoli collapses, as in atelectasis. Blood travels past these collapsed alveoli without oxygenation (shunting), without carbon dioxide transfer, and without oxygen uptake. This can result from **hypoventilation**, which can occur secondary to pain or inability to inspire (traumatic asphyxia). When the lung collapses, as in **pneumothorax**, **hemothorax**, or a combination of the two, less surface area is available for gas exchange. Alternately, a ventilation/perfusion mismatch can occur when blood is prevented from reaching the alveolar capillary membranes but alveolar ventilation remains adequate. This occurs when a blood clot travels to or is formed in the pulmonary arterial system, a condition known as *pulmonary thromboembolism*.

You can correct oxygen derangements by increasing ventilation, administering supplemental oxygen, using intermittent positive-pressure ventilation (IPPV), or administering medications to correct underlying problems such as pulmonary edema, asthma, or **pulmonary embolism**. The emergency being treated determines the desired fractional concentration of oxygen (**FiO$_2$**) to be delivered. It is crucial to remember not to withhold oxygen from any patient whose clinical condition indicates its need.

Carbon Dioxide Concentrations in the Blood

The blood transports carbon dioxide mainly in the form of bicarbonate ion (HCO$_3^-$). It carries approximately 70 percent as bicarbonate and approximately 23 percent combined with hemoglobin. Less than 7 percent is dissolved in the plasma. Unlike oxygen, when carbon dioxide binds with hemoglobin, it binds to an amino acid and not to the iron-containing heme binding site where oxygen binds (Figure 15-8). Several factors influence carbon dioxide's concentration in the blood, including increased CO$_2$ production and/or decreased CO$_2$ elimination:

- Hyperventilation lowers CO$_2$ levels and can be the result of an increased respiratory rate or deeper respiration, both of which increase the **minute volume**. (We discuss minute volume more completely later in this chapter.)

- Causes of increased CO$_2$ production include:
  - Fever
  - Muscle exertion
  - Shivering
  - Metabolic processes resulting in the formation of metabolic acids

- Decreased CO$_2$ elimination (increased CO$_2$ levels in the blood) results from decreased alveolar ventilation. Common causes include hypoventilation due to:
  - Respiratory depression by drugs
  - Airway obstruction
  - Impairment of the respiratory muscles
  - Obstructive diseases such as asthma and emphysema

Increased CO$_2$ levels (**hypercarbia**) are usually treated by increasing the rate and/or volume of ventilation and by correcting the underlying cause.

Regulation of Respiration

Voluntary and Involuntary Respiratory Controls

The number of times a person breathes in 1 minute, the **respiratory rate**, is unique in that both voluntary and involuntary nervous system mechanisms control it. We do not ordinarily need to make a conscious effort to breathe; our brains automatically regulate this function. However, we can voluntarily override our involuntary respirations until physical and chemical mechanisms signal the nervous system's respiratory centers to provide involuntary impulses and correct any breathing irregularities.

FIGURE 15-8 Respiratory gas exchange and transport at the alveolar/capillary membrane.

NERVOUS IMPULSES FROM THE RESPIRATORY CENTER The main respiratory center lies in the *medulla,* located in the brainstem. Various neurons within the medulla initiate impulses that result in respiration. A rise in the frequency of these impulses increases the respiratory rate. Conversely, a decrease in their frequency decreases the respiratory rate. The medulla is connected to the respiratory muscles primarily via the vagus nerve. This is an involuntary pathway. If the medulla fails to initiate respiration, an additional control center in the pons, called the *apneustic center,* assumes respiratory control to ensure the continuation of respirations. A third center, the *pneumotaxic center,* also in the pons, controls expiration (Figure 15-9).

STRETCH RECEPTORS During inspiration, the lungs become distended, activating stretch receptors. As the degree of stretch increases, these receptors fire more frequently. The impulses they send to the brainstem inhibit the medullary cells, decreasing the inspiratory stimulus. Thus, the respiratory muscles relax, allowing the elastic lungs to recoil and expel air from the body. As the stretch decreases, the stretch receptors stop firing. This process, called the *Hering-Breuer reflex,* prevents overexpansion of the lungs.

CHEMORECEPTORS Other involuntary respiration controls include central chemical receptors in the medulla and peripheral chemoreceptors in the carotid bodies and in the arch of the aorta. These chemoreceptors are stimulated by decreased PaO_2, increased $PaCO_2$, and decreased pH. (The pH scale expresses the degree of acidity or alkalinity. A lower pH indicates greater acidity; a higher pH indicates greater alkalinity; the chaper "Pathosphysiology" discusses pH in greater detail.) Cerebrospinal fluid (CSF) pH is the primary control of respiratory center stimulation. The CSF pH responds very quickly to changes in arterial PCO_2. Any increase in PCO_2 will decrease CSF pH, which will, in turn, stimulate the central chemoreceptors to increase respiration.

Conversely, low $PaCO_2$ levels will raise CSF pH, in turn decreasing chemoreceptor stimulation and slowing respiratory activity. Because $PaCO_2$ is inversely related to CSF pH, $PaCO_2$ is seen as the normal neuroregulatory control of respirations. Additionally, any increase in the arterial PCO_2 stimulates the peripheral chemoreceptors to signal the brainstem to increase respiration, thus speeding CO_2 elimination from the body.

HYPOXIC DRIVE The body also constantly monitors the PaO_2 and the pH. In fact, **hypoxemia** (decreased partial pressure of oxygen in the blood) is a profound stimulus of respiration in a normal individual. People with chronic respiratory disease such as emphysema and chronic bronchitis tend to retain CO_2 and, therefore, have a chronically elevated $PaCO_2$. Chemoreceptors in the periphery eventually become accustomed to this chronic condition, and the central nervous system stops using $PaCO_2$ to

Nervous Control & Respiration

- Stimulation
- Inhibition

Pneumotaxic center

Apneustic center

Pons

Respiratory rhythmicity center
- Ventral respiratory group (VRG)(expiratory center)
- Dorsal respiratory group (DRG)(respiratory center)

Medulla oblongata

Internal intercostal muscles

External intercostal muscles

Diaphragm

FIGURE 15-9 Nervous control of respiration.

regulate respiration. This activates a default mechanism called **hypoxic drive**, which increases respiratory stimulation when PaO_2 falls and inhibits respiratory stimulation when PaO_2 climbs. High-volume oxygen administration to people with this condition can cause respiratory arrest. Because high-concentration oxygen can quickly double or even triple the PaO_2, peripheral chemoreceptors stop stimulating the respiratory centers, causing **apnea** (cessation of breathing). Although this is a potential threat, it is never appropriate to withhold oxygen from a patient for whom oxygen therapy is indicated. However, you must be prepared to assist with ventilations if the patient's respiratory effort becomes inadequate.

Measures of Respiratory Function

The respiratory rate is the number of respiratory cycles per minute, normally 12 to 20 breaths per minute in adults, 18 to 24 in children, and 40 to 60 in infants. Several factors affect respiratory rate:

- *Fever*—increases rate
- *Emotion*—increases rate
- *Pain*—increases rate
- *Hypoxia* (inadequate tissue oxygenation)—increases rate
- *Acidosis*—increases rate
- *Stimulant drugs*—increase rate
- *Depressant drugs*—decrease rate
- *Sleep*—decreases rate

Paramedics must fully understand ventilatory mechanics and capacities for the average adult's respiratory system. This knowledge will enable you to adapt your mechanical ventilation techniques to your patient's size, lung compliance, need for hyperventilation, or other individual requirements. It is especially crucial in situations that call for advanced mechanical ventilator skills. Respiratory capacities and measurements with which you must be familiar include the following:

- *Total lung capacity (TLC)*. **Total lung capacity** is the maximum lung capacity—the total amount of air contained in the lung at the end of maximal inspiration. In the average adult male, this volume is approximately 6 liters.
- *Tidal volume (V_T)*. The **tidal volume** is the average volume of gas inhaled or exhaled in one respiratory cycle. In the adult male this is approximately 500 mL (5 to 7 mL/kg).
- *Dead space volume (V_D)*. The dead space volume is the amount of gas in the tidal volume that remains in air passageways unavailable for gas exchange. It is approximately 150 mL in the adult male. Anatomic dead space

includes the trachea and bronchi. Obstructions or diseases such as chronic obstructive pulmonary disease or atelectasis can cause physiologic dead space.

- *Alveolar volume (V_A)*. The alveolar volume is the amount of gas in the tidal volume that reaches the alveoli for gas exchange. It is the difference between tidal volume and dead-space volume (approximately 350 mL in the adult male):

$$V_A = V_T - V_D$$

- *Minute volume (V_{min})*. The minute volume is the amount of gas moved in and out of the respiratory tract in 1 minute:

$$V_{min} = V_T \times \text{respiratory rate}$$

- *Alveolar minute volume (V_{A-min})*. The alveolar minute volume is the amount of gas that reaches the alveoli for gas exchange in 1 minute:

$$V_{A-min} = (V_T - V_D) \times \text{respiratory rate or}$$
$$V_{A-min} = V_A \times \text{respiratory rate}$$

- *Inspiratory reserve volume (IRV)*. The inspiratory reserve volume is the amount of air that can be maximally inhaled after a normal inspiration.
- *Expiratory reserve volume (ERV)*. The expiratory reserve volume is the amount of air that can be maximally exhaled after a normal expiration.
- *Residual volume (RV)*. The residual volume is the amount of air remaining in the lungs at the end of maximal expiration.
- *Functional residual capacity (FRC)*. The functional residual capacity is the volume of gas that remains in the lungs at the end of normal expiration:

$$FRC = ERV + RV$$

- *Forced expiratory volume (FEV)*. The forced expiratory volume is the amount of air that can be maximally expired after maximum inspiration.

Respiratory Problems

Respiratory emergencies can pose an immediate life threat to the patient. You must calmly and quickly assess the severity of his illness or injury while considering the potential causes of and treatment for his respiratory distress. Often, he will give you little help, because of either anxiety or difficulty speaking. His respiratory difficulty may be due to airway obstruction, injury to upper or lower airway structures, inadequate ventilation caused by worsening of an underlying lung disease and fatigue, or central nervous system problems that threaten the airway or respiratory effort.

Airway Obstruction

Blockage of the airway is an immediate threat to the patient's life and a true emergency. **Upper airway obstruction** may be defined as an interference with air movement through the upper airway.

Airway obstruction may be either partial or complete. Partial obstruction allows either adequate or poor air exchange. Patients with adequate air exchange can cough effectively; those with poor air exchange cannot. They often emit a high-pitched noise while inhaling (stridor), and their skin may have a bluish appearance (cyanosis). They also may have increased breathing difficulty, which can manifest as choking, gagging, dyspnea, or dysphonia (difficulty speaking). When you cannot feel or hear airflow from the nose and mouth, or when the patient cannot speak (aphonia), breathe, or cough, his airway is completely obstructed. He will quickly become unconscious and die if you do not relieve the obstruction. In the absence of breathing, difficulty ventilating the patient will indicate complete airway obstruction.

Causes of Airway Obstruction

The tongue, foreign bodies, teeth, spasm or edema, vomitus, and blood can all obstruct the upper airway.

THE TONGUE The tongue is the most common cause of airway obstruction (Figure 15-10). Normally, the submandibular muscles directly support the tongue and indirectly support the epiglottis. However, without sufficient muscle tone, the relaxed tongue falls back against the posterior pharynx, thus occluding the airway. This may produce snoring respiratory noises. At the same time, the epiglottis also

FIGURE 15-10 The tongue as airway obstruction. Note that the tongue has fallen backward, totally obstructing the airway.

may block the airway at the larynx. This at least diminishes airflow into the respiratory system, and the patient's breathing efforts may inadvertently suck the base of his tongue into an obstructing position. The patient's tongue can block his airway whether he is lateral, supine, or prone; however, the blockage depends on the position of the patient's head and jaw, so simple airway maneuvers such as the jaw-thrust can usually open his airway.

FOREIGN BODIES Large, poorly chewed pieces of food can obstruct the upper airway by becoming lodged in the hypopharynx. These cases often involve alcohol consumption and denture dislodgement. Because they frequently occur in restaurants and are mistaken for heart attacks, they are commonly called "café coronaries." The patient may clutch his neck between the thumb and fingers, a universal distress signal. Children, especially toddlers, often aspirate foreign objects, as they have the tendency to put objects into their mouths.

TRAUMA In trauma, particularly when the patient is unresponsive, loose teeth, facial bone fractures, and avulsed or swollen tissue may obstruct the airway. Secretions such as blood, saliva, and vomitus may compromise the airway and risk aspiration. Additionally, penetrating or blunt trauma may obstruct the airway by fracturing or displacing the larynx, allowing the vocal cords to collapse into the tracheal **lumen** (channel).

LARYNGEAL SPASM AND EDEMA Because the glottis is the narrowest part of an adult's airway, edema (swelling) or spasm (spasmotic closure) of the vocal cords is potentially lethal. Even moderate edema can severely obstruct airflow and cause asphyxia (the inability to move air into and out of the respiratory system). Just beneath the mucous membrane that covers the vocal cords is a layer of loose tissue where blood or other fluids can accumulate. This tissue may swell following injury, and the swelling will be slow to subside. Causes of laryngeal spasm and edema include trauma, anaphylaxis, epiglottitis, and inhalation of superheated air, smoke, or toxic substances. The most common cause of spasm is overly aggressive intubation. In addition, it often occurs immediately on **extubation**, especially when the patient is semiconscious. Some authors propose that laryngeal spasm can sometimes be partially overcome by strengthening ventilatory effort, forceful upward pull of the jaw, or the use of muscle relaxants, although the success of these maneuvers is quite variable.

ASPIRATION Vomitus is the most commonly aspirated material. Patients most at risk for this are those who are so obtunded (drowsy) that they cannot adequately protect their airways. This can occur with hypoxia, central nervous system toxins, or brain injury, among other causes. In addition to obstructing the airway, aspiration's other effects also significantly increase patient mortality. Vomitus consists of food particles, protein-dissolving enzymes, hydrochloric acid, and gastrointestinal bacteria that have been regurgitated from the stomach into the hypopharynx and oropharynx. If this mixture enters the lungs, it can result in increased interstitial fluid and pulmonary edema. The consequent marked increase in alveolar/capillary distance seriously impairs gas exchange, thus causing hypoxemia and hypercarbia. Aspirated materials can also severely damage the delicate bronchiolar tissue and alveoli. Gastrointestinal bacteria can produce overwhelming infections. These complications occur in 50 to 80 percent of patients who aspirate foreign matter.

Inadequate Ventilation

Insufficient minute volume respirations can compromise adequate oxygen intake and carbon dioxide removal. Additionally, oxygenation may be insufficient when conditions increase metabolic oxygen demand or decrease available oxygen. A reduction of either the rate or the volume of inhalation leads to a reduction in minute volume. In some cases, the respiratory rate may be rapid but so shallow that little air exchange takes place. Among the causes of such decreased ventilation are depressed respiratory function as from impairment of respiratory muscles or nervous system, bronchospasm from intrinsic disease, fractured ribs, pneumothorax, hemothorax, drug overdose, renal failure, spinal or brainstem injury, or head injury. In some conditions, such as sepsis, the body's metabolic demand for oxygen can exceed the patient's ability to supply it. Additionally, the environment may contain a decreased amount of oxygen, as in high-altitude conditions or a house fire, which also produces toxic gases such as cyanide and carbon monoxide. These situations of inadequate ventilation can lead to hypercarbia and hypoxia.

Respiratory System Assessment

Vigilance is the key to airway management in every patient. The trauma patient whose airway and breathing initially looked fine on exam may become symptomatic with the pneumothorax that was not initially evident. The asthma patient who initially responded to nebulizer treatment may have a sudden bronchospasm and worsen acutely. Minute-by-minute reassessment of the adequacy of every patient's airway and breathing is essential. The changes may be subtle increases in rate, worsening or onset of irregularity, or increased difficulty speaking. Assessment of the respiratory system begins with the primary assessment and should continue through the secondary assessment and the reassessment. (The chapters titled "Primary Assessment," "History Taking," "Secondary Assessment," "Patient Monitoring Technology," and "Patient Assessment in the Field" discuss in detail the steps of patient assessment that are summarized next.)

Primary Assessment

The purpose of the primary assessment is to identify any immediate threats to the patient's life, specifically **a**irway, **b**reathing, and **c**irculation problems (**ABCs**). For patients in cardiac arrest, compressions come before airway and breathing (CAB). However, as discussed in the introduction, airway assessment, management, and ventilation should be considered and can occur together.

First, assess the airway to ensure that it is patent. Snoring or gurgling may indicate potential airway problems. Next, determine the adequacy of breathing. If the patient is comfortable, with a normal respiratory rate, alert, and speaking without difficulty, you may generally assume that his airway is patent and breathing is adequate.

Patients with altered mental status warrant further evaluation. Feel for air movement with your hand or cheek (Figure 15-11). Look for the chest to rise and fall normally with each respiratory cycle (Figure 15-12). Listen for air movement and equal bilateral breath sounds (Figure 15-13). The absence of breath sounds on one side may indicate a pneumothorax or hemothorax in the trauma patient. In an adult patient, the respiratory rate generally ranges between 12 and 20 breaths per minute. Breathing should be spontaneous, effortless, and regular. Irregular breathing suggests a significant problem and usually requires ventilatory support. Observe the chest wall for any asymmetrical movement. This condition, known as **paradoxical breathing**, may suggest a **flail chest**. Patients showing increased respiratory effort; insisting on upright, sniffing, or semi-Fowler's positioning; or refusing to lie supine should be considered to be in significant respiratory distress.

FIGURE 15-11 Feel.

FIGURE 15-12 Look.

FIGURE 15-13 Listen.

If the patient is not breathing, or if you suspect airway problems, open the airway using the head-tilt/chin-lift or jaw-thrust maneuver, as described later in this chapter. If trauma is possible, use the jaw-thrust maneuver while stabilizing the cervical spine in the neutral position. Once the airway is open, reevaluate the breathing status. If breathing is adequate, provide supplemental oxygen and assess circulation. Consider the use of airway adjuncts, as discussed later. If breathing is inadequate or absent, begin artificial ventilation (Figure 15-14). When assisting a patient's breathing with a ventilatory device (bag-valve mask or other positive-pressure device), or after placing an airway adjunct (nasopharyngeal airway or oropharyngeal airway), or endotracheally intubating, monitor the chest's rise and fall to determine correct usage and placement. (We discuss these ventilatory devices and mechanical airways in detail later in this chapter.)

Secondary Assessment

After you complete the primary assessment and correct any immediate life threats, conduct the secondary assessment while continuously monitoring the patient's airway, breathing, and circulation.

FIGURE 15-14 Bag-valve-mask ventilation.

History

The time when the patient and his family noted the onset of symptoms is important information, as is whether the acute event occurred suddenly or gradually. Identifying possible triggers such as allergens or heat also can help the patient avoid them in the future. Additionally, the symptoms' course of development since onset will help direct diagnosis and treatment. Have they been progressively worsening, recurrent, or continuous? Associated symptoms will further help to assess the cause of the patient's problem. Has he had fever or chills, productive cough, chest pain, nausea or vomiting, or diaphoresis? Does he think his voice sounds normal?

The patient's past medical history will put his present complaints into perspective and help to identify the risk factors for a variety of likely diagnoses. Determine whether the present episode is similar to any past episodes of shortness of breath, what medical evaluations have been done, and what they have found. Has the patient ever been admitted to the hospital for his complaints? Has he ever been intubated?

The recent history leading to the onset of symptoms is also important. Did the patient run out of medication? Has he been noncompliant with (not taken) his medications? Did he drink too much fluid or alcohol? Did he have a seizure or vomit? Did he eat something that might induce an allergic reaction? Did he receive any trauma? If an injury is involved, evaluate the mechanism of injury. Keep in mind that blunt trauma to the neck may have injured the larynx. Anything that makes the patient's condition better (ameliorates) or worse (exacerbates, aggravates) is also significant.

Physical Examination

Your physical examination of a patient with respiratory problems should continue the evaluation of his airway, breathing, and circulation begun during your primary assessment. Now you will use the physical examination techniques of inspection, auscultation, and palpation to evaluate his injury or illness in more detail and determine your plan of action. (The chapter "Primary Assessment" explains these techniques in detail.)

INSPECTION Begin the physical assessment by inspecting the patient. Evaluate the adequacy of his breathing. Note any obvious signs of trauma. Always remember to assess skin color as an indicator of oxygenation status. Early in respiratory compromise, the sympathetic nervous system will be stimulated to help offset the lack of oxygen. When this happens, the skin will often appear pale and diaphoretic. **Cyanosis** (bluish discoloration) is another sign of respiratory distress. When oxygen binds with the hemoglobin, the blood appears bright red. Deoxygenated hemoglobin, however, is blue and gives the skin a bluish tint. This is not a reliable indicator, however, as severe tissue hypoxia is possible without cyanosis. In fact, cyanosis is considered a late sign of respiratory compromise. When it does appear, it usually affects the lips, fingernails, and skin. A red skin rash, especially if accompanied by hives, may indicate an allergic reaction. A cherry-red skin discoloration may, on rare occasions, be associated with carbon monoxide poisoning, as can bullae (large blisters).

Observe the patient's position. Tripod positioning (seated, leaning forward, with one arm forward to stabilize the body) may indicate COPD or asthma exacerbation; orthopnea (increased difficulty breathing while lying down) may indicate congestive heart failure, or asthma.

Next, inspecting for **dyspnea**—an abnormality of breathing rate, pattern, or effort—is essential. Dyspnea may cause or be caused by **hypoxia**. Prolonged dyspnea without successful intervention can lead to **anoxia** (the absence or near-absence of oxygen), which without intervention is a premorbid (occurring just before death) event, as the brain can survive only 4 to 6 minutes in this state. Remember that all interventions are useless if you do not establish a patent airway.

Also observe for the following modified forms of respiration:

- *Coughing*—forceful exhalation of a large volume of air from the lungs. This performs a protective function in expelling foreign material from the lungs.
- *Sneezing*—sudden, forceful exhalation from the nose. It is usually caused by nasal irritation.
- *Hiccoughing (hiccups)*—sudden inspiration caused by spasmodic contraction of the diaphragm with spastic closure of the glottis. It serves no known physiologic purpose. It has, occasionally, been associated with acute myocardial infarctions on the inferior (diaphragmatic) surface of the heart.

- *Sighing*—slow, deep, involuntary inspiration followed by a prolonged expiration. It hyperinflates the lungs and reexpands atelectatic alveoli. This normally occurs about once a minute.
- *Grunting*—a forceful expiration that occurs against a partially closed epiglottis. It is usually an indication of respiratory distress.

Note any decrease or increase in the respiratory rate, one of the earliest indicators of respiratory distress. Also, look for use of the accessory respiratory muscles—intercostal, suprasternal, supraclavicular, and subcostal retractions—and the abdominal muscles to assist breathing. This indicates increased respiratory effort secondary to respiratory distress. In infants and children, nasal flaring and grunting indicate respiratory distress. COPD patients having difficulty breathing will purse their lips during exhalation. Monitor the patient's blood pressure, including any differences noted during expiration versus inspiration. Patients with severe chronic obstructive pulmonary disease may sustain a drop in blood pressure during inspiration. This drop is due to increased pressure within the thoracic cavity that impairs the ability of the ventricles to fill. Thus, decreased ventricular filling leads to decreased blood pressure. A drop in blood pressure of greater than 10 torr is termed **pulsus paradoxus** and may be indicative of severe obstructive lung disease.

Determine whether the pattern of respirations is abnormal—deep or shallow in combination with a fast or slow rate. Some common abnormal respiratory patterns include:

- *Kussmaul's respirations*—deep, slow or rapid, gasping breathing, commonly found in diabetic ketoacidosis
- *Cheyne–Stokes respirations*—progressively deeper, faster breathing alternating gradually with shallow, slower breathing, indicating brainstem injury
- *Biot's respirations*—irregular pattern of rate and depth with sudden, periodic episodes of apnea, indicating increased intracranial pressure
- *Central neurogenic hyperventilation*—deep, rapid respirations, indicating increased intracranial pressure
- *Agonal respirations*—shallow, slow, or infrequent breathing, indicating brain anoxia

Finally, observing altered mentation may be key in determining whether breathing is adequate or if significant hypoxia may be present. If the patient's mental status is not normal, you must determine his usual baseline mental status before you can make this assessment.

AUSCULTATION Following inspection, listen at the mouth and nose for adequate air movement. Then listen

FIGURE 15-15 Positions for auscultating breath sounds.

to the chest with a stethoscope (auscultate) (Figure 15-15). In a prehospital setting, you should auscultate the right and left apex (just beneath the clavicle), the right and left base (eighth or ninth intercostal space, midclavicular line), and the right and left lower thoracic back or right and left midaxillary line (fourth or fifth intercostal space, on the lateral aspect of the chest). When the patient's condition permits, you can monitor six locations on the posterior chest, three right and three left. The posterior surface is preferable because heart sounds do not interfere with auscultation at this location. However, because patients are usually supine during airway management, the anterior and lateral positions usually prove more accessible. Breath sounds should be equal bilaterally. Sounds that point to airflow compromise include:

- *Snoring*—results from partial obstruction of the upper airway by the tongue
- *Gurgling*—results from the accumulation of blood, vomitus, or other secretions in the upper airway
- *Stridor*—a harsh, high-pitched sound heard on inhalation, associated with laryngeal edema or constriction
- *Wheezing*—a musical, squeaking, or whistling sound heard in inspiration and/or expiration, associated with bronchiolar constriction
- *Quiet*—diminished or absent breath sounds are an ominous finding and indicate a serious problem with the airway, breathing, or both

CONTENT REVIEW
➤ Beware of the quiet chest.

Sounds that may indicate compromise of gas exchange include:

- *Crackles (rales)*—a fine, bubbling sound heard on inspiration, associated with fluid in the smaller bronchioles
- *Rhonchi*—a coarse, rattling noise heard on inspiration, associated with inflammation, mucus, or fluid in the bronchioles

When you assess the effectiveness of ventilatory support or the correct placement of an airway adjunct, remember that air movement into the epigastrium may sometimes mimic breath sounds. Thus, listening to the chest should be only one of several means that you use to assess air movement. Another method of checking correct placement of an airway adjunct is to auscultate over the epigastrium; it should be silent during ventilation. When you provide ventilatory support, watch for signs of gastric distention. They suggest inadequate hyperextension of the neck, undue pressure generated by the ventilatory device, or improper placement of airway adjuncts.

PALPATION Finally, palpate. First, using the back of your hand or your cheek, feel for air movement at the mouth and nose. (If an endotracheal tube is in place, you can check for air movement at the tube's adapter.) Next, palpate the chest for rise and fall. In addition, palpate the chest wall for tenderness, symmetry, abnormal motion, crepitus, and subcutaneous emphysema.

When ventilating with a bag-valve device, gauge airflow into the lungs by noting compliance. **Compliance**

Table 15-2 Comparison of Pulse Oximetry and Capnography

	Pulse Oximetry (SpO$_2$)	Capnography (ETCO$_2$)
Gas measured	Oxygen (O$_2$)	Carbon dioxide (CO$_2$)
Parameter evaluated	Oxygenation	Ventilation
Speed of information provided	• Reflects changes in oxygenation <5 minutes • Delayed detection of hypoventilation or apnea	• Reflects changes in ventilation <10 seconds • Immediate detection of hypoventilation and apnea
Compatibility	Should be used with capnography	Should be used with pulse oximetry

refers to the stiffness or flexibility of the lung tissue, and it is indicated by how easily air flows into the lungs. When compliance is good, airflow meets minimal resistance. When compliance is poor, ventilation is harder to achieve. Compliance is often poor in diseased lungs and in patients suffering from chest wall injuries or tension pneumothorax. If a patient shows poor compliance during ventilatory support, look for potential causes. Upper airway obstructions, which cause difficulty with mechanical ventilation, can mimic poor compliance. If ventilating the patient is initially easy but then becomes progressively more difficult, repeat the primary assessment and look for the development of a new problem, possibly related to the mechanical airway maneuvers. The following questions will aid this assessment:

- Is the airway open?
- Is the head properly positioned in extension (nontrauma patients)?
- Is the patient developing tension pneumothorax?
- Is the endotracheal tube occluded (a mucus plug or aspirated material)?
- Has the endotracheal tube been inadvertently pushed into the right or left mainstem bronchus?
- Has the endotracheal tube been displaced into the esophagus?
- Is the mechanical ventilatory equipment functioning properly?

Pulse rate abnormalities may also suggest respiratory compromise. Tachycardia (an abnormally fast pulse) usually accompanies hypoxemia in an adult, whereas bradycardia (an abnormally slow pulse) hints at anoxia with imminent cardiac arrest.

Noninvasive Respiratory Monitoring

CONTENT REVIEW

➤ A fall in the pulse rate in a patient with airway compromise is an ominous finding.

Several available devices will help you measure the effectiveness of oxygenation and ventilation and maintain parameters at the appropriate levels. Those measurements used most commonly in prehospital care are pulse oximetry, CO oximetry, and capnography. Peak expiratory flow testing can also be useful in the prehospital setting for some respiratory diseases, although it is not widely employed. These measurements use various devices and methodologies that, when used alone, have their limitations. However, when used together, they can provide a fairly comprehensive and reliable picture of the patient's respiratory status. Table 15-2 details some of the advantages and limitations of pulse oximetry and capnography.

Pulse Oximetry

Pulse oximetry is widely used in prehospital emergency care and often referred to as the "fifth vital sign." A pulse oximeter measures hemoglobin oxygen saturation in peripheral tissues (Figure 15-16). It is noninvasive (does not require entering the body), rapidly applied, and easy to operate. Pulse oximetry readings are generally accurate measures of arterial oxygen saturation and continually reflect any changes in peripheral oxygen delivery. In fact, pulse oximetry often detects problems with oxygenation

FIGURE 15-16 Pulse oximeter.

faster than assessments of blood pressure, pulse, and respirations. When available, you should use it in virtually any situation to determine the patient's baseline value, to guide patient care, and to monitor the patient's responses to your interventions.

To determine peripheral oxygen saturation, you place a sensor probe over a peripheral capillary bed such as a fingertip, toe, or earlobe. In infants, you can wrap the sensor around the heel and secure it with tape. The sensor contains two light-emitting diodes and two sensors. One diode emits near-red light, a wavelength specific for oxygenated hemoglobin; the other emits infrared light, a wavelength specific for deoxygenated hemoglobin. Each hemoglobin state absorbs a certain amount of the emitted light, preventing it from reaching the corresponding sensor. Less light reaching the sensor means more of its type of hemoglobin is in the blood. The oximeter then calculates the ratio of the near-red and infrared light it has received to determine the **oxygen saturation percentage (SpO$_2$)**.

Pulse oximeters display the SpO$_2$ and the pulse rate as detected by the sensors. They show the SpO$_2$ either as a number or as a visual display that also shows the pulse's waveform and heart rate. The latter helps the provider ensure that the SpO$_2$ reading is based on good data. If the patient's pulse is 120 but the pulse oximetry waveform is detecting only 60, or the waveform is nearly flat, then the saturation reading is unlikely to be accurate. The relationship between SpO$_2$ and the partial pressure of oxygen in the blood (PaO$_2$) is very complex. However, the SpO$_2$ does correlate with the PaO$_2$. The greater the PaO$_2$, the greater will be the oxygen saturation. Because hemoglobin carries 98 percent of oxygen in the blood, whereas plasma carries only 2 percent, pulse oximetry accurately analyzes peripheral oxygen delivery.

As a guide, normal SpO$_2$ varies between 96 and 99 percent at sea level. Readings between 91 and 95 percent indicate mild hypoxemia and warrant further evaluation and supplemental oxygen administration. Readings between 86 and 90 percent indicate moderate hypoxemia. You should generally give these patients high-concentration supplemental oxygen using a nonrebreather. Readings of 85 percent or lower indicate severe hypoxemia and warrant immediate intervention, including the administration of high-concentration oxygen, ventilatory assistance, or CPAP (discussed later). Your goal is to maintain the SpO$_2$ in the normal range (Table 15-3).

Recent studies show that oxygen administration is not without risk. Excess oxygen can cause the body to manufacture toxic chemicals called **free radicals**. (Free radicals were also discussed in the chapter "Pathophysiology.") These toxic chemicals can damage body tissues—especially in areas that are highly oxygen dependent, such as the brain and heart. Because of this, oxygen should be administered only to patients who are found to be hypoxic by pulse

Table 15-3 Interpretation of Pulse Oximetry Readings and Recommended Actions

SpO$_2$ Reading (%)	Interpretation	Intervention
95–100	Normal	Change FiO$_2$ to maintain saturation.
91–94	Mild hypoxemia	Increase FiO$_2$ to increase saturation.
86–90	Moderate hypoxemia	Increase FiO$_2$ to increase saturation. Assess and increase ventilation.
<85	Severe hypoxemia	Increase FiO$_2$ to increase saturation. Increase ventilation.

oximetry. Then, only enough supplemental oxygen should be administered to correct hypoxia and restore **normoxia** (increase it to within a normal range). Trying to fully saturate hemoglobin with oxygen can cause the formation of free radicals and result in what is called *oxidative stress.* Excess concentrations of oxygen (**hyperoxia**) should be avoided. The production of toxic free radicals from oxygen administration has been associated with worsened outcomes in patients with brain trauma and stroke, and in post-cardiac arrest victims. It can cause numerous problems in neonates. Thus, always administer the lowest flow of oxygen that will restore normoxia (without causing hyperoxia) as evidenced by dynamic pulse oximetry readings.[1–3]

False readings with pulse oximetry are infrequent and vary with the type of device used. When they do occur, the heart rate on the pulse oximeter may not correlate with the patient's true heart rate, the waveform may be flat or nearly flat, and/or the oximeter will generate an error signal or a blank screen. Causes of false readings include carbon monoxide poisoning, high-intensity lighting, nail polish, poor perfusion, and certain hemoglobin abnormalities. Fortunately, second-generation pulse oximeters have eliminated many of these problems. In hypovolemia and in severely anemic patients, however, the pulse oximetry reading may be misleading. Although the SpO$_2$ reading may be normal, the total amount of hemoglobin available to carry oxygen may be so markedly decreased that the patient will remain hypoxic at the cellular level.

Pulse oximetry provides key information about the patient and is an important part of emergency care, including prehospital care. However, it is only one assessment tool and does not replace other physical assessment or monitoring tools or skills. Do not depend solely on pulse oximetry readings to guide care. Always consider and treat the whole patient.

Pulse CO Oximetry

Pulse CO oximeters are devices that detect abnormal hemoglobins such as carboxyhemoglobin (from carbon monoxide poisoning) and methemoglobin (as seen in methemoglobinemia). Some devices can also detect total hemoglobin. Until recently, these devices were found only in hospital laboratories and required a blood sample. Recently, noninvasive CO oximeters have been developed that will detect and measure carboxyhemoglobin in the same manner that standard pulse oximeters detect and report oxygen saturation. These devices may prove useful when screening patients with potential exposures or vague unexplained symptoms.

Pulse CO oximeters use multiple wavelengths of light to detect various forms of hemoglobin found in humans (Figure 15-17). Like a pulse oximeter, they detect hemoglobin with oxygen bound (oxyhemoglobin), and they detect hemoglobin without oxygen (deoxyhemoglobin). Depending on the device, they can also detect the following:

- *Carboxyhemoglobin.* When carbon monoxide (CO), a toxic gas, is inhaled, it will displace oxygen from the iron-containing heme molecules in hemoglobin. There are four heme binding sites on each hemoglobin molecule. CO will displace oxygen molecules that are already present on the heme, allowing the CO to bind and form carboxyhemoglobin. As the heme molecules are bound with CO, the oxygen-carrying capacity of the hemoglobin is reduced. Pulse CO oximeters can detect increased carboxyhemoglobin. The amount of carboxyhemoglobin detected is reported as a percentage of total hemoglobin and abbreviated SpCO.[4–6]

- *Methemoglobin.* Methemoglobin is a form of hemoglobin in which the iron molecules in the heme units are in the ferric (Fe^{3+}) state. Thus, methemoglobin can neither bind nor transport oxygen. Methemoglobin has a bluish-brown color. Normally, there are enzyme systems (e.g., methemoglobin reductase) that can restore methemoglobin to the ferrous (Fe^{2+}) state,

FIGURE 15-18 Total hemoglobin by pulse CO oximetry.

(© Dr. Bryan E. Bledsoe)

forming deoxyhemoglobin, so it can again transport oxygen. Typically, less than 2 percent of the hemoglobin in the body is in the form of methemoglobin, which cannot bind or transport oxygen. However, several conditions and drugs can cause abnormal elevations of methemoglobin (methemoglobinemia). Selected pulse CO-oximeters can measure methemoglobin and report it as a percentage of total hemoglobin (SpMET).[7–8]

- *Total hemoglobin.* Pulse CO oximetry now allows for noninvasive measurement of total hemoglobin in the prehospital setting (Figure 15-18). This reading is reported as SpHb. This now allows for the prehospital detection of anemia and blood loss and can serve as a surrogate indicator of the blood's oxygen-carrying content. When coupled with standard pulse oximetry readings (based on the arterial oxygen content formula discussed earlier), it is possible to noninvasively estimate oxygen content in the blood (SpOC).

Noninvasive monitoring technology is evolving rapidly. Many of the parameters discussed here are available on many of the popular commercial patient monitors used in EMS (Figure 15-19). Like any other technology, prehospital personnel should not solely rely on monitoring technology. Instead, they should look at the entire patient picture and make treatment decisions based on multiple findings and parameters.

Capnography

Exhaled carbon dioxide (CO_2) monitoring, also called end-tidal carbon dioxide ($ETCO_2$) monitoring, or capnometry, is a noninvasive method of measuring the levels of carbon dioxide (CO_2) in the exhaled breath. **Capnography** is a recording or display of the exhaled carbon dioxide levels measured by capnometry. When first introduced

FIGURE 15-17 Pulse CO oximetry.

(© Dr. Bryan E. Bledsoe)

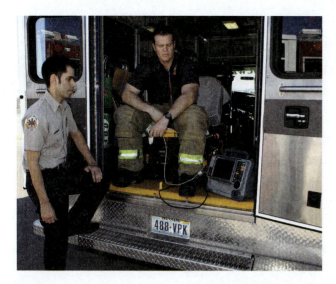

FIGURE 15-19 Multiple noninvasive parameters in a single display monitor.

(© Dr. Bryan E. Bledsoe)

into prehospital care, capnometry was used exclusively to verify proper endotracheal tube placement in the trachea. The detection of adequate levels of exhaled CO_2 following intubation confirms the tube is in the trachea (or above) and not in the esophagus. More robust technology provides accurate noninvasive measurements of exhaled CO_2 levels, thus providing medical personnel with information about the status of systemic metabolism, circulation, and ventilation. The use of capnometry and capnography has become commonplace in the operating room, in the emergency department, and in the prehospital setting.[9–10]

Various terms have been applied to capnography, and a review of them may help you to understand the material in this section. These terms include:

- *Capnometry.* Capnometry is the measurement of expired CO_2. It typically provides a numeric display of the partial pressure of CO_2 (in Torr or mmHg) or the percentage of CO_2 present.
- *Capnography.* Capnography is a graphic recording or display of the capnometry reading over time.
- *Capnograph.* A capnograph is a device that measures expired CO_2 levels.
- *Capnogram.* A capnogram is the visual representation of the expired CO_2 waveform.
- *End-tidal CO_2 (ETCO$_2$).* End-tidal CO_2 is the measurement of the CO_2 concentration at the end of expiration (maximum CO_2).
- *PETCO$_2$.* PETCO$_2$ is the partial pressure of end-tidal CO_2 in a mixed gas solution.
- *PaCO$_2$.* The PaCO$_2$ represents the partial pressure of CO_2 in the arterial blood.

- *End-tidal gradient.* The end-tidal gradient is the difference between the partial pressure of arterial CO_2 (PaCO$_2$) and the end-tidal CO_2 (ETCO$_2$). It is calculated as:

$$PaCO_2 - ETCO_2 = End - tidal\ gradient$$

This value is normally less than 5 mmHg. However, an increase in dead space ventilation (ventilation of nonperfused lung tissue) reflects a ventilation/perfusion mismatch (V/Q mismatch). This occurs in pulmonary embolism and similar processes. As dead space ventilation increases, the ETCO$_2$ falls, thus widening the end-tidal gradient.

CO_2 is a normal end product of metabolism and is transported by the venous system to the right side of the heart and on to the lungs where it diffuses into the alveoli and is removed from the body through exhalation. When circulation is normal, exhaled CO_2 levels change proportionally with ventilation and are a very reliable estimate of the partial pressure of carbon dioxide in the arterial system (PaCO$_2$). Normal PaCO$_2$ is approximately 40 and a normal exhaled CO_2 is just 1 to 2 mm less, or 38 mmHg (Table 15-4).

When perfusion decreases, as occurs in shock or cardiac arrest, exhaled CO_2 levels reflect pulmonary blood flow and cardiac output, not ventilation. Decreased levels of exhaled CO_2 can be found in shock, cardiac arrest, pulmonary embolism, bronchospasm, and with incomplete airway obstruction (such as mucus plugging). Increased levels of exhaled CO_2 are found with hypoventilation, respiratory depression, and hyperthermia (Table 15-5).

CO_2 is detected by using either a colorimetric or an infrared device. It can be reported as a percentage (the amount of CO_2 in a given volume of gas) or as a partial pressure (mmHg).

COLORIMETRIC DEVICES The colorimetric device is a disposable ETCO$_2$ detector that contains pH-sensitive, chemically impregnated paper encased within a plastic chamber (Figure 15-20). It is placed in the airway circuit between the patient and the ventilation device. When the paper is exposed to CO_2, hydrogen ions (H$^+$) are generated (change in pH), causing a color change in the paper. The color change is reversible and changes breath to breath. A color scale on the device estimates the ETCO$_2$ level.

Table 15-4 Comparison of PaCO$_2$ and ETCO$_2$

	Arterial CO$_2$ (PaCO$_2$) Arterial Blood Gases	End-Tidal CO$_2$ (ETCO$_2$) Capnography
Partial Pressure (mmHg)	35–45 mmHg	30–43 mmHg
Percentage (%)	4.6–5.9%	4.0–5.6%

Table 15-5 Basic Rules of Capnography

Symptom	Possible Cause
Sudden drop of $ETCO_2$ to zero	• Esophageal intubation • Ventilator disconnection or defect in ventilator • Defect in CO_2 analyzer
Sudden decrease of $ETCO_2$ (not to zero)	• Leak in ventilator system; obstruction • Partial disconnect in ventilator circuit • Partial airway obstruction (secretions)
Exponential decrease of $ETCO_2$	• Pulmonary embolism • Cardiac arrest • Hypotension (sudden) • Severe hyperventilation
Change in CO_2 baseline	• Calibration error • Water droplet in analyzer • Mechanical failure (ventilator)
Sudden increase in $ETCO_2$	• Accessing an area of lung previously obstructed • Release of tourniquet • Sudden increase in blood pressure
Gradual lowering of $ETCO_2$	• Hypovolemia • Decreasing cardiac output • Decreasing body temperature; hypothermia; drop in metabolism
Gradual increase in $ETCO_2$	• Rising body temperature • Hypoventilation • CO_2 absorption • Partial airway obstruction (foreign body); reactive airway disease

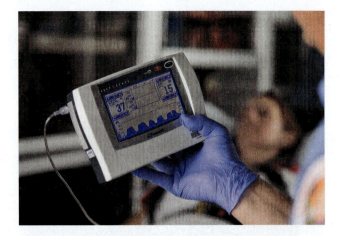

FIGURE 15-21 Handheld capnography unit.

FIGURE 15-20 Colorimetric end-tidal CO_2 detector.

(© Edward T. Dickinson, MD)

Colorimetric devices cannot detect hyper- or hypocarbia (increased or decreased CO_2 levels). If gastric contents or acidic drugs (e.g., endotracheal epinephrine) contact the paper in the device, subsequent readings may be unreliable.

INFRARED DEVICES Electronic exhaled CO_2 detectors use an infrared technique to detect CO_2 in the exhaled breath (Figure 15-21). A heated element in the sensor generates infrared radiation. The CO_2 molecules absorb infrared light at a very specific wavelength and can thus be measured. Electronic exhaled CO_2 detectors may be either qualitative (i.e., they simply detect the presence of CO_2) or quantitative (i.e., they determine how much CO_2 is present). Quantitative devices are now routinely used in prehospital care. Exhaled $ETCO_2$ readings can be monitored both in patients who are not intubated and in those who are intubated (Figures 15-22 and 15-23). Most modern capnometers can both display a number and provide a digital waveform (capnogram) that reflects the entire respiratory cycle (Figure 15-24).

There are two major types of capnography—mainstream and sidestream. Each has its advantages and disadvantages. With mainstream capnography, the infrared light is shone through the gas within the patient circuit. With sidestream capnography, a sample of the gas is aspirated from the main gas flow circuit, using a separate sample line. This sample line is attached to a sensor unit that is

FIGURE 15-22 End-tidal carbon dioxide monitoring in a non-intubated patient.

(© Edward T. Dickinson, MD)

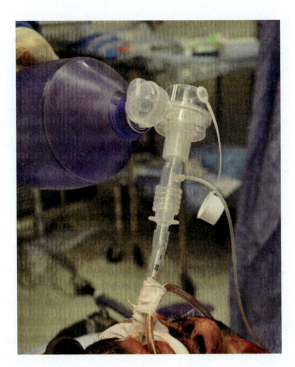

FIGURE 15-23 End-tidal carbon dioxide monitoring in an intubated patient.

(© Edward T. Dickinson, MD)

FIGURE 15-24 Some CO_2 detectors can display both a waveform and a number.

typically housed in the patient monitor. The differences are illustrated in Table 15-6.

CAPNOGRAM The capnogram reflects exhaled CO_2 concentrations over time. It is typically divided into four phases (Figure 15-25).

- *Phase I.* Phase I (AB in Figure 15-25) is the respiratory baseline. It is flat when no CO_2 is present and corresponds to the late phase of inspiration and the early part of expiration (in which dead-space gases without CO_2 are released).

- *Phase II.* Phase II (BC in Figure 15-25) is the respiratory upstroke. This reflects the appearance of CO_2 in the alveoli.

Table 15-6 Comparison of Mainstream and Sidestream Capnography

Mainstream Capnography	Sidestream Capnography
CO_2 sensor located between ET tube and breathing circuit	CO_2 aspirated from a sampling tube and analyzed in an analyzer/sensor away from the patient
Advantages	
• Provides real-time information • More accurate • No sampling tube • Not affected by water vapor pressure changes	• Lightweight • Less expensive • Can be used in non-intubated patients (including CPAP) • Easy to connect • Disposable tubing • Can be used with simultaneous oxygen administration • Calibration automatic
Disadvantages	
• Bulkiness/weight of sensor • Can be used only in intubated patients • Expensive probe • Requires calibration	• Small sampling tube easily obstructed (e.g., by water vapor) • Slightly less accurate • Delay of several seconds analyzing sample • Water vapor may affect ETCO2 reading • Pressure drop along sampling tube may affect ETCO2 reading

- *Phase III.* Phase III (CD in Figure 15-25) is the respiratory plateau. It reflects the airflow through uniformly ventilated alveoli with a nearly constant CO_2 level. The highest level of the plateau (point D in Figure 15-25) is called the $ETCO_2$ and is recorded as such by the capnometer.

- *Phase IV.* Phase IV (DE in Figure 15-25) is the inspiratory phase. It is a sudden downstroke and ultimately returns to the baseline during inspiration. The respiratory pause restarts the cycle (EA in Figure 15-25).

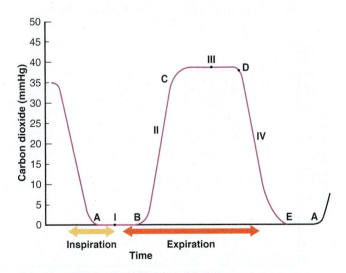

FIGURE 15-25 Normal capnogram. AB = *Phase I:* late inspiration, early expiration (no CO_2). BC = *Phase II:* appearance of CO_2 in exhaled gas. CD = *Phase III:* plateau (constant CO_2). D = highest point ($ETCO_2$). DE = *Phase IV:* rapid descent during inspiration. EA = respiratory pause.

CLINICAL APPLICATIONS At its most basic, qualitative capnography may be used to assess correct initial and periodic endotracheal tube placement. Continuous quantitative capnography may be used in intubated patients to confirm initial tube placement and to constantly monitor for tube misplacement. Continuous waveform capnography may also be used to ensure proper exhaled CO_2 levels for head trauma and stroke patients. Continuous waveform capnography adds the ability to help troubleshoot hypoxemia and difficult ventilation and assess for bronchospasm, pulmonary embolus, and so on. Continuous waveform capnography also has utility in monitoring nonintubated patients. By following trends in the capnogram, prehospital personnel can continuously monitor the patient's condition, detect trends, and document the response to medications.

Several medical conditions and mechanical ventilation problems can be readily detected by capnography when compared to the normal capnogram (Figure 15-26). These include:

- *Obstructive disease.* Obstructive pulmonary diseases, such as asthma and chronic obstructive pulmonary disease (COPD), obstruct air entry and alter the shape of the capnogram. These diseases give the typical "shark fin" shape to the capnogram (Figure 15-27).

- *Rebreathing.* Rebreathing of gas can result in failure of the capnogram to reach the baseline. This can be due to hyperventilation or to problems in the breathing circuit (Figure 15-28).

- *Curare cleft.* Appears when neuromuscular blockers begin to subside. The depth of the cleft is inversely proportional to the degree of drug activity (Figure 15-29).

- *Esophageal intubation.* The absence of a waveform, or the presence of a small disorganized waveform, is indicative of esophageal intubation (Figure 15-30).

FIGURE 15-27 Capnogram pattern showing classic "shark fin" waveform consistent with obstructive pulmonary disease (asthma and COPD).

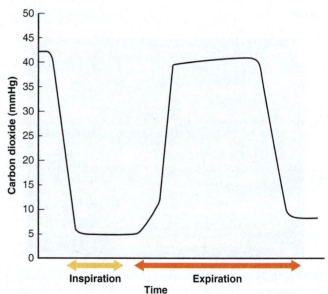

FIGURE 15-28 An elevation in the baseline indicates rebreathing of CO_2 and is generally seen with hyperventilation.

- *Endotracheal tube or circuit leak.* Waveform variations are seen when there is a leak in the endotracheal tube cuff or if the airway is too small for the patient (Figure 15-31).

- *Ventilation/perfusion (V/Q) mismatch.* With a ventilation/perfusion mismatch, as occurs in pulmonary embolism and similar conditions, the increase in dead space ventilation causes a decrease in ETCO$_2$ levels throughout the respiratory cycle (Figure 15-32).

- *Apnea.* A fall of the waveform to the baseline indicates apnea (Figure 15-33).

FIGURE 15-26 Normal capnogram. Capnography provides immediate information about the patient's ventilatory status.

FIGURE 15-29 So-called curare notch or curare cleft seen in mechanically ventilated patients as neuromuscular blocker levels fall.

FIGURE 15-30 Capnogram showing absent waveform consistent with esophageal intubation.

- *Hyperventilation.* Hyperventilation leads to elimination of CO_2 and a progressively lower exhaled CO_2 level (Figure 15-34).

- *Hypoventilation.* Hypoventilation results in CO_2 retention and a progressive elevation in exhaled CO_2 levels (Figure 15-35).

Exhaled CO_2 detection is also useful in CPR. During cardiac arrest, CO_2 levels fall abruptly following the onset of cardiac arrest. They begin to rise with the onset of effective CPR and return to near-normal levels with a return of spontaneous circulation. During effective CPR, exhaled CO_2 levels have been found to correlate well with cardiac

FIGURE 15-31 Waveform variations seen with leakage in the endotracheal tube cuff or in the breathing circuit.

FIGURE 15-32 Persistently low $ETCO_2$ levels consistent with significant dead space ventilation (V/Q mismatch) as seen in pulmonary embolism.

FIGURE 15-33 Apnea.

FIGURE 15-34 Progressive reduction in ETCO$_2$ levels consistent with hyperventilation.

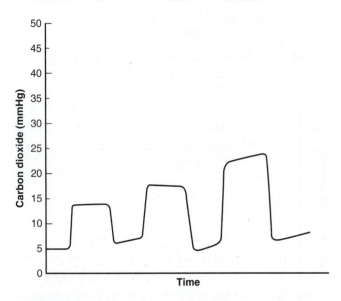

FIGURE 15-35 Progressive increase in ETCO$_2$ levels consistent with hypoventilation.

output, coronary perfusion pressure, and even with the effectiveness of CPR compressions.

Continuous waveform capnography is rapidly becoming a standard of care in EMS (Figure 15-36). Misplaced endotracheal tubes represent a significant area of liability

FIGURE 15-36 Most modern patient monitors allow the constant monitoring of numerous physiologic parameters.

in EMS and the documentation provided by this technology can provide irrefutable evidence of proper endotracheal tube placement.

Peak Expiratory Flow Testing

Peak expiratory flow testing uses a disposable plastic chamber into which the patient exhales forcefully after maximal inhalation. It can be used as a crude measure of respiratory efficacy. Improving measurements can indicate good response to treatment of acute respiratory illness.

PART 2: Basic Airway Management and Ventilation

Basic airway management and ventilation includes most airway maneuvers that have been shown to be lifesaving, including proper positioning, suctioning, oxygen administration, and bag-valve-mask (BVM) ventilation. Paramedics must continue to focus on these basic skills, despite their advanced training and techniques. It is easy to get tunnel vision when considering endotracheal intubation and other advanced procedures, yet these techniques are rarely lifesaving and are often worthless if not preceded by good basic management. As the senior member of most EMS teams, it is the responsibility of the paramedic to ensure that other providers on scene are performing optimal basic airway management. Lead by example whenever possible!

Proper Positioning

Trauma patients are often confined to the supine position as a result of spinal immobilization. However, some circumstances may warrant flexibility, if permitted by local protocols. For example, the patient with facial and airway trauma who is able to maintain his airway as long as he is sitting up may be placed in a cervical collar in a seated position rather than restricted to a supine position.

Conscious medical patients should be maintained in their position of comfort if they are not placed in cervical immobilization. Unconscious medical patients who do not require other interventions, such as BVM ventilation, should be placed on their side with the head elevated (if not contraindicated) to minimize the risk of aspiration.

Unconscious patients who do require airway and ventilation interventions, such as BVM ventilation or intubation, are usually best maintained in an **ear-to-sternal-notch position**, in which the supine patient's head is elevated to the point where the ear and the sternal notch are horizontally aligned (Figure 15-37). This position is often referred to as the **sniffing position** in non-obese patients and the

(a)

(b)

FIGURE 15-37 Airway management and ventilation is improved when the ear-to-sternal notch axis is aligned: (a) child, (b) adult.

ramped position in obese patients. With both the sniffing and ramped positions, the ear-to-sternal notch alignment is maintained. This positioning maximizes upper airway patency allowing for effective ventilation and, if required, endotracheal intubation. It also improves the mechanics of ventilation, both with spontaneous breathing and with BVM ventilation.

Sniffing Position

To place non-obese patients in the sniffing position, first achieve an ear-to-sternal notch horizontal alignment by slightly flexing the patient's neck and extending the head (assuming no cervical spine injury is suspected). This can be maintained by placing a towel or small pillow under the head (Figure 15-38).

Ramped Position

The strategy for positioning obese patients is different. It is often difficult or impossible to place them into the sniffing position by elevating just the head. Instead, you must elevate the entire upper portion of the body. This can be achieved with blankets, towels, and pillows or with a

FIGURE 15-38 The "sniffing position" provides adequate ear-to-sternal notch alignment in non-obese adults.

(© Edward T. Dickinson, MD)

FIGURE 15-39 (a) In the supine obese patient, the line from ear to sternal notch is not horizontal. (b) The "ramped position" with the upper body raised achieves horizontal ear-to-sternal notch alignment in obese patients.

commercial wedge pillow (Figure 15-39). When considering airway management in an obese patient, prepare a proper ramp (head and shoulder support) before transferring the patient. Lifting obese patients during airway management is often difficult.[11]

Oxygenation

Oxygen is an important drug, and you must thoroughly understand its indications and precautions. Providing supplemental oxygen to patients who are frankly hypoxemic will diminish the hypoxia's secondary effects on organs such as the brain and the heart and lessen subjective respiratory distress.

In some circumstances, oxygen administration is also indicated even though the patient's oxygen saturation may be normal. Keep in mind that oxygen may be carried both on hemoglobin and dissolved in the blood. Under normal circumstances, the dissolved portion of oxygen is relatively insignificant. When supplemental oxygen is administered, the dissolved portion of oxygen may increase many-fold. This relatively small amount of extra oxygen may be important to patients with tissue hypoxemia from any cause such as septic shock, myocardial infarction, cardiogenic shock, or severe trauma. Oxygen administration is also very important prior to intubation, regardless of the oxygen saturation. Finally, ill or injured pregnant patients may benefit from supplemental oxygen administration, regardless of their oxygen saturation, to enhance oxygen delivery to the fetus.

Never withhold oxygen from any patient for whom it is indicated. Caution is advised in patients with COPD, who may have developed a hypoxic drive to breathe (in which reduced oxygen levels trigger breathing), as opposed to a normal hypercarbic drive to breathe (in which breathing is triggered by chronic hypercarbia, or elevated

levels of carbon dioxide). In these patients there is a theoretical risk of depressing respirations as the body senses plentiful oxygen. This is rarely a clinical issue during all but the longest EMS transports. Thus, you should feel comfortable giving as much oxygen as necessary to maintain adequate oxygen saturations. Remember, however, that you do not necessarily need to return these patients to normal oxygen saturations, as their bodies are generally used to lower oxygen levels. Of course, you should monitor your patient closely for evidence of respiratory depression. You may also use capnography to assess for early signs of worsening hypercarbia.

As discussed earlier in this chapter, there is now evidence that high oxygen levels (hyperoxia) may be as dangerous as low levels (hypoxia) because of the possible formation of oxygen free radicals. This has been demonstrated in post-cardiac arrest patients, stroke patients, neonates, and head trauma patients. Therefore, oxygen saturation should always be maintained in the normal range, using the lowest necessary oxygen flow.

Oxygen Supply and Regulation

Oxygen is supplied either as a compressed gas or a liquid. Compressed gaseous oxygen is stored in an aluminum or steel tank in 400-liter (D), 660-liter (E), or 3,450-liter (M) volumes. To calculate how long the oxygen will last, use the appropriate formula below—the same formula but with a different constant for each type of cylinder: 0.16 for a D cylinder, 0.28 for an E cylinder, and 1.56 for an M cylinder:

D cylinder tank life in minutes = (tank pressure in psi × 0.16)
÷ liters per minute

E cylinder tank life in minutes = (tank pressure in psi × 0.28)
÷ liters per minute

M cylinder tank life in minutes = (tank pressure in psi × 1.56)
÷ liters per minute

Liquid oxygen is cooled to aqueous form and warmed back to its gaseous state for delivery. Although liquid oxygen requires less storage space than an equal amount of compressed oxygen, you must keep it upright and accommodate other special requirements for its storage and transfer.

A regulator for an oxygen tank is either a **high-pressure regulator**, which is used to transfer oxygen at high pressures from tank to tank, or a **therapy regulator**, which is used for delivering oxygen to patients. The default pressure for therapy regulators is 50 psi, which is controlled within the regulator to allow for adjustable low-flow oxygen delivery.

Oxygen Delivery Devices

Oxygen delivery to patients is measured in liters of flow per minute (L/min). A number of delivery devices are available; the patient's condition will dictate which method you use. You must continually reassess the patient who requires oxygen therapy to be certain that the method of delivery and flow rate are adequate. Some patients may require positive pressure ventilation rather than a passive delivery device.

Nasal Cannula

The **nasal cannula** is a catheter placed at the nares. It provides an optimal oxygen supplementation of up to 40 percent when set at 6 L/min flow. At flow rates above 6 L/min, the nasal mucous membranes become very dry and easily break down. Patients generally tolerate the nasal cannula well. It is indicated for low-to-moderate oxygen requirements and long-term oxygen therapy.

Venturi Mask

The **Venturi mask** is a high-flow face mask that uses a Venturi system to deliver relatively precise oxygen concentrations, regardless of the patient's rate and depth of breathing. As oxygen passes into the mask through a jet orifice in the base of the mask, it entrains room air. The device then delivers the resulting mixture to the patient. Some Venturi masks have dial selectors to control the amount of ambient air taken in; others have interchangeable caps. Either type can deliver concentrations of 24 percent, 28 percent, 35 percent, or 40 percent oxygen. The liter flow depends on the oxygen concentration desired. The Venturi mask is particularly useful for COPD patients, who benefit from careful control of inspired oxygen concentration. These masks are rarely placed by EMS providers, but you will encounter them during transfers.

CONTENT REVIEW
➤ Continually reassess the patient who requires oxygen therapy to be sure the method of delivery and flow rate are adequate.

Simple Face Mask

The simple face mask is indicated for patients requiring moderate oxygen concentrations. Side ports allow room air to enter the mask and dilute the oxygen concentration during inspiration. Flow rates generally range from about 6 to 10 L/min, providing 40 to 60 percent oxygen at the maximum rate, depending on the patient's respiratory rate and depth. Delivery of volumes beyond 10 L/min does not enhance oxygen concentration. These devices are rarely carried by EMS providers but will be encountered during transfers.

Partial Rebreather Mask

The partial rebreather mask is indicated for patients requiring moderate-to-high oxygen concentrations when satisfactory clinical results are not obtained with the simple face mask. One-way disks that cover the partial rebreather mask's side ports prevent the inspiration of room air. Minimal dilution occurs with inspiration of residual expired air along with the supplemental oxygen. Maximal flow rate is 10 L/min.

Nonrebreather Mask

The nonrebreather mask has one-way side ports as well, but also has an attached reservoir bag to hold oxygen ready to inhale. It provides the highest oxygen concentration of all oxygen delivery devices available, or about 80 percent when set at 15 L/min of oxygen and the mask is fit tightly to the face. These masks are commonly used by EMS for initial management of patients with high oxygen requirements. Any patient who requires a nonrebreather should be closely monitored for refractory hypoxemia that requires invasive or noninvasive positive pressure ventilation.

Small-Volume Nebulizer

Nebulizer chambers containing 3 to 5 mL of fluid are attached to a face mask that allows for delivery of medications in aerosol form (nebulization) that is more likely to pass through the upper airway to the lower airways. Pressurized oxygen or air enters the chamber to create a mist, which the patient then inspires. Oxygen is the usual carrier but air is occasionally used in COPD patients, and a helium–oxygen mixture may be used in patients with upper airway obstruction.

Oxygen Humidifier

You can provide humidified oxygen to the patient by attaching a sterile water reservoir to the oxygen outlet. Humidified oxygen is often given to pediatric patients with upper airway problems such as croup, although there is no evidence that it improves outcomes. Humidification is also useful for patients receiving long-term oxygen therapy to prevent the complications of drying out the mucous membranes. Humidification is rarely necessary in the EMS setting.

Positive Airway Pressure

Positive airway pressure (PAP) is delivered via a face mask to maintain a constant level of pressure within the airway, which assists a patient in breathing by preventing collapse of the airway during inhalation. **Continuous positive airway pressure (CPAP)** maintains a steady level of pressure during both inhalation and exhalation. **Bilevel positive airway pressure (BiPAP)** maintains a higher level of pressure during inhalation and a lower level of pressure during exhalation. CPAP and BiPAP devices can be used to administer oxygen in conjunction with increased airway pressures.

Manual Airway Maneuvers

Manual maneuvers are the simplest airway management techniques. They require no specialized equipment, are safe, and are noninvasive. They are highly effective but are often neglected in prehospital care.

In the patient who is unconscious or has a decreased level of consciousness, posterior displacement of the tongue is often the cause of airway obstruction. The head-tilt/chin-lift and the jaw-thrust are safe and dependable maneuvers for relieving this obstruction. You should perform one of these techniques on all unconscious patients, but do not perform them on responsive patients.

If you suspect cervical spine injury, perform the modified jaw-thrust with in-line stabilization of the cervical spine. Always follow Standard Precautions and use a mask and face shield during airway management maneuvers.

Head-Tilt/Chin-Lift

In the absence of cervical spine trauma, the head-tilt/chin-lift is the best technique for opening the airway in an unresponsive patient who is not protecting his own airway (Figure 15-40). This maneuver is potentially hazardous to patients with cervical spine injuries. To perform the head-tilt/chin-lift:

1. Place the patient supine and position yourself at the side of the patient's head.
2. Place one hand on the patient's forehead and, using firm downward pressure with your palm, tilt the head back.
3. Put two fingers of the other hand under the bony part of the chin and lift the jaw anteriorly to open the airway.

Caution: Avoid compressing the soft tissues of the neck and chin, which could cause airway obstruction.

Jaw-Thrust Maneuver without Head Extension

A jaw-thrust is acceptable for any unresponsive patient and recommended for any patient at risk for cervical spine injury who cannot protect his airway. It may be necessary to remove the cervical collar to advance the jaw sufficiently to open the airway; however, the provider performing the jaw-thrust is usually able to maintain manual in-line immobilization simultaneously. To perform the jaw-thrust:

- Lift the jaw using fingers behind the mandibular angles; do not tilt the head (Figure 15-41). It usually helps to prop the thumbs on the cheekbones to provide some counterforce.

Although they are simple and effective, none of these manual airway maneuvers protects the airway from aspiration. Additionally, the jaw-thrust is difficult to maintain for an extended time. Placing an oral and/or nasopharyngeal airway, if tolerated and not contraindicated, may open the airway sufficiently that a strong jaw-thrust is no longer required until the airway can be more definitively managed.

FIGURE 15-40 Head-tilt/chin-lift maneuver.

FIGURE 15-41 Modified jaw-thrust without head extension in trauma.

Basic Airway Adjuncts

CONTENT REVIEW

➤ Always attempt any appropriate manual maneuvers before placing a mechanical airway.

In the absence of trauma, secretions, foreign bodies, and edema, basic manual airway maneuvers should succeed in clearing the tongue from the air passages. However, the tongue often falls back, subsequently, to block the airway again. Two available airway adjuncts, the nasopharyngeal airway and the oropharyngeal airway, prevent this. These adjuncts cannot replace good head positioning, but they do help to lift the base of the tongue forward and away from the posterior oropharynx, establishing and maintaining a patent airway.

Nasopharyngeal Airway

The **nasopharyngeal airway (NPA)**, or "nasal trumpet," is an uncuffed tube made of soft rubber or plastic. The nasopharyngeal airway follows the natural curvature of the nasopharynx, passing through the nose and extending from the nostril to the posterior pharynx just below the base of the tongue. It varies from 17 to 20 cm in length, and its diameter ranges from 20 to 36 Fr (**French**). A funnel-shaped projection at its proximal end helps prevent the tube from slipping inside a patient's nose and becoming lost or aspirated. The distal end is beveled to facilitate passage. Nasopharyngeal airways are generally underutilized. They are well tolerated in most patients and are very effective at maintaining the airway. Specific indications for the use of the nasopharyngeal airway include obtunded patients (those with reduced mental acuity, with or without a suppressed gag reflex) and unconscious patients. If the patient does not tolerate the nasopharyngeal airway, you should remove it.

Advantages of the Nasopharyngeal Airway

- It can be rapidly inserted and safely placed blindly.
- It bypasses the tongue, providing a patent airway.
- You may use it in the presence of a gag reflex.
- You may use it when the patient has suffered injury to his oral cavity.
- You may suction through it.
- You may use it when the patient's teeth are clenched.

Disadvantages of the Nasopharyngeal Airway

- It is smaller than the oropharyngeal airway.
- It does not isolate the trachea.
- It is difficult to suction through.
- It may cause severe nosebleeds if inserted too forcefully.
- It may cause pressure necrosis of the nasal mucosa.

FIGURE 15-42 Nasopharyngeal airway.

- It may kink and clog, obstructing the airway.
- Inserting it is difficult if nasal damage (old or new) is present.
- You may not use it if the patient has or is suspected to have a basilar skull fracture, as the tube could inadvertently pass into the cranium.

The properly sized nasopharyngeal tube is slightly smaller in diameter than the patient's nostril, and in adults it is equal to or slightly longer than the distance from the patient's nose to his earlobe. Selecting the appropriate size is important. Too small a tube will not extend past the tongue; too long a tube may pass into the esophagus and result in hypoventilation of the lungs and distention of the stomach when positive pressure is applied (Figures 15-42 and 15-43).

Inserting the Nasopharyngeal Airway

To insert a nasopharyngeal airway:

1. Ensure or maintain effective ventilation with supplemental oxygen.

FIGURE 15-43 Nasopharyngeal airway, inserted.

2. Lubricate the exterior of the tube with a water-soluble gel to decrease trauma during insertion. Lidocaine gel may be used to increase tolerance of the device after insertion.

3. Select the naris that appears largest. Push gently up on the tip of the nose and pass the tube gently into the nostril with the bevel oriented toward the septum and the airway directed straight back along the nasal floor, parallel to the mouth. Avoid pushing against any resistance, because this may cause tissue trauma and airway kinking.

4. Verify the appropriate position of the airway. Resolution of noisy breathing and improved compliance during BVM ventilation support correct positioning. Also, feel at the airway's proximal end for airflow on expiration.

5. Provide supplemental oxygen and/or ventilate the patient as indicated.

Oropharyngeal Airway

The **oropharyngeal airway (OPA)** is a noninvasive semicircular plastic or rubber device designed to follow the palate's curvature. It holds the base of the tongue away from the posterior oropharynx, thus preventing it from obstructing the glottis. Its use is indicated in patients with no gag reflex.

Advantages of the Oropharyngeal Airway

- It is easy to place using proper technique.
- Air can pass around and through the device.
- It helps prevent obstruction by the teeth and lips.
- It helps manage profoundly unconscious patients who are breathing spontaneously or need mechanical ventilation.
- It makes suction of the pharynx easier, as a large suction catheter can pass on either side of the device.
- It serves as an effective bite block in case of seizures or to protect the endotracheal tube.

Disadvantages of the Oropharyngeal Airway

- It does not isolate the trachea or prevent aspiration.
- It cannot be inserted when the teeth are clenched.
- It may obstruct the airway if not inserted properly.
- It is easily dislodged.
- Return of the gag reflex may produce vomiting.

Do not use an oropharyngeal airway in conscious or semiconscious patients who have a gag reflex, because it may cause vomiting (by stimulating the posterior tongue gag reflexes) or laryngospasm. As is often said, "If a patient tolerates an oral airway, then he needs an oral airway." The converse is also true: If a patient resists placement of the airway, then his gag reflex is intact and an oral airway is not indicated.

Oropharyngeal airways are available in sizes ranging from #0 (for neonates) to #6 (for large adults). Selecting the proper size is important. If the airway is too long, it can press the epiglottis against the entrance of the larynx, resulting in airway obstruction. If it is too small, it will not adequately hold the tongue forward. To measure for the appropriate oropharyngeal airway, place the flange beside the patient's cheek, parallel to the front of the teeth (Figure 15-44). A properly sized airway will extend from the patient's mouth to the angle of his jaw (Figure 15-45).

Inserting the Oropharyngeal Airway

To insert the oropharyngeal airway:

1. Open the mouth and remove any visible obstructions.

2. Ensure or maintain effective ventilation with supplemental oxygen.

3. Grasp the patient's jaw and lift anteriorly.

4. With your other hand, hold the airway device at its proximal end and insert it into the patient's mouth. Make sure the curve is reversed, with the tip pointing toward the roof of the mouth.

5. Once the tip reaches the level of the soft palate, gently rotate the airway 180° until it comes to rest over the tongue.

FIGURE 15-44A Insert the oropharyngeal airway with the tip facing the palate.

FIGURE 15-44B Rotate the airway 180° into position.

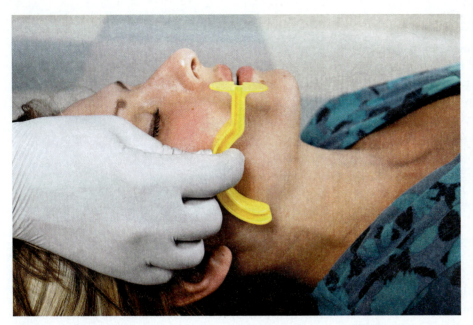

FIGURE 15-45 Measure the oropharyngeal airway externally to ensure proper sizing.

6. Verify appropriate position of the airway. Clear breath sounds and chest rise indicate correct placement.

7. Apply supplemental oxygen and/or positive pressure ventilation if indicated.

An alternative insertion method useful in both pediatric and adult patients is to press the tongue upward and forward with a tongue blade. Then, the airway can be advanced until the flange is seated at the teeth. This is the preferred method of airway insertion in infants and children.

Oral and/or nasal airways should be considered in all obtunded older pediatric and adult patients and are mandatory whenever the patient has signs of airway obstruction ("noisy breathing is obstructed breathing") or BVM ventilation is difficult. These airways may also be used in combination, such as two nasal airways, one nasal and one oral, or even two nasal and one oral airway in extreme circumstances.

Ventilation

Many of your cases in the field will call for ventilatory support. These situations range from apneic (nonbreathing) patients to less obvious instances when patients are experiencing depressed respiratory function. Remember that an unconscious patient's respiratory center may not function adequately. A significant decrease in the patient's rate or depth of breathing will lead to decreased respiratory minute volume with subsequent hypercarbia and respiratory acidosis. This will result in further decreases in mental status, creating a vicious cycle. Hypoxemia may also result if the decrease in breathing is significant or oxygen demand is substantial. Acidosis and/or hypoxemia may eventually lead to respiratory or cardiac arrest.

Effective ventilatory support requires a tidal volume of 6 to 8 mL/kg of ideal body weight at a rate of 12 breaths per minute. Note that these volumes are significantly less than the 10 to 15 mL/kg that was formerly recommended.

When providing ventilatory support, you must generate enough force to overcome the elastic resistance of the lungs and chest wall, as well as the frictional resistance in the respiratory passageways, without overinflating the lungs. This is similar to blowing up a balloon; you must overcome the balloon's resistance in order to inflate it.

Keep in mind that air will travel the path of least resistance. If you do not maintain a tight seal between the ventilation mask and your patient's face, air will flow out of the gaps rather than through the respiratory passageways. If you do not keep the airway maximally open with proper manual positioning and use of airway adjuncts to facilitate an open passage into the trachea, the airway pressure generated with PPV can open the esophagus and allow air to flow into the stomach. Therefore, effective artificial ventilation requires a patent airway, an effective seal between the mask and the patient's face, and delivery of appropriate ventilatory volumes directed into the lungs and not into the stomach. Exercise care when you attempt to generate enough pressure to ventilate the lungs. Too much pressure may lead to gastric distention and regurgitation. Also, be certain that you allow the patient to exhale between delivered breaths.

Mouth-to-Mouth/ Mouth-to-Nose Ventilation

Mouth-to-mouth and mouth-to-nose ventilation are the most basic methods of rescue ventilation, but their use is limited by exposure to body fluids and by limited oxygen delivery, as expired air contains only 17 percent oxygen. These methods are indicated only in the presence of apnea when no other ventilation devices are available. When using one of these methods, take care not to hyperinflate the patient's lungs nor to hyperventilate yourself.

CONTENT REVIEW

▶ Remember that an unconscious patient's respiratory center may not function adequately.

Mouth-to-Mask Ventilation

The pocket mask is a clear plastic device with a one-way valve that you place over an apneic patient's mouth and nose. It prevents direct contact between you and your patient's mouth and expired air, thus reducing the risk of contamination and subsequent infection. A pocket mask also has an inlet for supplemental oxygen. Mouth-to-mask ventilation combined with an oxygen flow rate of 10 L/min can deliver an inspired oxygen concentration of approximately 50 percent. However, pocket masks are much less effective than bag-valve-mask devices and are very tiring for the rescuer.

To perform the mouth-to-mask technique, position the head to open the airway by one of the previously discussed methods (head-tilt/chin-lift or jaw-thrust), position the mask to obtain a good seal, and provide adequate ventilatory volumes. As with mouth-to-mouth and mouth-to-nose methods, hyperinflation of the patient's lungs, gastric distention in the patient, and hyperventilation in the rescuer are potential complications.

Bag-Valve-Mask Ventilation

The first technique employed for most patients who are not breathing or not breathing adequately is **bag-valve-mask (BVM)** ventilation with a self-inflating bag and reservoir attached to high-concentration oxygen. Many patients may be entirely managed with BVM ventilation whereas, in other cases, it is a bridge to more invasive techniques. BVM ventilation is one of the most important and challenging EMS skills and must be mastered. Even though the paramedic may need to delegate BVM ventilation to other providers, the paramedic is still responsible for ensuring good technique.

The BVM consists of an oblong, self-inflating silicone or rubber bag with two one-way valves (an air/oxygen-inlet valve and a patient valve), a detachable transparent plastic face mask, and an oxygen reservoir. Both the bags and the masks come in variable sizes to fit patients from neonates to large adults. The valve must be open for oxygen to flow to the patient. Some devices have a built-in colorimetric end-tidal CO_2 detector (Figure 15-46) or positive-pressure valves. Because of the risk of transmitting infectious diseases, BVMs should be disposable. Do not reuse them.

Some BVM devices have a pop-off valve to limit the risk of lung injury from overaggressive ventilation. However, some patients with high airway resistance and/or poor lung compliance require high pressures for ventilation, so a mechanism to override the pop-off valve is essential.

Another variety of BVM bag is the anesthesia bag, more commonly called a *flow-inflating bag*, which does not self-inflate but instead relies on an adequate flow of oxygen. Oxygen flow into the bag and flow out of the bag may

FIGURE 15-46 Bag-valve-mask unit.

be adjusted to maintain appropriate volumes in the bag so the bag is neither overinflated nor subject to collapsing entirely with each ventilation. Because they are more complicated to use, flow-inflating-bag devices are rarely used in EMS except in critical care transport of neonates and infants.

Any patient who requires assisted ventilation needs supplemental oxygen, so high-flow oxygen (10 to 15 L/min) should always be used. Because of the attached reservoir, a bag-valve device can deliver 90 to 95 percent oxygen with these flow rates and a tight mask seal.

One, two, or three rescuers may perform BVM ventilation. One-person BVM ventilation is the most difficult method to master, because obtaining and maintaining the mask seal while simultaneously delivering ventilations can be challenging, especially if there are secretions, facial hair, or the need for high airway pressures, and/or the rescuer has small hands. Therefore, BVM ventilation should generally be performed with at least two providers, one to squeeze the bag and one to open the airway and maintain the mask seal.

Observe the patient for chest rise, development of gastric distention, and changes in compliance of the bag with ventilation. Complications of BVM ventilation include inadequate volume delivery if there is a poor mask seal or improper technique, barotrauma from overinflation of the lungs, and gastric distention.

Cricoid Pressure

Posterior pressure on the cricoid cartilage is referred to as cricoid pressure. Because the cricoid ring is the only complete ring in the trachea, posterior pressure on the front of the ring will be transmitted to the back of the ring and will hopefully compress the esophagus between the back of the cricoid ring and the front of the spinal column.

This maneuver became popular with the advent of **rapid sequence intubation (RSI)** as a means to limit regurgitation and subsequent aspiration. (RSI is discussed in detail later in this chapter.) Recent evidence suggests that the risk-to-benefit ratio may not actually favor cricoid pressure during intubation, because cricoid pressure applied correctly to compress the esophagus often obscures the intubator's view of the larynx. Additionally, the esophagus does not always lie directly behind the cricoid ring, and the pressure itself causes a reflex decrease in lower-esophageal sphincter tone (actually working against the intended aspiration-sparing effect).

Cricoid pressure use during BVM ventilation specifically (and not as a technique to improve laryngoscopic view), may still be of some benefit according to clinical research despite the skill falling into disfavor.[12] Due to this conflict on the efficacy of the skill, in any instance where cricoid pressure may attempted, the paramedic should ensure the skill is still approved by protocol, or at very least, approved by online medical direction.

Since cricoid pressure may still be used by some providers under specific criteria, the skill to do so properly will now be discussed. To locate the cricoid cartilage, first palpate the thyroid cartilage and feel the depression just below it (cricothyroid membrane). The prominence inferior to this depression is the cricoid ring. Apply firm downward pressure to the anterolateral aspect of the cartilage, using the thumb, index, and middle finger of one hand.

Use caution not to apply so much pressure as to deform and possibly obstruct the trachea; this is a particular danger in infants. The necessary pressure has been estimated as the amount of force that will compress a capped 50-mL syringe from 50 mL to the 30 mL marking. In the event that the patient actively vomits, it is imperative to release the pressure to avoid esophageal rupture.

Optimal BVM Ventilation Using the Rule of Threes

The *rule of threes* was developed to help providers recall the components of optimal BVM ventilation. Many patients can be easily oxygenated and ventilated without using all components of the rule of threes. Whenever BVM ventilation is difficult, however, the rule of threes should be employed.

- *Three providers.* One provider on the mask, one on the bag, and one for external laryngeal manipulation.
- *Three inches.* A reminder to place the patient in the sniffing position (elevate the head three inches) if not contraindicated.
- *Three fingers.* Three fingers on the larynx to perform external laryngeal manipulation (Figure 15-47).
- *Three airways.* In a worst-case scenario, the airway can be maintained, if necessary, with an oropharyngeal airway and two nasopharyngeal airways (one in each nostril).
- *Three PSI.* A gentle reminder to use the lowest pressure necessary to see the chest rise.
- *Three seconds.* A reminder to ventilate slowly and allow time for adequate exhalation.
- *Three PEEP.* Or up to 15 cm/H_2O positive-end expiratory pressure (PEEP) as needed to improve oxygen saturations.

Bag-Valve Ventilation of the Pediatric Patient

The differences in the pediatric patient's anatomy require some variation in ventilation technique. First, the child's relatively flat nasal bridge makes achieving a mask seal more difficult. Pressing the mask against the child's face to improve the seal can actually obstruct the airway, which is more compressible than an adult's. You can best achieve the mask seal with the two-person BVM technique, using a jaw-thrust to maintain an open airway.

For BVM ventilation, the bag size depends on the child's age. Full-term neonates and infants will require a pediatric BVM with a capacity of at least 450 mL. For children up to 8 years of age, the pediatric BVM is preferred, although for patients in the upper portion of that age range you can use an adult BVM with a capacity of 1,500 mL if you do not maximally inflate it. Children older than 8 years require an adult BVM to achieve adequate tidal volumes. Additionally, be

> **CONTENT REVIEW**
> ➤ The Rule of Threes for Optimal BVM Ventilation
> - Three providers
> - Three inches
> - Three fingers
> - Three airways
> - Three PSI
> - Three PEEP

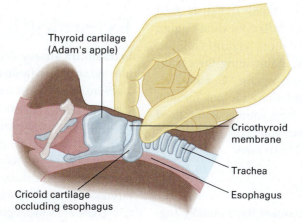

Thyroid cartilage (Adam's apple)
Cricothyroid membrane
Trachea
Esophagus
Cricoid cartilage occluding esophagus

FIGURE 15-47 External laryngeal manipulation.

FIGURE 15-48 Demand valve and mask.

certain that the mask fits properly, from the bridge of the nose to the cleft of the chin. If a length-based resuscitation tape (Broselow tape) is available, you can use it to help determine the proper mask size.

To achieve a proper mask seal, place the mask over the patient's mouth and nose. Avoid compressing the eyes. Using one hand, place your thumb on the mask at the apex and your index finger on the mask at the chin (C-grip). Apply gentle pressure downward on the mask to establish an adequate seal. Maintain the airway by lifting the bony prominence of the chin with the remaining fingers forming an *E* under the jaw. Avoid placing pressure on the soft area under the chin. You may use the one-rescuer technique, although the two-rescuer technique will be more effective.

Ventilate according to current standards, obtaining chest rise with each breath. Begin the ventilation and say, "squeeze," providing just enough volume to initiate chest rise—being very careful not to overinflate the child's lungs. Allow adequate time for exhalation, saying, "release, release." Continue ventilations, maintaining the correct timing by saying, "squeeze, release, release." Use three criteria to assess adequacy of ventilations: (1) look for adequate chest rise; (2) listen for lung sounds at the third intercostal space, midaxillary line; and (3) assess for clinical improvement (skin color and heart rate).

Demand-Valve Device

The **demand-valve device**, also called the manually triggered, oxygen-powered ventilation device or flow-restricted,

oxygen-powered ventilation device, will deliver 100 percent oxygen to a patient at its highest flow rates (40 liters per minute maximum). Flow is restricted to 30 cm H_2O or less to diminish gastric distention that can occur with its use (Figure 15-48). Demand-valve devices have fallen out of favor because of the risks of gastric distension and barotrauma in unconscious patients.

PART 3: Advanced Airway Management and Ventilation

Advanced airway management has historically meant just endotracheal intubation and surgical airways (which will be discussed later in the chapter). Now, however, advanced airway management includes placement of other invasive airways that do not pass through the vocal cords, such as extraglottic airways.[13–16]

Extraglottic Airway Devices

Extraglottic airway (EGA) devices are inserted blindly into the airway to facilitate oxygenation and ventilation via a self-inflating bag or transport ventilator, but do not enter the glottis (the space between the vocal cords). Hence the term *extraglottic*, meaning "outside the glottis." Because EGAs do not enter the glottis, these devices do not require the use of a laryngoscope to visualize the glottic opening, although some of them permit it. Their insertion without laryngoscopy is described as "blind."

There are subcategories of EGAs, depending on where they actually "sit." Some sit in the esophagus, which places them behind the vocal cords (**retroglottic airways**); others sit above the vocal cords (**supraglottic airways**).[17]

An EGA may be used as a primary or secondary device depending on the provider's scope of practice and protocols and the clinical scenario. Use as a primary device means immediate use of the EGA without first trying to achieve endotracheal intubation; secondary use means use of the EGA only after an attempt at endotracheal intubation has failed. Accumulating evidence and experience suggest that EGAs are faster and easier to insert than endotracheal tubes and may be associated with fewer complications. It is very likely that these devices will play a growing role in prehospital airway management.

Retroglottic Airway Devices: Dual Lumen

Dual-lumen devices are designed to be inserted blindly into the esophagus but may still be used in the event of fortuitous tracheal placement. Clinical assessment is required to be sure that the correct port is used for ventilation. EGAs in this category include the Esophageal Tracheal Combitube™ (ETC) and the Pharyngeal Tracheal Lumen Airway™ (PTL).

Esophageal Tracheal Combitube (ETC™)

The Esophageal Tracheal Combitube (ETC™), also called simply the *Combitube™*, is a dual-lumen retroglottic airway available in two sizes for patients over 4 feet tall. The ETC is inserted blindly through the mouth into the posterior oropharynx and then gently advanced—although directed esophageal placement using a laryngoscope is often employed in the operating room and may be employed by EMS providers if it is within their scope of practice. The tube may enter either the trachea or the esophagus (Figures 15-49 and 15-50), but esophageal placement is most common. Because placement is nearly always esophageal, the port that ventilates in this position is longer, numbered 1, and is blue.[18–19]

Advantages of the ETC

- Insertion is rapid and highly successful.
- It is time tested.
- Insertion does not require visualization.
- It will provide ventilation with either esophageal or tracheal placement.
- The large pharyngeal balloon may tamponade oral bleeding.
- It will generate high airway pressures for ventilation when necessary.
- It offers reasonable aspiration protection in either the esophageal or tracheal position.

FIGURE 15-49 The Esophageal Tracheal Combitube (ETC) is a dual-lumen airway with a ventilation port for each lumen. The longer, blue port (#1) is the proximal port; the shorter, clear port (#2) is the distal port, which opens at the distal end of the tube. The ETC has two inflatable cuffs—a 100-mL cuff just proximal to the distal port and a 15-mL cuff just distal to the proximal port. First, ventilate through the longer, blue port (#1). Ventilation will be successful if the tube has been placed (as is most common) in the esophagus.

FIGURE 15-50 If ventilation through tube #1 is not successful, then ventilate through the shorter clear tube (#2). Ventilation will be successful if the tube has been placed in the trachea.

- In the esophageal position, gastric decompression is possible through the #2 port.
- When intubating around the ETC, the proximal balloon may be deflated and the distal balloon left inflated to seal off the esophagus.

Disadvantages of the ETC

- Trauma, including esophageal perforation, has been reported.
- It cannot be placed in patients with an intact gag reflex.
- High cuff volumes may result in tissue ischemia.
- It cannot be placed in patients under 4 feet tall.
- Clinical assessment is necessary to ensure ventilation through the correct port.
- It does not completely isolate the trachea in the esophageal position.
- Placement is not 100 percent foolproof.

Inserting the ETC

To place the ETC:

1. Perform optimal BVM ventilation with high-concentration oxygen.
2. Place the patient supine in a neutral position if possible.
3. Prepare and check equipment. Select a *Regular size* for patients 6 feet tall or taller. Select a *Small-Adult size* for patients less than 6 feet tall. Note that this sizing instruction is evidence based but is different from the manufacturer's instructions.
4. Stabilize the cervical spine if cervical injury is possible.
5. Perform the **Lipp maneuver** (or modified Lipp maneuver) to preshape the ETC (Figure 15-51).
6. Grab and lift the jaw or, if within your scope of practice, use a laryngoscope to create a channel and visualize the esophagus. Insert the ETC gently in midline and advance it past the hypopharynx to the depth indicated by the markings on the tube. The black rings on the tube should be between the patient's teeth.

7. Inflate the pharyngeal cuff with 100 mL of air and the distal cuff with 10 to 15 mL of air.
8. Ventilate through the longer, blue, #1, proximal port with a bag-valve device connected to 100 percent oxygen, while auscultating over the chest and stomach. If you hear bilateral breath sounds over the chest and none over the stomach (indicating that the device is sitting in and occluding the esophagus while directing oxygen flow into the trachea), secure the tube and continue ventilating.
9. If you hear gastric sounds over the epigastrium and no breath sounds (indicating that the device is sitting in and occluding the trachea while directing oxygen flow into the esophagus), change ports and ventilate through the clear, shorter, #2, distal port to direct oxygen into the trachea. Confirm breath sounds over the chest with absent gastric sounds.
10. Use multiple confirmation techniques. End-tidal CO_2 is reliable with an ETC as long as the patient is producing CO_2. An esophageal detector device (EDD) may be used on an ETC by attaching it to the #2 port that is open on the distal end. Note that failure to inflate indicates appropriate esophageal positioning and you should continue ventilation through the #1 port. This is somewhat backward compared to using an EDD to confirm endotracheal intubation. (The EDD will be explained in detail later.)
11. Secure the tube and continue ventilating with 100 percent oxygen.
12. Frequently reassess the airway and adequacy of ventilation.

(a)

(b)

FIGURE 15-51 Lipp maneuver. (a) The Lipp maneuver and (b) the modified Lipp maneuver will aid in ETC placement and will help to minimize associated trauma to the airway.

Pharyngeo-Tracheal Lumen Airway (PtL™)

The Pharyngeo-Tracheal Lumen Airway (PtL™) is a two-tube system (Figure 15-52). The first tube is short, with a large diameter; its proximal end is green. A large cuff encircles the tube's lower third. When inflated, the cuff seals the entire oropharynx. Air introduced at this tube's proximal end will enter the hypopharynx. The second tube is long, with a small diameter, and clear. It passes through and extends approximately 10 cm beyond the first tube. This second tube may be inserted blindly into either the trachea or the esophagus. A distal cuff, when inflated, seals off whichever anatomical structure the tube has entered. When the second tube enters the trachea, you will ventilate the patient through it.

Each of the PtL's tubes has a 15/22-mm connector at its proximal end, allowing the attachment of a standard ventilatory device. A semirigid plastic stylet in the clear plastic tube allows redirection of the oropharyngeal cuff while the other cuff remains inflated. An adjustable cloth neck strap holds the tube in place. When the long, clear tube is in the esophagus, deflating the cuff in the oropharynx allows you to move the device to the left side of the patient's mouth. This may permit endotracheal intubation while continuing esophageal occlusion. However, placement of an endotracheal tube with a PtL already in place is difficult at best.

Advantages of the PtL

- It can function in either the tracheal or esophageal position.
- It has no face mask to seal.

FIGURE 15-52 Pharyngo-tracheal lumen (PtL) airway.

- It does not require direct visualization of the larynx and, thus, does not require the use of a laryngoscope or additional specialized equipment.
- It can be used in trauma patients, as the neck can remain in neutral position during insertion and use.
- It helps protect the trachea from upper airway bleeding and secretions.

Disadvantages of the PtL

- It does not isolate and completely protect the trachea from aspiration.
- The oropharyngeal balloon can migrate out of the mouth anteriorly, partially dislodging the airway.
- Intubation around the PtL is extremely difficult, even with the oropharyngeal balloon deflated.
- It cannot be used in conscious patients or those with a gag reflex.
- It cannot be used in pediatric patients.
- It can only be passed orally.

Inserting the PtL

To insert the pharyngeo-tracheal lumen airway:

1. Complete basic manual and adjunctive maneuvers and provide supplemental oxygen and ventilatory support with a BVM and hyperventilation.
2. Place the patient supine and kneel at the top of his head.
3. Prepare and check the equipment.
4. Place the patient's head in the appropriate position. Hyperextend the neck if there is no risk of cervical spine injury. Maintain neutral position with stabilization of the cervical spine if cervical spine injury is possible.
5. Insert the PtL gently, using the tongue-jaw-lift maneuver.
6. Inflate the distal cuffs on both PtL tubes simultaneously with a sustained breath into the inflation valve.
7. Deliver a breath into the green oropharyngeal tube. If the patient's chest rises and you auscultate bilateral breath sounds, the long clear tube is in the esophagus. Inflate the pharyngeal balloon and continue ventilations via the green tube.
8. If the chest does not rise and you auscultate no breath sounds, the long clear tube is in the trachea. Remove the stylet from the clear tube and ventilate the patient through that tube.
9. Attach the bag-valve device to the 15-mm connector, secure the tube, and continue ventilatory support with 100 percent oxygen.
10. Multiple placement confirmation techniques are again essential, as are good assessment skills. Misidentification of placement has been reported. Frequently reassess the airway and adequacy of ventilation.

If the patient regains consciousness or if the protective airway reflexes return, remove the PtL. It is best to remove the PtL before endotracheal intubation.

Complications of PtL placement include the following:

- Pharyngeal or esophageal trauma from poor technique
- Unrecognized displacement of the long tube from the trachea into the esophagus
- Displacement of the pharyngeal balloon

Retroglottic Airway Devices: Single Lumen

King LT™ Airway

The King LT™ Airway is an airway with a large silicone cuff that disperses pressure over a large mucosal surface area (Figure 15-53). This serves to stabilize the airway at the base of the tongue, thus minimizing the risk of injury to the vocal cords and trachea. The King LT airway allows up to 30 cm H_2O ventilation pressures. It is supplied in three sizes: one for adults less than 61 inches (5 feet, 1 inch) in height, one for adults taller than 61 inches but less than 71 inches (5 feet, 11 inches) in height, and one for adults taller than 71 inches. The device can be cleaned, sterilized, and reused. A disposable latex-free version (King LT-D™) is also available.[20–22]

The King LT-D is a disposable single-lumen retroglottic airway available in three adult and two pediatric sizes. (The "D" in LT-D means "disposable.") The adult sizes are also available in a King LTS-D model that has a channel to facilitate gastric decompression. The King has a large pharyngeal balloon and smaller esophageal balloon like other

retroglottic airways, but both balloons are inflated through a single port with a single syringe. The King is able to generate significant airway pressures when needed and offers substantial aspiration reduction.

Esophageal Obturator Airway (EOA®) and Esophageal Gastric Tube Airway (EGTA®)

These devices were among the first extraglottic airways introduced. The Esophageal Obturator Airway (EOA®) is a hollow, closed-ended tube with air holes at the level of the hypopharynx for ventilation, a distal cuff intended to block air from the esophagus, and a proximal end that fits into a mask. Ventilation, therefore, requires creation of a tight mask seal rather than relying on a large pharyngeal balloon. The Esophageal Gastric Tube Airway (EGTA®) adds the ability to place a gastric tube through the distal port into the stomach for decompression of contents. These devices are now obsolete, because superior extraglottic airways have subsequently been introduced, although they still may be found in some areas.

Supraglottic Airway Devices

A number of supraglottic airway devices have been introduced, including the S.A.L.T. and various LMA devices.

Supraglottic Airway Laryngopharyngeal Tube (S.A.L.T.®)

The Supraglottic Airway Laryngopharyngeal Tube™ (S.A.L.T.®) is an extraglottic airway. It contains a central tube with a fenestrated (with an opening) end that overlies the larynx in the laryngopharynx (Figure 15-54). It can serve two purposes. First, it can be used as a simple mechanical airway adjunct—much like an oropharyngeal airway. It has a collar on the proximal end and can be used with a BVM device. Alternatively, the S.A.L.T. can be used as a blind endotracheal tube introducer when laryngoscopy is difficult or impossible.[23]

FIGURE 15-53 King LT Airway.

(© Edward T. Dickinson, MD)

FIGURE 15-54 S.A.L.T.® Airway.

Laryngeal Airways

Laryngeal airways are supraglottic airways. They are available in a variety of specific types, including the original LMA, the LMA Supreme™, the LMA Fastrach™, the CookGas air-Q™, and the Ambu Laryngeal Mask.

Laryngeal Mask Airway (LMA™)

The laryngeal mask airway (LMA™) was the first laryngeal airway (Figure 15-55). As this device is now off patent, there are multiple similar devices on the market. The LMA is commonly used in the operating room (OR) setting for selected cases. EMS use was becoming widespread when this was the only supraglottic airway available. Even though the original LMA is easily inserted, EMS use of it is now limited because the LMA does not offer the features available in other, more recently introduced extraglottic devices.[24–26]

LMA Supreme™

The LMA Supreme™ is an updated version of the LMA. The LMA Supreme has several features that are very appealing for EMS use. The Supreme has a rigid design that makes for easy insertion without the need to place fingers in the mouth. The Supreme offers a very good seal against aspiration and facilitates gastric decompression through a separate channel. The Supreme can also generate high airway pressures when necessary to ventilate an obese patient or a patient with lung disease. Additionally, the Supreme has a built-in bite block and a fixation tab that makes it easy to secure the device with a single strip of tape

FIGURE 15-56 LMA Supreme airway.

(Figure 15-56). The primary disadvantages of the Supreme are that the decompression channel will not accommodate a gastric tube larger than 14 Fr, and blind intubation through the device is not possible.

LMA Fastrach

The LMA Fastrach™ was the first intubating laryngeal airway designed to facilitate blind endotracheal intubation with a special tube or a regular tube reverse loaded (i.e., with the curvature of the tube opposite to the curve of the device) (Figure 15-57). The Fastrach is a rigid, anatomically curved airway tube that is wide enough to accept an 8.0-mm cuffed endotracheal tube (ETT) and is short enough to ensure passage of the ETT cuff beyond the vocal cords. It has a rigid handle to facilitate insertion and adjustment of the device's position to enhance oxygenation and alignment with the glottis. There is an epiglottic elevating bar in the mask aperture that elevates the epiglottis as the ETT is passed through and a ramp that directs the tube centrally and anteriorly to reduce the risk of arytenoid trauma or esophageal placement. The Fastrach has been shown to

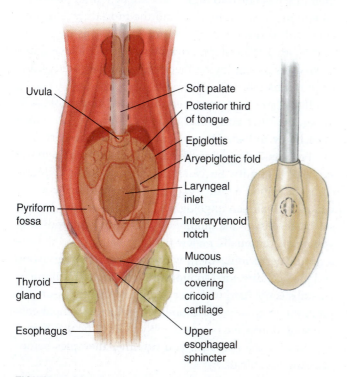

- Uvula
- Soft palate
- Posterior third of tongue
- Epiglottis
- Aryepiglottic fold
- Laryngeal inlet
- Pyriform fossa
- Interarytenoid notch
- Mucous membrane covering cricoid cartilage
- Thyroid gland
- Esophagus
- Upper esophageal sphincter

FIGURE 15-55 Laryngeal mask airway (LMA).

FIGURE 15-57 LMA Fastrach intubating laryngeal mask airway (LMA).

FIGURE 15-58 CookGas air-Q airway

(© Dr. Bryan E. Bledsoe)

FIGURE 15-59 Ambu® laryngeal mask.

have an excellent seal to protect against aspiration and generate high airway pressures when necessary. Extensive studies in the operating suite setting have demonstrated extremely high success rates with minimal training, even in obese patients and those with spinal precautions. Disadvantages include the inability to decompress the stomach, absence of sizes for patients less than 30 kg ideal body weight, and somewhat temperamental positioning for sustained bag-valve-device ventilation.

CookGas air-Q®

The air-Q® is another intubating laryngeal airway (Figure 15-58). In contrast to the Fastrach, the air-Q is available in pediatric sizes and looks much more like a traditional laryngeal airway. This shape allows intubation to be performed with an endotracheal tube introducer as well as with direct tube placement. The major disadvantages of the air-Q include the inability to decompress the stomach and the absence of literature validating the seal and success rates with blind intubation.

Ambu® Laryngeal Mask

The Ambu® laryngeal mask is a supraglottic, single-use, disposable airway (Figure 15-59). It features a special curve that replicates the natural human airway anatomy. This curve is molded directly into the tube so that insertion is easy, without abrading the upper airway. The curve ensures that the patient's head remains in a neutral position when the mask is in use.

Legal Considerations

Have a Backup. Every EMS system should have at least one backup mechanical airway device in the event endotracheal intubation fails. You must be familiar and proficient with any backup airway device used in your system.

Endotracheal Intubation

Endotracheal intubation involves inserting an endotracheal tube into the trachea, usually with direct visualization of the vocal cords—typically via direct laryngoscopy.

Endotracheal intubation provides optimal aspiration protection and ventilation, but it comes at a high cost. These costs include prolonged scene times, potential airway trauma, and potential hypoxemia and aspiration. Furthermore, with this method you are bypassing important physiologic functions of the upper airway: warming, filtering, and humidifying the air before it enters the lower airway. As already noted, many extraglottic airways now provide excellent ventilation and significant aspiration protection with the benefit of much faster, easier, and less traumatic insertion. Because the majority of literature has failed to find a survival benefit to prehospital endotracheal intubation, and the procedure is associated with serious potential complications, as discussed next, many EMS systems are moving entirely to extraglottic airways or employing them earlier in the event of difficult intubation.[27–30]

If you are performing endotracheal intubation, it is imperative that you select patients carefully (i.e., those most likely to benefit), perform the procedure correctly, practice regularly, and move early to a backup plan in the event of difficulty. Successfully accomplishing endotracheal intubation requires extensive training. Furthermore, you must maintain ongoing proficiency to ensure patient safety. To ensure the quality of your judgment and skill, you must continually review field intubations and the criteria for performing them with your peers, supervisors, and medical director. Monitoring success rates for particular skills is not hard with an appropriate quality assurance program. Evaluating your ability to judge which patients you should intubate is considerably more difficult. Often it is better for the patient if you try other therapies before deciding to intubate.[31–33]

Oral Endotracheal Intubation Indications—Non–Medication-Assisted

Oral endotracheal intubation (OETI) is generally restricted to patients in cardiac or respiratory arrest or to patients in extreme respiratory failure, which will allow such an invasive procedure to be performed. Intubation is particularly helpful in patients with anticipated airway swelling that may potentially go on to occlude the airway, such as anaphylaxis and airway burns.

Advantages of Endotracheal Intubation

- It isolates the trachea and permits complete control of the airway.
- It impedes gastric distention by channeling air directly into the trachea.
- It eliminates the need to maintain a mask seal.
- It offers a direct route for suctioning of the respiratory passages.
- It permits administration of the medications **l**idocaine, **e**pinephrine, **a**tropine, and **n**aloxone via the endotracheal tube. (Use the mnemonic LEAN or NAVEL [if vasopressin is added] to remember these medications.)

Disadvantages of Endotracheal Intubation

- The technique requires considerable training and experience.
- It requires specialized equipment.
- It requires direct visualization of the vocal cords.
- It bypasses the upper airway's function of warming, filtering, and humidifying the inhaled air.
- It is time consuming.
- It is associated with many potential complications including aspiration, hypoxemia, airway trauma, increased intracranial pressure, and others.
- It has not been shown to improve survival.

Equipment

The equipment needed for traditional oral endotracheal intubation includes a functioning laryngoscope (handle and blade), an appropriate-size endotracheal tube with stylet, a 10-mL syringe, a bag-valve mask, a suction device, a bite block, Magill forceps, a means to confirm tube placement, and a means to secure the tube in place. An endotracheal tube

CONTENT REVIEW

➤ Endotracheal Intubation Indicators
- Respiratory arrest
- Cardiac arrest
- Airway swelling (anaphylaxis; airway burns)

FIGURE 15-60 Airway roll and necessary airway management equipment and supplies.

introducer (gum-elastic bougie) and backup airways should also be available (Figure 15-60).

Laryngoscope

The **laryngoscope** is an instrument for lifting the tongue and epiglottis out of the line of sight so that you can see the vocal cords. You will typically use it to place an endotracheal tube, but you may also use it in conjunction with Magill forceps to retrieve a foreign body obstructing the upper airway or to place retroglottic airways such as the ETC.

A laryngoscope consists of a handle and a blade. The handle may be either reusable or disposable. It houses batteries that power a light in the blade's distal tip. This light illuminates the airway, making it easier to see upper airway structures. The point attaching the handle and the blade is called the fitting; it locks the blade in place and provides electrical contact between the batteries and the bulb (Figure 15-61).

FIGURE 15-61 Engaging the laryngoscope blade and handle.

FIGURE 15-62 Activating the laryngoscope light source.

FIGURE 15-64 Curved blades in a variety of sizes.

FIGURE 15-65 Straight blades in a variety of sizes.

To prepare for intubation, attach the indentation on the proximal end of the laryngoscope's blade to the bar of the handle. It will click into place when properly seated. To determine whether the laryngoscope is functional, raise the blade to a right angle with the handle until it clicks into place (Figure 15-62). The light should turn on and be bright and steady. A yellow, flickering light will not sufficiently illuminate the anatomical structures. If the light fails to go on, the problem may be either dead batteries or a loose bulb. Every airway kit should include spare parts. Infrequently, the contact points or the wire that runs through the blade to the bulb will fail.

Like the handle, the blade may be reusable or disposable. Blades may be divided into two types: curved and straight. The major variety of curved blades are called Macintosh; there are several varieties of straight blades including, but not limited to, the Miller, Philips, and Wisconsin. Each has various advantages and proponents. Laryngoscope blades range in size from 00 for premature infants to 4 for large adults (Figure 15-63).

The curved blade has a large flange for sweeping the tongue from the right side of the mouth to the left side and is generally inserted slowly, looking progressively for the base of the tongue and epiglottis. The curved blade is designed to fit into the vallecula (Figure 15-64) and trigger a ligament that connects the epiglottis to the base of the

tongue: the hyoepiglottic ligament. This will raise the epiglottis so that you can see the glottic opening.

The straight blades are designed to fit under the epiglottis and manually lift it out of the way (Figure 15-65). The straight blade has no flange for sweeping the tongue and is best used by placing and maintaining it in the right side of the mouth, between the tongue and teeth (hence sometimes called "paraglossal" or "retromolar"), and directing the distal tip toward the midline. The straight blade may either be inserted progressively, as with a curved blade, or with a "hub technique," in which the entire blade is gently inserted into the esophagus all the way to the hub and then withdrawn slowly until the epiglottis pops into view. Because the blade and handle are on the right side of the mouth, there is limited working room, so an endotracheal tube introducer (described later) is often helpful to facilitate tube placement.

Several newer laryngoscope blades have been developed to aid in adequately visualizing the anterior airway, such as the ViewMax®, Grandview™, and articulating tip blades (Figures 15-66 and 15-67).

The choice of straight or curved blade is often a matter of experience and provider preference. In most patients, either will be adequate. Many providers find a curved blade easier to use, although this is often because straight-blade training has been limited. The straight-blade technique is worth mastering, however, as a straight blade

FIGURE 15-63 Laryngoscope blades in various sizes.

FIGURE 15-66 ViewMax® laryngoscope blade.

(© Viewmax™, Rüsch Inc. a division of Teleflex Medical)

FIGURE 15-67 Grandview laryngoscope blade.

FIGURE 15-69 Endotrol ETT.

combined with a bougie is often the "go-to technique" among experienced intubators for managing the difficult airway, particularly when only the epiglottis can be visualized. A straight blade is often better for endotracheal intubation in infants, because it helps to lift the relatively large and floppy epiglottis, although a curved blade may be useful to control a large infant tongue.

Endotracheal Tubes

The **endotracheal tube (ETT)** is a flexible translucent tube open at both ends and available in lengths ranging from 12 to 32 cm, with centimeter markings along its length (Figure 15-68). The distal end has a beveled tip to facilitate smooth movement through airway passages. The proximal end has a standard 15-mm inside diameter and 22-mm outside diameter connector that attaches to the ventilatory device, usually either a self-inflating bag or a mechanical ventilator. The ETT is available with internal tube diameters ranging from 2.5 to 9.0 mm, which is clearly marked on the tube and packaging. The typical tube size is 7.0 to

7.5 mm for average-sized females and 7.5 to 8.0 mm for average-sized adult males. (We discuss endotracheal intubation of children in detail later in this chapter.)

Adult tubes come with an inflatable cuff at the distal end to provide a seal between the tube and the trachea. Pediatric tubes are available with or without a cuff. Historically, only uncuffed tubes were placed in pediatric patients, but now it is common practice to use a cuffed tube in infants and older children. A thin inflation tube runs the length of the main tube from the distal cuff to a syringe. A one-way valve at the proximal end of the inflation tube permits the syringe to push air into the distal cuff or pull it out but prevents air from escaping the cuff when the syringe is removed. A pilot balloon at the inflation tube's proximal end helps indicate whether the distal cuff is properly inflated, although evidence has shown that this is highly unreliable. Because overinflation may lead to tracheal mucosal damage, it is suggested that a manometer be used to ensure proper pressures, especially during longer transports. Alternatively, paramedics should learn to listen for air leakage and place only enough air in the cuff to inflate it without causing a leak. Always check the distal cuff for leaks before insertion.

Suppliers typically prewrap an ETT in a gently curved shape. This is because the trachea lies anteriorly in the neck, and the tube must be directed upward to enter the glottic opening. Stylets may be used to make further shape enhancements. Another variation is the Endotrol ETT, which has a proximal O-shaped ring attached to a plastic wire that runs the length of the tube and terminates distally (Figure 15-69). Pulling the ring bends the distal end of the tube upward and directs it into the glottic opening. This can facilitate placement of the tube without the need for a stylet, primarily during nasotracheal intubation.

Open end
(top)

15mm adaptor

Inflation
valve

Pilot
balloon

10cc
syringe

Cuff

Open end
(bottom)

FIGURE 15-68 ETT and syringe.

FIGURE 15-70 ETT, stylet, and syringe, unassembled.

(© Dr. Bryan E. Bledsoe)

Stylet

The malleable **stylet** is a plastic-covered metal wire that may be placed inside the ETT, stopping just short of the distal end, to allow the tube to be stiffened and maintained in the optimal shape for intubation (Figure 15-70). Research has now shown that the optimal shape in most cases is "straight-to-cuff" with the distal tip angulated less than 35 degrees (Figure 15-71). Anesthesiologists and anesthetists often avoid using stylets, as they may increase the chance of airway trauma. Stylets are frequently used in EMS and emergency medicine to enhance control of the ETT and potentially improve intubation success, particularly in patients with challenging anatomy, but you need to use the stylet gently to minimize the possibility of airway trauma. Alternatively, you may attempt intubation without a stylet and have a tracheal tube introducer at the ready in case you encounter difficulty.

Endotracheal Tube Introducer

The **endotracheal tube introducer**, commonly called a *gum-elastic bougie*, is a 60- or 70-cm straight, semi-rigid, stylet-like device with a distal bent tip that is covered with a protective resin (Figure 15-72). It is used to facilitate endotracheal

FIGURE 15-71 ETT, stylet, and syringe, assembled for intubation with "straight-to-cuff" configuration of stylet and tube.

(© Dr. Bryan E. Bledsoe)

FIGURE 15-72 Gum elastic bougie.

(© Dr. Bryan E. Bledsoe)

intubations when only the epiglottis may be visualized—that is, "semi-blind" intubations or Cormack and LeHane Class 3 views (discussed later in this chapter). Tactile feedback is used to determine the correct intratracheal positioning; once that positioning is achieved, an endotracheal tube can be passed over the introducer into the trachea. This is discussed further under "Objective Techniques" later in this chapter.

10-mL Syringe

The syringe allows you to inflate the distal cuff to avoid air leaks around the tube. Although a 10-mL syringe is commonly used, this much air is rarely, if ever, necessary and may cause tracheal ischemia. Use a manometer to gauge the correct volume, or listen for air leakage with ventilation. Assessment of the pilot balloon has been shown to be inadequate for determining safe cuff volumes.

Tube-Holding Devices

The reasons for securing the ETT are twofold. First, moving the patient about during resuscitation or transportation can easily dislodge the tube and cause cardiovascular stimulation, an elevation in intracranial pressure, or injury to the tracheal mucosa. Second, the person providing ventilatory support may inadvertently push down on the ETT, forcing it into the right or left mainstem bronchus. The tube may be secured with tape, cloth, or a commercial device (Figure 15-73). If not using a commercial device that has an integral bite block, an oral airway should be inserted to prevent the patient from biting down on the tube and obstructing ventilation. Note that the airway need not be correctly sized nor inserted in a rotary manner when used in this manner.

Magill Forceps

The **Magill forceps** are scissor-style clamps with circular tips used primarily to remove foreign bodies in the airway (Figure 15-74).

Lubricant

Water-soluble lubricants facilitate inserting the ETT. Do not use petroleum-based lubricants, as they may damage the ETT and cause tracheal inflammation.

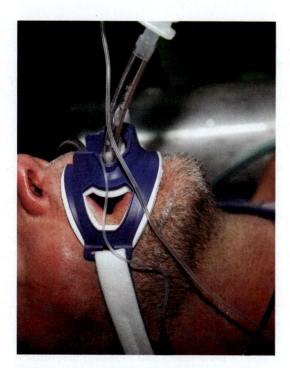

FIGURE 15-73 Commercial ET tube holder.

(© Dr. Bryan E. Bledsoe)

FIGURE 15-74 Magill forceps.

Suction Unit

A suction unit helps to remove secretions and foreign materials from the oropharynx during intubation attempts. It is a vital element that you must never forget. (This will be discussed in more detail later in this chapter.)

End-Tidal CO_2 Detector or Esophageal Detector Device

It is imperative that all tube placements be confirmed objectively using an end-tidal CO_2 detector or an esophageal detector device. It is not adequate to rely on subjective measures such as direct visualization, misting, lung sounds, or an absence of epigastric sounds.

Protective Equipment

Endotracheal intubation, like many airway procedures, carries the risk of exposure to body substances. Because of this, it is essential to employ Standard Precautions. These include, but are not limited to, gloves, mask, protective eyewear, and possibly a gown. Remember, personal safety comes first! Always use Standard Precautions.

Legal Considerations

Negligence and Malpractice Suits. Although negligence and malpractice lawsuits against EMS personnel are relatively uncommon, many of those that do arise involve airway management. Airway issues may result in death or serious disability, so paramedics must take great care to ensure that airway management procedures are performed properly. In systems not using medication-assisted intubation, the most common source of airway-related claims is unrecognized esophageal intubation. Systems performing medication-assisted intubation also expose themselves to claims related to inappropriate intubation and failed intubations in patients who arguably might have done better without intubation in the first place.

Your best line of defense is to be highly competent in these procedures. This starts with your initial paramedic education but must continue after school is completed. If you work in a system where there is limited opportunity to use your airway skills, then you should increase your in-service education and arrange to spend some time in the operating suite if this is available. When there, do not overlook opportunities to place extraglottic airways and to practice bag-valve-mask ventilation.

Always make sure that all airway equipment is functioning properly at the beginning of each shift and after each call. After performing endotracheal intubation, it is essential to confirm and document proper tube placement by at least three methods, including at least one objective means such as an esophageal detector device or capnography. Following intubation, periodically and *obsessively* check and confirm continued proper tube placement, especially after any patient movement. If there is a doubt in regard to tube placement, the tube should be checked or removed and mechanical ventilation continued by other means.

You must have at least one extraglottic airway available at all times as a backup and have a clear plan of when to use it based on your experience, patient condition, service or regional protocols, and local convention. Persisting in attempts to intubate with resulting hypoxemia, airway trauma, and aspiration is a common source of EMS airway litigation. If you are using medication-assisted intubation, you should carefully weigh the risks and benefits, including any predicted difficulties in airway management, before proceeding, and consider calling medical control in borderline cases.

Finally, clear and accurate documentation is imperative. Be especially mindful of documenting your indication for airway management, other options considered, tube confirmation, and any noted complications.

Complications of Endotracheal Intubation

Intubation presents a number of potential complications. Properly attending to detail and taking appropriate precautions will help you to avoid many of these problems.

Equipment Malfunction

Equipment malfunctions consume valuable time when you are establishing an airway. Having a preassembled airway kit that is checked regularly will lessen the chances of this occurring. Ideally, someone should check the airway kit daily to be sure that all needed supplies are present and that the laryngoscope bulb, batteries, and blade are in good working condition.

Tooth Breakage and Soft-Tissue Laceration

Endotracheal intubation can easily injure the lips and teeth, but you can eliminate this hazard by carefully using the laryngoscope as an instrument, not a tool. Guide the blade gently into the mouth and avoid pressure on the teeth. When manipulating the jaw anteriorly, keep your wrist straight while lifting with your shoulder, using gentle traction upward and toward the feet rather than rotating and flexing your wrist (i.e., levering). All levers require a fulcrum—and the only fulcrums available in your patient's mouth will be his upper incisors. Having an assistant apply a jaw-thrust during laryngoscopy and paying attention to precise triggering of the hyoepiglottic ligament in the vallecula when using a curved blade will also minimize trauma.

If you use the laryngoscope too roughly, you can also traumatize the patient's tongue, posterior pharynx, glottic structures, and trachea. This can also happen if you direct the tube away from the midline into the pyriform sinuses, allow the stylet to protrude from the distal end of the ETT, or merely apply too much pressure to a styletted tube. In some cases, the trauma may be so substantial that the patient can no longer be ventilated with an extraglottic airway device or bag-valve mask. A gentle technique, attention to detail, and moving early to alternative strategies in the event of difficulty are the keys to avoiding these traumatic complications.

Aspiration

Aspiration is the entry of stomach contents, blood, or secretions into the lungs. A common cause of aspiration during non–medication-facilitated airway management is placing a laryngoscope (or tongue blade or oropharyngeal airway) into the mouth of a patient who has just enough gag reflex to vomit but is too obtunded to fully protect his airway. Therefore, you need to be very gentle in placing anything into the mouth when you are not sure whether the patient has an intact gag reflex. Rapid sequence intubation, discussed later, is intended to minimize the risk of aspiration

through the use of a neuromuscular blocking agent that eliminates the gag reflex and prevents active vomiting. Use of a sedative alone to facilitate intubation without a neuromuscular blocker potentially creates a high risk for aspiration, as these drugs will depress the patient's ability to protect his airway without eliminating the gag reflex.

Elevated Intracranial Pressure

Intracranial pressure (ICP) can become elevated during intubation from the reflex response to stimulation of the airway with a laryngoscope and endotracheal tube, whether or not the patient is sedated and/or paralyzed. In most patients, this elevation is of no clinical significance. In a few rare patients with intracranial bleeding or masses who are on the brink of brain herniation, however, this increase can have significant repercussions. In such patients, you can either avoid the procedure altogether, use medications to attempt to blunt the reflex response, and/or use a very gentle technique. The possibility of increasing ICP is one of the reasons that nasotracheal intubation is relatively contraindicated in head injury and stroke.

Transport Delays

Whenever an airway procedure is performed on scene rather than en route, it will add to the total out-of-hospital time. In some cases there may be no choice, but in other cases it may be possible to defer the intubation until transport or to perform a bridge procedure, such as placing an extraglottic airway or providing BVM ventilation. The paramedic needs to look at the big picture and decide whether the underlying problem can be treated adequately in the prehospital setting by airway management or whether the patient requires an emergency lifesaving procedure that is available only at the hospital, such as a catheterization or surgery.

Hypoxemia

Delays in oxygenation from prolonged intubation attempts can produce profound, life-threatening hypoxemia. If the patient has a measurable oxygen saturation, it is simple to monitor and abort the attempt as soon as the saturation reaches a predetermined cutoff level, usually 90 percent for patients with head trauma or stroke. For patients without a detectable oxygen saturation, it is much more difficult to know when to abort the attempt, although it is safe to assume that such patients have very little reserve. One basic rule is to limit each intubation attempt to no more than 20 seconds before stopping to reoxygenate the patient. To gauge this interval, some paramedics were once taught to hold their breath from the time they stop ventilating the patient until they start again; this is no longer recommended, as it is very difficult to perform a complex procedure while holding your breath.

A new strategy, called **apneic oxygenation**, supplies oxygen to the apneic (non-breathing) patient during endotracheal intubation to minimize the likelihood of hypoxemia occurring during intubation. To achieve apneic oxygenation in endotracheal intubation, place the patient's head in a reverse Trendelenburg position at a 20° to 30° angle. Then, insert a nasal oxygen cannula with the flow rate set at 5 liters per minute (or more). If possible, the patient should be pre-oxygenated with 3 minutes of normal tidal volume breathing or eight vital capacity breaths (BVM-assisted ventilation). With mechanical ventilation, the nasal cannula can be placed under the BVM mask (Figure 15-75). This effectively pre-oxygenates the patient prior to intubation and increases the physiologic reserve of oxygen, thus mitigating the possible effects of hypoxia during intubation.

If you cannot pass the tube through the vocal cords on the first attempt, at least identify your landmarks and note any unique or difficult features that may be modifiable. For example, if you can identify only the epiglottis, this will warrant use of a bougie, or a very anterior larynx will prompt use of external laryngeal manipulation or better positioning. The absence of any identifiable landmarks should prompt placement of an extraglottic airway.

Esophageal Intubation

Misplacement of the ETT into the esophagus deprives the patient of oxygenation and ventilation. It is potentially lethal, resulting in severe hypoxemia and brain death if you do not recognize it immediately. It also directs air into the stomach, encouraging regurgitation, which can lead to aspiration. Indicators of esophageal intubation include the following:

- An absence of chest rise and absence of breath sounds with mechanical ventilation

FIGURE 15-75 To improve oxygenation during apneic intubation, the nasal cannula can be placed under the BVM mask.

- Gurgling sounds over the epigastrium with each breath delivered
- Distention of the abdomen
- An absence of breath condensation in the endotracheal tube
- A persistent air leak, despite inflation of the tube's distal cuff
- Cyanosis and progressive worsening of the patient's condition
- Phonation (noise made by the vocal cords)
- No color change with colorimetric exhaled CO_2 detector
- An absent waveform on capnography
- A falling pulse oximetry reading

If you have any suspicion that the tube is in the esophagus, remove it immediately. Perform BVM ventilation with 100 percent oxygen and either initiate transport, place an extraglottic airway, or repeat endotracheal intubation with another tube.[34–35]

Endobronchial Intubation

If you pass the endotracheal tube successfully through the vocal cords and advance it too far, it likely will enter either the right or left mainstem bronchus, although it is far more likely to pass into the right mainstem, which angles away from the trachea less acutely than does the left. In either case, the ETT then ventilates only one lung, and the result is hypoventilation and hypoxia from inadequate gas exchange. Also, when the bag-valve device **insufflates** enough air for two lungs into the smaller area of only one lung, it can create enough pressure to cause barotrauma, such as a pneumothorax, worsening the patient's condition. Findings in endobronchial intubation include breath sounds present on one side of the chest but diminished or absent on the other, poor compliance (resistance to ventilations with the bag-valve device), and evidence of hypoxemia.

You may avoid inserting the ETT too far by following these guidelines:

1. Advance the proximal end of the cuff no more than 1 to 2 cm past the vocal cords.
2. Once the tube is positioned, hold it in place with one hand to prevent it from being pushed any farther.
3. Inflate the cuff and firmly secure the tube in place with tape or a commercial tube-holding device.
4. Note the number marking on the side of the ETT where it emerges from the patient's mouth at the teeth, gums, or lips. This will allow you to quickly recognize any changes in tube placement. Approximate ETT depth for the average adult is 21 cm at the teeth for women and 23 cm at the teeth for men, although this will vary.

To resolve the problem, loosen or remove any securing devices and withdraw the ETT until breath sounds are present and equal bilaterally. Be certain to deflate the cuff when pulling back on the ETT.

Tension Pneumothorax

Any tear in the lung parenchyma can cause a pneumothorax. This may occur from excessive pressure being applied to a healthy lung or normal pressures applied to abnormal lungs such as occurs in COPD patients or patients who have suffered recent chest trauma. If this is allowed to progress untreated, a tension pneumothorax may develop. A tension pneumothorax will adversely affect the other lung, the heart, and the structures of the mediastinum. Tension pneumothorax is marked by progressively worsening compliance (more difficulty in ventilating), diminished unilateral breath sounds, hypoxemia with hypotension, and distended neck veins. If you suspect tension pneumothorax, needle decompression of the chest is indicated, as described in the chapter "Chest Trauma."

Orotracheal Intubation Technique

Two paths for intubation are the orotracheal path (through the mouth) and the nasotracheal path (through the nose). The most widely used path for endotracheal intubation is the orotracheal route (through the mouth), because it allows direct visualization of the vocal cords and a clear view of the ETT's passage through them. Nasotracheal intubation will be discussed later in the chapter.

To perform orotracheal intubation in the absence of suspected trauma (Procedure 15–1):

1. Use Standard Precautions.
2. Place the patient supine and properly position the patient's head and neck. To visualize the larynx, you must align the three axes of the mouth, the pharynx, and the trachea. To do this, place the patient's head in a "sniffing position" by elevating the head and flexing the neck forward and the head backward. The ear and sternal notch should be on the same horizontal level. (Review Figure 15-38.) In obese patients it is necessary to place padding under the upper back, shoulders, and head to achieve the same position. This is called the "ramped position." (Review Figure 15-39.)
3. Perform BVM ventilation with 100 percent oxygen using the "rule of threes," as mentioned earlier in the chapter under the discussion of BVM ventilation. Avoid aggressive hyperventilation, as this is likely to fill the stomach with air and predispose to aspiration.
4. Prepare your intubation equipment as already discussed.
5. Turn on the suction and attach an appropriate tip.
6. Remove any dentures or partial dental plates.

7. Hold the laryngoscope in your left hand, whether you are right- or left-handed. Insert the laryngoscope blade gently into the right side of the patient's mouth. If using a curved blade, gently sweep the tongue to the left and work in the midline. If using a straight blade, remain on the right side of the mouth. Your primary goal at this point is to visualize the epiglottis.
8. Advance the curved blade until the distal end is at the base of the tongue in the vallecula (Figure 15-76a). Advance the straight blade until the distal end is under the epiglottis (Figure 15-76b). Alternatively, with a

FIGURE 15-76A The curved blade is placed into the vallecula and indirectly lifts the epiglottis.

FIGURE 15-76B The straight blade is placed under the epiglottis and directly lifts the epiglottis upward to expose the vocal cords and glottic opening.

Procedure 15–1   Endotracheal Intubation

15-1A Ventilate the patient.

15-1B Prepare the equipment.

15-1C Apply external laryngeal manipulation to assist in vocal cord visualization.

15-1D Visualize the larynx and insert the ETT.

15-1E Inflate the cuff, ventilate, and auscultate.

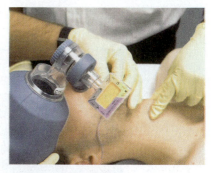

15-1F Confirm placement with an ETCO$_2$ detector.

15-1G Secure the tube.

15-1H Reconfirm ETT placement.

straight blade, you may fully advance until the distal tip is in the esophagus and then visualize while slowly withdrawing the blade. If you cannot visualize the epiglottis, withdraw the blade, reposition the patient, and repeat.

9. Keeping your left wrist straight, use your left shoulder and arm to continue lifting the mandible and tongue to a 45° angle to the ground (up and toward the feet) until landmarks are exposed (Figure 15-77). Be careful not to put pressure on the teeth. Consider having an assistant perform the jaw-thrust simultaneously. At this point, you may need to suction any large amounts of emesis, blood, or secretions in the posterior pharynx.

10. Quickly but carefully visualize the airway structures to assure you can visualize the vocal cords. If you still cannot visualize the posterior cartilages, perform external laryngeal manipulation. You may not see the entire glottis or even part of it, but you should at least clearly visualize the posterior cartilages and interarytenoid notch.[36]

11. Hold the ETT in your right hand with your fingertips as you would a dart or a pencil. This gives you control to gently maneuver the ETT. Advance the tube through the right corner of the patient's mouth, and direct it toward the midline. Pass the ETT gently through the glottic opening until its distal cuff

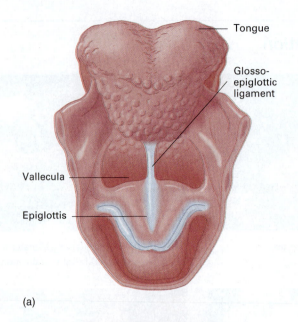

Tongue

Glosso-
epiglottic
ligament

Vallecula

Epiglottis

(a)

(b)

FIGURE 15-77 (a) The epiglottis. (b) Laryngoscope view of the glottis, closed during the act of swallowing.

(Source (b): Gastrolab/Science Source)

disappears beyond the vocal cords; then advance it another 1 to 2 cm. Hold the tube in place with your hand to prevent its displacement. Do not let go under any circumstance until it is taped or tied securely in place.

12. Remove the stylet (if used) and attach a bag-valve device to the 15/22-mm connector on the tube.

13. Objectively confirm tube placement with capnography. In addition, check for equal breath sounds to be sure the tube is not too deep.

14. Ventilate the patient with 100 percent oxygen.

15. Gently insert an oropharyngeal airway to serve as a bite block, and secure the ETT with umbilical tape, adhesive tape, or a commercial tube-holding device.

16. Place the patient on the transport ventilator and monitor the continuous capnography waveform.

17. Reconfirm appropriate tube placement periodically, especially after any major patient movement or if there is any deterioration of patient status.

Verification of Proper Tube Placement

It is absolutely imperative that endotracheal placement of the tube be objectively confirmed immediately after placement and continuously throughout care, particularly if the patient is moved or deteriorates. You should employ a number of methods in the field to confirm correct ETT placement, but do not become overly reliant on technology. The patient's clinical condition should be the deciding factor in your patient management decisions. There have been countless EMS airway disasters related to unrecognized esophageal intubation. The common theme in these situations is excessive confidence and inappropriate reliance on subjective measures.

Subjective Techniques

Subjective methods of tube placement confirmation include direct visualization, tube misting, and auscultation for breath sounds. Well-performed EMS studies have demonstrated that reliance on subjective means alone results in a 10 to 20 percent rate of missed esophageal intubations. Therefore, subjective observations, although they are important, should not be relied on solely for confirmation of correct tube placement.

- **Direct visualization.** Although seeing the tube pass through the cords should be considered the gold standard, this method of tube confirmation has failed. There are at least three possible explanations. First, in the emergency situation, visualization of the tube's passage through the cords is often unsatisfactory as a result of patient immobilization, positioning, or blood/vomitus in the airway. Second, the tube itself often obscures visualization. Third, even if the tube is observed to pass through the cords, it may become dislodged when the stylet is removed and/or if the end-tidal CO_2 detector and BVM are attached before the tube has been secured. For these reasons direct visualization alone cannot be relied on to confirm tube placement.

- **Tube misting.** Observing mist or condensation in the tube, or a "vapor trail," has long been held out as a means of confirming tracheal placement of the tube, but it is not reliable. There have been many cases of a vapor trail noted with an esophageal intubation as well as cases when the vapor trail is missing with a correctly placed tracheal tube. Never make any decisions on tube placement based solely on tube misting.

- *Auscultation.* After intubation, breath sounds should be checked bilaterally and compared to pre-intubation breath sounds, unless ambient noise (e.g., in an aircraft) makes this impossible. Sounds should be present bilaterally if they were present bilaterally before intubation. Newly diminished sounds on the left with strong breath sounds on the right strongly suggest right mainstem intubation. Absence of sounds over the epigastrium should be confirmed. (Epigastric sounds suggest esophageal placement.) It is important to recognize that breath sounds have proved unreliable many times. This is particularly common in children (sounds are easily transmitted throughout the pediatric thorax), obese patients, and those with lung pathology. Like the other subjective means of tube confirmation, breath sounds should be neither relied on entirely nor ignored.

FIGURE 15-78 Bulb-type and syringe-type esophageal detector devices.

Objective Techniques

Objective methods of tube confirmation include capnography, esophageal detector device (EDD), endotracheal tube introducer, pulse oximetry, chest rise and fall, and presence or absence of gastric distention. Remember that objective methods such as these must be used, in addition to subjective observations, to confirm proper tube placement.

- *Capnography.* Detection of end-tidal CO_2 (capnography) is the gold standard for tube confirmation—if the patient is producing enough CO_2 to detect. As detailed previously, there are two types of end-tidal CO_2 detection: qualitative (indicating only whether CO_2 is present or absent) and quantitative (providing a measure, usually with a waveform for analysis, of how much CO_2 is present). Either type is acceptable for initial tube verification. The quantitative detectors are better for ongoing monitoring, especially during air medical transport, where clinical means are limited. There are virtually no false positive readings with these detectors. This means that if the detector says that CO_2 is present, then you are not in the esophagus, but you may be above the trachea in the hypopharynx. On the other hand, false negatives may occur in the setting of cardiac arrest. During cardiac arrest, CO_2 production and transfer eventually cease. Therefore, you may have the tube correctly in the trachea without evidence of CO_2 being present.

- *Esophageal detector device.* Use of an esophageal detector device (EDD) is another means of objective tube verification. A syringe device or bulb is placed on the end of the endotracheal tube to create suction (Figure 15-78). If the tube is correctly placed in the trachea, the cartilaginous rings keep the trachea patent when suction is applied, so there is rapid air return into the device. If the tube is incorrectly placed in the esophagus, the soft distensible tissues occlude the end of the tube when suction is applied, so air return does not occur or occurs very slowly. These devices are inexpensive and are almost as accurate as capnography for detecting esophageal placements. In settings where most intubations are performed for cardiac arrest—that is, most EMS systems without rapid sequence intubation (RSI) capability—EDDs may be preferred to capnography, as there is little point in measuring exhaled CO_2 in a cardiac arrest patient. These devices are FDA approved down to 20-kg patients and have been well studied down to 10 kg. It is important, however, to use the "off-deflate" method in children—that is, squeeze the air out of the device before it is placed on the tube. Generally speaking, capnography ($ETCO_2$) monitoring has replaced EDD use for tube placement verification.

- *Endotracheal tube introducer.* Though principally used to facilitate difficult intubations, an endotracheal tube introducer (bougie) may also be used to confirm tube placement. When a well-lubricated introducer is passed through an endotracheal tube that is correctly placed in the trachea, you should be able to feel it "hold up" (meet resistance) in the smaller airways within approximately 40 cm of the teeth or about 50 cm from the tube end. (It has been said that you should also be able to feel "clicks" as the introducer passes over the tracheal rings. However, clicks may not be detectable because the tube bypasses most of the large rings of the trachea.) Absence of hold-ups at the depth where you would expect to feel them with a tracheal placement is an indication of incorrect esophageal placement.

- *Pulse oximetry and other findings.* As another objective finding, an increase in the oxygen saturation will help confirm proper placement of the endotracheal tube. Similarly, a rise and fall of the chest indicates correct endotracheal intubation. Worsening gastric distention may indicate esophageal placement. Any gastric distention should be investigated. Remember, though, that it is not uncommon for gastric distention to develop prior to endotracheal intubation from mechanical ventilation. Even in experienced hands, it is very difficult to avoid gastric distention with mechanical ventilation until an endotracheal tube is placed.

Retrograde Intubation

Retrograde intubation is a technique in which a needle is inserted into the airway through the cricoid membrane from the outside, much like a needle cricothyrotomy, except it is directed superiorly rather than inferiorly. Once the needle is in the airway, a guidewire is passed through the needle and hopefully retrieved in the oral cavity and withdrawn through the mouth. An endotracheal tube is then passed over the wire into the airway.

One difficulty is that the guidewire must be withdrawn before the tube can be passed distal to the cricoid membrane, and that does not leave a lot of margin for error. Overall, the technique is not very rapid, so the patient must be quite stable. Although some EMS services have embraced this technique over the years and used it successfully, there are not many cases in which this would be the only viable approach. Retrograde intubation will probably be replaced by newer technology and simpler techniques, such as those making use of external laryngeal manipulation (ELM) and the gum-elastic bougie, which are discussed under "Improving Endotracheal Intubation Success."

Optical Laryngoscopes

Several devices allow visualization of the glottic opening and associated anatomy using fiber-optic technology. Among these is the AirTraq™, a disposable device, available in a variety of adult and pediatric sizes, that transmits the view from the end of the device to a small attached screen via a prism mechanism (Figure 15-79). The endotracheal tube is preloaded into a channel on the side of the device. Once the cords are visualized on the screen, the tube is advanced into the glottis through the channel. The tube is directable by redirecting the entire device rather than the tube itself. A video monitor that can be attached to project the obtained view onto a screen is also available. Studies and clinical experience have found the AirTraq to be very successful, although the cost advantage of a disposable device is offset somewhat by having multiple sizes to stock with expiration dates and needing to use them regularly to maintain skills.

FIGURE 15-79 AirTraq.

Video Laryngoscopy

Video laryngoscopes have a camera on the distal end of the device that transmits a high-quality magnified image to a video screen that is attached to the device either directly or by a cable. The screen is held by an assistant, mounted in the ambulance, or placed on the patient's chest or bedside. The technique is considered indirect in that the intubator looks at the screen while intubating, not directly in the patient's mouth, much like a video game. Studies with this technology demonstrate that it is superior to traditional direct laryngoscopy unless the pharynx is completely full of blood, emesis, or secretions. A number of devices are now available with a wide range of prices. None of these devices has been shown to be clearly superior to the others. This technology will likely replace traditional direct laryngoscopy in the years to come as prices come down (Figures 15-80 and 15-81).[37]

FIGURE 15-80 McGrath® video laryngoscope.

(© Dr. Bryan E. Bledsoe)

FIGURE 15-81 GlideScope® Ranger.

(© *Kevin Link*)

Improving Endotracheal Intubation Success

Most studies of prehospital intubation show relatively poor success rates when using first-attempt and overall successful endotracheal tube placement as the marker of success. It is now clear, however, that physiologic parameters, such as maintenance of oxygen saturation and avoidance of aspiration and airway trauma during the intubation process, are far more important markers of success than the percentage of times an endotracheal tube is successfully placed within three attempts. It has also been demonstrated that success rates rapidly plateau after two or three attempts, whereas complications go up exponentially. Therefore, paramedics should strive to make their first attempt rapidly successful. How do we maximize the chance of rapid success on the first attempt? These include good initial training, ongoing practice, using the endotracheal tube introducer, managing neck pressure, ensuring optimal positioning, using video laryngoscopy and other technology, and using rapid sequence intubation.

> **CONTENT REVIEW**
>
> ➤ Maximizing Rapid Success with Endotracheal Intubation
> - Good initial training
> - Ongoing practice
> - Using the endotracheal tube introducer
> - Managing neck pressure
> - Optimal positioning
> - Video laryngoscopy
> - Other technology
> - Rapid sequence intubation

Good Initial Training

There is no substitute for being well trained from the beginning of your career. Bad habits are very difficult to break, and in times of stress we all naturally revert to what we learned first. Take your airway education very seriously and take advantage of every learning opportunity.

Ideally, you will be able to intubate a number of live patients under the watchful eye of an anesthesiologist or nurse anesthetist in the operating suite. Here you should focus on perfect technique and close observation of airway anatomy. You should also try to place as many extraglottic airways as possible if the opportunity presents itself.

During your field internship, hopefully, you will be able to intubate a number of patients under the supervision of an experienced paramedic, where you can learn the ins and outs of managing airways in bad light, with lots of secretions, and with awkward positioning. The evidence suggests that at least 15 intubations are necessary for most providers to achieve at least 90 percent success in the operating suite, but more than 30 are necessary to achieve the same success in the field. Unfortunately, opportunities for operating suite practice for paramedics are very limited in some locales. You cannot expect optimal performance if you have not had sufficient experience, and your threshold for placing an extraglottic airway device should be lower, in that case, to prevent patient complications.

Ongoing Practice

Nearly as important as your initial training is the seriousness with which you maintain your skills. One study has demonstrated that patients cared for by a paramedic who had intubated more than 25 patients in the past 5 years did better than patients cared for by paramedics with lesser experience. If you do not intubate frequently in your practice setting, you should practice the basic motor skills and checklists routinely on a mannequin/simulator and visit the operating suite if possible.

Using the Endotracheal Tube Introducer

The endotracheal tube introducer (gum-elastic bougie) is a simple device that helps facilitate intubation when only the epiglottis is visible. It is a flexible device, 60 to 70 cm in length, that is stiff enough to be directable and to transmit tactile information (that is, you can feel its movements and responses) but flexible enough to allow a tube to be passed over it. There are disposable and nondisposable products of this kind, and each brand has a different balance of these properties, creating a unique feel and different performance for each, especially at temperature extremes. Some operators prefer to preshape the bougie by holding it in a curved shape for several seconds before insertion.

Once the intubator identifies a difficult airway—despite optimal positioning, removal of the cervical collar with in-line immobilization and jaw-thrust maneuver, and external laryngeal manipulation—an introducer is placed into the pharynx with the *coude* tip (bent end) distal and anterior (Figure 15-82).

If the introducer enters the airway, the operator may be able to feel "clicks" as the *coude* tip passes over each cartilaginous ring of the trachea. Because clicks cannot be felt

FIGURE 15-82 Preshaping the bougie prior to use will improve insertion. Note the *coude* tip.

(© Dr. Bryan E. Bledsoe).

FIGURE 15-83 External laryngeal manipulation (ELM) can assist with better visualization of the glottis and airway structures.

(© Dr. Bryan E. Bledsoe)

in all cases, tracheal positioning should also be confirmed by hold-up, the resistance felt when the introducer passes into the smaller airways. If hold-up does not occur by the time the device has been inserted 40 cm beyond the teeth (introducers have a mark to indicate this distance), then it is safe to assume that you are in the esophagus.

Once tracheal position is ensured, an endotracheal tube may be passed over the introducer while the intubator maintains an open channel with the laryngoscope. The scope is not removed until the tube is passed. A gentle counterclockwise rotation of the tube over the introducer may be necessary to avoid its getting stuck on cartilages or cords. Once the tube is passed to the appropriate depth, the introducer is removed and the tube placement confirmed with the usual methods.

Many programs have introducers at the patient's side during all intubations. Some EMS programs have even adopted use of the introducer in place of a stylet for all intubations instead of waiting to use it only for difficult intubations. The introducer may also be used as a "place saver" if the glottic opening is swollen or smaller than anticipated, rather than withdrawing completely while preparing a smaller tube.

Managing Neck Pressure

As previously discussed, well-intended cricoid pressure can actually obscure the laryngeal view. If the intubator is having difficulty during normal visual laryngoscopy seeing appropriate landmarks, it is not recommended to just attempt a 'blind' insertion into the trachea. If the view is still limited, the assistant should slide his hand up to the thyroid cartilage, and the intubator should move the larynx into an optimal position using his own right hand on top of the assistant's hand—a procedure called

external laryngeal manipulation (ELM) (Figure 15-83). A third option is to have the assistant apply **b**ackward, **u**pward, **r**ightward **p**ressure on the larynx (the BURP maneuver) (Figure 15-84). ELM affords the intubator the opportunity to use immediate hand-eye feedback to obtain the optimal view and is now generally preferred over the BURP maneuver.

Optimal Positioning

There is no substitute for a well-positioned patient. Unless contraindicated or impossible for reasons such as patient entrapment, all patients should be in a sniffing position or, if obese, in the ramped position.

Video Laryngoscopy

This technology is clearly changing how we intubate. Except in patients with excessive oral secretions, video laryngoscopy is superior to traditional direct laryngoscopy.

Rightward

Backward

Upward

FIGURE 15-84 BURP airway maneuver.

As these devices become more affordable, they will likely take over EMS airway management. A number of devices are on the market, and none has been shown to be clearly superior to the others. Each device uses a different technique, but they are all very different from traditional direct laryngoscopy. If you have one of these devices, you will need specific training and regular practice in using it.

Other Technology

Other devices that may prove valuable in certain circumstances are specialized blades, lighted stylets, intubating laryngeal airways, and fiber-optic stylets. Most of these devices are much more affordable at this point than video laryngoscopes and will probably see greater use in EMS.

A number of different blades are available, including different shapes, different lighting mechanisms (e.g., IntuBrite™), articulating tips, and attached prisms (Figure 15-85).

Lighted stylets, such as the Trachlight™, allow for intubation with a high degree of success despite oral secretions and cervical precautions (Figure 15-86). The device is placed blindly into the airway with an endotracheal tube preloaded, and the intubator observes for a bright glow in the midline of the anterior neck, indicating tracheal placement. The tube is then slid over the device into the trachea. Unfortunately, this technique is more difficult in bright ambient light, with obese patients, and patients with very dark skin.

Intubating laryngeal airways allow for intubation with a high degree of success despite oral secretions, cervical precautions, and obesity.

Fiber-optic stylets combine the visualization common in flexible bronchoscopes seen in hospital operating suites and intensive care units with a rigid delivery device to simplify placement.

FIGURE 15-86 Trachlight™ lighted stylet in use.

(© Dr. Bryan E. Bledsoe)

Most EMS services with a substantial budget are choosing video devices over fiber optics.

Using Rapid Sequence Intubation

Success rates with rapid sequence intubation (RSI) are routinely higher than success rates without RSI, although this may be offset by the increased potential for devastating complications. The balance of the literature to date has not shown improved survival with prehospital RSI. RSI is discussed in more detail later.

Blind Nasotracheal Intubation

As previously noted, the oral route is usually preferred over the nasal route for prehospital intubation. The **nasotracheal route** (through the nose and into the trachea) used to be very common in EMS, emergency medicine, and anesthesia but has generally fallen out of favor. In a few circumstances, however, the nasal route may be the best or only option, such as in the patient with trismus or with an anticipated difficult laryngoscopy, so this remains an important paramedic skill. When done by EMS, nasotracheal intubation is a "blind" procedure performed without direct visualization of the vocal cords; in the hospital setting, it may be performed with direct visualization or fiber-optic guidance. It is important to remember that blind nasotracheal intubation (BNTI) requires a cooperative or unresponsive spontaneously breathing patient.

Relative Contraindications

- Suspected nasal fractures
- Suspected basilar skull fractures
- Suspected elevation of intracranial pressure
- Combative/uncooperative patient

FIGURE 15-85 Intubrite™ laryngoscope system.

(© Dr. Bryan E. Bledsoe)

- Coagulopathy, including therapeutic warfarin or heparin
- Significantly deviated nasal septum or other nasal obstruction
- Hypoxemia

Absolute Contraindications

- Cardiac or respiratory arrest

Disadvantages of Nasotracheal Intubation

The following disadvantages of nasotracheal intubation discourage its use unless clearly indicated by the patient's condition:

- It is often more difficult and time consuming to perform than orotracheal intubation.
- There is a significant risk of epistaxis (nosebleed).
- Smaller-diameter tubes must be placed, which makes ventilation more difficult.
- There is a significant risk of sinusitis, so these tubes must generally be changed out in the hospital.

FIGURE 15-87 Blind nasotracheal intubation.

The fact that there are so many contraindications and disadvantages means that many patients are not good candidates for this procedure.

Blind Nasotracheal Intubation Technique

To perform blind nasotracheal intubation (Figure 15-87):

1. Use Standard Precautions.
2. Using basic manual and adjunctive maneuvers, open the airway and ventilate the patient with 100 percent oxygen.
3. Prepare your equipment.
4. Place the patient in his position of comfort. If the patient is unconscious or if you suspect cervical spine injury, place the patient supine and use manual in-line stabilization as appropriate.
5. Inspect the nose and select the larger nostril as your passageway.
6. Select the correct size endotracheal tube. Normally use a tube one-half to one full size smaller than for oral intubation. For an average adult male, a size 7 mm is appropriate. For an average adult female, a size 6.5 mm is appropriate. Tubes with a directable tip may make

the procedure easier, if available. Attach an end-tidal CO_2 detection device to the proximal end of the tube. Alternatively, a device to enhance audible detection of breath sounds, such as the Beck Airway Airflow Monitor (BAAM®) whistle or the Burden nasoscope, may be used (Figures 15-88 and 15-89).

7. Lubricate the tube generously. Topical lidocaine may be preferred for long-term comfort but probably does not affect the initial attempt.
8. Insert the ETT into the nostril with the bevel along the floor of the nostril or facing the nasal septum, directed posteriorly. This will help avoid damage to the turbinates. There is some tendency to direct the tube upward, but recall that the nasopharynx runs directly anterior to posterior.

FIGURE 15-88 Beck Airway Airflow Monitor (BAAM®) for blind nasotracheal intubations.

this point. Continue passing the ETT until the distal cuff is just past the vocal cords, which should occur at a depth of approximately 26 cm in an average adult female and 28 cm in an average adult male. Coughing or bucking and anterior displacement of the larynx generally indicate tracheal placement, whereas gagging or vocal sounds indicate esophageal placement.

11. Holding the ETT with one hand to prevent displacement, inflate the distal cuff with enough air to eliminate any audible leak, connect a bag-valve device, ventilate the patient with 100 percent oxygen, and confirm proper placement of the ETT using multiple techniques, including bilateral breath sounds, absent epigastric sounds, and capnography.

12. Secure the ETT and reconfirm proper placement. Continue to observe the patient's condition, maintain ventilatory support, and frequently recheck ETT placement. Use continuous waveform capnography to monitor tube placement and ventilation.

Digital Intubation

Digital intubation is another old technique that has largely been replaced by newer extraglottic airways and devices such as lighted stylets. However, digital intubation still may be a viable option in certain circumstances, such as a patient in a position that does not allow direct visualization, when there are copious secretions obscuring the airway, and in the event of equipment failure (Figure 15-90). Digital intubation is risky for the paramedic; it may stimulate even

FIGURE 15-89 The Burden nasoscope, a commercial nasotracheal tube auscultation device.

(© Brant Burden, EMT-P)

9. As you feel the tube drop into the posterior pharynx, listen closely at its proximal end for the patient's respiratory sounds, and observe for end-tidal CO_2. Sounds are loudest when the ETT is proximal to the epiglottis. When the ETT tip reaches the posterior pharyngeal wall, you must take care to direct it toward the glottic opening. This may be done with a directable-tip tube or by inflating the cuff, as the Endotrol tracheal tube. At this point, the tip of the ETT may catch in the pyriform sinus. If it does, you will feel resistance, and the skin on either side of the Adam's apple will tent. To resolve pyriform sinus placement, slightly withdraw the ETT and rotate it to the midline.

10. With the patient's next inhaled breath, advance the ETT gently but quickly into the glottic opening, observing exhaled CO_2. If you inflated the tube cuff to help with anterior displacement, the cuff must be deflated at

FIGURE 15-90 Blind orotracheal intubation by digital method.

FIGURE 15-91 Digital intubation. Insert your middle and index fingers into the patient's mouth.

a deeply comatose patient to clamp down and bite your finger. Do not use it with any patient who may have an intact gag reflex.

To perform digital intubation:

1. Use Standard Precautions.

2. Continue oxygenation with bag-valve mask and high-concentration oxygen.

3. Prepare and check your equipment. You will need the following items: an appropriately sized ETT, a malleable stylet, water-soluble lubricant, a 5- to 10-mL syringe, a bite block, and umbilical tape or a commercial anchoring device. Insert the stylet into the endotracheal tube and bend the ETT/stylet into a J shape.

4. Remove the front of the collar and have an assistant stabilize the neck as appropriate.

5. Place a bite block device between the patient's molars to help protect your fingers.

6. Insert your left middle and index fingers into the patient's mouth (Figure 15-91). By alternating fingers, "walk" your hand down the midline while simultaneously tugging gently forward on the tongue. You may also use gauze to hold and extend the tongue more effectively, which lifts the epiglottis up and away from the glottic opening so that it is within reach of your probing fingers.

7. Palpate the arytenoid cartilage posterior to the glottis and the epiglottis anteriorly with your middle finger (Figure 15-92). Press the epiglottis forward, and insert the endotracheal tube into the mouth, anterior to your fingers (Figure 15-93).

8. Advance the tube, pushing it gently with your right hand. Use your left index finger to keep the tip of the ETT against your middle finger. This will direct the tip to the epiglottis.

9. Use your middle and index fingers to direct the tip of the ETT between the epiglottis (in front) and your fingers (behind). Then, with your right hand, advance the ETT through the cords while simultaneously maneuvering it forward with your left index and middle fingers. This will prevent it from slipping posteriorly into the esophagus.

10. Hold the tube in place with your hand to prevent its displacement, remove stylet, and inflate cuff.

11. Confirm placement with multiple techniques.

12. Ventilate the patient with 100 percent oxygen. Gently insert an oropharyngeal airway to serve as a bite block. Secure the ETT with umbilical tape. Repeat steps to confirm proper ETT placement and maintain ventilatory support. Continue your airway assessment periodically.

FIGURE 15-92 Digital intubation. Walk your fingers and palpate the patient's epiglottis.

FIGURE 15-93 Digital intubation—insertion of the ETT.

Special Intubation Considerations

Trauma Patient Intubation

Airway management and ventilatory support in the trauma patient are essential for a successful outcome. Appropriate treatment of all other injuries is meaningless if you do not ensure a patent airway and adequate oxygenation and ventilation.

The trauma patient, however, presents a number of obstacles to effective airway management and ventilation. These include difficult access, the need for extrication, blood in the oropharynx, distorted anatomy due to injury, and the need to protect the cervical spine. Getting an adequate seal on a mask is very difficult when the patient is being extricated or has significant facial trauma. You must keep the cervical spine in a neutral, in-line position throughout your management of all patients with known or suspected cervical spine trauma.

Options for airway management include BVM ventilation, extraglottic devices, and intubation. Intubation may

be performed with simple modifications of standard laryngoscopy techniques or others, using equipment such as lighted stylets or video laryngoscopy. Occasionally digital intubation or nasotracheal intubation may be employed.

To perform direct laryngoscopy with in-line stabilization (Procedure 15–2):

1. Use Standard Precautions.

2. Perform basic airway management, including BVM ventilation with simple mechanical airways as needed.

3. Remove the front of the collar and have an assistant maintain in-line stabilization.

4. Immediately before laryngoscopy, have the assistant perform a jaw-thrust and release cricoid pressure.

5. Perform external laryngeal manipulation as needed to help with glottic visualization, and have the assistant maintain this optimal position of the larynx.

The trauma patient may present a number of obstacles to effective airway management and ventilation, including the need for extrication, blood in the oropharynx, distorted anatomy, and/or the need to protect the cervical spine. In addition, patients with nervous system trauma are very intolerant of hypoxemia. Therefore, you must have a plan to optimize your intubation attempts and must make early use of extraglottic airway devices.[38–42]

When a patient presents in a nontraditional position, the patient may still undergo direct laryngoscopy using an alternative approach, such as a face-to-face technique. Alternatively, extraglottic airways may be used as a bridge until the patient can be positioned better, or they may be used all the way to the receiving hospital.

To perform orotracheal intubation on a trauma patient, you need an assistant who will both maintain in-line stabilization and simultaneously perform a jaw-thrust. Maintaining in-line stabilization of the cervical spine is, of course, critical for the trauma patient who may have suffered spinal injury. The jaw-thrust maneuver will not only open the airway but also will assist with direct laryngoscopy, as the patient cannot be placed into the optimal ear-to-sternal notch position.

It is imperative that the front of the cervical collar be removed during direct laryngoscopy to allow forward movement of the jaw. When using alternative techniques such as video laryngoscopy, intubating laryngeal airways, and lighted stylets, it may not be necessary to remove the front of the cervical collar.

Procedure 15–2   Endotracheal Intubation with In-Line Stabilization

15-2A Ventilate the patient and apply manual C-spine stabilization.

15-2B Apply extra laryngeal manipulation to assist with glottic visualization.

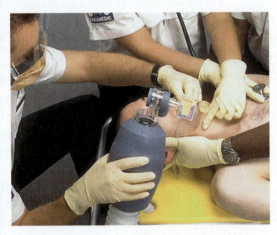

15-2C Ventilate the patient and confirm placement.

15-2D Secure the ETT and place a cervical collar.

15-2E Reconfirm placement.

Foreign Body Removal under Direct Laryngoscopy

When confronted with a patient who has apparently choked, you should initially carry out basic maneuvers for airway obstruction that are appropriate to the patient's age and mental status, such as abdominal thrusts or chest thrusts. If these fail to alleviate the obstruction, direct visualization of the airway with a laryngoscope may enable you to remove an obstructing foreign body using Magill forceps or a suction device (Figure 15-94). The procedure for visualizing the airway is identical to that used for orotracheal intubation.

Pediatric Intubation

Pediatric airway emergencies generally produce more anxiety than adult emergencies among both medical care providers and the family, although many airway procedures themselves are often easier to perform in this patient population. Historically, we have separated the parents and the child during resuscitation and critical procedures, but recent experience in the emergency department has shown it to be beneficial to have parents present. As difficult as it may be for the providers, children who are conscious usually benefit from having their parents present, and parents benefit from seeing all the efforts made to save their children, even if these efforts are unsuccessful. The final decision on separation must be made on a case-by-case

basis, by individual paramedics, in light of local protocols and customs.

A randomized controlled study in a large urban area comparing non–drug-facilitated intubation in children with BVM ventilation of children showed no improvement in outcomes with intubation over outcomes with BVM ventilation. Recent evidence also shows that extraglottic airway devices can be very effective in children. For now, the decision on whether pediatric intubation is part of the paramedic scope of practice, and for what circumstances, is determined locally.[43]

Airway management in children is similar to that for adults, but there are a few important differences based on pediatric anatomy and physiology:

- *Structures are smaller.* The airway structures in children are proportionally smaller and more flexible than an adult's.
- *Nasal openings are small and adenoids are large.* Inserting any tube or device into a child's nose often causes trauma and bleeding because of the size and the presence of enlarged adenoid tissues.
- *Nasal airway diameters are inadequate.* Nasal pharyngeal airways and nasotracheal intubations are generally too large to be useful in the child.
- *Cricoid pressure can worsen the situation.* Because a child's cricoid is less rigid than an adult's, aggressive cricoid pressure can compress the cricoid and obstruct the airway.
  - *Surgical airways are unavailable.* Surgical airway use is restricted to patients older than 6 to 10 years.
  - *Tube size is critical.* Selecting the appropriate tube diameter for children is critical. Too large a tube can cause tracheal edema and/or damage to the vocal cords, whereas too small a tube may not allow exchange of adequate ventilatory volumes. Table 15-7 lists general guidelines for selecting ETT size according to the child's age, and many tables or devices based on the child's age, weight, or length are available. Another guide for children's sizes is this formula:

    $$ETT\ size\ (mm) = (Age\ in\ years + 16) \div 4$$

    The correct tube size for an 8-year-old, for instance, would be $(8 + 16) \div 4$, or 6 mm. You can also determine correct tube size by matching the diameter of the child's smallest finger.
  - *Depth of ETT insertion is different.* The depth of insertion of the distal tip for

FIGURE 15-94 Foreign body removal with direct visualization and Magill forceps.

Table 15-7 Approximate Size of ETT for Pediatrics

Patient's Age	ETT Size	Type	Depth of ETT Insertion	Laryngoscope Blade Size
Premature infant	2.5–3.0	Uncuffed	8 cm	0 straight
Full-term infant	3.0–3.5	Uncuffed	8–9.5 cm	1 straight
Infant to 1 year	3.5–4.0	Uncuffed	9.5–11 cm	1 straight
Toddler	4.0–5.0	Uncuffed	11–12.5 cm	1–2 straight
Preschool	5.0–5.5	Uncuffed	12.5–14 cm	2 straight
School age	5.5–6.5	Uncuffed	14–20 cm	2 straight
Adolescent	7.0–8.0	Cuffed	20–23 cm	3 straight or curved

pediatric endotracheal tubes should be 2 to 3 cm below the vocal cords, as deeper insertion may result in mainstem intubation or injury to the carina. The uncuffed ETT has a black glottic marker at its distal end that should be placed at the level of the vocal cords. The cuffed ETT should be placed so that the cuff is just below the vocal cords. For detailed guidelines regarding the depth of insertion for different age groups, refer to Table 15-7. Alternatively, you can use the formula described earlier.

- **The occiput is relatively large.** Infants will often require a towel roll behind the shoulders to maintain an open airway, much the same way that older children and adults may require a towel roll behind the head.

- **The epiglottis is floppy and round ("omega" shaped).** A straight blade is usually preferred initially to control the epiglottis. An introducer may be useful if the glottis cannot be viewed.

- **The tongue is larger in relation to the oropharynx.** A curved blade may be useful to control the tongue during intubation.

- **The glottic opening is higher and more anterior in the neck.** Thus, it is easy to place the blade and tube too deep. External laryngeal manipulation (ELM) is useful to bring the glottis into view.

- **The narrowest part of the airway is the cricoid cartilage, not the glottic opening as in adults.** Uncuffed tubes were traditionally mandated on the theory that the narrow cricoid made the cuff unnecessary, although many current management protocols have changed, and cuffed tubes are being used more commonly. For now, most EMS services are still using uncuffed tubes for pediatric patients under the age of 8 years.

- **Greater vagal tone.** Infants and children are much more prone to bradycardia with hypotension during airway management, caused by hypoxemia or direct stimulation with the laryngoscope, or from succinylcholine. To prevent this complication, avoid long intubation attempts and be as gentle as possible during laryngoscopy. You must monitor heart rate throughout the procedure and stop the procedure to provide 100 percent oxygen by BVM ventilation or extraglottic airway device if the heart rate falls below 60 beats per minute in a child or below 80 beats per minute in an infant. You should also be prepared to give atropine (0.02 mg/kg, 0.1 mg minimum) by IV bolus, although this is never a substitute for oxygenation.

- **Higher basal metabolism combined with less functional residual capacity (smaller volume of air present in the lungs).** Children are more prone to a decrease in oxygen saturation during intubation attempts. Ensuring adequate preoxygenation, keeping intubation attempts short, and moving early to an extraglottic device are helpful precautions.

To perform endotracheal intubation on a pediatric patient (Procedure 15–3):

1. Use Standard Precautions.

2. Continue BVM ventilation with 100 percent oxygen while using a towel roll under the shoulders of an infant or towels under the head in older children (if not in cervical spine precautions) to achieve a sniffing position.

3. Prepare and check your equipment. As stated earlier, a straight blade is usually preferred in infants and small children, but it is suggested to have an age-appropriate curved blade available as well, in case tongue control becomes critical. With children younger than 8 years, you will either use an uncuffed endotracheal tube or a cuffed tube that is a half size smaller than calculated with standard formulas. Because of the short distance between the mouth and the trachea, you rarely need a stylet to position the tube properly. Remember to lubricate the ETT with water-soluble gel.

Procedure 15–3   Endotracheal Intubation in the Child

15-3A Ventilate the child.

15-3B Prepare the equipment.

15-3C Insert the laryngoscope.

15-3D Visualize the child's larynx and insert the ETT.

15-3E Ventilate, inflate the ETT cuff (if it is a cuffed tube), and auscultate.

15-3F Confirm placement with an ETCO$_2$ detector or waveform capnography.

(Continued)

15-3G Secure the tube.

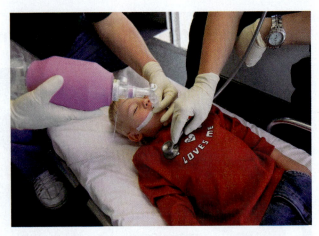

15-3H Reconfirm proper ETT placement.

4. In case of trauma, remove the front of the cervical collar and have an assistant maintain manual in-line stabilization of the cervical spine.

5. Hold the laryngoscope in your left hand and insert it gently into the right side of the patient's mouth. Do not attempt to sweep the tongue with a straight blade.

6. Advance the straight blade on the right side of the tongue with the tip directed toward the midline until the distal end reaches the base of the tongue. Alternatively, you may use the "hub technique" by initially advancing the straight blade gently into the esophagus as far as it will go without resistance, then withdrawing while performing ELM. If using a curved blade, sweep the tongue from right to left and advance in the midline.

7. Look for the tip of the epiglottis and gently lift with the tip of the blade while simultaneously performing ELM with an assistant's hand until the glottis or posterior cartilages are visualized. Keep in mind that a child—particularly an infant—has a shorter airway and a higher glottis than an adult. Because of this, you may see the cords much sooner than you expect.

8. If you cannot see the epiglottis, you are likely too deep. Gently and slowly withdraw while continuing to visualize until the vocal cords fall into view.

9. Grasp the endotracheal tube in your right hand and, under direct visualization of the vocal cords or posterior cartilages, insert it through the right corner of the patient's mouth into the glottic opening. Pass it through until the vocal cord marking on the tube is at the level of the cords or until the distal cuff of the ETT just disappears beyond the vocal cords. In some cases, advancing an endotracheal tube will be difficult at the level of the cricoid. Do not force the ETT through this region, as it may cause laryngeal edema and bleeding.

Confirm correct placement of the ETT. Hold the tube in place with your left hand, attach an age-appropriate bag-valve device to the 15/22-mm connector, and deliver several breaths with an end-tidal CO_2 detector in-line. For additional confirmation, observe for symmetrical chest rise and fall with each ventilation. Also auscultate for equal, bilateral breath sounds at the lateral chest wall, high in the axilla, and absent breath sounds over the epigastrium. An esophageal detector device may also be used for patients over 10 kg as long as you squeeze the bulb before attaching it to the tube.

10. If the tube has a distal cuff, do not inflate it unless there is a detectable air leak. If a leak is audible, inflate the distal cuff with just enough air to stop the leak.

11. Secure the ETT with tape or a commercial device, being very careful not to compress the tube. Note placement of the distance marker at the teeth/gums, recheck for proper placement, and continue ventilatory support. Periodically reassess ETT placement and watch the patient carefully for any clinical signs of difficulty. Continue ongoing waveform capnography monitoring if possible.

12. Place a gastric tube if allowed by protocol.

Monitoring Cuff Pressure

Several recent studies have shown that even experienced paramedics are unable to judge the pressure in an endotracheal tube cuff accurately by palpating the pilot balloon, and that cuff pressures may be way in excess of the recommended ranges. Similarly, we now know that excessive pressures can cause tracheal damage much sooner than previously thought. Combining these two pieces of information tells us that we must use extreme caution and vigilance regarding cuff pressures, because even if the prehospital transport time is short, it is unlikely that the hospital staff will assess cuff pressures in the initial management of a critically ill patient.

Ideally, cuff pressures would be assessed with a cuff manometer, but this is often not available. Second best is to place only enough air into the cuff to eliminate an audible leak. Providers may be surprised to find out that only 3 or 4 mL of air may be necessary to create an appropriate seal in some adults. A third option is to place only half the cuff volume, but this may leave the patient at risk for both aspiration and tissue damage. Finally, some providers will inflate the cuff with 10 mL of air but leave the syringe attached for 10 to 20 seconds to allow any back-pressure to release.[44]

Post-Intubation Agitation and Field Extubation

Occasionally, an intubated patient will awaken and be intolerant of the ETT. This happens most often with patients who undergo rapid sequence intubation and then awaken from the sedative agent and paralytic. This occurrence usually indicates inadequate sedation/analgesia and/or inappropriate ventilator settings. Paralytics alone should never be given to treat agitation, as the patient will be fully aware of the paralysis (a harrowing feeling), even though his outward signs of agitation will resolve.

Only rarely should extubation be considered in the field, because this may be associated with serious complications such as aspiration, laryngospasm, and negative-pressure pulmonary edema—not to mention that the patient may deteriorate again and be difficult to reintubate. If the patient is clearly able to maintain and protect his airway, is intolerant of the tube and ventilator, no medications are available to make him comfortable, and reassessment indicates that the problem that led to endotracheal intubation is resolved (such as a narcotic overdose), extubation may be indicated.

To perform field extubation:

1. Use Standard Precautions.
2. Ensure adequate oxygenation. A crude method for accomplishing this in the field is to be certain that the patient's mental status, skin color, and pulse oximetry are optimal on room air with the ETT in place.
3. Prepare intubation equipment and suction.
4. Confirm patient responsiveness.
5. Position patient on his side if possible.
6. Suction the patient's oropharynx.
7. Deflate the ETT cuff.
8. Remove the ETT upon cough or expiration.
9. Provide supplemental oxygen as indicated.
10. Reassess the adequacy of the patient's ventilation and oxygenation.

Cricothyrotomy

With proper training and frequent practice, including the use of rapid sequence procedures and newer technologies such as video laryngoscopy, you will be able to manage most airways in the field with BVM ventilation, an extraglottic airway device, or endotracheal intubation. Occasionally, though, extreme circumstances require a more invasive approach. In these situations, performing a cricothyrotomy may be the only way to ensure your patient's best chance for survival. Overall, however, the incidence of these procedures being performed in both the prehospital and hospital settings has fallen precipitously in the past five to ten years with the more widespread use of EGAs and RSI.

Two different techniques, **needle cricothyrotomy** (also called *transtracheal jet ventilation* or *transtracheal jet insufflation*) and **open cricothyrotomy**, both provide access to the airway through the cricothyroid membrane. A needle cricothyrotomy is generally the easier procedure but makes providing adequate ventilation more difficult; this approach is generally reserved for pediatric patients. The open cricothyrotomy technique is the more difficult procedure but allows for more effective oxygenation and ventilation. The open approach often takes longer than anticipated and has been associated with complications in up to 50 percent of cases. Therefore, you must master these techniques and reserve their use for situations in which you have exhausted your other options and have decided that no other means will establish an airway. Even when performed correctly, these procedures are highly invasive and prone to long-term complications, such as tracheal **stenosis**.

Indications that may warrant cricothyrotomy include situations that prevent adequate BVM ventilation, EGA placement, and endotracheal tube placement by the oral and nasal routes. An example is a patient with trismus (masseter muscle spasm that prevents opening the mouth), who cannot be oxygenated with a BVM ventilation, is also not a candidate for blind nasotracheal intubation, and presents in an EMS system that does not permit drug-facilitated airway management. Another example is a hypoxemic patient who has such severe facial trauma that BVM ventilation, EGA placement, and endotracheal intubation are not viable options. Other possible indications include total upper airway obstruction from epiglottitis or a foreign body, severe anaphylaxis, and burns to the face and respiratory tract.

Relative contraindications to performing cricothyrotomy in the field include inability to identify anatomical landmarks (including trauma and

> **CONTENT REVIEW**
> ► The only indication for a surgical airway is the inability to establish an airway by any other method.

short, fat necks), crush injury to the larynx, suspected tracheal transection, and underlying anatomical abnormalities such as tumor or subglottic stenosis. There are no absolute contraindications to cricothyrotomy.

Needle Cricothyrotomy

Needle cricothyrotomy involves placing a large-bore needle with plastic cannula, such as a 14-gauge intravenous catheter, through the cricothyroid membrane into the trachea. Oxygen must then be forced through this small-caliber device, using a bag-valve device or a high-pressure oxygen source. Ventilation by this route is called *transtracheal jet ventilation* or *transtracheal jet insufflation*. (*Insufflation* is blowing something into the body.)

Because very high pressures may insufflate large volumes of oxygen, **barotrauma**, including pneumothorax, is a potential complication. Exhalation is limited if it must take place through the same small-diameter catheter, which results in rising carbon dioxide levels. In some cases, the anatomy that required the needle cricothyrotomy for oxygenation does not impede normal exhalation.

In general, needle cricothyrotomy is considered a temporizing technique to be used for 30 minutes or less and restricted to pediatric patients in whom open cricothyrotomy is contraindicated. This technique has been removed from the paramedic scope of practice in some states because it is rarely used and there are few, if any, reports of it saving a life.

The potential complications of needle cricothyrotomy with jet ventilation include:

- Barotrauma from overinflation if using transtracheal jet insufflation
- Excessive bleeding due to improper catheter placement
- Subcutaneous emphysema from improper placement into the subcutaneous tissue, excessive air leak around the catheter, or laryngeal trauma
- Bleeding
- Hypoventilation and respiratory acidosis
- Aspiration, as the airway is unprotected

Needle Cricothyrotomy with Jet Ventilation Technique

To perform needle cricothyrotomy with jet ventilation:

1. Use Standard Precautions, including face mask and shield.

2. Manage the patient's airway as well as possible with basic maneuvers and supplemental oxygen while you prepare your equipment. Attach a large-bore IV needle with a catheter (adults: 14- or 16-gauge; children: 18- or 20-gauge) to a 10- or 20-mL syringe. If time permits

FIGURE 15-95 Anatomic landmarks for cricothyrotomy.

you may fill the syringe with sterile water or saline to facilitate detection of air when aspirating.

3. Place the patient supine and hyperextend the head and neck. (Maintain neutral position if you suspect cervical spine injury.) Position yourself at the patient's side.

4. Palpate the inferior portion of the thyroid cartilage and the cricoid cartilage. The indention between the two is the cricothyroid membrane (Figures 15-95 and 15-96).

5. Prepare the anterior neck with antiseptic solution.

6. Firmly grasp the laryngeal cartilages and reconfirm the site of the cricothyroid membrane.

7. Carefully insert the needle into the cricothyroid membrane at midline, directed 45° caudally (toward the feet) (Figure 15-97). Often you will feel a pop as the needle penetrates the membrane.

FIGURE 15-96 Locate/palpate the cricothyroid membrane.

FIGURE 15-97 Proper positioning for cricothyroid puncture.

8. Advance the needle while aspirating with the syringe. If air returns easily, the catheter is in the trachea. If blood returns or you feel resistance to return, reevaluate needle placement.

9. After you confirm proper placement, hold the needle steady and advance the catheter. Then withdraw the needle (Figure 15-98).

10. Reconfirm placement by again withdrawing air from the catheter with the syringe. Secure the catheter in place (Figure 15-99).

11. Attach the jet-ventilation device to the catheter and a 50-psi oxygen supply. If this is unavailable, you may connect a bag-valve device to the catheter using the inner adapter from a 7.5-mm endotracheal tube. The bag-valve device must be connected to oxygen.

FIGURE 15-98 Advance the catheter with the needle.

12. Open the release valve to introduce an oxygen jet into the trachea (Figure 15-100). Then adjust the pressure to allow adequate lung expansion (usually about 50 psi, compared with about 1 psi through a regulator).

13. Watch the chest carefully, turning off the release valve as soon as the chest rises. Exhalation then occurs passively through the glottis as a result of elastic recoil of the lungs and chest wall. Deliver at least 20 breaths per minute, keeping the inflation-to-deflation time approximately 1:3. Keep in mind that you may need to adjust this to the patient's needs, particularly in COPD and asthma patients, who often require a longer expiration time.

FIGURE 15-99 Cannula properly placed in the trachea.

FIGURE 15-100 Jet ventilation with needle cricothryotomy.

14. Continue ventilatory support, assessing for adequacy of ventilations and looking for the development of any potential complications.

15. You should be anticipating the need for an alternative means of oxygenation and ventilation within approximately 30 minutes.

Open Cricothyrotomy

An open, or surgical, cricothyrotomy involves placing an endotracheal or tracheostomy tube directly into the trachea through a surgical incision at the cricothyroid membrane. Open cricothyrotomy is preferred to needle cricothyrotomy in older pediatric patients and adult patients, because it allows for enhanced oxygenation and ventilation and protects the airway against aspiration. The greater potential complications of open cricothyrotomy mandate even more training and skills monitoring than for the needle method.

Indications are the same as for needle cricothyrotomy. Contraindications are the same as for needle cricothyrotomy with the addition that open cricothyrotomy is contraindicated in children under the age of 8 because the cricothyroid membrane is small and underdeveloped.

The potential complications of open cricothyrotomy with jet ventilation include:

- Incorrect tube placement into a false passage
- Cricoid and/or thyroid cartilage damage
- Thyroid gland damage
- Severe bleeding
- Laryngeal nerve damage
- Subcutaneous emphysema
- Vocal cord damage
- Infection

Open Cricothyrotomy Traditional Technique

To perform open cricothyrotomy by the traditional technique (Procedure 15–4):

1. Use Standard Precautions, including face mask and shield.

2. Use BVM ventilation and supplemental oxygen to maintain oxygenation and ventilation as well as possible while preparing supplies.

3. Locate the thyroid cartilage and the cricoid cartilage. Identify the cricothyroid membrane between these two cartilages.

4. Clean the area with antiseptic solution.

5. Stabilize the cartilages with one hand, while using a scalpel in the other hand to make a 2- to 4-cm vertical skin incision in the midline over the membrane.

6. Locate the cricothyroid membrane again, using blunt dissection if necessary.

7. Make a 1- to 2-cm incision in the horizontal plane through the membrane.

8. Insert a tracheal hook on the inferior portion of the thyroid cartilage to help maintain the opening. This may also be improvised with an adult or pediatric stylet.

9. Insert curved hemostats into the membrane incision and spread it open.

10. Insert either a cuffed endotracheal tube or a tracheostomy tube into the opening, directing the tube distally into the trachea. Ideally a 6-mm tube will fit, although smaller patients may require a smaller size.

11. Inflate the cuff and ventilate.

12. Confirm placement with multiple methods as available and appropriate.

13. Secure the tube in place.

Procedure 15–4   Open Cricothyrotomy

15-4A Locate the cricothyroid membrane.

15-4B Stabilize the larynx and make a 1- to 2-cm skin incision over the cricothyroid membrane.

15-4C Make a 1-cm horizontal incision through the cricothyroid membrane.

15-4D Using a curved hemostat, spread the membrane incision open.

15-4E Insert an ETT (6.0 or 7.0) or Shiley (6.0 or 8.0).

(Continued)

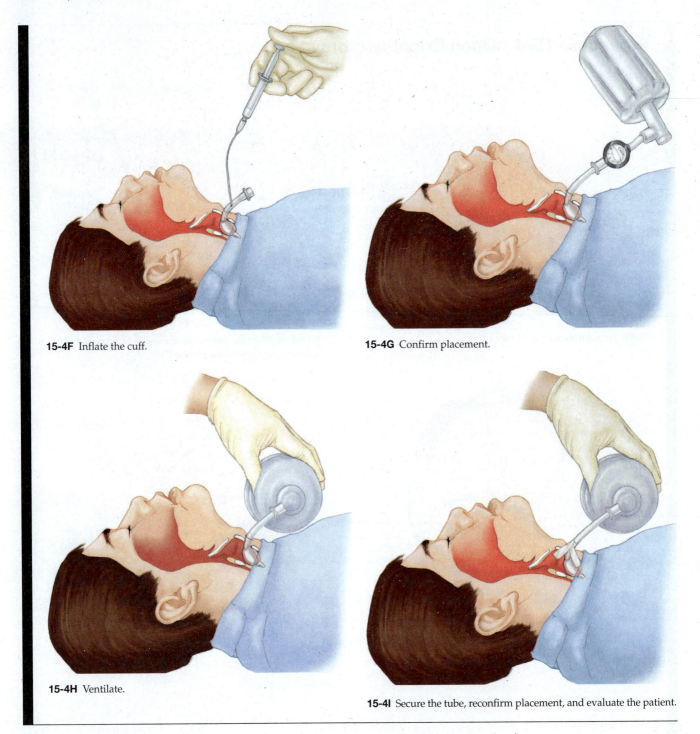

15-4F Inflate the cuff.

15-4G Confirm placement.

15-4H Ventilate.

15-4I Secure the tube, reconfirm placement, and evaluate the patient.

Open Cricothyrotomy Technique Variations

Variations on the traditional open cricothyrotomy technique include the rapid four-step technique and the bougie-aided technique.

- *Rapid four-step.* In this technique, a single incision is made horizontally through the skin and cricoid membrane, then a tracheal hook is held in the left hand and traction is applied against the cricoid membrane, directed toward the feet, and the tube is inserted with the right hand, mimicking endotracheal intubation.

This technique has been associated with more complications in some studies.

- *Bougie-aided.* An endotracheal tube introducer (bougie) may be used with either the traditional or the rapid four-step technique to minimize the risk of placement in a false passage, to allow the operator to let go without losing critical landmarks, and to ease threading of the tube. In the simplest version of this technique, an adult bougie is passed into the trachea through the incision in the cricothyroid membrane, directed distally, and intratracheal placement is confirmed with palpation of clicks as the bougie passes over the cartilage rings and/or palpation of hold-up within 20 cm. Note that the distance to hold-up is much shorter than when using the introducer/bougie through the mouth. Once placement is confirmed, the endotracheal or tracheostomy tube is threaded over the bougie into the trachea.

Minimally Invasive Percutaneous Cricothyrotomy

A number of hybrid techniques are available to perform a cricothyrotomy using a needle but allowing for a much larger diameter ventilation catheter. Some of these techniques involve devices that are placed blindly and that consist of the needle, a dilator, and a catheter, all in one. Other methods are based on the Seldinger technique (the same technique used for central line insertion), in which a guidewire is placed through a needle, which is then removed so that dilators and the ventilation tube may be placed into the trachea over the guidewire.

In general, there is no advantage to these needle techniques over the open techniques, and complications may actually be higher, although there is substantial variation among devices and techniques. Individual agencies should consult their medical director and evaluate each device and technique on a case-by-case basis. We cannot stress enough that you must continually practice this skill with the medical director's involvement to maintain proficiency.

Medication-Assisted Intubation

Medication-assisted intubation (MAI), which is also called drug-assisted or pharmacologically assisted intubation, is becoming more common. MAI may take several forms, including rapid sequence intubation (RSI) and sedation-facilitated intubation.

MAI techniques give you the option of managing airways that you could not otherwise manage because the patient is too awake or has trismus, and they are used early in the clinical course when the procedure may be easier and the patient has more reserve to tolerate complications.

The flip side is that these procedures come with great risk, as you are employing very powerful medications that may result—and have resulted—in severe morbidity and death when the paramedic is unable to intubate and cannot maintain adequate oxygenation through other means. In the setting of cardiac arrest, of course, you cannot realistically make the situation any worse. MAI, however, is employed in patients who are alive and sometimes conscious, when both the potential benefits and the potential harms are greater.[45–51]

The current evidence has not found a survival benefit to prehospital RSI outside the air-medical setting, and in some cases survival rates are notably worse with RSI. Despite this literature, some EMS services have been able to employ these techniques safely and with apparent advantage to their patients, but it takes a great deal of initial and ongoing training, active medical director involvement, a thorough quality assurance program, and the maturity to select patients carefully and move early to backup devices.

Rapid Sequence Intubation

Your immediate concern with every patient you treat is to maintain a patent airway and adequate oxygenation and ventilation (except for patients in cardiac arrest, in whom chest compressions would come first). Clearly, if a patient is in cardiac arrest (once circulation has been attended to) or is in respiratory arrest, or is unconscious or obtunded and not protecting his airway, airway management with BVM ventilation, an EGA, or intubation is indicated.

Occasionally, however, you may encounter an awake patient with an airway disorder who is hypoxemic despite high-concentration oxygen via a nonrebreather or CPAP and therapy directed at the underlying problem. This patient is working hard to breathe but does not have adequate gas exchange to support life. Subtle altered mental status may indicate that some level of significant hypoxemia is putting essential brain functions at risk.

Assisting respirations with a BVM on such a patient is challenging because of patient anxiety. Nasal intubation is difficult and often exacerbates hypoxemia. You cannot perform oral intubation on this patient until he fatigues enough to have respiratory failure, with resultant unconsciousness and decreased muscle tone leading to loss of a gag reflex. By then, however, the patient will have suffered prolonged hypoxemia, possibly accompanied by myocardial infarction, brain or kidney damage, or vomiting with aspiration.

If a patient clearly is precipitously failing maximal aggressive medical management, or if the history of his problem clearly indicates that he will not be able to, or already cannot, protect his airway, then active intervention is appropriate to control the airway and provide adequate ventilation.

One potential solution to this problem is rapid sequence intubation (RSI). Classic rapid sequence *induction* is a procedure borrowed from anesthesia

> **CONTENT REVIEW**
>
> ➤ If a patient is precipitously failing maximal aggressive medical management and will be or already is unable to protect his airway, active intervention—such as RSI—is appropriate.

and modified in emergency medicine and EMS to become rapid sequence *intubation*.

RSI involves a series of steps that includes administration of a neuromuscular blocking drug to a critically ill or injured patient, who is presumed to have a full stomach, to facilitate oral intubation without aspiration or other complications. The procedure is called "rapid" because the individual steps are performed in "rapid succession," one right after the other, not because the entire procedure is fast. In fact, RSI can take quite a bit of time in some cases.

The entire RSI procedure is intended to minimize the risk of aspiration in a high-risk population. This requires preoxygenation and avoiding positive pressure ventilation when possible. The risks of RSI are very substantial, since a patient undergoing the procedure is, by definition, breathing, yet you are giving the patient medications that will eliminate his respiratory drive and his ability to protect his own airway from aspiration.

Potential indications include those listed next. Note, however, that the fact that a patient meets a stated indication for RSI does not mean that this is the best thing to do for that individual patient.

Indications

- Impending or actual respiratory failure from any cause
- Impending or actual inability to protect the airway from any cause
- Combativeness secondary to presumed head trauma
- Hypoxemia despite maximal therapy

Relative Contraindications

- Predicted difficult airway
- Short ETA to hospital or more experienced providers
- Only one paramedic on scene
- Ability to manage the patient with less risky procedures
- When the only indication is airway protection

Absolute Contraindications

- Respiratory arrest
- Cardiac arrest

Preoxygenation

The air we are all breathing at this very moment is only 21 percent oxygen, regardless of your location or altitude; the remaining 79 percent is nearly all nitrogen. If all the nitrogen in your lungs were replaced with oxygen, you would have nearly five times the oxygen present now. This is what occurs with preoxygenation. Hence, preoxygenation is sometimes called "denitrogenation" or "nitrogen washout." This fivefold increase in oxygen in the lungs creates an oxygen reserve that the body can

draw on once a patient has been administered a paralytic agent and ceases to breathe.

Patients with healthy lungs and adequate functional residual capacity may develop enough reserve from preoxygenation to survive up to 8 minutes of medication-induced apnea without desaturation (loss of blood oxygen saturation). Thus, preoxygenation allows us to chemically paralyze a patient yet withhold positive pressure ventilation, thereby limiting the risk of gastric insufflation and subsequent aspiration, without the patient becoming hypoxemic.

Unfortunately, many critically ill or injured patients cannot tolerate 8 minutes of apnea. Common clinical variables that affect the amount of apnea time a patient can withstand before becoming hypoxic include age, obesity, pregnancy, lung disease, baseline saturations, acute illness, and more (Table 15-8). Children, for instance, have shorter apnea times in large part because of their increased basal metabolism. Some patients, such as those with fever, shock, alcohol withdrawal, and cocaine/amphetamine intoxication, have substantially increased oxygen demand and "chew through" their reserve very quickly. Obese and pregnant patients have less reserve in large part because of limited functional residual capacity.[52]

In most cases, preoxygenation will be accomplished with a tight-fitting nonrebreather mask with 10–15 lpm flow for at least 3 minutes. Such a system delivers 70 to 90 percent oxygen and is sufficient for most patients. A bag-valve mask may be used *without* positive pressure to deliver 100 percent oxygen if desired. If positive pressure must be used due to patient hypoxia, concentrate on good technique to minimize air entry into the stomach.

After preoxygenation, patients may be roughly categorized as having "adequate," "limited," or "no" reserve, which generally dictates the preoxygenation preparations

Table 15-8 High-Risk Characteristics That Decrease Oxygen Reserve

Characteristics That Decrease Oxygen Reserve
Decreased Oxygen Storage Capacity
• Elderly • Obesity • Pregnancy • Lung disease: acute, chronic, acute-on-chronic • Chest trauma • Baseline hypoxemia
Increased Oxygen Consumption
• Fever/sepsis • Severe pain • Alcohol withdrawal • Cocaine/methamphetamine intoxication • Tachycardia • Shock • Children

Table 15-9 Patient Categorization and Preparations Following Preoxygenation

Preoxygenation Categories and Preparations

Adequate Reserve—Oxygen Saturation Near 100%

- Positive pressure ventilation usually not necessary
- Potential false sense of security if patients have high-risk characteristics

Limited Reserve—Oxygen Saturation 90–97%

- Some patients will require careful BMV ventilation
- Be prepared to abort intubation attempt
- Have rescue airway immediately available: not necessary to remove from package in advance

No Reserve—Oxygen Saturation Below 90%

- Positive pressure ventilation is unavoidable
- Consider CPAP/BiPAP or assisted respirations before medication
- Consider planned PPV with BVM or SGA after medication and before intubation
- Have rescue airway immediately ready for insertion: out of package and lubricated

that should be made (Table 15-9). Patients with underlying lung disease, especially acute or acute-on-chronic disease resulting in hypoxemia, are a particularly scary group to intubate because they are hypoxic to begin with, and they are prone to very rapid desaturation after medication.

Patho Pearl

Importance of Head Elevation. Research has demonstrated that preoxygenation is more successful for most patients with at least 20 degrees of head elevation; this is especially true for obese patients. This is yet another reason that all trauma patients in spinal precautions should be considered difficult intubations. The inability to elevate the patient's head limits preoxygenation, and that, in turn, limits the amount of time you will have to perform the procedure. This also emphasizes the importance of keeping patients, particularly those with respiratory distress, in their position of comfort as long as their mental status allows.

Patients with a saturation of 100 percent after preoxygenation have an "adequate reserve," those with less than 100 percent but above 90 percent have "limited reserve," and those with less than 90 percent have "no reserve." In the first group (adequate reserve), the goal should be no positive pressure ventilation, although some patients, particularly those with any of the high-risk characteristics listed in Table 15-8, may still desaturate quickly.

In the second group (limited reserve), the clinician should plan to optimize first-pass success and anticipate that some patients will require careful positive pressure ventilation if the intubation attempt is prolonged.

In the last group (no reserve), positive pressure ventilation is unavoidable; the clinician should consider CPAP/BiPAP or assisted respirations before medication and be prepared to provide immediate optimal BVM ventilation and to place a rescue airway if saturations cannot be maintained. Many inexperienced providers faced with a patient who is desaturating make the mistake of waiting too long to abort the procedure, trying even harder or trying "just one more time," only to face critical hypoxia and cardiac arrest.

Airway Pharmacology

PREMEDICATIONS Premedications are drugs given early in the course of RSI to mitigate anticipated complications. Examples are lidocaine (to blunt the rise in intracranial pressure [ICP] associated with succinylcholine and laryngoscopy) and atropine (to prevent the bradycardia associated with succinylcholine in children).

As it turns out, none of these agents are required. Few have been proven to do what they were hoped to do, and all are associated with some potential adverse effects. The movement in the last few years has been away from the routine use of premedications.

The following are agents that might still be considered if time and protocols permit:

- *Fentanyl.* At routine doses, fentanyl is an excellent analgesic (pain reliever) that may keep a patient more comfortable during a painful procedure such as intubation. At higher doses, fentanyl is a sympatholytic agent that blunts the hypertension, tachycardia, and ICP elevation associated with laryngoscopy. It is reasonable to consider giving all patients analgesic doses of fentanyl at least 3 minutes before the procedure and higher doses to patients at risk for life-threatening elevations of ICP. Although fentanyl is highly regarded for its hemodynamic (blood flow/blood pressure) stability, it may occasionally cause hypotension (a drop in blood pressure) in patients who are dependent on their sympathetic drive for blood pressure maintenance, especially at higher doses.

- *Atropine.* Succinylcholine is associated with bradycardia (slow heartbeat) in younger children and in any patient receiving a second dose. Historically, atropine was recommended routinely 2 to 3 minutes before administration of succinylcholine to children less than 6 to 8 years of age to reduce the risk of bradycardia. Evidence now shows that this is optional, although atropine must always be at the bedside.

- *Lidocaine.* Although lidocaine is commonly used in head injury patients to blunt an increase in ICP, there has been a movement away from this practice in some circles because of limited evidence for benefit and the potential risk of hypotension as well as time delays.

There is evidence that lidocaine is useful in asthmatic patients to avoid or lessen bronchospasm triggered by airway manipulation.[53]

INDUCTION AGENTS The purpose of an induction agent is to render the patient unaware during the procedure. Some EMS RSI protocols call for the use of induction agents only in awake patients. Because it is impossible to know how aware an unconscious patient might be, we recommend routine use for any patient who requires RSI (Table 15-10). Common induction agents used in EMS include the following:

- *Etomidate.* Etomidate is a great agent for induction because it rarely causes any rise or drop in blood pressure or pulse. It also works extremely fast, with a relatively consistent dose response. There has been concern about suppression of adrenal gland function in septic patients, but thus far there is no evidence that this is a significant enough safety concern to cause EMS to avoid it.
- *Midazolam.* Midazolam is a benzodiazepine sedative/hypnotic. The major advantage of midazolam is amnesia. That is, the patient is unlikely to recall the procedure. The major disadvantage is that the dose required for induction is commonly associated with hypotension. It is also hard to predict the dose that will make any particular patient unaware.
- *Ketamine.* Ketamine is a dissociative agent that is being used more in emergency medicine and critical care transport with some use in EMS as well. The advantages of ketamine are that it has a predictable dose response, does not cause hypotension, and provides analgesia as well as sedation. The major disadvantage is hypertension and tachycardia in some

patients. There used to be concern about using ketamine in patients with head trauma and stroke, but that has largely been disproved as long as the patient is not hypertensive.

- *Propofol.* Propofol is commonly used in the hospital for induction, but its use is limited in EMS by potentially profound hypotension.

NEUROMUSCULAR BLOCKING AGENTS (PARALYTICS) Paralytics, or neuromuscular blocking agents, are drugs that temporarily stop skeletal muscle function without affecting cardiac or smooth muscle. The two primary categories are competitive and noncompetitive agents. The competitive agents have a dose response such that the higher the dose, the quicker the paralysis takes place but the longer it lasts. Competitive agents are nondepolarizing; that is, they do not cause fasciculations (muscle twitches) and generally have fewer adverse effects and contraindications. Noncompetitive agents have a much more limited dose response such that the onset time and duration are somewhat fixed as long as a reasonable dose is used. The noncompetitive agents are also called depolarizing agents because they cause fasciculations before the onset of paralysis.[54–56]

- *Succinylcholine.* Succinylcholine is the prototype noncompetitive depolarizing neuromuscular blocker. Because of its fast onset (about 45 seconds) and short duration (about 8 minutes), this is the preferred agent for most EMS services. Unfortunately, succinylcholine has a host of potential adverse effects (Table 15-11) that result in a number of contraindications that must be considered in all patients. Succinylcholine is not routinely recommended for maintaining paralysis, so a second competitive agent must usually be carried as well.

Table 15-10 Guidelines for Sedative (Induction) Agents

Induction Agent	Dose	Onset	Duration (min)	Advantages	Disadvantages
Midazolam (Versed)	0.1–0.3 mg/kg	1–3 min	20–30 min	Amnesia effects, good sedative	Hypotension
Diazepam (Valium)	0.2–0.5 mg/kg	2–3 min	30–40 min	Amnesia effects	Hypotension, respiratory depression
Etomidate (Amidate)	0.3 mg/kg	1–2 min	5 min	Little effect on blood pressure, decreases intracranial pressure (ICP)	Suppresses cortisol, not good for head-injured patients
Ketamine (Ketalar)	1–2 mg/kg	1 min	10–20 min	Decreases bronchospasm, little hypotension, amnesia	Increases ICP
Sodium thiopental	3–5 mg/kg	1 min	5 min	Blunts ICP changes	Significant hypotension, bronchospasm
Propofol (Diprivan)	1–1.5 mg/kg	1 min	3–5 min	Rapid onset, good sedative effects	Significant hypotension
Fentanyl	3–5 mcg/kg	1–2 min	30–40 min	Little effect on blood pressure; blunts ICP changes	Can cause muscle rigidity in chest wall

Table 15-11 Contraindications to Succinylcholine

Contraindications to Succinylcholine (may exaggerate hyperkalemia)
Disease/Injury
Neuromuscular diseases • Muscular dystrophies • Myopathies • Guillain-Barré
Stroke
Parkinson's disease (severe)
Tetanus
Botulism
Rhabdomyolysis
Burns >24–28 hours old
Spinal cord injury (>72 hours and <9 months old)
Prolonged immobility/paralysis
Severe infection (abdominal and neurologic)
Severe trauma (especially musculoskeletal)

- *Rocuronium.* Rocuronium is now the most commonly used competitive agent in emergency medicine and EMS. The onset time with rocuronium is only slightly longer than with succinylcholine (60 seconds) as long as higher doses are used. At the recommended intubation doses, rocuronium may last 30 minutes or longer. Although this is often used as an argument against rocuronium for EMS use, it is used successfully by many services that argue that even 8 minutes is too long with succinylcholine before moving on to a rescue airway. Rocuronium has few adverse effects and may be used for initial and ongoing paralysis.

- *Vecuronium.* Vecuronium is a competitive agent that is commonly used to maintain paralysis after succinylcholine. Vecuronium is a second- or third-line agent for RSI because of its long onset time. Although there are tricks that may be used to shorten the onset time, they add complexity and a very long duration of action.

SEDATIVES AND ANALGESICS Sedatives and analgesics are essential for keeping a patient comfortable after intubation. Both analgesia and sedation should be provided to every patient who is chemically paralyzed, unless contraindicated by hypotension, and to all other patients, unless you are confident that the patient is comfortable, such as an un-paralyzed post–cardiac-arrest patient who is completely unresponsive.

- *Narcotics.* Narcotics are critical to provide analgesia. Fentanyl is used most commonly because it has a rapid onset and minimal effects on blood pressure unless the patient is sympathetic dependent. Other narcotics such as morphine may also be used cautiously.

- *Benzodiazepines.* Benzodiazepines are optimal for keeping patients sedated while intubated. Midazolam is a favorite among critical care transport crews because of its rapid onset and short duration. Lorazepam and diazepam may also be used. All benzodiazepines must be used cautiously in volume depleted and hypotensive patients.

- *Propofol.* Propofol infusions are commonly used in the intensive care unit and during critical care transport to maintain sedation. The very short duration of action facilitates neurologic examination when the infusion is stopped. Propofol is even more prone to cause hypotension than the benzodiazepines and must be used cautiously.

RSI Procedure

To perform a typical rapid sequence intubation, there are 10 steps, as listed next. As with other airway procedures, be sure to begin with Standard Precautions.

1. *Preoxygenate* to achieve nitrogen washout and create an oxygen reserve (as discussed earlier). Use a nonrebreather mask with high-concentration oxygen for at least 3 minutes, if possible. Consider CPAP, assisted respiration, and BVM ventilation as indicated. Avoid positive pressure if the patient is not hypoxemic.

2. *Protect the C-spine* if indicated. The front of the cervical collar should be removed and manual in-line stabilization performed by an assistant who is also ready to perform a jaw-thrust maneuver.

3. *Position optimally* if possible. Patients not in cervical precautions should be placed in sniffing or ramped position.

4. *Assign provider to initiate external laryngeal manipulation* if sufficient assistance is available, upon request. Until the laryngoscopy blade is introduced, maintain the larynx in its normal position. External laryngeal manipulation should be implemented as directed by the intubator.

5. *Ponder* whether intubation is really necessary. Are there other management options, if this is likely to be a difficult airway? Use a checklist, if possible.

6. *Premedicate* if time permits and allowed by protocol and scope of practice. Consider regular-dose fentanyl for most patients, high-dose fentanyl for suspected critical ICP, and lidocaine for severe asthmatics.

7. *Prepare equipment,* using a checklist to ensure that all supplies are ready. This includes intubation, BVM ventilation, rescue, and post-intubation supplies.

8. *Sedate and paralyze,* using appropriate medications and doses. Most patients should receive both an induction

agent and paralytic. The induction agent should routinely be given before the paralytic.

9. *Pass the tube* with direct or indirect visualization or an endotracheal tube introducer. Use all available adjunctive techniques including external laryngeal manipulation (ELM). Monitor oxygenation and be ready to abort the attempt *before* the oxygen level reaches critical point. In most cases, where the patient is adequately preoxygenated and has a saturation of 100 percent beforehand, the attempt should be stopped when the saturation reaches about 93 percent.

10. *Post-intubation management* begins with objective tube confirmation, using capnography. Lung sounds should be used to help guide tube depth. A bite block should be inserted, and the tube should be secured in place and the cervical collar replaced if indicated. The patient should be placed on the transport ventilator including in-line continuous capnography. The patient should then receive analgesia and sedation. Ongoing paralysis should be administered only if absolutely necessary to manage the patient on the ventilator and never without analgesia and sedation. Monitor oxygen saturation (SpO_2), end-tidal CO_2, blood pressure, clinical exam, and ventilator parameters.

Rapid Sequence Airway

Rapid sequence airway (RSA) is a new airway management technique in which the preparation and pharmacology of RSI is paired with intentional placement of an extraglottic airway device, without prior attempt at direct laryngoscopy, in selected patients. The theoretical advantages to RSA over RSI include less hypoxemia, less airway trauma, and no risk of tube misplacement. The major risks are aspiration and ineffective ventilation. The risk of aspiration is offset by fewer airway attempts and new gastric-isolation EADs that achieve an excellent seal pressure and also allow for gastric decompression. The risk of ineffective ventilation is offset through careful patient and device selection.

RSA Indications

- Same as RSI

Absolute RSA Contraindications

- Upper airway pathology known or suspected
- Blunt or penetrating anterior neck trauma
- Inhalation injury
- Angioedema
- Anaphylaxis
- Upper airway tumor
- Obstructing upper airway infection—croup, epiglottitis, parapharyngeal abscess
- Caustic ingestion

Relative RSA Contraindications

- Patient's airway may be managed by other means
- Anticipated inability to ventilate by BVM
- Anticipated need for very high airway pressures
- Very high aspiration risk
- Short ETA to hospital or arrival of help with more resources
- Only one paramedic on scene

The Difficult Airway

As a paramedic, you will be expected to be able to effectively manage patients when establishing and maintaining an airway may be difficult. It has been estimated that 1 out of 10 endotracheal intubations can be classified as "difficult," and intubation may be impossible in 1 out of 100 patients when conventional techniques (including straight-blade, ELM, and introducers) are attempted.[57–58]

It is important, however, to think globally in terms of the difficult airway rather than considering only difficult intubation. The concept of the difficult airway includes difficult BVM ventilation, difficult extraglottic airway placement and ventilation, difficult intubation, and difficult cricothyrotomy.

- *Difficult bag-valve-mask ventilation:* a clinical situation in which a paramedic anticipates or experiences difficulty maintaining an adequate saturation (usually >90%) using high-concentration oxygen, basic airway adjuncts, and two-person technique.

- *Difficult extraglottic airway:* a clinical situation in which a paramedic anticipates or experiences difficult inserting or ventilating with an extraglottic airway device.

- *Difficult intubation:* a clinical situation in which a paramedic anticipates or experiences difficulty visualizing the vocal cords or posterior cartilages within one optimal attempt and without the patient developing hypoxemia.

- *Difficult cricothyrotomy:* a clinical situation in which a paramedic anticipates or experiences difficulty obtaining a surgical airway in less than 60 seconds.

- *Difficult airway:* a clinical situation in which a paramedic anticipates or experiences difficulty with any critical portion of airway management, including BVM ventilation, extraglottic airway placement, endotracheal intubation, or surgical cricothyrotomy.

> **CONTENT REVIEW**
> ➤ Difficult Airway Factors
> - Difficult BVM ventilation
> - Difficult extraglottic airway placement
> - Difficult intubation
> - Difficult cricothyrotomy

Predictors of a Difficult Airway or Ventilation

It would be useful if we could reliably predict which airways are likely to cause difficulty and which will not (Table 15-12). This is particularly important if you are considering a medication-facilitated airway procedure. For patients for whom we anticipate difficulty, we could call for help in advance, consider deferring the procedure, consider managing the airway with BVM ventilation or an extraglottic device, or simply be better prepared, such as having different blades or devices, an introducer, a backup airway, and cricothyrotomy supplies immediately available. In most emergency situations, however, a detailed airway assessment may not be practical. In many such cases, management must proceed, even when airway assessment predicts difficulty, because of patient acuity and a favorable risk-to-benefit analysis.

Table 15-12 Predictors of Difficult Airway and Ventilation

Predictors of Difficult Airway and Ventilation
Difficult Bag-Valve-Mask Ventilation Predictors
• Facial trauma   • Facial hair   • Obesity   • Lack of teeth (and without dentures)   • History of snoring   • Mallampati grade 3 or 4   • Severely limited jaw protrusion   • Thyromental distance less than 6 cm
Difficult Extraglottic Airway Insertion or Ventilation Predictors
• Limited mouth opening   • Massive secretions   • Morbid obesity   • Severe pulmonary disease   • Pathology below the device (e.g., inhalation burns, laryngeal trauma, angioedema)
Difficult Laryngoscopy and Orotracheal Intubation Predictors
• Facial trauma or anomalies   • Increasing Mallampati grade   • Short thyromental distance   • Short sternomental distance   • Limited mouth opening   • Limited neck mobility   • Obesity   • Buckteeth
Difficult Surgical Airway (Cricothyrotomy) Placement

• Cricothyroid membrane cannot be located:
   • Morbid obesity
   • Anterior neck trauma
   • Prior radiation therapy
   • Ludwig's angina (skin infection to anterior neck)
 • Tube insertion prevented by conditions within airway lumen:
   • Tumor
   • Infection
   • Swelling
   • Foreign body

Predictors of difficult BVM ventilation include facial trauma, facial hair, obesity, and lack of teeth (assuming you don't have the dentures to replace during BVM ventilation). Other risk factors for difficult BVM ventilation demonstrated in the anesthesia literature include age over 55, history of snoring, Mallampati class 3 or 4 (discussed later), severely limited jaw protrusion, and thyromental distance (the distance between the thyroid notch and the bony point of the chin) less than 6 cm.

Predictors of difficult extraglottic airway (EGA) device placement include limited mouth opening. Situations in which an EGA may be inserted easily but where it may be difficult to ventilate the patient include massive secretions, morbid obesity, severe pulmonary disease, and pathology below the device, such as inhalation burns, laryngeal trauma, and angioedema.

Commonly used predictors of difficult laryngoscopy and intubation include facial trauma/anomalies, increasing Mallampati class (discussed later), short thyromental distance, short sternomental distance (distance between the suprasternal notch and the bony point of the chin), limited mouth opening, limited neck mobility, obesity, and buckteeth.

Predictors of difficult surgical airway placement include situations in which the cricothyroid membrane cannot be located—such as morbid obesity, anterior neck trauma, prior radiation therapy, and infection such as Ludwig's angina (a very serious skin infection that tracks down into the anterior neck, usually from a dental infection)—and situations in which a tumor, infection, swelling, or foreign body within the airway lumen prevents tube insertion, even when the membrane can be located.

Difficult Airway Scoring Systems

Various difficult airway scoring systems have been developed to aid the clinician in detecting and managing the difficult airway. The most frequently used system of pre-intubation airway assessment is the **Mallampati classification system** (Figure 15-101). With this system, the tonsillar pillars and the uvula are assessed. The more concealed the tonsillar pillars and the uvula, the more difficult the intubation. Based on these features, the patient's airway is classified into four classes. The higher the class, the more difficult the airway is expected to be.

Class I: Entire tonsil clearly visible

Class II: Upper half of tonsil fossa visible

Class III: Soft and hard palate clearly visible

Class IV: Only hard palate visible

CONTENT REVIEW

➤ Difficult Airway Scoring Systems
  • Mallampati classification system
  • Cormack and LeHane grading system
  • POGO scoring system

Class I   Class II   Class III   Class IV

Grade I   Grade II   Grade III   Grade IV

FIGURE 15-101 Airway scoring systems. Mallampati classification system (top); Cormack and LeHane classification system (bottom).

Rarely will a paramedic have time to assess the Mallampati class prior to intubation attempts. The Mallampati assessment is done with the patient awake and sitting up. The patient opens his mouth and sticks his tongue out. Recognizing that the Mallampati system is of little use in the unconscious patient, Cormack and LeHane adapted the system to classify the view one sees with a laryngoscope. The **Cormack and LeHane grading system** is similar to Mallampati's (see Figure 15-101).

Grade 1: Entire glottic opening and vocal cords may be seen.

Grade 2: Epiglottis and posterior portion of glottic opening may be seen with a partial view of vocal cords.

Grade 3: Only epiglottis and (sometimes) posterior cartilages seen.

Grade 4: Neither epiglottis nor glottis seen.

A similar system used in EMS is the percentage of glottic opening (POGO) system. With the **POGO scoring system,** the percentage of the glottis that can be visualized is scored. The score ranges from 0 (none of the glottis visualized) to 100 (vocal cords fully visualized). This system also helps to predict the difficulty of endotracheal intubation (Figure 15-102).

As you may already have figured out, airway classification systems such as Mallampati, Cormack and LeHane, and POGO, though very helpful in more controlled or leisurely environments, have little application to emergency medicine. This is especially so in the case of the austere prehospital environment. However, knowing the features of these classification systems can help you to better anticipate the difficult airway.

"LEMONS"

"LEMONS" is an acronym that can be used to remember assessments and findings associated with a difficult airway. Factors that have been assembled into the LEMONS mnemonic can encompass the entire difficult airway assessment, including difficult bag-valve-mask ventilation, EGA insertion and ventilation, endotracheal intubation, and cricothyrotomy (Table 15-13). Unfortunately, most of these clinical assessments cannot be realistically performed in the austere prehospital environment. For example, the Mallampati score, as already noted, relies on having a cooperative patient sit up, open his mouth fully, and stick out his tongue so the hard palate, uvula, and posterior pharynx can be visualized. The astute paramedic will still look into the mouth before committing to intubation in order to assess overall working room—a modified Mallampati score.

Percentage of glottic opening (POGO) scale.

FIGURE 15-102 POGO scoring system.

Table 15-13 LEMONS Mnemonic Used to Evaluate Difficult Airway

LEMONS	
L	Look externally
E	Evaluate 3-3-2 rule
M	Mallampati score
O	Obstruction
N	Neck mobility
S	Saturations

The 3–3–2 Rule

Keep in mind that the measurements are based on the *patient's* fingers, not yours! (For example, two of your fingers might equal three of the patient's.)

Check that the mouth opening equals at least 3 patient-sized fingers.

Check that there is room for 3 patient-sized fingers between the tip of the chin and the hyoid bone.

Check that there is room for 2 patient-sized fingers between the hyoid bone and the top of the thyroid cartilage.

FIGURE 15-103 The 3-3-2 rule.

LOOK EXTERNALLY Look for factors that will make BVM ventilation, EGA, intubation, or surgical airway difficult. This includes facial hair, secretions, massive obesity, facial trauma, upper airway pathology, and gross face/neck anatomic deformities.

EVALUATE 3-3-2 RULE The 3-3-2 rule is one tool to help estimate the difficulty of laryngoscopy by assessing anatomic limitations to visualizing the larynx—for example, small mouth opening, short chin (no room to displace the tongue), and superior/anterior location (Figure 15-103). Criteria evaluated are as follows (using the patient's finger measurements):

- Check that the mouth opening is at least **3** patient-sized fingers.
- Check that there is room for **3** patient-sized fingers between the tip of the chin and the hyoid bone.
- Check that there is room for **2** patient-sized fingers between the hyoid bone and the top of the thyroid cartilage.

MALLAMPATI SCORE The Mallampati score assesses the working space available within the mouth (review Figure 15-101 and see Table 15-14). To be done correctly, the patient must be able to sit up and stick out his tongue. A crude estimate may be substituted by manually opening the mouth and looking, although this technique has never been validated. A tongue blade may be used cautiously to avoid stimulating a gag reflex. The most important thing is to make sure you look into the mouth before committing to intubation to assess mouth opening, size of tongue, dentures/dentition, edema, trauma, and secretions.

OBSTRUCTION The airway may be obstructed by a foreign body, the tongue, secretions, blood, or vomitus and/or edema. Edema may result from trauma, infectious causes such as epiglottitis and abscess, or from allergic reactions. Consider the age and history to predict possible obstruction. Intubating a pediatric patient with retropharyngeal abscess or an adult with Ludwig's angina is a scary proposition.

Table 15-14 Mallampati Score

Mallampati Score
Class I = visualization of the soft palate, fauces, uvula, and anterior and posterior pillars = "Easy"
Class II = visualization of the soft palate, fauces, and uvula = "Mildly Difficult"
Class III = visualization of the soft palate and the base of the uvula = "Moderately Difficult"
Class IV = soft palate is not visible at all = "Difficult"

NECK MOBILITY Neck mobility is most often limited by cervical spine immobilization, although patients with rheumatoid arthritis or spinal fusions, and elderly patients with severe degenerative disease, may also have restricted range of motion. This is another reminder that any patient in spinal precautions should be considered to have a difficult airway. It is important in these cases that the front of the cervical collar be removed and manual stabilization with a jaw-thrust applied during intubation to allow forward movement of the chin.

SATURATIONS One of the most critical elements in airway management is the time allowed to successfully complete the procedure. The primary determinant of time in these procedures is the oxygen saturation and, in turn, your ability to preoxygenate and create an oxygen reserve. As noted earlier, a patient whose oxygen saturation is near 100 percent following preoxygenation has "adequate reserve," above 90 percent but less than 100 percent has "limited reserve," and less than 90 percent despite appropriate preoxygenation has "no reserve."

Effects of Obesity

The airway effects of obesity are complex but, overall, negative. Much of the anatomic problem with intubation in the morbidly obese may be overcome with proper positioning—that is, the ramped position, which was described earlier in the chapter. Obesity also limits the effects of preoxygenation due to reduced functional residual capacity as well as increased oxygen demand so that time to perform the intubation before critical hypoxemia may be limited. Obesity definitely makes BVM ventilation more difficult, and some extraglottic rescue devices

may not generate enough airway pressure to lift a very heavy chest. Finally, obesity may make identification of landmarks for a surgical airway very difficult.

Predicting Difficulty: An Imperfect Science

Prediction of difficult intubation is an imperfect science at best with limited applicability to most patients undergoing emergency airway management (Figure 15-104). Prediction of difficult BVM ventilation is somewhat more reliable. Nonetheless, providers should look for and heed obvious warning signs of a difficult intubation or BVM ventilation and prepare accordingly. Do not,

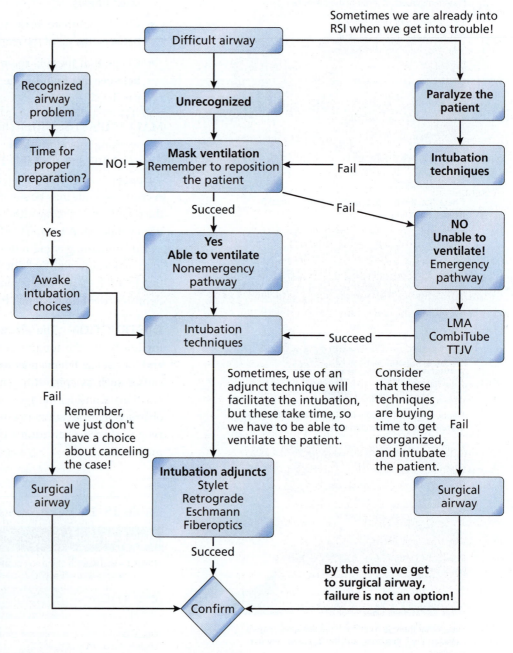

FIGURE 15-104 Difficult airway management algorithm.
(From Stewart, C. E. Advanced Airway Management, Upper Saddle River, NJ; Pearson/Prentice Hall, 2002)

however, let the absence of any predicted difficulties create a sense of complacency. Any patient, no matter how favorable his airway appears, may prove difficult or impossible to intubate. If you have not encountered such a patient you have not yet intubated enough!

PART 4: Additional Airway and Ventilation Issues

Managing Patients with Stoma Sites

Patients who have had a laryngectomy (removal of the larynx) or tracheostomy (surgical opening into the trachea) may breathe through a **stoma**, an opening in the anterior neck that connects the trachea with the ambient air. These patients frequently have tracheostomy tubes, which consist of an inner and outer cannula, in place to keep the soft-tissue stoma open (Figure 15-105). Patients with longstanding stomas may not use a tracheostomy tube.

Although providers often have anxiety about managing a patient with a stoma, this anxiety is usually unwarranted, because these patients have a secure airway. Potential problems include clogging of the tracheostomy tube with secretions, a dislodged tube, bleeding, and respiratory distress.

Tube clogging is a common problem because a laryngectomy produces a less-effective cough, making it more difficult to clear secretions. If these secretions organize, they form a mucus plug that can occlude the stoma. A clogged tube can usually be managed easily by removing the inner cannula from the fixed external cannula and cleaning it. The external cannula should not be removed, because the stoma may begin closing and it may be difficult to replace.

If a tracheostomy tube becomes completely dislodged, it should be replaced as soon as possible. This is particularly critical if the tracheostomy is less than a few weeks old. If another tube is not available, an endotracheal tube may be used temporarily. In this case, choose the largest diameter ETT that will pass through the stoma to maintain the airway before complete obstruction occurs. Lubricate the ETT, instruct the patient to exhale, and gently insert the ETT to about 1 to 2 cm beyond the distal cuff. Inflate the cuff, then confirm comfort, patency, and proper placement. Be certain to suspect and check for improper placement

FIGURE 15-105 Tracheostomy cannulae.

into the surrounding subcutaneous tissue, which will produce a false lumen. Subcutaneous emphysema, as well as the lack of clinical improvement in the patient, indicates a false lumen. If difficulty persists and the patient is in extremis, an endotracheal tube introducer may be passed into the stoma to gently confirm proper intratracheal positioning and the tracheostomy or endotracheal tube passed over the introducer, much as with a bougie-aided cricothyrotomy.

Bleeding may come from irritation of the skin externally around the stoma site or internally. External bleeding is usually minor, although it may scare the patient, especially if the tracheostomy is new or bleeding has not occurred previously. Internal bleeding, on the other hand, may be catastrophic. This warrants very expeditious transport and contact with medical direction.

If the patient is complaining of respiratory distress, you must first make sure the tracheostomy is patent. If it is, then the distress is probably unrelated to the tracheostomy, and you should perform your usual history and physical exam.

Other stoma-related problems to consider are excessive secretions that are not obstructing the lumen of the tube but are nevertheless causing respiratory problems. You may suction the airway through the stoma, but you must use extreme caution as this process can, itself, cause soft-tissue

Table 15-15 Advantages and Disadvantages of Various Suction Types

Type	Advantages	Disadvantages
Hand-powered	Lightweight, portable, inexpensive, simple to operate	Limited volume, manually powered, fluid contact components are not disposable
Oxygen-powered	Small, lightweight	Limited suction power, uses a lot of oxygen
Battery-operated	Lightweight, portable, excellent suction power, simple to operate and troubleshoot in the field	Battery memory decreases with time; mechanically more complicated than hand-powered, some fluid contact components are not disposable
Mounted	Strong suction, adjustable vacuum power, disposable fluid contact components	Not portable, cannot be serviced in the field, no substitute power source

swelling. Begin by preoxygenating the patient with 100 percent oxygen and then inject 3 mL sterile saline down the trachea through the stoma. Gently insert a sterile catheter until resistance is met. While the patient coughs or exhales, suction the airway during withdrawal of the catheter.

Supplemental oxygen may be delivered by placing an oxygen mask over the stoma or tracheostomy tube. If this is insufficient or if the patient requires positive pressure ventilation, it is very easy to attach a bag-valve device to the tracheostomy tube. If the patient has a stoma but no tracheostomy tube, then gently insert a lubricated endotracheal or tracheostomy tube to perform ventilation.

Suctioning

Anticipating and being prepared for complications when managing airways is the key for successful outcomes. You must anticipate that a patient may vomit and be prepared to turn the patient and **suction** in order to remove blood, mucus, and emesis. The first line of defense against aspiration should be gravity: Turning the patient or just his head to the side (if not in cervical precautions) is faster and more effective than any suction device. However, suctioning equipment still must be readily available for all patients if repositioning is not possible or as an adjunct to rotation.

Suctioning Equipment

Many kinds of suctioning devices are available. They may be handheld, oxygen-powered, battery-operated, or mounted (nonportable). Table 15-15 details the advantages and disadvantages of each.

To suit the prehospital environment, your equipment should be lightweight, portable, and durable; generate a vacuum level of at least 300 mmHg when the distal end is occluded; and allow a flow rate of at least 30 liters per minute when the tube is open. In addition to a portable device, the ambulance should have a mounted, vacuum-powered suction device that can generate stronger suction and that can be a backup device in case of equipment failure (Figure 15-106).

FIGURE 15-106 Oropharyngeal suctioning.

Table 15-16 Types of Suctioning Catheters

Hard/Rigid Catheter	Soft Catheters
A large tube with multiple holes at the distal end	Long, flexible tube; smaller diameter than hard-tip catheters
Suctions larger volumes of fluid rapidly	Cannot remove large volumes of fluid rapidly
Standard size	Various sizes
Used in oropharyngeal airway only	Can be placed in the oropharynx, nasopharynx, or down the endotracheal tube
Removes larger particles	Suction tubing without catheter (facilitates suctioning of large debris)

The most commonly used suction catheters are hard/rigid catheters ("Yankauer" or "tonsil tip") and soft catheters ("whistle tip"). Table 15-16 summarizes their differences.

Because suctioning also removes oxygen, and because you must interrupt oxygen delivery to suction, you should limit each suctioning attempt to 10 seconds. If possible, hyperventilate the patient with 100 percent oxygen before and after each effort. Do not apply suction while inserting the catheter. Apply suction only as you withdraw the catheter after properly positioning it.

Complications of suctioning are usually related to hypoxemia from prolonged suctioning attempts without proper ventilation. The decrease in myocardial oxygen supply can cause cardiac dysrhythmias. Suctioning can also stimulate the vagus nerve, causing bradycardia and hypotension, or the anxiety of being suctioned can cause hypertension and tachycardia. Stimulation of the cough reflex will cause a patient to cough, causing an increase in intracranial pressure and reducing cerebral blood flow.

Suctioning Techniques

You must have suction equipment by any patient who has airway compromise and will need airway management. Do not forget this basic and important skill. To suction a patient:

1. Use Standard Precautions, including protective eyewear, gloves, and face mask.

2. Preoxygenate the patient; this may require brief hyperventilation.

3. Determine the depth of catheter insertion by measuring from the patient's earlobe to his lips.

4. With the suction turned off, insert the catheter into your patient's pharynx to the predetermined depth.

5. Turn on the suction unit and place your thumb over the suction control orifice; limit suction to 10 seconds.

6. Continue to suction while withdrawing the catheter. When using a whistle-tip catheter, rotate it between your fingertips.

7. While maintaining ventilatory support, hyperventilate the patient with 100 percent oxygen.

In many cases, you will suction extremely viscous, or thick, secretions that can obstruct the flow of fluid through the tubing. To reduce this problem, suction water through the tubing between suctioning attempts. This dilutes the secretions and facilitates flow to the suction canister. Most suction units have small water canisters for this purpose.

Tracheobronchial Suctioning

Suctioning is normally applied to the oropharynx. However, you may occasionally need to suction a patient through an endotracheal tube or a tracheostomy tube to remove secretions or mucus plugs from the tracheobronchial airway that can cause respiratory distress. Tracheobronchial suctioning risks hypoxemia, so ensuring adequate oxygenation before and after the procedure is essential. Sterile technique should be used to avoid contaminating the pulmonary system. Use only the soft-tip catheter intended for endotracheal use to avoid damaging any structures, and be certain to lubricate well. Once you have preoxygenated the patient with 100 percent oxygen, gently insert the lubricated tube, using sterile gloves, until you feel resistance (Figure 15-107). Then apply suction for only about 10 seconds while withdrawing the catheter. You may need to inject 3 to 5 mL of sterile water or saline down the endotracheal tube before suctioning to help loosen thick secretions.

Gastric Distention and Decompression

A common problem during BVM ventilation is the entry of air into the stomach (gastric insufflation), which increases the risk of vomiting and regurgitation with subsequent aspiration. The enlarged stomach also pushes against the diaphragm, inhibiting the lungs' expansion and increasing resistance to ventilation. Pediatric patients are prone to bradycardia from vagal stimulation that may result. Ideally, gastric insufflation will be prevented rather than treated, as it is much less likely to occur with optimal BVM

FIGURE 15-107 Tracheostomy suction technique.

ventilation technique, as discussed earlier in this chapter. Gastric insufflation is even less likely to occur with an extraglottic airway (EGA) device.

Unfortunately, even with optimal BVM ventilation technique, gastric insufflation is inevitable with prolonged ventilation, and poor BVM ventilation technique is still rampant in prehospital care. Therefore, paramedics will need to be able to treat this condition with gastric decompression, which involves the placement of a gastric tube into the stomach via the mouth (orogastric) or the nose (nasogastric) or through an EGA.

Nasogastric tube placement is generally preferred in awake patients, as it is more comfortable than orogastric placement and does not interfere with speech. However, placement in an awake patient is rarely necessary in prehospital care, except during some air medical transports, and is not discussed here.

Orogastric tube placement is recommended in most unconscious patients to minimize the risk of epistaxis and sinusitis. It is also recommended with facial fractures, to avoid placing the tube through a skull fracture into the brain, and in patients who are at increased risk for nasal bleeding. If the patient has an EGA in place that has a dedicated channel for gastric tube insertion, this should be used.

Contrary to popular belief, gastric tubes may be gently placed in patients who have gastric or esophageal varices unless they have undergone a banding or cautery procedure within the past two weeks. However, gastric intubation should be avoided if esophageal obstruction or perforation is suspected.

All three routes—nasogastric, orogastric, and EGA—carry the risk of misplacement into the lungs, although this is much less likely using an EGA. Both the oral and nasal routes put the patient at risk for vomiting and bleeding during insertion. For this reason, gastric tubes should not be placed in obtunded patients unless they are already intubated or have an EGA in place.

As for any other invasive procedure, you should always wear protective eyewear, gloves, and a face shield whenever you place a gastric tube. To place an orogastric tube in the unconscious patient:

1. Take Standard Precautions.
2. Place the patient's head in a neutral position while ventilating via the endotracheal tube or EGA.
3. Select the correct size gastric tube. Most adults take a 16 Fr when placed orally. Some EGAs will accommodate only larger or only smaller sizes, and this should be checked in advance.
4. Determine the approximate length of tube insertion by measuring from the epigastrium to the angle of the jaw, then to the mouth opening or to the proximal end of the EGA.

5. Generously lubricate the distal tip of the gastric tube and gently insert it into the oral cavity at midline.

6. Advance the tube gently to the length you determined prior to insertion.

7. Check that the tube has not curled in the mouth.

8. Confirm placement by injecting 30 to 50 mL of air while listening to the epigastric region for air entry into the stomach. In addition, end-tidal CO_2 detectors are now available that will attach to a gastric tube. In this case the detection of CO_2 indicates incorrect placement in the lungs, rather than correct placement in the stomach. Coughing also suggests malposition in the lungs, although this is unreliable in unconscious patients.

9. Apply gentle suction to the tube to evacuate gastric fluids and gas.

10. Secure the tube in place.

11. Document the indication for gastric decompression, the size tube placed, the technique, means of confirmation, any complications incurred, the type and volume of gastric contents evacuated, and the clinical response.

Transport Ventilators

Mechanical ventilation, as by a transport ventilator mounted in the ambulance, is designed to assist or replace the patient's own breathing. In a patient who is not breathing spontaneously, the mechanical ventilator provides "controlled" ventilations. Some mechanical ventilators are designed to provide intermittent "mandatory" ventilation; that is, the ventilator will assist a patient's own spontaneous breaths but will revert to controlled ventilations if the patient stops breathing.

There is accumulating evidence that mechanical ventilation is superior to manual ventilation except in the crashing patient, for whom assessment of compliance and elimination of the ventilator as a source of the problem becomes essential. Mechanical ventilation frees up provider hands and, when used correctly, is less likely to cause hemodynamic impairment or CO_2 fluctuations that have been associated with worse outcomes in head trauma patients. It is recommended that all patients with an invasive airway (ETT or EGA) be maintained on a ventilator all the way to patient turnover in the hospital when a ventilator is available and not contraindicated.

There are two general varieties of ventilators for prehospital use: simple compact devices with a minimum of options for general use and more complicated devices for critical care transport.

The simple out-of-hospital ventilator devices are designed for convenience and ease of use during short transports of relatively uncomplicated adult and older pediatric patients. These devices generally allow for control of ventilatory rate and tidal volume only. Most of these units deliver controlled ventilation only (will breathe only for patients who are not breathing on their own), whereas other units will function as intermittent mandatory ventilators (assisting spontaneously breathing patients), which revert to controlled mechanical ventilation in patients who are not breathing.

The inspired oxygen concentration is usually fixed at 100 percent, but it may be adjustable. Oxygen consumption on longer transports may be substantial. Most of these devices do not provide CPAP. These devices also offer little ability to monitor airway pressures or delivered volumes and usually do not have warning alarms, but instead have a pop-off valve that prevents pressure-related injury. When airway pressure exceeds a preset level (typically 60 cm H_2O), the valve opens, venting some of the tidal volume. This safety feature may actually hinder ventilation in patients who require greater positive pressure, such as those with significant lung pathology (e.g., cardiogenic pulmonary edema, adult respiratory distress syndrome [ARDS], pulmonary contusion, and bronchospasm). Consider using a bag-valve device if this problem occurs.

Critical care transport ventilators, in contrast to the simple units just described, offer a host of features such as different ventilator modes, enhanced monitoring, alarms, and more (Figure 15-108). The increased adjustability allows for keeping the patient more comfortable with less sedation, analgesia, and paralysis. Some of these devices can be used to provide mask CPAP as well. Inspired oxygen concentration can usually be adjusted. These critical transport devices can be used on most pediatric patients and some neonates. The trade-off for these features is much higher cost, and their greater complexity requires much more extensive training. These advanced ventilators are worth considering if you have long transports, do a lot of interfacility transports, or have a large pediatric population.

FIGURE 15-108 Transport ventilators.

Documentation

Accurate and thorough documentation of airway management is critical for clinical care after the patient is transported, for quality assurance, and for medical–legal defense. Documentation should include not only what was done but also the thought process of why it was done and any complications that occurred. A significant percentage of claims and lawsuits that are filed against prehospital providers involve airway issues, and often these cases are won or lost based on the field documentation. Therefore, it is crucial that the provider learn to document in medically correct and legally sufficient terms exactly what was done in managing the airway.

AMERICAN MEDICAL RESPONSE OF EL PASO COUNTY
AIRWAY REPORTING FORM

Turn in this form attached to a copy of your PCR to CES mailbox immediately

DEMOGRAPHICS

PCR #:_____ Date:_____ Time called:_____ Time arrived:_____

Pt. Age:_____ Gender:_____ Patient Initials:_____ Pt. Weight:_____Kg

Attending Emp ID#_____ Attending Emp Name:_____

Hosp MR #:_____ Receiving ED Physician:_____

INDICATIONS FOR AIRWAY MANAGEMENT

☐ Apnea or agonal respiration   ☐ Injury or illness involving airway

☐ Airway reflexes compromised   ☐ Anticipated compromise or decompensation

☐ Ventilation Compromised   ☐ Other: (describe) _____

ALL PROCEDURES PERFORMED (select all performed)

☐ BVM   ☐ OETT (no medications)   ☐ NETT   ☐ LMA

☐ OPA   ☐ OETT (awake)   ☐ Digital Intubation ☐ Cricothyrotomy (surgical)

☐ NPA   ☐ OETT (RSI)   ☐ Combitube   ☐ Cricothyrotomy (needle)

STATE OF AIRWAY PRIOR TO INTERVENTION

☐ Clear   ☐ Blood   ☐ Gag Reflex: ABSENT   ☐ Combative/Resistive

☐ Emesis   ☐ Teeth/Foreign objects ☐ Gag Reflex: PARTIAL   ☐ Burns

☐ Sputum/Secretions ☐ Trismus -OR- Biting ☐ Gag Reflex: PRESENT   ☐ Other:_____

BASIC INTERVENTIONS

Procedure	Size:	Done By:(emp # or agency)	Time
☐ NPA			
☐ OPA			
☐ BVM Vent	--- N/A ---		

INTUBATION INTERVENTIONS

*AN **ETI** ATTEMPT IS DEFINED AS INSERTING THE TUBE INTO THE NOSTRIL OR INSERTING THE BLADE PAST THE TEETH/GUMS AMR PROTOCOL IS A MAXIMUM TOTAL OF THREE ATTEMPTS.*

Pulsox pre-attempt: ☐   Pulsox drop < 90 during attempt? ☐ Yes ☐ No ☐ N/A (unable to get pulsox > 90 pre-attempt)

Cricoid pressure used: ☐ Yes ☐ No   Was Surevent used: ☐ Yes ☐ No

Attempt	Intubation Method: nett, oett,digital,RSI, etc.	Performed By (emp#)	Successful: (yes/no)	Time Performed:
# 1				
# 2				
# 3				
# 4				

PLACEMENT CONFIRMATION STEPS PERFORMED (Check only those actually performed)

YES/NO		YES/NO		YES/NO	
☐ ☐ Visualized Through Cords		☐ ☐ ETCO2 Colormetric Used (color): _____		☐ ☐ Lung Sounds PRESENT	
☐ ☐ Negative EDD (In Trachea)		☐ ☐ ETCO2 Capnography Used (peak #)_____		☐ ☐ Gastric Sounds ABSENT	
☐ ☐ Positive EDD (In Esophagus)		☐ ☐ Capnography Waveform Present		☐ ☐ Chest Rise/ Fall	
☐ -- Equivocal EDD (unsure placement)					

Tube Size: ☐   Tube Depth: ☐   How Secured: ☐

FIGURE 15-109 Airway reporting form.

(Courtesy of American Medical Response of El Paso County, Colorado and David Ross, DO, FACEP)

The documentation sample shown in Figure 15-109 is by no means the only way to document airway management. It is, however, provided as an example. One may be tempted to say that the example is "over-documentation." However, few practitioners who have been called to testify under oath about their airway management would agree. Because patients who require prehospital airway management are at high risk for a bad outcome from the outset, and because airway management literally determines whether the patient lives or dies, it stands to reason that the greatest emphasis should be placed on detailed documentation of these issues.

MEDICATIONS USED: (check mark all meds used)

Medication	Dosage	Given By	Time Given	Medication	Dosage	Given By	Time Given
☐ Etomidate				☐ Fentanyl			
☐ Succinylcholine				☐ Morphine			
☐ Vecuronium				☐ Valium			
☐ Atropine				☐ Neosyn.			
☐ Lidocaine				☐ Viscous			
☐ Topical Spray				☐ Other			

IF FAILED INTUBATION, INDICATE SECONDARY (RESCUE) AIRWAY / VENTILATION TECHNIQUE USED (check all that apply)

Procedure	Done By:	Ventilation Yes/ No	Time	Procedure	Done By:	Ventilation Yes/ No	Time
☐ BVM (rescue)				☐ Cric (surgical)			
☐ Combitube				☐ Cric (needle)			
☐ LMA				☐ Other			

IF COMBITUBE WAS USED:

☐ Ventilation successful with # 1 blue tube (esophageal placement)　**Peak ETCO2:** [   ] (from the tube used)

☐ Ventilation successful with #2 white tube (tracheal placement)

IF ALL ATTEMPTS AT INTUBATION FAILED, INDICATE SUSPECTED REASONS FOR FAILURE (check all that apply)

☐ Unable to visualize glottic opening　　　　　☐ Difficult anatomy: (anterior, overbite, obesity, edema, tumor, etc.)

☐ Unable to pass vocal cords　　　　　　　　☐ Secretions / Blood / Vomit

☐ Complete obstruction; unable to clear　　　　☐ Unable to locate anatomical landmarks

☐ Inadequate patient or muscular relaxation　　☐ Poor patient access: (extrication, spinal immob., confined space, etc.)

☐ Poor jaw/ neck mobility　　　　　　　　　☐ Arrival at hospital prior to completion of procedure

☐ Severe trauma　　　　　　　　　　　　　☐ Other: _____

ED PHYSICIAN CONFIRMATION OF PROPER ETT / CRICOTHYROIDOTOMY PLACEMENT:

　　　　☐ Correct Placement　　　　　☐ Incorrect Placement

Comments:_____

_____

_____

PHYSICIAN SIGNATURE:

MEDICAL DIRECTOR EVALUATION:

　　　　☐ Appropriate Intervention　　　☐ Confirmation criteria MET

　　　　☐ Inappropriate Intervention　　☐ Confirmation criteria NOT met

MEDICAL DIRECTOR COMMENTS:

_____

_____

MEDICAL DIRECTOR SIGNATURE:　　　　　　　　DATE REVIEWED:

TURN IN THIS FORM ATTACHED TO A COPY OF YOUR PCR TO CES MAILBOX IMMEDIATELY

FIGURE 15-109 (*Continued*)

Summary

Airway assessment and maintenance is the most critical step in managing any patient. If you do not promptly establish a definitive airway and provide proper ventilation, the patient's outcome will be poor. Frequently reassessing the airway is mandatory to ensure that the patient has not decompensated, requiring additional airway procedures. Successful management of all airways requires the paramedic to follow the proper management sequence.

Basic airway and management skills can make the difference between a successful outcome and a poor patient prognosis. Once you have mastered these basic skills and made them a part of airway management in every patient, you should learn and use advanced skills such as intubation, RSI, and cricothyrotomy. You must maintain proficiency in all airway skills, especially the more advanced techniques, through ongoing continuing education, physician medical direction, and testing with each EMS service. If you cannot do this, it is in the patient's best interest to focus on less sophisticated airway skills. If you anticipate that every airway will be complicated, apply basic airway skills before using advanced procedures, and perform frequent reassessments, you will give the patient his best chance for meaningful survival.

You Make the Call

You and your paramedic partner, Preston Connelly, are assigned to District 4, a quiet suburban neighborhood, on a warm Saturday in June. At 2:00 P.M., you are dispatched to care for a choking child at the Happy Hotdog Restaurant on Main Street. On your way to the location, the dispatcher advises you that they are currently giving prearrival choking instructions to the bystanders at the scene. On arrival, you find a frantic mother who tells you that her 6-year-old son was eating a hot dog and drinking a soda when he started coughing and gasping for air. She keeps yelling for you to do something. Bystanders surround the child and are attempting to perform the Heimlich maneuver without success. On your primary assessment, you find a 6-year-old boy lying on the floor, unconscious and apneic, with a pulse rate of 130. There is cyanosis surrounding his lips and fingernail beds, with a moderate amount of secretions coming from his mouth. There are no signs of trauma. You and Preston immediately start management of this child.

1. What is your primary assessment and management of this child?

2. What are your first actions?

3. What are your options for managing the airway after the obstruction is relieved?

4. What are the major anatomic differences between pediatric and adult patients in terms of airway management?

See Suggested Responses at the back of this book.

Review Questions

1. The depression between the epiglottis and the base of the tongue is called the _____
   a. naris.
   b. glottis.
   c. larynx.
   d. vallecula.

2. The average volume of gas inhaled or exhaled in one respiratory cycle is the_____
   a. minute volume.
   b. tidal volume.
   c. respiratory rate.
   d. total lung capacity.

3. A drop in blood pressure of greater than 10 torr during inspiration is called_____
   a. compliance.
   b. laryngeal spasm.
   c. pulsus paradoxus.
   d. paradoxical breathing.

4. To avoid hypoxia during intubation, limit each intubation attempt to no more than _____ seconds before reoxygenating the patient.
   a. 10
   b. 20
   c. 30
   d. 40

5. Which medication is *not* a preferred neuromuscular blocking agent for emergency RSI?
   a. Atracurium
   b. Vecuronium
   c. Pancuronium
   d. Succinylcholine

6. The_____ is the most superior part of the airway.
   a. pharynx
   b. larynx
   c. oral cavity
   d. nasal cavity

7. The _____ is the only bone in the axial skeleton that does not articulate with any other bone.
   a. femur
   b. hyoid
   c. stapes
   d. patella

8. The _____ comprise(s) the key functional unit of the respiratory system.
   a. hilum
   b. alveoli
   c. bronchi
   d. respiratory bronchioles

9. The paramedic can correct oxygen derangements by_____
   a. increasing the ventilatory rate in a spontaneously breathing patient.
   b. administering supplemental oxygen.
   c. using negative CPAP pressure.
   d. all of the above.

10. The _____ is the amount of gas in the tidal volume that remains in air passageways unavailable for gas exchange.
    a. base tidal volume
    b. minute volume
    c. dead-space volume
    d. total lung capacity

11. "Difficulty speaking" defines_____
    a. aphagia.
    b. aphonia.
    c. dysphonia.
    d. dysphagia.

12. "An irregular pattern of rate and depth with sudden, periodic episodes of apnea, indicating increased intracranial pressure" describes_____
    a. agonal respirations.
    b. Biot's respirations.
    c. Kussmaul's respirations.
    d. Cheyne-Stokes respirations.

13. _____ is often called the "fifth vital sign."
    a. Heart rate
    b. Blood pressure
    c. Pulse oximetry
    d. Blood glucose level

14. The visual representation of the expired CO_2 waveform is the_____
    a. capnogram.
    b. capnograph.
    c. capnometry.
    d. capnography.

15. Which of the following is an advantage of the nasopharyngeal airway?
    a. It isolates the trachea from aspiration.
    b. It is designed to be suctioned through.
    c. It can be used in a patient with a gag reflex.
    d. It cannot cause any type of soft tissue trauma during insertion.

16. Advantages of endotracheal intubation include which of the following?
    a. It eliminates the need to maintain a mask seal.
    b. It isolates the trachea and permits complete control of the airway.
    c. It impedes gastric distention by channeling air directly into the trachea.
    d. All of the above.

17. Which medication is generally the second-line paralytic when succinylcholine is contraindicated?
    a. Atracurium
    b. Fentanyl
    c. Rocuronium
    d. Pancuronium

18. Relative contraindications for blind nasotracheal intubation include_____
    a. suspected elevation of intracranial pressure.
    b. suspected basilar skull fracture.
    c. a combative patient.
    d. all of the above.

19. Which airway can work properly regardless of the tip being in the esophagus or the trachea?
    a. ET
    b. ETC
    c. LMA
    d. PLA

20. Open cricothyrotomy is contraindicated in children under the age of _____ because the cricothyroid membrane is small and underdeveloped.
    a. 8
    b. 10
    c. 12
    d. 14

See Answers to Review Questions at the back of this book.

References

1. Austin, M. A., K. E. Wills, L. Blizzard, E. H. Walters, and R. Wood-Baker. "Effect of High Flow Oxygen on Mortality in Chronic Obstructive Pulmonary Disease Patients in Prehospital Setting: Randomised Controlled Trial." *BMJ* 341 (2010): c5462.

2. Body, R. and K. Hogg. "Best Evidence Topic Reports. Oxygen in Acute Uncomplicated Myocardial Infarction." *Emerg Med J* 21 (2004): 75.

3. Moradkhan, R. and L. I. Sinoway. "Revisiting the Role of Oxygen Therapy in Cardiac Patients." *J Am Coll Cardiol* 56 (2010): 1013–1016.

4. Barker, S. J., J. Curry, D. Redford, and S. Morgan. "Measurement of Carboxyhemoglobin and Methemoglobin by Pulse Oximetry: A Human Volunteer Study." *Anesthesiology* 105 (2006): 892–897.

5. Bledsoe, B. E., K. Nowicki, J. H. Creel, D. Carrison, and H. W. Severance. "Use of Pulse CO-Oximetry as a Screening and Monitoring Tool in Mass Carbon Monoxide Poisoning." *Prehosp Emerg Care* 14 (2010): 131–133.

6. Rucker, J., J. Tesler, L. Fedorko et al. "Normocapnia Improves Cerebral Oxygen Delivery during Conventional Oxygen Therapy in Carbon Monoxide-Exposed Research Subjects." *Ann Emerg Med* 40 (2002): 611–618.

7. Camp, N. E. "Methemoglobinemia." *J Emerg Nurs* 33 (2007): 172–174.

8. Abu-Laban, R. B., P. J. Zed, R. A. Purssell, and K. G. Evans. "Severe Methemoglobinemia from Topical Anesthetic Spray: Case Report, Discussion and Qualitative Systematic Review." *CJEM* 3 (2001): 51–56.

9. Kupnik, D. and P. Skok. "Capnometry in the Prehospital Setting: Are We Using Its Potential?" *Emerg Med J* 24 (2007): 614–617.

10. Silvestri, S., G. A. Ralls, B. Krauss et al. "The Effectiveness of Out-of-Hospital Use of Continuous End-Tidal Carbon Dioxide Monitoring on the Rate of Unrecognized Misplaced Intubation within a Regional Emergency Medical Services System." *Ann Emerg Med* 45 (2005): 497–503.

11. Collin, J. S., H. J. Lemmens, J. B. Brodsky et al., "Laryngoscopy and Morbid Obesity: A Comparison of the 'Sniff' and 'Ramped' Position." *Obes Surg* 14 (2004): 1171–1175.

12. Ellis, D. Y., T. Harris, and D. Zideman. "Cricoid Pressure in Emergency Department Rapid Sequence Tracheal Intubations: A Risk-Benefit Analysis." *Ann Emerg Med* 50 (2007): 653–665.

13. Hubble, M. W., L. Brown, D. A. Wilfong, A. Hertelendy, R. W. Benner, and M. E. Richards. "A Meta-Analysis of Prehospital Airway Control Techniques Part I: Orotracheal and Nasotracheal Intubation Success Rates." *Prehosp Emerg Care* 14 (2010): 377–401.

14. Hubble, M. W., D. A. Wilfong, L. H. Brown, A. Hertelendy, and R. W. Benner. "A Meta-Analysis of Prehospital Airway Control Techniques Part II: Alternative Airway Devices and Cricothyrotomy Success Rates." *Prehosp Emerg Care* 14 (2010): 515–530.

15. Colwell, C. B., K. E. McVaney, J. S. Haukoos, et al. "An Evaluation of Out-of-Hospital Advanced Airway Management in an Urban Setting." *Acad Emerg Med* 12 (2005): 417–422.

16. Guyette, F. X., M. J. Greenwood, D. Neubecker, R. Roth, and H. E. Wang. "Alternate Airways in the Prehospital Setting (Resource Document to NAEMSP Position Statement)." *Prehosp Emerg Care* 11 (2007): 56–61.

17. Bercker, S., W. Schmidbauer, T. Volk et al. "A Comparison of Seal in Seven Supraglottic Airway Devices Using a Cadaver Model of Elevated Esophageal Pressure." *Anesth Analg* 106 (2008): 445–448, Table of Contents.

18. Cady, C. E. and R. G. Pirrallo. "The Effect of Combitube Use on Paramedic Experience in Endotracheal Intubation." *Am J Emerg Med* 23 (2005): 868–871.

19. Cady, C. E., M. D. Weaver, R. G. Pirrallo, and H. E. Wang. "Effect of Emergency Medical Technician-Placed Combitubes on Outcomes after Out-of-Hospital Cardiopulmonary Arrest." *Prehosp Emerg Care* 13 (2009): 495–499.

20. Russi, C. S., L. Miller, and M. J. Hartley. "A Comparison of the King-LT to Endotracheal Intubation and Combitube in a Simulated Difficult Airway." *Prehosp Emerg Care* 12 (2008): 35–41.

21. Gaither, J. B., J. Matheson, A. Eberhardt, and C. B. Colwell. "Tongue Engorgement Associated with Prolonged Use of the King-LT Laryngeal Tube Device." *Ann Emerg Med* 55(4) (2010): 367–369.

22. Guyette, F. X., H. Wang, and J. S. Cole. "King Airway Use by Air Medical Providers." *Prehosp Emerg Care* 11 (2007): 473–476.

23. Bledsoe, B. E., D. Slattery, R. Lauver, W. Forred, L. Johnson, and G. Rigo. "Can Emergency Medical Services Personnel Effectively Place and Use the S.A.L.T. Airway?" *Prehosp Emerg Care* 15 (2011): 359–365.

24. Murray, M. J., M. J. Vermeulen, L. J. Morrison, and T. Waite. "Evaluation of Prehospital Insertion of the Laryngeal Mask Airway by Primary Care Paramedics with Only Classroom Mannequin Training." *CJEM* 4 (2002): 338–343.

25. Chen, L. and A. L. Hsiao. "Randomized Trial of Endotracheal Tube versus Laryngeal Mask Airway in Simulated Prehospital Pediatric Arrest." *Pediatrics* 122 (2008): e294–e297.

26. Choyce, A., M. S. Avidan, C. Patel et al. "Comparison of Laryngeal Mask and Intubating Laryngeal Mask Insertion by the Naïve Intubator." *Br J Anaesth* 84 (2000): 103–105.

27. Davis, D. P. "Should Invasive Airway Management Be Done in the Field?" *CMAJ* 178 (2008): 1171–1173.

28. Bochicchio, G. V. and T. M. Scalea. "Is Field Intubation Useful?" *Curr Opin Crit Care* 9 (2003): 524–529.

29. Wang H. E. and D. M. Yealy. "Out-of-Hospital Endotracheal Intubation: Where Are We?" *Ann Emerg Med* 47 (2006): 532–541.

30. Wang, H. E., G. K. Balasubramani, L. J. Cook, J. R. Lave, and D. M. Yealy. "Out-of-Hospital Endotracheal Intubation Experience and Patient Outcomes." *Ann Emerg Med* 55(6) (2010): 527–537.e6.

31. Wang, H. E. and D. M. Yealy. "How Many Attempts Are Required to Accomplish Out-of-Hospital Endotracheal Intubation?" *Acad Emerg Med* 13 (2006): 372–377.

32. Warner, K. J., D. Carlbom, C. R. Cooke, E. M. Bulger, M. K. Copass, and S. R. Sharar. "Paramedic Training for Proficient Prehospital Endotracheal Intubation." *Prehosp Emerg Care* 14 (2010): 103–108.

33. Wang, H. E., B. N. Abo, J. R. Lave, and D. M. Yealy. "How Would Minimum Experience Standards Affect the Distribution of Out-of-Hospital Endotracheal Intubations?" *Ann Emerg Med* 50 (2007): 246–252.

34. Katz, S. H. and J. L. Falk. "Misplaced Endotracheal Tubes by Paramedics in an Urban Emergency Medical Services System." *Ann Emerg Med* 37 (2001): 32–37.

35. Jones, J. H., M. P. Murphy, R. L. Dickson, G. G. Somerville, and E. J. Brizendine. "Emergency Physician-Verified Out-of-Hospital Intubation: Miss Rates by Paramedics." *Acad Emerg Med* 11 (2004): 707–709.

36. Levitan, R. M., W. C. Kinkle, W. J. Levin, and W. W. Everett. "Laryngeal View during Laryngoscopy: A Randomized Trial Comparing Cricoid Pressure, Backward-Upward-Rightward Pressure, and Bimanual Laryngoscopy." *Ann Emerg Med* 47 (2006): 548–555.

37. Wayne, M. A. and M. McDonnell. "Comparison of Traditional versus Video Laryngoscopy in Out-of-Hospital Tracheal Intubation." *Prehosp Emerg Care* 14 (2010): 278–282.

38. Cobas, M. A., M. A. De la Peña, R. Manning, K. Candiotti, and A. J. Varon. "Prehospital Intubations and Mortality: A Level 1 Trauma Center Perspective." *Anesth Analg* 109 (2009): 489–493.

39. Davis, D. P., J. Peay, M. J. Sise et al. "The Impact of Prehospital Endotracheal Intubation on Outcome in Moderate to Severe Traumatic Brain Injury." *J Trauma* 58 (2005): 933–939.

40. Shafi, S. and L. Gentilello. "Pre-Hospital Endotracheal Intubation and Positive Pressure Ventilation Is Associated with Hypotension and Decreased Survival in Hypovolemic Trauma Patients: An Analysis of the National Trauma Data Bank." *J Trauma* 59 (2005): 1140–1145; discussion 1145–1147.

41. Zink, B. J. and R. F. Maio. "Out-of-Hospital Endotracheal Intubation in Traumatic Brain Injury: Outcomes Research Provides Us with an Unexpected Outcome." *Ann Emerg Med* 44 (2004): 451–453.

42. Stockinger, Z. T. and N. E. McSwain. "Prehospital Endotracheal Intubation for Trauma Does Not Improve Survival over Bag-Valve-Mask Ventilation." *J Trauma* 56 (2004): 531–536.

43. Gausche, M., R. J. Lewis, S. J. Stratton et al. "Effect of Out-of-Hospital Pediatric Endotracheal Intubation on Survival and Neurological Outcome: A Controlled Clinical Trial." *JAMA* 283 (2000): 783–790.

44. Henning, J., P. Sharley, and R. Young. "Pressures within Air-Filled Tracheal Cuffs at Altitude—An In Vivo Study." *Anaesthesia* 59 (2004): 252–254.

45. Mizelle, H. L., S. G. Rothrock, S. Silvestri, and J. Pagane. "Preventable Morbidity and Mortality from Prehospital Paralytic Assisted Intubation: Can We Expect Outcomes Comparable to Hospital-Based Practice?" *Prehosp Emerg Care* 6 (2002): 472–475.

46. Bernard, S. A., V. Nguyen, P. Cameron, et al. "Prehospital Rapid Sequence Intubation Improves Functional Outcome for Patients with Severe Traumatic Brain Injury: A Randomized Controlled Trial." *Ann Surg* 252 (2010): 959–965.

47. Bulger, E. M., M. K. Copass, D. R. Sabath, R. V. Maier, and G. J. Jurkovich. "The Use of Neuromuscular Blocking Agents to Facilitate Prehospital Intubation Does Not Impair Outcome after Traumatic Brain Injury." *J Trauma* 58 (2005): 718–723; discussion 723–724.

48. Cudnik, M. T., C. D. Newgard, M. Daya, and J. Jui. "The Impact of Rapid Sequence Intubation on Trauma Patient Mortality in Attempted Prehospital Intubation." *J Emerg Med* 38 (2010): 175–181.

49. Davis, D. P., J. V. Dunford, J. C. Poste et al. "The Impact of Hypoxia and Hyperventilation on Outcome after Paramedic Rapid Sequence Intubation of Severely Head-Injured Patients." *J Trauma* 57 (2004): 1–8; discussion 8–10.

50. Davis, D. P., D. B. Hoyt, M. Ochs et al. "The Effect of Paramedic Rapid Sequence Intubation on Outcome in Patients with Severe Traumatic Brain Injury." *J Trauma* 54 (2003): 444–453.

51. Davis, D. P., M. Ochs, D. B. Hoyt, D. Bailey, L. K. Marshall, and P. Rosen. "Paramedic-Administered Neuromuscular Blockade Improves Prehospital Intubation Success in Severely Head-Injured Patients." *J Trauma* 55 (2003): 713–719.

52. Dunford, J. V., D. P. Davis, M. Ochs, M. Doney, and D. B. Hoyt. "Incidence of Transient Hypoxia and Pulse Rate Reactivity during Paramedic Rapid Sequence Intubation." *Ann Emerg Med* 42 (2003): 721–728.

53. Butler, J. and R. Jackson. "Towards Evidence Based Emergency Medicine: Best BETs from Manchester Royal Infirmary. Lignocaine Premedication before Rapid Sequence Induction in Head Injuries." *Emerg Med J* 19 (2002): 554.

54. Reid, C., L. Chan, and M. Tweeddale. "The Who, Where, and What of Rapid Sequence Intubation: Prospective Observational Study of Emergency RSI outside the Operating Theatre." *Emerg Med J* 21 (2004): 296–301.

55. Walls, R. M., C. A. Brown, A. E. Bair, and D. J. Pallin, of the NEAR II Investigators. "Emergency Airway Management: A Multi-Center Report of 8937 Emergency Department Intubations." *J Emerg Med* 41(4) (2010): 347–354.

56. Wang, H. E., D. P. Davis, M. A. Wayne, and T. Delbridge. "Prehospital Rapid-Sequence Intubation; What Does the Evidence Show?" *Prehosp Emerg Care* 8 (2004): 366–377.

57. Kheterpal, S., L. Martin, A. M. Shanks, and K. K. Tremper. "Prediction and Outcomes of Impossible Mask Ventilation: A Review of 50,000 Anesthetics." *Anesthesiology* 110 (2009): 891–897.

58. Vadeboncoeur, T. F., D. P. Davis, M. Ochs, J. C. Poste, D. B. Hoyt, and G. M. Vilke. "The Ability of Paramedics to Predict Aspiration in Patients Undergoing Prehospital Rapid Sequence Intubation." *J Emerg Med* 30 (2006): 131–136.

Further Reading

American College of Surgeons, Committee on Trauma. *Advanced Trauma Life Support Course: Student Manual.* 8th ed. Chicago: American College of Surgeons, 2008.

Bledsoe, Bryan E. and Dwayne Clayden. *Prehospital Emergency Pharmacology.* 7th ed. Upper Saddle River, NJ: Pearson/Prentice Hall, 2012.

Braude, D. *Rapid Sequence Intubation & Rapid Sequence Airway*, 2nd ed. Albuquerque, NM: University of New Mexico Press, 2009.

Stewart, Charles E. *Advanced Airway Management.* Upper Saddle River, NJ: Pearson/Prentice Hall, 2002.

Precautions on Bloodborne Pathogens and Infectious Diseases

Prehospital emergency personnel, like all health care workers, are at risk for exposure to bloodborne pathogens and infectious diseases. In emergency situations it is often difficult to take or enforce proper infection control measures. However, as a paramedic, you must recognize your high-risk status. Study the following information on infection control carefully.

Infection control is designed to protect emergency personnel, their families, and their patients from unnecessary exposure to communicable diseases. Laws, regulations, and standards regarding infection control include:

- *Centers for Disease Control and Prevention (CDC) Guidelines.* The CDC has published extensive guidelines on infection control. Proper equipment and techniques that should be used by emergency response personnel to prevent or minimize risk of exposure are defined.

- *The Ryan White Act.* The Ryan White Act of 1990 allows emergency personnel to find out if they were exposed to an infectious disease while rendering patient care. Employers are required to name a "designated officer" to coordinate communications with the treating hospital.

- *Americans with Disabilities Act.* This act prohibits discrimination against individuals with disabilities, including those with contagious diseases. It guarantees equal employment opportunities and job protection if the infected individual can perform essential job functions and does not pose a threat to the safety and health of patients and coworkers.

- *Occupational Safety and Health Administration (OSHA) Regulations.* OSHA has enacted a regulation entitled Occupational Exposure to Bloodborne Pathogens that classifies emergency response personnel as being at the greatest risk of occupational exposure to communicable diseases. This regulation requires employers to provide hepatitis B (HBV) vaccinations free of charge, maintain a written exposure control plan, and provide personal protective equipment. These requirements primarily apply to private employers. Applicability to local and state governmental employees varies by locality. Many states have developed their own OSHA plans.

- *National Fire Protection Association (NFPA) Guidelines.* This is a national organization that has established specific guidelines and requirements regarding infection control for emergency response agencies, particularly fire departments and EMS services.

Standard Precautions and Personal Protective Equipment

Emergency response personnel should practice Standard Precautions by which ALL body substances are considered to be potentially infectious. To practice Standard Precautions, all emergency personnel should utilize personal protective equipment (PPE). Appropriate PPE should be available on every emergency vehicle. The minimum recommended PPE includes the following:

- *Gloves.* Disposable gloves should be donned by all emergency response personnel BEFORE initiating any emergency care. When an emergency incident involves more than one patient, you should attempt to change gloves between patients. When gloves have been contaminated, they should be removed as soon as possible. To properly remove contaminated gloves, grasp one glove approximately 1 inch from the wrist. Without touching the inside of the glove, pull the glove halfway off and stop. With that half-gloved hand, pull the glove on the opposite hand completely off. Place the removed glove in the palm of the other glove, with the inside of the removed glove exposed. Pull the second glove completely off with the ungloved hand, only touching the inside of the glove. Always wash hands after gloves are removed, even when the gloves appear intact.

- *Masks and Protective Eyewear.* Masks and protective eyewear should be present on all emergency vehicles and used in accordance with the level of exposure encountered. Masks and protective eyewear should be worn together whenever blood spatter is likely to occur, such as during arterial bleeding, childbirth, endotracheal intubation, invasive procedures, oral suctioning, and cleanup of equipment that requires heavy scrubbing or brushing. Both you and the patient should wear masks whenever the potential for airborne transmission of disease exists.

- *HEPA and N-95 Respirators.* Due to the resurgence of tuberculosis (TB), prehospital personnel should protect themselves from TB infection through use of an N-95 or a high-efficiency particulate air (HEPA) respirator, as approved by the National Institute of Occupational Safety and Health (NIOSH). It should fit snugly and be capable of filtering out the tuberculosis bacillus. An N-95 or HEPA respirator should be worn when caring for patients with confirmed or suspected TB. This is especially true when performing "high-hazard" procedures such as administration of nebulized medications, endotracheal intubation, or suctioning on such a patient.

- *Gowns.* Gowns protect clothing from blood splashes. If large splashes of blood are expected, such as with childbirth, wear impervious gowns.

- *Resuscitation Equipment.* Disposable resuscitation equipment should be the primary means of artificial ventilation in emergency care. Such items should be used once, then disposed of.

Remember, the proper use of personal protective equipment ensures effective infection control and minimizes risk. Use ALL protective equipment recommended for any particular situation to ensure maximum protection.

Consider ALL body substances potentially infectious and ALWAYS practice Standard Precautions.

Suggested Responses to "You Make the Call"

The following are suggested responses to the "You Make the Call" scenarios presented in each chapter of Volume 1, Introduction to Advanced Prehospital Care. Each represents an acceptable response to the scenario but should not be interpreted as the only correct response.

Chapter 1—Introduction to Paramedicine

1. *Discuss the vast differences between EMS and paramedic care in the United States, Canada, and other economically developed nations compared with those that exist in some less-developed countries of the world. How should awareness of such differences affect your attitude about your work?*

While people in the United States, Canada, and other developed countries consider EMS a necessity and benefit from high standards of emergency care, people in some poorer or less-developed countries often do not expect anything more than a ride to the hospital. Rather than feeling smug about our "superiority," however, North American paramedics should feel both privileged and determined to work hard to live up to the high standards we enjoy. There is also an obligation to take part in any opportunities to participate in programs in which information is exchanged between nations and EMS systems in the ongoing effort to raise standards both in the United States and around the world. From those to whom much is given, much is expected.

Chapter 2—EMS Systems

1. *Which of the "ten system elements" identified by NHTSA are mentioned in this scenario?*

   - Transportation—two modes of transportation were used in this incident, air and ground.

   - Facilities—by designating special referral centers, prehospital personnel can make transport decisions to medical facilities based on specific patient's needs.

   - Communications—without a single system of communication, which allows all EMS personnel to communicate with each other, efficiently managing this type of incident would be impossible.

   - Trauma systems—by having a system of specialized care for trauma patients, patients involved in this incident can be assured of the appropriate care.

   - Medical direction—an active physician medical director provided on-line guidance to EMS providers.

2. *For what possible reason was the top-priority patient sent so far from the scene?*

   The top-priority patient was likely sent so far away because of the extent of injuries and/or need for specialty care. Local hospitals may not be the most effective facility to receive a patient when specialty care (burn care, trauma care, stroke, cardiac, etc.) is required. Sometimes it is in the patient's best interest to bypass a local facility for another facility that is better prepared to handle the situation/care.

3. *How important was the role played by the emergency medical dispatcher in this scenario? Explain.*

   The role the 911 dispatcher played was extremely important. He put the mass-casualty plan into effect and sent the appropriate law enforcement and fire personnel. That is, as a key member of a centralized communications system, he directed the movement of resources within the system, while maintaining enough available resources to provide for the rest of the community.

4. *How might the EMS system benefit from an evaluation of this incident?*

   Even if this incident went smoothly, the QI process should review it. If nothing else, the review of the event will prove to be a good opportunity to provide continuing education on how such an event should be handled. It is unlikely that the event was handled so perfectly that there is nothing to learn from it. It could be something as simple as a better staging location for the ambulances or landing zone for the helicopter. Either way, by reviewing the event in QI, the agency will be able to identify and improve areas that may have been overlooked during the heat of the moment.

Chapter 3—Roles and Responsibilities of the Paramedic

1. *What were your key responsibilities in the previously detailed scenario?*

Your primary responsibilities in this scenario, just like any other, are safety for you and your partner followed by patient care and safety of the patient and bystanders. After ensuring that neither you nor your partner is in any danger, assessment and treatment of the patient is your next responsibility. This scenario is complicated by the family's ignorance of the capabilities and roles of EMS within the health care system. If possible, your partner can use this teaching moment to briefly educate the family to your capabilities. Maintaining a professional demeanor and going out of the way to make sure the family is made aware of the patient's status are diplomacy skills used by a true professional.

Additionally, you have the responsibility to transport the patient to the most appropriate facility, notify medical control of the situation, and ensure the continuity of care by reporting and turning the patient over to someone of equal or higher training. Your final responsibilities with continuity of care involve timely and accurate documentation of your assessment and treatment for the patient and being sure the documentation has been submitted to the patient's chart at the receiving hospital. Finally, you must ensure your unit has been placed back in service as quickly as possible and made available for any additional calls.

2. *How should you have prepared yourself mentally and physically for this call?*

Preparing yourself for this call involves physical and mental fitness preparation. A good exercise and diet program helps to ensure good health which, in turn, helps you to deal with stressors of the job. Clearly, this situation is a stressful situation and one that is all too familiar. Mental preparation involves staying up to date with continuing education and familiarizing yourself with your protocols. When you are confident in your actions and care, stressors such as family or bystanders yelling at you will not sway your treatment

or confidence.* People will pick up on the slightest signal that you are not confident, which in turn can possibly escalate the situation.

3. *Did you and your partner act professionally? If so, explain how.*

Yes, the paramedics acted professionally. Initially, they had to respond to the patient, his wife, and his son. Although the family was being difficult, that did not change the patient-care routine. They did not become rude with the family, or take out their frustrations on the patient. They were self-confident, and showed inner strength, self-control, excellent communication skills, and excellent decision-making skills.

Chapter 4—Workforce Safety and Wellness

1. *Are your stress levels inappropriately high? What are the indications?*

Yes, your stress levels are inappropriately high. This is evidenced by your irritability and sour stomach. Your stress is compounded by a poor diet, financial and home troubles, and the death of a young person. Even worse, you knew this person, and you will see the continued effects of the loss. In this situation, you are not handling the stress appropriately. Instead of spending your time off doing stress-relieving activities such as exercise, hobbies, sports, or other relaxation activities, you took on yet another overtime shift.

2. *Might it be a good idea for you to go to the funeral? Why or why not?*

The answer to this question depends on the individual. Some individuals need to have final closure and can only find this by attending the funeral or at least visiting the family at the funeral home. Other people choose to avoid the funeral home and services, claiming that the lack of closure is easier to deal with. In any event, you should be aware of which method works best to help you deal with stressful events and follow through with them.

3. *How can you improve stress management in the future?*

Methods to manage stress include following through with a healthy diet, regular exercise (30+ minutes a day), avoiding additional stress when possible, relaxation exercises, and finding a hobby to relieve stress. Suggest and attend discussion meetings following any critical events such as the one mentioned in the scenario. Don't hesitate to contact a mental health professional and make an appointment.

---

*Confidence and arrogance (cockiness) are close cousins. It is imperative that you learn to be confident without being arrogant. Arrogance breeds dissention between you and coworkers, first responders, hospital personnel, and the public. On the other hand, self-confidence can be calming and build a sense of trust.

Chapter 5—EMS Research

1. What is your study's hypothesis?

The incidence of narcotic overdoses in our EMS system is low.

2. Did you prove or disprove your hypothesis?

Although the term "incidence" is not precise, overall the number of narcotic overdoses in the system is relatively low. To get a better handle on the issue, it would be appropriate, if possible, to compare your system's incidence of narcotic overdoses to systems of similar size and demographics.

3. What was the derived benefit from the study?

The increased awareness of the low incidence of narcotic overdoses in the system resulted in, at least temporarily, decreased overall usage of naloxone.

Chapter 6—Public Health

1. How will you counter the arguments the two paramedics made?

The fire service has been doing prevention and safety programs for years now, and they still have jobs. As long as there are people, there will always be a need for EMS. By doing prevention programs, we are offering another public service and making our community safer. Not to mention, if we can prevent slips, trips, falls, and other minor injuries, we will be more available for the truly life-threatening emergencies. The scope of practice for paramedics is constantly being expanded, but patient care and safety are still our number one priorities.

2. Why is prevention an important responsibility of being a paramedic?

As paramedics, we are part of the medical community. In order for us to be recognized as a profession within the medical community, we need to fully participate in the medical community. Part of medicine is preventive medicine, health education, and controlling communicable diseases. These are the basic principles of public health and an under-addressed area of EMS. Prevention strategies help prevent the spread of communicable diseases through Standard Precautions training. Additional prevention strategies help reduce injuries and long-term disability from injuries.

3. List ten ideas for an illness and injury prevention program that may be appropriate in your area. (Answers might include any of the following suggestions or others.)

1. Seat belt campaigns
2. First aid & CPR classes
3. Swimming lessons
4. Car seat safety classes
5. Helmet and protective padding initiatives for kids
6. Home assessments for the elderly
7. Carbon monoxide detector installing
8. Environmental assessments of homes of the elderly (heat or cold assessment)
9. Vial of life/file of life or other medical information programs
10. Stroke and heart attack awareness programs

Chapter 7—Medical/Legal Aspects of Out-of-Hospital Care

1. You believe that the child needs emergency care, but the child's parents are unavailable. What should you do?

Begin emergency care under the doctrine of implied consent.

2. If you decide to treat the child without consent, can you be sued for doing so?

You can be sued for anything. But, in this case, assuming a responsible family member could not be located, you would be rendering care for an apparent life-threatening injury or illness under the doctrine of implied consent.

3. What would you do if the parents returned home and refused to grant permission for treatment?

Make multiple and sincere attempts to convince the parents to accept care for their child; make certain that they are fully informed about the implications of their decision and the potential risks of refusing care; consult with on-line medical direction; have them and a disinterested witness, such as a police officer, sign a "release-from-liability" form; advise them that they may call you again for help if necessary; document the entire situation thoroughly on your patient care report.

Chapter 8—Ethics in Paramedicine

1. What potential benefits are there in yielding to the patient's request (beneficence)?

The potential benefits in yielding to the patient's request are those involving doing good (beneficence). In this case, that would mean possibly getting to the hospital faster and thereby lessening the time the patient has to suffer severe pain.

2. What potential harm is there in yielding to the patient's request (nonmaleficence)?

Nonmaleficence refers to the paramedic's obligation to "first, do no harm." In this case, staying within the service's policy restrictions could be described as causing the patient to suffer pain longer than may be necessary. However, if you consider why the policy restricts the use of lights and siren (because they increase the risk of vehicle collision), perhaps the obligation to do no harm is better met by staying within those restrictions and avoiding the risk of further injury or further delay.

3. *How does justice come into play in this situation?*

Justice refers to the paramedic's obligation to treat all patients fairly. If the paramedic were to use the emergency lights and siren for Phil Cornock, he would be making an exception to a policy restriction. If he makes this exception, and there are other patients who might benefit by getting to the hospital faster but do not because the paramedics are following the rules, then those patients are not being treated fairly.

4. *How should paramedics in general respond when a patient requests an intervention that is not medically indicated?*

In the absence of standards or protocols that fit the situation, the paramedic needs to reason out the problem. He must first state the action in a universal form, then consider the implications or consequences of the action and, finally, compare them to relevant values.

Chapter 9—EMS System Communications

1. *Based on the information provided, organize and prepare your radio report to inform the receiving hospital of your patient's condition.*

Rescue: Palermo Rescue to Davidson Medical Center.

Hospital: Davidson Medical, Doctor Stowe here, go ahead.

Rescue: Davidson Medical, this is Paramedic Kirk inbound to your facility with a 69-year-old male patient complaining of chest pain. How do you copy?

Hospital: I copy a 69-year-old male complaining of chest pain, go ahead.

Rescue: Doctor Stowe, this patient's pain began about 30 minutes ago while he was at rest. He describes it as a substernal pressure-type pain radiating into his arm and jaw. He has a history of heart disease and two prior MIs with bypass surgery two years ago. His current meds are Lanoxin, Lasix, Capoten, and aspirin, and he is allergic to Mellaril. His blood pressure is 210/110, pulse of 70, respirations of 20 mildly labored with a pulse oximetry of 93 percent with supplemental oxygen. He has become progressively more dyspneic in our presence. We have an ETA to your facility of 10 minutes. Do you have any further orders at this time?

Chapter 10—Documentation

1. *What is wrong with this narrative?*

What is a "10-48"? Is this the same in every EMS system?

Was the ambulance dispatched to the corner of Main and Spice?

Was the ambulance dispatched to the coroner, at Main and Spice?

Was the ambulance dispatched to the main coroner, whose name is Spice?

What is "PMD"?

"Patient is nasty and abusive" is judgmental.

"Looks like a drug abuser" is judgmental.

"Abnoctious" should be spelled "obnoxious."

"Obnoxious" is judgmental.

What exactly are the injuries?

Exactly what treatment, if any, was rendered?

Was EMS transport not needed because the patient was not hurt, or because the police transported him?

Did the patient go to the hospital or to jail?

2. *What will you do to make sure your documentation is better than this?*

Avoid using codes.

Practice spelling and use only words you can spell correctly.

Do not use abbreviations that are unclear; spell out terms the first time you use them, followed by the abbreviation in parentheses.

Do not be judgmental.

Describe the head-to-toe assessment completely.

Be particularly careful and complete in no-transport situations.

Chapter 11—Human Life Span Development

1. *Do you believe that this is normal behavior for a patient of this age and in this particular situation?*

Yes, it is exactly the type of behavior that should be expected from a patient this age and in this situation.

2. *What is a likely reason for this behavior?*

Adolescents are very concerned with modesty and privacy. The reason for her behavior is likely that her parents and younger sister are in the room with her. Additionally, the patient may have been hiding something from her parents, such as sexual activity, drug or alcohol use, birth control pills, or another issue, that she does not want to reveal to them or her sister.

3. *What might you do to make this patient more cooperative?*

If possible, have a "same sex" provider perform the patient assessment. If this is possible, then you might ask the parents and sister to leave the room. If there is no "same sex" provider available, then have the mother stay in the room for the protection of both the patient and the provider, but have her move to a point away from the bed so that answers to your questions cannot be heard. If possible, palpate the abdomen through a thin sheet to further protect the patient's modesty.

Chapter 12—Pathophysiology

1. Explain the physiologic basis for the patient's apparent dehydration.

As blood glucose levels start to rise, glucose is lost into the urine through the kidneys. This typically occurs when the blood glucose level exceeds 180 mg/dL. The glucose molecules have osmotic properties. Thus, they take water molecules with them into the urine. This phenomenon, called osmotic diuresis, ultimately causes a decrease in intravascular fluid volume resulting in dehydration. This causes tachycardia and ultimately a fall in blood pressure. Also, it is the pathophysiologic basis for the polyuria (excessive urination) and polydipsia (excessive thirst) associated with untreated diabetes.

2. Describe the role of insulin in glucose transport into the cell.

Insulin is necessary for the transport of the glucose molecule into the cell (except for cells in the brain). Insulin activates specialized glucose transport proteins present on the surface of the cell. If insulin levels are inadequate, then glucose cannot enter the cell to fuel the various metabolic processes. This causes the cells to shift to a less-effective form of metabolism (anaerobic metabolism and lipid metabolism), ultimately resulting in the accumulation of acids and ketones. As ketones rise, they are eliminated through the urine and the respiratory tract. When this occurs, the characteristic odor of ketones can often be detected on the breath and in the urine.

3. Prepare a prehospital treatment plan given the information provided.

Prehospital treatment should first address the airway and breathing. If necessary, provide airway and respiratory support. In most cases, the airway will be patent. Supplemental oxygen should be administered via a nonrebreather mask if the patient is hypoxic. Then, an IV should be started with an isotonic crystalloid solution such as normal saline. Often the patient will require several liters of fluid to replace lost volume. Later, the patient will require intravenous insulin to move the glucose into the cells for normal metabolic processes. This is often administered in the form of an insulin drip. Blood glucose levels must be constantly monitored to prevent iatrogenic hypoglycemia.

Chapter 13—Emergency Pharmacology

1. What is dopamine and what is its mechanism of action?

It is a catecholamine that stimulates alpha, beta, and, supposedly, dopaminergic receptors. It was given in moderate dosage, which stimulates the beta receptors more than the others. This increases the force of cardiac contraction, which may increase cardiac output and, subsequently, blood pressure.

2. What was the purpose of the dopamine infusion?

Dopamine was given to increase cardiac output. The patient is suffering from cardiogenic shock with pulmonary edema and needs to have his blood pressure increased. Raising his cardiac output with dopamine is preferable to increasing his peripheral vascular resistance (afterload), because his obvious difficulty overcoming existing afterload is causing the pulmonary edema.

3. What is atropine's mechanism of action?

Atropine is a parasympatholytic that blocks the effects of acetylcholine at the muscarinic receptors, specifically those at the heart's SA and AV nodes, which regulate heart rate. A side effect of succinylcholine administration is bradycardia (the physical act of intubation may also cause bradycardia). Atropine is therefore given as a prophylactic treatment against expected bradycardia. This bradycardic side effect is most notable in pediatric patients.

4. Why was midazolam administered before succinylcholine?

Midazolam is a sedative with amnesic properties. Succinylcholine is a neuromuscular blocker that induces muscular paralysis without affecting consciousness. This would be a very unpleasant sensation, so some type of sedation or anesthesia is given before any neuromuscular blockade.

5. What are succinylcholine's classification and mechanism of action?

Succinylcholine is a depolarizing (fasciculating) neuromuscular blocker that is given to induce paralysis. This is most frequently done to facilitate intubation in rapid sequence intubation. It acts by competing with acetylcholine at the nicotinic receptors. When succinylcholine binds with these receptors, it causes depolarization much like acetylcholine; however, it remains bound to the receptor and prevents repolarization and subsequent depolarization of the muscle. This in turn prevents muscle contraction and causes paralysis. Pseudocholinesterase, an enzyme similar to acetylcholinesterase, eventually breaks down succinylcholine.

Chapter 14—Intravenous Access and Medication Administration

1. Before administering aspirin or any other medication orally (p.o.), what major consideration must you be sure of?

When administering a medication orally, or by way of the mouth and enteral tract, you must make sure that the patient has an adequate level of consciousness and can support his airway. Administering a medication orally to a semiconscious or unresponsive patient who cannot support his airway can cause an airway occlusion and/or aspiration into the lungs. If aspiration occurs, the patient is at risk for an inflammatory response and deadly aspiration pneumonia.

2. *Of the following medications and routes of delivery, which will provide the fastest and most predictable rate of absorption?*

- *aspirin—enteral tract*
- *nitroglycerin—sublingual*
- *morphine sulfate—IV bolus*

The morphine sulfate delivered as an intravenous bolus will provide the most predictable and fastest rate of drug absorption. Any medication delivered directly into the venous circulation will be carried by the blood and quickly reach its target site.

Drug absorption in the enteral tract (aspirin given orally) can be affected adversely by physical activity, emotion, and the presence of food. Absorption via the sublingual route involves passage of the medication (nitroglycerin) through the mucous membranes beneath the tongue. Once it passes through these membranes, the drug can then be circulated via the venous circulation throughout the body. Even though passage is relatively fast, overall absorption does not occur as quickly as when the medication is injected directly into the venous circulation.

3. *When administered sublingually, how is the nitroglycerin absorbed into the body?*

When administering nitroglycerin via the sublingual route, the medication must be absorbed through the mucous membranes beneath the tongue. The area beneath the tongue is extremely rich with blood vessels. Once through the mucous membranes, the nitroglycerin is carried by the venous circulation and systemically distributed throughout the body.

4. *You elect to administer 3 mg of morphine sulfate to the patient. The medication is packaged as 10 mg in 5 mL of solution in a multidose vial. How many milliliters must you administer to give the 3 mg of morphine?*

Using the formula as discussed in the chapter, the drug dosage can be calculated as follows:

$$\frac{5 \text{ ml (volume on hand)} \times 3 \text{ mg (desired dose)}}{10 \text{ mg (dosage on hand)}} = 1.5 \text{ mL}$$

To deliver 3 mg of morphine sulfate, you must administer 1.5 mL of the medication solution.

Using the ratio and proportion method, the amount of drug to administer is calculated as follows:

$$5 \text{ mL}/10 \text{ mg} = x \text{ mL}/3 \text{ mg}$$
$$15/10 = x$$
$$x = 1.5 \text{ mL}$$

Chapter 15—Airway Management and Ventilation

1. *What is your primary assessment and management of this child?*

Your initial assessment always begins with making sure the scene is safe and donning PPE. Your next step is to determine if there is any suspected trauma and assess the child's LOC by gently tapping and calling the child's name. Quickly follow this with opening the airway (head-tilt/chin-lift if no trauma is suspected and jaw-thrust if trauma is suspected) and determine if the child is breathing. If the child is not breathing, give positive pressure ventilations ([×]2) by either BVM, FROPVD, or pocket mask and begin chest compressions. (Remember, these are done in lieu of abdominal thrusts for pediatric patients.) If you are the only ALS person on scene, these BLS maneuvers should be performed by your basic partner or another BLS-trained person while you prepare your equipment. Approximately every 2 minutes, you should stop the BLS compressions, assess the airway for a visible obstruction, and begin the compressions again.

Note: Even though the patient is not breathing, placing a nonrebreather mask over the patient's mouth and nose may help provide some oxygenation during the compressions. (If the airway is completely obstructed, this is less likely to help. However, if there is any air movement, no matter how small, the increased oxygenation provided by the NRB can do nothing but help.) Remember to remove the mask prior to attempting any type of ventilations.

If the airway obstruction is not relieved by BLS maneuvers within the first 2 minutes of your arrival, you should begin advanced airway procedures including the use of an appropriately sized extraglottic airway, direct laryngoscopy, and retrieving the occlusion with Magill forceps or placing an endotracheal tube. If the obstruction is still unrelieved, your last resort would be use of a surgical airway (cricothyrotomy) to create an airway until hospital doctors can remove the obstruction.

2. *What are your first actions?*

Your first actions are to gain control of the scene and call for any needed additional assistance, such as Emergency Medical Responders or other EMS units or law enforcement, to help with maintaining order. Additionally, you will want to attempt to determine the extent of the child's airway obstruction by opening the airway; listening, looking, and feeling for air movement and chest rise; and giving positive pressure ventilations with a BVM or pocket mask.

3. *What are your options for managing the airway after the obstruction is relieved?*

Upon relieving the airway obstruction, your first priority is to ventilate the patient and check for circulatory function or pulses. If pulses are present, you should proceed with securing the airway with whatever means necessary and available to maintain a secure, open airway. Options for this will include (in order from least invasive to most invasive):

- Oxygen delivery via nonrebreather mask
- Nasopharyngeal airway
- Oropharyngeal airway
- Blind insertion airway device
- Endotracheal tube

In addition to the airway device just mentioned, the patient should be placed on supplemental oxygen to maintain pulse oximetry levels of at least 90 percent. This may include nasal cannula, nonrebreather mask, or bag-valve mask.

4. *What are the major anatomic differences between pediatric and adult patients in terms of airway management?*

- Pediatric structures are smaller and more difficult to navigate.

- Pediatric tongues are larger in proportion.
- Nasal openings are smaller and adenoids are large on pediatric patients.
- The pediatric cricoid rings are pliable and may be compressed with overaggressive cricoid pressure.
- Distance from the vocal cords to the carina is closer in pediatrics, requiring the tube to be inserted only 2–3 cm below the cords.
- Large occiput in pediatrics makes positioning difficult.
- The pediatric epiglottis is floppy and round ("omega" shaped), making use of the straight (Miller) blades more popular for pediatric intubation.
- The pediatric glottic opening is higher and more anterior in the neck, making it easier to insert the laryngoscope blade too deeply.
- The narrowest part of the pediatric airway is the cricoid cartilage, not the glottic opening.
- Children will desaturate (oxygen) faster than an adult.

Answers to Review Questions

Below are answers to the Review Questions presented in each chapter of Volume 1.

Chapter 1—Introduction to Paramedicine

1. c
2. d
3. a
4. d
5. c

Chapter 2—EMS Systems

1. b
2. b
3. c
4. b
5. a
6. b
7. c
8. b
9. b
10. a

Chapter 3—Roles and Responsibilities of the Paramedic

1. b
2. c
3. a
4. a
5. d
6. d
7. c
8. a

Chapter 4—Workforce Safety and Wellness

1. a
2. c
3. c
4. d
5. d
6. c
7. b
8. b
9. a
10. d

Chapter 5—EMS Research

1. b
2. b
3. a
4. b
5. a
6. d
7. a

Chapter 6—Public Health

1. c
2. b
3. b
4. c
5. b
6. b

Chapter 7—Medical/Legal Aspects of Out-of-Hospital Care

1. a
2. d
3. b
4. a
5. c
6. c
7. d
8. c
9. d
10. d

Chapter 8—Ethics in Paramedicine

1. b
2. c
3. a
4. a
5. d

Chapter 9—EMS Systems and Communications

1. c
2. d
3. a
4. b
5. e
6. a
7. b

8. c
9. b
10. a

Chapter 10—Documentation

1. d
2. c
3. b
4. a
5. a
6. a
7. d
8. c

Chapter 11—Human Life Span Development

1. c
2. d
3. c
4. a
5. c
6. b
7. c
8. c
9. a
10. c

Chapter 12—Pathophysiology

1. a
2. b
3. c
4. b
5. d
6. d
7. d
8. b
9. c
10. c
11. b
12. d
13. b
14. b
15. d
16. d

17. b
18. c
19. a
20. d
21. d
22. c
23. c
24. b
25. c

Chapter 13—Emergency Pharmacology

1. c
2. b
3. b
4. c
5. b
6. b
7. a
8. b
9. d
10. c
11. c
12. d
13. a
14. c
15. b
16. d
17. d
18. b
19. b
20. b

Chapter 14—Intravenous Access and Medication Administration

1. a
2. c
3. c
4. b
5. b
6. b
7. d
8. c

9. c
10. c
11. b
12. d
13. c
14. a
15. b
16. d
17. a
18. c
19. d
20. d
21. a
22. b
23. b
24. b
25. c
26. a
27. c
28. c
29. d
30. b
31. e
32. b

Chapter 15—Airway Management and Ventilation

1. d
2. b
3. c
4. c
5. c
6. d
7. b
8. b
9. b
10. c
11. c
12. d
13. c
14. a
15. c
16. d
17. c
18. d
19. b
20. a

Glossary

10-code radio communications system using codes that begin with the word *ten*.

abandonment termination of the paramedic–patient relationship without assurance that an equal or greater level of care will continue.

ABCs airway, breathing, and circulation.

ABO blood groups four blood groups formed by the presence or absence of two antigens known as A and B. A person may have either (type A or type B), both (type AB), or neither (type O). An immune response will be activated whenever a person receives blood containing A or B antigen if this antigen is not already present in his own blood.

abstract a written summary of the key points, especially of a scientific paper; a report presented before publication of the entire paper.

accelerometers sensors in a vehicle that can measure a change in total velocity, forces applied to the vehicle, direction forces were applied, whether the vehicle rolled over, whether air bags were deployed, and the vehicle's final resting position.

accreditation a system ensuring that education programs for paramedics and other EMS personnel levels meet minimal guidelines for faculty, facilities, equipment, medical oversight, clinical affiliations, and financial stability.

acid–base reaction any chemical reaction that results in the transfer of protons.

acidosis a high concentration of hydrogen ions; a pH below 7.35; an excess of acids in the body.

acids substances that give up protons during chemical reactions.

acquired immunity protection from infection or disease that is (1) developed by the body after exposure to an antigen (active acquired immunity) or (2) transferred to the person from an outside source such as from the mother through the placenta or as a serum (passive acquired immunity).

active transport movement of a substance through a cell membrane against the osmotic gradient; that is, from an area of lesser concentration to an area of greater concentration, opposite to the normal direction of diffusion; requires the use of energy to move a substance.

actual damages compensable physical, psychological, or financial harm.

acute of sudden onset, as an acute disease.

ad hoc database database created each time a patient is encountered to include information about that patient such as vital signs, video, electronic health record, and voice-to-text medical findings that can be stored and then accessed as needed by rescuers, helicopter crew, and hospital physicians.

addendum addition or supplement to the original report.

adenosine triphosphate (ATP) a high-energy compound present in all cells, especially muscle cells; when split by enzyme action, it yields energy. Energy is stored in ATP.

adipocytes fat cells.

adipose tissue fat.

adjunct medication agent that enhances the effects of other medications.

administration tubing flexible, clear plastic tubing that connects the solution bag to the IV cannula.

administrative law law that is enacted by governmental agencies at either the federal or state level. Also called regulatory law.

adrenergic pertaining to the neurotransmitter norepinephrine.

advance directive a document created to ensure that certain treatment choices are honored when a patient is unconscious or otherwise unable to express his choice of treatment.

advanced automatic crash notification (AACN) data collection and transmission system that can automatically contact a national call center or local public safety answering point and transmit detailed crash data, such as the type of vehicle, speed and direction of impact, and probable severity of injury to occupants. The AACN call center can simultaneously dispatch a variety of responders, including rescue/extrication crews, fire service, and medical helicopter transport, and advise the most appropriate hospital or trauma center to prepare for arrival of patients.

Advanced Emergency Medical Technician (AEMT) the level of EMS practitioner who performs the responsibilities of an EMT with the addition of limited advanced emergency medical care.

aerobic metabolism the second stage of metabolism, requiring the presence of oxygen, in which the breakdown of glucose (in a process called the Krebs or citric acid cycle) yields a high amount of energy. *Aerobic* means "with oxygen."

affinity force of attraction between a medication and a receptor.

afterload the resistance a contraction of the heart must overcome in order to eject blood; in cardiac physiology, defined as the tension of cardiac muscle during systole (contraction).

against medical advice (AMA) your patient refuses care even though you feel he needs it.

agonist medication that binds to a receptor and causes it to initiate the expected response.

agonist–antagonist medication that binds to a receptor and stimulates some of its effects but blocks others. Also called *partial agonist.*

AIDS (acquired immunodeficiency syndrome) a group of signs, symptoms, and disorders that often develop as a consequence of HIV infection.

air embolism air in the vein.

albumin a protein commonly present in plant and animal tissues. In the blood, albumin works to maintain blood volume and blood pressure and provides colloid osmotic pressure, which prevents plasma loss from the capillaries.

alkalosis a low concentration of hydrogen ions; a pH above 7.45; an excess of base in the body.

allergy exaggerated immune response to an environmental antigen.

allied health professions ancillary health care professions apart from physicians and nurses, such as paramedics, respiratory therapists, and physical therapists.

alveoli microscopic air sacs where most oxygen and carbon dioxide gas exchanges take place.

amino acids molecules containing an amine group, a carboxylic acid group, and varying side chains; among other functions, amino acids are the building blocks of proteins.

ampule breakable glass vessel containing liquid medication.

amylopectin a highly branched polymer of glucose; one of two types of starch, the other being amylose.

amylose a linear, unbranched polymer of glucose; one of two types of starch, the other being amylopectin.

anabolism the constructive phase of metabolism in which cells convert nonliving substances into living cytoplasm; the synthesis of steroid compounds by the body.

anaerobic metabolism the first stage of metabolism, which does not require oxygen, in which the breakdown of glucose (in a process called glycolysis) produces pyruvic acid and yields very little energy. *Anaerobic* means "without oxygen."

analgesia the absence of the sensation of pain.

analgesic medication that relieves the sensation of pain.

analysis of variance (ANOVA) parametric statistic used to ascertain the extent to which significant group differences can be inferred to the population.

anaphylaxis a life-threatening allergic reaction; also called *anaphylactic shock.*

anchor time set of hours when a night-shift worker can reliably expect to rest without interruption.

anesthesia the absence of all sensations.

anesthetic medication that induces a loss of sensation to touch or pain.

anion an ion with a negative charge—so called because it will be attracted to an anode, or positive pole.

anoxia the absence or near-absence of oxygen in certain tissues or in the body as a whole.

antacid alkalotic compound used to increase the gastric environment's pH.

antagonist medication that binds to a receptor but does not cause it to initiate the expected response.

antiarrhythmic medication used to treat and prevent abnormal cardiac rhythms.

antibiotic agent that kills or decreases the growth of bacteria.

antibody a substance produced by B lymphocytes in response to the presence of a foreign antigen that will combine with and control or destroy the antigen, thus preventing infection.

anticoagulant medication that inhibits blood clotting.

antiemetic medication used to prevent vomiting.

antifibrinolytic medication that inhibits the activation of plasminogen to plasmin, prevents the breakup of fibrin (fibrinolysis), and maintains clot stability.

antigen a marker on the surface of a cell that identifies it as "self" or "non-self."

antigen–antibody complex the substance formed when an antibody combines with an antigen to deactivate or destroy it; also called *immune complex.*

antigen-presenting cells (APCs) cells, such as macrophages, that present (express onto their surfaces) portions of the antigens they have digested.

antigen processing the recognition, ingestion, and breakdown of a foreign antigen, culminating in production of an antibody to the antigen or in a direct cytotoxic response to the antigen.

antihistamine medication that arrests the effects of histamine by blocking its receptors.

antihyperlipidemic medication used to treat high blood cholesterol.

antihypertensive medication used to treat hypertension.

antineoplastic agent medication used to treat cancer.

antiplatelet medication that decreases the formation of platelet plugs.

antiseptic cleansing agent that is not toxic to living tissue.

antitussive medication that suppresses the stimulus to cough in the central nervous system.

anxious avoidant attachment a type of bonding that occurs when an infant learns that his caregivers will not be responsive or helpful when needed.

anxious resistant attachment a type of bonding that occurs when an infant is uncertain about whether or not his caregivers will be responsive or helpful when needed.

apnea temporary stop in breathing.

apneic oxygenation a method of providing oxygen to an apneic (non-breathing) patient during endotracheal intubation to minimize the possibility of hypoxia developing during the procedure.

apoptosis response in which an injured cell releases enzymes that engulf and destroy it; one way the body rids itself of damaged and dead cells.

arterial oxygen concentration (CaO_2) a measure of oxygen content in the arterial blood.

asepsis a condition free of pathogens.

aspiration inhaling foreign material such as vomitus into the lungs.

assault an act that unlawfully places a person in apprehension of immediate bodily harm without his consent.

assay test that determines the amount and purity of a given chemical in a preparation in the laboratory.

atelectasis alveolar collapse.

atom the fundamental chemical unit, which contains subatomic particles, including electrons, protons, and neutrons.

atomic number the number of protons in the nucleus of an atom; an element is defined by its atomic number.

atrophy a decrease in cell size resulting from a decreased workload.

aural medication medication administered through the mucous membranes of the ear and ear canal.

authoritarian a parenting style that demands absolute obedience without regard to a child's individual freedom.

authoritative a parenting style that emphasizes a balance between a respect for authority and individual freedom.

autoimmune disease failure of the immune system to recognize certain tissues normally present in the body resulting in an attack against those tissues by the immune system; autoimmune disease includes rheumatic heart disease and rheumatoid arthritis.

autoimmunity an immune response to self-antigens, which the body normally tolerates.

automatic crash notification (ACN) data collection and transmission system that can automatically contact a national call center or local public safety answering point and transmit limited specific crash data, such as that a crash has taken place and where it is located.

automatic location information (ALI) in computers at enhanced 911 communication centers, the ability to display the location of a caller's phone.

automatic number identification (ANI) in computers at enhanced 911 communication centers, the ability to display a caller's telephone number.

autonomic ganglia groups of autonomic nerve cells located outside the central nervous system.

autonomic nervous system the part of the nervous system that controls involuntary actions.

autonomy a competent adult patient's right to determine what happens to his own body.

B lymphocytes the type of white blood cells that, in response to the presence of an antigen, produce antibodies that attack the antigen, develop a memory for the antigen, and confer long-term immunity to the antigen.

bacteria (singular, bacterium) single-celled organisms with a cell membrane and cytoplasm but no organized nucleus. They bind to the cells of a host organism to obtain food and support.

bag-valve mask (BVM) ventilation device consisting of a self-inflating bag with two one-way valves and a transparent plastic face mask.

bandwidth (1) the width of a range of frequencies, measured in hertz; (2) a rate of data transmission, measured in bits per second (bps).

barotrauma injury caused by pressure within an enclosed space.

basement membrane a thin sheet of fibers that underlies the epithelia, the membranes that line or cover internal and external body surfaces.

bases substances that acquire protons during chemical reactions.

basophils granular white blood cells that, similarly to mast cells, release histamine and other chemicals that control constriction and dilation of blood vessels during inflammation.

battery the unlawful touching of another individual without his consent.

bench research research done in a controlled laboratory setting using nonhuman subjects.

beneficence the principle of doing good for the patient.

benign not cancerous; not able to spread to other tissues. *See also* malignant.

bias potential unintended or unavoidable effect on study outcomes.

bilevel positive airway pressure (BiPAP)   air or oxygen delivered under pressure that is higher during inhalation and lower during exhalation.

bioassay   test to ascertain a medication's availability in a biologic model.

bioavailability   amount of a medication that is still active after it reaches its target tissue.

bioequivalence   relative therapeutic effectiveness of chemically equivalent medications.

biologic half-life   time the body takes to clear one-half of a medication.

biotransformation   special name given to the metabolism of medications.

blood tube   glass container with color-coded, self-sealing rubber top.

blood tubing   administration tubing that contains a filter to prevent clots or other debris from entering the patient.

blood–brain barrier   tight junctions of the capillary endothelial cells in the central nervous system vasculature through which only non–protein-bound, highly lipid-soluble medications can pass.

bolus   concentrated mass of medication.

bonding   the formation of a close personal relationship (as between mother and child), especially through frequent or constant association.

breach of duty   an action or inaction that violates the standard of care expected from a paramedic.

bronchi   tubes from the trachea into the lungs.

bubble sheet   scannable run sheet on which you fill in boxes or "bubbles" to record assessment and care information.

buccal   between the cheek and gums.

buffer   a substance that tends to preserve or restore a normal acid-base balance by increasing or decreasing the concentration of hydrogen ions.

burette chamber   calibrated chamber of Berutrol IV administration tubing that enables precise measurement and delivery of fluids and medicated solutions.

burnout   when coping mechanisms no longer buffer job stressors, which can compromise personal health and well-being.

bystander   a family member, friend, or stranger to the patient who is present at the patient's medical emergency.

call routing   the process of transferring an emergency call to the nearest 911 center; occasionally technical problems cause such a call to be routed out of the call area.

cannula   hollow needle used to puncture a vein.

cannulation   *see* intravenous (IV) access.

CaO$_2$ *see* arterial oxygen concentration.

capnography   a recording or display of the measurement of exhaled carbon dioxide concentrations over time.

carbon dioxide   waste product of the body's metabolism.

carcinogenesis   the process of developing a cancer.

cardiac contractile force   the strength of a contraction of the heart.

cardiac output   the amount of blood pumped by the heart in 1 minute (computed as stroke volume × heart rate).

cardiogenic shock   shock caused by insufficient cardiac output; the inability of the heart to pump enough blood to perfuse all parts of the body.

carrier proteins   proteins involved in carrying solutes (ions or molecules) across a biologic membrane.

carrier-mediated diffusion   process in which carrier proteins transport large molecules across the cell membrane. *See* facilitated diffusion.

cartilage   a type of connective tissue that provides structure and support to other tissues.

cascade   a series of actions triggered by a first action and culminating in a final action—typical of the actions caused by plasma proteins involved in the complement, coagulation, and kinin systems.

case report   a structured study of a single unit, subject, event, or patient.

case series   observational study that tracks patients with a known exposure or examines their medical records for exposure and outcome.

catecholamines   epinephrine and norepinephrine, hormones that strongly affect the nervous and cardiovascular systems, metabolic rate, temperature, and smooth muscle.

catheter inserted through the needle/intracatheter   Teflon catheter inserted through a large metal stylet.

cation   an ion with a positive charge—so called because it will be attracted to a cathode, or negative pole.

cell membrane   *also* plasma membrane; the outer covering of a cell.

cell   the basic structural unit of all plants and animals. A membrane enclosing a thick fluid and a nucleus. Cells are specialized to carry out all of the body's basic functions.

cell-mediated immunity   the short-term immunity to an antigen provided by T lymphocytes, which directly attack the antigen but do not produce antibodies or memory for the antigen.

cells   regions into which a cell phone service is divided.

cellular adaptation   physiologic or structural changes to a cell in response to change or stress or a pathological condition.

cellular respiration   metabolic processes with a cell that convert nutrients to energy in the form of adenosine triphosphate (ATP) and that subsequently release waste products from the cell.

cellular telephone system   A type of wireless communication, called "cellular" because it is based on a complex of separate base stations, each covering one "cell" or geographic area. As a cell phone user travels, calls are transferred from base station to base station.

cellulose a polysaccharide polymer with glucose as its monomer that is the major structural material of plants.

central venous access surgical puncture of the internal jugular, subclavian, or femoral vein.

centrioles cylindrical structures within cells that play an important role in cell division.

certification the process by which an agency or association grants recognition to an individual who has met its qualifications.

chain of survival As defined by the American Heart Association, the five most important factors affecting survival of a cardiac arrest patient: (1) immediate recognition and activation of EMS; (2) early CPR; (3) rapid defibrillation; (4) effective advanced life support; (5) integrated post–cardiac arrest care.

chemoreceptors sensory receptors that detect and act on chemical signals—for example, sensing a change in carbon dioxide levels in the blood and responding by causing an increase in respiratory rate to expel the excess carbon dioxide from the body.

chemotactic factors chemicals that attract white cells to the site of inflammation, a process called chemotaxis.

chemotaxis *see* chemotactic factors.

chi square test nonparametric statistic used with nominal data to test group differences.

cholinergic pertaining to the neurotransmitter acetylcholine.

chromatin a combination of DNA and other proteins in the nucleus of a cell that condenses to form chromosomes.

chromosomes threadlike structures within the nuclei of cells that carry genetic information.

chronic slow in onset, persisting over a long period of time, as in a chronic disease.

cilia threadlike projections from the surface of cells that move back and forth and can sweep debris such as mucus or dust away from the cell.

circadian rhythms physiologic phenomena that occur at approximately 24-hour intervals.

circulatory overload an excess in intravascular fluid volume.

cisternae saclike structures within body cells that form part of the structure of rough endoplasmic reticulum (RER) and of the Golgi apparatus and act as carrier vessels that transport proteins from the RER to the Golgi apparatus for further processing.

citric acid cycle a key phase of glucose metabolism, requiring the presence of oxygen, in which pyruvic acid (a product of the breakdown of glucose) is oxidized, resulting in the release of energy in the form of ATP and carbon dioxide as waste. Also called the *Krebs cycle* or the *tricarboxylic acid (TCA) cycle*.

civil law division of the legal system that deals with noncriminal issues and conflicts between two or more parties.

civil rights the rights of personal liberty guaranteed to American citizens by the 13th and 14th amendments to the United States Constitution and by certain acts of Congress.

cleaning washing an object with cleaners such as soap and water.

clinical presentation the manifestation of a disease; the signs and symptoms of a disease.

clinical protocols the policies and procedures established by a medical director for all components of an EMS system, such as medical treatment protocols.

clonal diversity the development of receptors, by B lymphocyte precursors in the bone marrow, for every possible type of antigen.

clonal selection the process by which a specific antigen reacts with the appropriate receptors on the surface of immature B lymphocytes, thereby activating them and prompting them to proliferate, differentiate, and produce antibodies to the activating antigen.

coagulation system a plasma protein system that results in formation of a protein called fibrin. Fibrin forms a network that walls off an infection and forms a clot that stops bleeding and serves as a foundation for repair and healing of a wound. Also called the *clotting system*.

Code Green Campaign organization that works to raise awareness of mental health issues and care that can be provided for mental health challenges associated with EMS service. *See also* Tema Conter Memorial Trust.

coenzymes nonprotein substances that bind to enzyme proteins to assist them in biochemical transformations. Also called *cofactors*.

cofactors *see* coenzymes.

cognitive radio a "smart" device that is able to search the airwaves it covers for strong signals with no competing transmissions to provide the best possible channel of communication.

cohort study study of a group of subjects initially identified as having one or more characteristics in common who are followed over time.

collagen proteins that are the main component of connective tissue.

colloid intravenous solution containing large proteins that cannot pass through capillary membranes; also *colloid solution*.

common law law that is derived from society's acceptance of customs and norms over time. Also called case law or judge-made law.

common operating picture (COP) a single display of operational information, such as data about a traffic crash and emergency responses to it, that is simultaneously shared by all units involved in responding to the emergency so that all those involved are working with the same information.

communication the process of exchanging information between individuals.

communication protocols predetermined, written guidelines for the type of information you may communicate by various means of communication without breaching patient confidentiality and privacy.

community paramedicine health care performed by paramedics apart from customary emergency response and transport, such as in physicians' offices, outpatient clinics, or as part of paramedic crews specially trained to periodically assess and monitor high-risk patients receiving home care or elsewhere in the community. Also called *mobile integrated health care.*

compensated shock early stage of shock during which the body's compensatory mechanisms are able to maintain normal perfusion.

competent able to make an informed decision about medical care.

competitive antagonism one medication binding to a receptor and causing the expected effect while also blocking another medication from triggering the same receptor.

complement system a group of plasma proteins (the complement proteins) that are dormant in the blood until activated, as by antigen-antibody complex formation, by products released by bacteria, or by components of other plasma protein systems. When activated, the complement system is involved in most of the events of inflammatory response.

compliance the stiffness or flexibility of the lung tissue.

complications abnormalities or conditions that result from another, original disease or problem. Also called *sequelae.*

compound chemical union of two or more elements.

concentration weight per volume.

concentration gradient the gradual change in concentration of a solution over a distance within the solution.

confidence interval an expression of how closely the sample estimate matches the true value in the whole population.

confidentiality principle of law that prohibits the release of medical or other personal information about a patient without the patient's consent.

congenital metabolic diseases diseases affecting the metabolism that are present from birth.

connective tissue the most abundant body tissue; it provides support, connection, and insulation. Examples are bone, cartilage, fat, and blood.

consent the patient's granting of permission for treatment.

constitutional law law based on the U.S. Constitution.

continuous positive airway pressure (CPAP) air or oxygen delivered under pressure that is maintained at a steady level during both inhalation and exhalation.

contraction inward movement of wound edges during healing that eventually brings the wound edges together.

control group an experimental study group that does not receive a treatment or intervention that is given to the experimental group.

convenience sampling sampling in which the subjects or patients are selected, in part or in whole, at the convenience of the researcher.

conventional reasoning the stage of moral development during which children desire approval from individuals and society.

Cormack and LeHane grading system a system for evaluating and scoring airway difficulty based on the portion of the glottic opening and vocal cords that may be seen.

cortisol a steroid hormone released by the adrenal cortex that regulates the metabolism of fats, carbohydrates, sodium, potassium, and proteins and has an anti-inflammatory effect.

covalent bond force holding atoms together that results when atoms share electrons.

cricoid pressure pressure applied in a posterior direction to the anterior cricoid cartilage; occludes the esophagus.

cricothyroid membrane membrane between the cricoid and thyroid cartilages of the larynx.

criminal law division of the legal system that deals with wrongs committed against society or its members.

cristae folds within mitochondria that form shelves within the mitochondria.

critical care transport the transport of critically ill or injured patients.

cross-sectional study a study in which a statistically significant sample of a population is used to estimate the relationship between an outcome of interest and population variables as they exist at one particular time.

crystalloid intravenous solution that contains electrolytes but lacks the larger proteins associated with a colloid; also *crystalloid solution.*

cyanosis bluish discoloration.

cytokines proteins, produced by white blood cells, that regulate immune responses by binding with and affecting the function of the cells that produced them or of other, nearby cells.

cytoplasm the thick fluid, or protoplasm, that fills a cell.

cytoskeleton system of filaments, microtubules, and intermediate filaments that are part of the internal structure of a cell.

cytotoxic toxic, or poisonous, to cells.

data dictionary a source of information about a specific set of data that provides definitions of terms, explanations of interrelations among the separate data, and similar information.

data dredging   the inappropriate (sometimes deliberately so) use of data mining to uncover relationships in data that may be misleading.

data mining   the process of searching large amounts of data for patterns or relationships.

dead spot   an area where transmission and reception of a radio or other signal is poor.

debridement   the cleaning up or removal of debris, dead cells, and scabs from a wound, principally through phagocytosis.

decompensated shock   advanced stages of shock when the body's compensatory mechanisms are no longer able to maintain normal perfusion; also called *progressive shock*.

defamation   an intentional false communication that injures another person's reputation or good name.

degranulation   the emptying of granules from the interior of a mast cell into the extracellular environment.

dehydration   excessive loss of body fluid.

delayed hypersensitivity reaction   a hypersensitivity reaction that takes place after some time elapses following reexposure to an antigen. Delayed hypersensitivity reactions are usually less severe than immediate reactions.

demand-valve device   a ventilation device that is manually operated by a push button or lever.

denaturation   loss of a protein's three-dimensional shape caused by factors such as heat, chemicals, or pH; the change in the appearance and structure of an egg white when it is cooked is an example of denaturation.

deoxyribonucleic acid (DNA)   double-stranded, helical polymer chain within the nucleus of a cell that carries the genetic information that encodes proteins and enables the cell to reproduce and perform its functions.

Department of Homeland Security (DHS)   a department of the U.S. government charged with the protection of the country from threats and attacks.

dependent variable   variable assessed by the experimenter to determine whether there is a difference in it that is due to the independent variable.

descriptive statistics   statistics that summarize research data.

desired dose   specific quantity of medication needed.

diagnosis   the process of identifying and assigning a name to a disease in an individual patient or a group of patients with similar signs and symptoms.

diapedesis   movement of white cells out of blood vessels through gaps in the vessel walls that are created when inflammatory processes cause the vessel walls to constrict.

difficult child   an infant who can be characterized by irregularity of bodily functions, intense reactions, and withdrawal from new situations.

diffusion   the movement of atoms or molecules from an area of higher concentration to an area of lower concentration. *See also* facilitated diffusion; osmosis.

digital communications   data or sounds translated into a digital code for transmission, usually a binary code consisting of 1 and 0, the numbers corresponding to voltage values.

disaccharides   complex sugars, such as sucrose, lactose, and maltose.

disease   an abnormal structural or functional change within the body.

disinfectant   cleansing agent that is toxic to living tissue.

disinfection   cleaning with an agent that can kill some microorganisms on the surface of an object.

dissociate   separate; break down. For example, sodium bicarbonate, when placed in water, dissociates into a sodium cation and a bicarbonate anion.

dissociation reaction   any reaction in which a compound or a molecule breaks apart into separate components.

diuretic   an agent that increases urine secretion and elimination of body water; medication used to reduce circulating blood volume by increasing the amount of urine.

Do Not Resuscitate (DNR) order   legal document, usually signed by the patient and his physician, that indicates to medical personnel which, if any, life-sustaining measures should be taken when the patient's heart and respiratory functions have ceased.

dosage on hand   the amount of medication available in a solution.

dose packaging   medication packages that contain a single dose for a single patient.

double blind study   study comparing two or more treatments in which neither the investigators nor the subjects know which treatment group individual subjects have been assigned to.

down-regulation   binding of a medication or hormone to a target cell receptor that causes the number of receptors to decrease.

drip chamber   clear plastic chamber that allows visualization of the drip rate.

drip rate   pace at which the fluid moves from the bag into the patient.

drop   (Latin *guttae*, drops [*gutta*, drop]); quantity of a solution that falls in one spherical mass.

drop former   device that regulates the size of drops.

drug-response relationship   correlation of different amounts of a medication to clinical response.

drugs   foreign substances placed into the human body. *See also* medications.

duplex communications system that allows simultaneous two-way communications by using two frequencies for each channel.

duration of action length of time the amount of medication remains above its minimum effective concentration.

duty to act a formal contractual or informal legal obligation to provide care.

dynamic steady state homeostasis; the tendency of the body to maintain a net constant composition even though the components of the body's internal environment are always changing.

dysplasia a change in cell size, shape, or appearance caused by an external stressor.

dysplastic having an abnormal appearance, as with a cell seen under a microscope.

dyspnea an abnormality of breathing rate, pattern, or effort.

ear-to-sternal-notch position position in which a supine patient's head is elevated to the point where the ear and the sternal notch are horizontally aligned. In the non-obese patient, this position may be called the sniffing position. In the obese patient, this position may be called the ramped position.

easy child an infant who can be characterized by regularity of bodily functions, low or moderate intensity of reactions, and acceptance of new situations.

echo procedure immediately repeating each transmission received during radio communications.

ectoderm the outermost of three germ layers, primitive cell types that develop in the embryo and that will differentiate into the various tissues and organs of the body. *See also* endoderm; germ layers; mesoderm.

edema excess fluid in the interstitial space.

efficacy a medication's ability to cause the expected response.

electrolyte a substance that, in water, separates into electrically charged particles.

electron negatively charged particle that orbits the nucleus of an atom.

electron shells levels of orbitals within which electrons rotate around the nucleus of an atom. *See also* orbital.

electron transport chain carriers embedded on the cristae in the inner membrane of the mitochondria of cells that transfer electrons from one molecule to another, releasing energy in the process.

element a substance that cannot be separated into simpler substances. An element is defined by its atomic number, the number of protons in its nucleus.

emancipated minor a person under 18 years of age who is married, pregnant, a parent, a member of the armed forces, or financially independent and living away from home.

embolus foreign particle in the blood.

Emergency Medical Dispatcher (EMD) the person who manages an EMS system's response and readiness and is responsible for assignment of emergency medical resources to a medical emergency.

Emergency Medical Responder (EMR) the level of EMS practitioner who is likely to be the first person on the scene with emergency care training and the ability to initiate immediate lifesaving care.

Emergency Medical Services (EMS) system a comprehensive network of personnel, equipment, and resources established for the purpose of delivering aid and emergency medical care to the community.

Emergency Medical Technician (EMT) the level of EMS practitioner who provides basic emergency medical care and transportation.

employment laws laws that address employee/employer relationships.

endocrine secretions secreted substances that are released into the bloodstream or surrounding tissues without the aid of ducts.

endocytosis process by which substances can enter a cell when a section of the cell's plasma membrane encircles the substance, then pinches off into a vesicle that is released into the cell. *See also* exocytosis.

endoderm the innermost of three germ layers, primitive cell types that develop in the embryo and that will differentiate into the various tissues and organs of the body. *See also* ectoderm; germ layers; mesoderm.

endoplasmic reticulum organelle within a cell that is a network of tubules, vesicles, and sacs that interconnect with the plasma membrane, the nuclear envelope, and many of the other organelles of the cell.

endotoxins molecules in the walls of certain Gram-negative bacteria that are released when the bacterium dies or is destroyed, causing toxic (poisonous) effects on the host body.

endotracheal tube (ETT) a flexible plastic tube that is inserted into the trachea, usually under laryngoscopy, for the purpose of ventilating the lungs.

endotracheal tube introducer a device designed to facilitate the introduction of an endotracheal tube; commonly called a gum-elastic bougie. It is a stylet that can be pushed into the glottis and is flexible enough so that the operator can feel the entry. When entry is achieved, the endotracheal tube can then be passed over the introducer and into the glottis.

enema a liquid bolus of medication that is injected into the rectum.

enteral route delivery of a medication through the gastrointestinal tract.

enzymes substances that speed up chemical reactions without themselves being consumed in the process.

enzyme–substrate complex   an enzyme and the substance (substrate) it is bound to and working on.

eosinophils   granular white blood cells that attack parasites and also help to control and limit the inflammatory response.

epidemiology   the study of factors that influence the frequency, distribution, and causes of injury, disease, and other health-related events in a population.

epithelial tissue   the protective tissue that lines internal and external body tissues. Examples include skin, mucous membranes, and the lining of the intestinal tract.

epithelialization   growth of epithelial cells under a scab, separating it from the wound and providing a protective covering for the healing wound.

epithelium   *see* epithelial tissue.

erythrocytes   red blood cells, which contain hemoglobin, which transports oxygen to the cells.

ethics   the rules or standards that govern the conduct of members of a particular group or profession.

etiology   the study of disease causes; the occurrences, reasons, and variables of a disease.

eukaryotic cells   cells that contain a nucleus and organelles. The cells of most multicellular organisms, including humans, are eukaryotes. *See also* prokaryotic cells.

eustachian tube   a tube that connects the ear with the nasal cavity.

evidence-based medicine (EMB)   the conscientious, explicit, and judicious use of scientific evidence of effectiveness in decisions about the care of a patient or patients.

excited delirium syndrome (ExDS)   a condition that may result from abuse of stimulant drugs, typically presenting as a triad of effects: delirium, psychomotor agitation, and physiologic excitation.

exocrine secretions   secreted substances that are deposited on the surface of the skin or other epithelial surface through ducts.

exocytosis   process by which substances can exit after being encircled by a membrane vesicle. *See also* endocytosis.

exotoxins   toxic (poisonous) substances secreted by bacterial cells during their growth.

expectorant   medication intended to increase the productivity of cough.

experiment   study in which the researcher has control over some of the conditions in which the study takes place and control over some aspects of the independent variables being studied.

experimental group   the group in experimental design that receives the experimental condition or treatment.

experimental study   study in which subjects are randomly assigned to groups that experience carefully controlled interventions manipulated by the investigator according to a strict logic that allows causal inference about the effects of the interventions under investigation.

exposure   any occurrence of blood or body fluids coming in contact with nonintact skin, mucous membranes, or parenteral contact (e.g., a needlestick).

expressed consent   verbal, nonverbal, or written communication by a patient that he wishes to receive medical care.

extension tubing   IV tubing used to extend a macrodrip or microdrip setup.

external validity   the extent to which the findings of a study are relevant to subjects and settings beyond those in the study; a synonym for *generalizability*.

extracellular fluid (ECF)   the fluid outside the body cells. Extracellular fluid is composed of intravascular fluid and interstitial fluid.

extraglottic airway (EGA) device   airway device that does not enter the glottis.

extrapyramidal symptoms (EPS)   common side effects of antipsychotic medications, including muscle tremors and parkinsonism-like effects.

extravasation   leakage of fluid or medication from the blood vessel that is commonly found with infiltration.

extravascular   outside the vein.

extubation   removing a tube from a body opening.

exudate   substances that penetrate vessel walls to move into the surrounding tissues.

facilitated diffusion   process in which carrier proteins transport large molecules across the cell membrane. *Also called* carrier-mediated diffusion.

false imprisonment   intentional and unjustifiable detention of a person without his consent or other legal authority.

Federal Communications Commission (FCC)   agency that controls all nongovernmental communications in the United States.

fermentation   the breakdown of glucose without oxygen.

fibrinolytic   medication that acts directly on thrombi to break them down; also called *thrombolytic*.

fibroblasts   the most abundant cells in the connective tissue; cells that secrete collagen proteins that maintain a structural framework for many tissues and play an important role in wound healing.

Fick principle   principle stating that the overall movement and utilization of oxygen in the body is dependent on five conditions: adequate concentration of inspired oxygen; appropriate movement of oxygen across the alveolar/capillary membrane into the arterial bloodstream; adequate number of red blood cells to carry the oxygen; proper tissue perfusion; and efficient offloading of oxygen at the tissue level.

field diagnosis what you believe to be your patient's problem, based on the patient's history and physical exam.

filtration movement of water out of the plasma across the capillary membrane into the interstitial space; movement of molecules across a membrane from an area of higher pressure to an area of lower pressure.

FiO$_2$ concentration of oxygen in inspired air.

first-pass effect the liver's partial or complete inactivation of a medication before it reaches the systemic circulation.

flagella threadlike structures whose undulating movement provides motion to certain bacteria, protozoa, and spermatozoa.

flail chest defect in the chest wall that allows a segment to move freely, causing paradoxical chest wall motion.

free drug availability proportion of a medication available in the body to cause either desired or undesired effects.

free radicals atoms or molecules with an unpaired electron in the outer shell. Most free radicals are highly reactive and cause cell damage, especially oxidative damage.

free water water that is free of solute.

French unit of measurement approximately equal to one-third of a millimeter.

fructose a five-carbon monosaccharide sugar found in many plants and vegetables as well as in honey.

gag reflex mechanism that stimulates retching, or striving to vomit, when the soft palate is touched.

galactose a six-carbon monosaccharide sugar found primarily in dairy products.

gauge the size of a needle's diameter.

general adaptation syndrome (GAS) a sequence of stress response stages: stage I, alarm; stage II, resistance or adaptation; stage III, exhaustion.

geographic information system (GIS) an information system that stores and analyzes information about or within a specific geographic area for the purpose of aiding decision making within an organization or group for which the specific GIS has been developed.

germ layers the three primitive cell types (endoderm, ectoderm, mesoderm) that develop in the embryo and that will differentiate into the various tissues and organs of the body. *See also* ectoderm; endoderm; mesoderm.

global positioning system (GPS) a global navigational satellite system in which satellites orbiting the earth provide specific time and location information.

glottis liplike opening between the vocal cords.

glucagon substance that increases blood glucose level.

glucose a six-carbon monosaccharide sugar that is the principal energy source for the human body.

glycogen a glucose polymer that is primarily stored in the liver and skeletal muscle that can be converted by the body into glucose. *See also* glycogenolysis.

glycogenolysis a process controlled by the hormones glucagon and epinephrine in which stores of glycogen are broken down into glucose to meet a bodily need for glucose. *See also* glycogen.

glycolysis a series of reactions by which a molecule of glucose is converted into two molecules of pyruvic acid, a process that begins the conversion of glucose into energy and that also produces free hydrogen ions that determine the body's pH.

Golgi apparatus organelle within a cell that processes proteins for the cell membrane and other organelles.

Good Samaritan laws laws that provide immunity to certain people who assist at the scene of a medical emergency.

granulation filling of a wound by the inward growth of healthy tissues from the wound edges.

granulocytes white cells with multiple nuclei that have the appearance of a bag of granules; also called *polymorphonuclear cells*. Types of granulocytes are neutrophils, eosinophils, and basophils.

granuloma a tumor or growth that forms when foreign bodies that cannot be destroyed by macrophages are surrounded and walled off.

half-life a unit of rate of decay of radioactive isotopes; the time it takes for the decaying parent isotope to decrease by half.

hand-off the process of transferring patient care to receiving facility staff; the verbal report given by an EMT or paramedic to the receiving nurse or physician.

haptens molecules that do not trigger an immune response on their own but can become immunogenic when combined with larger molecules.

Health Insurance Portability and Accountability Act (HIPAA) law enacted by the United States Congress in 1996 that includes provisions for protecting the security and privacy of a person's health information.

helicopter air ambulances (HAA) emergency care provided by EMS personnel and helicopter flight crews who are trained in the preparation of patients for and the care of patients during helicopter transport.

hematocrit the percentage of the blood occupied by erythrocytes.

hemoconcentration elevated numbers of red and white blood cells.

hemoglobin an iron-based pigment present in red blood cells that binds with oxygen and transports it to the cells.

hemoglobin-oxygen saturation (SaO$_2$) the amount of oxygen bound to one gram of hemoglobin.

hemolysis the destruction of red blood cells.

hemostasis the stoppage of bleeding.

hemothorax   accumulation in the pleural cavity of blood or fluid containing blood.

heparin lock   peripheral IV cannula with a distal medication port used for intermittent fluid or medication infusions. Flushes of heparin solution, which inhibit blood coagulation, are used to maintain patency of the device.

hepatic alteration   change in a medication's chemical composition that occurs in the liver.

Hgb   the amount of hemoglobin present in arterial blood.

high-pressure regulator   regulator used to transfer oxygen at high pressures from tank to tank.

histamine   a substance released during the degranulation of mast cells and also released by basophils that, through constriction and dilation of blood vessels, increases blood flow to the injury site and also increases the permeability of vessel walls.

histology   the study of tissues.

histopathology   the study of diseased or abnormal tissues.

HIV (human immunodeficiency virus)   a virus that breaks down the immune defenses, making the body vulnerable to a variety of infections and disorders.

HLA antigens   antigens the body recognizes as self or non-self; present on all body cells except the red blood cells.

hollow-needle catheter   stylet that does not have a Teflon tube but is itself inserted into the vein and secured there.

homeostasis   the natural tendency of the body to maintain a steady and normal internal environment.

hotspot   relating to Internet access that is provided over a wireless local area network through a router to an Internet service provider.

Huber needle   needle that has an opening on the side of the shaft instead of the tip.

humoral immunity   the long-term immunity to an antigen provided by antibodies produced by B lymphocytes.

hydrogen bond   a weak bond formed by the attraction between a slightly positively charged hydrogen atom and a slightly negatively charged oxygen atom, as between H_2O (water) molecules.

hydrolysis   the breakage of a chemical bond by adding water, or by incorporating a hydroxyl (OH^-) group into one fragment and a hydrogen ion (H^+) into the other.

hydrophilic   attracted to water.

hydrophobic   repellent to water.

hydrostatic pressure   blood pressure or force against vessel walls created by the heartbeat. Hydrostatic pressure tends to force water out of the capillaries into the interstitial space.

hypercapnia   an elevated level of plasma CO_2.

hypercarbia   excessive level of carbon dioxide in the blood.

hyperoxia   excessive level of oxygen in certain tissues or in the body as a whole.

hyperplasia   an increase in the number of cells resulting from an increased workload.

hypersensitivity   an exaggerated and harmful immune response; an umbrella term for allergy, autoimmunity, and isoimmunity.

hypertonic   state in which a solution has a higher solute concentration on one side of a semipermeable membrane than on the other side; having a greater concentration of solute molecules; one solution may be hypertonic to another.

hypertrophy   an increase in cell size resulting from an increased workload.

hyperventilation syndrome   excessive CO_2 elimination resulting in respiratory alkalosis, caused by hyperventilation.

hyperventilation   rapid or deep breathing in excess of the body's needs.

hypnosis   instigation of sleep.

hypocapnia   a reduced level of plasma CO_2.

hypodermic needle   hollow metal tube used with the syringe to administer medications.

hypoperfusion   inadequate perfusion of the body tissues, resulting in an inadequate supply of oxygen and nutrients to the body tissues. Also called *shock*.

hypothesis   testable statement that indicates what the researcher expects to find, based on theory and knowledge of the literature.

hypotonic   state in which a solution has a lower solute concentration on one side of a semipermeable membrane than on the other side; having a lesser concentration of solute molecules; one solution may be hypotonic to another.

hypoventilation   reduced rate or depth of breathing that does not meet the body's needs.

hypovolemic shock   shock caused by a loss of intravascular fluid volume.

hypoxemia   decreased partial pressure of oxygen in the blood.

hypoxemia   decreased partial pressure of oxygen in the blood.

hypoxia   a general oxygen deficiency or oxygen deficiency to a particular tissue or organ.

hypoxic drive   mechanism that increases respiratory stimulation when PaO_2 falls and inhibits respiratory stimulation when PaO_2 climbs.

iatrogenic disease   a disease that results from a medical treatment given for another disease or condition.

idiopathic   of unknown cause, in reference to a disease.

immediate hypersensitivity reaction   a swiftly occurring secondary hypersensitivity reaction (one that occurs after reexposure to an antigen). Immediate hypersensitivity reactions are usually more severe than delayed reactions. The swiftest and most severe such reaction is anaphylaxis.

immune response the body's reactions that inactivate or eliminate foreign antigens.

immunity exemption from legal liability; a long-term condition of protection from infection or disease; the body's ability to respond to the presence of a pathogen.

immunogens antigens that are able to trigger an immune response.

immunoglobulins antibodies; proteins, produced in response to foreign antigens, that destroy or control the antigens.

implied consent consent for treatment that is presumed for a patient who is mentally, physically, or emotionally unable to grant consent. Also called emergency doctrine.

in vitro descriptive term for processes that are carried out outside the living body, usually in the laboratory, as distinguished from *in vivo* processes.

in vivo descriptive term for processes that are carried out within a living body.

incubation period the time between contact with a disease organism and the appearance of first symptoms.

independent variable presumed cause of the dependent variable.

induced therapeutic hypothermia (ITH) the administration of cold IV fluids to cardiac arrest patients to minimize subsequent secondary injury.

infectious disease any disease caused by the growth of pathogenic microorganisms that may be spread from person to person.

inferential statistics statistics used to determine whether changes in a dependent variable are caused by an independent variable.

inflammation the body's response to cellular injury; also called the *inflammatory response*. In contrast to the immune response, inflammation develops swiftly, is nonspecific (attacks all unwanted substances in the same way), and is temporary, leading to healing.

information communications technology (ICT) information technology blended with communications technology to provide for dissemination of information.

informed consent consent for treatment that is given based on full disclosure of information.

infusion liquid medication delivered through a vein.

infusion controller gravity-flow device that regulates fluid's passage through an electromechanical pump.

infusion pump device that delivers fluids and medications under positive pressure.

infusion rate speed at which a medication is delivered intravenously.

inhalation drawing of medication into the lungs along with air during breathing.

injection placement of medication in or under the skin with a needle and syringe.

injury intentional or unintentional damage to a person resulting from acute exposure to thermal, mechanical, electrical, or chemical energy or from the absence of such essentials as heat and oxygen.

injury risk a hazardous or potentially hazardous situation that puts people in danger of sustaining injury.

injury surveillance program the ongoing systematic collection, analysis, and interpretation of injury data essential to the planning, implementation, and evaluation of public health practice.

inorganic chemicals chemicals that do not contain the element carbon. *See also* organic chemicals.

insidious existing without symptoms or with mild symptoms, as a disease that does not seem as serious as it is or as it may become.

institutional review board (IRB) board of experts, established at all research institutions, that oversees the ethical conduct of research.

insufflate to blow into.

insulin substance that decreases blood glucose level.

intentional tort a civil wrong committed by one person against another based on a willful act. *See also* tort law.

internal validity ability of the research design to accurately answer the research question.

interoperability a feature of the emergency and public safety communications infrastructure that allows personnel from different jurisdictions and systems to communicate with one another effectively.

interstitial fluid the fluid in body tissues that is outside the cells and outside the vascular system.

intervener physician a physician at the scene of an emergency who is not affiliated with EMS or not affiliated with the EMS service that has been dispatched to the scene.

intracatheter *see* catheter inserted through the needle.

intracellular fluid (ICF) the fluid inside the body cells.

intradermal within the dermal layer of the skin.

intramuscular within the muscle.

intraosseous within the bone.

intravascular fluid the fluid within the circulatory system; blood plasma.

intravenous (IV) access surgical puncture of a vein to deliver medication or withdraw blood. Also called *cannulation*.

intravenous fluid chemically prepared solution tailored to the body's specific needs.

intubation passing a tube into a body opening.

invasion of privacy violation by one person of another person's personal life or personal information.

involuntary consent consent to treatment granted by the authority of a court order.

ion a charged particle; an atom or group of atoms whose electrical charge has changed from neutral to positive or negative by losing or gaining one or more electrons. (In an atom's normal, nonionized state, its positively charged protons and negatively charged electrons balance each other so that the atom's charge is neutral.)

ion channels hydrophilic pores through a membrane that open and allow certain types of solutes, usually inorganic ions, to pass through.

ionic bond a bond resulting from the attraction between an atom or molecule with a negative charge and an atom or molecule with a positive charge.

ionize become electrically charged or polar.

irreversible antagonism a competitive antagonist permanently binds with a receptor site.

irreversible shock shock that has progressed so far that no medical intervention can reverse the condition and death is inevitable.

ischemia a blockage in the delivery of oxygenated blood to the cells.

isoimmunity an immune response to antigens from another member of the same species—for example, Rh reactions between a mother and infant or transplant rejections; also called *alloimmunity*.

isometric exercise active exercise performed against stable resistance, where muscles are exercised in a motionless manner.

isotonic state in which solutions on opposite sides of a semipermeable membrane are in equal concentration; equal in concentration of solute molecules. Solutions may be isotonic to each other.

isotonic exercise active exercise during which muscles are worked through their range of motion.

isotopes variants of the same element, having the same number of protons but varying in the number of neutrons. *See also* element.

iterative process process for calculating a desired result by means of a repeated cycle of operations that comes closer and closer to the desired result.

IV catheter *see* over-the-needle catheter.

jargon language used by a particular group or profession.

justice the obligation to treat all patients fairly.

kinin system a plasma protein system that produces bradykinin, a substance that works with prostaglandins to cause pain. It also has actions similar to those of histamine (vasodilation and bronchospasm, increased permeability of the blood vessels, and chemotaxis) but acts more slowly than histamine, thus being more important during later stages of inflammation.

lactose the principal sugar in milk; a disaccharide, it is a combination of glucose and galactose.

laryngoscope instrument for lifting the tongue and epiglottis in order to see the vocal cords.

larynx the complex structure that joins the pharynx with the trachea.

laxative medication used to decrease stool's firmness and increase its water content.

legislative law law created by lawmaking bodies such as Congress and state assemblies. Also called statutory law.

leukocytes white blood cells, which play a key role in the immune system and inflammatory (infection-fighting) responses.

leukotrienes also called *slow-reacting substances of anaphylaxis (SRS-A)*; substances synthesized by mast cells during the inflammatory response that cause vasodilation, vascular permeability, and chemotaxis.

liability legal responsibility.

libel the act of injuring a person's character, name, or reputation by false statements made in writing or through the mass media with malicious intent or reckless disregard for the falsity of those statements.

licensure the process by which a governmental agency grants permission to engage in a given trade or profession to an applicant who has attained the degree of competency required to ensure the public's protection.

life expectancy based on the year of birth, the average number of additional years of life expected for a member of a population.

lipid bilayer plasma membrane consisting of two layers of phospholipids. Each phospholipid molecule has a hydrophilic head (that attracts water) and a hydrophobic tail (that repels water). In the outer layer, the hydrophilic heads face outward, in contact with the extracellular fluid (ECF). In the inner layer, the hydrophilic heads face inward, in contact with the intracellular fluid (ICF). The hydrophobic tails of both layers face each other and hold the layers of the membrane together.

lipids a broad group of chemicals, not soluble in water, that includes triglycerides, phospholipids, and steroids.

Lipp maneuver a procedure for manually preshaping an Esophageal Tracheal Combitube (ETC).

living will a legal document that allows a person to specify the kinds of medical treatment he wishes to receive should the need arise.

local limited to one area of the body.

logarithm a base number that is raised to a certain *power*. A common example is $2^3 = 8$, in which 2 is raised to the third power, meaning that 2 (the first power) is multiplied by itself (to the second power, which equals 4), then multiplied by itself again (to the third power, which equals 8)—which may be expressed as $2 \times 2 \times 2 = 8$. In 2^3, 2 is the *base number* and 3 is the *exponent*.

Luer sampling needle long, exposed needle that screws into the vacutainer and is inserted directly into the vein.

lumen   the channel through a tube.

lymphocyte   a type of leukocyte, or white blood cell, that attacks foreign substances as part of the body's immune response.

lymphokine   a cytokine released by a lymphocyte.

lysosome   organelle within a cell that degrades and removes products of ingestion and worn out parts of the cell and converts complex nutritional molecules into simple nutritional molecules; sometimes called the cell's "garbage disposal system."

macrodrip tubing   administration tubing that delivers a relatively large amount of fluid.

macrophages   large white blood cells (matured monocytes) that will ingest and destroy, or partially destroy, invading organisms.

Magill forceps   scissor-style clamps with circular tips.

major histocompatibility complex (MHC)   a group of genes on chromosome 6 that provide the genetic code for HLA antigens.

malfeasance   a breach of duty by performance of a wrongful or unlawful act.

malignant   cancerous; able to spread to other tissues. *See also* benign.

Mallampati classification system   a system for evaluating and scoring airway difficulty by assessing the tonsillar pillars and uvula.

maltose   a breakdown product of starch; a disaccharide, it is a combination of two glucose molecules.

margination   adherence of white cells to vessel walls in the early stages of inflammation.

mass number   the total number of neutrons and protons in an atom.

mast cells   large cells, resembling bags of granules, that reside near blood vessels. When stimulated by injury, chemicals, or allergic responses, they activate the inflammatory response by degranulation (emptying their granules into the extracellular environment) and synthesis (construction of leukotrienes and prostaglandins).

maturation   continuing processes of wound reconstruction that may occur over a period of years after initial healing, as scar tissue is remodeled and strengthened.

maximum life span   the theoretical, species-specific, longest duration of life, excluding premature or "unnatural" death.

mean   average obtained by adding the objects or items and dividing the sum by the number of objects or items present.

measured volume administration set   IV setup that delivers specific volumes of fluid.

measures of central tendency   numerical information regarding the most typical or representative scores in a group.

mechanism of injury (MOI)   the force or forces that caused an injury.

median   the middle score in a set of scores that have been ordered from lowest to highest.

medical director   a physician who is legally responsible for all clinical and patient care aspects of an EMS system.

medical oversight   the medical policies, procedures, and practices established by the medical director of an EMS system.

medically clean   careful handling to prevent contamination.

medicated solution   parenteral medication packaged in an IV bag and administered as an IV infusion.

medication injection port   self-sealing membrane into which a hypodermic needle is inserted for medication administration.

medications   agents used in the diagnosis, treatment, or prevention of disease. *See also* drugs.

memory cells   cells produced by mature B lymphocytes that "remember" the activating antigen and will trigger a stronger and swifter immune response if reexposure to the antigen occurs.

mesoderm   the middle of three germ layers, primitive cell types that develop in the embryo and that will differentiate into the various tissues and organs of the body. *See also* ectoderm; endoderm; germ layers.

meta-analysis   the process or technique of synthesizing research results by using various statistical methods to retrieve, select, and combine results from previous separate but related studies.

metabolic acid–base disorders   metabolic acidosis and metabolic alkalosis; disorders that result from changes in the production of acid or changes in bicarbonate levels within the body.

metabolic acidosis   acidity caused by an increase in acid, often because of increased production of acids during metabolism or from causes such as vomiting, diarrhea, diabetes, or medication.

metabolic alkalosis   alkalinity caused by an increase in plasma bicarbonate resulting from causes including diuresis, vomiting, or ingestion of too much sodium bicarbonate.

metabolism   the total changes that take place during physiologic processes; the body's breaking down of chemicals into different chemicals.

metallic elements   elements that tend to lose electrons. *See also* nonmetallic elements.

metaplasia   replacement of one type of cell by another type of cell that is not normal for that tissue.

metastasis   movement of cancer cells to other areas of the body from the original site.

metered dose inhaler   handheld device that produces a medicated spray for inhalation.

microdrip tubing   administration tubing that delivers a relatively small amount of fluid.

minimum effective concentration minimum level of medication needed to cause a given effect.

minor depending on state law, this is usually a person under the age of 18.

minute volume (V_{min}) the amount of air (gas) inhaled and exhaled in one minute.

minute volume the amount of air (gas) inhaled and exhaled in one minute.

misfeasance a breach of duty by performance of a legal act in a manner that is harmful or injurious.

mission-critical communications information that must get through without fail because a patient's well-being depends on it.

mitochondria organelles within the cells that are the principal site of conversion of food to energy.

mixed research a research design that contains both quantitative and qualitative properties.

Mix-o-Vial *see* nonconstituted medication vial.

mobile data unit (MDU) vehicle-mounted computer keyboard and display with broadband capacity via radio or wireless connection, capable of sending ambulance status and patient information to the hospital or ambulance quarters.

mobile integrated health care health care performed by paramedics apart from customary emergency response and transport, such as in physicians' offices, outpatient clinics, or as part of paramedic crews specially trained to periodically assess and monitor high-risk patients receiving home care or elsewhere in the community. Also called *community paramedicine.*

mode value that occurs most frequently in a data set.

modeling a procedure whereby a subject observes a model perform some behavior and then attempts to imitate that behavior. Many believe it is the fundamental learning process involved in socialization.

molarity moles of solute per liter of solution. A mole is the measure of mass or weight used in chemistry, sometimes defined as "molecular weight."

mole *see* molarity.

molecule a substance made up of atoms held together by one or more covalent bonds.

monoclonal antibody an antibody that is very pure and specific to a single antigen.

monocytes white cells with a single nucleus; the largest normal blood cells. During inflammation, monocytes mature and grow to several times their original size, becoming macrophages.

monokine a cytokine released by a macrophage.

monomer an atom or a small molecule that may bind chemically to other monomers to form a polymer. *See also* polymer.

monosaccharides simple sugars, such as glucose, fructose, and galactose.

morals social, religious, or personal standards of right and wrong.

morbidity the rate or incidence of a disease.

Moro reflex a reflex that occurs when a newborn is startled; arms are thrown wide, fingers spread, and a grabbing motion follows; also called *startle reflex.*

mortality the number of deaths in a given period.

mucolytic medication intended to make mucus more watery.

mucous membrane lining in body cavities that handle air transport; usually contains small, mucous-secreting cells.

mucus slippery secretion that lubricates and protects airway surfaces.

multiband radio radio or radio system that combines a wide range of radio bands, allowing services that operate on separate bands—such as police, fire, and EMS—to communicate across the separate systems.

multiple organ dysfunction syndrome (MODS) progressive impairment of two or more organ systems resulting from an uncontrolled inflammatory response to a severe illness or injury.

multiplex duplex system that can transmit voice and data simultaneously.

muscle tissue tissue that is capable of contraction when stimulated. There are three types of muscle tissue: cardiac (myocardium, or heart muscle), smooth (within intestines, surrounding blood vessels), and skeletal, or striated (allows skeletal movement). Skeletal muscle is mostly under voluntary, or conscious, control; smooth muscle is under involuntary, or unconscious, control; cardiac muscle is capable of spontaneous, or self-excited, contraction.

nares (*sing.* naris) nostrils.

nasal cannula catheter placed at the nares.

nasal medication medication administered through the mucous membranes of the nose.

nasolacrimal ducts tubular vessels that drain tears and debris from the eyes into the nasal cavity.

nasopharyngeal airway (NPA) uncuffed tube that follows the natural curvature of the nasopharynx, passing through the nose and extending from the nostril to the posterior pharynx.

nasotracheal route through the nose and into the trachea.

National Emergency Medical Services Education Standards: Paramedic Instructional Guidelines Guidelines developed and published in 2009 by the U.S. Department of Transportation for the education of the various levels of EMS practitioner—Emergency Medical Responders, Emergency Medical Technicians, Advanced Emergency Medical Technicians, and Paramedics.

National EMS Information System (NEMSIS) national repository formed to collect and store EMS data from every state in the United States, to create a national

EMS database and to create a data dictionary that can be accessed and used by individual EMS systems.

National EMS Research Agenda document describing the history and current status of EMS research and proposing a strategy to guide the research component of EMS into the future; commissioned by the National Highway Traffic Safety Administration and the Maternal and Child Health Bureau of the United States government; published in 2001.

National Highway Traffic Safety Administration (NHTSA) An agency of the U.S. government established by the Highway Safety Act of 1970 to carry out safety programs to improve motor vehicle and highway safety, particularly to prevent vehicular crashes.

National Incident Management System (NIMS) a system administered by the U.S. Secretary of Homeland Security to provide a consistent approach to disaster management by all local, state, and federal employees who respond to such incidents.

National Transportation Safety Board (NTSB) an independent U.S. government investigative agency responsible for civil transportation accident investigation, including investigation of aviation accidents and incidents, certain types of highway crashes, ship and marine accidents, pipeline incidents, and railroad accidents.

natriuretic peptides (NPs) peptide hormones synthesized by the heart, brain, and other organs with effects that include excretion of large amounts of sodium in the urine and dilation of the blood vessels.

natural immunity inborn protection against infection or disease that is part of the person's or species' genetic makeup.

nature of the illness (NOI) a patient's general medical condition or complaint.

nebulizer inhalation aid that disperses liquid into aerosol spray or mist.

necrosis cell death; the sloughing off of dead tissue; a pathological cell change. Four types of necrotic cell change are coagulative, liquefactive, caseous, and fatty. Gangrenous necrosis refers to tissue death over a wide area.

needle adapter rigid plastic device specifically constructed to fit into the hub of an intravenous cannula.

needle cricothyrotomy surgical airway technique that inserts a 14-gauge needle into the trachea at the cricothyroid membrane.

negative feedback loop body mechanisms that work to reverse, or compensate for, a pathophysiologic process (or to reverse any physiologic process, whether pathological or nonpathological).

negligence deviation from accepted standards of care recognized by law for the protection of others against the unreasonable risk of harm. In medical practice,

negligence is often considered to be synonymous with malpractice. The four elements that must be present to prove negligence in a court of law are duty to act, breach of duty to act, actual damages, and proximate cause. *See also* negligence *per se*.

negligence *per se* negligence committed as a result of violating a statute with resultant injury; automatic negligence. *See also* negligence.

neoplasia abnormal or uncontrolled cell growth. *See also* neoplasm.

neoplasm a tumor that results from neoplasia. *See also* neoplasia.

nerve tissue tissue that transmits electrical impulses throughout the body.

net filtration the total loss of water from blood plasma across the capillary membrane into the interstitial space. Normally, hydrostatic pressure forcing water out of the capillary is balanced by oncotic force pulling water into the capillary for a net filtration of zero.

neuroeffector junction specialized synapse between a nerve cell and the organ or tissue it innervates.

neurogenic shock shock resulting from brain or spinal cord injury that causes an interruption of nerve impulses to the arteries with loss of arterial tone, dilation, and relative hypovolemia.

neuroglia glial cells that support, insulate, and protect neurons.

neuroleptanesthesia anesthesia that combines decreased sensation of pain with amnesia while the patient remains conscious.

neuroleptic antipsychotic (literally, affecting the nerves).

neuron nerve cell; cell that transmits electrical impulses.

neurotransmitter chemical messenger that conducts a nervous impulse across a synapse.

neutron electrically neutral particle within the nucleus of an atom.

neutrophil a type of white blood cell; a phagocyte that has the ability to ingest other cells and substances.

nominal data categorical data in which the order of the categories is arbitrary (e.g., 1 = male, 2 = female).

noncompetitive antagonism the binding of an antagonist causes a deformity of the binding site that prevents an agonist from fitting and binding.

nonconstituted medication vial/Mix-o-Vial vial with two containers, one holding a powdered medication and the other holding a liquid mixing solution.

nonfeasance a breach of duty by failure to perform a required act or duty.

nonmaleficence the obligation not to harm the patient.

nonmetallic elements elements that tend to gain electrons. *See also* metallic elements.

nonrandomized controlled trial research protocol in which the subjects are assigned to the study groups by a method other than randomization.

normoxia   normal level of oxygen in certain tissues or in the body as a whole.

nuclear envelope   double membrane that encloses the nucleus of a cell.

nuclear pores   openings in the nuclear envelope. *See also* nuclear envelope.

nucleolus   a specialized region of DNA within the nucleus of a cell that is active in the production of ribosomal RNA.

nucleoplasm   the materials on the inside of the nucleus of a cell.

nucleotides   the fundamental building blocks of the nucleic acids, DNA and RNA; nucleotides consist of five-carbon sugar molecules bound to a nitrogen base and a phosphate group.

nucleus   the organelle within a cell that contains the DNA and RNA, or genetic material, proteins, and other components; in the cells of higher organisms, the nucleus is surrounded by a membrane.

null hypothesis   a hypothesis that predicts that an observed difference is due to chance alone and not to a systematic cause.

observational study   study in which a phenomenon is described but no attempt is made to analyze the effects of variables on the phenomenon; also called a descriptive study.

ocular medication   medication administered through the mucous membranes of the eye.

odds ratio   a measure of association in a case-control study that quantifies the relationship between an exposure and health outcome from a comparative study.

off-line medical oversight   medical policies, procedures, and practices established by a system medical director in advance of a call.

oncotic force   a form of osmotic pressure exerted by the large protein particles, or colloids, present in blood plasma. In the capillaries, the plasma colloids tend to pull water from the interstitial space across the capillary membrane into the capillary. Oncotic force is also called *colloid osmotic pressure*.

on-line medical direction   orders directly provided to a prehospital care provider by a qualified physician by either radio or telephone.

onset of action   the time from administration until a medication reaches its minimum effective concentration.

Ontario Prehospital Life Support Study (OPALS)   a study conducted in the province of Ontario, Canada, of prehospital practices and outcomes.

open access journals   scientific publications, typically Internet based, that allow unrestricted access to the contents.

open cricothyrotomy   surgical airway technique that places an endotracheal or tracheostomy tube directly into the trachea through a surgical incision at the cricothyroid membrane.

orbital   a specific region within which an electron rotates around the nucleus of an atom. Each orbital has a specific shape and can hold two or more electrons. *See also* electron shells.

ordinal data   a type of data containing limited categories with a ranking from the lowest to the highest (e.g., mild, moderate, severe).

organ system   a group of organs that work together. Examples are the cardiovascular system, formed of the heart, blood vessels, and blood; and the gastrointestinal system, comprising the mouth, salivary glands, esophagus, stomach, intestines, liver, pancreas, gallbladder, rectum, and anus.

organ   a group of tissues functioning together. Examples are heart, liver, brain, ovary, and eye.

organelles   structures that perform specific functions within a cell.

organic chemicals   chemicals that contain the element carbon. *See also* inorganic chemicals.

organic nitrates   potent vasodilators used to treat all forms of angina.

organism   the sum of all the cells, tissues, organs, and organ systems of a living being. Examples include the human organism and a bacterial organism.

oropharyngeal airway (OPA)   semicircular device that follows the curvature of the palate.

osmolality   the concentration of solute per kilogram of water. *See also* osmolarity.

osmolarity   the concentration of solute per liter of water (often used synonymously with *osmolality*).

osmosis   movement of solvent in a solution from an area of lower solute concentration to an area of higher solute concentration.

osmotic diuresis   greatly increased urination and dehydration due to high levels of glucose that cannot be reabsorbed into the blood from the kidney tubules, causing a loss of water into the urine.

osmotic gradient   the difference in concentration between solutions on opposite sides of a semipermeable membrane.

osmotic pressure   the pressure exerted by the concentration of solutes on one side of a membrane that, if hypertonic, tends to "pull" water (cause osmosis) from the other side of the membrane.

osteocytes   cells that reside in the lacunae, or cavities, within mature bone and are responsible for the turnover of mineral content of the surrounding bone.

outcomes-based research   research designed to understand the end results of particular health care practices and interventions.

overhydration   the presence or retention of an abnormally high amount of body fluid.

over-the-needle catheter/IV catheter semiflexible catheter enclosing a sharp metal stylet.

oxidation the loss of hydrogen atoms or the acceptance of an oxygen atom. This increases the positive charge (or lessens the negative charge) of the molecule; the loss of electrons from one atom to another. *See also* reduction.

oxygen gas necessary for energy production.

oxygen saturation percentage (SpO_2) the saturation of arterial blood with oxygen as measured by pulse oximetry expressed as a percentage.

P **value** the probability of obtaining by chance a result at least as extreme as that observed, even when the null hypothesis is true and no real difference exists; if it is ≤0.05, the sample results are usually deemed statistically significant and the null hypothesis is rejected.

PA alveolar partial pressure.

Pa arterial partial pressure.

$PaCO_2$ partial pressure of carbon dioxide in the blood.

palmar grasp a reflex in the newborn, which is elicited by placing a finger firmly in the infant's palm.

paradoxical breathing asymmetrical chest wall movement that lessens respiratory efficiency.

Paramedic the level of EMS practitioner who provides the highest level of prehospital care, including advanced assessments and care, formation of a field impression, and invasive and drug interventions.

paramedicine the totality of the roles and responsibilities of paramedic practice involving health care, public health, and public safety; the highest level of Emergency Medical Systems practice.

parameter a value that specifies one of the members of a family of probability distributions, such as the mean or the standard deviation.

parasympatholytic medication or other substance that blocks or inhibits the actions of the parasympathetic nervous system (also called *anticholinergic*).

parasympathomimetic medication or other substance that causes effects like those of the parasympathetic nervous system (also called *cholinergic*).

parenchyma principal or essential parts of an organ.

parenteral route delivery of a medication outside the gastrointestinal tract, typically using needles to inject medications into the circulatory system or tissues.

partial agonist *see* agonist–antagonist.

partial pressure the pressure exerted by each component of a gas mixture.

passive transport movement of a substance without the use of energy.

pathogen a microorganism capable of producing infection or disease, such as an atom or a virus.

pathogenesis the sequence of events in the development of a disease.

pathologist a physician who specializes in pathology.

pathology the study of disease and its causes.

pathophysiology the study of the functional changes that occur within living cells and tissues that are associated with or that result from disease or injury.

peer review a process of self-evaluation by a profession such as EMS in which qualified individuals within the profession or service assess ongoing practices to maintain standards and improve performance.

peptide a protein chain containing less than 10 amino acids. *See also* polypeptide.

peptide bond the force that holds amino acids together; the primary linkage of all protein structures.

perfusion the supplying of oxygen and nutrients to the body tissues as a result of the constant passage of blood through the capillaries.

peripheral vascular resistance the resistance of the vessels to the flow of blood: increased when the vessels constrict, decreased when the vessels relax.

peripheral venous access surgical puncture of a vein in the arm, leg, or neck.

peripherally inserted central catheter (PICC) line threaded into the central circulation via a peripheral site.

permissive a parenting style that takes a tolerant, accepting view of a child's behavior.

peroxisome organelle within a cell within which hydrogen peroxide is degraded.

personal protective equipment (PPE) equipment used by EMS personnel to protect against injury and the spread of infectious disease.

pH scale *pH* is the abbreviation for potential of hydrogen, a measure of relative acidity or alkalinity. The pH scale is inverse to the concentration of acidic hydrogen ions; therefore, the lower the pH, the greater the acidity, and the higher the pH, the greater the alkalinity. The pH scale ranges from 0 to 14. A normal pH range is 7.35 to 7.45.

phagocytes cells that have the ability to ingest other cells and substances, such as bacteria and cell debris. All granulocytes and monocytes are phagocytes.

phagocytosis the process whereby a cell engulfs large particles or bacteria.

pharmacodynamics how a medication interacts with the body to cause its effects.

pharmacokinetics how a medication is absorbed, distributed, metabolized (biotransformed), and excreted; how medications are transported into and out of the body.

pharmacology the study of medications and their interactions with the body.

pharynx a muscular tube that extends vertically from the back of the soft palate to the superior aspect of the esophagus.

phospholipids class of lipids that form the membrane that surrounds cells.

physician orders for life-sustaining treatment (POLST) a set of orders regarding care for a terminally ill patient, signed by a physician, to be honored by health care providers who deal with the patient.

physiologic stress a chemical or physical disturbance in the cells or tissue fluid produced by a change in the external environment or within the body.

pinocytosis the process whereby a cell engulfs droplets of fluid.

placebo a substance or intervention having no effect but administered or provided as a control in testing — experimentally or clinically — the efficacy of a biologically active preparation.

placental barrier biochemical barrier at the maternal–fetal interface that restricts certain molecules.

plasma the liquid part of the blood.

plasma membrane the membrane that surrounds a cell. *See also* cell membrane.

plasma protein systems complex sequences of actions triggered by proteins present in the blood. For example, immunoglobulins (antibodies) are plasma proteins. Three plasma protein systems involved in inflammation are the complement system, the coagulation system, and the kinin system.

plasma-level profile describes the lengths of onset, duration, and termination of action, as well as the medication's minimum effective concentration and toxic levels.

platelet aggregation inhibitor medication that decreases the formation of platelet plugs.

platelets fragments of cytoplasm that circulate in the blood and work with components of the coagulation system to promote blood clotting. Platelets also release serotonin, a vasoconstrictive substance.

pleura membranous connective tissue covering the lungs.

pneumothorax accumulation of air or gas in the pleural cavity.

POGO scoring system a system for evaluating and scoring airway difficulty by the percentage of the glottis that can be visualized.

pOH scale the number of hydroxide ions present in a solution. The pOH is the opposite of the pH. *See also* pH scale.

polar bond an unequal covalent bond; a bond in which the sharing of electrons is unequal. *See also* covalent bond.

polar molecule a molecule formed with a polar bond, in which different parts of the same molecule have a different and unequal charge. *See also* polar bond.

polymer a large organic molecule formed by combining many smaller molecules (monomers). An example is the polymer starch, which is largely made up of smaller glucose molecules. *See also* monomer.

polypeptide a protein chain containing more than 10 amino acids. *See also* peptide.

polysaccharides a type of carbohydrate that includes starches, cellulose, and glycogen.

population group of persons, elements, or both that share common characteristics that are being studied by the investigator.

positional asphyxia lack of oxygen resulting in unconsciousness or death that occurs in a person who is being restrained. Also called *restraint asphyxia.*

post hoc taking place after the fact, as in a review of data after the experiment has concluded.

postconventional reasoning the stage of moral development during which individuals make moral decisions according to an enlightened conscience.

postganglionic nerves nerve fibers that extend from the autonomic ganglia to the target tissues.

post-traumatic stress disorder (PTSD) anxiety disorder that develops after exposure to traumatic events.

prearrival instruction instructions from a medically trained dispatcher to a person at the scene of an emergency on how to initiate lifesaving first aid with the dispatcher's help while waiting for the on-scene arrival of emergency personnel.

preconventional reasoning the stage of moral development during which children respond mainly to cultural control to avoid punishment and attain satisfaction.

predisposing factors factors that may lead to or increase the chance of contracting a disease.

prefilled/preloaded syringe syringe packaged in a tamperproof container with the medication already in the barrel.

preganglionic nerves nerve fibers that exit the central nervous system and terminate in the autonomic ganglia.

prehospital care report (PCR) the written record of an EMS response.

preload the amount of blood delivered to the heart during diastole (when the heart fills with blood between contractions); in cardiac physiology, defined as the tension of cardiac muscle fiber at the end of diastole.

primary care basic health care provided at the patient's first contact with the health care system.

primary immune response the initial development of antibodies in response to the first exposure to an antigen in which the immune system becomes "primed" to produce a faster, stronger response to any future exposures.

primary intention simple healing of a minor wound without granulation or pus formation.

primary prevention keeping an injury from ever occurring.

principal investigator (PI) the scientist or scholar with primary responsibility for the design and conduct of a research project.

priority dispatching system that uses medically approved questions and predetermined guidelines to determine the appropriate level of response.

prodrug (parent drug) medication that is not active when administered, but whose biotransformation converts it into active metabolites.

profession a specialized body of knowledge or skills.

professional boundaries ethical and societal limits to the interactions between members of a profession, such as doctors or paramedics, and the clients or patients they serve.

professionalism the conduct or qualities that optimally characterize a practitioner in a particular field or occupation.

prognosis the expected outcome of a disease or injury.

prokaryotic cells cells that do not contain a nucleus and do not contain organelles. Most prokaryotes are surrounded by a rigid cell wall. The cells of most single-celled organisms, such as bacteria, are prokaryotes. *See also* eukaryotic cells.

prospective medical oversight guidelines established by a medical director in advance of emergency calls, such as those regarding selection of personnel and supplies, training and education, and protocol development.

prospective study study designed to observe outcomes or events that will occur subsequent to the identification of the group of subjects to be studied.

prostaglandins substances synthesized by mast cells during the inflammatory response that cause vasodilation, vascular permeability, and chemotaxis and also cause pain.

proteins nitrogen-based complex compounds that are the basic building blocks of cells and are essential for the growth and repair of living tissues.

proton positively charged particle within the nucleus of an atom.

prototype medication that best demonstrates the class's common properties and illustrates its particular characteristics.

proximate cause action or inaction of the paramedic that immediately caused or worsened the damage suffered by the patient.

psychoneuroimmunological regulation the interactions of psychological, neurologic/endocrine, and immunologic factors that contribute to alteration of the immune system as an outcome of a stress response that is not quickly resolved.

psychotherapeutic medication medication used to treat mental dysfunction.

public health the science and practice of protecting and improving the health of a community through the use of preventive medicine, health education, control of communicable diseases, application of sanitary measures, and monitoring of environmental hazards.

public safety answering point (PSAP) any agency that takes emergency calls from citizens in a given region and dispatches the emergency resources necessary to respond to individual calls for help.

PubMed computerized database operated by the National Libraries of Medicine that allows one to search many of the world's science resources.

pulmonary embolism blood clot that travels to the pulmonary circulation and hinders oxygenation of the blood.

pulse oximetry a measurement of hemoglobin oxygen saturation in the peripheral tissues.

pulsus paradoxus drop in blood pressure of greater than 10 torr during inspiration.

pus a liquid mixture of dead cells, bits of dead tissue, and tissue fluid that may accumulate in inflamed tissues.

pyrogen foreign protein capable of producing fever.

qualitative research research in which the researcher explores relationships using textual, rather than quantitative, data. Case study, observation, and ethnography are forms of qualitative research.

qualitative statistics the analysis of nonnumeric data.

quality improvement (QI) an evaluation program that emphasizes service and uses customer satisfaction as the ultimate indicator of system performance.

quality of life the general well-being of individuals and society.

quantitative research a study type that quantifies relationships between variables, using numeric terms.

quantitative statistics statistics that involve analysis of numeric data and are used to make conclusions and future predictions.

quasiexperimental study study that does not use random assignments to place the subjects into the various study groups.

radio band a range of radio frequencies.

radio frequency the number of times per second a radio wave oscillates.

radioactive decay the breakdown of the nucleus of an unstable atom, resulting in the emission of radiation. *See also* radioactive isotopes.

radioactive isotopes atoms with unstable nuclei that break down and emit radiation, in a process called radioactive decay.

ramped position the ear-to-sternal-notch position in an obese patient. *See also* ear-to-sternal-notch position.

random sampling sampling in which subjects are chosen by random chance. *See* randomized controlled trial (RCT).

randomized controlled trial (RCT) study in which subjects are assigned to different treatments, interventions, or conditions according to chance, rather than with reference to some aspect of their condition, history, or prognosis.

rapid sequence intubation (RSI) giving medications to sedate (induce) and temporarily paralyze a patient and then performing orotracheal intubation.

reasonable force the minimal amount of force necessary to ensure that an unruly or violent person does not cause injury to himself or others.

recall bias an error caued by differences in the accuracy or completeness of the recollections retrieved by study participants regarding events or experiences from the past.

receptor specialized protein that combines with a medication resulting in a biochemical effect.

reciprocity the process by which an agency grants automatic certification or licensure to an individual who has comparable certification or licensure from another agency.

reduction the gain of atoms by one atom from another. *See also* oxidation.

regeneration regrowth through cell proliferation.

registration the process of entering one's name and essential information within a particular record, done in EMS to verify the provider's initial certification and to monitor recertification.

repair healing of a wound with scar formation.

repeaters electronic devices that receive a signal and rebroadcast it at a higher power.

res ipsa loquitur a legal doctrine invoked by plaintiffs to support a claim of negligence; it is a Latin term that means "the thing speaks for itself."

research a systematic investigation, including development of the research design, testing, and evaluation, intended to develop or contribute to generalizable knowledge.

resolution the complete healing of a wound and return of tissues to their normal structure and function; the ending of inflammation with no scar formation.

respiration the exchange of gases between a living organism and its environment.

respiratory acid–base disorders respiratory acidosis and respiratory alkalosis; disorders that result from an inequality between carbon dioxide generation in the peripheral tissues and carbon dioxide elimination by the respiratory system.

respiratory acidosis acidity caused by abnormal retention of carbon dioxide resulting from impaired ventilation.

respiratory alkalosis alkalinity caused by excessive elimination of carbon dioxide resulting from increased respirations.

respiratory rate number of times a person breathes in 1 minute.

response time time elapsed from when a unit is alerted until it arrives on the scene.

restraint asphyxia lack of oxygen resulting in unconsciousness or death that occurs in a person who is being restrained. Also called *positional asphyxia*.

retroglottic airways extraglottic airway devices that are placed in the esophagus (behind the vocal cords).

retrospective medical oversight actions of a medical director intended to evaluate ongoing calls or calls that have already taken place, such as auditing a call, directing peer review, conflict resolution, and other quality assurance or improvement processes.

retrospective study research conducted by reviewing records (e.g., birth and death certificates, medical records, school or employment records) or information about past events elicited through interviews with persons who have, and controls who do not have, the disease or condition, or another characteristic under investigation.

Rh blood group a group of antigens discovered on the red blood cells of rhesus monkeys that is also present to some extent in humans.

Rh factor an antigen in the Rh blood group that is also known as antigen D. About 85 percent of North Americans have the Rh factor (are Rh positive), whereas about 15 percent do not have the Rh factor (are Rh negative). Rh positive and Rh negative blood are incompatible; that is, a person who is Rh negative can experience a severe immune response if Rh positive blood is introduced, as through a transfusion or during childbirth.

ribonucleic acid (RNA) a chemical similar to deoxyribonucleic acid (DNA) that serves as a template for protein synthesis.

ribosome organelle within a cell that synthesizes polypeptides and proteins.

rooting reflex a reflex that occurs when an infant's cheek is touched by a hand or cloth; the hungry infant turns his head to the right or left.

rough endoplasmic reticulum (RER) parts of the endoplasmic reticulum that contain ribosomes during protein synthesis. *See also* endoplasmic reticulum; ribosome.

rules of evidence guidelines that must be followed for permitting a new medication, process, or procedure to be used in EMS.

SafeCom a communications program of the U.S. Department of Homeland Security that provides research and guidance to emergency response agencies regarding the development of interoperable communications systems.

saline lock peripheral IV cannula with a distal medication port used for intermittent fluid or medication infusions. Saline is injected into the device to maintain its patency.

sampling error difference between the values obtained from the sample and those that actually exist in the total population.

SaO$_2$ *see* hemoglobin-oxygen saturation.

saturated fatty acids a class of triglycerides that have a single bond between carbon atoms, leaving room for two hydrogen atoms.

scaffolding a teaching/learning technique in which one builds on what has already been learned.

science the systematic study of the nature and behavior of the material and physical universe, based on observation, experiment, and measurement, and the formulation of laws to describe these facts in general terms.

scientific method a method of investigation in which a problem is first identified and observations, experiments, or other relevant data are then used to construct or test hypotheses that purport to solve it.

scope of practice the range of duties and skills paramedics and other levels of EMS certification are allowed and expected to perform.

second messenger chemical that participates in complex cascading reactions that eventually cause a medication's desired effect.

secondary immune response the swift, strong response of the immune system to repeated exposures to an antigen.

secondary intention complex healing of a larger wound involving sealing of the wound through scab formation, granulation or filling of the wound, and constriction of the wound.

secondary prevention medical care after an injury or illness that helps to prevent further problems from occurring.

secretory immune system lymphoid tissues beneath the mucosal endothelium that secrete substances such as sweat, tears, saliva, mucus, and breast milk; also called the *external immune system* or the *mucosal immune system*.

secure attachment a type of bonding that occurs when an infant learns that his caregivers will be responsive and helpful when needed.

sedation state of decreased anxiety and inhibitions.

selection bias the selection of individuals, groups, or data for analysis in such a way that proper randomization is not achieved, thereby ensuring that the sample obtained is not representative of the population intended to be analyzed.

semantic related to the meaning of words.

semipermeable referring to a membrane that allows unrestricted movement of some substances across the membrane while restricting the movement of other substances. Also called *selectively permeable*.

septic shock shock that develops as the result of infection carried by the bloodstream, eventually causing dysfunction of multiple organ systems.

septicemia the systemic spread of toxins through the bloodstream. Also called *sepsis*.

septum cartilage that separates the right and left nasal cavities.

sequelae *see* complications.

serotonin a substance released by platelets that, through constriction and dilation of blood vessels, affects blood flow to an injured or affected site.

serum solution containing whole antibodies for a specific pathogen.

sharps container rigid, puncture-resistant container clearly marked as a biohazard.

shock *see* hypoperfusion.

side effect unintended response to a medication.

sign objective finding that can be identified through physical examination.

simple diffusion the passive movement of molecules through a membrane from an area of greater concentration to an area of lesser concentration. *See also* facilitated diffusion; osmosis.

simplex communications system that transmits and receives on the same frequency.

single blind study a study in which the investigator, but not the subject, knows the treatment assignment.

sinus air cavity that conducts fluids from the Eustachian tubes and tear ducts to and from the nasopharynx.

situational awareness (SA) perception of all aspects of a scene or situation.

slander act of injuring a person's character, name, or reputation by false or malicious statements spoken with malicious intent or reckless disregard for the falsity of those statements.

slow-to-warm-up child an infant who can be characterized by a low intensity of reactions and a somewhat negative mood.

smart phone devices that combine the voice capability of a basic cell phone with the ability to perform a variety of data messaging functions such as e-mail and Internet connections as well as taking and sending photos and video.

smooth endoplasmic reticulum (SER) portion of the endoplasmic reticulum without ribosomes; it provides surface area of the action or storage of key enzymes and their products. *See also* endoplasmic reticulum; enzymes.

sniffing position the ear-to-sternal-notch position in a non-obese patient. *See also* ear-to-sternal-notch position.

sodium–potassium pump an enzyme (Na^+-K^+-ATPase); a mechanism of active transport in the plasma membrane, powered by adenosine triphosphate (ATP), that moves sodium ions out of a cell and potassium ions into the cell to help maintain cell potential and regular cellular volume.

solute a substance dissolved in a solvent, forming a solution. *See also* solvent.

solvent a substance that dissolves other substances, forming a solution. *See also* solute.

spike sharp-pointed device inserted into the IV solution bag's administration set port.

standard deviation (SD, σ) a statistic representing the degree of dispersion of a set of scores around their mean.

standard of care the degree of care, skill, and judgment that would be expected under like or similar circumstances by a similarly trained, reasonable paramedic in the same community.

Standard Precautions a strict form of infection control that is based on the assumption that all blood and other body fluids are infectious.

standing orders treatment procedures preauthorized by a medical director.

starches polymers of glucose; carbohydrates.

statistics mathematical techniques used to summarize research data or to determine whether the data support the researcher's hypothesis.

statuatory law law created by lawmaking bodies such as Congress and state assemblies. Also called *legislative law*.

stem cells undifferentiated cells in the bone marrow from which all blood cells, including thrombocytes, erythrocytes, and various types of leukocytes, develop; stem cells are also called *hemocytoblasts*.

stenosis narrowing or constriction.

sterile free of all forms of life.

sterilization use of a chemical or physical method such as pressurized steam to kill all microorganisms on an object.

steroids an organic compound, a class of lipid. The dietary fat cholesterol and the sex hormones estradiol and testosterone are examples of steroids.

stock solution standard concentration of routinely used medications.

stoma opening in the anterior neck that connects the trachea with ambient air.

stress response changes within the body initiated by a stressor.

stress a hardship or strain; a physical or emotional response to a stimulus.

stressor a stimulus that causes stress.

stroke volume the amount of blood ejected by the heart in one contraction.

stylet plastic-covered metal wire used to bend the ETT into a J or hockey-stick shape.

subcutaneous the layer of loose connective tissue between the skin and muscle.

sublingual beneath the tongue.

substrate a substance an enzyme acts on.

sucking reflex a reflex that occurs when an infant's lips are stroked.

sucrose common table sugar; a disaccharide, it is a combination of glucose and fructose.

suction to remove with a vacuum-type device.

sugars a class of carbohydrate that can be further classified as simple sugars (monosaccharides) or complex sugars (disaccharides). *See also* disaccharides; monosaccharides.

suppository medication packaged in a soft, pliable form for insertion into the rectum.

supraglottic airways extraglottic airway devices that are placed above the vocal cords (above the glottis).

surfactant substance that decreases surface tension.

sympatholytic medication or other substance that blocks the actions of the sympathetic nervous system (also called *antiadrenergic)*.

sympathomimetic medication or other substance that causes effects like those of the sympathetic nervous system (also called *adrenergic*).

symptom subjective complaint; what the patient is experiencing and, possibly, can describe.

synapse space between nerve cells.

syndrome a constellation of signs and symptoms commonly found in association with a particular disease or condition.

syringe plastic tube with which liquid medications can be drawn up, stored, and injected.

systemic throughout the body.

systematic sampling statistical sampling technique in which there is order to the selection of samples for the study. The most common form is where every kth sample is taken (e.g., every 10th name from the phone book).

T cell receptor (TCR) a molecule on the surface of a helper T cell that responds to a specific antigen. There is a specific TCR for every antigen to which the human body may be exposed.

T lymphocytes the type of white blood cell that does not produce antibodies but, instead, attacks antigens directly.

***t* test** a statistical test used to determine if the scores of two groups differ on a single variable.

teachable moment a time shortly after an injury when the patient and observers remain acutely aware of what has happened and may be especially receptive to teaching about how a similar injury or illness could be prevented in the future.

Tema Conter Memorial Trust Canadian organization that works to raise awareness of mental health issues and care that can be provided for mental health challenges associated with EMS service. *See also* Code Green Campaign.

teratogenic drug medication that may deform or kill a fetus.

teratogens external factors that can affect the development of a fetus.

terminal-drop hypothesis a theory that death is preceded by a five-year period of decreasing cognitive functioning.

termination of action time from when the medication's level drops below its minimum effective concentration until it is eliminated from the body.

terrestrial-based triangulation a system of location based on the use of three land-based points of observation, such as using the strengths of signals from three cell phone towers to locate a given cell phone signal, or more traditional methods such as the use of sextants in surveying.

tertiary prevention rehabilitation after an injury or illness that helps to prevent further problems from occurring.

therapeutic index ratio of a medication's lethal dose for 50 percent of the population to its effective dose for 50 percent of the population.

therapy regulator pressure regulator used for delivering oxygen to patients.

thrombocytes platelets, which are important in blood clotting.

thrombophlebitis inflammation of the vein.

thrombus blood clot.

tidal volume (T_V) the average volume of gas inhaled or exhaled in one respiratory cycle.

tiered response multiple levels of emergency care personnel responding to the same incident.

time sampling statistical sampling technique in which the samples are chosen by a given time interval or time span (e.g., what the subjects were thinking about at intervals of three hours, or what they were doing during the same half-hour each day).

tissue a group of cells that perform a similar function.

tonicity solute concentration or osmotic pressure relative to the blood plasma or body cells.

topical medications material applied to and absorbed through the skin or mucous membranes.

tort law division of the legal system that deals with civil wrongs committed by one individual against another. *See also* intentional tort.

total body water (TBW) the total amount of water in the body at a given time.

total lung capacity (TLC) maximum lung capacity.

trachea 10- to 12-cm-long tube that connects the larynx to the mainstem bronchi.

transdermal absorbed through the skin.

trauma center a medical facility that has the capability of caring for the acutely injured patient. A trauma center must meet strict criteria to use this designation.

trauma a physical injury or wound caused by external force or violence.

treatment group the study group in an experimental design that will receive the treatment or intervention being studied.

triage tags tags containing vital information, which are affixed to the patient during a multiple-patient incident.

triglycerides lipids consisting of one molecule of glycerol and three fatty acid molecules that are a rich source of energy for the body.

trocar a sharp, pointed instrument.

trunking communications system that pools all frequencies and routes transmissions to the next available frequency.

trust vs. mistrust refers to a stage of psychosocial development that lasts from birth to about 1½ years of age.

tumor a mass of uncontrolled cell growth. A tumor may be benign (noncancerous) or malignant (cancerous).

turgor normal tension in a cell; the resistance of the skin to deformation. (In a normally hydrated person, the skin, when pinched, will quickly return to its normal formation. In a dehydrated person, the return to normal formation will be slower.)

turnover the continual synthesis and breakdown of body substances that results in the dynamic steady state.

ultrahigh frequency (UHF) radio frequency band from 300 to 3,000 megahertz.

ultrasound use of high frequency sound waves to produce images of internal body structures.

unit predetermined amount of medication or fluid.

unsaturated fatty acids a class of triglycerides that have a double bond between carbon atoms, leaving room for only one hydrogen atom.

upper airway obstruction an interference with air movement through the upper airway.

up-regulation when a medication causes the formation of more receptors than normal.

vaccine solution containing a modified pathogen that does not actually cause disease but still stimulates the development of antibodies specific to it.

vacuole organelle within a cell that provides temporary storage or transport of substances such as food sources.

vacutainer device that holds blood tubes.

valence electrons electrons found in the outermost shell (valence shell) of an atom.

valence shell the outermost electron shell of an atom. *See also* electron shells.

validity extent to which an investigator's findings are accurate or reflect the underlying purpose of the study.

vallecula depression between the epiglottis and the base of the tongue.

variance measure of variability indicating the average of the squared deviations from the mean.

venous access device surgically implanted port that permits repeated access to central venous circulation.

venous constricting band flat rubber band used to impede venous return and make veins easier to see.

ventilation the mechanical process that moves air into and out of the lungs.

Venturi mask   high-concentration face mask that uses a Venturi system to deliver relatively precise oxygen concentrations.

very high frequency (VHF)   radio frequency band from 30 to 300 megahertz.

vial   plastic or glass container with a self-sealing rubber top.

virus   an organism much smaller than a bacterium, visible only under an electron microscope. Viruses invade and live inside the cells of the organisms they infect.

voice over Internet protocol (VOIP)   technology that provides voice communications through Internet access from a computer or mobile device.

volume on hand   the available amount of solution containing a medication.

years of productive life   a calculation made by subtracting the age at death from 65.

Index